Pathology
of
Drug-Induced
and
Toxic Diseases

Pathology
of
Drug-Induced
and
Toxic Diseases

Edited by

Robert H. Riddell
M.B., B.S., M.R.C.Path.

Associate Professor
Department of Pathology
University of Chicago
Chicago, Illinois

With 28 Contributors

Churchill Livingstone
New York, Edinburgh, London, and Melbourne 1982

Distributed in the United Kingdom by Churchill Livingstone, Robert Stevenson House, 1-3 Baxter's Place, Leith Walk, Edinburgh EH1 3AF and by associated companies, branches and representatives throughout the world.

First published 1982
Printed in U.S.A.

ISBN 0-443-08083-6

7 6 5 4 3 2 1

Library of Congress Cataloging in Publication Data
Main entry under title:

Pathology of drug-induced and toxic diseases.
Bibliography: p.
Includes index.
1. Drugs—Toxicology. 2. Drugs—Side effects. I. Riddell, Robert H. [DNLM: 1. Drugs—Adverse effects. 2. Poisoning—Pathology. QZ 42 P297]
RA1238.P37 616 82-4230
ISBN 0-443-08083-6 AACR2

To my parents, Joyce and Harry,
my wife, Gillian,
and my children, Juliet and Mark.

Contributors

Robert E. Fechner, M.D.
Professor and Director of Surgical Pathology, University of Virginia School of Medicine, Charlottesville, Virginia

Cecilia M. Fenoglio, M.D.
Professor, Department of Pathology, Columbia University College of Physicians and Surgeons, New York, New York

Robert A. Goepp, D.D.S., Ph.D.
Director and Professor, Walter G. Zoller Memorial Dental Clinic, University of Chicago, Chicago, Illinois

Raul Hinojosa, M.D.
Research Associate and Associate Professor, Section of Otolaryngology, University of Chicago, Chicago, Illinois

Nelson S. Irey, M.D.
Chairman, Department of Environmental and Drug-Induced Pathology, Armed Forces Institute of Pathology, Washington, D.C.

Kamal G. Ishak, M.D., Ph.D.
Chairman, Department of Hepatic Pathology, Armed Forces Institute of Pathology, Washington, D.C.

Wellington Jao, M.D.
Vice Chairman, Department of Pathology, Michael Reese Hospital and Medical Center; Associate Professor of Pathology, University of Chicago, Chicago, Illinois

Byron A. Kakulas, A.O., M.D., (Hon. Athens), M.D. (W.A.) F.R.A.C.P., F.R.C.Path., F.R.C.P.A.
Professor of Neuropathology, University of Western Australia; Head of Department of Neuropathology, Royal Perth Hospital, Perth, Western Australia

John R. Lindsay, M.D.
Professor, Department of Surgery (Otolaryngology), University of Chicago, Chicago, Illinois

Gregory J. Matz, M.D.
Professor, Department of Surgery; Chairman, Section of Otolaryngology, University of Chicago, Chicago, Illinois

Maria Medenica, M.D.
Associate Professor, Department of Medicine, University of Chicago, Chicago, Illinois

Hugh A. McAllister, Jr., M.D., F.A.C.C.
Chairman, Department of Cardiovascular Pathology, Armed Forces Institute of Pathology; Professor of Pathology and Clinical Professor of Surgery, Uniformed Services University of the Health Sciences; Clinical Professor of Medicine (Cardiology), Georgetown University School of Medicine, Washington, D.C.

Florabel G. Mullick, M.D.
Associate Chairman, Department of Environmental and Drug-Induced Pathology, Armed Forces Institute of Pathology; Clinical Associate Professor of Pathology, Uniformed Services University of the Health Sciences; Clinical Associate Professor of Pathology, Georgetown University School of Medicine, Washington, D.C.

Ralph F. Naunton, M.D.
Professor Emeritus, Department of Surgery, University of Chicago, Chicago, Illinois

Henry J. Norris, M.D.
Chairman, Department of Gynecologic and Breast Pathology, Armed Forces Institute of Pathology, Washington, D.C.

Eugene V. D. K. Perrin, M.D.
Professor of Pathology, Associate in Pediatrics, Obstetrics and Gynecology, and Anatomy, Wayne State University School of Medicine; Director of Histopathology, Children's Hospital of Michigan; Associate in Pathology, Hutzel and Sinai Hospitals, Detroit, Michigan

Wanda de Poitiers, B.Sc.
Formerly, Research Assistant, Department of Morbid Anatomy, King's College Hospital Medical School, London, England

Jaime Prat, M.D.
Assistant Professor of Pathology, Massachusetts General Hospital, Harvard Medical School, Boston, Massachusetts

Robert H. Riddell, M.B., B.S., M.R.C.Path.
Associate Professor, Department of Pathology, University of Chicago, Chicago, Illinois

Stanley J. Robboy, M.D.
Associate Professor of Pathology, Massachusetts General Hospital, Harvard Medical School, Boston, Massachusetts

Barbara F. Smith, M.D.
Consultant Neuropathologist, Department of Pathology, St. Bartholomew's Hospital, London, England

Francis H. Straus II, M.D.
Professor, Department of Pathology, University of Chicago, Chicago, Illinois

Brenda J. Tripathi, Ph.D.
Research Associate and Assistant Professor, Department of Ophthalmology, University of Chicago, Chicago, Illinois

Ramesh C. Tripathi, M.D., Ph.D., M.R.C.Path.
Professor, Department of Ophthalmology, University of Chicago, Chicago, Illinois

James W. Vardiman, M.D.
Associate Professor, Department of Pathology, University of Chicago, Chicago, Illinois

Daina Variakojis, M.D.
Associate Professor, Department of Pathology, University of Chicago, Chicago, Illinois

William R. Welch, M.D.
Assistant Professor of Pathology, Brigham and Women's Hospital, Harvard Medical School, Boston, Massachusetts

W. F. Whimster, M.R.C.P., M.R.C.Path.
Senior Lecturer, Department of Morbid Anatomy, King's College Hospital Medical School, London, England

Barbara Winkler, M.D.
Chief Resident, Department of Pathology, Columbia University College of Physicians and Surgeons, New York, New York

Preface

Drug-induced disease is a rapidly expanding field that has become increasingly well recognized. Unwanted effects of drugs and side-effects caused by drug interaction are taught routinely in medical school. While many of these are of a pharmacologic nature that modify normal responses, others cause distinct lesions that may result in clinical disease. However, the pathology of the underlying disease is often poorly documented. Furthermore, when information does exist it is often difficult to obtain by conventional library searching techniques because the details are often buried within papers that were not written primarily to discuss side-effects. For example, the toxicity following treatment of leukemia is often stated in a few paragraphs of the discussion in a paper primarily describing the comparative effectiveness of a new chemotherapeutic regimen. Even when mentioned, such side-effects are often not described morphologically.

Pathologists as a group tend not to share the same awareness of possible effects of drugs as clinicians, particularly with the increasing numbers of therapeutic agents available. Further, even when faced with the possibility of a drug-induced disease, many pathologists feel daunted by the maze of polypharmacy with which they are often confronted and from which they are supposed to pluck the offending drug. The chance of establishing possible drug-induced disease is therefore all too frequently lost, and with it the chance to relate it to the underlying pathology. These problems are addressed in the first chapter.

This book was therefore undertaken for a variety of reasons. Perhaps the most important was to provide the pathologist with a comprehensive well-referenced work that answers the questions of whether a particular drug can cause a specific disease or histologic reaction and whether the underlying pathology has any features that distinguish it from similar lesions occurring in patients not taking the drug.

The lack of knowledge regarding the underlying morphology in many instances of drug-induced disease is all too often apparent. It is hoped that this book will act as a stimulus for pathologists to become increasingly aware of the need to establish a relationship between drug or toxin and subsequent disease and then document fully the nature of the underlying morphology and if possible suggest the mechanisms involved. The need for clinical awareness and suspicions by both clinician and pathologist cannot be overemphasized. Some diseases included have virtually no pathology, yet serve to make pathologists aware of potential associations; indeed making pathologists aware of associations between drug or toxin and disease is a further major function of the book. Others, such as those following the use of diethylstilbestrol (DES), have been allotted a small section out of proportion to the frequency with which the effects are seen. Nevertheless, the underlying pathology is deemed sufficiently interesting to warrant such a section.

Although toxins are included, the book is not meant to be a comprehensive textbook of toxicology. In each chapter the space devoted to toxins has been left entirely up to the authors. Some include single case reports, usually because of their potential importance, but sometimes to point out the lack of evidence concerning a suggested association. Sometimes entire topics, such as dust-related diseases, have been deliberately omitted because they are so well described in conventional textbooks of pathology.

Stylistically, the authors have been given absolute freedom. While it would have been satisfying and possibly advantageous to use a standard format throughout, it is apparent that each system or organ is not suited to such rigidity. Some are best covered using an anatomic framework (e.g., glomeruli, tubules, collecting system, interstitium); others are best considered by either the diseases caused or on a drug by drug basis. Combinations of these are also utilized. Occasionally small sections on normal histology are included when this is deemed appropriate as an aid in understanding the interpretation of abnormal findings.

While the text is primarily a reference work, it is also hoped that some will enjoy reading it just because it opens up a fascinating new corner of pathology with which they were previously unfamiliar.

Robert H. Riddell

Contents

1

When Is a Disease Drug Induced?

Nelson S. Irey

Drugs and chemicals can produce in the human body the same spectrum of tissue changes that occur in diseases not caused by drugs and chemicals. Nor, with rare exceptions, are there any clinical or pathologic "markers" that, per se, differentiate adverse drug reactions (ADRs) from other diseases. For orientation in evaluating ADRs, the following questions are raised and discussed:

1. What findings should make one suspect the presence of an ADR?
2. If an ADR is suspected, are there ways of confirming or denying its existence?
3. Are the methods used for diagnosing an ADR during life the same as those used at autopsy?
4. Is there difficulty in differentiating a basic disease from an ADR?
5. What are the major difficulties in diagnosing an ADR?
6. Should a judgment be made on the degree of certainty of an ADR diagnosis?
7. Are there differences in the circumstances generating ADRs, and if so, should the ADRs be subgrouped accordingly?

From the Department of Environmental and Drug-Induced Pathology, the Armed Forces Institute of Pathology, Washington, D.C. 20306.

The Department of Environmental and Drug-Induced Pathology is sponsored by the Food and Drug Administration (under contract FDA 224-77-3001) of the Department of Health, Education, and Welfare; and by the Armed Forces Institute of Pathology.

The opinions or assertions contained herein are the private views of the author and are not to be construed as official or as reflecting the views of the Department of the Army or of Defense or of the sponsors of the Department of Environmental and Drug-Induced Pathology.

Before developing answers to these questions, a few points of guidance are in order.

There are three reasons why it is important to recognize an ADR:

1. For immediate therapy. Besides discontinuation of the drug, which is usually followed by remission of the ADR, there may be the indication for antidotes, symptomatic therapy (steroids and other treatment), or both.
2. Recognition of the responsible agent will point to future avoidance (prophylaxis). This is true not only for the particular patient, but may be broadened to the general patient population. It took over 60 years to recognize the relationship between chronic hypochromic microcytic anemia and gastrointestinal blood loss in chronic salicylate users; it took 30 years for general recognition that aminopyrine can cause leukopenia or agranulocytosis.
3. For medicolegal purposes. Failure to recognize an ADR may allow an initially mild reaction to progress to serious morbidity or to a lethal conclusion. This may be regarded as negligence in subsequent litigation.

There are three major elements in an ADR; namely the specific drug, the site, and the pathologic change.

1. With regard to the first element, there is hardly a drug or chemical that will not cause an adverse reaction in someone, at some time, at some place, and the number of these agents is legion. Many of these drugs and commercial chemicals have been developed in the very recent past, and represent new chemical experiences for the human biologic system. The

1979 *Drug Nomenclature Printout*[5] published by the American Medical Association lists more than 50,000 designations for 11,200 individual compounds and 500 mixtures. The most recent *AMA Drug Evaluations*[1] contains approximately 1,200 drugs, including "all nationally distributed products that are dispensed exclusively or principally by prescription"; it is estimated that these 1,200 drugs make up 90% of the medications used by physicians. Another standard reference for drug and chemical information is the *Merck Index*[14]; this contains monographs on approximately 10,000 of the more important chemicals, drugs, pesticides, and biologically active substances currently in use. *Clinical Toxicology of Commercial Products*[7] lists over 17,500 trade names or products that might be ingested either accidentally or with suicidal intent. Lastly, the number of "over the counter" drugs available to the public numbers several hundred thousand.

2. The second major element in an ADR is the site. There is no organ or tissue that may not be the site of an ADR. Particularly likely locations for ADRs are organs or tissues related to the absorption, metabolism, storage, and excretion of drugs and chemicals: the gastrointestinal system, the liver, and the kidney. However, no organ, organ system, or tissue is exempt from the possibility of being an ADR site.

3. The third major consideration in ADRs are the types of pathologic changes that may be induced by drugs or chemicals. These run the gamut of the morphologic alterations that have long been recognized in general pathology: congenital and developmental abnormalities; benign and malignant tumors; hyperplasias, hypoplasias, and aplasias; acute, subacute, chronic, and granulomatous inflammations; vascular alterations and coagulopathies; hypersensitivity reactions; and functional changes without evident morphologic changes. These relatively few reaction patterns are well-known final common paths into which all causes of human disease funnel, whether the etiologic agent is in the physical, chemical, or biologic category. Likewise, the same clinical findings (symptoms, signs, and clinical laboratory findings) are shared by drug- and non-drug-related illnesses. By not usually producing distinctive or unique clinicopathologic changes, ADRs may be difficult to recognize, identify, and diagnose, and may be missed if the possibility of an ADR is not included in the differential diagnosis along with infectious, metabolic, neoplastic, and other well-established major categories of human illness. To put ADRs in perspective, it is estimated that about 70% are of a minor nature, while the remaining 30% are associated with serious morbidity or with mortality.

Now, back to the seven questions initially raised.

WHAT FINDINGS SHOULD MAKE ONE SUSPECT THE PRESENCE OF AN ADR?

There are a number of circumstances, warnings, or "red flags" that should lead one to suspect that an ADR is occurring:

1. When there is a clinical or laboratory finding that is atypical for the patient's basic disease. Example: Jaundice developing in a patient with pulmonary tuberculosis being treated with isoniazid.

2. When an anatomic site becomes the seat of pathologic change that is not usually involved in the basic disease for which the patient is being treated.

Example: Aplasia or hypoplasia of the bone marrow, and an associated decrease in one or more of the formed elements of the peripheral blood in a patient being treated with a sulfonamide for an upper respiratory infection.

3. When a pathologic process develops that is foreign to the basic disease of the patient.

Example: Pulmonary fibrosis developing in a leukemic patient being treated with busulfan.

4. When a clinical illness develops that doesn't fit any of the more common clinical entities.

Example: An epileptic patient inadvertently received twice the usual dosage of diphenylhydantoin. This was followed by a severe, bizarre, and "unusual syndrome": fever (to 103°F), shaking chills, weakness, fatigue, vertigo, anorexia, nausea, and vomiting, cough, hypoactive tendon reflexes, ataxia, nystagmus, slurred speech, visual and auditory hallucinations, confusion, and somnolence. Twelve hours after discontinuing the double dosage of the anticonvulsant, her symptoms and signs began to abate, and by day 13 she had completely recovered.

5. When an autopsy fails to reveal an anatomic cause of death.

Example: Drug overdose cases, in which the anatomic findings are usually limited to pulmonary edema and congestion, and generalized visceral congestion. In our "drug-culture" society, such cases should have toxicologic examination of the blood, urine, and viscera (liver, kidney, and brain particularly).

Example: Electrolyte imbalance and drug–drug interaction cases.

6. When a pathologic process occurs at an unusual age.

Example: Bilateral gangrene of the feet requiring below-knee amputations in a 21-year-old woman who persisted in secretly taking ergotamine tartrate for several years for relief of severe migraine.

Example: A fatal cerebral hemorrhage in a 17-year-old drug addict who used methamphetamine. (He was not known to be previously hypertensive, nor did he have a congenital "berry" aneurysm).

IF AN ADR IS SUSPECTED, ARE THERE WAYS OF CONFIRMING OR DENYING ITS EXISTENCE?

There are methods and tools that are of use in analyzing and diagnosing cases of suspected ADR. They include a broad base of time-related clinical and laboratory information; a viewpoint that shifts from "pattern" to "etiologic" diagnosis; utilization of the chemistry and toxicology laboratory as appropriate; and the microscope. These "ways and means" of confirming or denying the possibility of an ADR constitute a validation process that removes suspected cases from the merely anecdotal category.

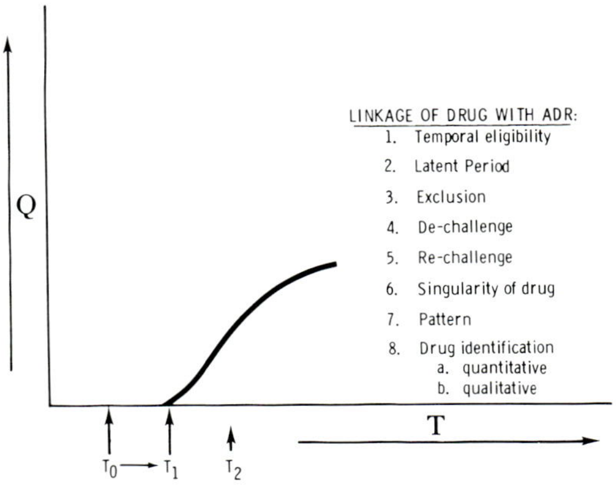

Fig. 1-1. Time-flow chart representing an adverse drug reaction, with a listing of key points to be considered in evaluating ADR cases.

Figure 1-1 lists eight methods of linkage of a drug with an ADR; these will be taken up in turn, with illustrative cases.

Temporal Eligibility

To be responsible for an adverse reaction, a drug must be administered at some interval of time before the reaction occurs. Temporal eligibility is the first criterion to be met in establishing a drug-based etiology for an illness. In Figure 1-1, a drug given at T_2 could not have initiated the curve of the ADR.

Example: Figure 1-2 represents the time-flow chart of a 61-year-old man with myelogenous leukemia treated with busulfan, who died in renal failure. The question raised by the contributing pathologist was whether or not the busulfan caused the kidney dysfunction. It is clear that the marker (NPN) was already twice normal upon admission of the patient, before the drug was first administered. Further, the slope of the NPN curve after busulfan therapy was begun was essentially unaltered.

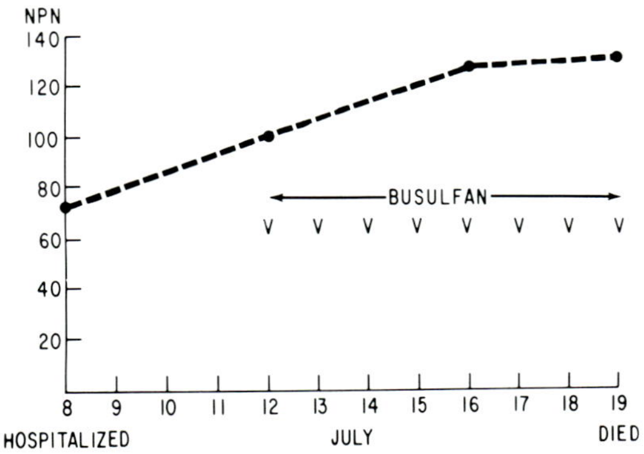

Fig. 1-2. Time-flow chart demonstrating the temporal ineligibility of busulfan to have initiated the non-protein nitrogen (NPN) elevation (upper limit of normal is 35). The latter was already present on admission to the hospital, and prior to the first administration of the drug. (From Irey, N. S.: Diagnostic Problems in Drug-Induced Diseases. In: Meyler, L. and Peck, H. M. (Eds): Drug-Induced Diseases. Vol. 4. Excerpta Medica, Amsterdam, 1972, by permission of the publishers.)

Autopsy revealed heavy leukemic infiltration of the kidneys, and severe arterial and arteriolar nephrosclerosis. In this instance the drug is ineligible to have initiated the elevation in NPN; the combination of leukemic involvement and vascular disease of the kidney reasonably account for the renal dysfunction.

Example: Jaundice in a 33-year-old white male was initially alleged to have been caused by a phenothiazine medication. Further information revealed that his jaundice preceded the first pill of prochlorperazine by 3 days, clearly establishing the temporal ineligibility of this agent to have caused the jaundice. The jaundice was later found to be due to viral hepatitis.

Latent Period

This is the interval from the time at which a drug is first administered to the beginning of the ADR. (T_0 to T_1, Fig. 1-1). This interval varies within wide limits from drug to drug: from seconds to minutes for death from cyanide; from minutes to approximately an hour for the first manifestations of a drug overdose; from 1 to 3 months for the fatal pancytopenia following chloramphenicol; and from one to three decades for thorium-induced hepatic angiosarcoma. The latent period may also vary for a particular drug—sometimes rather widely—as with isoniazid; here the latent period for the appearance of liver damage may vary from 2 weeks to 12 months. For many drugs the latent period range is sufficiently small to be of some diagnostic assistance, and is particularly valuable in a negative sense if it is either too short or too long.

Example: Fatal pancytopenia developed in a 52-year-old woman receiving sulfamethoxazole for a urinary tract infection. This drug was initially implicated in the dyscrasia. However, only a 10-day interval separated the beginning of the sulfonamide therapy and the finding of a hemoglobin level of 6.6 grams. Considering the half-life of the red cell, and without evidence of either hemorrhage or hemolysis to explain the decrease in the hemoglobin level, the 10-day latent period was too short to account for the anemia on the basis of bone marrow toxicity and subsequent hypoplasia. The cause of the pancytopenia was never determined, but the sulfamethoxazole was disqualified as a possible cause on the basis of a latent period that was too short.

Example: An illustration of an excessively long latent period is that of a 44-year-old arthritic woman who took a muscle relaxant (chlorzoxazone) for 6 months without untoward effect. After discontinuing this agent for 1 month, she developed nausea, fever, and pain in the right upper quadrant of the abdomen. There was "marked elevation" of the serum transaminases, and the serum bilirubin rose to 17.9 mg percent. A liver biopsy 2 weeks after the onset of symptoms revealed submassive necrosis. The long latent period of 6 months, plus a drug-free period of an additional month, makes it unreasonable to ascribe the patient's subsequent submassive liver necrosis to the chlorzoxazone.

Exclusion

This method of linking an illness with its causative drug involves elimination of other drug candidates on the basis of time relationships. A selected "marker" of the ADR—a specific clinical or laboratory parameter—is plotted against time. The exclusion method requires detailed and time-related information on the particular marker of the ADR, as well as on the drugs administered. The exclusion method is not applicable in all cases of possible ADR, either because of insufficient data or because of simultaneous eligibility of more than one drug.

Example: Figure 1-3 is a time-flow chart on a 15-year-old black male with pulmonary blastomycosis. He was treated with five drugs and developed acute renal failure; a kidney biopsy revealed acute and chronic interstitial nephritis. It is evident from the graph that the only drug that could have initiated the patient's BUN increase was stilbamidine, and that after this drug was stopped there was a rapid return of the BUN to normal. The other four drugs are excluded by their temporal ineligibility.

Figure 1-4 represents the case of a 56-year-old white male, diabetic and hypertensive, who received a total of 11 drugs over a 5-year period. Midway in this period he developed a progressive decrease in hemoglobin and white cell count—the two markers in this case—as seen in the time-flow chart. As is evident from this chart, four drugs were given continuously for several years prior to the fall in hemoglobin and total white cell count. These drugs were therefore disqualified because of the lengths of their latent periods. Two other drugs (Lasix and probanthene) were given prior to the fall in hematologic markers; but both were given for very short periods and thus are extremely unlikely to have had an effect for over a year after they were discontinued. Indocin may have been eligible even though it was given for only a short period of time, but it was administered after what appeared to be the first major fall in the white cell count. Three of the agents (Elavil, quinine, and chlorthalidone) were clearly ineligible temporally. Thus hydralazine was the only drug that was given continuously during the time the markers fell. This fact and the exclusion of the other ten drugs led to the conclusion that hydralazine was the agent responsible for the anemia and leukopenia. On the basis of these findings and their interpretation, it was recommended that hydralazine be discontinued. Word was later received that this drug had been discontinued as recommended; subsequently, hemoglobin and white count levels were received. These are plotted

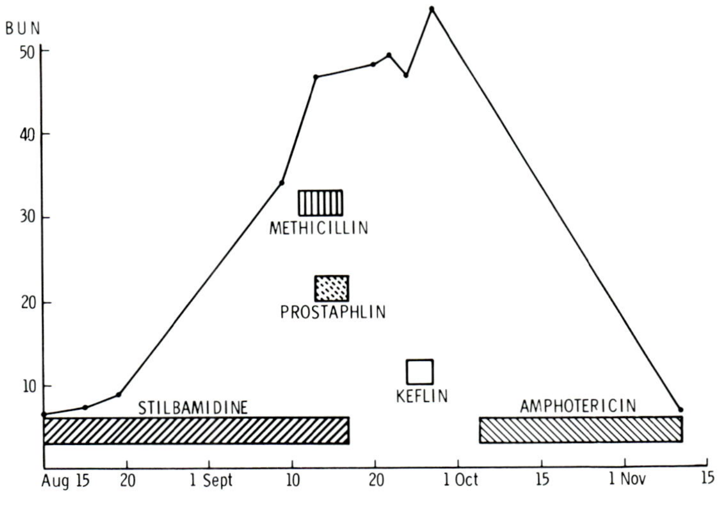

Fig. 1-3. Time-flow chart showing temporal eligibility of stilbamidine to have produced the BUN elevation, and the ineligibility of the other four drugs to have initiated the renal dysfunction. (From Irey, N. S.: Diagnostic Problems in Drug-Induced Diseases. In: Meyler, L. and Peck, H. M. (Eds): Drug-Induced Diseases. Vol. 4. Excerpta Medica, Amsterdam, 1972, by permission of the publishers.)

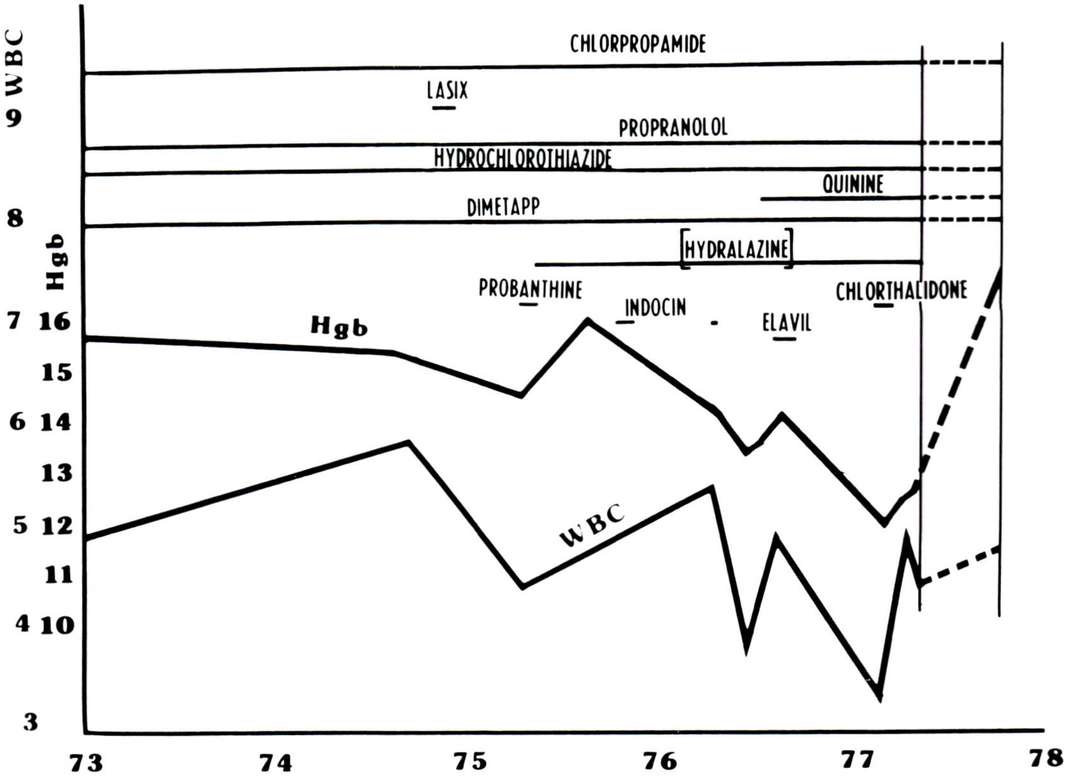

Fig. 1-4. Time-flow chart demonstrating the correction of the anemia after hydralazine was discontinued. Other drugs were eliminated because they were given for too short a time (Lasix, probanthine and Indocin), were temporally ineligible (quinine, Elavil and chlorthalidone), or were given continuously (chlorpropamide, propranolol, hydrochlorothiazide, and Dimetapp).

in dotted lines in Figure 1-4; the hemoglobin had returned to a normal level, and the white count was on the rise. The diagnosis of an hydralazine-related ADR was based on exclusion plus the results of de-challenge.

De-challenge and Re-challenge

These are discussed together because they are related to the same principle: namely, that many ADRs are reversible after discontinuance of the responsible drug, rendering de-challenge a valuable diagnostic procedure in cases of suspected ADR. Re-challenge with a responsible drug may be dangerous; it is sometimes done inadvertently.

Example: The hydralazine case illustrating the exclusion method (Fig. 1-4) also serves as an example of the principles of de-challenge: when the presumed cause (hydralazine) of the anemia and leukopenia was removed, the anemia was corrected and the white count went on an upswing.

Example: Another de-challenge illustration is that of a 58-year-old white male, with alcoholism and a manic-depressive reaction, who developed a severe lichenoid dermatitis that was particularly severe on his exposed skin. During the preceding 3 years, he had received numerous drugs (laxatives, antispasmodics, analgesics, tranquilizers, antipsychotics, antibiotics, antacids, vasodilators, and cold remedies). A prominent feature of this drug "cocktail" was that it included seven members of the phenothiazine group; throughout this

3-year period continued to take at least one of these phenothiazine tranquilizers. They constituted a common thread over the 3-year interval before the patient's presentation, and they have a known association with skin rashes; it was therefore recommended that all phenothiazine-type drugs be discontinued. Six months after the phenothiazines were discontinued, the patient's severe skin rash had disappeared.

Example: The value of re-challenge as a diagnostic aid, as well as its danger, is illustrated by the case of a 59-year-old black woman who was treated with phenylbutazone for arthritis. This was followed by pancytopenia and hypoplasia of the bone marrow. The drug was discontinued, and the woman recovered. Several months later, under the care of another physician, phenylbutazone was again started; this was followed by a recurrence of the blood dyscrasia, dominated by a severe hemorrhagic diathesis. The woman died with cerebral and pulmonary hemorrhages. The initial association between the drug and the dyscrasia was apparently not communicated to the second physician.

Singularity of the Drug

In this age of polypharmacy, it is unusual to find a patient taking only one drug. Such a circumstance makes for a relatively easy ADR diagnosis.

Example: A 21-year-old white female with severe migraine used ergotamine tartrate suppositories for a 3-year period. She developed pain and coolness in both lower legs and feet, and was hospitalized and studied for the possibility of having Reynaud's disease. No history of the use of an ergot preparation was obtained during this hospitalization, and the woman's physicians were unaware that she was using ergot suppositories even during her hospitalization. It was not until gangrene had developed in both legs, months later—requiring bilateral below the knee amputation—that her prolonged use of ergot became known.

There is little doubt that this case represents an instance of an adverse reaction to a single drug. The patient was not diabetic, and sections revealed no evidence of arteritis or atherosclerosis. Vascular insufficiency related to ergot is a well-established association.

Pattern

The use of "pattern" in evaluating ADRs shifts the diagnostic emphasis from a drug-related etiology to the results of the drug action. Pattern may refer to a total clinicopathologic picture having similarities to cases in the literature (literature precedent), or it may refer to a morphologic pattern in a target organ that suggests an association with a particular drug or group of drugs.

Example: A 40-year-old white female underwent a kidney homotransplant because of congenital polycystic kidneys and uremia. The procedure was followed by immunosuppresive therapy with azathioprine and prednisone. After a year of this therapy, the woman developed a complex of neurologic symptoms, deteriorated rapidly, and died. Autopsy revealed multiple foci of malignant lymphoma in the brain, and in multiple sites in the lungs. A major basis for linking her posttransplant therapy with her malignant lymphoma is the precedent of a marked increase in the incidence of neoplasia in immunosuppressed individuals.[16]

Examples: The coagulation necrosis in the central and midzonal areas of liver lobules that occurs with acetaminophen toxicity (also seen in tannic acid toxicity, mushroom poisoning, and hypoxia); the peripheral necrosis of liver lobules associated with iron toxicity; the distinctive intracytoplasmic inclusions, in pancreatic acini, that are associated with boric acid poisoning[4]; and the aldactone bodies in the adrenal cortex that are related to spironolactone therapy[10] are all illustrations of tissue patterns suggesting particular drug associations.

Example: A 59-year-old white female was

on chronic warfarin therapy following cardiac surgery. Some months prior to her death, she was also put on allopurinol because of an elevated blood uric acid level. A few days before death she became weak and dyspneic, and had black, tarry stools, a hematocrit of 15.9, a hemoglobin of 5 grams, and prothrombin time of 14 percent. Terminally, the patient was in shock, and had a massive gastrointestinal hemorrhage. The mechanism of the hemorrhage in this case was probably related to the prolongation of the half-life of the warfarin the patient was receiving by the allopurinol she also received. The key in this case is knowing that such a drug–drug interaction may occur.[18]

Example: A 70-year-old white woman with a manic-depressive psychosis was treated, in sequence, with phenelzine sulfate (an MAO inhibitor) and imipramine (a tricylic antidepressant). On the same day that the MAO inhibitor was discontinued, the woman was started on the imipramine. Within half an hour she had a seizure and developed opisthotonos; her blood pressure rose (220/110 mm Hg); she became hyperthermic (temperature to 108°F); her pulse became rapid; and her breathing became sterterous. She died 5 hours later. Her ADR is another example of a drug–drug interaction. If a tricylic compound is given without a waiting period of about 2 weeks after discontinuing a MAO inhibitor, a severe and sometimes fatal reaction may occur characterized by hyperpyrexia, convulsions, and delirium.[1]

Example: A 61-year-old obese, diabetic woman, with hypertension and suspected pulmonary embolism, was treated with dicumarol. On the eighth day of this therapy, she developed discoloration of the skin over one breast, which proceeded to necrosis of the underlying tissue. Examination of the excised specimen of breast revealed infarction and necrosis of skin and subcutaneous tissue, associated with multiple organizing and organized thrombi in arterial and venous channels in the subcutaneous tissues. There was no evidence of vasculitis. The pattern of findings and associations in this woman is similar to the pattern of induced skin necrosis seen with coumarin congeners, as described in the literature.[15]

Drug Quantitation

Drug quantitation shifts our diagnostic attention back to the drug; it involves the determination of drug levels in body fluids and viscera. This method has its major utility in overdose cases, and requires the availability of toxicologic data on previously validated overdose cases for comparison.

Determining blood and body fluid levels of a drug is of little diagnostic value in cases that fall into the categories of hypersensitivity, idiosyncratic, or pharmacogenetic reactions, because in these instances drugs are given in therapeutic doses. Thus, while determination of drug levels in the three foregoing categories does confirm the presence of the agents being administered, we are still left with the problem of identifying the causative drug.

Example: A young soldier in Vietnam reported, in acute respiratory distress, to a medical unit. He stated that he was sensitive to chloroquine, and that he had just taken one chloroquine-primaquine tablet (for malarial prophylaxis). He died shortly thereafter. Autopsy revealed no anatomic cause of death. Fortunately, the autopsy prosector had chloroquine levels determined in the blood and viscera, with the following results: blood, 6.5 mg percent; liver, 23 mg percent; brain, 2.5 mg percent; lung, 23 mg percent; kidney, 24 mg percent; and stomach contents, 12.5 mg in the total sample. These levels are within the lethal range for chloroquine, as found in 13 chloroquine overdose deaths previously reported.[11]

The quantitative drug determinations in this case were responsible for the recognition of an instance of toxicity, not of hypersensitivity, as it first appeared from the history.

In fatal overdose cases, although the history may give a lead as to a single responsible drug, toxicologic screening should be requested on autopsy samples since multiple drug exposure is very common. Since sublethal levels of several drugs (combined effect) may cause death, toxicologic screening may bring to light one or more additionally responsible agents, and may account for a death in which the initially identified drug was present at levels below its minimum lethal range.

Example: A 1-year-old black female was given syrup of ipecac to induce vomiting, on the suspicion that she had accidentally ingested aspirin. She subsequently developed symptoms consistent with emetine toxicity, and died in less than 24 hours. Autopsy showed no anatomic cause of death. Analysis of the ipecac-labeled bottle revealed a concentration of emetine 29 times greater than in the usual formulation.

This case illustrates the point that quantitation of a drug should not be limited only to body fluids and viscera.

Drug Qualitation

Sometimes the qualitative identification of a drug in the tissues is of sufficient diagnostic assistance in a case of suspected ADR as to obviate the need for determining the quantity of drug present.

Example: A 3-year-old white male infant died after ingesting ferrous sulfate. His serum iron reached 810 μg/100 ml (normal: 40 to 140 μg/100 ml). Iron stains on small-intestine sections were strongly positive for iron in the mucosal tissues. If serum iron levels had not been available, iron stains on the intestinal mucosa would have been helpful in correlating with the history of iron ingestion.

Example: A 25-year-old white male drug addict died of an overdose of methadone. The blood level of methadone was 0.05 mg percent (within the lethal range); in addition, the lungs of the deceased were the seat of multiple granulomas associated with birefringent material. A portion of the wet tissue was digested with NaOH. The resulting sediment was examined by the powder method of x-ray diffraction. The pattern obtained indicated the presence of talc. Methadone, clandestinely produced, may have talc, lactose, or starch as excipients or filler. The granulomas in this case were associated with talc, demonstrated qualitatively, indicating probably chronic, intravenous drug usage.

ARE THE METHODS USED FOR DIAGNOSING AN ADR DURING LIFE THE SAME AS THOSE USED AT AUTOPSY?

All of the methodologic considerations heretofore considered (temporal eligibility, latent period, exclusion, de-challenge, re-challenge, singularity of the drug, pattern, and quantitation and qualitation of the drug) are equally applicable to autopsy and biopsy cases. The only provision specifically concerning fatal ADRs is that the use of de-challenge and re-challenge have occurred—of necessity—in the retrospective time frame.

Example: A 64-year-old woman with rheumatoid arthritis, hypothyroidism, and Reynaud's disease was treated recurrently with chlorambucil and prednisone for 6 years. She died with progressive liver failure, pancytopenia, and necrotizing bronchitis.

As seen in Figure 1-5, chlorambucil was given over a 6-year period, with two intervals of discontinuation. The markers (SGOT, LDH, and alkaline phosphatase) rose each time chlorambucil was reinstituted (two re-challenges), while the SGOT and alkaline phosphatase decreased during the two de-challenges, and the LDH decreased during the second de-challenge. The final elevations in these markers were associated with an increase in the bilirubin. The liver at autopsy weighed 800 grams, and was the seat of moderate cholestasis, multiple foci of necrosis, portal fibrosis, and acute and chronic triaditis. Because liver biopsies were unavailable, the status of the liver prior to chlorambucil therapy is unknown. Whether or not there was initial basic

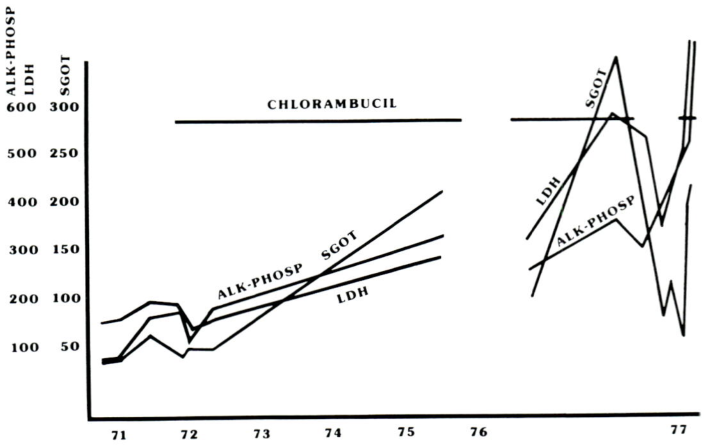

Fig. 1-5. Time-flow chart showing fluctuations in SGOT, LDH, and alkaline phosphatase during a succession of de-challenges and re-challenges with chlorambucil.

liver disease, the time-flow chart presents strong circumstantial evidence for a relationship between the chlorambucil and the successive changes in the markers of liver disease in this case. In addition to the circumstantial evidence provided by de-challenge and re-challenge, there is a precedent (pattern) for a relationship between chlorambucil and liver damage.[13, 17]

Example: A second illustration of the use of time relationships in a retrospective manner in an autopsy case is that of a 59-year-old white male who had an elective transurethral prostatectomy, the procedure taking 2 hours. After a brief period in the recovery room, and upon return to the ward, the patient became progressively drowsy, then unresponsive and cyanotic, and then went into respiratory arrest. After resuscitation he remained in a deep coma, with flat EEG waves.

Table 1-1. Medications During Elective Prostatectomy

11:00 AM (pre-operative):	
	Meperidine, 75 mg IM
	Promethazine, 25 mg
	Atropine, 0.4 mg
11:25 AM (during surgery):	
	Meperidine, 25-25-25 mg, IV
	Thiopental, 300-100-100 mg, IV
	Nitrous oxide
	Diazepam
12:55 PM (recovery room):	
	Meperidine, 75 mg, IM
	Promethazine, 25 mg
1:00 PM (on the ward):	
	Meperidine, 75 mg IM

Listing of medications received in a 2-hour period during an elective prostatectomy. (Note that meperidine was administered four times, the last two being within 5 minutes of one another.)

This man, during the 2 hour operative period, received a total of seven drugs (Table 1-1). A critical factor in this case is the meperidine: it was given four times in a 2-hour period (the 300 mg administered over the 2-hour period is an amount ordinarily given over a 6 to 9 hour period): and the last two doses of meperidine were given within 5 minutes of one another. This case is interpreted as being a fatal central depression from multiple drugs—their administration compressed into too short a time—with particular emphasis on the meperidine. In the context of methodology, the ADR diagnosis was made on the basis of a qualitative-quantitative drug identification from the patient's history, without benefit of the toxicology laboratory, and is put in the category of overdose. The diagnostic requirement was the availability of detailed and time-related information.

IS THERE DIFFICULTY IN DIFFERENTIATING A BASIC DISEASE FROM AN ADR?

This differentiation may be relatively easy if the target organ for the ADR differs from the site of the basic disease, and if the morphologic changes or other markers of the ADR are distinct from those of the basic disease. This differentiation is also simplified if there is no precedent for an adverse reaction to the particular drug in the site of the basic disease. This distinction becomes difficult when the organ or site of the basic disease is also the location of the alleged ADR, or when there is a morphologic similarity between the tissue alterations caused by the basic disease and the drug-induced changes.

Example: A 36-year-old sailor, with chronic alcoholism, developed jaundice while receiving chlorpromazine. A liver biopsy revealed prominent and predominantly centrilobular, intracanalicular and intracellular cholestasis (a finding not incompatible with a phenothiazine-induced jaundice). However, several other liver changes pointed to the likelihood of an extrahepatic cause of the cholestasis; among these changes were periductal lamellar fibrosis involving the larger interlobular ducts, and an acute and chronic inflammatory infiltrate in the portal triads, with polynuclear leukocytes within the walls and lumens of some of the interlobular ducts. A nondrug cause of the jaundice was confirmed by a later laparotomy that revealed stones in the common bile duct. In this case, the site (liver) and the pathologic change (cholestasis) were the same for both the drug and nondrug etiologies. Differentiation was aided by microscopic findings that predicted a nondrug causation, later confirmed by a surgical procedure.

Example: A 54-year-old white man developed right upper quadrant pain, a 20-pound weight loss, and a spiking fever unresponsive to antibiotics. His condition deteriorated progressively, until death occurred 3 months after his initial symptoms. His liver weighed 4,700 grams and contained multiple hemorrhagic nodules due to angiosarcoma. In addition, the portal fibrous tissues contained heavy deposits of brown pigment that were negative with the iron stain, nonbirefringent, and associated with alpha tracks by autoradiography. These findings are consistent with, if not diagnostic of, the presence of thorium dioxide, and correlated with a history of the patient having received intravenous thorotrast 16 years before while being studied for a possible liver abscess. Even though the liver may be the site of idiopathic angiosarcoma, the history and the microscopic findings in this case, along with autoradiography, put the tumor in a drug- or chemical-related category.

WHAT ARE THE MAJOR DIFFICULTIES IN DIAGNOSING AN ADR?

There are four major difficulties.

Incomplete Information

Time-related drug and disease-marker data are essential if the methods of confirming or denying drug linkage (temporal eligibility, latent period, exclusion, de-challenge, and re-challenge), as listed in Figure 1-1, are to be used. In order to achieve diagnostic success in ADR cases, the data base furnished by the microscopic findings alone (so dominant in general pathology) must be enlarged to include historical, clinical, and clinical laboratory information. The lack of adequate information to supplement the morphologic findings usually leads to diagnostic uncertainty or failure.

Polypharmacy

The numerous drugs received by many patients complicate the analytic problem in ADRs tremendously. The cases illustrated in Figures 1-3 and 1-4 illustrate the application of the time-flow chart to the analysis of polypharmacy problems. Nevertheless, in many instances the lack of adequate data, or the failure of the time-flow chart to "select-out" a single drug, results in diagnostic uncertainty.

The Lack of Objective Means of Demonstrating Linkage of the Drug with the Reaction

Even though we have instrumental methods (with autoanalyzers, spectrophotometers, chromatographs, x-ray diffraction devices, and other instruments) and histochemical techniques for identifying and demonstrating drugs and chemicals, these, except in overdose cases, do not have the diagnostic significance that the special stains and culture methods have for demonstrating specific causative organisms in granulomatous inflammation. At present, we must use time-flow charts and morphologic and clinicopathologic patterns to establish the causation of drug-related illnesses.

The Limited Number of Reaction Patterns of the Body to All Causes of Disease

Since the tissue changes produced by all etiologic agents in ADRs funnel into a limited number of "final common paths," these morphologic changes alone will seldom be diagnostic.

Of the four difficulties in the diagnosis of an ADR, only the first—incomplete information—is subject to a degree of immediate control. An illustration of the value of efforts to improve the information base is afforded in a study of 104 cases of jaundice and liver damage in patients taking one or another of the phenothiazine group of tranquilizers.[9] Figure 1-6 has two graphs. The one on the left represents the results of case evaluations using the information initially available. Note that confirmation of a drug reaction was made in 22 percent, was denied in 35 percent, and was uncertain in 43 percent of the cases. The graph on the right represents the results of evaluation after more adequate information was obtained on these same cases. Note that the "possible" or uncertain group was reduced to 13 percent, and that confirmation of a drug reaction was raised from 22 to 37 percent. The group in which a drug relationship to illness was denied was increased to 50 percent. This latter represents a large overdiagnosis by contributing pathologists, in view of the fact that most cases were submitted for evaluation because they were considered as likely ADRs.

SHOULD A JUDGMENT BE MADE ON THE DEGREE OF CERTAINTY OF AN ADR DIAGNOSIS?

After making a diagnosis in a case of suspected ADR, it is advisable to make a judgment on the certainty of the link between the drug and the alleged drug-induced illness. This judgment can be divided into five degrees of certainty: causative, probable, possible, coincidental, and negative. The causative and probable categories taken together mean "yes"; coincidental and negative mean "no"; and the possible category admits uncertainty as to drug causation. Definitions and illustrations of these five degrees of certainty follow:

Causative

Cases in this group are essentially limited to those of drug overdose (toxicity), with the diagnosis established primarily by a report of a lethal level of drug in body fluids, tissues, or both. A second criterion for this category is the absence of morphologic cause of death. An example is the chloroquine overdose case discussed previously.

Probable

This term is equivalent to "consistent with," a phrase frequently used in the practice of pathology. Cases in this group are considered to be drug-related, but are separated from "causative" because they lack the objective and quantitative laboratory finding that is the main basis for the "causative" diagnosis. The

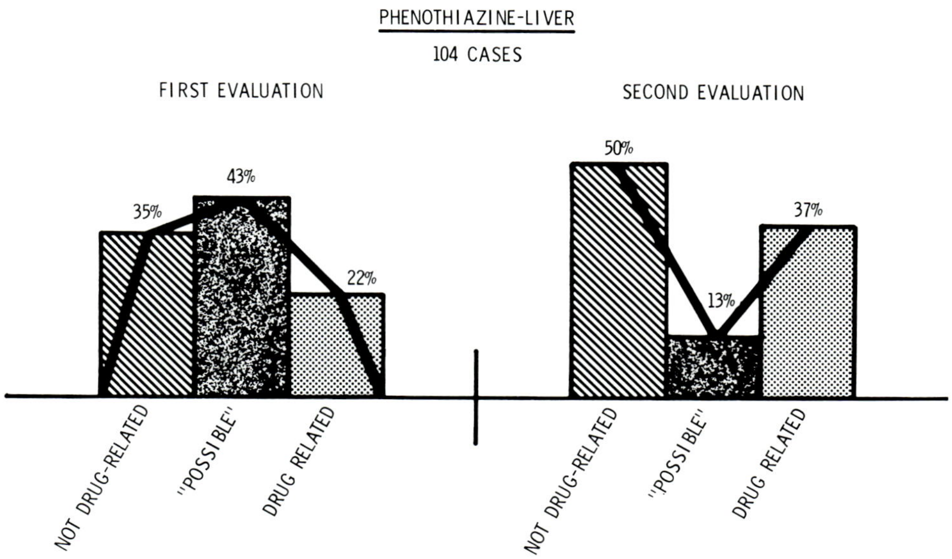

Fig. 1-6. Graphs illustrating the value of more complete case information, in a study of 104 cases of phenothiazine-associated hepatoses. First evaluation on left; second on right after obtaining additional data. Note inversion of the curve, reduction of the "possible" category, and large overcall group (50 percent) after the second evaluation. (From Irey, N. S.: Diagnostic Problems in Drug-Induced Diseases. In: Meyler, L. and Peck, H. M. (Eds): Drug-Induced Diseases. Vol. 4. Excerpta Medica, Amsterdam, 1972, by permission of the publishers.)

"probable" category may include any type of adverse reaction: toxicity, hypersensitivity, idiosyncratic, pharmacogenetic, exaggeration of therapeutic action, secondary pharmacologic action, and potentiation of one drug by the action of another.

Cases put in the "probable" category have the following characteristics: (1) The criteria of temporal eligibility and an appropriate latent period are met. (2) The clinical and morphologic findings are consonant with previous experience and literature precedent for the drug in question. (3) Other causes have been reasonably eliminated (the basic disease, comorbid states, other modalities of therapy). (4) One or several of the means of linking the drug to the reaction have been utilized (exclusion, de-challenge, re-challenge, singularity of drug, and "pattern" as previously defined and illustrated).

Example: The hydralazine case illustrated in Figure 1-4 serves as an example of a "probable" drug reaction. In this instance the drug was temporally eligible, and a positive de-challenge response was the basis for linking the hydralazine with the anemia and the leukopenia. The other 10 drugs were excluded either on the basis of temporal ineligibility, too long a latent period, or having been given continuously.

Possible

Cases are placed in this group when the relationship between a drug and an ADR can be neither confirmed nor denied. These cases may be divided into three types, having the following characteristics:

1. Cases with other potential causes: (1) The criteria for temporal eligibility and latent period in an ADR are met. (2) There is a precedent in the literature for an association between the clinicopathologic features of the illness and the drug in question. (3) The drug

candidates have been narrowed down to one by appropriate considerations (exclusion, dechallenge, re-challenge, and so forth.) (4) However, the clinicopathologic picture could have equally well been produced by the basic disease of the patient, a co-morbid state, or by other modalities of therapy.

2. Cases that meet some of the criteria for drug linkage, but in which there is insufficient information to meet all of these criteria. As an example, the phenothiazine study illustrated in Figure 1-6 had a large group (43 percent) of cases that had to be initially placed in the "possible" group because of inadequate data.

3. A third group in the "possible" category includes instances in which all the criteria for the "probable" class have been met except for a literature precedent. When such a case may constitute a new, emergent entity, it is put in the "possible" category, awaiting further confirmatory experience or a more extensive search of the literature.

Example: A 16-year-old white female drug-abuser developed pulmonary distress following a "pot" party, and was later admitted to the hospital with "extremely abnormal blood gases" and a diffuse bilateral pneumonic process identified by chest films. She suffered progressive pulmonary distress and died 1 month later. At autopsy, the lungs weighed 1,020 and 900 grams, respectively, and were the site of interstitial and intraalveolar fibrosis.

The history suggests a relationship between the "pot" party and the lung changes. While marijuana itself has not been implicated in pulmonary fibrosis, growing marijuana plants are sometimes sprayed with the herbicide paraquat, and there is precedent for paraquat-induced lung fibrosis in animal inhalation experiments, and in humans following skin absorption, parenteral injection, and ingestion.[2, 3, 19] While inhaled paraquat has not as yet been associated in humans with lung fibrosis, this still remains a possibility, and demonstration of paraquat in the lung tissues of this girl would strengthen this possible association. However, even if this herbicide was to be found in the pulmonary tissues, the case would still have to remain in the "possible" category, awaiting further confirmatory experience in humans.

Coincidental

Cases in this category represent instances in which the patient was indeed exposed to a drug or chemical, but in which analysis of the case reveals a nondrug cause, or cases in which the allegedly causative drug clearly was ineligible for an etiologic relationship.

Example: A 34-year-old Asian female was admitted to the hospital in coma with areflexia, with a history of possible overdose of glutethimide. The glutethimide blood level on admission was 2.5 mg percent (in toxic–lethal range). The patient was maintained on a Bird respirator and had two hemodialyses. She died on the fifth hospital day. Autopsy revealed and angiomatous malformation of the cerebellum that had bled into the posterior fossa and around the upper spinal cord; flattened gyri from edema; and hypoxic microscopic changes in the brain tissues. In view of the demonstration of an acceptable anatomic cause of death relating to a preexisting vascular anomaly, the role of the glutethimide was judged to be coincidental in this death.

Negative

This category is reserved for alleged ADR cases in which the drug was not in the patient's system at the time of onset of illness. This circumstance arises if the patient either did not take the drug (as assumed), or if the drug taken by the patient was incorrectly labeled.

Example: A diabetic supposedly taking tolbutamide developed renal dysfunction associated with a granulomatous interstitial nephritis. Since there is a precedent in the literature for an occasional association between sulfonylurea compounds (of which tolbutamide is one) and visceral granuloma formation, and there was also apparent temporal eligibility and apparent singularity of drug in this instance, the case was initially coded in the "possible" category, awaiting follow-up, and particularly the results of a de-challenge. We were later told that the patient had never taken the tolbutamide, though successive prescriptions for this drug had been filled over a 2-year period. The final coding was in the "negative" category, since the drug was not taken.

Example: A patient taking "ascorbic acid" developed urticaria, dyspnea, nausea, and vomiting. On analysis, the "ascorbic acid" was identified as benzyl penicillin.[6]

Using the criteria for the five degrees of certainty just described, the AFIP experience with 3,800 cases yielded the results shown in Fig. 1-7. Confirmation of the presence of an ADR was made in slightly less than half the cases (47 percent), denial of the presence of an ADR was made in about one-fifth (19.3 percent), and there remained an uncertain group of 33.7 percent of cases in which an ADR could be neither confirmed nor denied.

ARE THERE DIFFERENCES IN THE CIRCUMSTANCES GENERATING ADRs, AND IF SO SHOULD THE ADRs BE SUBGROUPED ACCORDINGLY?

In analyzing a group of 827 deaths in which validated ADRs occurred, it was found necessary to divide them into seven groups, in recognition of a variety of circumstances and factors that led to their occurrence,[8] as shown in Table 1-2. Fifty percent of the deaths (group I) were related to the nonmedicinal use of drugs (accidental or suicidal overdose cases). Twenty-five percent of the 827 deaths (groups II to VI) included cases in which drugs known to have high risk/benefit ratios were taken, those in which the ADRs were minor and nonlethal, those ADRs generated by errors committed by the medical team, and those in which responsibility for death from the drug could not be determined because of concomitant serious and potentially lethal basic diseases. Only 25 percent of the 827 cases (group VII) met the criteria for ADRs in the usual

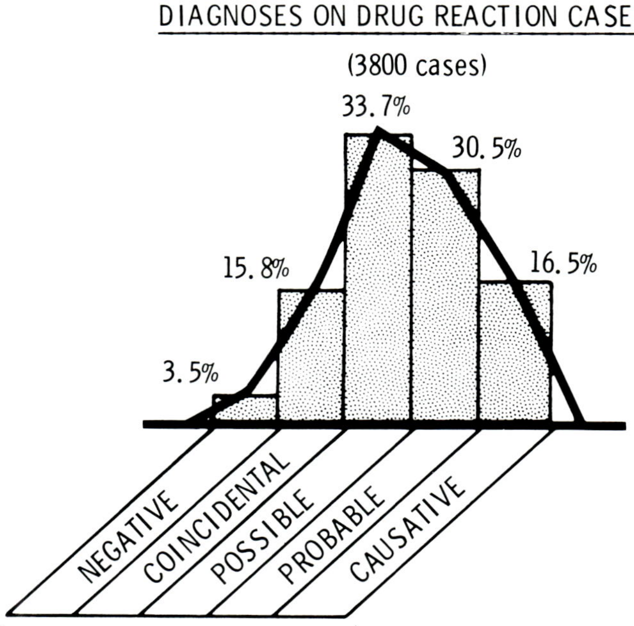

Fig. 1-7. Graph showing distribution of degrees of certainty as to the relationship between the drug and the alleged ADR in 3,800 cases.

Table 1-2. Adverse Drug Reactions & Death (827 Cases)

Group		No. Cases	Percent
I	Overdose	428	51.8
II	Malignancies Rx with cytostatics	48	5.7
III	Reactions to occupational chemicals	19	2.3
IV	ADRs present but minor and non-lethal	65	7.9
V	Coexistance of lethal ADR & lethal basic disease	22	2.6
VI	Lethal ADR associated with Dx or Rx errors	25	3.0
VII	ADRs in strict definitional sense	220	26.6
	Total	827	99.9

Subdivision of ADR cases into groups with recognition of special factors and circumstances relating to their genesis. (Note that Group VII (ADRs in the strict definitional sense) make up only 25 percent of the 827 cases.)

definitional sense, in that there was proper indication for the use of the drug, that the drug was given in recommended doses by the medical team and was properly administered, but in which an unintended and harmful reaction followed.

Putting an ADR case into one of the seven groups noted above is valuable when attempting to identify correctable factors in the genesis of ADRs, and may be useful to hospital drug-reaction committees in their assessment of the responsibility for and control of ADRs that occur within their jurisdiction.

SUMMARY

The emphasis in this introductory chapter on the pathology of drug-induced and toxic diseases has been on methods of analyzing and diagnosing cases of ADR. Our interest has been primarily on pinpointing the responsibility of a drug or chemical agent for an illness, and in identifying the drug or chemical. Put in another way the issue is *how* to diagnose, not *what* to diagnose. The use of this methodology should assist in confirming, denying, or admitting uncertainty as to the role of a drug in a patient's illness. The lack of application of an adequate methodology in evaluating alleged ADRs may be the basis for the wide disparity in estimates of mortality from ADRs. These estimates vary from 30,000 to 140,000 per year in the United States.[12] An estimate with this magnitude of difference indicates the lack of consistent diagnostic criteria.

In brief review, the successive steps in validating ADRs are:

1. To confirm the temporal eligibility of the drug and establish that the latent period is reasonably consonant with past experience.
2. To link the drug with the marker(s) of the reaction by one or several means: exclusion, de-challenge, re-challenge, singularity of drug, pattern (combined clinicopathologic features as well as morphologic pattern), and quantitation or qualitation of the drug.
3. If a drug etiology appears likely at this point, be sure that the patient's basic disease or co-morbid state is not linked with the marker(s) or indicator(s) selected for the analysis.
4. Make a judgement as to the degree of certainty of drug etiology.
5. Put the case into one of the seven categories listed in Table 1-2, so that the part played by other-than-drug factors may be recognized, thus avoiding clustering of cases with uncommon denominators.

Finally, a few comments on the "degree of certainty" categories:

1. In general pathology, diagnoses are sometimes made with qualifications, that is, a tumor may be so rare for a particular site, or the microscopic findings so borderline, that neither a diagnosis of benign nor malignant disease can be made with certainty. Usually, however, diagnoses in general pathology are made in unequivocal terms: cancer of the breast, tuberculous lymphadenitis, bronchopneumonia, and so forth. In contrast, owing to the complexity of the subject and the present state of our knowledge, it seems advisable in the field of ADRs to qualify each case with one of the five previously described and

defined "degrees of certainty." This is in parallel with reporting some serologic tests (+, ++, +++, or ++++), and with weather predictions made in terms of percentages of probability (such as a 90 percent chance of rain).

2. The "causative" category is essentially limited to drug overdose deaths, in which the key diagnostic factor is an objective and laboratory-derived finding (the drug level in body fluids, tissues, or both). This level is, of course, supplemented with a compatible history and clinical picture, and the failure to find an anatomic cause of death.

3. The "probable" category is the second strongest degree of certainty in the context of the methodology previously described; cases so designated are considered to be drug-related with the information that is available. This caveat leaves the way open for later reconsideration of such cases if additional information comes to light. This additional information may take two forms: (1) additional new data; or (2) correction of original information. The first diagnosis might therefore either be strengthened or invalidated. In any event, the use of "probable" would allow diagnostic flexibility in reacting to any new facts, and the evaluator would not be "painted into a corner" with regard to the diagnosis. This flexibility is important in both clinical and medicolegal settings.

4. If a case has all the requisites for "probable" except for a literature precedent, and if a further literature search fails to uncover similar cases, consideration should be given to publishing the single case. Since many ADRs are rare occurrences, there may be other, similar single cases that are also awaiting literature precedent. It is not unusual for a single case report of a "new" ADR to be followed by a succession of similar cases appearing in the journals—the result of others having taken courage from the initial report. If such a "possible" case is reported, it is important to leave no doubt that the ADR is as yet unproven, though the data appears to support such an allegation.

5. The "coincidental" and "negative" categories of certainty can usually be made with more assurance than can the other three categories, because they are eliminative in principle. They are not, however, immune from the impact of new or corrective information at a later date.

It is evident from the foregoing considerations that it is important to have a written or implied understanding with the recipients of diagnostic reports that the diagnoses on ADR cases are made on the basis of the data then available.

REFERENCES

1. AMA Drug Evaluations. AMA Department of Drugs. 3rd Ed. PSG Publishing Company, Inc., Littleton, Massachusetts, 1977.
2. Cross, C. E., & Last, J. A.: Paraquat goes to pot. Chest 74:358, 1978.
3. Fairshter, R. D., & Wilson, A. F.: Paraquat and marijuana: Assessing the Hazard (Editorial). Chest 74:357, 1978.
4. Fisher, R. S.: Intracytoplasmic inclusions in the pancreas due to boric acid poisoning. Am. J. Pathol. 28:745, 1951.
5. Fuerst, S. V.: Drug Nomenclature Printout. Department of Medical Terminology and Nomenclature, American Medical Association, Chicago, 1979.
6. Golbert, T. M., & Patterson, R.: Recurrent anaphylaxis caused by a misidentified drug. Ann. Intern. Med. 68:621, 1968.
7. Gosselin, R. E., Hodge, H. C., Smith, R. P., & Gleason, M. N.: Clinical Toxicology of Commercial Products, 4th Ed. Williams & Wilkins Co., Baltimore, 1976.
8. Irey, N. S.: Adverse drug reactions and death: A review of 827 cases. J.A.M.A. 236:575, 1976.
9. Ishak, K. G., & Irey, N. S.: Hepatic injury associated with the phenothiazines. Arch. Pathol. 93:283, 1972.
10. Janigan, D. T.: Cytoplasmic bodies in the adrenal cortex of patients treated with spironolactone. Lancet 1:850, 1963.
11. Kiel, F. W.: Chloroquine suicide. J.A.M.A. 190:398, 1964.
12. Koch-Weser, J.: Fatal reactions to drug therapy. N. Engl. J. Med. 291:302, 1974.

13. Koler, R. D., & Forgren, A. L.: Hepatotoxicity due to chlorambucil: Report of a case. J.A.M.A. 167:316, 1958.
14. The Merck Index. 9th Ed. Merck & Company, Inc., Rahway, New Jersey, 1976.
15. Nalbandian, R. M., Mader, I. J., Barrett, J. L., Pearce, J. F., & Rupp, E. C.: Petechiae, ecchymoses, and necrosis of skin induced by coumarin congeners. J.A.M.A. 192:603, 1965.
16. Penn, I.: Malignant disease in immunodeficient states in man. p. 96. In Grundmann, E., and Gross, R., Eds.: The Ambivalence of Cytostatic Therapy. Springer-Verlag, Berlin, Heidelberg, New York, 1975.
17. Schiff, L.: Diseases of the Liver. 4th Ed. p. 662. J. B. Lippincott Company, Philadelphia, Toronto, 1975.
18. Vesell, E. S., Passananti, G. T., & Greene, F. E.: Impairment of drug metabolism in man by allopurinol and nortriptyline. N. Engl. J. Med. 283:1484, 1970.
19. Zavala, D. C., & Rhodes, M. L.: An effect of paraquat on the lungs of rabbits: Its implications in smoking contaminated marijuana. Chest 74:418, 1978.

2

The Fetus, Infant, and Young Child

Eugene V.D.K. Perrin

INTRODUCTION

The knowledge of adverse reactions to drugs and environmental toxic substances is old. The code of Hammurabi of 2200 B.C. ordained that a physician who caused a patient's death should lose his hands, and the Hermetic books of Thoth outlined therapeutic paths from which the physician strayed only at his peril. In the "Odyssey," Homer wrote that there are many drugs that are excellent when mingled, and many fatal. Hippocrates pleaded—in its later, Latin equivalent—"per primam non nocere," Galen warned against the dangers of badly written and obscure prescription, and Rhazes advised "if simple remedies are effective, do not prescribe compound remedies."[1] Adverse effects of mercury, lead, cadmium, zinc, and a wide variety of other substances have been cited since earliest times. This study is largely concerned with the response to drugs and foreign substances of *Homo sapiens,* in the extremely limited period of intrauterine life, infancy, and early childhood. Rarely, substances that "should" cause damage in infants and fetuses, but that have not been recorded to do so, will be cited from examples encountered in older children.

Although many physicians had written about remedies with disastrous visible side effects, it was not until the turn of this century that critical studies were suggested; specifically, these were the first formal inquiries into such suspected adverse reactions to drugs as sudden deaths from chloroform anesthesia in 1880 and jaundice following the arsenic treatment of syphilis. In 1929, John Leake drew attention to the inadequacy of existing testing procedures for new drugs, writing that "many drug firms make the mistake of believing that their chemists can furnish trustworthy pharmacologic opinion."

The only shortcut from the chemical laboratories to the clinic is one that passes too close to the morgue. In 1937, 107 people died from poisoning by an elixir of sulphanilamide that contained diethylene glycol as a solvent. The manufacturer did not trouble to inquire whether the solvent was safe for its purpose. In France, a disaster of similar magnitude occurred when 100 people died from poisoning by Stalinon, an organic compound of tin used in the treatment of boils. Unfortunately, although major catastrophes focused attention on the toxicity of the drug at fault, awareness and concern were only transient. The profession's threshold of stimulation remained too high, and its latent period before reaction remained too long. It had taken some 47 years to discover that amidopyrine was a potent marrow poison. Fifteen years had passed before it was determined that cincophen caused jaundice. Aspirin had been in use for 40 years before it was incriminated in 1938 as a cause of gastric hemorrhage, and was used for another 20 years before the news spread adequately. The dangers of chloramphenicol were first appreciated in the early 1950s, yet some two decades later the chairman of a U.S. Senate Subcommittee had good cause to complain that warnings of these dangers had gone unheeded.

Until the 1950s, textbooks of medicine and pharmacy devoted comparatively little space to adverse drug reactions, and even that was given over unto the ill effects of one or two drugs. In 1952, Meyler's first book on adverse drug reactions was published, and in 1960, the U.S. Food and Drug Administration began to collect reports of adverse reactions. Following the disaster with thalidomide which had been prescribed as a safe hypnotic, basic research on adverse drug reactions (ADRs) took an upswing. Furthermore even though the reported incidence of such reactions varies from 1 percent or less to 28 percent, in most studies the figure has been between 10 and 20 percent. The type of reaction that occurs most frequently is an unwanted pharmacologic action of a drug; the next most common is an excessive effect of the required pharmacologic action of a drug; the third is an allergic reaction to a drug.

According to a 1974 study, one-third of all ADRs were attributed to eight types of drugs, the first five of which were aspirin, antimicrobials, digoxin, anticoagulants and diuretics. A 1967 study found that 90 percent of ADRs were caused by digitalis, antimicrobials, insulin, and diuretics. Miller, in 1974, reported that the drugs most commonly causing or strongly influencing admission to hospitals were digoxin, aspirin, prednisone, warfarin, and guanethidine; while heparin, prednisone, spironolactone, hydrochlorothizide and digoxin had the highest reaction rates.

Further descriptions of much of the information mentioned in this introduction can be found in Davies's *Textbook of Adverse Drug Reactions* (see General References).

PREDISPOSITION

According to one study, ADRs of all types are more common in white than in dark peoples; other studies have not shown this result. The rate at which drugs are acetylated varies considerably, with "rapid acetylators" predominating among Eskimos and Japanese, and "slow acetylators" among Mediterranean Jews. Compared with fast acetylators, all slow acetylators are likely to develop peripheral neuropathy from isoniazid, and lupus associated either with treatment with this drug or with hydralazine. Interestingly, fast acetylators may be more susceptible than slow acetylators to the type of lupus associated with procainamide therapy.

In the neonate, especially when premature, some of the enzymes involved in drug metabolism may be poorly developed, thus increasing the risk of ADR. The most hazardous drugs in this regard are chloramphenicol, sulfonamides, novobiocin, barbiturates, morphine and its derivatives, and vitamin K and its analogues. In the very young child, chloramphenicol may induce the "grey syndrome" characterized by abdominal distention, vomiting, peripheral cyanosis, profound shock, respiratory failure, and death. Sulfonamides, novobiocin, and vitamin K analogues may induce or aggravate kernicterus. Barbiturates and morphine, as well as other narcotics, may cause severe respiratory depression.

Some ototoxic antibiotics, such as streptomycin, are cleared by the kidney more slowly in the young child than the adult, and toxic effects may occur unless the dose is suitably altered; an increased sensitivity to digoxin in the first 2 weeks of life may be explained by a similar mechanism. The increased sensitivity of the newborn to morphine and its derivities has been attributed to a poorly developed glucuronidation process. A poorly developed oxidation reaction and possibly inadequate renal function, or both, may also account for the poor tolerance of the newborn to some barbiturates.

THE EFFECT OF ENVIRONMENTALLY ENCOUNTERED CHEMICALS AND DRUGS ON THE EMBRYO, FETUS, AND SMALL INFANT

Much of the material to be studied in this chapter is based upon case reports (see Tables 2-1, 2-2, and 2-3). No animal work will be cited. In most cases, as for instance in poisoning from acetylsalicylic acid, the physical alterations produced are not specific, and such phenomena as those related to edema of the brain will be cited. In other cases, as with use of certain anesthetics, there will be listed such effects as respiratory failure, the morphologic features of which are simply those related to prolonged anoxia. In general, there is insufficient pathologic data on ADRs in the embryo, fetus, and infant for the creation of a large body of knowledge. An attempt to collect such information has been vigorously pursued by the Registry of Untoward Reactions to Drugs at the Armed Forces Institute of Pathology.

When fetal damage is considered, this must include, by inference, the damage that inhibits the development of the fertilized egg beyond the first few cell divisions. The consequences of some chemical agents and environmental insults may be the loss of a fertilized early conceptus with no specific clinical evidence that such an event has occurred.

The current major reference on the intrauterine tissue response to material ingestion or exposure to medication or toxic substances is the catalogue of Shepard,[103] in which morbid anatomy is not delineated in detail. All relevant references may be found in that text and in the current edition of Smith,[108] as well as in Martin,[62] Warkany,[121] Schardein,[99] Schwarz et al.,[100] Tuchmann-Duplessis,[118] Nishimura et al.,[76a] and Pomerance et al.[88] Wilson and Fraser,[124] in their four-volume *Handbook of Teratology,* have summarized most of the existing knowledge, and have pointed out the directions for appropriate research.

A common belief is that the placenta is a barrier behind which the conceptus is protected. There is considerable information that virtually all unbound chemicals in the maternal plasma have access to the conceptus. Many small molecules, of less than 600 molecular weight and low ionic charge, cross the placenta by simple diffusion; others cross by facilitated diffusion, through transport mechanisms or by other mechanisms; thus the question is not whether a given molecule of iron crosses the placenta, but that the rate at which it crosses is determined by a variety of physical and chemical factors. The chemical agents or their breakdown products that cross the placenta usually reach the embryo or fetus in some fraction of their maternal concentration; therefore even though there may be high dosage and absorption in the mother, this does not mean that a significant dosage will reach the fetus.

As is well known, the general principles of teratology related to drugs and chemicals, and in part the transplacental toxic alterations that are not specifically malformation-producing in the fetus, continue to hold.

To paraphrase Wilson[124]:

(1) Susceptibility to such action of a drug or chemical depends upon the genetic makeup of the conceptus and the way in which this reacts and interacts with the environment.

(2) Susceptibility to such chemical agents varies with the stage of development of the embryo or fetus at the time of exposure. There is considerable knowledge about teratogenesis in this regard, but not much is known about toxic effects that are not teratogenic.

(3) The responsible drugs and chemical agents act through specific mechanisms on developing tissues and cells to initiate abnormal development. This phenomenon may not necessarily lend itself to morphologic analysis; by the time the microscopist or quantitative biologist can examine the damaged conceptus, reparative mechanisms may have removed such evidences of disturbed morphogenesis as hemorrhage, necrotic cells, and aberrant structures. Several authors in the Wilson and Fraser handbook suggest that one of the most frequently observed signs of abnormal embryogenesis is cell death in excess of that normally associated with development. Cellular interaction in the form of induction is not always qualifiable morphologically. The same is true of morphogenetic movements, with which chemical substances may interfere. One of the more interesting observations is that some agents which are initially destructive of developing cells may cause cellular depletion

Table 2-1. Morphology of Drug- and Environmental Substance-Associated Intrauterine Disease*

Thyroid drugs	
Iodine	Fetal goiter, hyperplasia of acinar epithelium
Tapazol	Same
Tumor therapy agents	
Methotrexate	Abortion, anomalies (see text), cleft palate
Busulfan	Oral clefts
Cyclophosphamide	Defects of extremities, intrauterine growth retardation, fetal death
Chlorambucil	Abortion, possible cause of agenesis of kidney and ureter
Antibiotics	
Chloramphenicol	No data (fetal death?)
Streptomycin	No morphology, clinical hearing loss, controversial
Tetracyclines	Deciduous tooth staining, controversial bone abnormalities
Analgesics	
Acetaminophen	Renal failure without description, no malformations[14]
Salicylates	Reduced fetal size, increased stillbirth, no malformations. ?Metanephric adenoma[13]
Drugs of abuse[32]	
Cannabis	Not known teratogenic in humans
Codeine, morphine	Same
Heroin	Same
Methadone	Same
Cocaine	Same
Mescaline	Not proved teratogenic in humans
Caffeine	Not proved teratogenic in humans
Barbiturates	Same
Lysergic Acid (LSD)	Same, (see text)
Methylqualone	Same
Phencyclidine	Controversial[33]
Dextroamphetamine	Ventricular and atrial septal defects (?) Biliary atresia (?)[55,80]
Anaesthetics	
Volatile anesthetics	No morphologic data, increased fetal loss.
Local anesthetics	Inadvertent injection into fetus, central nervous system depression, gliosis[24,66]
Antineurotics, antipsychotics, tranquilizers	
Diazepam	Oral clefts, controversial
Meclizine, phenothiazines, benzodiazapines	Not proved teratogenic in humans
Chlorpromazine	Same
Haloperidol, imipramine	Same
Chloroquine	In a single case,[103,107] a woman on heavy doses during four pregnancies had two children congenitally deaf with vestibular dysfunction; a third child had hemihypertrophy and Wilms' tumor [significance (?)]
Chlorbiphenyls	PCB. No anatomic data. Skin staining. PBB. No anatomic data, no known malformations. PCP. No anatomic data, no known malformations. PCB[29]
Metals (see text)	
Cortisone and related compounds	Controversial association with oral clefts[11,98]
Digitalis	No convincing anatomic data in fetus.
Methyldopa	One malformation recorded in offspring of 122 mothers [significance (?)]

Continued

Table 2-1. *Continued*

Diethylstilbestrol (see text)	
Hyperthermia (sauna baths)	Conjectural, controversial[109]
Carbon monoxide	Controversial. Central nervous system.[59,103,121]
Transplacental carcinogenesis	Highly controversial. No clear evidence of nitrosourea or vinyl chloride transplacental carcinogenesis. Case of poorly differentiated liver tumor in infant whose mother worked with paints, possibly vinyl chloride (Perrin, unpublished study). Long latent period (?)
Hexachlorophene	Not known to be fetotoxic or teratogenic in humans
Monosodium glutamate	Same
Oral contraceptives	Controversial[103]
Phenmetrazine	Controversial case of multiple anomalies[103]
Doxylamine (Bendectin)	Controversial, limb anomalies, most studies not convincing
Vitamin excesses	
Vitamin A	"Cerebral palsy," eye damage, syndactyly. No good morphologic data, controversial
Vitamin D	Hypercalcemia, ??mental retardation
Anticoagulants	
Bishydroxycoumarin	Fetal death, intrauterine hemorrhage
Ethyl biscoumacetate	Same
Warfarin sodium	Characteristic facies, flat nasal bridge, intrauterine hemorrhage;[103,108] punctate epiphyses (?)[103,108] Asplenia syndrome (?)[52]
Antiepileptics (see text)	
Diphenylhydantoin	Highly variable syndrome, little detailed anatomy available, variable risk[108]
Tridione	More severe cardiac anomalies and mental retardation, characteristic facies[108]
Ethyl alcohol (see text)	Highly variable syndrome, of most significance in heavy drinkers; possible significance in others
Pesticides, herbicides	
2,4-D	Of this ubiquitous substance and its contaminant "dioxin" (TCDD) little save anecdotal material is known. This is also true of 2,4,5,-T; eldrin, aldrin, DDT, and breakdown products in humans.

* (See refs. 99, 103, 121). Some substances are mentioned in which effect has been expected but not recorded, some mentioned in which no frank, detailed anatomic data is yet recorded, but may be.

in a single locus, but may ultimately result in excessive tissue, such as an extra finger.

(4) Death of the embryo or fetus, malformation, growth retardation, and functional disorder are the final manifestations of abnormal development. The cause of death may not be clear, and resorption frequently occurs. Nor is malformation always accompanied by identifiable specific cellular changes other than reduction in cells, absence of cells, or aberrant position of cells.

To the four principles concerning the effects of drugs or chemicals on the developing organism that have been listed above, we may add two more:

(5) That the access of these abnormal environmental influences depends upon the nature of the influences themselves; with regard to this, we have already discussed the failure of the placenta to protect the fetus.[85]

(6) That there is probably a dose dependent relationship from no effect to a lethal effect with most compounds. It may be stated that there exist some situations in which cells are destroyed but in which there is no obvious manifestation of abnormality within the fetus or the conceptus in life. Damage to large numbers of cells by a larger than normal dosage of a drug or chemical would logically lead to some embryotoxicity. An organized embryo

Table 2-2. A List of Selected Morphologic Reactions in Infancy and Early Childhood[62, 117]

Acetaminophen	Liver necrosis[77] Renal tubular necrosis Cerebral edema
Ampicillin	Pseudomembranous enterocolitis[5]
Aminophyllin	Cerebral and pulmonary edema[78]
Arsenic	Squamous cell skin carcinomas, other[4]
Aspirin	Hepatotoxicity[86, 125] Gastrointestinal hemorrhage[9] Cerebral edema Focal necrosis: liver, pancreas (see Fig. 2-1).
Barbiturates	Cerebral edema (seizures)
Boric acid	Pancreatic acinar intracytoplasmic inclusions[119]
Carbon monoxide	Acute cerebral hemorrhages Chronic focal necrosis, globus pallidus; gliosis
Chloramphenicol	Marrow depression
Dicloxacillin	Hepatotoxicity Gastrointestinal bleeding
Digitalis	No morphology
Diphenylhydantoin	Stevens-Johnson syndrome Liver necrosis Atypical lymphoid hyperplasia[97] Calvarial thickening[45] Gingival hyperplasia Rickets[12] Lupus erythematosus-like syndrome[8]
Ethanol	Hypoglycemia and convulsions Cerebral edema Chronic pancreatitis
Glucocorticoids	Pancreatitis Myopathy Osteoporosis Compression fractures Atherosclerosis Adrenal depression
Gold	Intrahepatic cholestasis[30] Neutropenia
Hexachlorophene	Spongy cerebral degeneration, infants[105]
Hydrochlorthiazide	Neutropenia
Imipramine	Cerebral edema[70]
Iron compounds	Fatal poisoning[60] Gastrointestinal iron incrustation, ulcer, hemorrhage Liver necrosis[110]
Isoniazid	Liver necrosis[120]
Kerosene ingestion	Lipid pneumonia[111]
Lead	Cerebral edema[71, 72] Lead line in gums Lead line in bones
(With gasoline sniffing)[10]	Nuclear inclusions in liver, renal tubules[35]
Lomotil	Respiratory depression, gliosis in fatal cases
Organic mercury[6, 28, 63, 114]	Acute: Renal tubular necrosis Liver and myocardial necrosis Chronic: atrophy of calcarine area, loss of granular layer, cerebellum, peripheral nerve degeneration-regeneration, fetal, infantile (Minimata, see p. 34 and Ch. 6)

Continued

Table 2-2. *Continued*

Methadone	Sudden death, asphyxial changes
Sodium hydroxide (lye)	Burn, esophagus
Sodium hypochlorite (Clorox)	Rare erosion, ulceration, esophageal scarring
Parenteral nutrition, prolonged	Cholestatic liver disease
Sulfonamides Sulfamethoxazole-Trimethaprim	Pancytopenia
Tetracycline	Discoloration and hypoplasia, teeth Bone growth changes (?) Pseudotumor cerebri Hepatotoxicity[57]
Thallium	Alopecia Hepatic necrosis, fatty metamorphosis Gastrointestinal hemorrhage[94]
Tumor therapy agents (in addition to marrow/tumor effect)	Second tumors [56]
Cyclophosphamide	Pulmonary fibrosis[1] and chest deformity; bladder ulcers
Amethopterin (methotrexate)	Intestinal mucosal nuclear enlargement, ulceration Fatty liver, fibrosis of liver
6-Mercaptopurine	Fibrosis of liver
Actinomycin D	Acute hepatic necrosis
Adriamycin	Cardiomyopathy
Velban (vinblastine)	Epilation, vesiculation of the mouth, nuclear/cytoplasmic ratio changes as in folic acid deficiency; testicular atrophy; acute cerebral edema, chromatolysis of neurons
Valproic acid	Pancreatitis[7]
Vitamin A (excess)	Cerebral edema Cortical hyperostosis
Vitamin D (excess)	Diffuse calcification, heart, kidneys, soft tissue, other
Special, miscellaneous	Lactobezoars in the low-birth-weight infant[20,21] Antacid bezoars in newborns[90]
Glue-sniffing (n-hexanes)	Cerebral edema Pulmonary edema Fatty metamorphosis, liver Degeneration, peripheral nerve[48]
Contrast medium	Renal glomerular thrombosis, other[3]

repairs itself better than do individual cells, and the destruction of a number of cells in excess of the reparative ability of the embryo produces malformations.

The mechanisms of malformation and toxicity in the fetus are only partially helpful in understanding morphologic alterations. Mutation is among the most frequently discussed mechanisms, followed by chromosomal nondisjunction and breakage, mitotic interference, altered nucleic acid integrity or function, changes in the precursors and substrates needed for biosynthesis, altered energy sources, enzyme inhibition, imbalance of an osmolar nature, and altered membrane characteristics; however, none of these necessarily assist in our understanding of the problem. The work of Kurent and Sever[69] on infectious disease in the fetus is one type of a model for the effects of drugs and chemicals. At the cellular level, mechanisms of malformation produced by viruses include acute cell death, persistent infection without cell death, and immune-mediated cellular damage. Mitotic inhibition with decreased numbers of cells, chromosomal abnormalities invisible at the light-microscopic level, vascular inflammatory alterations, and nonspecific alterations men-

(Text continues on p. 29)

Table 2-3. Typical Fatal Poisonings Seen in a Children's Hospital Among Infants and Small Children, 1960–1980

Misc. Substance	Age	Race/Sex	Details of Exposure	Autopsy Findings
Salt	2 months	Black/male	Dietary, inadvertent, 8 gm/day (!), patient with salt-losing adreno-genital syndrome	Renal vein thrombosis with tubular casts, glomerular damage
Ellipten (aminoglutethide)	1½ years	White/male		"Lissencephaly" Portal fibrosis Hyperplasia of thyroid Hyperplasia, adrenal cortex
Amitryptylene (dibenzazepine)	1 year	White/male	Took 7-12 pills from drawer, cardiac arrest	Nonspecific features of shock
Chloromycetin	12 days	Black/female		Cardiac dilatation, biventricular Hepatocellular necrosis, piecemeal Massive atelectasis (?) Astrocytic swelling, slight gliosis, brain
Tumor therapy drugs				
Actinomycin D	6 years	White/female		Toxic enterocolitis with ulceration Agranulocytosis with marrow hypoplasia, sepsis
Vincoleukoblastine	3 years and 18 years	White/female and Mexi-can-Ameri-can/female		Alopecia, granulocytic ulcers of skin Exfoliative dermatitis Hemorrhagic pneumonia Marrow hypoplasia Massive ulceration of small bowel
Nicotine	1 year	White/male	Less than ½ cc	Perivascular "cuffing" in brain, cord; lymphocytic infiltration in sympathetic ganglia
Aminophylline	19 months	White/female	Five 250 mg suppositories	Acute neuron necrosis Necrotizing bronchiolitis Interstitial pneumonia
Imipramine (Tofranil)	1 year	White/male	15 tablets (375 mg)	Massive pulmonary edema Toxic gastroenterocolitis
Kerosene and petroleum distil-lates, exemplary (several cases)	2 years	Black/male	3 cc	Acute hemorrhagic broncho-pneumonia followed by lipid pneumonia Chemical tracheobronchitis
Quinine	1½ years	White/female	12 tablets	No specific findings
Salicylates, many examples, e.g.:	5 months	Black/female		None significant
	11 years	White/female	80 mg%	Brain swelling
	26 hours	White/female	Mother took 110 grains ASA in 4th week, then 2 gr. phenobar-bitol and 800 mg Equanil throughout pregnancy	Massive aspiration, amniotic sac contents Pyknosis and hyperplasia of pancreatic islets (Fig. 2-1) Fatty metamorphosis, liver. Renal tubular necrosis (Fig. 2-5)

	19 months	White/female	Level: 30 mg%	Lipid depletion, adrenal; thymic involution Inclusions (viral), lymph nodes Anoxic changes, brain
	2 years	White/female	38 mg%	Pulmonary edema Chronic pneumonitis Anoxic changes, brain (Liver *Toxocara*)
	6½ years	White/male	85 mg%	Pulmonary edema "Idiopathic" cardiac hypertrophy Toxic nephropathy Brain swelling
	23 months	White/male	70 mg%	Lobular (broncho-) pneumonia Fatty liver
	5 months	White/female	78 mg%	Fatty metamorphosis (parents on several antipsychotics), liver
	18 months	White/male	53 mg% phenol salicylate "Salol" 1.8 mg% phenol	Acute enteritis Fatty metamorphosis, microvesicular, liver Focal necrosis, pancreas
Urokon	2½ years	Black/female		Renal glomerular infarcts (Fig. 2-6) and tubular necrosis Neuron necrosis, brain stem Severe tetralogy of Fallot
	9 weeks	Black/male		Tubular necrosis, kidney Left hypoplasia, heart
Dilantin	4 years	Black/male	Dilantin and Mellaril given for hyperkinetic state	Erythema multiforme bullosum (Stevens-Johnson syndrome), involving esophagus, pharynx, trachea
	2½ years	White/male	Dilantin and phenobarbitol	Erythema multiforme bullosum, involving tracheobronchial tree Aplastic anemia
Fetal Dilantin syndrome	2 cases	White/female Black/female		Characteristic facies Hypoplastic distal phalanges, nails [cause of death unrelated(?)]
Alcohol	3 fatal cases			Characteristic facies Hypoplastic distal phalanges, nails
Acetaminophen	6 months	White/female	6 doses, twice prescribed amount	Liver: acute massive centrolobular necrosis Microvesicular fatty metamorphosis, liver Acute encephalopathy with cerebral edema, neuron necrosis Virologic studies, negative on lung, heart, liver
	2½ years	White/female	3 doses, as expected	Liver: massive necrosis
Metals				
Mercury	3 months	White/male	Given ½ cc mercurial diuretic and theophylline; urine level 0.48 mg/L of Hg	Mucosal necrosis, ulcerations, stomach, small bowel Fatty metamorphosis, liver (Fig. 2-4) Severe renal tubular necrosis (Fig. 2-7)
	9 weeks	White/male	Mercurial diuretic	Myocardial necrosis, papillary muscle (Fig. 2-2) Renal tubular necrosis "Toxic splenitis"

Continued

Table 2-3. *Continued*

Misc. Substance	Age	Race/Sex	Details of Exposure	Autopsy Findings
Boron (boric acid)	1 year	White/female	Boric acid to diaper rash for 8 months, infant hypotonic	Pneumonia Many intracytoplasmic inclusions, pancreatic acinar cells
	18 months	White/male	Chlorox burns of buttocks, boric acid solution applied to raw areas	No anatomic cause of death, no inclusions
Copper (copper cyanide)	2 years	White/male	Accidental ingestion, father an engraver	Methemoglobinemia secondary to treatment Cerebral edema
Iron (4 cases)	16 months	Black/female		Iron incrustation, ileum (Fig. 2-3), colon Transmural hemorrhagic necrosis, ileum, rectum, bladder Minimal siderosis, liver, kidneys, mesenteric lymph nodes Haemorrhagic necrosis, massive, adrenals Cerebral edema, toxic neuron necrosis
Lead (7 cases, ages 2½ to 7 years)				
Exemplary cases	3 years	White/male		Brain swelling, perivascular edema Neuronal necrosis Cerebral vascular calcification (Fig. 2-9) Growth arrest and lead line; long bones Toxic hepatitis; nuclear inclusions in liver, kidney tubules (Fig. 2-8)
	2⅔ years	Black/female		Confluent pneumonia, *Klebsiella* Fatty metamorphosis, liver Cerebral edema, neuron necrosis Cortical necrosis, cerebellum Lead line, growth arrest, long bones
	3½ years	White/male		Acute necrotizing enteritis Nuclear inclusions, liver, renal tubules Cerebral and cerebellar edema; neuron necrosis, dentate

tioned elsewhere are those that have been described. Insertion of viruses into the genetic mcehanism has also been described.

Agenesis resulting from tissue repair of intrauterine damage is a model for other forms of transplacental injury, producing such abnormalities as scarring of the cerebral aqueduct with apparent agenesis. This model also holds for the loss of limb structures. Other abnormalities are hypoplasia, such as is seen when immature cells are attacked by a virus, and defects of normal ear organogenesis, such as defects of neural tube closure, produced by viruses and chemical agents alike. Frank necrotic and cavitary changes, with inhibition of cell movement, are well known features.

The many mutagenic agents—some of which produce postnatal abnormalities—are reviewed in the contribution of Malling and Wassom[61] and in the several volumes edited by Hollander;[43] many of the most devastating are tumor therapy agents, but others in the environment have been studied. Environmental mutagens have also been studied by the Environmental Mutagen Society, and there is now a center at Oak Ridge, Tennessee for obtaining information on environmental mutagens and environmental toxicology.

The general effects of mutation can occasionally be morphologically discerned. In mammals, there may be found dominant lethal mutations that can result in preimplantation and loss or resorption of the embryo after implantation; implantation sites or stunted embryos may be seen. Point mutations, usually recessive, have little or no effect on the individual; the carrier is also not usually affected. Some mutations result in disease, and fortuitous matings can result in expression of the mutation in the offspring. Some believe that the repair mechanism has much to do with the type of abnormality that is expressed.

Agricultural chemicals, mainly pesticides, have been isolated from the fat of fetuses and stillborns; these have included 2,4-D with its early contaminant TCDD, one of the dioxins about which much concern has been expressed. In addition, DDT, 2,4,5-T, dieldrin, captan, and carbaryl, producing malformations in experimental animals but not known to produce recognizable malformation patterns in humans, have been studied. Industrial compounds are of concern both as environmental contaminants producing damage in the infant and child, and also in crossing the placenta as a result of maternal exposure; these areas have been extremely poorly studied. Such agents as dimethylnitrosamine and ethylnitrosourea are suspected of having the ability to cause human cancer when crossing the placenta, but no such evidence yet exists.[95,124] Compounds of mercury and lead also encountered in industry are known to be teratogens and transplacental toxic substances,[103] and the same is true of food and feed additives, particularly diethylstilbestrol, a compound used for many years as an antiabortion agent and now found to be associated with rare cases of clear-cell adenocarcinoma in female offspring, vaginal "adenosis" and cervical "eversion," and distinct alterations of normal sperm production and maintenance in males.[64,69] The ability of diethylstilbestrol to produce such abnormalities as a result of its use as a food additive is not yet clear.

Pollutants and drugs have also been studied as mutagens. Population studies of the effects on the embryo, fetus, neonate, and child have yet to be completed. Nitrosamines, formaldehyde, such compounds of partially burned fossil fuels as benzanthracines and benzo-*a*-pyrene, and mercury, lead, cadmium, ozone, 2,4-D, 2,4,5-T, and benzene are the best known of these pollutants.[2a,103]

Wilson[124] has suggested that perhaps 4 to 5 percent of all developmental defects in humans are associated with drugs and environmental chemicals. Wilson lists, as those proven to have shown a distinct deleterious effect, androgenic hormones, tumor therapy drugs—with folic acid antagonists in particular—thalidomide, oral anticoagulants, maternal alcoholism, anticonvulsants, organic mercury, perhaps oral hypoglycemics, and a few neurotrophic anorectics. He further mentions that teratogenic effects, by which is meant nonspecific structural malformation induced by these chemicals, are usually seen in experimental animals in doses well above therapeutic levels or above likely exposure levels to the environmental chemicals cited. In addition to those chemicals described above, Wilson also lists salicylates, certain alkaloids such as caffeine and nicotine, antihistamines, antibiotics, corticosterids, antimalarials, anesthetics, solvents, pesticides, and industrial effluents, which he includes in addition to mercury, lead, arsenic, lithium, cadmium, some plants, and miscellaneous substances such as trypan blue, Triparonol, and Diamox.

In his book on environment and birth defects, Wilson[123] has set forth criteria for recognizing new teratogenic agents in humans. He feels that one must have rigid criteria including:

(1) an abrupt increase in the incidence of a particular defect or association of defects;

(2) a coincidence of this increase with a known environmental change, such as the widespread use of a new drug;

(3) known exposure to the environmental change early in pregnancy, yielding characteristically defective infants; and

(4) the absence of other factors.

Categories of drugs known to produce abnormalies can be classified in a similar manner to the categories given by Irey of drugs to which an adverse response has been recorded (see Chapter 1). In their embryotoxic potential such drugs may be considered as: (1) established; (2) suspected; (3) possibly embryotoxic; and (4) not embryotoxic.

SUBSTANCES KNOWN OR SUSPECTED OF PRODUCING EMBRYOTOXICITY (see Table 2-1)

Antibiotics

Infants whose mothers were treated with tetracyclines after the third month of gestation have been reported to have hypoplasia and yellow or brown discoloration of their deciduous teeth. Histologically, one can see vivid autofluorescence on an appropriate ground section of the teeth. The tetracyclines are incorporated into fetal bones after maternal administration, and have been implicated as the cause of a depression of normal skeletal growth which is totally reversible after the drugs are discontinued. Two cases of congenital cataracts have been reported with tetracycline drugs, and one case of digit defects has been reported in an infant born to a woman treated with 250 mg of tetracycline over a 12-day period. Clearly, single reports are not productive of causative relationships.[99, 100, 103] Streptomycin and dihydrostreptomycin have been associated with hearing loss and eighth nerve damage in infants following their administration to mothers during pregnancy; there did not appear to be a dose-effect relationship in these cases, and several observers regard them as instances of individual susceptibility. Histologically, no studies have been done on the fetal effects of the streptomycins.[103]

Erythromycin has been reported by one author to be associated with extensive malformation. The infant in the case was small for its gestational age, and there was anencephaly with the placenta attached to the head and a major craniofacial defect. This was an isolated finding.[103]

For the intrauterine effects of the antitubercular drugs, a number of incomplete reports can be found in the European literature. Varbela (in ref. 103) is said to have found cases of congenital malformation in the offspring of mothers taking antitubercular drugs of a variety of kinds during the first 3 months of gestation. Lowe reported two cases, one with multiple defects and the other with hypospadias, but did not regard this as an increased incidence of defects. There is a report of the harmful effects of isoniazid from France, (in ref. 103), stating that encephalopathy was induced in a fetus by this drug, but no morphologic information is given. Ethambutol does not appear to be a teratogen (in ref. 103).

Antineoplastic Agents

Folic acid antagonists have produced distinct collections of abnormalities. Aminopterin in particular gives rise to individuals with severe growth retardation, a large head, a small mandible, deformed ears, abnormal facies, webbing of the neck, club hands, and club feet; hydrocephalus has occasionally also been observed, as well as failure of formation of the cerebral hemispheres, retardation of ossification of the skull bones, malformed ears, cleft palate, and micrognathia.[108] Mild mental retardation has been observed in survivors. Other tumor therapy drugs have been associated with various malformations but there are too few cases to allow definite conclusions to be drawn.[18, 103, 104, 121]

Cardiovascular Drugs

Digitalis compounds pass readily across the placenta. Little is known about the effect of these preparations on the fetus, but there is no known deleterious effect of digitalis and its preparations. Quinidine, although productive of fatal arrhythmias in the infant, has not been associated with specific defects. Quinine, however, has been linked over the last 40 years with congenital malformations, although the drug was not taken in therapeutic doses, but as an abortifacient. The malformations produced were specific auditory nerve hypoplasias, although other anomalies such as those involving the limbs, and mental deficiency, ambiguous genitalia, and multiple anomalies have also been described. The other antimalarial drugs are apparently well tolerated by the fetus when given in therapeutic doses.[103, 121, 124]

Although a number of diuretic agents are teratogenic in laboratory animals, no acceptable reports of teratogenicity have been reported in humans.[103]

Hypnotics and Sedatives

Of the drugs established for being embryotoxic in humans, those characteristically productive of morphologic abnormalities include such substances as thalidomide, first produced as an anti-influenza agent and then as a sedative. In 1961, the striking incidence of severe limb deformities in newborns of mothers taking this drug aroused the attention of several geneticists and pediatricians to its dangers.[121] When taken in the first trimester, thalidomide (alpha-phthalimino glutarimide) produces a distinct spectrum of abnormality. There is a reduction of skeletal elements in size and number, with 5 percent of affected newborns having total amelia, 65 percent having total or subtotal aplasia of the proximal part of the humerus combined with total aplasia of the radius and of digits 1 to 3; and 15 percent having total or partial aplasia of the radius, with hypoplasia or dysplasia of the ulna and absence of digits 1 and 3. The ears are deformed in 30 percent of cases, and colobomas of the iris and retina and microphthalmia of various degrees have also been described.

With the exception of thalidomide, none of the hypnotic or sedative drugs produces any apparent significant anomalies. This drug group includes the barbiturates, chloral hydrates, and paraldehyde.[103]

Tranquilizers and Antidepressants

Chlordiazepoxide (Librium) and diazepam (Valium) cross the human placenta and appear in the cord blood in concentrations similar to those in the mother. No consistent pattern of malformation has been described in the offspring of mothers taking these drugs, although one unusual malformation, with complete absence of the thumbs and metacarpal bones, has been described in an infant exposed in the first trimester.[99, 103]

The phenothiazines are widely used tranquilizers; most exhibit characteristic placental transfer. Among these are chloropromazine, promazine, promethazine, and others. Malformations have been reported on rare occasions in the infants of mothers taking a variety of antipsychotic agents; these malformations have ranged from limb defects to cataracts,[75] but are not constant. In general, it is believed[99] that, given appropriate circumstances, some tranquilizers—particularly trifluoperizine, haloperidol, and prochlorperizine, and perhaps others—may present teratogenic hazards to the human fetus.

Lithium salts have recently been introduced into the therapeutic armamentarium as antidepressants, and lithium toxicity in the infants of lithium-treated mothers has been reported; however, there has been no morphologic study of these individuals. Although two infants of mothers taking lithium during pregnancy have been reported as having congenital anomalies, these affected different organ systems, and do not appear to be related.[122] The incidence of cardiac anomalies remains to be studied (see Metals).[80,122]

Tridione[22,103,108] and hydantoin[41,103,108] may produce characteristic developmental abnormalities (see Table 2-1). The possible association between ganglioneuroblastoma and fetal hydantoin-alcohol syndromes is discussed by Seeler et al.[101] Our cases of fetal hydantoin syndrome have not yielded constant anatomic anomalies.

Diabetes and Insulin

Diabetes is associated with an increased incidence of fetal malformations and with several malformation syndromes, including caudal regression syndrome, a cerebral dysgenesis syndrome, and an increased incidence of certain congenital heart defects, including transposition of the great vessels. Although injection of insulin can produce malformations in experimental animals, particularly chickens, it is not known to produce malformations in humans, although most of the diabetics studied were insulin-dependent.[103]

Hypotensive Drugs

The morphology of the effects of hypotensive drugs on the fetus is little understood and has been little studied. Except for a diazoxide study, in which treated infants developed alopecia with hypoplasia of the hair follicles, and one had hypertrichosis—which is also seen in children given this drug—no other significant abnormalities were observed.[67a] Hydralazine is known to produce a generally reversible lupus erythematous-type syndrome, but this has not been reported in the fetus. Magnesium sulfate, although producing a hypermagnesemia syndrome, does not affect the fetus.[103] Redman et al.[93] have reviewed the antihypertensive agents.

Drugs of Abuse in Addition to Opiates

Lysergic Acid Diethylamide. The transplacental passage of lysergic acid diethylamide (LSD) has not been documented in humans, although it has been confirmed in the mouse. Chromosomal anomalies are surely present to an increased extent among LSD users, and several cases of defects have been found in the offspring of individuals who took this drug before or during pregnancy. The collection of chromosomal anomalies is startlingly mixed, including one case of unbalanced D–D translocation and three with a recognized genetic-defect type of family history such as pyloric stenosis, cystic fibrosis and an unusual form of neonatal dwarfism. Also seen were limb deficiencies, a case of megacolon, and bladder extrophy. The most striking finding was limb deficiency in 5 of 161 children examined and reported by Long. In her excellent review,[58] Long makes clear that there is no strong evidence for the teratogenecity of LSD in humans, but that the positive cases found thus far suggest that the survey must be continued. The limb defects seen were striking, and included phalangeal deficiencies and syndactyly of both hands. Another child was described with multiple defects including anencephaly, facial deformities, aplasia of the upper limb, cleft palate and lip, and attachment of the placenta to the edge of the anencephaly.

Alcohol. One substance suspected of embryotoxicity is alcohol, in heavy maternal usage. The dosage question is now controversial because of the belief that even small amounts of alcohol, equivalent to 1 ounce of absolute alcohol per day, are associated with mild evidence of the so-called fetal alcohol syndrome. The original and current references are cited in Smith,[108] Hanson et al.,[38, 39] Shepard.[103] Qazi et al.[91] observed renal anomalies, i.e., hypoplasia, in two infants of severely alcoholic mothers.

Of severely alcoholic mothers, about one-third give birth to infants with a small birth weight, microcephaly, a characteristic face with narrow palpebral fissures, a flat nasal bridge and "ironed-out" philtrum, and micrognathia; some have cleft plates, and a few have had evidence of extreme structural damage of the brain, with severe, persistent immaturity of hemispheric development and, rarely, hydrocephalus.[103, 108]

Smoking. Extensive reviews have been done on the relationship of maternal cigarette smoking and pregnancy outcome. In general, smokers have had infants of significantly lower than normal birth weight, but no specific collections of abnormalities have been found. Some authors have seen excessive perinatal loss of the babies of smokers, most marked among the poor and among blacks. Morphologic studies of the offspring of smokers have not found consistent abnormalities. The issue of carbon monoxide concentrations in the blood of smokers being higher than in that of nonsmokers has been of much importance, and carbon monoxide has been shown to cross the placental barrier.

In the nonsurviving infants of mothers who have been smokers, there was no frank evidence of reduced cell number in the forebrains studied. In one unconfirmed study, there was twice the incidence of congenital heart disease among infants of mothers who smoked as among those of nonsmoking mothers. In another, similar study, an increased incidence of cleft lip and palate was found among infants of smoking mothers. The numbers of cases studied are too small to provide definite conclusions in most of these studies, but it is generally thought that there is no clear association between smoking during pregnancy and congenital malformation of the fetus.[16, 51, 62, 74, 103] Cannabis has not been confirmed as a human teratogen.

Steroids

The maternal administration of androgens during pregnancy resulting in masculinization of the female fetus is well known. Estrogens and estrogenic types of compounds administered for use in threatened abortion remains a highly controversial and questionably useful therapeutic approach, having several major complications, including adenocarcinoma of the vagina after a latent period of 14 to 22 years, adenosis in the vagina, cervical glandular "erosion," and transverse cervical or vaginal ridges (see Chapter 13). Abnormalities, probably benign malformations, are hoods of the upper vagina, vascular abnormalities such as "strawberry cervix" or a cervical "cockscomb," and endocervical adenoma. The male offspring of mothers taking androgens have an increased incidence of abnormal penises and epididymal cysts; sperm counts are decreased, and the number of abnormal sperm is elevated.[103]

Synthetic progesterone use once led to masculinization of female fetuses; masculinization was also seen in fetuses whose mothers had been given androgenic hormones for the treatment of breast cancer. These phenomena occured before the 12th week of gestation, since differentiation of the external genitalia is largely complete at that time.[103, 121]

Thyroid and Anti-thyroid Drugs

Neonatal goiter, with a hyperplastic pattern of follicles having a moderate columnar-to-cuboidal epithelium and a tortuous follicular pattern without significant lymphocytic infiltration, has been described as a result of both maternal iodide treatment and of treatment with such antithyroid drugs as propylthiouracil and its congeners. Neonatal goiter as a result of maternal cobalt administration is no longer seen, since this trace metal has been removed from hematinics.[103]

Other Drugs

Schardein[99] lists the nonteratogenic effects of drugs on the human fetus; most of these have no specific morphologic effect. Those producing morphologic abnormality include drugs associated with bleeding—the salicylates in large amounts and excessive phenobarbital. Warfarin (Coumadin) may produce characteristic developmental abnormalities[103, 108] (see Table 2-1). Other drugs causing morphologic abnormalities include those producing platelet dysfunction or decrease in numbers, such as tolbutamide, alphaprodine, and quinine; and those producing hemolysis, particularly, nitrofurantoin, Primaquine, and Pentaquine.

Metals

Mercury. Several episodes of severe cerebral damage have been reported in infants whose mothers were exposed to food contaminated with mercury. The best known cases are those from Minimata in Japan, and from a second episode in Niigata, the morbid anatomy of which is reviewed by Takeuchi[114] and also by Friberg and Vostal.[28] Since the occurrence of these episodes, similar reports of "cerebral palsy" and microcephaly have been recorded in association with the ingestion of bread made from wheat contaminated with a methylmercury fungicide,[2] and as a result of the ingestion of porcine meat similarly contaminated.[103] The cases that may have occurred as a result of the ingestion of similarly contaminated fish from Canadian rivers have not yet been analyzed.

Acute poisoning from the Minimata disaster, which occurred over a number of years, was nonspecific in its anatomic pattern, and is not germane to a discussion of the fetal effects of mercury. Chronically affected children, with severe spastic quadriparesis and mental retardation, had atrophic brains, with severe calcarine convolutional atrophy and occasional atrophic foci in other areas. There was atrophy of the white matter and severe disturbance of cerebellar architecture, with loss of granular cells and rarely Purkinje cell loss. The fetal cases in particular were affected by atrophy, widely distributed neuronal and cortical degeneration, hypoplasia of most of the normally developing structures in the cerebellum and hindbrain, and extensive neuronal vacuolar and chromatolytic degeneration. The other features of mercury poisoning, both fetal and infantile, were nonspecific, including marrow depression, hypoplasia of lymph nodes, and fatty metamorphosis of the liver and renal tubules.[6]

Lead. The evidence of specific effects of lead on the fetus is far less convincing than it is for mercury.[103] In the older literature, there is evidence that maternal lead poisoning is associated with an increased incidence of stillbirth and abortion. The evidence of central nervous system damage from fetal exposure to lead is inconclusive.[2a, 76, 81, 82]

Other Metals. Cadmium, a most toxic substance, has been associated with a decreased birth weight of the infants of mothers working in the cadmium industry; however no specific fetopathy has yet been recorded with this metal.[103, 116] To date, aluminum, beryllium, boron, arsenic, antimony, chromium, and zinc have not been associated with specific fetal disease. Lithium, as noted above, is a controversial teratogen. Of the malformations described among the infants of mothers taking lithium, a small number consisted of Ebstein's malformation, a rare disorder of the tricuspid valve. Gold, molybdenum, and nickel are not known fetotoxic or teratogenic substances. Cobalt, as noted elsewhere, has been goitrogenic. Copper is not a known teratogen.

Nonmetallic Elements. The long controversy over the association of fluoride in low-

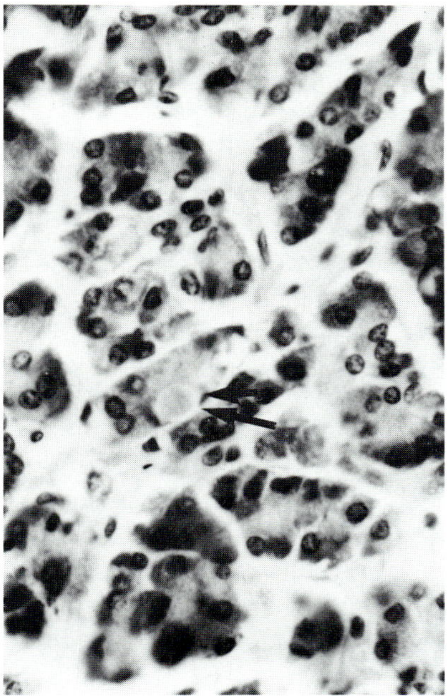

Fig. 2-1. Focal necrosis, pancreatic islets, aspirin poisoning, ? maternal in patient referred to in Table 2-2. H & E, × 250.

doses with Down's syndrome remains unsettled, but most teratologists do not regard any such association as significant. Iodine is a goitrogen.

INFANCY AND EARLY CHILDHOOD

A brief listing of the morphologic manifestations of the effects of drugs and toxic substances is appended (Tables 2-2 and 2-3); in a few cases this is given by organ, and when many systems are involved it is given by substance. Standard texts of pediatric pathology and pediatric surgical pathology contain a few examples of such phenomena, but biopsies—save for those of the liver or skin—are rare, and autopsies are the major source of information. Many of these are in the files of medical examiners and have not been corroborated, at least in the case of fetal and neonatal disease, except for occasional papers in journals of forensic science, clinical toxicology, and pediatrics.

Irey and his colleagues at the Armed Forces Institute of Pathology have been among the first to list, observe, and classify the morbid anatomy of untoward reactions to drugs (see Chapter 1). In the case of intrauterine damage from drugs or inadvertently encountered environmental toxins, the morphology that is given is limited to gross descriptions of abnormal faces, grotesquely distorted or malformed limbs, oral clefts, and cardiovascular malformations; the microscopic anatomy of toxic drug and chemical reactions in infancy and childhood is largely limited to ablations or gross alterations of normal cells. Mullick et al.[73] describe inflammation, degeneration and infiltration, hypoplasia, aplasia, hyperplasia, necrosis, circulatory disturbances, vascular abnormalities, and teratogenic effects produced by foreign substances. The greatest of these are degeneration and infiltration, and the organ most frequently damaged according to Mullick et al.[73] is the liver.

The experience in one children's tertiary care institution is recorded in Table 2-3. Until 1972, this institution had less than 140 beds; it now has 320. Only autopsy cases recorded during a 20 year period as having been poisonings were reviewed, and some such cases were undoubtedly lost. The most remarkable aspect of the study was the absence of specific data. Most of the features seen were the result of shock, collapse, hypoxia, therapy with toxic substances, acute nutritional disturbances, and prolonged maintainance of "life systems" beyond likely retrieval of function. What is clearly needed in autopsy cases of adverse drugs and chemical effects is careful recording of anatomic data, correlated with levels of toxic substances in individual organs and appropriate studies of fine structure and intracellular function—the obvious "extended autopsy"—with the treatment of each tragedy as an opportunity to extract maximal information from the tissue in an appropriate manner. When that occurs, this text can be rewritten with less speculation and fewer blank spaces and embarassing deficiencies in data. There are serious methodologic difficulties in achieving this goal, however. For example, what is the morbid anatomy of an orofacial cleft, craniosynostosis, ventricular septal defect, or a limb ablation other than its gross classification at present? Is the fatty liver metamorphosis in one kind of systemic poisoning really different from that in another?

Organ-based Morbid Anatomy of Selected Toxic Substances in Infancy and Childhood

Teeth. Little careful anatomic material is present on such specimens as the ground sections of affected teeth in fatal cases of poisoning. Texts of oral pathology give gross descriptions in most cases, with little or no microscopic detail (see also Chapter 7).

Eye. What was said for the teeth is also true of the toxic effects of drugs and chemicals on the eye, which are fully described clinically[15,36] but on which little detailed anatomy is available, even in specialty journals; and in the case of fetus and infant, even less (see also Chapter 16).

Skin (see also Chapter 6). This easily biopsied target organ for many toxic reactions has been well studied, and reliable texts of dermatopathology, such as those of Pinkus et al.[87] and Lever et al.[54] contain detailed information and documentation of the effects of a variety of toxic substances, with some speculation. Martin,[62] among others, lists a number of "life-threatening drug-induced skin eruptions" which the pathologist may encounter at the autopsy table or the surgical desk.

Exfoliative Dermatitis. In children, we have seen this response, also called a generalized eczematoid tissue response with extensive reddening, swelling and scaling, to antibiotics, antituberculosis drugs, antiepileptic substances, especially Dilantin and carbamazepine (Tegretol), and immunizing substances, such as diphtheria and tetanus toxoids, pertussis vaccine, poliomyelitis vaccine of the killed virus variety, and measles vaccine, among others. There may be spongiotic disease or characteristic drug eruption.

Erythema Multiforme Bullosum. If it involves the respiratory mucosa of tracheo-bronchial tree this condition can be devastating. Its appearance varies from epidermal edema to the classic three-region type, with massive dermal edema, vasodilatation, and severe epidermodermal necrosis with bulla formation. We have seen this with Dilantin, sulfasoxizole, Kynex (sulfamethoxypyridazine), trimethadione, and some tetracyclines; several deaths ensued. As in the experience of others, we have seen a diphenylhydantoin case with erythema multiforme bullosum (Stevens-Johnson syndrome) in which the patient had a lupus erythematosus-like episode, with antinuclear antibodies and even a slight degree of renal mesangial proliferation.

Toxic Epidermal Necrolysis. Both the infantile type of this condition—which is also known as Lyell's syndrome—with necrosis of the upper epidermal layers, and the adult variety have been observed, most often with infections rather than drugs or environmental toxic substances. Again, diphenylhydantoin, barbiturates, ipecac, sulfonamides, some tetracyclines, synthetic penicillins, and Benadryl have been productive of this reaction in our clinics (see Chapter 6).

Lupus Erythematosus-like Syndromes. These syndromes, produced by a number of substances in adults and usually wholly reversible, have been seen infrequently in children. The characteristic skin alterations of the basal layer, and the usual plugs of keratin are not usually seen on biopsy. We have seen this syndrome with diphenylhydantoin, trimethadione, para-aminosalicylic acid, and in a child on gold therapy for rheumatoid disease.

Heart. Except for the peculiar cardiomyopathy of Adriamycin therapy (see Chapter 10) and two cases of myocardial necrosis associated with mercury poisoning (Fig. 2-2), we have seen little other than secondary phenomena of drug or chemical intoxication following shock or acute heart, liver, or renal failure. Other substances known to produce cardiac necrosis or cardiomyopathy in childhood are barium, the toxin of poisoning with the mushroom *Amanita phalloides,* carbon tetrachloride, and salicylates.

Lung. We have seen a number of cases of interstitial fibrosis and toxic alterations of the alveolar lining cells in patients on tumor therapy agents, usually for such reticuloendothelial diseases as Hodgkin's disease, leukemia, poorly differentiated lymphoma and occasionally associated with secondary exotic infections such as with *Pneumocystis* or cytomegalovirus (see also Chapter 9).[96] The effect of radiation in this regard is well known. Bleo-

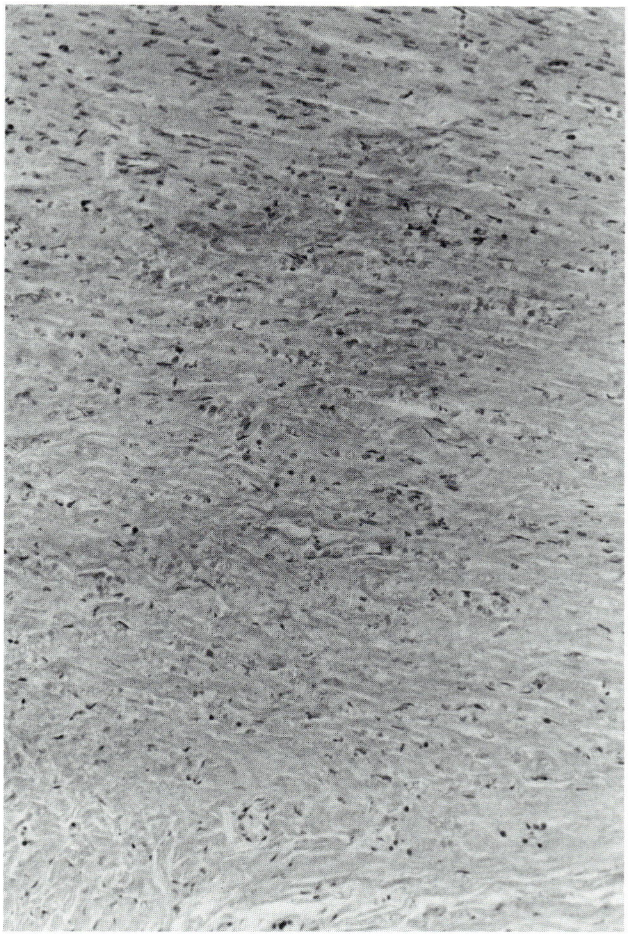

Fig. 2-2. Myocardial necrosis, diffuse. Mercury poisoning. H & E, × 100.

mycin, capable of producing interstitial fibrosis in the lung, is rarely used in infancy and early childhood. Phenytoin, paraquat, and nitrofurantoin are not fibrogenic in the fetus, infant, or child. Other causes of interstitial lung disease other than infection are smoke inhalation and the inhalation of more specific noxious fumes, such as chlorine—should the person recover. Kerosene aspiration following ingestion, of this substance, and the vomiting or ingestion of substances containing light petroleum distillates may produce—in addition to central nervous system depression occasionally ending in severe hypoxia and gliosis—a massive chemical pneumonia. Pulmonary edema is a feature in many kinds of toxic reactions.

Gastrointestinal Tract. Gastrointestinal bleeding, scarring, stenosis, and the like are known complications of the ingestion of numbers of corrosive substances, including those with other systemic toxic effects, such as bichloride of mercury and phenolics. The antifolic acid agents may produce a pernicious anemia-like alteration of the upper gastrointestinal tract mucosa, with large atypical nuclei and unchanged patterns of cytoplasmic growth. In association with cerebral edema or toxic encephalopathy following the ingestion of corrosive substances, there may be a "trophic blowout" of the greater curvature of the stomach, with little seen on microscopic examination other than "accelerated autolysis," one of the so-called Cushing-Rokitansky-type "ulcers." Various forms of iron in poisoning cases may be associated with gastric or intestinal ulceration. Iron encrustation is also a well-known feature of this variety of accident (Fig. 2-3).

Liver. Mikhael et al.[66] has reviewed drug-induced liver injury in infancy and childhood (see also Chapter 17). The liver has a limited repertory of morphologic responses, although some of its most interesting toxic responses are the results of progressive maturation of vital detoxication systems or the unavailability of a mature system at the time of the untoward event. A general form of "toxic hepatosis" or "hepatitis" is well recognized, and may be seen in a variety of responses to tumor therapy agents: This reaction includes (1) pleomorphism or hepatic cord cells, with apparent polyploidy; (2) a variable degree of fatty metamorphosis, usually macrovesicular; (3) pigment deposition, usually of iron, in Kupffer cells; (4) bile stasis; and (5) "piecemeal necro-

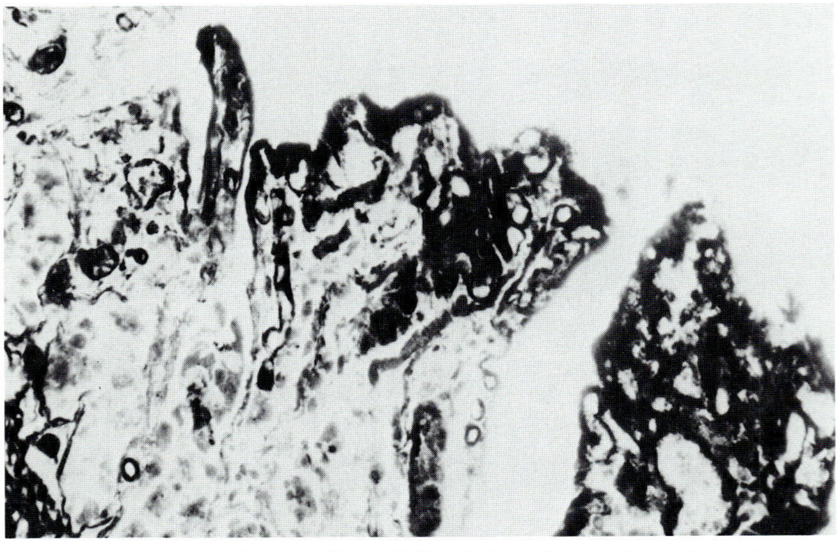

Fig. 2-3. Iron encrustation, small bowel. The dark surface, perivascular and macrophage staining is iron-positive. Iron poisoning. H & E, × 75.

sis" or necrobiosis. Cholestasis alone is a feature in childhood of treatment with allopurinol, PAS, anabolic steroids, some arsenicals, chlorothiazide, chlorpromazine, ethacrynic acid, griseofulvin, phenazopyridine, and other agents, and of "cholestatic hepatitis." Not described in detail by most authors or by Mikhael et al.[66] this cholestasis apparently includes focal necrosis and overlaps with "toxic liver reaction." Massive necrosis or a syndrome resembling a viral-like hepatitis with a poor prognosis has been seen in response to acetaminophen, actinomycin D, amethopterin, PAS, and *Amanita phalloides* ingestion; with barium enemas, owing to the now omitted tannic acid component; and with carbon tetrachloride, chlorambucil, copper sulfate, DDT, dimethylnitrosamine, iron poisoning, Tofranil (imipramine), iproniazid, methotrexate, mitomycin C, monoamine oxidase inhibitors, arsenic compounds, phenoxypropazine and related compounds, phosphorus ingestion, chlorinated hydrocarbons, thioguanine, tromethamine, urethane, and zoxazolamine, to mention but a few substances.

Less severe forms of focal liver necrosis are seen with a wide and, alas, unpredictable variety of therapeutic and toxic substances. Included are such easily available and ubiquitous substances as aspirin ("aspirin hepatitis"), amphotericin B, azathioprine, ethacrynic acid, iopanoic acid (Telepaque), isoniazid, a variety of antitumor drugs, phenbutazone, diphenylhydantoin, probenecid, propylthiouracil, rifampin, *Senecio* alkaloids, many sulfonamides, trichlorethylene, trimethadione, and trimethobenzamide. Massive fatty changes may be seen with any of the cytotoxic agents, antimony poisoning, asparaginase, carbon tetrachloride, chlorinated hydrocarbon poisoning, various corticosteroids, ether, ethyl alcohol, iron salts, tetracyclines, phenoxypropazine, phosphorus, tannic acid, thallium, and mercury (Fig. 2-4). Finally, fibrosis or serious impairment of the liver can be seen in any of the few massive necrosis sufferers who survive, in some of the lesser necrotic events, and with some regularity in persons exposed to methotrexate, imuran, and chlorambucil, again to select out a few of the guilty agents.

The issue of induced liver tumors has been

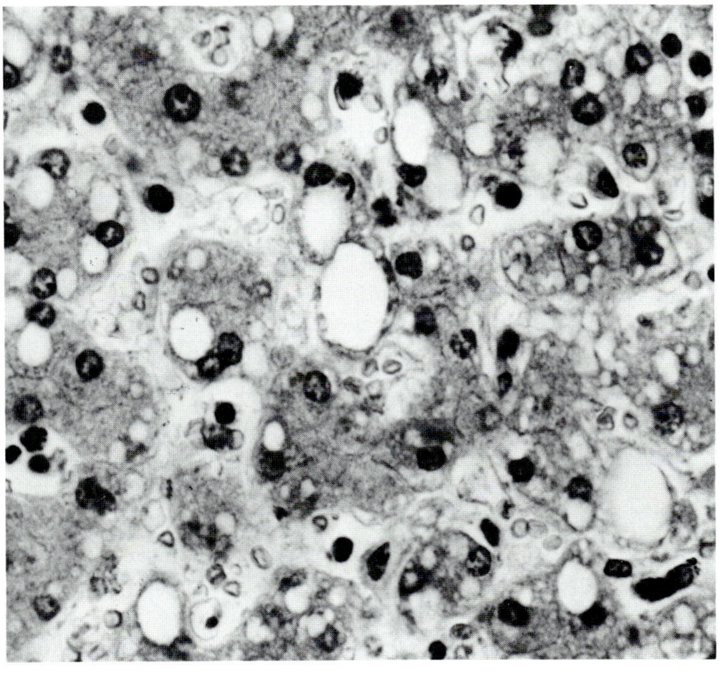

Fig. 2-4. Fatty metamorphosis, severe, liver, in mercury poisoning. H & E, × 255.

reviewed by Nunnerley et al.,[84] and there does not appear to be such an event recorded in fetuses or the very young. The adenomas recorded in association with certain oral contraceptives have not been seen in very young, sexually active girls. The issue of latent periods is probably the key to surveillance for potential liver neoplasms. Thorotrast, for instance, has not been associated with neoplasm in childhood, despite occasional exposures. Further, if the mother was exposed, it is likely that Thorotrast did not cross the placenta.

The role of aflatoxin exposure in the genesis of hepatic tumors is discussed in Chapter 17. Finally, the effects of copper raise serious theoretical issues in the special case of Indian childhood cirrhosis, which may be encountered in infancy. Copper concentrations are higher in such livers than in controls.[89,113]

Kidney. In standard texts of renal pathology, such as that by Lant,[50] and in the review by Schreiner and Maher[99a] a variety of toxic agents are described, few of which apply to the fetus, infant, or young child. It must be remembered that renal tubular necrosis, as a feature of either hypoperfusion of any cause or of direct toxicity, is nonspecific. The most frequently encountered nephrotoxic agents have been bichloride of mercury, which produces coagulative necrosis of the proximal convoluted tubules and then of other renal tubular structures; ethylene glycol, with its distinctive tubular necrosis, vacuolation, degeneration, and occasional oxalate deposition; and tubular degeneration in carbon tetrachloride accidents. The rich blood supply of the kidney, accounting for up to one-quarter of the cardiac output, means that this organ is readily exposed, even if only transiently, to a large variety of ingested substances. Sulfonamides have been associated with acute tubular necrosis, hypersensitivity vasculitis, a lupus-like nephrosis and, in the past, with obstructive crystallization episodes.

The well-recorded Fanconi-like disorder seen following the ingestion of tetracyclines whose structure has degraded to produce toxic epimers is not histologically understood, nor is the evanescent nephrogenic diabetes insipidus observed with doxycycline. Polymyxins have occasionally produced acute tubular necrosis in children, and in much higher doses have enlarged the juxtaglomerular apparatus. Some cases of penicillin-related interstitial nephritis and focal glomerular necrosis are recorded, but not with benzyl or semisynthetic homologues of this antibiotic. Occasionally, proximal tubular damage has been recorded with aminoglycoside antibiotics, such as gentamycin, streptomycin, and neomycin. The use of amphotericin B has been associated with nephrocalcinosis. Solvent-sniffing, rarely encountered in young children, has been associated with renal tubular necrosis, and also with liver necrosis and cerebral edema. Drug-induced nephrotic syndromes, with the classic fine-structural foot-process fusion visible upon electron microscopy, have been recorded in response to D-penicillamine. Examples of renal damage secondary to aspirin, Urokon, mercury and lead are shown in Figures 2-5 through 2-8.

Bone. Stamp[112] has reviewed the issue of drug- and chemical-induced rickets or osteomalacia. In children in the developed countries, the forms of these conditions other than those stemming from dietary deficiency or sunlight-lack are few. Purgative abuse, cholestyramine use interfering with small intestinal calcium absorbtion, and the effects of antacid phosphate binders may be associated with osteomalacia. Anticonvulsants are known to be associated with vitamin D-resistant rickets, morphologically identical to rickets in the young child; phenytoin, pheneturide, and carbamazepine have all been implicated. Questionable maternal exposure and possible infantile exposure to a few heavy metals have resulted in bone changes, probably secondary to renal toxicity; cadmium, mercury, gold, and lead, as well as other metals, have been cited, but the evidence is not convincing. The Japanese cadmium poisoning or "itai-itai" disease is not known in infants. Irregular alignment of vacuolating cartilage cells, imperfect formation of secondary spongiosa, and poor calcifi-

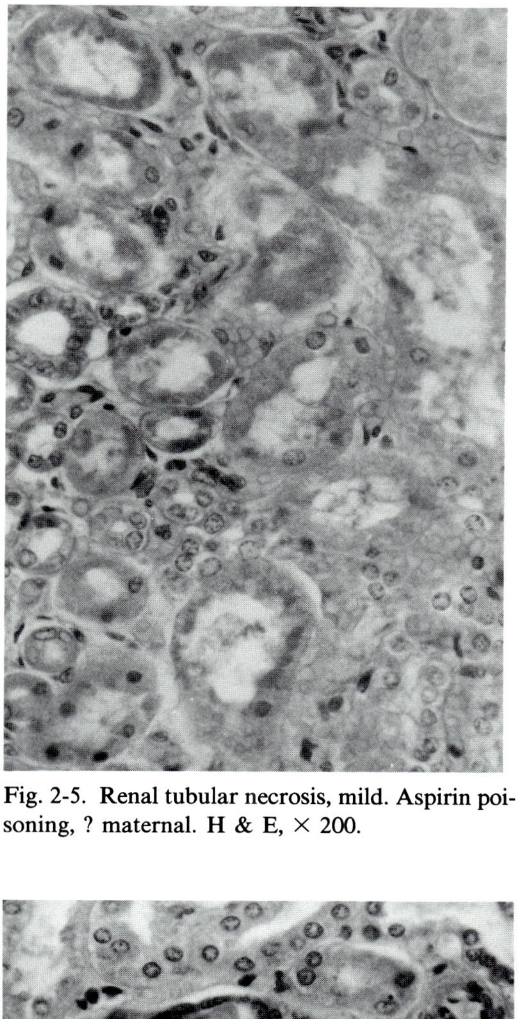

Fig. 2-5. Renal tubular necrosis, mild. Aspirin poisoning, ? maternal. H & E, × 200.

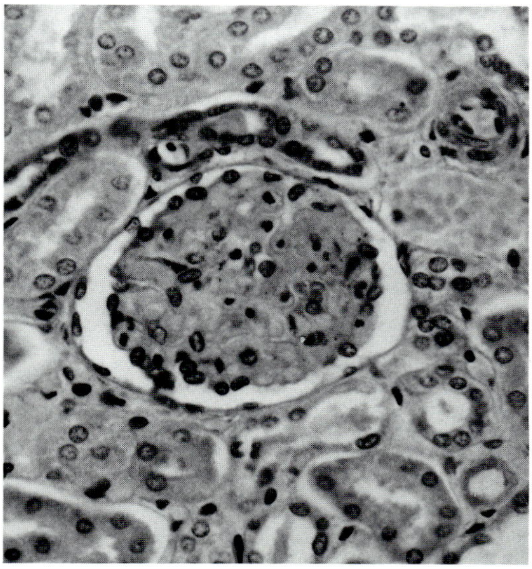

Fig. 2-6. Glomerular thrombosis and early necrosis, kidney, in Urokon reaction, untoward. H & E, × 185.

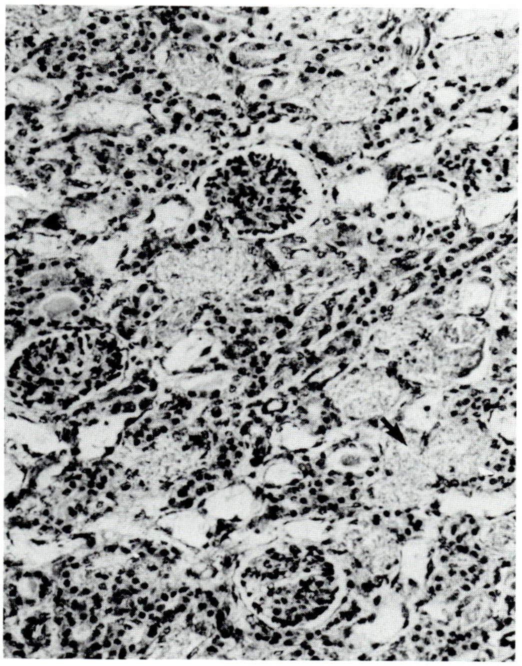

Fig. 2-7. Massive tubular necrosis, kidney. Mercury poisoning. H & E, × 185.

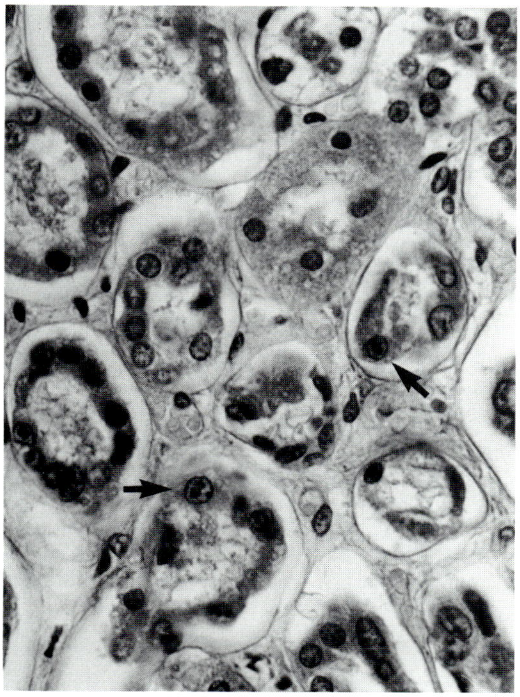

Fig. 2-8. Lead poisoning. Classical intranuclear inclusions, renal tubules. H & E, × 250.

cation of secondary trabeculae are seen in all of the foregoing, toxic forms of rickets. Osteomalacia is a feature of steroid therapy. The nutritional diseases induced by toxic substances in childhood, including the megaloblastic anemias and the marrow inhibition and hypoplasia phenomena, can be reviewed in standard texts of pediatric hematology, in Martin,[62] and in Chapter 5.

Lymph Nodes and Thymus. Little systematic study has been done in this area. Depletion is well-known, as a feature of stress from endogenous steroid effects on lymphoid populations and in association with fever, infection, or a generalized toxic response; and as a specific feature of the cytotoxic effects of tumor therapy agents. The hematologic effects of toxic substances are discussed in Chapter 5, and are also well reviewed in Martin;[62] these effects include the effects of such substances as diphenylhydantoin on the lymph nodes. Although we have not encountered this in infancy, older children receiving antiepileptic medication have had gross alterations of lymph node architecture, with loss of cortical and medullary pattern and striking cytologic atypicality of individual lymphocytes, resembling neoplastic transformation.[97]

Central Nervous System

As with the liver, study in this area is handicapped by the confusion of direct toxic effects with the result of prolonged supportive efforts, hypoxia, underperfusion, and similar nonspecific phenomena. With regard to the peripheral nervous system, texts dealing with peripheral neuropathy are mainly concerned with unusual occupational exposures and the inadvertent or suicidal ingestion of obviously toxic substances.

Cerebral edema is best seen grossly, since its microscopic confirmation is difficult. Weight, water content, and the pallor of stained sections, as well as secondary ischemic or angular neuron necrosis, are the elements to be sought. In infants, save for hypoglycemia and carbon monoxide effects, little is known of the toxic effects of drugs and chemicals on the nervous system. In older children, the effects of mercury poisoning of the chronic variety have been described by the observers of the Minimata disaster[114] (see also Chapter 15); the glial disorders and neuronal degeneration in this disease are also described on page 34. In chronic lead intoxication, usually only edema is seen in infants although occasionally other effects are seen (Fig. 2-9); the peripheral neuropathies of this intoxication are not seen in children. Also to be considered are those cases of kernicterus associated with the maternal ingestion of those substances that displace bilirubin from its binding with albumin, or compete for the binding site, to mention two mechanisms.[65,68]

As is now well-known, bathing of the whole body of premature infants on several occasions, using a 3 percent hexachloraphene-con-

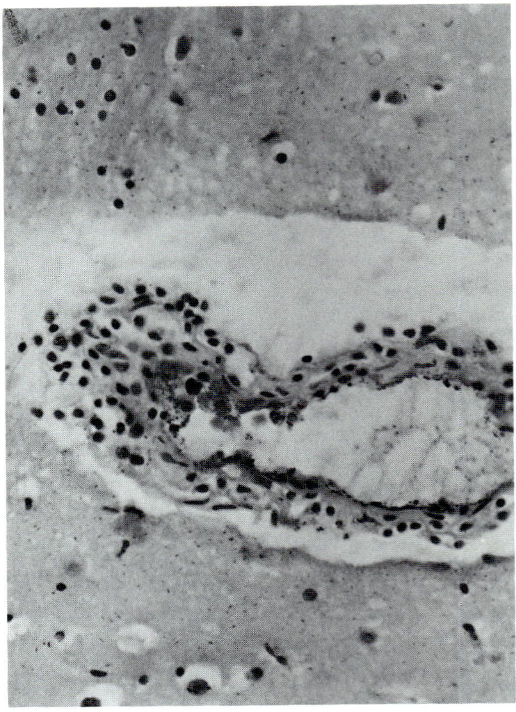

Fig. 2-9. Lead poisoning. Perivascular edema, perivascular "cuffing," early vascular calcification, represented by the fine dark stippling or smudging. H & E, × 170.

taining soap (pHisoHex), has been followed by a neurological degenerative disorder, with a more-or-less characteristic morphological disorder of the central nervous system, best discussed by Shuman, et al. (1974). The abnormalities, characterized as vacuolar encephalopathy of the brainstem reticular formation has been produced in the experimental animal on several occasions.[105] In most cases distinct vacuoles were seen in the reticular formation, in clusters between glial nuclei, neurons or blood vessels. In addition, in some cases, when neurons are damaged and edema is present, from causes not necessarily related to the hexachlorophene, the vacuolar alterations of anoxia, ischemia and edema must be differentiated from that of the vacuoles associable with repeated applications of the hexachlorophene soap. The changes of hexachlorophene toxicity do not extend into the neuropil of the defined brainstem, nuclei, but does involve the heavily myelinated long tracts of the brainstem, e.g., medial longitudinal fasciculus, medial lemniscus, and cerebellar peduncles. This alteration more or less varies in severity with the number of exposures to the soap and is seen in its full-blown form and in significant frequency only in those infants weighing less than 1400 grams.

CONCLUSION

In this brief discussion, we have attempted to list a few exemplary results of the effects of drugs and toxic substances on the developing fetus and the very young human. Much information on the morbid anatomy of such conditions is superficial, incomplete, or lacking. We know nothing of the effect of many potentially deleterious substances on the sperm of the potential father or on the reproductive system of the mother-to-be. The irregular association of specific features of toxicity and teratogenicity in readily available nonprimate experimental animals with human disease makes our screening task more difficult.

The development of an awareness of the need for screening techniques, and the progressive sophistication and seriousness of those governmental and industrial experts responsible to the public for appropriate surveillance will ensure the avoidance of the disasters and callous carelessness of the past. The lack of availability of primate models and lack of seriousness of large-scale "megamouse" experiments, not to mention their prohibitive cost, will result in a new generation of alternative screening methods. The use of fish, invertebrate, and plant models in the fields of teratology and mutagenesis research is well under way;[67] moreover the superb series of such prospectuses as Wilson and Fraser's *Handbook of Teratology,*[124] Hollaender and de Serres's series on chemical mutagens,[43] and Meyler's (and later Dukes's) *Side Effects of Drugs* (see general references) are encouraging, as are the new journals of toxicology, teratology, and environmental mutagenesis. We have not yet educated medical and other scientific professionals—not to mention the concerned lay public or responsible government bodies—to the nature of these problems.

GENERAL REFERENCES

Teratology

Heinonen, O. P., Slone, D., & Shapiro S.: Birth Defects and Drugs in Pregnancy. Publishing Science Group, Inc., Littleton, Massachusetts, 1977.

Nishimura, H., & Tanimura, A. T. (Eds.): Clinical Aspects of the Teratogenicity of Drugs. Excerpta Medica, Elsevier, Amsterdam, 1976.

Tuchmann-Duplessis, H.: Teratogenic Actions of Drugs. Pergamon Press, New York, 1975.

Warkany, J. Congenital Malformations. Year Book Publishers, Chicago, 1971.

Wilson, J. G. Environment and Birth Defects. Academic Press, New York, 1973.

Wilson, J. G. & Fraser, F. C.: Handbook of Teratology. Vol. 1. General Principles and Etiology; Vol. 3. Comparative, Maternal and Epidemiologic Aspects. Plenum Press, New York, 1977, 1979.

Toxicology

Davies, D. M. (Ed.): Textbook of Adverse Drug Reactions. Foreword and Ch. 1, pp. vii-ix and pp. 1-7. Oxford, New York, 1977.

Hunter, D.: Diseases of Occupations. 4th Ed. English University Press, London, 1969.

Martin, E. W. (Ed.): Types of Hazardous drug reactions and their etiologies. In: Hazards of Medication. 2nd Ed. pp. 307-338. J.B. Lippincott, Philadelphia, 1978.

Meyler, L. (Ed.): Side Effects of Drugs. Vols. 1-7, 1957 to 1975. Same series: Side Effects of Drugs Annual. No. 4. Dukes, M.N.G. (Ed.): Excerpta Medica, Amsterdam, 1980.

Thienes, C. H. & Haley, T. J.: Clinical Toxicology. 5th Ed. Lea & Febiger, Philadelphia, 1972.

REFERENCES

1. Alvarado, C. S.; Boat, T. F., & Newman, A. J.: Late-onset pulmonary fibrosis and chest deformity in two children treated with cyclophosphamide. J. Pediatr. 92:443-445, 1978.
2. Amin-Zaki, L., Elhassani, S., Majeed, M. A. et al: Intrauterine methylmercury poisoning in Iraq. Pediatrics 54:587-595, 1974.

2a. Angle, C. R., & McIntyre, M. S.: Lead poisoning during pregnancy Am. J. Dis. Child. 108:436-439, 1964.

3. Ansell, G: Fatal overdose of contrast medium in infants. Br. J. Radiol. 43:395-396, 1970.
4. Armando, V. L., Angel, A. O: Arsenicismo cronico. Bol. Med. Hosp. Infant 36:849-861, 1979.
5. Aurett, W. A., Hervada, A. R., & Fendrick, G.: Fatal pseudomembranous enterocolitis following oral ampicillin therapy. J. Pediat. 93:882-883, 1978.
6. Baker, F., Damluji, S. F., & Amin-Zaki, L. et al. Methylmercury Poisoning in Iraq. Science 181:230-241, 1973.
7. Batalden, P. B., VanDyne, B. J., & Cloyd, J.: Pancreatitis associated with valproic acid therapy. Pediatrics 64:520-522, 1979.
8. Beernink, D. H., & Miller, J. J.: Anticonvulsant-induced antinuclear antibodies and lupus-like disease in children. J. Pediatr. 82:113-117, 1973.
9. Bergman, G. E., Philippidis, P., & Naiman, J. L.: Severe gastrointestinal hemorrhage and anemia after therapeutic doses of aspirin in normal children. J. Pediatr. 88:501-503, 1976.
10. Boeckx, R. L., Postl, B., & Coodin, F. J.: Gasoline sniffing and tetraethyl lead poisoning in children. Pediatrics 60:140-145, 1977.
11. Bongiovanni, A. M., & McPadden, A. J.: Steroids during pregnancy and possible fetal consequences. Fertil. Steril. 11:181-186, 1960.
12. Borgstedt, A. D., Bryson, M. F., Young, L. W., & Forbes, G. B.: Long-term administration of antiepileptic drugs and the development of rickets. J. Pediatr. 81:9-15, 1972.
13. Bove, K. E., Bhathena, D, Wyatt, R. J., et al: Diffuse metanephric adenoma after in utero aspirin intoxication: Unique case of progressive renal failure. Arch. Pathol. 103: 187-190, 1979.
14. Chai, V. C., Chandra, R., Fletcher, A. B. et al: Polyhydramnios and neonatal renal failure: A possible association with maternal acetaminophen ingestion.
15. Chan, G. H. (Jr.): Durg induced ocular slide effects. In: Harley, R. D., Ed. Pediatric Ophthalmology. pp. 714-715. Saunders, Philadelphia, 1975.
16. Coleman, S., Pietrow, P. T., & Rinehard, W.: Hazards of tobacco smoking in human reproduction. Population Reports Series L, No. 1, 1979.
17. D'Arcy, P. F., & Griffin, J. P.: Iatrogenic Diseases. pp. 48-56. Oxford Univ. Press, 1972.
18. Diamond, I., Anderson, M. M., & McCreadie, S. R.: Transplacental transmission of busulfan in a mother with leukemia. Pediatrics 25:85-90, 1960.
19. Dipaolo, J. A., & Kotin, P.: Teratogenesis–oncogenesis: A study of possible relationships. Arch. Pathol. 81:3-23, 1966.
20. Duritz, G., & Oltorf, C.: Lactobezoar formulation associated with high-density caloric formula. Pediatrics 63:647-649, 1979.
21. Erenberg, A., Shaw, R. D., & Yousefzadeh, O.: Lactobezoar in the low birth weight infant. Pediatrics 63:642-646, 1979.
22. Feldman, G. L., Weaver, D. D., & Lovrien, E. W.: Fetal trimethadione syndrome: Report of an additional family and further delineation of this syndrome. Am. J. Dis. Child. 131:1389-1392, 1977.
23. Finitzo-Hieber, T., McCrackan, G. H.,

Roeser, R. J., Allen, D. A., Chrane, D. F., & Morrow, J.: Ototoxicity in neonates treated with gentamicin and kanamicin. Pediatrics 63:443-450, 1979.

24. Finster, M., Poppers, P. J., Sinclair, J. C., et al: Accidental intoxication of the fetus with local anesthetic drug during caudal anesthesia. Am. J. Obstet. Gynecol. 92:922, 1965.
25. Fox, H. A.: Effects of maternal analgesics on neonatal morbidity. In: Adamsons, K., & Fox, H. A., Preventability of Perinatal Injury. Liss, A. R. New York. 1977.
26. Freeman, R.: Chronic lead poisoning in children: Reviw of 90 children diagnosed in Sydney, 1948–1967. Aust Paediat. J. 5:27-35, 1969.
27. Friberg, L., Poscator, M., & Nordberg, G.: Cadmium in the Environment. Chemical Rubber Co., Cleveland, 1971.
28. Friberg, L., & Vostal, J.: Mercury in the Environment. Chemical Rubber Co., Cleveland, 1972.
29. Funatsu, H., Yamashita, F., Ito, Y. et al: Polychlorobiphenyls (PCB)-induced fetopathy. I. Kurume Med. J. 19:43-50, 1972.
30. Ghedan, F. K., LaBreque, D. R., & Younoszai, K.: Intrahepatic cholestasis after gold therapy in juvenile rheumatoid arthritis. J. Pediatr. 93:1042-1043, 1978.
31. Gill, W. B., Schumacher, G. F. B., & Bibb, M.: Structural and functional abnormalities in the sex organs of male offspring of mothers treated with diethylstilbestrol. J. Reprod. Med. 16:147-153, 1976.
32. Glass, L: Effects of narcotics on the fetus. In Morselli, P. L., Garattini, S., & Sereni, F. (Eds.) Basic and Therapeutic Aspects of Perinatal Pharmacology. Raven Press, New York, 1975.
33. Golden, N. L., Sokol, R. J., & Rubin, I. L.: Angel dust: Possible effects on fetus. Pediatrics 65:18-20, 1980.
34. Goodman, R. M., Bat, M., Katznelson, M., Hertz, M., Katznelson, D., & Rotem, Y.: Congenital malformations in four siblings of a mother taking anticonvulsant drugs. Am. J. Dis. Child. 130:884-887, 1976.
35. Goyer, R. A., & Chisholm, J. J.: Lead. In: Lee, D. H., Ed. Metallic Contaminants and Human Health: Fogarty International Center Proceedings. Academic Press, New York, 1972.
36. Grant, W. M.: Toxicology of the Eye. 2nd Ed. Charles C. Thomas, Springfield, Illinois, 1974.
37. Guillozet, N.: The risks of paracervical anesthesia: Intoxication and neurological injury of the newborn. Pediatrics 55:533-536, 1975.
38. Hanson, J. W., Jones, K. L., & Smith, D. W.: Fetal alcohol syndrome: Experience with 41 patients. J.A.M.A. 235:1458-1460, 1976.
39. Hanson, J. W., Stressguth, A. P., & Smith, D. W.: The effects of moderate alcohol consumption during pregnancy on fetal growth and morphogenesis. J. Pediatr. 92:457-460, 1978.
40. Heinonen, O. P., Slone, D., & Shapiro, S.: Birth Defects and Drugs in Pregnancy. Publishing Science Group Inc., Littleton, Massachusetts, 1977.
41. Hill, R. M., Verniaud, W. M., Horning, M. G., McCulley, L. B., & Morgan, N. F. Infants exposed in utero to antiepileptic drugs: Prospective study. Am. J. Dis. Child 127:645-653, 1974.
42. Himmelberger, D. U., Brown, B. W., & Ghan, W. N.: Cigarette smoking during pregnancy and the occurrence of spontaneous abortion and congenital abnormality. Am. J. Epidemiol. 108:470-479, 1978.
43. Hollaender, A.: Chemical Mutagens—Principles and Methods for Their Detection—Vols. 1–5 (Vol. 5, et seq., with de Serres, F. J.) From 1970–1978, Plenum, New York.
44. Hunter, W. J., & Smeets, J. G. P. M.: The Evaluation of Toxicological Data for the Protection of Public Health. Pergamon, Oxford, 1977.
45. Kattan, K. R.: Calvarial thickening after dilantin therapy. Am. J. Roentgenol. 110:102-105, 1970.
46. Kim, W. Y., Pomerance, J. J., & Miller, A. A.: Lidocaine intoxication in a newborn following local anesthesia for epesiotomy. Pediatrics 64:643-645, 1979.
47. Kissane, J. M.: Pathology of Infancy and Childhood. 2d Ed. C. V. Mosby, St. Louis, 1975.
48. Korobkin, R., Asbury, A. K., Sumner, A. J.,

et al: Glue-sniffing neuropathy. Arch. Neurol. 32:158-162, 1975.
49. Kurent, J. E., & Sever, J. L.: Infectious diseases. In: Wilson, J. L., & Fraser, F. C., Eds. Handbook of Teratology. pp. 225-259. Vol. I. Plenum Press, New York, 1977.
50. Lant, A. F.: Renal excretion and toxicity of drugs. In: Black, D., & Jones, N. F., Eds. Renal Disease. pp. 627-639. 4th Ed. Blackwell, 1979.
51. Landesman-Dwyer, S., & Emanuel, I.: Smoking during pregnancy. Teratology 19:119-126, 1979.
52. Laros, R. K., Hage, M. L., & Hayashi, R. H.: Pregnancy and heart valve prosthesis. Obstet. Gynecol. 35:241-247, 1970.
53. Lefebvre, E. B., Haining, R. C., & Labbe, R. F.: Coarse facies, calvarial thickening and hyperphosphatasia associated with long-term anticonvulsant therapy. N. Engl. J. Med. 286:1301-1302, 1972.
54. Lever, W. F., Lever, G.: Histopathology of the Skin. Lippincott, Philadelphia, 1975.
55. Levin, J. N.: Amphetamine ingestion with biliary atresia. J. Pediatr. 79:130-131, 1971.
56. Li, F. P., Cassady, J. R., & Jaffe N.: Risk of second tumors in survivors of childhood cancer. Cancer 35:1230-1235, 1975.
57. Lloyd-Still, J. D., Grand, R. J., & Vawter, G. F.: Tetracycline hepatotoxicity in differential diagnosis of postoperative jaundice. J. Pediatr. 84:366-370, 1974.
58. Long, S. Y.: Does LSD induce chromosomal damage and malformations? Teratology 6:75-90, 1972.
59. Longo, L. D.: The biological effects of carbon monixide in the pregnant woman, fetus and newborn infant. Am J. Obstet. Gynecol. 129:69-103, 1977.
60. Luongo, M. A., & Bjornson, S. S.: The liver in ferrous sulfate poisoning. N. Engl. J. Med. 251:995-999, 1954.
61. Malling, H. V., & Wassom, J. S.: Action of mutagenic agents. In: Wilson, J. G., & Fraser, F. C., Eds. Handbook of Teratology. Vol. 1. pp. 99-152. Plenum Press, New York, 1977.
62. Martin, E. W. (Ed.): Types of hazardous drug reactions and their etiologies. In: Hazards of Medication. Ed 2. pp. 307-338. J. B. Lippincott, Philadelphia, 1978.
63. Matthes, F. T., Kerschner, R., Yow, M. D., et al: Acute poisoning associated with inhalation of Hg vapor. Pediatrics 22:675, 1958.
64. McLachan, J. A., & Dixon, R. L.: Teratologic comparisons of experimental and clinical exposures to diethylstilboestrol during gestation. In Thomas, J. A., & Singhal, R. L., Eds. Regulatory Mechanisms Affecting Research pp. 309-336. University Park Press, Baltimore, 1977.
65. Meyer, A.: Intoxications. In Blackwood, A., et al., Eds. Greenfield's Neuropathology. 2nd Ed. Williams and Wilkins, Baltimore, 1963.
66. Mikhael, N. Z., Campbell, J. S., Napke, E., et al: Drug induced liver injury. In: R. K., Chandra, Ed. The liver and Biliary System in Infants and Children. pp. 234-239. Churchill Livingstone, Edinburgh, 1979.
67. Miller, R. W.: The discovery of human teratogens, carcinogens and mutagens: lessons for the future. In: Hollaender, A. & de Serres, F. J., Eds. Chemical Mutagens. Vol. 5. pp. 101-126. (Volumes 1-4 edited by A. Hollaender) Plenum, New York, 1978.
67a. Milner, R. D., Chouksey, S. K.: Effects of fetal exposure to diazoxide in man. Arch. Dis. Child. 47:537–543, 1972.
68. Minckler, J.: Pathology of the Nervous System. Vol. 2. Part XIX. Intoxications. (Various authors) pp. 1618-1704. McGraw-Hill, New York, 1971.
69. Mills, J. L., & Bongiovanni, A. M.: Effect of prenatal estrogen exposure on male genitalia. Pediatrics (Suppl.) 62:1160-1165, 1978.
70. Monnet, P., Fayard, C., Guilhot, J. et al: Intoxication by imipramine and its derivatives in children. Rev. Lyon Med. 19:845-847, 1970.
71. Moore, M. R., Campbell, B. C., & Goldberg, A.: Lead. In Lenchan, J., & Fletcher, W. W., Eds. Environment and Man. Vol. 6. pp. 64-92. Blackie, Glasgow, 1978.
72. Moore, M. R., & Meredith, P. A.: The carcinogenicity of lead. Arch. Toxicol. 42:87-94, 1979.
73. Mullick, F., Drake, R. M., & Irey, N. S.: Morphologic changes in adverse drug reactions in infants and children. Hum. Pathol. 8:361-378, 1977.
74. Naeye, R. L.: Relationship of cigarette smoking to congenital anomalies and perinatal death. Am. J. Pathol. 90:289-293, 1978.
75. Nahas, G., & Goujaro, J.: Phenothiazines, benzodiazepines and the fetus. In: Scarpelli, E. M., & Cosmi, E. V., Eds. "Reviews in Peri-

natal Medicine. Raven Press, New York, 1977.

76. Newberne, P. M. (Ed.): Trace Substances and Health. Part I. Marcel Dekker, New York, 1976.

76a. Nishimura, H. & Tanimura, A. T. (Eds.): Clinical Aspects of the Teratogenicity of Drugs. Excerpta Medica, Elsevier, Amsterdam, 1976.

77. Nogen, A. G., & Brenner, J. E.: Fatal acetaminophen overdosage in a young child. J. Pediatr. 92:832-833, 1978.

78. Nolke, A.: Aminophylline poisoning deaths in children. J.A.M.A. 161:693-695, 1956.

79. Nora, J. J., Vargo, T. A., Nora, A. H., et al: Dexamphetamine: A possible environmental trigger in cardiovascular malformations. Lancet 1:1290-1291, 1970.

80. Nora, J. J., Nora, A. H., & Toews, W. H.: Lithium, Ebstein's anomaly and other congenital heart defects. Lancet 2:594-595, 1974.

81. Nordberg, G. F. Ed.: Effects and Dose Response Relationship of Toxic Metals. Elsevier, Amsterdam, 1976.

82. Nordberg, G. F. (Ed.): Factors influencing metabolism and toxicity of metals: A consensus report. Environ. Health Perspect. 25:3-41, 1978.

83. Nordstrom, S., Beckman, L., & Nordenson, I.: Occupational and environmental risks in and around a smelter in northern Sweden. III. Frequencies of spontaneous abortion. Hereditas 88:51-54, 1978.

84. Nunnerley, H., Laws, J. W., Davis, M., et al: Chemical and drug induced liver tumors. In: Preger, L., Ed. Induced Disease. pp. 3-26. Grune & Stratton, New York, 1980.

85. Pelkonen, O., Korhonen, P., Jouppila, P. et al: Placental transfer and fetal metabolism of drugs. In Morselli, P. L., Garattini, S., & Sereni, F., Eds. Basic and Therapeutic Aspects of Perinatal Pharmacology. pp. 65-74. Raven Press, New York, 1975.

86. Petty, B. G., Zahka, U. G., & Bernstein, M. T.: Aspirin hepatitis associated with encephalopathy. J. Pediatr. 93:881-882, 1978.

87. Pinkus, H. and Mehregan, A. H.: A Guide to Dermatohistopathology. 2d Ed. Appleton-Century-Crofts, 1976.

88. Pomerance, J. J., & Yaffe, S.: Maternal medication and its effect on the fetus. Curr. Prob. Pediatr. 4:1-60, 1973.

89. Popper, H., Goldfischer, S., Sternlieb, I., et al.: Cytoplasmic copper and its toxic effects. Lancet 1:1205-1208, 1979.

90. Portugez-Malavasi, A., & Aranda, J. V.: Antacid bezoar in a neonate. Pediatrics 63:679-680, 1979.

91. Qazi, Q., Masakawa, A., Milman, D. McGann, B., Chua, D., & Halley, J.: Renal anomalies in fetal alcohol syndrome. Pediatrics 63:886-889, 1979.

92. Raivio, K. O., Ikonen, E., & Saarikoski, S.: Fetal risks due to warfarin therapy during pregnancy. Acta Paediatr. Scand. 66:735-739, 1977.

93. Redman, C. W. G., Beilin, L. J., Bonnar, J. et al.: Fetal outcome of antihypertensive treatment in pregnancy. Lancet 2:753-756, 1976.

94. Reed, D., Crawley, J., Faro, S. N. et al.: Thallotoxicosis, J.A.M.A. 183:516-522, 1963.

95. Rice, J. M.: An overview of transplacental chemical carcinogenesis. Teratology 8:113-126, 1973.

96. Rodin, A. E., Haggard, M. E., & Travis, L. B.: Lung changes and chemotherapeutic agents in childhood. Am. J. Dis. Child. 12:337 1970.

97. Saltzstein, S. L., & Ackerman, L. V.: Lymphadenopathy produced by anticonvulsant drugs and mimicking clinically and pathologically malignant lymphomas. Cancer 12:164-182, 1959.

98. Saxen, I.: Associations between oral clefts and drugs taken during pregnancy. Int. J. Epidemiol. 4:37-44, 1975.

99. Schardein, J. L.: Drugs as Teratogens. Chemical Rubber Company Press, Cleveland, 1976.

99a. Schreiner, G. E., Maher, J. F.: Toxic nephropathy. Am. J. Med. 38:409-449, 1965.

100. Schwarz, R. H., & Yaffe, S. J.: Drug and Chemical Risks to the Fetus and Newborn. Alan R. Liss, New York 1980.

101. Seeler, R. A., Israle, J. N., Royal, J. E., et al.: Ganglioneuroblastoma and fetal hydantoin-alcohol syndromes. Pediatrics 63:524-527, 1979.

102. Shaw, E. B.: Fetal damage due to maternal aminopterin. Am. J. Dis. Child. 124:93-94, 1972.

103. Shepard, T.: A Catalog of Teratogenic Agents. 3rd Ed. Johns Hopkins University Press, Baltimore, 1980.

104. Shotton, D., & Monie, I. W.: Possible teratogenic effects of chlorambucil on a human fetus. J.A.M.A. 186:74-75, 1963.

105. Shuman, R. M., Leech, R. W., & Ellsworth, C. A., Jr.: Neurotoxicity of hexachlorophene in the human. I. Clinicopathologic study of 248 children. Pediatrics 54:689-695, 1974.
106. Smialek, J. E., Monforte, J. R., Aronow, R., & Spitz, W. U.: Methadone deaths in children: Continuing problem. J.A.M.A. 238:2516-2517, 1977.
107. Smith, D. W.: Dysmorphology (teratology) J. Pediatr. 69:1150-1169, 1966.
108. Smith, D. W.: Recognizable patterns of human malformation—2nd Ed. p. 211, p. 336-347. W. B. Saunders, Philadelphia, 1976.
109. Smith, D. W., Clarren, S. K., & Harvey, M. A. S.: Hyperthermia as a possible teratogenic agent. J. Pediatr. 92:881-883, 1978.
110. Smith, J. P.: The pathology of ferrous sulphate poisoning. J. Pathol. Bacteriol. 64:467-472, 1952.
111. Soule, A. B., & Foley, J. C.: Poisoning from petroleum distillates. J. Maine Med. Assoc. April 1957.
112. Stamp, T. C. B.: Drug and Chemical-Induced rickets. In: Preger, L., Ed. Induced Disease. pp. 27-43. Grune & Stratton, New York, 1980.
113. Stromeyer, F. W., & Ishak, N. G.: Histology of the liver in Wilson's disease. Am. J. Clin. Pathol. 73:12-24, 1980.
114. Takeuchi, T.: Biological reactions and pathological changes in human beings and animals caused by organic mercury contamination. In Hartung, R. and Dinman, B. D., Eds. Environmental Mercury Contamination. pp. 257-274. Ann Arbor Science, Ann Arbor, Michigan, 1972.
115. Tanner, M. S., Portmann, B., Mowat, A. P., et al.: Increased hepatic copper concentration in Indian childhood cirrhosis. Lancet 1:1203-1205, 1979.
116. Therault, J., Schaller, R. H., Engelhardt, E. et al.: The cadmium content of the human Placenta. Int. Arch. Occup. Environ. Health 36:19-27, 1975.
117. Thienes, C. H., & Haley, T. J.: Clinical Toxicology. 5th Ed. Lea & Febiger, Philadelphia, 1972.
118. Tuchmann-Duplessis, H.: Fetal damage. In Finckh, E. S., Clayton-Jones, E., Eds. The Effects of Environment on Cells and Tissues pp. 58-82. Excerpta Medica, Amsterdam, 1976.
119. Valdes-Dapena, M. A., & Arey, J. B.: Boric acid poisoning. J. Pediatr. 61:531-546, 1962.
120. Vanderhoof, J. A., & Ament, M. E.: Fatal hepatic necrosis due to isoniazid chemoprophylaxis. J. Pediatr. 88:867-870, 1976.
121. Warkany, J.: Congenital Malformations. Year Book Publishers, Chicago, 1971.
122. Weinstein, M. R., & Goldfield, M.: Cardiovascular malformation with lithium use during pregnancy. Am. J. Psychiatry 132:529-531, 1975.
123. Wilson, J. G.: Environment and Birth Defects. Academic Press, New York, 1973.
124. Wilson, J. G. & Fraser, F. C.: Handbook of Teratology. Vol. I. General Principles and Etiology; Vol. 3. Comparative, Maternal and Epidemiologic Aspects. Plenum Press, New York, 1977, 1979.
125. Zucker, P., Daum, F., & Cohen, M. I.: Aspirin hepatitis. Am. J. Dis. Child. 129:1433-1434, 1975.

3

Skeletal Muscle

Byron A. Kakulas

Skeletal muscle forms by far the greatest quantity of tissue in the human body; apart from its role in locomotion, it also serves a major secondary function in maintaining metabolic homeostasis and a store of protein.[28] In its primary role, skeletal muscle is often required to undergo sudden and extreme contraction, with total recruitment of its full metabolic and mechanical power at short notice. The apparent ease of injury to skeletal muscle by a great variety of drugs and toxins is probably related to its specialized metabolism, and to the associated effects on these metabolic processes by the physiologic demands.

The term myopathy describes any pathologic change in skeletal muscle. When regarding the effects of drug and toxic myopathies, an anatomic approach, according to the site of action of the agent, is probably more useful than any other. Thus the drug myopathies can be grouped according to whether they involve the peripheral nerve, and thus produce denervation atrophy in the muscle; the motor end-plate, causing a myasthenia-like state; the muscle membrane, producing myotonia; or the actual sarcoplasm of the muscle fiber, in which case the myopathy is usually manifest as a polyfocal myonecrosis.

Because of the special features of muscle innervation, which predispose the motor end-plate to a great variety of pathophysiologic or "functional" disorders, there are no obvious structural changes in many of the toxic and drug myopathies. It is for this reason also that there are many drug-induced myasthenic and pseudomyasthenic states. The other "physiologic" disorder caused by toxins and drugs, owing to their effect on the muscle membrane, is associated with a failure of relaxation known as myotonia or pseudomyotonia, depending upon the electromyography. An irritant may also quite subjectively cause pain by stimulating the intramuscular, pain-mediating nerve fibers; drug-induced myalgias are very common.[67]

In those cases in which a drug or toxin causes polyfocal muscle necrosis, the site of maximal involvement is partly determined by the degree of metabolic activity at the time of action of the agent. This is one of the principles of toxicology; it is simply stated as: "The greater the metabolic acitivity of the target organ at the time of action of a toxin (or drug), the greater is its harmful effect." Furthermore, some time must lapse before the cumulation of polyfocal lesions is sufficiently great for muscle weakness to become clinically significant.

The muscles most often involved by polyfocal toxic lesions and subsequent weakening are the large proximal muscles of the shoulder and pelvic girdles. This is so because these muscles contain both a greater bulk of muscle, and are more powerful and more active overall than the other muscles in these areas. These necrobiotic proximal myopathies will therefore cause their greatest symptomatic difficulty when the patient attempts to climb stairs or arise from a chair. Raising the arms above the head may also be very difficult or impossible. This proximal weakness is in contrast to the distribution of weakness fround in a peripheral neuropathy, in which case the weakness is more severe in the distal extremities, with the hands and feet being the most affected.

In the motor end-plate disorders, the most used muscles are always the most affected. In this case the weakness appears rapidly, and with consecutive contractions of the involved muscles, they become weaker and weaker. In these situations external opthalomoplegia and wrist drop are common.

In addition to the clinical assessment of the patient, including a review of the history and the findings on physical examination, a muscle biopsy, electromyography (EMG), and serum creatine kinase (CK) assay are the standard diagnostic procedures when a myopathy is suspected. EMG is very useful in detecting denervation, myasthenia, and myotonia, and will also give a characteristic pattern in the primary necrobiotic myopathies. The CK is greatly elevated when there is necrosis because of the release of muscle enzymes from necrotic foci into the serum. Because it helps to differentiate a primary muscle condition from the denervation and end-plate disorders that are associated with low or relatively low levels of serum CK, this is the basis of a useful clinical test.

In the "wasting diseases" there is in reality an associated myopathy in which there is "brown atrophy" of skeletal muscle. This is a common feature of many final illnesses as in the muscle wasting of disseminated malignancy, with loss of muscle bulk due to the protein store being given up. In these cases the corresponding reduction in muscle strength is appropriate, and the CK is not elevated unless there is associated polymyositis; however, the latter can be the situation, since polymyositis is often present subclinically in terminal malignancy. In cachexia, weakness is usually a lesser feature than the visible loss of muscle tissue. This appearance is accentuated by the associated loss of subcutaneous fat. In simple and disuse atrophy the EM changes consist of myofibrillar loss, the fragmentation and infolding of basement membranes, and other changes.[30]

In patients with peripheral neuropathy, muscle denervation causes distal weakness some days before the atrophy becomes clinically apparent. At the bedside, disorders of neuromuscular transmission are detected by their effect on sustained or repeated muscle contraction, because of the easy fatiguability or "myasthenia" which they produce. Myotoxicity causing myotonia may be clinically silent; when well developed, this phenomenon is detectable as a failure of relaxation of the grip. The patient may complain of "stiff" joints or "sticky" fingers.

Suspected myotonia, motor end-plate disorders and early denervation are better demonstrated by physiologic methods, especially EMG, than by morphologic techniques. Although the intravital staining of end-plates and EM may give some positive findings in the "myasthenic" and "myotonic" conditions, these techniques are difficult and time consuming relative to the information gained; they are therefore more in the realm of "research" than in that of routine pathology laboratory testing. On the other hand, muscle biopsy is an essential adjunct in the clinical work-up for those conditions that cause morphologic changes, often providing information of diagnostic importance. Certain guidelines for muscle biopsy should be noted from the outset.[60] It must also be understood that because of the stereotyped nature of the muscle fiber reaction to injury, a precise clinicopathologic diagnosis is usually achieved only when the clinical, EMG, and enzyme studies are considered together. Beyond this, it must be kept in mind that because of the focal nature of most myopathies, a negative muscle biopsy has very little clinical value.

Handling of Muscle Biopsies. In choosing the site for biopsy, a clinically involved (that is, a weak) muscle must be selected; however, this muscle should not be totally paralyzed, because the histopathology may then be at the "end-stage" and no longer helpful. The best results are obtained by an open surgical method. After infiltration with a short-acting local anesthetic, a number of specimens are removed, as follows: for light microscopy (LM), a block of muscle at least $1 \times 1.5 \times 1$ cm is required. Following removal, the specimen, because of its irritability and in order to avoid artifact, is laid out in its natural orientation on a piece of cardboard, and left in the air for 3 to 5 minutes before being fixed by immersion in 10 percent buffered formol saline. Formalin is advocated because it allows a wide range of staining methods; however, for phosphotungstic acid hematoxylin (PTAH) staining, Susa fixative gives much better results. The most useful muscle tissue stains are hematoxylin and eosin (H & E), trichrome, and periodic acid Schiff (PAS) (before and after diastase) for glycogen content. PTAH is a useful connective tissue stain and gives particularly deep and almost specific staining of myofibrils.

Following the removal of a biopsy specimen for staining, a second piece of muscle is removed for EM. In order to minimize artifact, this specimen is best tied to an applicator (orange) stick after removal, although some prefer a special clamp for this purpose. A specimen of about 1.5 cm length and 2 mm diameter is usually adequate. The muscle to be removed must be carefully cut away from the remaining bulk of muscle. It is very important that the piece of muscle between the sutures not be handled or touched; this precaution is necessary to avoid mechanical artifact. The EM specimen is fixed in about 10 ml of cacodylate buffered 2.5 percent glutaraldehyde at room temperature. Separation from the stick and further dissection and trimming are undertaken as soon as the specimen reaches the laboratory. Fixation continues for 2 hours, and the biopsy is then washed in buffer, trimmed, and blocked. These steps are necessary because of the poor penetrating power of the fixatives. Postfixing in osmium tetroxide for a further 2 hours is then undertaken, and the blocks are dehydrated in graded alcohols and embedded in a resin such as Araldite or Epon. Semithin cross and longitudinal sections should be examined and selected for further cutting prior to EM viewing. These ultrathin sections are stained for 30 minutes in saturated aqueous uranyl acetate and then in lead citrate for 3 minutes. For the electron micrographs, longitudinal sections are more informative than cross sections.

The next step in the biopsy procedure is the selection of a third piece of muscle for histochemistry. A muscle fascicle 1 cm in length and about 4 mm in width is the minimum required. For ease of handling, some laboratory technologists prefer this piece to also be tied to a short piece of applicator stick, as described above. On removal the specimen is immediately quenched by immersion in isopentane in liquid nitrogen, and after a few minutes it is placed directly into liquid nitrogen.

A battery of histochemical methods is recommended for identification of the oxidative enzymes (type I muscle fibers) and anaerobic pathways (type II muscle fibers), in a muscle tissue specimen, since technical difficulties are often encountered with any one method. For type I muscle fibers, the identification of lactic dehydrogenase (LDH), succinic dehydrogenase (SDH), and the reduced nicotinamide adenine dinucleotide tetrazolium reductase (NADH-TR) method are standard. "Routine" adenosine triphosphatase (ATPase incubated at pH 9.4) and phosphorylase methods demonstrate the type II (glycolytic) fibers. ATPase preincubated at pH 4.6 and pH 4.2 provides information that permits a subdivision of the type II fibers. An oil-red-O-stained frozen section is useful in assessing the neutral fat content of the muscle.

If further pieces of muscle are required, such as for immunologic studies, a biopsy technique similar to that used for the histochemical procedures is recommended. Quite often in a research department, a larger piece, perhaps 5 to 10 grams of muscle, is also required for biochemistry; in this case the specimen is also deep frozen.

Despite the advantages of an open surgical biopsy technique for convenience and for organizational reasons, more myopathologists are obtaining samples of muscle by a needle method.[124] Although much less satisfactory because of the smallness of the muscle sample and associated mechanical artifacts, clinically useful interpretations may be made from such specimens by experienced myopathologists. However, if the result is unsatisfactory, the clinician should revert to the open method for diagnostic accuracy, which is in the patient's interest.

A knowledge of the elements of myopathology is necessary for the understanding of toxic and drug effects on muscle.[2,61,62] One principle concerns the regenerative potential of skeletal muscle. Human skeletal muscle has great powers of regeneration, and complete restoration of architecture is the rule, provided that the supporting framework of the muscle is not disturbed. For this reason, in other than mechanical injuries to muscle, complete regeneration can be expected when the noxious agent ceases to act. This is relevant to the clinician because the main treatment of a drug or toxic myopathy is the simple withdrawal of the offending agent. For the pathophysiologic end-plate disorders, a specific pharmacologic antidote may be known, and if so should be given. The same is true for the snakebite antivenins.

Rest and passive physiotherapy are recommended as part of the treatment of a toxic myopathy. Clinical progress is monitored by serial serum CK measurements as well as by the bedside assessment of muscle power, with regular charting. Regeneration can be expected to proceed very rapidly under these conditions. Bed rest is also advisable because of the possible involvement of the myocardium. Indeed, it should be expected as a general rule that whenever skeletal muscle is diseased, the cardiac muscle may also be affected, even though this is subclinical or silent. The heart is often found at necropsy to be involved in fatal cases of any skeletal muscle condition, polyfocal necrosis or interstitial fibrosis.

Useful clinical reviews listing the common drug-induced myopathies[67] and those drugs that cause neuromuscular blockade,[5] as well as drugs and toxins causing peripheral neuropathy,[6,15] have recently appeared.

DRUGS AND TOXINS CAUSING DENERVATION

There is a large number of drugs and toxins that damage the peripheral nerves and so cause a peripheral neuropathy. Some of these are diphtheria toxin, heavy metals (lead, arsenic, gold, thallium, and mercury), hexane, alcohol, gasoline, carbon tetrachloride, trichlorethylene, isoniazid, furans clioquiniol, sulfonamides, monoamine oxidase (MAO) inhibitors, and nitrogen mustards.[15]

In denervation, apart from the changes in the nerve, there is atrophy of the several hundred muscle fibers that the affected motor nerve supplies. The result is therefore known as motor unit atrophy. Although in a given human skeletal muscle, both type I and type II fibers are usually present throughout admixed in a checkerboard fashion, all of the muscle fibers supplied by a single motor nerve are of the same histochemical type. Generally, in a peripheral neuropathy, only a proportion of all the motor fibers in a peripheral nerve are affected, and some motor units are therefore spared. At first a histochemical, and later a morphologic distinction, develops between the intact and affected motor units.

The late morphologic change known as "grouped atrophy" becomes apparent only after a few weeks have passed, because a sequence of events is required before it becomes manifest. The first event to occur is new cross-innervation of the atrophied fibers by the unaffected, neighboring nerves supplying an adjoining motor unit. Because of the histochemical consistency of motor units in the early stages of denervation, histochemical methods are very useful in the diagnosis of a toxic peripheral neuropathy, since they reveal the loss of the checkerboard pattern that is normal to the muscle, and its replacement by a histochemical type-grouping (Fig. 3-1). The appearance of atrophic and hypertrophic groupings depends upon the progression of the neuropathy to the point at which it involves the motor nerve responsible for the reinnervation. At that point, the total combined population of two or more motor units undergoes atrophy, giving rise to the highly characteristic appearance of grouped atrophy (Fig. 3-2).

Improvements in the biopsy diagnosis of denervation are based on recognition of the physiologic relationship between motor nerve and muscle,[18] and the discovery of the histo-

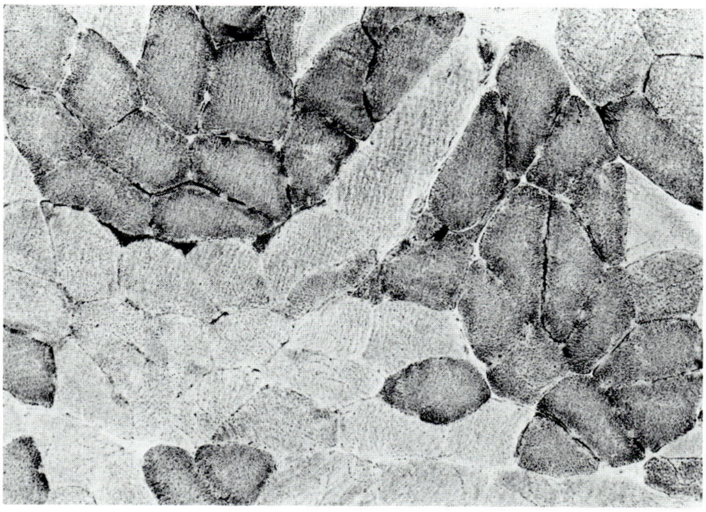

Fig. 3-1. Succinic dehydrogenase stain showing loss of the normal checkerboard admixture of type I and type II muscle fibers, which are replaced by histochemical type-grouping—an early sign of denervation. × 100.

chemical specificity of the muscle fiber types in individual motor units.[65] It is believed that the particular histochemical fiber type is governed by the physiologic function of the motor unit, rather than by particular, anterior horn-cell specificity.[92]

It is out of the realm of this chapter to further describe the effects of toxins and drugs that act on the peripheral nerves. Broad considerations of these topics are available in the standard texts.[7,15,77]

DRUGS AND TOXINS THAT BLOCK NEUROMUSCULAR TRANSMISSION

The classic drugs and toxins in this group are natural curare and its derivatives. However, a wide range of drugs, and especially the antibiotics, are known to cause a neuromuscular blockade. Postoperative respiratory depression may occur with clindamycin, colistin, kanamycin, lincomycin, neomycin, strep-

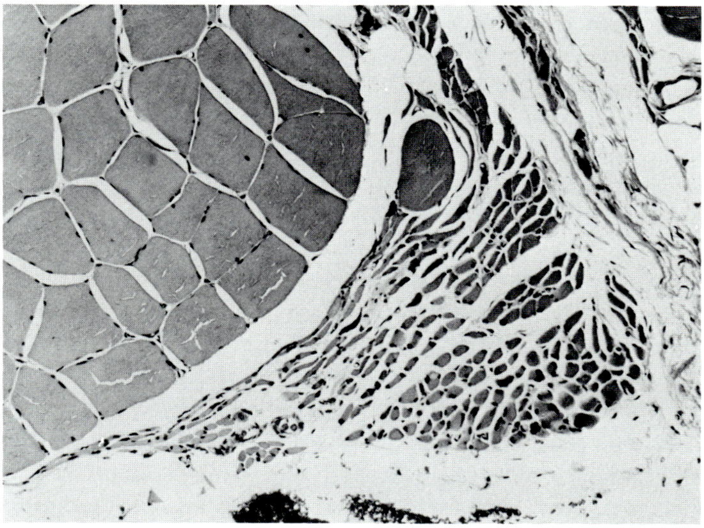

Fig. 3-2. Distinctive grouped-atrophy of muscle fibers in long-standing denervation. H & E, × 100.

tomycin, and tobramycin. It has also been found to occur with lidocaine, quinidine, and trimethaphan, while chloroquine, lithium, phenelzine and promazine, aprotinin, cholinesterase inhibitors, and oxytocin may also depress respiration.[5] Other drugs are known to aggravate or unmask myasthenia gravis, a muscle end-plate disorder. These are colistin, kanamycin, streptomycin, tetracyclines, procainamide, propranolol, quinidine, chloroquine, chlorpromazine, lithium, phenytoin, ACTH, corticosteroids, thyroid hormones, acetylcholinesterase inhibitors, and methoxyflurane.[5]

A drug-induced myasthenic syndrome may be caused by colistin, gentamicin, kanamycin, neomycin, polymyxin B, streptomycin, oxprenolol, practolol, trimethaphan, D-penicillamine, phenytoin, trimethadoine, oral contraceptives, and tetanus antitoxin.[5] These will not be considered further, since little is known of the morphologic counterpart—if any—of the condition, and the toxic effect is usually reversed upon removal of the drug.

DRUGS THAT CAUSE MYOTONIA

Inhibitors of cholesterol biosynthesis are known to cause myotonia.[122] Among these inhibitors, 20,25-diazocholesterol is often used for the experimental investigation of myotonia[34]; the effects of the inhibition are related to the accumulation of desmosterol in the muscle fiber. The myotonia is due to a membrane disorder in which there is excessive permeability of the chloride ion, as a result of aberrant membrane synthesis (lipid) from interruption of cholesterol biosynthetic pathways.

Myotonia induced by 2,4-dichlorphenoxyacetate (2,4-D) has also been widely studied.[101] Because of its metabolic effect,[53] 2,4-D has also been used to study the pathogenesis of experimental myopathies, and even human muscular dystrophy. The first observed changes in the effect of 2,4-D on muscle are histochemical, because this agent, like fluoro- and iodoacetate, acts by inhibiting glucose-3-phosphate dehydrogenase. The histochemical changes involve the white or type II muscle fibers, and are accompanied by mitochondrial changes. Vacuolation leading to muscle fiber necrosis occurs in advanced lesions. In other EM studies, 2,4-D given in high doses to guinea pigs has been shown to cause a proliferation of tubular profiles.[29]

A series of nine related monocarboxylic acids previously known to inhibit membrane chloride conductance were studied for their ability to produce myotonia.[44] All induced a characteristic myotonia that could be duplicated by the simple removal of chloride ion. Calcium ion concentration and ambient temperature were modifying factors, while diphenylhydantion inhibited the myotonia. Myotonia is also produced by indoleacetic acid in mice[43] and by clofibrate in rats.[66] Additionally, clofibrate will directly affect the muscle fiber. The myopathology of this agent in humans includes the breakdown of contractile material, derangement of mitochondria, dilation of the sarcoplasmic reticulum, and the accumulation of membrane dense bodies.[1]

DRUGS AND TOXINS THAT CAUSE POLYFOCAL MYONECROSIS

A very large number of toxins, drugs, and metabolic derangements will cause polyfocal myonecrosis. These are conveniently grouped under the headings that follow.

Drugs

Steroids. Steroid hormones have long been known to cause muscle fiber necrosis under suitable experimental conditions.[27,36] Necrosis with associated regeneration is easily induced experimentally with glucocorticoids; the synthetic analogues of these substances (fludrocortisone[72] and triamcinolone[121]) are even more potent in this respect. Furthermore, a steroid myopathy is clinically well known. In cases of this condition, in addition to polyfocal necrosis, muscle biopsies reveal type II fiber atrophy. In fact, histochemical changes are more frequently found overall in cases of steroid myopathy than is necrosis. Electron microscopically, cortisone causes atrophy with loss of myofilaments, as well as necrosis visible on light microscopy.[47] Vacuolation of muscle fibers, especially in EM preparations, is another feature of the corticosteroid myopathies. In 7 patients taking 17-hydroxycorticosteroids who developed a myopathy, vacuolation and muscle fiber necrosis were observed.[91] In another report, 50 patients with rheumatoid arthritis and 1 with ankylosing spondylitis all developed a corticosteroid (prednisolone) myopathy; in these patients, however, the main parameter of measurement was the mean potential duration (MPD).[25] Other physiologic parameters of steroid myopathy include enhancement of the specific twitch tension, which is thought to possibly reflect structural and functional differences in fast or slow muscle membrane systems.[45]

In rabbits, the combination of methylchlorocortisol and NaH_2PO_4 administration[10] may produce an acute paralytic condition. The condition—which resembles familial periodic paralysis—is prevented by chlorides.[106] In experimental animals with $NaClO_4$-induced motor disturbances, the predominantly mineralocorticoid steroids greatly enhance the disturbance, while glucocorticoids prevent it.[10]

Other Hormones. In addition to the therapeutic drug-induced steroid myopathies, an associated myopathy is well known in Cushing's syndrome.[81] Acromegaly is also sometimes associated with a myopathy which causes weakness and atrophy. Hypothyroidism[8] and hyperthyroidism[2] are both associated with serious muscle disorders; hypothyroid myopathy causes proximal muscle weakness with a polyfocal necrosis seen in muscle biopsies. There is also a characteristic "delay" in tendon reflexes (Hoffman's syndrome), and EMG reveals pseudomyotonia. In hyperthyroidism, external ophthalmoplegia is frequent, while an associated myasthenia gravis is a common clinical hazard. Again, necrosis, rather than simple atrophy, is the more significant histopathologic change in thyrotoxic myopathy. Less commonly, periodic paralysis may be associated with thyrotoxicosis.

In Addison's disease there is often severe muscular weakness, and hypokalemia due to primary aldosteronism will cause a necrotizing myopathy which has been studied both light microscopically[103] and by EM[9]; the ultrastructural changes seen in this condition are similar to those in experimental hypokalemia, with vacuolation and dilation of the sarcoplasmic reticulum.[32]

Immunosuppressive and Cytotoxic Drugs. Muscle fiber degeneration caused by vincristine is well known; spheromembranous structures are described in this condition.[109] The drug is also known to cause a peripheral neuropathy. Human vincristine neuromyopathy has been extensively studied clinically, physiologically, and pathologically.[17] Adriamycin, another cytotoxic drug, is known to occasionally cause a myocardiopathy; although there is no documentation of skeletal muscle involvement with use of this drug, it would be surprising were muscle fibre necrosis not to be associated with it. Hypokalemic rhabdomyolysis and myoglobinuria have followed amphotericin-B therapy.[35] Other cytotoxic drugs are known to produce muscle pain and cramps,[67] and azathioprine also causes an experimental muscle fiber necrosis (Fig. 3-3).

Antibiotics. Systemic lupus erythematosus (SLE) and dermatomyositis are reported as complications of the sulfacetamide treatment of conjunctivitis.[71] Thiabendazole, a broad spectrum antibiotic, may cause myalgia. Another antimicrobial agent, nitroxoline, causes neuromyopathic changes in the mouse[85]; the muscle changes consist of swollen fibers with central nuclei, but there is little necrosis. Histochemically, phosphorylase is less active in the affected muscle fibers.

Intramuscular injections of chloramphenicol and oxytetracycline produce severe muscle

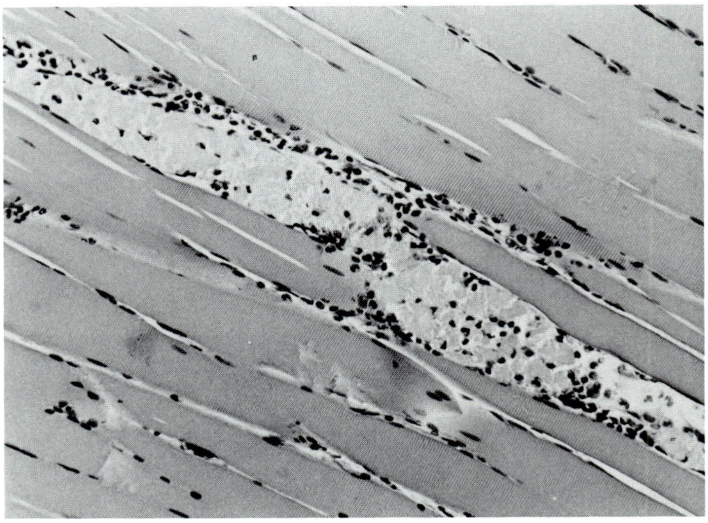

Fig. 3-3. Segmental necrosis of sarcoplasm (center field), with flocculation and beginning infiltration by macrophages and polymorphs. This lesion was induced in a rat by the intramuscular injection of azothioprine, 1 mg/day, for 10 days. H & E, × 200.

damage with fibrosis in mice; streptomycin, cephalothine, and aminobenzyl penicillin cause similar but less severe changes. EM reveals degeneration of muscle fibers, motor end-plates, and peripheral nerves 1 day following a single injection with chloramphenicol; in animals injected on three occasions, localized fibrosis and degenerating myotubes attributed to peripheral nerve damage were also produced.[123]

Diuretics. Although diuretics per se are not known to produce muscle fiber necrosis, the dysionic state, with hypokalemia, caused by these agents will be associated with such necrosis (see electrolyte disorders, below).

Analgesics. In two patients, the analgesic pentazocine caused muscle fibrosis when given by injection over a long period.[33] Paracetamol and salicyclate intoxication, causing coma and hyperthermia in a young woman, are also described as having given rise to muscle fiber necrosis.[108] Dimethylsulfoxide (DMSO), which was once introduced as an anti-inflammatory agent, is known to specifically injure plasma membranes, and causes a neuropathy and myopathy in experimental animals.[62]

Halothane and many other general anesthetic agents may precipitate the malignant hyperpyrexia syndrome (MHP) in susceptible individuals. In MHP there is profound muscle rigidity and myonecrosis with myoglobinuria; death due to metabolic acidosis, is frequent. The muscle relaxant dantrolene is useful in treatment of MHP caused by general anesthetics.[67] The Landrace pig, which is predisposed to a similar disorder provides a convenient experimental model for the human condition.[61] Marcaine, a long acting local anesthetic, is said to have a specific myotoxic effect[12]; however, when injected into an experimental animal, marcaine produces severe pannecrosis involving connective tissue as well as muscle.

Antimalarials. The antimalarial drugs have a well-known history of causing a clinical myopathy. Quinine injected experimentally into rats produces severe necrosis (Figs. 3-4 and 3-5), and plasmocid has the same effect. In plasmocid myopathy, serum glutamic oxalacetic transaminase (SGOT) activity is greatly elevated with in 8 to 12 hours of administration of the drug, and large quantities of the amino acid taurine are excreted in the urine.[14] Plasmocid causes mitochondrial swelling, diminution of cristae, and dilation of sarcotubules,[26] and also destroys actin filaments.[95]

Among the antimalarial drugs, emetine is an especially notorious cause of a sometimes fatal[40] polyfocal necrosis in skeletal and car-

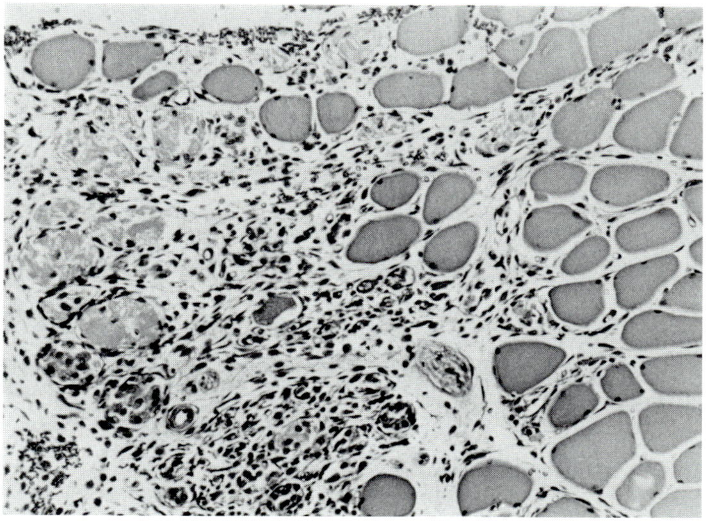

Fig. 3-4. Severe muscle fiber necrosis with myophagia and beginning regeneration induced by the intramuscular injection of quinine, 3 mg/day, for 10 days in a rat. H & E, × 150.

diac muscle. Experimental emetine myopathy in the rat causes pronounced structural changes when the drug is given in high doses[16]; these changes consist mainly of a polyfocal muscle fiber necrosis similar to that observed in the human patient.[40] Rod formation, myofilament loss, membrane proliferation, and Z-line streaming are other changes that have been described in experimental emetine myopathy in the rat.[13]

Chloroquine, widely used as an anti-inflammatory agent especially in rheumatology practice, is another antimalarial drug associated with a necrotizing myopathy.[3,96,119] The predominant changes in this condition are in the red fibers[111]; a focal myocardial necrosis may also occur.[3] EM studies of chloroquine myopathy include experimental[69] and clinical observations. In a patient with SLE who underwent chloroquine therapy for many years after the onset of the illness, muscle weakness developed 9 years after continuous chloroquine administration, and biopsy revealed inflammatory changes and distinctive cytosomes with curvilinear profiles.[83] Although the mechanism of action of chloroquine is not fully known, disturbances of lipid metabolism in turkey erythrocytes and heart

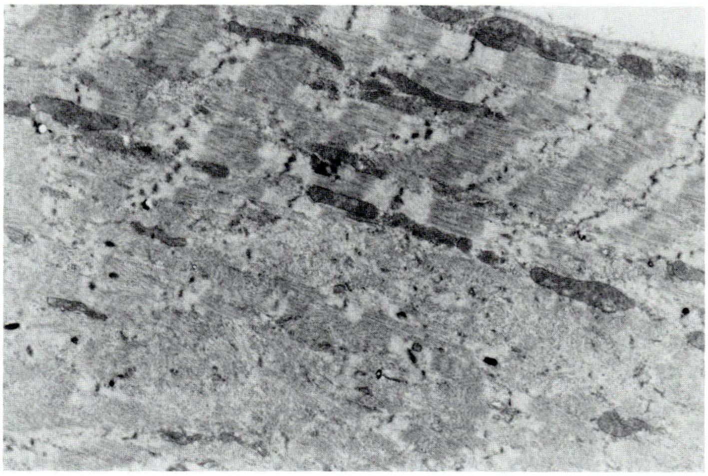

Fig. 3-5. Electron micrograph of the quinine lesion, showing disorganization of sarcomeres with disappearance of Z-bands (lower field), mitochondrial loss, and disorganization of myofibrils. These necrotic changes were induced in a rat by the injection of 6 mg of quinine twice daily for 7 days. Uranyl acetate and lead citrate stains, × 6,000.

muscle homogenates have been found.[51] The therapeutic effect of chloroquine is believed to be due to a lysosome stabilizing function and to the inhibition of antigen-antibody reactions.

Other Drugs. Intraperitoneal injection of colchicine in rats causes paralysis within 1 to 2 days after the injection.[73] Athough EM shows all organelles to be affected, the most conspicuous finding is the accumulation of large sarcoplasmic membranous bodies, which correlate with overt weakness. The broad spectrum antihelminthic agents thiabendazole (mintezol), colchicine, and clofibrate cause a painful myopathy in some patients.[67] Many other drugs, including lithium carbonate, cimetidine, danazol, isoetherine, and some diuretics and cytotoxic agents will also cause muscle pain, weakness, or myokymia by yet unexplored mechanisms.[67] Clofibrate-induced myopathy in the rat is marked by the formation of vesicular bodies and the swelling and dilation of mitochondria and sarcoplasmic reticulum.[115]

Narcotics are also known to be associated with a myopathy. Acute myoglobinuria has been reported in a heroin addict,[97] muscle fibrosis and contractures have been reported in a pethidine addict,[76] and "muscular dystrophy" was induced in mice by subcutaneous injections of cannabinoids.[46]

Other drugs reported in the literature as causes of drug myopathy are as follows: Epsilon aminocaproic acid (EACA) in the treatment of hereditary periodic edema[64]; EACA also produced a severe, painful proximal myopathy in two female patients who received this drug as an antifibrinolytic agent following subarachnoid hemorrhage. In these patients, muscle biopsy revealed an acute monophasic necrotizing myopathy.[68] Perhexiline maleate is another drug that has been associated with a myopathy.[117] Pencillamine, in addition to its neuromuscular blocking effect, is believed to have caused dermatomyositis in two patients.[93]

When given by intramuscular injection,[67] amphetamine will cause acute rhabdomyolysis (Fig. 3-6). Phencyclidine is also known to cause acute rhabdomyolysis.[24] The membrane alterations in chlorphentermine myopathy in rats were studied by freeze fracturing, for comparison with similar changes in the muscle membrane in human dystrophy.[104] *p*-Phenylinediamine (PPD) is a potent cause of muscle fiber necrosis (Fig. 3-7), and the experimental myopathy caused by this drug has been extensively studied.[75] An interesting finding is the experimental production of nemaline rods by neostigmine.[86] Injections of serotonin are said to produce "muscular dystrophy changes" in experimental animals, but these effects are

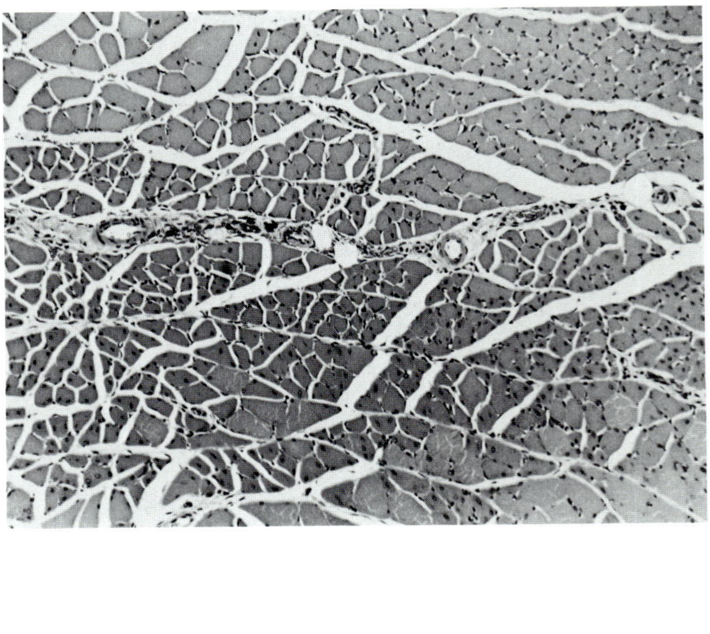

Fig. 3-6. Amphetamine-induced muscle lesions in which many myonuclei have migrated toward the center of the muscle fibers. There is also some shrinkage of muscle fibers. The amphetamine was injected in a rat daily, at 1 mg/day, for 10 days. H & E, × 120.

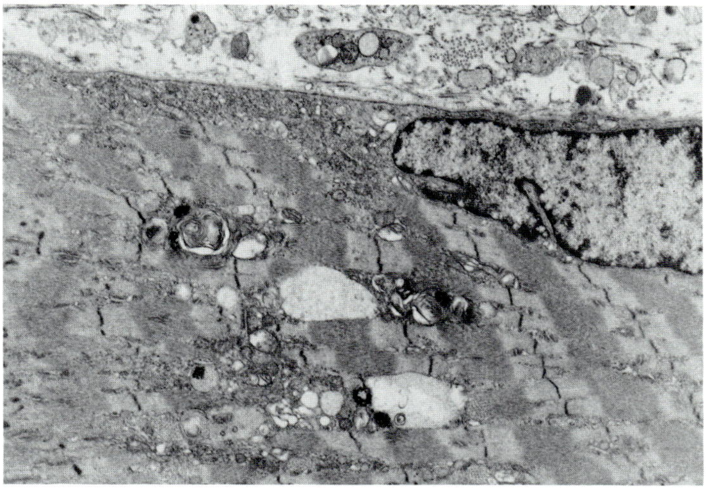

Fig. 3-7. Electron micrograph of *p*-phenylenedamine (PPD)-induced muscle lesions. Myofibrils are disorganized, and there are a number of multilaminated myelin figures, vesicles filled with amorphous material, and mitrochondrial swellings and dilations of the sarcoplasmic reticulum. The PPD was given by injection to a rat, at 6 mg twice daily, for 7 days. Uranyl acetate and lead citrate stains, × 6,000.

considered to be due to vascular changes caused by this agent.[89,105] Other catecholamines also induce muscle weakness in rabbits; in this work, changes resembling "human dystrophy" were produced by the monoamine oxidase (MAO) inhibitor pargyline hydrochloride, and excessive levels of catecholamine were detected in the tissues and urine of the "dystrophic" animals.[38] In yet other work, in which imipramine and serotonin were given together, the muscle changes were shown to be due solely to the serotonin; there was preferential damage to type I muscle fibers. However, it was considered that the myopathic effect was due to primary ischemia rather than to specific myotoxicity.[82]

The serotonin antagonist methysergide, a drug useful in migraine prevention, is known to cause myalgia, and a muscle biopsy from a patient with this myalgic myopathy has shown mitochondrial inclusions (Fig. 3-8). The chronic administration of methysergide is known to cause a serious cardiomyopathy, with an endocardial fibrosis resembling the cardiac changes that occur in the malignant carcinoid syndrome.

Intramuscular injections of diphenylhydantoin produce histologic changes in the muscle

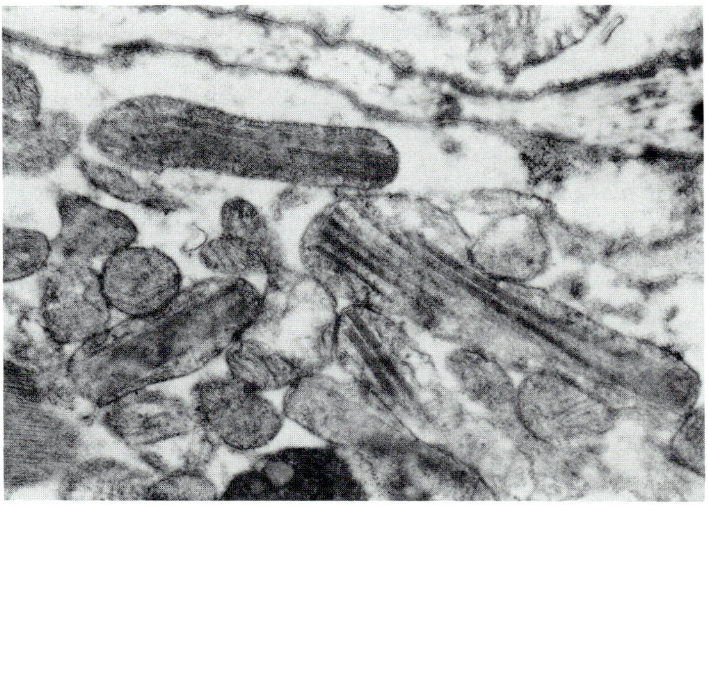

Fig. 3-8. Muscle biopsy of a patient with methysergide myalgia, showing enlarged mitochondria containing laminated crystalline inclusions within the cristae. Uranyl acetate and lead citrate stains, × 20,250.

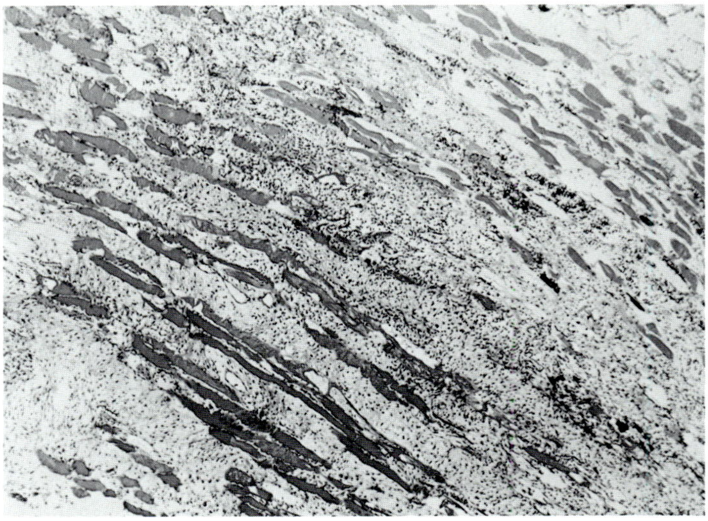

Fig. 3-9. Severe muscle necrosis caused by diphenylhydantoin. There is diffuse infiltration by macrophages and round cells within the areas of disintegrating sarcoplasm. The lesions were caused by 10 mg injections given daily to a rat for 10 days. H & E, × 40.

of cats; these consist of hemorrhage and necrosis, with crystallization of the diphenylhydantoin occurring in association with the necrosis.[107] Figure 3-9 shows severe muscle fibre necrosis produced by the experimental injection of diphenylhydantoin. Acute muscle necrosis has also been described after chronic overdosage of phenformin and fenfluramine.[88]

Toxins

Alcohol. Alcoholic myopathy, now a well-known human condition, is manifest as proximal limb-girdle weakness. Biopsy reveals polyfocal muscle fiber necrosis, and the serum CK is usually greatly elevated, thus distinguishing the condition from alcoholic peripheral neuropathy.[63, 90]

Studies of chronic alcoholic myopathy undertaken in human volunteers reveal dilated sarcoplasmic reticulum, osmiophilic particles, disordered mitochondria, and an increase in glycogen and fat.[110] Other reports include biochemical changes (a decrease in ATPase activity) and a reduced contractibility of actomyosin in vitro; isolated muscle membranes have shown a reduced calcium uptake.[100] Widespread muscle fiber necrosis is produced by the intramuscular injection of ethanol in rats (Fig. 3-10).

Oxygen and Glucose. In suicides by carbon monoxide, acute muscle fiber necrosis in the gastrocnemius and other muscles is commonly found; it is likely that this is due to pressure during the period of coma, rather than being a direct affect of the anoxia.[56] A myopathy has also been reported in status asthmaticus; again, this was probably due to the associated hydrocortisone treatment rather than to anoxia.[70] However, oxygen-produced cytotoxic effects on striated muscle are known.[21] Insulin, by causing hypoglycemia, has been associated with muscle fiber necrosis in both the heart and in skeletal muscle.[114]

Organic and Inorganic Poisons. Organophosphates, which are known to cause myeloneuropathies, are also described as giving rise to muscle fiber necrosis.[4] Besides this, organophosphate poisoning will cause extraocular muscle myopathy.[80] Organophosphate neuropathy has been used as a model to study the pathogenesis of central core, multicore, target, and cytoplasmic bodies.[118] Rhabdomyolysis and renal failure are described with acute mercuric chloride poisoning.[23]

Snakebite. The venom of many poisonous snakes will cause severe myonecrosis, myoglobinuria, and renal failure; of these, the sea snakes are the most notorious.[22, 56] One sea snake toxin is a phospholipase which causes

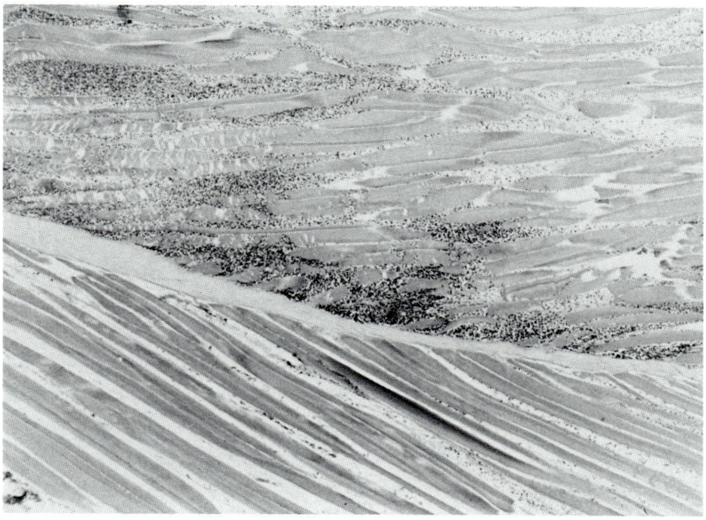

Fig. 3-10. In the upper field, muscle fiber necrosis due to ethanol is prominent. There is loss of architectural detail and beginning disintegration of muscle fibers, with vertical splitting and infiltration by inflammatory cells. The supporting tissues are also necrotic. Ethanol was injected into a rat, at 1 ml daily, for 10 days. H & E, × 40.

myoglobinuria in mice.[41] The Australian mulga snake produces an extremely powerful myotoxin,[99] and tiger snake toxin causes skeletal muscle degeneration when injected into the rat.[94]

Recently, it was found that the activity of a myotoxin consisting of a 39 amino-acid polypeptide, isolated from prairie rattlesnake venom, depended on the intactness of the two disulphide bridges that the polypeptide contained.[20]

Bacterial Toxins. Among the bacterial toxins, clostridial toxin causes severe skeletal muscle necrosis and also destroys connective tissue.[79] *Clostridium botulinum* toxin mainly causes denervation.[59] Diphtheria toxin produces fatty degeneration of cardiac muscle in guinea pigs; however, no consistent changes are found in skeletal muscle.[2]

Hornet Venom. The oriental hornet produces a toxin that causes both light- and electron microscopically visible muscle lesions, including a disturbance of the transverse tubular system of muscle.[57]

Metabolic Poisons. Powerful metabolic poisons, such as iodo- and fluroacetate, which block lactate production, cause massive rhabdomyolysis. Because of this, these agents are popularly used in experimental myopathology.[62] Imidazole, which accelerates phosphodiesterase activity,[74] causes myopathic changes in the gastrocnemius muscle of rats.[39] The foregoing chemicals are considered to be specific myotoxins because they cause pure sarcoplasmic necrosis, sparing the sarcolemmal and endomysial fibrous tissue sheaths. For this reason, when the toxin is withdrawn and if the animal survives, connective tissue proliferation is minimal in the recovery phase, and muscle regeneration is complete.

Triethyltinsulphate (TET) produces muscle cores under experimental conditions. The changes, which affect only the type I fibers, are observed in the soleus muscle of rats intoxicated with TET for up to 23 days following the intoxication.[48]

Recently, 2,4-dinitrophenol, an uncoupler of oxidative phosphorylation, was shown to produce ragged red fibers and mitrochondrial inclusions in the muscle of experimental animals.[102] These ultrastructural changes are similar to those in the human oculocraniosomatic syndrome (ragged red fiber myopathy), suggesting a common pathogenesis for the two conditions.

With regard to conditions that disturb endogenous metabolism—in addition to the well known uremic neuropathy[7]—rhabdomyolysis with myoglobinuria was found, during a 3-year period, in 15 patients who presented with renal failure. Myoglobinuria in these cases resulted from "myopathies, seizures, prolonged coma, strenuous exercise or viral illness"; it was invariably accompanied by a triad of orthotolidine-positive urine, pigmented granular casts in the urine sediment, and elevation of the serum CPK levels.[50] Uremic myopathy can also be produced experimentally in rats, in which case the main lesion seems to be type I muscle fiber atrophy.[19]

Miscellaneous

Nutritional Disorders. Nutritional deficiencies as a cause of muscle fiber necrosis, sometimes with cardiac involvement and myoglobinuria, are well known in the veterinary literature. The most common cause of the necrosis is vitamin E deficiency,[52] which might be aggravated by lack of dietary antioxidants; because of this, a similar effect is readily produced by the administration of rancid fats or oxidative agents (such as ferric chloride) in the diet. Experimental vitamin E deficiency in the Rottnest Island quokka is a particularly good model for the study of muscle fiber necrosis, and some of the principles of myopathology were originally derived from this animal.[61] Muscle fiber necrosis, regeneration, and cellular infiltrates similar to those found in the quokka occur in α-tocopherol-deficient guinea pigs[55]; in the guinea pigs—which revived after treatment with α-tocopherol—CPK levels decreased.

Of interest is the report of a reversible human myopathy due to vitamin E deficiency. In this case a 7-year-old boy with severe malabsorption presented with muscle weakness and an elevated CPK, and showed atrophy of type I and especially of type II muscle fibers. EM revealed occasional Z-band smearing. The child recovered upon treatment with vitamin E.[116]

Selenium in trace quantities is another factor known to be essential for the maintenance of muscle. In sheep, selenium deficiency is associated with an acute myopathy resembling that caused by vitamin E deficiency. In different animals, vitamin E and selenium may or may not act interchangeably in preventing muscle degeneration.[112] Yet other nutritionally induced myopathies include the thiamine, choline, and vitamin C deficiencies in guinea pigs (low protein and raw egg white myopathies).[11] Iodine deficiency is also known to cause muscle weakness[98]; vitamin D deficiency results in defective calcium uptake in the sarcoplasmic reticulum and, when combined with protein deficiency, will cause pseudomyopathic changes.[42] In protein malnutrition, the response of different muscle fiber types to changes in the activity pattern has been reported.[120] When given in excess, vitamin A, vitamin C and vitamin D may cause a myopathy.[2]

Electrolyte Disorders. Potassium deficiency causing muscle fiber necrosis was first known to veterinarians.[54] Hypokalemic myopathy is often associated with steroid myopathy and is one of the mechanisms involved in producing steroid myopathy. However, corticosteroids will cause a myopathy even when serum electrolyte levels are normal. Hypokalemia also occurs in association with treatment with other drugs. A flaccid paralysis and myoglobinuria due to hypokalemia caused by carbonoxolone has been reported,[78] and a hypokalemic myopathy occurs during treatment with diuretics. In the latter condition vacuoles and the destruction of sarcomeres are revealed by both light- and electron microscopy.[58] Hypokalemic myopathy with myoglobinuria is also associated with excessive licorice ingestion. In one such case, licorice in large quantities was ingested by an obese patient striving to reduce. This led to severe potassium depletion and an acute, rapidly progressive myopathy and myoglobinuria. The serum potassium level was 1.6 MEq/L. Muscle biopsy, with both light- and EM study, revealed myopathic changes, with the observation of spherical concentric lamellar bodies. The patient improved after potassium was administered.[49]

Calcium deficiency, which causes tetany,

has not been associated with morphological changes in muscle, although an osteomalacic myopathy is known to occur with both human vitamin D deficiency[31] and under experimental conditions.[113]

Other Toxic Myopathies. A muscle condition known as Haff disease (named from a district of East Prussia) occurred as an epidemic in 1924 and has occurred on several occasions since. The patients, who had all consumed a fish meal on the previous day, developed severe muscle pains and myoglobinuria. Death from renal failure resulted in some cases. Widespread myonecrosis was present histologically. However, the cause of Haff disease has never been found.[56] Another mystery is quail myopathy, which occurs on the Greek island of Lesvos. The condition is reversible, and is believed to be due to a variety of hemlock seeds eaten by the quails.[56] The condition is currently under further study (Papapetropoulos, personal communication).

Nonspecific Effects of Intramuscular Injections. Focal muscle fiber necrosis can be expected for mechanical reasons following intramuscular injections,[37] and can cause spurious elevations in serum CK levels. Because the concentration of an injected drug is very high at the site of injection, some damage can also be predicted on this basis, and the process may lead to fibrosis and even to contracture.[84] Beyond this, a wide range of injectable medical preparations, with greatly variable pH and osmotic ratios, will cause muscle damage.[87]

CONCLUSIONS

A very wide range of drugs and toxins may be associated with myopathic changes of various types. These changes are readily categorized according to their main manifestation, such as denervation atrophy as a result of peripheral neuropathy caused by the drug, endplate disorder when the drug or toxin affects the neuromuscular junction, or a "primary" myopathy, in which event there is polyfocal muscle fiber necrosis.

Generally, there are two distinct categories of effect in toxicology: (1) those cases where there is a predictable and dose-related toxic reaction that will occur in most of the exposed individuals; and (2) rare individuals in whom the toxic effect is unpredictable and the reaction occurs with very small doses. In the latter instances, a genetic predisposition is to be postulated. This possibility is suggested to explain the malignant hyperpyrexia syndrome which is known to occur in pedigrees as either a dominant or a recessive factor.[67] By far the majority of toxic and drug myopathies show a dose-related toxic effect, belonging to the first category, in which case the intoxication will reverse rapidly upon withdrawal of the drug.

For those conditions in which there is myonecrosis, the period of action of the noxious agent, and the topographic distribution of the lesions, determine the histopathologic appearance of the muscle at any particular time. The variability of the microscopic lesions in a drug or toxic myopathy is therefore usually due only to the strength of the agent and the time over which it acts. This, together with the anatomic extent of the injury, determines the architectural outcome.

Through recognition of the inherent biologic capacity of muscle to regenerate after injury, the histopathology of the drug-induced necrotizing lesions becomes readily understood by the system described below. If the term *focal* is used to represent the anatomic aspect of the lesion, and if the term *phasic* refers to the time factor and the prefixes *mono* and *poly* are added, then the full spectrum of possible histopathologic changes can be described precisely for the necrobiotic conditions. For instance, a monofocal and monophasic disorder results from an isolated mechanical injury to muscle. Such a lesion could be due, for instance, to a single insertion of a needle into a muscle. The second possibility is a polyfocal and monophasic histopathologic change. This occurs, for example, when a single sublethal dose of a powerful myotoxin is given. Such lesions are widespread, with polyfocal necrosis produced throughout the musculature; however, the changes are all in phase. If the experimental animal survives the insult, regeneration will also be in phase. The same result occurs in a possible drug myopathy in which rhabdomyolysis is acute, but the drug is withdrawn quickly, so that histologic events in the muscle are again in phase.

When a disorder is monofocal and polyphasic, the lesion is at one anatomic site but continues over a period of time. Such is the case with recurring mechanical injury, such as from repeated intramuscular injections. The last of the theoretical examples may be seen when the myopathologic changes are both polyfocal and polyphasic. Lesions of this type are found in the aggressive human dystrophies and in chronic polymyositis. They are much less common in the drug or toxic myopathies because the noxious effect is either rapidly lethal or the drug is withdrawn soon after the myopathy is recognized, permitting regeneration to proceed to complete restoration of the muscle well before more chronic architectural changes develop. However, polyfocal and polyphasic lesions can be induced experimentally.[62] Although the clinical disorder and morphology in many of the drug or toxic myopathies are similar, the pharmacobiochemical mechanisms must differ considerably; however, very little is known of this. The pursuit of the molecular toxicology of the drug myopathies is a challenging area for further research. Not only would such studies elucidate the exact mechanisms of action of the drug myopathies, but much useful information on the normal structure and function of muscle could be derived. In addition, clues helpful in the understanding of the natural human muscle diseases might be forthcoming.

For the clinician, the basic principles of toxicomyopathology as outlined above should be useful in the planning of treatment for the patient, while an understanding of the reaction of muscle in these states will greatly improve the consultant role of the pathologist when dealing with these problems.

ACKNOWLEDGMENTS

The experimental myopathies used in the illustrations were produced by Ian K. Passmore, B.Sc. The photographs were prepared by Philip J. Morling, B.Sc. (Hons); Trudy J. Parker, B.Sc., prepared the electron micrographs.

REFERENCES

1. Abourizk, N., Khalil, B. A., Bahuth, N., & Afifi, A. K.: Clofibrate-induced muscular syndrome. Report of a case with clinical, electromyographic and pathologic observations. J. Neurol. Sci. 42:1, 1979.
2. Adams, R. D.: Diseases of Muscle. A Study in Pathology. 3rd Ed. Harper & Row, New York, 1975.
3. Aguayo, A. J., & Hudgson, P.: Observations on the short-term effects of chloroquine on skeletal muscle. An experimental study in the rabbit. J. Neurol. Sci. 11:301, 1970.
4. Ahlgren. J. D., Manz, H. J., & Harvey, J. C.: Myopathy of chronic organophosphate poisoning: A clinical entity? South Med. J. 72:555, 1979.
5. Argov, Z., & Mastaglia, F. L.: Medical intelligence—Drug therapy. Disorders of neuromuscular transmission caused by drugs. N. Engl. J. Med. 301:409, 1979.
6. Argov, Z., & Mastaglia, F. L.: Side effects of drugs. Drug-induced peripheral neuropathies. Br. Med. J. 1:663, 1979.
7. Asbury, A. K., & Johnson, P. C.: Pathology of peripheral nerve. In: Bennington, J. L., Ed. Major Problems in Pathology. Vol. 9. p. 2. W. B. Saunders Co., Philadelphia, 1978.
8. Aström, K.-E., Kugelberg, E., & Muller, R.: Hypothyroid myopathy. Arch, Neurol. 5:472, 1961.
9. Atsumi, T., Isikawa, S-e, Miyatake, T., & Yoshida, M.: Myopathy and primary aldosteronism: electronmicroscopic study. Neurology 29:1348, 1979.
10. Bajusz, E.: Experimental myopathies: influence of various factors as reflected by histochemical and morphological studies. In: Beckmann, R., Ed. Myopathien. p. 121. Georg Thieme, Stuttgart, 1965.

11. Banker, B. Q.: The experimental myopathies. Res. Publ. Assoc. Nerv. Ment. Dis. 38:197, 1960.
12. Benoit, P. W., & Belt, W. D.: Destruction and regeneration of skeletal muscle after treatment with a local anaesthetic, bupivacaine (Marcaine). J. Anat. 1:547, 1970.
13. Bindoff, L., & Cullen, J. J.: Experimental emetine myopathy. Ultrastructural and morphometric observations. J. Neurol. Sci. 39:1, 1978.
14. Bowden, D. H., & Goyer, F. A.: Drug-induced muscle necrosis with massive taurinuria. Arch. Pathol. 74:137, 1962.
15. Bradley, W. G.: Disorders of Peripheral Nerves. Blackwell Scientific Publications, Oxford, 1974.
16. Bradley, W. G., Fewings, J. D., Harris, J. B., & Johnson, M. A.: Emetine myopathy in the rat. Br. J. Pharmacol. 57:29, 1976.
17. Bradley, W. G., Lassman, L. P., Pearce, G. W., & Walton, J. N.: The neuromyopathy of vincristine in man. Clinical, electrophysiological and pathological studies. J. Neurol. Sci. 10:107, 1970.
18. Buller, A. J., Eccles, J. C., & Eccles, R. M.: Interaction between motoneurones and muscles in respect of the characteristic speeds of their response. J. Physiol. (Lond.) 150:417, 1960.
19. Bundschu, H. D., Pfeilsticker, H., Suchenwirth, R., Matthews, C., & Ritz, E.: Experimental uremic myopathy. Abstract 330 In: Abstracts of papers presented 3rd International Congress on Muscle Diseases, Newcastle-upon-Tyne. (International Congress Series No. 334). Excerpta Medica, Amsterdam, 1974.
20. Cameron, D. L., & Tu, A. T.: Characterization of myotoxin venom of prairie rattlesnake (*Crotalus viridis* viridis). Biochemistry 16:2546, 1977.
21. Caulfield, J. B., Shelton, W., & Burke, J. F.: Cytotoxic effects of oxygen on striated muscle. Arch. Pathol. 94:127, 1972.
22. Chen-Yuan, L. Ed.: Handbook of Experimental Pharmacology. Vol. 52. Springer, Berlin, 1979.
23. Chugh, K. S., Singhal, P. C., & Uberoi, H. S.: Rhabdomyolysis and renal failure in acute mercuric chloride poisoning. Med. J. Aust 2:125, 1978.
24. Cogen, F. C., Rigg, G., Simmons, J. L., & Domino, E. F.: Phencyclidine-associated acute rhabdomyolysis. Ann. Intern. Med. 88:210, 1978.
25. Coomes, E. N.: Corticosteroid myopathy. Ann Rheum. Dis. 24:465, 1965.
26. D'Agostino, A. N.: An electron microscopic study of skeletal and cardiac muscle of the rat by plasmocid. Lab. Invest. 12:1060, 1963.
27. D'Agostino, A. N., & Chiga, M.: Cortisone myopathy in rabbits. A light and electron microscopic study Neurology (Minneap.) 16:257, 1966.
28. Daniel, P. M., Pratt, O. E., & Spargo, E.: The metabolic homoeostatic role of muscle and its function as a store of protein. Lancet 2(8035):446, 1977.
29. Danon, J. M., Karpati, G., & Carpenter, S.: Subacute skeletal myopathy induced by 2,4-dichlorophenoxyacetate in rats and guinea pigs. Muscle Nerve 1:89, 1978.
30. Dastur, D. K., Gagrat, B. M., & Manghani, D. K.: Fine structure of muscle in human disuse atrophy: Significance of proximal muscle involvement in muscle disorders. Neuropathol. Appl. Neurobiol. 5:85, 1979.
31. Dastur, D. K., Gagrat, B. M., & Wadia, N. H., et al.: Nature of muscular change in osteomalacia: Light and electron microscope observations. J. Pathol. 117:211, 1975.
32. De Coster, W. J.: Experimental hypokalemia: Ultrastructural changes in rat gastrocnemius muscle. Acta Neuropathol. (Berl.) 45:79, 1979.
33. de Lateur, B. J., & Halliday, W. R.: Pentazocine fibrous myopathy: Report of two cases and literature review. Arch. Phys. Med. Rehabil. 59:394, 1978.
34. Dobosz, I., Mrozek, K., & Kwiecinski, H.: Biochemical studies of sarcoplasmic reticulum and muscle plasma membranes on myotonic rats. Abstract 354. In: Abstracts of papers presented 3rd International Congress on Muscle Diseases, Newcastle-upon-Tyne. International Congress Series No. 334. Excerpta Medica. Amsterdam, 1974.
35. Drutz, D. J., Fan, J. H., & Tai, T. Y., et al.: Hypokalemic rhabdomyolysis and myoglobinuria following amphotericin B therapy. J.A.M.A. 211:824, 1970.
36. Ellis, J. T.: Necrosis and regeneration of skele-

tal muscle in cortisone-treated rabbits. Am. J. Pathol. 32:993, 1956.
37. Engel, W. K.: Focal myopathic changes produced by electro-myographic and hypodermic needles. "Needle myopathy." Arch. Neurol. 16:509, 1967.
38. Felmus, M. T., Patten, B. M., Hart, A., & Martinez, C.: Catecholamine-induced muscle weakness. Arch. Neurol. 34:280, 1977.
39. Fenichel, G. M., & Martin, J. T.: An experimental myopathy in rats produced with imidazole. Abstract 331. In: Abstracts of papers presented 3rd International Congress on Muscle Diseases, Newcastle-upon-Tyne. International Congress Series No. 334. Excerpta Medica, Amsterdam, 1974.
40. Fewings, J. D., Burns, R. J., & Kakulas, B. A.: A case of acute emetine myopathy. In: Kakulas, B. A., Ed. Clinical Studies in Myology. p. 594. Proceedings of the 2nd International Congress on Muscle Diseases, 1971. Part 2, Excerpta Medica, Amsterdam, 1973.
41. Fohlman, J., & Eaker, D.: Isolation and characterization of a lethal myotoxic phospholipase A from the venom of the common sea snake *Enhydrina schistosa* causing myoglobinuria in mice. Toxicon 15:385, 1977.
42. Francis, M. J. O., Curry, O. B., & Smith, R.: Vitamin D and muscle: A defect of calcium uptake by sarcoplasmic reticulum in vitamin D deficient rabbits. Abstract 324. In: Abstracts of papers presented 3rd International Congress on Muscle Diseases, Newcastle-upon-Tyne. International Congress Series No. 334. Excerpta Medica, Amsterdam, 1974.
43. Fuller, R. W., Lacefield, W. B., & Kattau, R. W., et al.: Myotonia produced by indoleacetic acid. Studies with related compounds and correlation with drug levels in tissues. Arch. Int. Pharmacodyn. Ther. 193:48, 1971.
44. Furman, R. E., & Barchi, R. L.: The pathophysiology of myotonia produced by aromatic carboxylic acids. Ann. Neurol. 4:357, 1978.
45. Gardiner, P. F., & Edgerton, V. R.: Contractile responses of rat fast-twitch and slow-twitch muscles to glucocorticoid treatment. Muscle Nerve 2:274, 1979.
46. Giusti, G. V., Chiarotti, M., & Passatore, M., et al.: Muscular dystrophy in mice after chronic subcutaneous treatment with cannabinoids. Forensic Sci. 10:133, 1977.
47. Golding, D. N., Murray, M., Pearce, G. W., & Thompson, M.: Corticosteroid myopathy. Ann. Phys. Med. 6:171, 1961.
48. Graham, D. I., Bonilla, E., Gonatas, N. K., & Schotland, D. L.: Core formation in the muscles of rats intoxicated with triethyltin sulfate J. Neuropathol. Exp. Neurol. 35:1, 1976.
49. Gross, E. G., Dexter, J. D., & Roth, R. G.: Hypokalemic myopathy with myoglobinuria associated with licorice ingestion. N. Engl. J. Med. 274:602, 1966.
50. Grossman, R. A., Hamilton, W., & Morse, B. M., et al.: Nontraumatic rhabdomyolysis and acute renal failure. N. Engl. J. Med. 291:807, 1974.
51. Gutierrez, J.: Effect of the antimalarial chloroquine on the phospholipid metabolism of avian malaria and heart tissue. Am. J. Trop. Med. Hyg. 15:818, 1966.
52. Hadlow, J. J.: Diseases of skeletal muscle. In: Innes, J. R. M. and Saunders, L. Z., Ed. Comparative Neuropathology. p.147. Academic Press, New York, 1962.
53. Heene, R.: Experimental myopathies and muscular dystrophy. In: Bauer, H., Ed. Studies in the Formal Pathogenesis of the Myopathy of 2,4-Dichlorophenoxyacetate. Neurology Series, Band 16. Springer, Berlin, 1975.
54. Hove, E. L., & Herndon, J. F.: Potassium deficiency in the rabbit as a cause of muscular dystrophy. J. Nutr. 55:363, 1955.
55. Howell, J. McC., & Buxton, P. H.: α-tocopherol responsive muscular dystrophy in guinea pigs. Neuropathol. Appl. Neurobiol. 1:49, 1975.
56. Hughes, J. T.: Pathology of Muscle. In: Bennington, J. L., Ed. Major Problems in Pathology. Vol. 4. p.151. W. B. Saunders Company, Philadelphia, 1974.
57. Ishay, J., Lass, Y., & Sandbank, U.: A lesion of muscle transverse tubular system by oriental hornet (*Vespa orientalis*) venom: Electron microscopic and histological study. Toxicon 13:57, 1975.
58. Jensen, O. B., Mosdal, C., & Reske-Nielsen, E.: Hypokalemic myopathy during treatment with diuretics. Acta Neurol. Scand. 55:465, 1977.
59. Johnston, D. M., & Drachman, D. B.: Neurotropic regulation of dynamic properties of skeletal muscle: Effects of botulinum toxic and denervation. Abstract 21. In: Abstracts of papers presented 3rd International Congress on

Muscle Diseases, Newcastle-upon-Tyne. International Congress Series No.334. Excerpta Medica, Amsterdam, 1974.

60. Kakulas, B. A.: Muscle biopsy. Royal College of Pathologists of Australia Broadsheet, No.19, 1975.
61. Kakulas, B. A.: Experimental muscle diseases. Methods Achiev. Exp. Pathol. 7:109, 1975.
62. Kakulas, B. A.: Experimental myopathies. In: Walton, J. N., Ed. Disorders of Voluntary Muscle. 4th Ed. Churchill Livingstone, Edinburgh, 1980.
63. Klinkerfuss, G., Bleisch, V., Dioso, M. M., & Perkoff, G. T.: A spectrum of myopathy associated with alcoholism. II. Light and electron microscopic observations. Ann. Intern. Med. 67:393, 1967.
64. Korsan-Bengtsen, K., Ysander, L., Blohme, G., & Tibblin, E.: Extensive muscle necrosis after long-term treatment with amino-caproic acid (EACA) in a case of hereditary periodic edema. Acta Med. Scand. 185:341, 1969.
65. Kugelberg, E., Edstrom, L., & Abbruzzese, M.: Mapping of motor units in experimentally reinnervated rat muscle. Interpretation of histochemical and atrophic fibre pattern in neurogenic lesions. J. Neurol. Neurosurg. Psychiatry 33:319, 1970.
66. Kwiecinski, H.: Myotonia induced with clofibrate in rats. J. Neurol. 219:107, 1978.
67. Lane, R. J. M., & Mastaglia, F. L.: Drug-induced myopathies in man. Lancet 2(8089):562, 1978.
68. Lane, R. J. M., McLelland, N. J., Martin, A. M., & Mastaglia, F. L.: Epsilon aminocaproic acid (EACA) myopathy. Postgrad. Med. J. 55:282, 1979.
69. MacDonald, R. D., & Engel, A. G.: Experimental chloroquine myopathy. J. Neuropathol. Exp. Neurol. 29:479, 1970.
70. MacFarlane, I. A., & Rosenthal, F. D.: Severe myopathy after status asthmaticus. Lancet 2(8038):615, 1977.
71. Mackie, B. S., & Mackie, L. E.: Systemic lupus erythematosus-dermatomyositis induced by sulphacetamide eye drops. Australas. J. Derm. 20:49, 1979.
72. MacLean, K., & Schurr, P. H.: Reversible amyotrophy complicating treatment with fludrocortisone. Lancet 1(7075):701, 1959.
73. Markand, O. N., & D'Agostino, A. N.: Ultrastructural changes in skeletal muscle induced by colchicine. Arch. Neurol. 24:72, 1971.
74. Martin, J. T., Laskowski, M. D., & Fenichel, G. M.: Imidazole myopathy: Production of the myopathy and its dependence on acetycholine. Neurology (Minneap.) 27:484, 1977.
75. Mascres, C., & Jasmine, G.: Changes in the muscle fibre induced by p-phenalinedranine in the rat. Pathol. Biol. (Paris) 23:193, 1975.
76. Mastaglia, F. L., Gardner-Medwin, D., & Hudgson, P.: Muscle fibrosis and contractures in a pethidine addict Br. Med. J. 4:532, 1971.
77. McComas, A. J.: Neuromuscular Function and Disorders. Butterworths, London, 1977.
78. Mohamed, S. D., Chapman, R. S., & Crooks, J.: Hypokalemia, flaccid quadraparesis, and myoglobinuria with carbenoxolone (Biogastrone). Br. Med. J. 25:1581, 1966.
79. Morita, H.: An experimental study on the pathology of the black-leg. J. Jpn. Soc. Vet. Sci. 5:1, 1926.
80. Mukuno, K., & Imai, H.: Study on extraocular muscles of chronic organophosphate intoxication in beagle dogs. Acta Soc. Ophthalmol. Jap. 77:1246, 1973.
81. Muller, R., & Kugelberg, E.: Myopathy in Cushing's syndrome. J. Neurol. Neurosurg. Psychiatry 22:314, 1959.
82. Munsat, T. L., Hudgson, P., Johnson, M. A.: Experimental serotonin myopathy. Neurology (Minneap.) 27:772, 1977.
83. Neville, H. E., Maunder-Sewry, C. A., & McDougall, J., et al.: Chloroquine-induced cytosomes with curvilinear profiles in muscle. Muscle Nerve, 2:376, 1979.
84. Norman, M. G., Temple, A. R., & Murphy, J. V.: Infantile quadriceps-femoris contracture resulting from intramuscular injections. N. Engl. J. Med. 282:964, 1970.
85. O'Grady, F., & Smith, B.: Neuromyopathy in the mouse produced by the antimicrobial agent nitroxoline. J. Pathol. Bacteriol. 92:43, 1966.
86. Osame, M., Kawabuchi, M., Igata, A., & Sugita, H.: Experimental nemaline rods induced by anticholinesterase drug (neostigmine methylsulfate). Proc. Jpn. Acad. 51:598, 1975.
87. Oshida, S., Degawa, K., Takabashi, Y., & Akaishi, S.: Physico-chemical properties and local toxic effects of injectables. Tohoku J. Exp. Med. 127:301, 1979.
88. Palmucci, L., Bertolotto, A., & Schiffer, D.: Acute muscle necrosis after chronic overdosage of phenformin and fenfluramine. Muscle Nerve 1:245, 1978.

89. Patten, B. A., & Oliver, K. L.: Serotonin induced muscle weakness. Abstract 335. In: Abstracts of papers presented 3rd International Congress on Muscle Diseases, Newcastle-upon-Tyne. International Congress Series No.334. Excerpta Medica, Amsterdam, 1974.
90. Perkoff, G. T., Dioso, M. M., Bleisch, V., & Klinkerfuss, G. L.: A spectrum of myopathy associated with alcoholism. I. Clinical and laboratory features. Ann. Intern. Med. 67:481, 1967.
91. Perkoff, G. T., Silber, R., & Tyler, F. H., et al.: Studies in disorders of muscle. XII. Myopathy due to the administration of therapeutic amounts of 17-hydroxycorticosteroids. Am. J. Med. 1:891, 1959.
92. Peter, J. B.: Skeletal muscle: diversity and mutability of its histochemical electron microscopic, biochemical and physiologic properties. In: Pearson, C. M., & Mostofi, F. K., Eds. The Striated Muscle. Williams and Wilkins, Baltimore, 1973.
93. Petersen, J., Halberg, P., & Hojgaard, K., et al.: Penicillamine-induced polymyositis-dermatomyositis. Scand. J. Rheumatol. 7:113, 1978.
94. Pluskal, M. G., Pennington, R. J., Johnson, M. A., & Harris, J. B.: Some effects of tiger snake toxin upon skeletal muscle. Abstract 327. In: Abstracts of papers presented 3rd International Congress on Muscle Diseases, Newcastle-upon-Tyne. International Congress Series No. 334. Excerpta Medica, Amsterdam, 1974.
95. Price, H. M., Pease, D. C., & Pearson, C. M.: Selective actin filament and Z-band degeneration induced by plasmocid. An electron microscopic study. Lab. Invest. 11:549, 1962.
96. Rewcastle, N. B., & Humphren, J. G.: Vacuolar myopathy, clinical histo-chemical and microscopic study. Arch. Neurol. 12:570, 1965.
97. Richter, R. W., Challenor, Y. B., & Pearson, J., et al.: Acute myoglobinuria associated with heroin addiction. J.A.M.A. 216:1172, 1971.
98. Rosman, N. P., Schapiro, M. B., & Haddow, J.: Muscle weakness caused by an iodine-deficient diet: investigation of a nutritional myopathy. J. Neuropathol. Exp. Neurol. 37:192, 1978.
99. Rowlands, J. B., Mastaglia, F. L., Kakulas, B. A., & Hainsworth, D.: Clinical and pathological aspects of a fatal case of mulga (pseudechis australis) snakebite. Med. J. Aust. 1:226, 1969.
100. Rubin, E., Katz, A. M., & Lieber, C. S., et al.: Muscle damage produced by chronic alcohol consumption. Am. J. Pathol. 83:499, 1976.
101. Rudel, R., & Keller, M.: Intracellular recording of myotonic runs in dantrolene-blocked myotonic muscle fibres. In: Bradley, W. G., Gardner-Medwin, D., & Walton, J. N., Eds. Recent Advances in Myology. p. 441. Excerpta Medica, Amsterdam, 1975.
102. Sahgal, V., Subramani, V., & Hughes, R., et al.: On the pathogenesis of mitochondrial myopathies. An experimental study. Acta Neuropathol. (Berl.) 46:177, 1979.
103. Sambrook, M. A., Heron, J. R., & Aber, G. M.: Myopathy in association with primary hyperaldosteronism. J. Neurol. Neurosurg. Psychiatry 35:202, 1972.
104. Schmalbruch, H.: Early changes in chlorphentermine myopathy of rat studied by freeze fracturing. Muscle Nerve 1:421, 1978.
105. Selye, H.: Eine durch Serotonin erzeugte Muskeldystrophie. Naturwissenschaften 52: 519, 1965.
106. Selye, H., & Bajusz, E.: The prevention of experimental myopathies by various chlorides. J. Nutr. 72:37, 1960.
107. Serrano, E. E., & Wilder, B. J.: Intramuscular administration of diphenylhydantoin: Histologic follow-up studies. Arch. Neurol. 31:276, 1974.
108. Skjoto, J., & Reikvam, A.: Hyperthermia and rhabdomyolysis in self-poisoning with paracetamol and salicylates. Report of a case. Acta Med. Scand. 205:473, 1979.
109. Slotwiner, P., Song, S. K., & Anderson, P. J.: Sheromembranous degeneration of muscle induced by vincristine. Arch. Neurol. 15:172, 1966.
110. Song, S. K., & Rubin, E.: Ethanol produced muscle damage in human volunteers. Science 175:327, 1972.
111. Smith, B., & O'Grady, F.: Experimental chloroquine myopathy. J. Neurol. Neurosurg. Psychiatry 29:255, 1966.
112. Swash, K., Schwartz, K., & Foltz, C.: Selenium as an integral part of factors against dietary necrotic liver degeneration. J. Am. Chem. Soc. 79:3292, 1957.
113. Swash, M., Schwartz, M. S., & Sargeant, M. K.: Osteomalacic myopathy: An experi-

mental approach. Neuropathol. Appl. Neurobiol. 5:295, 1979.

114. Tannenberg, J.: Pathological changes in the heart, skeletal musculature and liver in rabbits treated with insulin in shock dosage. Am. J. Pathol. 15:25, 1939.

115. Teravainen, H., Larsen, A., & Hillbom, M.: Clofibrate-induced myopathy in the rat. Acta Neuropathol. (Berl.) 39:135, 1977.

116. Tomasi, L. G.: Reversibility of human myopathy caused by vitamin E deficiency. Neurology 29:1182, 1979.

117. Tomlinson, I. W., & Rosenthal, F. D.: Side effects of drugs. Proximal myopathy after perhexiline maleate treatment. Br. Med. J. 2:1319, 1977.

118. Tsubaki, T., Fukuhara, N., Hoshi, M., & Mori, S.: The pathogenesis of central core multicore, target and cytoplasmic bodies. In: Current Research In Muscular Dystrophy, Japan: Proceedings of the Annual Meeting of the Muscular Dystrophy Research Group, Tokyo, 1977.

119. Vartanian, G. A., & Chinyanga, H. M.: The mechanism of acute neuromuscular weakness induced by chloroquine. Can. J. Physiol. Pharmacol. 50:1099, 1972.

120. Ward, P., & Goldspink, G.: Response of difference fibre types to changes in activity pattern and to protein malnutrition. Abstract 16. In: Abstracts of papers presented 3rd International Congress on Muscle Diseases, Newcastle-upon-Tyne. International Congress Series No. 334. Excerpta Medica, Amsterdam, 1974.

121. Williams, R. S.: Triamcinolone myopathy. Lancet, 1(7075):698, 1959.

122. Winer, N., Klachko, D. M., & Baer, R. D., et al.: Myotonic response induced by inhibitors of cholesterol biosynthesis. Science 153:312, 1966.

123. Yamamura, S.: An experimental study on the mechanism of fibrous myopathy produced by intramuscular injections of chloramphenicol. Clin. Neurol. (Tokyo) 17:344, 1977.

124. Young, A., Wiles, C. M., & Edwards, R. H. T.: University college hospital muscle-biopsy needle. Lancet 2(8103):1285, 1978.

4

Bone and Joints

Robert E. Fechner

The pathologist regularly sees bone or joint tissue showing the effects of drug-related abnormalities or previous surgery. The most frequent bone alterations resulting from drug therapy are osteoporosis and osteomalacia; these are followed by aseptic necrosis, radiation damage, and changes secondary to the use of prosthetic devices. In most instances, there is no diagnostic problem; indeed, the pathologist may not even be notified that the material is, for example, from a patient with a drug-related bone disease, such as in a femoral head removed for aseptic necrosis produced by corticosteroid therapy.

OSTEOPOROSIS

Osteoporosis is a decrease in the mass of normally mineralized bone. Corticosteroids, of either natural or synthetic derivation, are by far the most common cause of drug-induced osteoporosis. The process in this disease is radiologically similar to that in the osteoporosis occuring in Cushing's disease.[80] The loss of bone is clinically manifest by pain and fractures. In such cases, steroid therapy has usually been given for 6 months or more, although in a few instances fractures have been reported within 5 to 8 weeks after the beginning of therapy.[10] Trabecular bone is more rapidly depleted than cortical bone, rendering corticosteroid-induced osteoporosis different from spontaneous osteoporosis, at least as measured in the radius by Hahn et al.[48] The most common sites of fractures in corticosteroid-induced osteoporosis are the lower thoracic and lumbar spine, the ribs, the distal radius, and the intertrochanteric region of the femur. Fractures of the wrist, ribs, and vertebra are seen earlier in the course of therapy than fractures of the femoral neck, owing to a relative predominance of trabecular bone in the former sites compared to the dense cortical bone of the femur. The effect of corticosteroids is most prominent in women beyond age 50,[99] but has also been seen in children.[28] In the latter, the high turnover rate of bone is apparently a predisposing factor, while in the former group the low initial bone mass seems to be more easily reduced to clinically detectable osteoporosis.

During corticosteroid therapy, bone formation is profoundly depressed; resorption is also depressed, but to a lesser degree; the net result is a loss of bone. The depression of bone growth activity appears to occur through a decrease in the total number of the foci at which bone formation or resorption take place. This indicates that the steroids decrease the ability of bone progenitor cells to divide and differentiate into osteoblasts or osteoclasts.[117] There may be some variation in the histologic pattern in steroid-induced osteoporosis, perhaps relating to the duration of therapy; Jowsey found an increased number of resorption sites and osteoclasts in osteoporotic bones.[59]

Methotrexate appears to cause osteoporosis when it is used to maintain remission in acute childhood leukemia.[90] Furthermore, although osteoporosis can be seen in leukemic patients prior to therapy, it seems to be accentuated during steroid therapy.[55] In most instances, radiographically detectable osteoporosis, accompanied by pain, occurs after 6 months of methotrexate therapy, although it is sometimes seen within 2 months; fractures are a complication.[90] Both clinical and radiographic improvement are seen after cessation of methotrexate.

The diminished osteoblastic response in patients taking corticosteroids delays the healing of pathologic fractures. Radiographically, there is a "cotton wool" appearance around the fractures, due to amorphous calcification. This has been referred to as a pseudocallus because it represents only an abortive attempt at healing.

In 1965, Griffith et al. described the first cases of heparin-induced osteoporosis.[45] Doses of up to 100 mg of heparin daily seem to cause no skeletal complications, regardless of the duration of therapy[105]; doses of more than 200 mg daily result in severe osteoporosis, including vertebral fractures, with men being as susceptible as women. The lesions usually become symptomatic only after several years of therapy, but in one case the symptoms had their onset 4 months after therapy began.[79] Most cases of heparin-induced osteoporosis have been in adults, but one patient was a teenager.[97] All of the fractures have been in the vertebral column or ribs; fractures in the long bones have never been reported.[58]

It is likely that partial gastrectomy may predispose to osteoporosis just as it does to osteomalacia. Aaron et al. had three patients (two of them males) with femoral neck fracture who had undergone partial gastrectomy.[1]

OSTEOMALACIA

Osteomalacia is characterized histologically by the accumulation of nonmineralized or poorly mineralized osteoid over the surface of cortical and medullary bone. The trabeculae of the bone may be of fairly uniform size, and the osteoid seams may be more or less uniform in width. In other fields, however, the trabeculae are more irregular in distribution and configuration, and there is greater variation in the widths of the osteoid layer. These same variable appearances are seen in both drug-induced osteomalacia and in osteomalacia unassociated with drug therapy.

There are several points at which drugs can act on vitamin D metabolism to produce osteomalacia. Vitamin D_2 (ergocalciferol). and vitamin D_3 (cholecalciferol) are present in the normal diet, and the latter is also synthesized in the skin by the action of ultraviolet light on 7-dehydrocholesterol. Both vitamin D_2 and D_3 are transported first to the liver and then to the kidney. Hydroxylation at the 25 position of these molecules takes place in the liver; a second hydroxylation, which occurs in the kidney, involves either the 1 or 24 position.

The first point at which drugs can interrupt the metabolism of vitamin D is in the intestine, where they prevent the absorption of its precursors. One such agent, cholestyramine, binds bile acids, hindering the absorption of fat soluble vitamins (including vitamin D) when given over a long period.[52] Another group of drugs that apparently impair the absorption of vitamin D and calcium are commercially available laxatives. These agents can include ricinoleic acid, senna, or phenolpthalein.[35] In one patient with purgative-induced osteomalacia, a peculiar deforming arthropathy occurred in addition to the osteomalacia.[36] The malabsorption of vitamin D as well as of calcium also occurs in approximately 25 percent of patients who have had partial gastrectomy.[29] Some authors have reported that vitamin D absorption is impaired in these patients[106]; others believe that the absorption of vitamin D is normal, but that the dietary intake of the vitamin is poor.[38] A similar phenomenon occurs in patients who have had intestinal bypass operations for obesity.[85]

Another point at which drugs may act is the liver, where 25-hydroxylation on the vitamin D precursors takes place. Minor and major tranquilizers, as well as anticonvulsants, can induce hepatic microsomal oxidase enzyme activity, and this induction leads to the increased catabolism of 25-hydroxyvitamin D to biologically inactive products that are rapidly excreted in the bile or urine. Diphenylhydantoin and phenobarbital have been most often implicated in this enzyme induction, probably because of their wisespread use[47]; a variety of other drugs, such as primidone, phensuximide, and mephobarbital, probably also contributes to the problem.[70] In addition to their effect on the liver, anticonvulsant drugs may also have a direct inhibitory effect on the membrane calcium transport mechanism; this could act directly at the level of the target organs.[46] Anticonvulsant associated osteomalacia can mask hyperparathyroidism.[13] Osteoclastic activity may be a part of the histologic pattern of anticonvulsant-induced osteomalacia.[16]

Another way that anticonvulsants contribute to osteomalacia in epileptics is suggested by the studies of Stamp et al. and Jubiz et al.[61, 107] The data of these authors raise the possibility that anticonvulsants may impair the action of 1,25-dihydroxyvitamin D on bone. It might be mentioned at this point that one anticonvulsant, acetazolamide, has produced ostomalacia by a different mechanism; this particular agent apparently acts to increase the urinary excretion of calcium that eventually results in osteomalacia.[72]

One patient taking glutethimide for 10 years developed osteomalacia. This drug structurally resembles phenobarbitone, and probably interferes with hepatic vitamin D metabolism in a manner similar to that of the anticonvulsants.[43]

Several patients have developed osteomalacia secondary to hypophosphatemia, owing to the ingestion of phosphate-binding antacids.[23] Hypophosphatemia with osteomalacia is also found in renal dialysis patients, whether or not they are taking antacids. In one study of dialysis patients, the thickness and arrangement of trabeculae were normal on bone biopsy, except for the unmineralized osteoid seams; in other patients the trabeculae were thicker and had a more irregular configuration. Both groups of patients showed osteoclastic resorption of varying degrees.[3] Renal dialysis patients are subject to hypophosphatemia due to malabsorption, loss of phosphate during dialysis, and low dietary intake.

Okita and Block noted the formation of osteomalacic bone during therapy for acute granulocytic leukemia.[84] The osteoid deposition was maximal at the time at which the leukemic infiltrate of the marrow was depleted.

HYPEROSTOSIS AND OSTEOSCLEROSIS

Hyperostosis—a thickening of cortical bone—occurs with the chronic ingestion of excessive quantities of vitamin A. Children are the usual victims, either because of misunderstandings of vitamin dosage or adherence to the concept that "more is better." Radiographically, there is periosteal bone growth, especially in the tubular bones and metatarsals. In infants, there may be changes in the skull that closely mimic the cortical hyperostosis of Caffey. The epiphyseal plates may close prematurely.[88] Extraosseous calcifications in the articular capsules, tendons, and ligaments are also found. One adult, taking massive doses of vitamin A for 8 years, developed osseous and soft-tissue lesions similar to those described in children[37]; biopsies of bone showed appositional new bone formation in the subperiosteal region.

Hypervitaminosis D is also mainly a disease of children. Radiographically, there are narrow, band-like zones of radio-opacity at the epiphyseal ends of the long tubular bones, reflecting the heavy calcification of matrix of the actively proliferating cartilage. Further along the bone shafts, the bone is radiolucent and osteoporotic. The original cortex becomes thin, while at the same time there is periosteal new bone formation. In adults, massive doses of vitamin D produce osteoporosis; in such cases, there are, in addition to bone changes, smoothly lobulated masses of calcium deposition in the soft tissues of joint capsules, bursae, and tendons.[21] Histologically, such areas show a foreign-body giant cell reaction surrounding calcified debris.[19]

Osteosclerosis, an increase primarily in the medullary bone mass, is most frequently seen in patients receiving excessive fluoride, either in the diet or therapeutically. Fluoride stimulates osteoblastic activity, and sometimes leads to a radiographically increased density of bone when used therapeutically in patients with generalized osteoporosis; in other patients, the bone is not increased in its strength, and fractures may occur.[56] The bone from patients receiving fluoride therapy has wide, unmineralized osteoid seams, which are seen even when there is an increase in the radiodensity of the bone. This microscopic appearance sometimes persists despite the addition of calcium to the diet.[44] If large doses of vitamin D are given in addition to calcium, there appears to be a better chance for proper calcium deposition and avoidance of the histologic findings of osteomalacia.[60] Regimens of fluoride and calcium, given either with or without vitamin D, also cause the reossification of lytic lesions in multiple myeloma.[68]

Generalized osteosclerosis has been reported in patients with the milk-alkali syndrome. Presumably, this reflects a chronic uptake of large quantities of absorbable alkaline salts.[91]

ASEPTIC NECROSIS

Corticosteroids have been implicated in the pathogenesis of aseptic necrosis. The development of aspectic necrosis in patients with diseases that are not ordinarily associated with this condition gives considerable weight to the argument that the steroid therapy is causative. Patients with diseases such as pemphigus, multiple sclerosis, and thrombotic thrombocytopenic purpura have developed aseptic necrosis while on steroid therapy.[9] Further support for a steroid effect in aseptic necrosis is suggested by the occurrence of such necrosis in steroid-treated children and young adults, in whom it is otherwise rarely encountered.[108] The necrosis generally occurs from 4 to 18 months after the advent of therapy.[109]

Aseptic necrosis is often seen in bones that are rarely the site of this condition from other causes. In one patient, necrosis of the navicular bone occurred bilaterally; in another patient, the capitate bone was affected.[2] Stern et al. noted that the femoral condyle was the most common site of necrosis in steroid-treated children with renal transplants. These authors also saw the radiographic changes characteristic of osteochondritis dissecans, which can be considered a radiographically distinctive form of aseptic necrosis.[108]

In corticosteroid-induced aseptic necrosis, multiple bone involvement is the rule. Klippel et al. found that 90 percent of their patients with aseptic necrosis had polyostotic involvement, and that it was symmetric in 83 percent.[65] Ruderman et al. reported a patient with six bones involved.[94] Milgram and Riley saw aseptic necrosis in 18 different bones in a patient who had taken high-dose steroids for 10 years because of idiopathic thrombocytopenic purpura[77]; there was spontaneous revascularization of some lesions even as new lesions were forming.

The controversy that surrounds the pathogenesis of idiopathic aseptic necrosis can be applied equally well to patients taking steroids. One can find proponents for the concept that aseptic necrosis develops as an accumulation of microfractures in osteoporotic bone, with a secondary compromise of the capillary blood flow because of the incompressible, fatty marrow,[31,92,103] altered mechanisms of coagulation,[8] and fat embolism.[33] Although there is evidence to support each of these possibilities, the inconsistencies between different studies—and even within individual studies—leaves the pathogenesis (or pathogeneses) of steroid-induced aseptic necrosis uncertain. Indeed, the causes of this condition may be multifactorial and variable in different patients, depending on underlying diseases, age, and sex.[120] In a disease such as systemic lupus erythematosus (SLE), it is unclear whether the vasculitis of SLE produces necrosis or whether the bone disease develops secondary to steroid therapy. Velayos et al. found vasculitis in the femoral heads of two patients with SLE who developed aseptic necrosis.[115] On the other hand, Leventhal and Dorfman found no vasculitis in 13 femoral heads resected from patients with lupus who had aseptic necrosis.[69] All but one of the patients was taking steroids, and Leventhal and Dorfman felt that the steroids were an important contributing cause of the necrosis.

Several studies of aseptic necrosis have included necrotic femoral heads from both steroid-treated patients and nontreated patients. There has been no mention of histologic differences between the two groups.[76,87] Moreover, Fisher and Bickel had three patients with Cushing's disease in their series of aseptic necrosis cases, and these three cases were apparently indistinguishable from cases of idiopathic lesions and steroid-related cases.[33] Hastings and MacNab, however, felt that their steroid-treated group of aseptic necrosis cases was more rapidly progressive clinically, and that histologically the bone was more osteoporotic.[51] Similarly, Springfield and Enneking have noted that the aseptic necrosis that occurs in steroid-treated patients has some features that differ from aseptic necrosis of the femoral head due to other causes.[104] They noted that steroid-treated cases had marked osteoporosis around the infarct, less density in the infarct, a "gentle sinking" of the articular cartilage rather than a subchondral fracture, slender trabeculae with little progress toward repair within the infarct, and less reaction of the bone at the periphery of the infarct.

The results of studies dealing with the total dose and duration of steroid therapy in cases of steroid-induced aseptic necrosis have been conflicting. Fisher and Bickel described two patients who received steroids for less than 6 weeks and developed bilateral femoral head necrosis 3 and 6 months later, respectively.[33] Bergstein et al. found that patients with SLE who developed aseptic necrosis had had higher doses of steroids, but could not correlate this with the duration of therapy.[6] Conversely, Hurley et al. found that a long duration of steroid therapy was associated with aseptic necrosis, but that there was no difference in the total dosage administered as compared to a control group.[54] Abeles et al. felt that aseptic necrosis was increased when patients were given either a high initial steroid dosage or high steroid pulses at any time during treatment.[2] Harrington et al. found that the incidence of aseptic necrosis was dose related in renal transplant patients[49]; aseptic necrosis occurred in 16 of 68 patients receiving high-dose therapy, but in only 2 of 136 patients receiving low-dose therapy. The aseptic necrosis is not related to the azothioprine that many transplant patients receive.

Aseptic necrosis has been reported in patients receiving cytotoxic agents for malignant disease.[112] Most of these regimens include steroids, and it is difficult to know the relative roles of the cytotoxic agents compared with those of the steroids. In one case, however, necrosis of the humeral head occurred in a patient taking cyclophosphamide and methotrexate but no steroids.[83] The lesion was fractured, and biopsy showed necrotic bone with secondary reactive changes. Another patient, taking only methotrexate for psoriasis, developed aseptic necrosis of the femoral head after receiving 10,000 mg of methotrexate.[93]

Catto has recently described medullary bone necrosis in a 21-year-old girl who had received two renal transplants within 2 years.[17] There was an area of necrosis several centimeters in length in the distal femoral metaphysis. The girl also had aseptic necrosis of the femoral heads.

Bullough et al. illustrated an infarction of the medullary part of the lower femur and upper end of the tibia in a woman who died with lupus erythematosus after cortisone therapy.[14] The lesions were not detectable before death, and the bone had been removed because of a history of arthralgias. The lesions were outlined by a hemorrhagic border, and failed to show evidence of repair or cellular reaction at the margin. Vasculitis was not present. The infarcts are identical to those described by Jackson et al. in a patient with anaplastic anemia treated with steroids.[57] The severe anemia in the patient of Jackson et al. may have been a major factor in the necrosis. Aseptic necrosis has been thought to occur in patients taking oral analgesics or anti-inflammatory agents such as phenylbutazone.[81]

EFFECTS OF RADIATION THERAPY

Normal bone that is in the field of radiation of malignant disease may undergo several alterations, including osteoporosis[12, 66] and aseptic necrosis.[71] Irradiated bone sometimes shows impaired callus formation and nonunion of pathologic fractures.[11]

Osteoporosis secondary to therapeutic radiation usually does not become clinically apparent until more than a year after the completion of such therapy, and often not until more than 2 years have passed.[53] The osteoporotic bone is, of course, susceptible to fracture that may occur more than 20 years after therapy. The most common site of fracture is the femoral neck, after radiation for cervical carcinoma[7]; other common sites are the ribs and clavicle after radiation for breast cancer. Fractures may occur even if there is no radiographic osteoporosis.[41]

Necrosis of bone following radiation therapy is a complication that is seen after 2,000 or more rads have been given.[25] The necrosis that occurs secondary to radiation has also been called radiation osteitis, but this is a misnomer, since inflammation is an inconspicuous component unless there is concomitant infection. Osteonecrosis can occur within several months after radiation therapy, especially in areas susceptible to infection, such as the mandible. On the other hand, necrosis may not become apparent until 5 to 10 years later.[100] The necrosis occurs either because of a direct effect of radiation on the osteocytes and connective tissue, or secondary to vascular damage, from both cases. The arteries in the ligamentum teres have been found to be completely occluded in some patients with postradiation necrosis of the femoral head, but this also occurs in nonirradiated vessels.[17]

Whether or not the necrosis following radiation therapy occurs acutely or as a late complication, the changes are similar. Fragmented trabeculae of the bone have empty lacunae, and the intervening marrow is necrotic. Small foci of a peculiar, disorganized, hypercalcified bone may occur.[41] As with aseptic necrosis of any etiology, there is a secondary fibrotic proliferation and new bone formation at the edges. There may be appositional bone growth on the dead trabeculae. Unlike nonirradiated fibrous tissue, the fibroblasts seen in postradiation necrosis can have bizarre nuclear forms (the so-called radiation fibroblasts). The marrow may be calcified.

Radiation of bones in children can result in epiphyseal injury with arrested growth. This is clinically most apparent in the spine, although deformities of nearly every skeletal component have been reported.[86] Injury to the facial bones in children who are irradiated for embryonal rhabdomyosarcoma can lead to severe deformity. The younger the patient, the greater is the risk for subsequent deformities.

Adult cartilage is relatively insensitive to radiation. The area of greatest clinical risk for radiation damage is the cartilage in the larynx, which may become necrotic and sequestrated, leading to airway obstruction.

Approximately 150 sarcomas have been reported at sites of irradiated benign bone lesions; about three-fourths of these cases received what are now considered unacceptably high radiation doses. The majority of the postradiation tumors have been osteosarcomas, but fibrosarcomas and chondrosarcomas have also been reported.[4] The latent period has varied from slightly less than 3 years to 30 years, with an average of 6 years for tumors occurring in weight-bearing bones and 14 years for those in non-weight-bearing bones.[96] About half of the cases have evidence of radiation osteonecrosis at the edge of the tumor.[4]

A new complication appears to be emerging

as a result of successful treatment of Ewing's sarcoma by irradiation of the primary tumor site, coupled with systemic chemotherapy: as reported in one study, 4 of 10 patients who lived 5 or more years after initial therapy for Ewing's sarcoma developed an osteosarcoma at the site of the original tumor.[18]

The occurrence of postradiation sarcoma in previously normal bone is rare. Phillips and Sheline reviewed about 6,000 patients treated for malignant disease, and found 2 cases of osteosarcoma arising in bone that was normal at the time of treatment, 5 and 11 years previously, respectively[89]; this represents only 0.03 percent of all of the patients treated, or 0.1 percent of the 5 year survivors. In another study, Tountas et al. found 10 cases of postradiation sarcoma, representing 0.03 percent of 5 year survivors.[113]

Benign osseous tumors occurring in the field of high dose radiotherapy have all been osteochondromas; these have arisen in the flat bones and vertebra of irradiated children, as well as in the long bones.[64, 95] No case of malignant transformation has yet been reported in this group.

Internal radiation from thorium dioxide (Thorotrast) has been associated with the development of osteosarcoma.[102] Thorotrast is visible microscopically in the form of brown, shiny granules lying free in fibrous tissue, or within macrophages. In cases of Thorotrast-induced osteosarcoma, the bone, in addition to neoplastic transformation, may undergo reactive changes. Two such cases were described by Teplick et al., who saw the "ghosts" of childhood bone in radiographs on two adults who had received Thorotrast as children[111]; the radiodense outlines of all of the vertebra and the pelvis were of the size expected at the age of 2 or 3 years, which was the age that Thorotrast had been given to the patients. In one case, histologic examination of autopsy material showed numerous Thorotrast-laden macrophages in the region of the dense bone. Presumably, the Thorotrast had been concentrated in the zone of original deposition, and had provoked a continuing reaction manifest as dense bone.

JOINTS

Effects of Orthopedic Hardware

Orthopedic prostheses and the tissue surrounding them constitute surgical specimens that are frequently removed when the device becomes loosened, either because of infection or mechanical failure. Prosthetic materials fall into one of three major categories; metallic, plastic, and the acrylic cement, methylmethacrylate, that is used to form a bond between prostheses and bone. The metals of which prostheses are made include stainless steel or the alloy Vitallium, which consists mainly of chromium and cobalt. The polmyers used to make prostheses include polyethylene, silicone elastomer, and proplast, which is a polymer of Teflon and carbon.

There are major changes in the bone adjacent to prosthetic substances even in the absence of recognizable infection. Initially, the bone next to the prosthesis develops a necrotic zone a few millimeters wide that persists for up to 2 years.[119] The death of bone at the bone–cement interface may be due to the trauma generated by the physical reaming of bone for the insertion of the device, or it may be secondary to the heat generated by the polymerization of the methylmethacrylate, which may reach 70° C.[118] Eventually, this dead bone is revascularized; later, a fibrous zone may occur at the interface, and may contribute to the later loosening of the prosthesis. Fragments of the acrylic cement can be found in the fatty marrow of the bone at the prosthesis site, either free in the tissue or within histiocytes, some of which may be multinucleated. A variety of appearances in this bone have been described, including spherules[116] and elongated sharp edged shreds[20]; the material retaining a spherule configuration may be the prepolymerized cement.[116] Cement has also

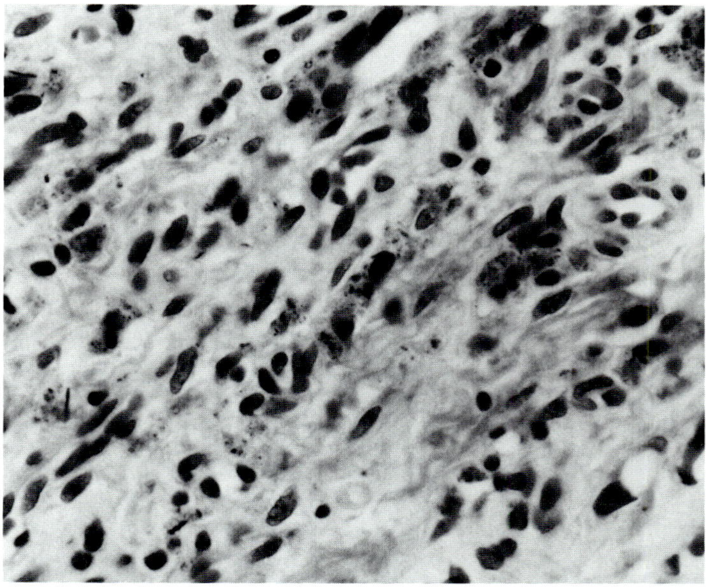

Fig. 4-1. Metallic debris is a black powder within mononuclear macrophages and is also free in the collagen. H & E, × 200.

been seen within the lumens of the arterioles and venules.[20]

The synovium accumulates material that is worn off from every type of prosthesis. Within a few months after their insertion, the metallic devices wear sufficiently to give the synovium a grey or black color. Microscopically, metallic debris is seen as a black powder lying free in fibrous tissue or within macrophages (Fig. 4-1); giant cells are rarely formed. The material is birefingent, and ranges from tiny rounded granules to cigarette-shaped rods up to 4 μm long.

The polyethylene devices provoke a much greater giant-cell response[32] (Fig. 4-2) These particles are colorless, and range up to 50 μm in greatest dimension. They are birefringent and form splinters and sheets as well as tiny punctate particles. Silicone elastomer is a yellow, refractile globular substance that elicits a multinucleated histiocyte response (Fig. 4-3); the elastomer has also been found in the regional lymph nodes draining the involved joints.[22]

Most of the methylmethacrylate particles deposited in the periarticular soft tissue of prosthesis wearers are dissolved out during tissue processing. The particles that persist are almost invisible optically because of their transparency, and are best identified with po-

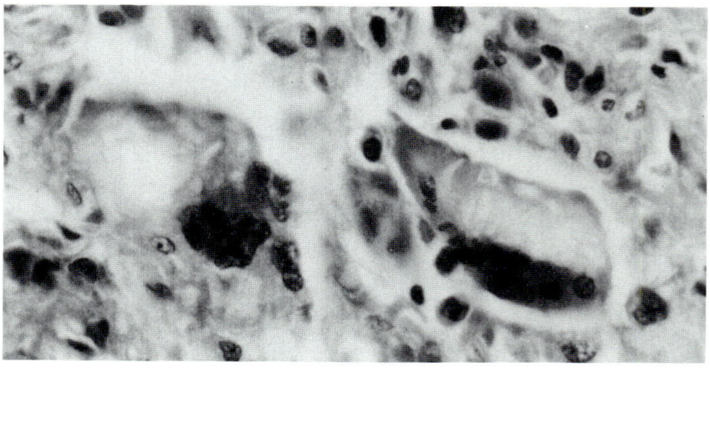

Fig. 4-2. Polyethylene forms irregular aggregates of colorless material that is barely discernible within the cytoplasm of multinucleated histiocytes. (Slide obtained through courtesy of J. M. Corson, M. D). H & E, × 325.

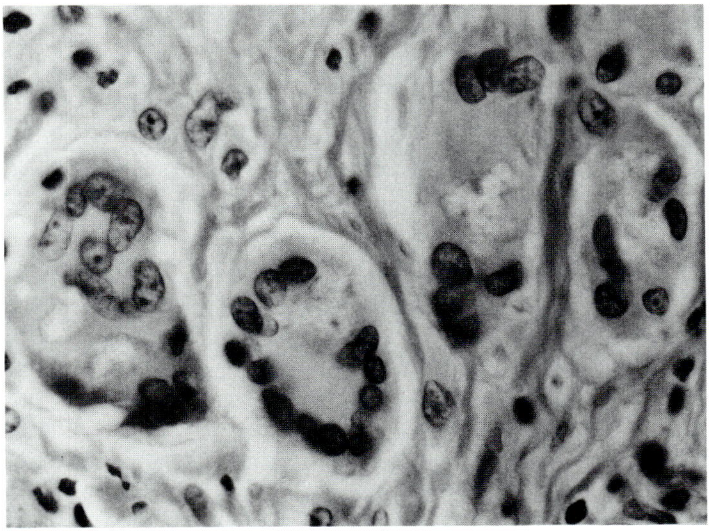

Fig. 4-3. Silicone elastomer is a highly refractile, yellow globular substance within multinucleated histiocytes. (Slide obtained through courtesy of A. J. Christie, M. D). H & E, × 365.

larized light, under which they appear as polyhedral fragments. Some authors have stated that the particles are uncommonly intracellular and do not excite a giant cell response,[20] whereas others have demonstrated a marked histiocytic reaction, including multinucleated giant cells.[116] In some methylmethacrylate preparations, barium sulfate is used as a radioopaque marker, and is seen as a fine granular material in tissue sections (Fig. 4-4).[15] Heating of tissue slides can help distinguish polyethylene from methylmethacrylate; the former reappears after the slide cools to room temperature.[24]

The long-term use of prosthestic materials raises concern for their possible carcinogenic action. To date, there have been no reports of neoplasms associated with joint prostheses. However, there have been four cases of neoplasms arising in bone or soft tissue adjacent to metal plates used to repair bone fractures. In two of these cases, the period between the initial operation and the development of the neoplasm was more than 30 years; in one of

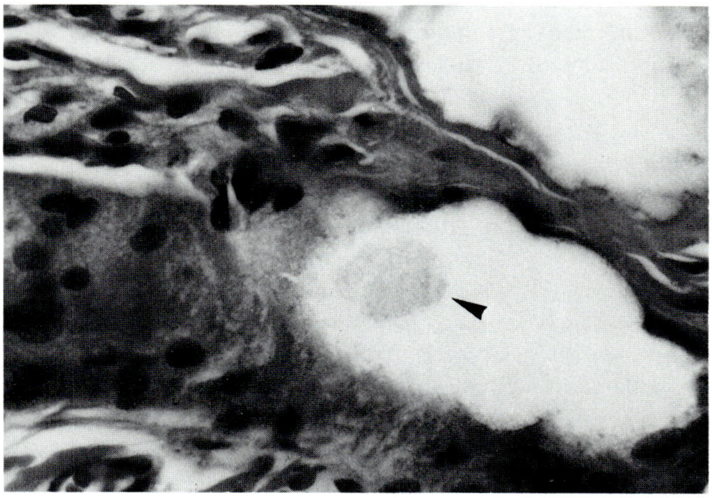

Fig. 4-4. Giant-cell response to methylmethacrylate. The methylmethacrylate is dissolved out and the sparse, finely granular material that remains is barium sulfate (arrow). H & E, × 340.

these two cases, a sarcoma of unclear histologic type developed in soft tissue near the plate, and the patient died of pulmonary metastases.[74] Dube and Fisher illustrate an angiosarcoma including the bone as well as soft tissues around a metal plate; their patient also died of metastases.[27] In two other patients, neoplasms developed 3 and 7 years, respectively, after the insertion of metal plates and screws. In one instance, the tumor was an osteosarcoma[26]; in the other case it was a Ewing's sarcoma that developed in an 11-year-old girl.[110]

Intra-articular Corticosteroid Injection

The intra-articular injection of corticosteroids suppresses symptoms of many disorders, including degenerative joint disease, gout, pseudogout, rheumatoid arthritis, and traumatic arthritis. The symptomatic relief probably occurs in the synovium, but changes are produced in the articular cartilage as well. In the latter, protein synthesis is decreased. The resultant weakness of the matrix is reversible, however, after the effects of the steroids have worn off.[34] Multiple injections of corticosteroids can lead to a rapidly progressive degenerative change, with the destruction of articular surfaces and the deposition of calcified debris into the soft tissues; furthermore, the destruction not only includes the cartilage, but the underlying bone, with the complete loss of a functional joint over a period of a few months. The changes are similar to those seen in neuropathic arthropathy.[5,78] Histologic examination of the edges of the bone remnants shows fractured trabeculae set in a dense fibrotic reaction that is surrounded by secondary new bone formation and granulation tissue.

It is of interest that the injection of commercially available corticosteroid preparations into the joints of volunteers without arthritis produces acute inflammation. The inflammatory response includes phagocytosis of crystalline steroid particles within 6 hours.[73] Kahn et al. have illustrated the appearance of crystals from several different steroid preparations in the synovial fluid in such cases.[62] These crystals include short and long rod shapes as well as more globular configurations with varying degrees of birefringence; they must be distinguished from endogenous crystals that may be found in synovial fluid aspirates.

Hemarthrosis

Hemorrhage into a joint may complicate anticoagulant therapy. There is indirect evidence that such hemorrhage may be more common in abnormal joints, but it certainly occurs in joints without previously recognized disease.[75] Hemarthrosis has been reported in patients receiving either heparin or warfarin.[50]

Drug-Induced Arthralgia and Arthritis

Arthralgia or arthritis frequently occurs secondary to alterations in uric acid metabolism. Large amounts of nuclear urates are released through the destructive effect of cytotoxic drugs on tumor cells. Kriegel and Müller listed 34 different agents that had been incriminated in at least one patient as causing hyperuricemia, and as therefore having the potential to produce gouty arthritis.[67] Diuretics, including thiazides, frusemide, ethacrynic acid, and chorthalidone are the drugs most commonly producing hyperuricemia; however, the list includes many other groups of drugs, such as hormones, antibiotics, antituberculous drugs, cholesterol-lowering drugs, and levodopa.

The list of drugs that have induced arthralgias is endless. It seems likely that a drug capable of inducing an allergic manifestation in any other organ can also produce arthralgia or signs of arthritis. The diverse agents that have been implicated include antibiotics, anticonvulsants, antithyroid agents, cytotoxic drugs, local anesthetics, cardiotropic drugs, oral contraceptives, and vaccines.[67] One well-studied case provides clear evidence of a cause and effect relationship of such a drug with arthralgia. The patient developed polyarthralgia 5 days after beginning isoniazid therapy, and this was followed by swelling and stiffness of the joints. Improvement occurred rapidly after cessation of therapy. The patient was then rechallenged with isoniazid, and the drug precipitated symptoms within a few hours, followed by morning stiffness.[98]

Isoniazid has also been implicated as the cause of more disabling symptoms, especially involving the joints of the upper extremity (shoulder-hand syndrome). The symptoms may appear gradually and progress during the first 8 weeks of therapy, with impairment of joint function and atrophy of soft tissues.[39] Other drugs have also been implicated in the shoulder-hand syndrome. A review of many patients with this condition disclosed a striking frequency of phenobarbital usage, especially in patients with bilateral disease. The duration of drug usage ranged from several weeks to more than 10 years, mainly in epileptic patients.[114] There is some regression of the changes after the phenobarbital therapy is stopped, but if the changes are severe, some functional defects may persist. The pathogenesis is unknown.

Miscellaneous

Many cases of arthritis or osteomyelitis have occurred following vaccination. In Europe, osteomyelitis from which mycobacteria can be grown is a complication of vaccination with BCG.[63] Silby et al. decribed a 65-year-old woman who received a smallpox vaccination and developed a monarticular arthritis of abrupt onset 12 days later.[101] The joint effusion was cultured and vaccinia virus was recovered. The patient had no previous history of arthritis or other joint abnormality. Osteomyelitis has also occurred from 10 to 14 days after vaccination. There is a rapid, prominent destruction of the metaphyseal portion of long bones, and the destruction may cross the epiphyseal plate. Periosteal new bone formation accompanies the cortical destruction. If the epiphysis is damaged, permanent limb shortening may occur.[30]

A complication of successful therapy for gouty tophi was reported by Gottlieb and Gray.[42] The patient had massive tophaceous deposits on the fingers, with subchondral bone erosions. The tophi disappeared during 3 years of allpurinol therapy, but there also occurred telescoping of the phalanges with the loss of several interphalangeal joints. The mechanism of this destructive complication is unclear, but it may have been related to impaired vascularity of the soft tissues owing to the original tophaceous deposits.

Several drugs have been implicated in the disturbance of growth in children. Corticosteroids, for example, inhibit the closure of epiphyseal plates.[82] Conversely, androgens accelerate epiphyseal closure, usually after a transient acceleration of growth.[40]

REFERENCES

1. Aaron, J. E., Gallagher, J. C., Anderson, J. et al.: Frequency of osteomalacia and osteoporosis in fractures of the proximal femur. Lancet 1:229, 1974.
2. Abeles, M., Urman, J. D., & Rothfield, N. F.: Aseptic necrosis of bone in systemic lupus erythematosus. Relationship to corticosteroid therapy. Arch. Intern. Med. 138:750, 1978.
3. Ahmed, K. Y., Wills, M. R., Skinner, R. K. et al.: Persistent hypophosphatemia and osteomalacia in dialysis patients not on oral phosphate-binders: Response to dihydrotachysterol therapy. Lancet 2:439, 1976.
4. Arlen, M., Higinbotham, N. W., Huvos, A. G., et al.: Radiation-induced sarcoma of bone. Cancer 28:1087, 1971.
5. Bentley, G., & Goodfellow, J. W.: Disorganisation of the knees following intra-articular hydrocortisone injections. J. Bone Joint Surg. 51B:498, 1969.
6. Bergstein, J. M., Wiens, C., & Fish, A. J.: Avascular necrosis of bone in systemic lupus erythematosus. J. Pediatr. 85:31, 1974.
7. Bickel, W. H., Childs, D. S., & Porretta,

C. M.: Post-irradiation fractures of the femoral neck. Emphasis on the results of treatment. J.A.M.A. 175:204, 1961.

8. Boettcher, W. G., Bonfiglio, M., Hamilton, H. H., et al.: Non-traumatic necrosis of the femoral head. Part I. Relation of altered hemostasis to etiology. J. Bone Joint Surg. 52A:312, 1970.
9. Boksenbaum, M., & Mendelson, C. G.: Aseptic necrosis of the femoral head associated with steroid therapy. J.A.M.A. 184:262, 1963.
10. Boland, E. W.: Prolonged uninterrupted cortisone therapy in rheumatoid arthritis. Br. Med. J. 2:191, 1951.
11. Bonarigo, B. C., & Rubin, P.: Nonunion of pathologic fracture after radiation therapy. Radiology 88:889, 1967.
12. Bonfiglio, M.: The pathology of fracture of the femoral neck following irradiation. Am. J. Roentgenol. 70:449, 1953.
13. Broadus, A. E., Hanson, T. A. S., Bartter, F. C., et al.: Primary hyperparathyroidism presenting as anticonvulsant-induced osteomalacia. Am. J. Med. 63:298, 1977.
14. Bullough, P. G., Kambolis, C. P., Marcove, R. C., et al.: Bone infarctions not associated with caisson disease. J. Bone Joint Surg. 47A:477, 1965.
15. Bullough, P. G.: Pathologic changes associated with the common arthritides and their treatment. Pathol. Ann., 14:69, 1979.
16. Campbell, J. E., Tam, C. S., & Sheppard, R. H.: "Brown Tumor" of hyperparathyroidism induced with anti-convulsant medication. J. Can. Assoc. Radiol. 28:73, 1977.
17. Catto, M.: Pathology of aseptic necrosis. In: Davidson, J. K., Ed. Aseptic Necrosis of Bone. p.3. Excerpta Medica. Amsterdam, 1976.
18. Chan, R. C., Sutow, W. W., Lindberg, R. D., et al.: Management and results of localized Ewing's sarcoma. Cancer 43:1001, 1979.
19. Chaplin, H. Jr., Clark, L. D., & Ropes, M. W.: Vitamin D intoxication. Am. J. Med. Sci. 221:369, 1951.
20. Charosky, C. B. Bullough, P. G., & Wilson, P. D., Jr.: Total hip replacement failures. A histological evaluation. J. Bone Joint Surg. 55A:49, 1973.
21. Christensen, W. R., Liebman, C., & Sosman, M. C.: Skeletal and periarticular manifestations of hypervitaminosis D. Am. J. Roentgenol. 65:27, 1951.
22. Christie, A. J., Weinberger, K. A., & Dietrich, M.: Silicone lymphadenopathy and synovitis. Complications of silicone elastomer finger joint prostheses. J.A.M.A. 237:1463, 1977.
23. Cooke, N., Teitelbaum, S., & Avioli, L. V.: Antacid-Induced osteomalacia and nephrolithiasis. Arch. Intern. Med. 138:1007, 1978.
24. Crugnola, A., Lowell, A. S., & Radin, E.: Polymeric debris in synovium after total joint replacement: Histological identification. J. Bone Joint Surg. 59A:860, 1977.
25. Dalen, N., & Edsmyr, F.: Bone mineral content of the femoral neck after irradiation. Acta. Radiol. Ther. 13:97, 1974.
26. Delgado, E. R.: Sarcoma following a surgically treated fractured tibia. A case report. Clin. Orthop., 12:315, 1958.
27. Dube, V. E., & Fisher, D. E.: Hemangioendothelioma of the leg following metallic fixation of the tibia. Cancer 30:1260, 1972.
28. Eberlein, W. R., Bongiovanni, W. M., & Rodriguez, C. S.: Diagnosis and treatment: the complications of steroid treatment. Pediatrics 40:279, 1967.
29. Eddy, R. L.: Metabolic bone disease after gastrectomy. Am. J. Med. 50:442, 1971.
30. Elliott, W. D.: Vaccinial osteomyelitis. Lancet 2:1053, 1959.
31. Evarts, C. M., & Phalen, G. S.: Osseous avascular necrosis associated with renal transplantation. Clin. Orthop. 78:330, 1971.
32. Ewald, F. C., Sledge, C. B., Corson, J. M., et al.: Giant cell synovitis associated with failed polyethylene patellar replacements. Clin. Orthop. 115:213, 1976.
33. Fisher, D. E., & Bickel, W. H.: Corticosteroid-induced avascular necrosis: A clinical study of 77 patients. J. Bone Joint Surg. 53A:859, 1971.
34. Fitzgerald, R. H., Jr.: Intrasynovial injection of steroids. Uses and abuses. Mayo Clin. Proc. 51:655, 1976.
35. Frame, B., Guiang, H. L., Frost, H. M., et al.: Osteomalacia induced by laxative (phenolphthalein) ingestion. Arch. Int. Med., 128:794, 1971.
36. Frier, B. M., & Scott, R. D. M.: Osteomalacia and arthropathy associated with prolonged abuse of purgatives. Br. J. Clin. Pract. 31:17, 1977.
37. Gerber, A., Raab, A. P., & Sobel, A. E.: Vitamin A poisoning in adults with description of a case. Am. J. Med. 16:729, 1954.

38. Gertner, J. M., Lilburn, M., & Domenech, M.: 25-hydroxycholecalciferol absorption in steatorrhea and postgastrectomy osteomalacia. Br. Med. J. 1:1310, 1977.
39. Good, A. E., Green, R. A., & Zarafonetis, C. J. D.: Rheumatic symptoms during tuberculosis therapy. A manifestation of isoniazid toxicity? Ann. Intern. Med. 63:800, 1965.
40. Good, T. A., & Bessman, S. P.: Anabolic steroids in cystic fibrosis of the pancreas. Am. J. Dis. Child. 111:272, 1966.
41. Goodman, A. H., & Sherman, M. S.: Postirradiation fractures of the femoral neck. J. Bone Joint Surg. 45A:723, 1963.
42. Gottlieb, N. L., & Gray, R. G.: Allopurinol-associated hand and foot deformities in chronic tophaceous gout. J.A.M.A. 238:1663, 1977.
43. Greenwood, R. H., Prunty, F. T. G., & Silver, J.: Osteomalacia after prolonged glutethimide administration. Br. Med. J. 1:643, 1973.
44. Grennan, D. M., Palmer, D. G., Malthus, R. S., et al.: Iatrogenic fluorosis. Aust. New Z. J. Med. 8:528, 1978.
45. Griffith, C. G., Nichols, G., Jr., Asher, J. D., et al.: Heparin osteoporosis. J.A.M.A. 193:91, 1965.
46. Hahn, T. J., Birge, S. J., Scharp, C. R., et al.: Phenobarbital-induced alterations in vitamin D metabolism. J. Clin. Invest. 51:741, 1972.
47. Hahn, T. J.: Anticonvulsant osteomalacia. Arch. Intern. Med. 135:997, 1975.
48. Hahn, T. J.: Corticosteroid-induced osteopenia. Arch. Intern. Med. 138:882, 1978.
49. Harrington, K. D., Murray, W. R., Kountz, S. L., et al.: Avascular necrosis of bone after renal transplantation. J. Bone Joint Surg. 53A:203, 1971.
50. Hasselbacher, P., Schimmer, B. M., & Weinberger, A.: Hemarthrosis with sodium warfarin and heparin. Arth. Rheum. 21:740, 1978.
51. Hastings, D. E., & MacNab, I.: Spontaneous avascular necrosis of the femoral head. A clinical and pathological review. Can. J. Surg. 8:68, 1965.
52. Heaton, K. W., Lever, J. V., & Barnard, D.: Osteomalacia associated with cholestyramine therapy for postileectomy diarrhea. Gastroenterology 62:642, 1972.
53. Howland, W. J., Loeffler, R. K., Starchman, D. E., et al.: Postirradiation and atrophic changes of bone and related complications. Radiology 117:677, 1975.
54. Hurley, R. M., Steinberg, R. H., Patriquin, H., et al.: Avascular necrosis of the femoral head in childhood systemic lupus erythematosus. Can. Med. Assoc. J. 111:781, 1974.
55. Ihde, D. C., & DeVita, V. T.: Osteonecrosis of the femoral head in patients with lymphoma treated with intermittent combination chemotherapy (including corticosteroids). Cancer 36:1585, 1975.
56. Inkovaara, J., Heikinheimo, R., Jarvinen, K., et al.: Prophylactic fluoride treatment and aged bones. Br. Med. J. 3:73, 1975.
57. Jackson, J. M., Pinkerton, P. H., & Wilson, I. R.: Infarction of femoral marrow in a case of anaplastic anaemia. J. Pathol. Bacteriol. 83:562, 1962.
58. Jaffee, M. D., & Willis, P. W.: Multiple fractures associated with long term sodium heparin therapy. J.A.M.A. 193:158, 1965.
59. Jowsey, J., & Riggs, B. L.: Bone formation in hypercortisonism. Acta Endocrinol. 63:21, 1970.
60. Jowsey, J., Riggs, B. L., Kelly, P. J., et al.: Effect of combined therapy with sodium fluoride, vitamin D and calcium in osteoporosis. Am. J. Med. 53:43, 1972.
61. Jubiz, W., Haussler, M. R., McCain, T. A., et al.: Plasma 1,25-dihydroxyvitamin D levels in patients receiving anticonvulsant drugs. J. Clin. Endocrinol. Metab. 44:617, 1977.
62. Kahn, C. B., Hollander, J. L., & Schumacher, H. R.: Corticosteroid crystals in synovial fluid. J.A.M.A 211:807, 1970.
63. Kallesoe, O., & Jesperson, A.: Metastatic osteomyelitis following BCG vaccination. Acta. Orthop. Scand. 49:134, 1978.
64. Katzman, H., Waugh, T., & Berdon, W.: Skeletal changes following irradiation of childhood tumors. J. Bone Joint Surg. 51A:825, 1969.
65. Klippel, J. H., Gerber, L. H., Pollak, L., et al.: Avascular necrosis in systemic lupus erythematosus. Silent symmetric osteonecroses. Am. J. Med., 67:83, 1979.
66. Kok, G.: Spontaneous fractures of the femoral neck after the intensive irradiation of carcinoma of the uterus. Acta. Radiol. 40:511, 1953.
67. Kriegel, W. & Müller, W.: Drug-induced diseases of the bones, joints and connective tissue. p. 423. In: Meyler, L. and Peck, H. M.,

Eds.: Drug-induced Disease. Vol. 4. Excerpta Medica, Amsterdam, 1972.

68. Kyle, R. A., & Jowsey, J.: Effect of sodium fluoride, calcium carbonate, and vitamin D on the skeleton in multiple myeloma. Cancer 45:1669, 1980.
69. Leventhal, G. H., & Dorfman, H. D.: Aseptic necrosis of bone in systemic lupus erythematosus. Semin. Arth. Rheum. 4:73, 1974.
70. Lifshitz, F., & Maclaren, N.: Vitamin D dependent ricketts in institutionalized mentally retarded children on long term anticonvulsant therapy. I. A survey of 288 patients. J. Pediatr. 83:612, 1973.
71. MacDougall, J. T., Gibson, A., & Williams, T. H.: Irradiation necrosis of the head of the femur. Arch. Surg. 61:325, 1950.
72. Mallette, L. E.: Acetazolamide-accelerated anticonvulsant osteomalacia. Arch. Intern. Med. 137:1013, 1977.
73. McCarty, D. J., Jr., & Hogan, J. M.: Inflammatory reaction after intrasynovial injection of microcrystalline adrenocorticosteroid esters. Arth. Rheum. 7:359, 1964.
74. McDougall, A.: Malignant tumor at site of bone plating. J. Bone Joint Surg. 38B:709, 1956.
75. McLaughlin, G. E., McCarty, D. J., Jr., & Segal, B. L.: Hemarthrosis complicating anticoagulant therapy. Report of three cases. J.A.M.A. 196:1020, 1966.
76. Merle d'Aubigné, R., Postel, M., Mazabraud, A., et al.: Idiopathic necrosis of the femoral head in adults. J. Bone Joint Surg. 47B:612, 1965.
77. Milgram, J. W., & Riley, L. H., Jr.: Steroid induced avascular necrosis of bones in eighteen sites. A case report. Bull. Hosp. Joint. Dis. 37:11, 1976.
78. Miller, W. T., & Restifo, R. A.: Steroid arthropathy. Radiology 86:652, 1966.
79. Miller, W. E., & DeWolfe, V. G.: Osteoporosis resulting from heparin therapy. Cleve. Clin. Q. 33:31, 1966.
80. Murray, R. O.: Radiological bone changes in Cushing's syndrome and steroid therapy. Br. J. Radiol. 33:1, 1960.
81. Murray, R. O., & Jacobson, H. G.: The Radiology of Skeletal Disorders. 2nd Ed. p. 837. Churchill Livingstone, London, 1977.
82. Niermann, W. A., & Van Metre, T. E. Jr.: Efficacy of medrol in treatment of bronchial asthma in children. Metabolism 7:473, 1958.
83. Obrist, R., Hartmann, D., & Obrecht, J. P.: Osteonecrosis after chemotherapy. Lancet 1:1316, 1978.
84. Okita, H., & Block, M.: Osteomalacic new bone formation during chemotherapy of acute granulocytic leukemia. Am. J. Clin. Pathol. 71:645, 1979.
85. Parfitt, A. M., Miller, M. J., Frame, B., et al.: Metabolic bone disease after intestinal bypass for treatment of obesity. Ann. Intern. Med. 89:193, 1978.
86. Parker, R. G., & Berry, H. C.: Late effects of therapeutic irradiation on the skeleton and bone marrow. Cancer 37:1162, 1976.
87. Patterson, R. J., Bickel, W. H., & Dahlin, D. C.: Idiopathic avascular necrosis of the head of the femur. A study of fifty two cases. J. Bone Joint Surg. 46A:267, 1964.
88. Pease, C. N.: Focal retardation and arrest of growth of bones due to vitamin A intoxication. J.A.M.A. 182:980, 1962.
89. Phillips, T. L., & Sheline, G. E.: Bone sarcomas following radiation therapy. Radiology 81:992, 1963.
90. Ragab, A. H., Frech, R. S., & Vietti, T. J.: Osteoporotic fractures secondary to methotrexate therapy of acute leukemia in remission. Cancer 25:580, 1970.
91. Rifkind, B. M., Chazan, B. J., & Aitchison, J. D.: Chronic milk-alkali syndrome with generalized osteosclerosis after prolonged excessive intake of "Rennies" tablets. Br. Med. J. 1:317, 1960.
92. Riniker, P., & Huggler, A.: Idiopathic necrosis of the femoral head (A further patho-anatomical study). In: Zinn, W. M. Ed.: Idiopathic Ischemic Necrosis of the Femoral Head in Adults. p. 67. University Park Press, Baltimore, 1971.
93. Roenigk, H. H., Jr., Bergfeld, W. F., St. Jacques, R., et al.: Hepatotoxicity of methotrexate in the treatment of psoriasis. Arch. Dermatol. 103:250, 1971.
94. Ruderman, M., & McCarty, D. J. Jr.: Aseptic necrosis in systemic lupus erythematosus: Report of a case involving six joints. Arth. Rheum. 7:709, 1964.
95. Rutherford, H., & Dodd, G. D.: Complications of radiation therapy: Growing bone. Semin. Roentgenol. 9:15, 1974.
96. Sabanas, A. O., Dahlin, D. C., & Childs, D. S., Jr.: Postradiation sarcomas of bone. Cancer 9:528, 1956.

97. Sackler, J. P., & Liu, L.: Heparin-induced osteoporosis. Br. J. Radiol, 46:548, 1973.
98. Saslaw, S., & Klainer, A. S.: Rheumatoid syndrome during isoniazid therapy. Am. Rev. Resp. Dis. 100:221, 1969.
99. Saville, P. D., & Kharmosh, O.: Osteoporosis of rheumatoid arthritis. Influence of age, sex and corticosteroids. Arth. Rheum. 10:423, 1967.
100. Sengupta, S., & Prathap, K.: Radiation necrosis of the humerus: A report of three cases. Acta Radiol Ther. 12:313, 1973.
101. Silby, H. M., Farber, R., O'Connell, C. J., et al.: Acute monarticular arthritis after vaccination. Report of a case with isolation of vaccinia virus from synovial fluid. Ann. Intern. Med. 62:347, 1965.
102. Sindelar, W. F., Costa, J., & Ketcham, A. S.: Osteosarcoma associated with Thorotrast administration. Report of two cases and literature review. Cancer 42:2604, 1978.
103. Solomon, L.: Drug-induced arthropathy and necrosis of the femoral head. J. Bone Joint Surg. 55B:246, 1973.
104. Springfield, D. S., & Enneking, W. F.: Idiopathic aseptic necrosis. In Ackerman, L. V. and Spjut, H. J., Ed.: Bones and Joints. p. 61. Williams and Wilkins Co., Baltimore, 1976.
105. Squires, J. W., & Pinch, L. W.: Heparin-induced spinal fractures. J.A.M.A. 142:2417, 1979.
106. Stamp, T.C.B.: Intestinal absorption of 25-hydroxycholecalciferol. Lancet 2:121, 1974.
107. Stamp, T. C. B., Flanagan, A., Richens, J. M., et al.: Anti-convulsant osteomalacia. In: Copp, D. H. and Talmage, R. V. Ed.: Endocrinology of Calcium Metabolism. p. 16. Excerpta Medica, Amsterdam-Oxford, 1978.
108. Stern, P. J., & Watts, H. G.: Osteonecrosis after renal transplantation in children. J. Bone Joint Surg. 61A:851, 1979.
109. Susan, L. P., Braun, W. E., Banowsky, L. H., et al.: Avascular necrosis following renal transplantation. Experience with 449 allografts with and without high-dose steroid therapy. Urology 11:225, 1978.
110. Tayton, K. J. J.: Ewing's sarcoma at the site of a metal plate. Cancer 45:413, 1980.
111. Teplick, J. G., Head, G. L., Kricun, M. E., et al.: Ghost infantile vertebrae and hemipelves within adult skeleton from Thorotrast administration in childhood. Radiology 129:657, 1978.
112. Timothy, A. R., Tucker, A. K., Malpas, J. S., et al.: Osteonecrosis after intensive chemotherapy for Hodgkin's disease. Lancet 1:154, 1978.
113. Tountas, A. A., Fornasier, V. L., Harwood, A. R., et al.: Postirradiation sarcoma of bone. A perspective. Cancer, 43:182, 1979.
114. Van der Korst, J. K., Colenbrander, H., & Cats, A.: Phenobarbital and the shoulder-hand syndrome. Ann. Rheum. Dis. 25:553, 1966.
115. Velayos, E. E., Leidholt, J. D., Smyth, C. J., et al.: Arthropathy associated with steroid therapy. Ann. Intern. Med., 64:759, 1966.
116. Vernon-Roberts, B., & Freeman, M. A. R.: The tissue response to total joint replacement prostheses. In: Swanson, S. A. V. and Freeman, M. A. R., Eds.: The Scientific Basis of Joint Replacement. p. 86. John Wiley & Sons, New York, 1977.
117. Villanueva, A. R., Klein, M., & Frost, H. M.: Effect of adrenalcorticoid hormones on human lamellar bone: quantitative histological measurements of resorption and formation indices. Henry Ford Hosp. Med. Bull. 12:63, 1954.
118. Wile, A. H., & Greenwald, A.S.: Acrylic bone cement. In: American Academy of Orthopedic Surgeons: Symposium on Osteoarthritis. p. 86. C. V. Mosby, St. Louis, 1976.
119. Willert, H-G., Ludwig, J., & Semlitsch, M.: Reaction of bone to methacrylate after hip arthroplast. A long-term growth, light microscopic, and scanning electron microscopic study. J. Bone Joint. Surg. 56 A:1368, 1974.
120. Zinn, W. M.: Introduction. In: Zinn, W. M., Ed.: Idiopathic Ischemic Necrosis of the Femoral Head in Adults. p. 1. University Park Press Baltimore, 1971.

5

The Hematopoietic System

James W. Vardiman and Daina Variakojis

Drug-induced blood dyscrasias are among the most common and serious of adverse drug reactions. The toxic dyscrasia most often seen is granulocytopenia, with thrombocytopenia, hemolytic anemia, and aplastic anemia following in that order.[13,14,37] These disorders account for almost 10 percent of all cases of reported, unexpected drug reactions, but they are responsible for as many as 48 percent of drug-related deaths.[13,14,37,50] If the suppressive effects of cancer chemotherapy and irradiation are also included, the incidence of iatrogenic hematopoietic disorders would be even greater.

In addition to producing life-threatening cytopenias, medications are increasingly implicated in a variety of other abnormal hematopoietic responses. Atypical immune responses in the lymph nodes, some nonlymphocytic leukemias, malignant lymphomas, and various inflammatory lesions may comprise the response of the hematopoietic system to drug-induced injury.

In this chapter, we will briefly describe the mechanisms by which drugs may damage hematopoietic tissue, and discuss the patterns of injury seen with the agents that are the most common offenders. We will also attempt to demonstrate some of the histologic and pathologic features of the blood cells, bone marrow, and lymphoid system in drug-induced hematopoietic disorders.

PATHOGENESIS OF ADVERSE DRUG REACTIONS

Adverse reactions to drugs may result from a variety of mechanisms, most of which are yet to be discovered. Drugs may interfere at any one of the various levels of growth and development of a cell, or may alter the microenvironment in which the cell develops. Inhibition of one group of cells by a medication may allow another group to proliferate unregulated, therefore changing the balance of helper and suppressor activities required for normal blood cell development and function. The specific mechanisms of adverse drug reactions will be given; at this point, however, some general remarks concerning the development of blood cells and the possible sites and patterns of interaction between these cells and drugs is useful.

Normal Hematopoiesis

Several excellent reviews of normal hematopoiesis are available[4,25,52,130,135,136,137,181]; however, the following paragraphs summarize the production of normal blood cells in the bone marrow.

Infusion of bone marrow into lethally irradiated mice leads to the reconstitution of hematopoiesis in the spleen.[112,181] Each colony of hematopoietic cells arises from a single progenitor cell, capable of self-renewal, which produces granulocytic, megakaryocytic, and erythroid colonies. This pluripotent stem cell is known as a CFU-S (colony-forming unit in spleen). Indirect evidence exists for a similar cell in humans: Philadelphia-chromosome positive chronic myelogenous leukemia (CML) shows the abnormal chromosome in the myeloid, erythroid, megakaryocytic, and macrophage series,[51,148] and the demonstration of Ph[1] chromosome-positive lymphoblasts during the blast crisis of CML[94,177] indicates that there exists a stem cell capable of differentiating toward both the lymphoid and myeloid series.

Erythropoiesis was first studied in a murine system, in which bone marrow in plasma clot, in the presence of erythropoietin, formed colonies composed of from 8 to 64 erythroid cells.[165] The committed stem cells responsible for these colonies were called the CFU-E (colony-forming unit erythroid). In those colonies examined later, large clusters or "bursts" of erythroid cells were seen, and the progenitor cells for these colonies were known as BFU-E (burst-forming units, erythroid).[73] The presence of CFU-Es and BFU-Es in human marrow and peripheral blood has been documented.[24,57,74,170] CFU-Es grow in the presence of low concentrations of erythropoietin, while BFU-Es require higher concentrations.[4]

Committed stem cells capable of forming granulocyte-monocyte cultures in soft agar culture (CFU-C) have been demonstrated in both human peripheral blood and bone marrow.[21,140] From these stem cells, neutrophils, eosinophils, monocytes, and macrophages develop in the presence of various colony-stimulating factors (CSF).

Colony-forming units for megakaryocytes in the mouse,[115] and for lymphoid cells in humans,[145] have also been documented.

In the bone marrow, the CFU-S is probably at rest during the ordinary steady state,[7,78,135] while the CFU-E, CFU-C, and other committed stem cells are in active, dividing cycles to maintain the hematopoietic system. For normal hematopoiesis to occur, these cells must exist in a favorable microenvironment, with humoral and cellular inhibitors and stimulators working in a balanced fashion. There is evidence that T-lymphocytes may be required for the differentiation of hematopoietic cells,[121] and may also increase the CFU-S proliferation rate.[135]

Classification of Drug Reactions

Dose-related, Expected Reactions. Some medications are expected to produce toxic changes in the hematopoietic system. These effects, usually suppressive in nature, are often the limiting factors in therapy with these medications, and are explained on the basis of the known pharmacologic actions of the drug.

The classic examples of dose-related, predictable drug toxicities are those caused by the cytostatic agents used for cancer chemotherapy. These medications may act directly on dividing, cycling cells (cycle-active drugs) or on both dividing and nondividing cells (non-cycle-active drugs). Cycle-active drugs tend to have a greater effect on committed, more differentiated cells such as CFU-Es and CFU-Cs, whereas non-cycle-active drugs affect dividing cells as well as such nondividing cells as the CFU-S. In general, non-cycle-active agents should produce the most protracted marrow damage, whereas the effects of cycle-specific agents should be more readily reversible.[63] This supposition would be true if only one course of a single drug were given, but since the pluripotent stem cell may be activated, and therefore "recruited," during the course of therapy, this distinction between cycle-active and non-cycle active agents is not always appreciated. Antimetabolites tend to be cycle-active drugs, whereas alkylating agents are non-cycle-active.

The morphologic features observed following the administration of a particular drug may depend upon which of the stem cells or differentiating cells is affected. For example, a primary effect on a multipotential stem cell would lead to a hypoplastic marrow, an effect on the CFU-E would lead to isolated erythroid hypoplasia and anemia, and a primary effect on differentiated erythroid cells would lead to a hyperplastic marrow with megaloblastic features.[42] Variations in susceptibility of the various committed stem cells to a given drug are demonstrated by the fact that there is often a dissociation in the production of reticulocytopenia, leukopenia, and thrombocytopenia by antitumor agents.[96]

Dose-dependent reactions may also be seen with drug classes other than the cytostatic agents. Chloramphenicol produces two patterns of toxicity which are probably not pathophysiologically related. The most serious is the development of aplastic anemia, a reaction which is not dose-dependent. Besides this, chloramphenicol administration is often followed by a dose-related, reversible hematologic suppression, often associated with a normocellular bone marrow with vacuolated erythroid and granulocytic precursors, reticulocytopenia, and a variable degree of anemia.[15,76,188] This reversible toxicity is probably produced by blockade of the binding of messenger RNA to ribosomes, and hence by the inhibition of mitochondrial protein synthesis.[179,188] Bone marrow cells from normal individuals are susceptible to chloramphenicol in culture systems,[70] and it has therefore been concluded by some that the reversible reaction seen with this drug is a function of the total duration and degree of marrow exposure to chloramphenicol.[37,62,77]

Idiosyncratic Reactions. These reactions are unpredictable, occur in only a small percentage of patients receiving the drug, and may or may not be dose-related. The pathophysiology of some of the reactions is well-known; for the vast majority of offending agents, however, the mechanism producing the idiosyncratic reaction is unclear. De Gruchy[37] has grouped the mechanisms for these unanticipated drug reactions into three types: (1) hypersensitivity reactions, in which the untoward effect is due to an antigen-antibody reaction, and for which prior sensitization is required; (2) pharmacogenetic reactions, in which the toxic effects are often related to the pharmacologic actions of the drug, but in which a genetically determined metabolic abnormality leads to accentuation of the drug effect; and (3) idiosyncratic reactions, which are not related to the known pharmacologic action of the drug, which may occur with the first dose, and the mechanism of which is unclear.

The best-known examples of hypersensitivity reactions would be the thrombocytopenia induced by sedormid, the cinchona alkaloids quinidine and quinine, and by stibophen and salicylamide; the agranulocytosis induced by aminopyrine, and the hemolysis of red cells due to penicillin, methyldopa, quinine, quinidine, stibophen, and salicylamide.

The actual immunologic mechanism involved in these reactions is varied and in some cases unknown. The initial concept of the mechanism of blood cell injury by immune mechanisms involved the attachment of drug to the cell to form an autoantigen which would induce an antibody against the drug-cell complex.[1] However, there are probably multiple mechanisms possible for drug-associated, immune-mediated injury. In the case of penicillin and red cells, the cells react with a penicillin derivative to form a firm cell-drug complex, with anti-penicillin antibodies then agglutinating the drug-coated cells. With quinine, salicylamide, and stibophen, the drug combines with a soluble plasma protein—a macromolecule—to form an antigen which induces an antibody specific for the drug-protein complex; the immune reaction involves the combination of drug with the antibody, with the resulting antibody-antigen complex being adsorbed onto the cell secondarily, leading to its destruction.[157,158] Methyldopa, on the other hand, leads to the formation of autoantibodies resembling those of spontaneous, idiopathic autoimmune hemolytic anemia, and which often show Rh-related blood-group specificity.[167] The actual mechanism underlying this effect of methyldopa may be the inhibition of suppressor T-cell function, leading to unregulated antibody production by B-cells.[84]

The best known examples of immune-mediated damage involve peripheral blood cells, but there is evidence accumulating that the marrow cells may be damaged as well. Kelton et al.[81] have reported drug-dependent suppression of CFU-Cs and CFU-Es in a patient with pancytopenia associated with quinidine therapy; Barret et al.[6] noted suppression of marrow colony growth in the presence of a serum factor and drug from a patient with aminopyrine-induced agranulocytosis; and Taetle et al.[169] have recently reported drug-dependent depression of granulopoiesis by non-complement-dependent antibody in a patient with dilantin-induced agranulocytosis. There also exist other possibilities for drug-induced immune injury to the hematopoietic system. Immunologic damage to the sinusoidal microcirculation might well lead to alterations of the microenvironment necessary for normal hematopoiesis.[90] As noted earlier, T-cells are necessary for proliferation of peripheral blood BFU-Es,[121, 135] and it is therefore possible that an antibody directed against a T-lymphocyte population could lead to impairment of hematopoiesis,[127] as well as to impairment of the regulation of other lymphoid elements. Hoffman et al.[67] demonstrated suppression of erythroid-colony formation by normal human bone marrow when the culture system was exposed to peripheral blood lymphocytes from patients with drug-induced aplastic anemia.

The development of aplastic anemia following treatment with chloramphenicol is an example of an idiosyncratic reaction that may well have a pharmacogenetic basis as well. Yunis[188] found that this antibiotic inhibits the uptake of formate into DNA and that, although chloramphenicol levels in excess of 100 μg/ml were required to inhibit DNA synthesis from normal subjects, significant inhibition occurred at 25 μg/ml in those patients who developed aplastic anemia. That there may be a genetic predisposition to chloramphenicol-induced aplastic anemia was illustrated by the finding that DNA synthesis was inhibited, and also at low levels of the drug, in the marrow cells of relatives of those patients who had chloramphenicol-induced aplastic anemia,[188] and by the reports of chloramphenicol-induced aplasia in identical twins.[120] Yunis postulated that the pluripotent stem cell was the cell most affected in these patients, and there is support for this concept in the work of others[70, 118] who have found that the stem cells in patients who have recovered from chloramphenicol-induced damage are more resistant to chloramphenicol, with less proliferative ability than normal, indicating elimination of sensitive cells and the selection of a resistant stem cell with reduced proliferative capacities.

PATTERNS OF DRUG REACTIONS IN BONE MARROW AND PERIPHERAL BLOOD

Drugs having some effect on the hematopoietic system are so numerous, and the possible patterns of reactions so diverse, that only those most likely to be encountered by the morphologist while reviewing bone marrow and peripheral blood will be discussed. Some drug reactions, such as the hemolysis of red cells in patients with G-6-PD deficiency, are well described in standard hematology texts, and will only be briefly mentioned.

Aplastic Anemia

At least half of all cases of aplastic anemia are drug-induced.[37, 169] Chloramphenicol, sulfonamides, oxyphenbutazone, and acetazolamide lead the list of offending drugs producing idiosyncratic aplastic anemia. Other drugs causative of idiosyncratic aplastic anemia are listed in Table 5-1.

Aplastic anemia is defined as having at least two of the three following peripheral blood abnormalities: granulocytes less than 500/mm^3, platelets less than 20,000/mm^3, and reticulocytes less than 1 percent; additionally, the bone marrow must be hypocellular.[4] The best means of ascertaining marrow cellularity is with a trephine biopsy, although it must be recognized that such a specimen represents a very small piece of a large organ, and the findings from a single biopsy may not always be representative. Usually in aplastic anemia, the bone core biopsy will show the marrow cellularity to be less than 10 percent (Fig. 5-

1), with erythropoiesis, myelopoiesis, and thrombopoiesis severely reduced; occasionally, only two of the three cell lines will be depressed. In a few cases of aplastic anemia, the biopsy may hit a "hot spot," which is a residual area of intense hematopoietic proliferation.[42] In such cases, a repeat biopsy or ferrokinetic studies may be required to differentiate the findings from a refractory anemia. In general, there is poor correlation between marrow cellularity and the prognosis for the patient with aplastic anemia, whether drug-induced or not.[171,183]

Erythropoiesis is most usually normoblastic, but occasionally nuclear irregularities, karyorrhexis, pyknosis, multinucleation, and cytoplasmic vacuolation can be seen.[98] There may also be intramedullary phagocytosis of erythroid cells and other nucleated hematopoietic cells.[171] Hemosiderin is increased. There may also be a relative as well as an absolute increase in lymphocytes, plasma cells, and supportive connective tissue elements.[151] Te Velde and Haak,[171] in a study of methacrylate-embedded bone marrow biopsies from patients with aplastic anemia, some of which were drug-induced, noted disruption of sinus walls and necrosis of capillary walls. Osteoblasts and osteoclasts were increased. In addition, these investigators found an increased amount of inflammatory infiltrate, consisting of lymphocytes, plasma cells, and foamy macrophages in all patients, and they correlated an increased amount of such an infiltrate with a poorer prognosis. Similarly, Li et al.[99] proposed that bone marrow lymphocytosis (in excess of 85 percent of the differential count), together with a relative lack of hematopoietic elements, indicates a poor prognosis. Occasional patients with drug-induced aplastic anemia may develop the erythroid abnormalities of paroxysmal nocturnal hemoglobinuria.[134,147]

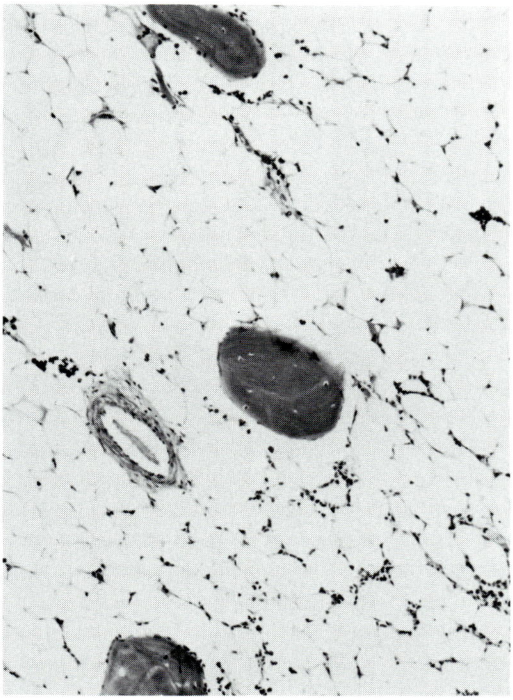

Fig. 5-1. Drug-induced aplastic anemia with markedly hypocellular bone marrow in the bone core biopsy. H & E, × 100.

Pure Red Cell Aplasia

As noted earlier, chloramphenicol is commonly associated with a transient, selective depression of erythropoiesis, characterized by vacuolated erythroid precursors in the marrow, with little evidence of maturation of these precursors past the pronormoblast stage. A few other drugs, cited in Table 5-1, may also cause selective depression of the erythroid series in the bone marrow. Some of these drugs effect dose-related responses, with remission following cessation of therapy, whereas others are not dose-related. Yunis et al.[189,190] described a case of anemia due to diphenylhydantoin (Dilantin) in which nucleated erythroid percursors were completely absent from the marrow, while the granulocytic elements and megakaryocytes (except for an increase in eosinophils) were normal. Yunis et al. demonstrated inhibition of DNA synthesis at the step of deoxyribotide formation in that particular patient.

Table 5-1. Some Drugs Implicated in Idiosyncratic Cytopenias

	Aplastic Anemia	Pure Red Cell Aplasia	Selective Granulo-cytopenia	Selective Thrombo-cytopenia
Acetaminophen				+
Acetazolamide	+		+	+
Acetysalicylic acid	+			+
Allopurinol	+			
Aminopyrine	+	+	+	
Amitryptiline	+		+	+
Amodiaquine	+		+	
Ampicillin	+		+	+
Antihistamines	+		+	+
Apronalide			+	+
Arsenicals	+			
Arsphenamine		+		
Azathioprine	+	+	+	+
Barbiturates	+	+		+
Calomel		+		
Carbimazole	+		+	
Cephalothin			+	+
Chlordiazepoxide	+		+	
Chloramphenicol	+	+	+	+
Chloroquine	+			+
Chlorothiazide			+	+
Chlorpromazine	+	+	+	+
Chlorthalidone	+		+	+
Colchicine	+			
Desipramine			+	+
Diazoxide			+	+
Digitoxin				+
Estrogen				+
Furosemide	+		+	+
Gold	+		+	+
Halothane		+		
Heparin				+
Hydantoins	+	+	+	+
Hydrochlorothiazide	+	+	+	+
Imipramine				+

(Continued)

Table 5-1. *(Continued)*

	Aplastic Anemia	Pure Red Cell Aplasia	Selective Granulo-cytopenia	Selective Thrombo-cytopenia
Indomethacin	+	+	+	+
Isoniazid	+	+	+	+
Lithium	+			
Meprobamate	+		+	+
Methicillin	+		+	+
Methyldopa	+		+	+
Oxytetracycline	+		+	+
Para-amino salicylic acid				+
Penicillamine	+		+	+
Penicillin		+		+
Phenothiazines	+		+	
Phenylbutazone	+	+	+	+
Potassium perchlorate	+			
Procainamide			+	
Pyrazinamide	+		+	
Pyrimethamine	+		+	+
Quinacrine	+			
Quinidine, quinine	+			+
Ristocetin	+			+
Salicylamide	+			+
Spironolactone			+	+
Stibophen	+		+	+
Streptomycin	+			+
Sulphamyl	+			
Sulfathiazole		+		
Sulfonamides	+	+	+	+
Sulfonylureas	+		+	+
Thiazides	+			+
Thiocarbamates	+			
Thiocyanates	+			
Thioridazine	+	+	+	+
Thiouracils	+			
Tolbutamide		+	+	+
Trimethadione	+		+	+
Trimethoprim				

Selective Agranulocytosis

In some drug toxicities, the granulocytic series alone is selectively involved. Drugs causing isolated granulocytopenia are included in Table 5-1. The morphology of the reactions to such drugs may vary, depending to some extent on the mechanisms of action of the causative drug, as well as the point in time at which the marrow is examined; usually the morphology is of little help in determining the pathophysiology. In agranulocytosis induced by immunologic methods or by drugs directly toxic to the cells, the bone marrow is usually hypocellular in the early phase and hypercellular during recovery. Examples of immune-mediated injuries are those due to aminopyrine and the pyrazoles, in which peripheral granulocytes are destroyed and the marrow precursors are also affected. With phenylbutazone, the morphologic changes in the marrow may vary from complete absence of granulocyte precursors to so-called "maturation arrest."[38] Idiosyncratic reactions involving drugs which directly interfere with cell division of the myeloid cells in susceptible individuals, such as the phenothiozines,[132] will lead to hypoplasia of the granulocytic series. Some of the more commonly used drugs, such as the phenothiozines, antithyroid drugs,[2] allopurinol,[21,56] and propranolol[122] are commonly reported to produce absence or severe hypoplasia of the marrow granulocytic cells, whereas others, such as cimetidine[86] and amodiaquine,[101] are reported to cause "maturation arrest." Dapsone is said to produce either morphologic picture.[19,125] However, it is probable that in most cases, the finding of a "maturation arrest" is related to the taking of a specimen at the early stage of recovery; care must be taken not to confuse this morphologic picture, in which myeloblasts and promyelocytes are numerous, with acute leukemia (Fig. 5-2).

Selective Thrombocytopenia

Thrombocytopenia resulting from drugs may be due to two mechanisms: (1) impaired platelet production owing to suppression of the megakaryocytic series; or (2) peripheral destruction of platelets. Usually, the latter effect is due to immune-mediated destruction of platelets, but a few drugs, such as ristocetin and probably alcohol, are directly toxic to circulating platelets. Occasionally, drugs such as

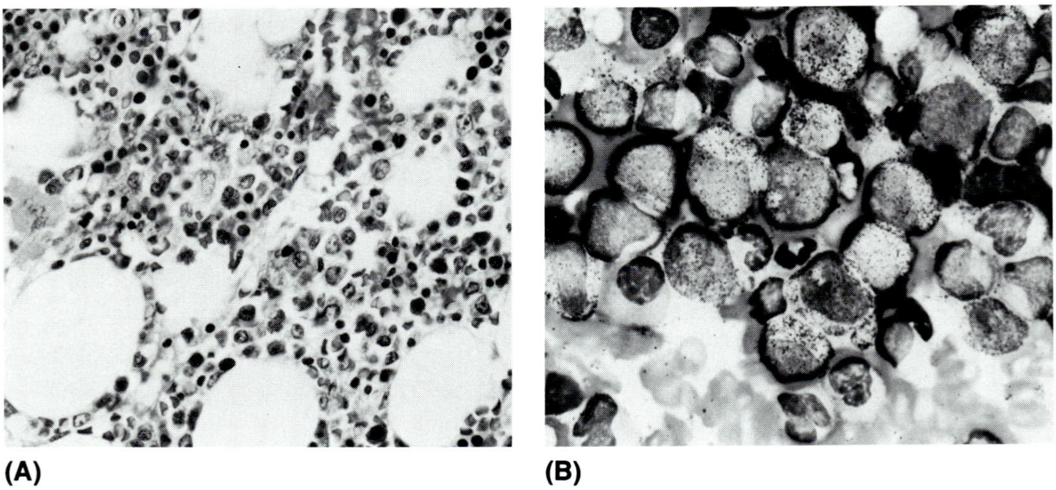

(A) (B)

Fig. 5-2. (A) Drug-induced maturation arrest showing granulocytic immaturity in bone core biopsy. H & E, × 320. (B) An aspirate from the same patient shows this maturation arrest to be predominantly at the promyelocyte stage. It can easily be mistaken for a promyelocytic leukemia. Wright-Giemsa, × 640.

the thiazide diuretics may produce thrombocytopenia through either of the preceding mechanisms, although we could find no reports of a drug leading to decreased platelets through both mechanisms simultaneously.

Drugs implicated in thrombocytopenia are listed in Table 5-1. The vast majority of drugs that lead to decreased platelet counts do so by inducing antibody formation, with ensuing destruction of platelets in the peripheral blood by the mechanisms described earlier in this chapter. Usually, the bone marrows of these patients are normal, or show megakaryocytic hyperplasia with increased numbers of immature forms.

Megakaryocytic hypoplasia or aplasia may be seen in conjunction with depression of the other cell series when cytostatic agents are used. Specific megakaryocytic hypoplasia or aplasia may be seen with a variety of drugs, as shown in Table 5-1, but the drugs most frequently producing this condition are phenylbutazone, indomethacin, gold salts, tolbutamide, chlorothiazide, hydralazine, chloramphenicol, streptomycin, sulfonamides, isoniazid, chlorpromazine, meprobamate, methylhydantoin, trimethadione, paramethadione, and estrogens.[63,162]

Evaluation of megakaryocytic numbers is not difficult if they are completely or almost completely absent, but minor deviations from normal must be carefully evaluated, since there is variation in the information available about the normal numbers of megakaryocytes per unit area of hematopoietic marrow[151]; the values of 67 megakaryocytes per 100 oil power fields (×100) in children and 40 per 100 oil power fields in the elderly seems most appropriate.[10] Many more drugs affect platelet function, but the discussion of hemorrhagic tendencies due to this type of drug-platelet interaction is beyond the scope of this chapter.

Changes Induced by Cytostatic Agents

The morphologist is presented with increasing numbers of bone marrow specimens, particularly biopsies, for evaluation of the effects and efficacy of chemotherapy for hematopoietic and nonhematopoietic malignancies. Several detailed reviews of the mechanisms of action of the cytostatic drugs are available,[33,43,78] and knowledge of the principles of how these drugs are thought to work is important. The morphologic features of the hematopoietic system in patients treated with these agents depend upon the pharmacologic action at varying points of cell maturation, as well as upon the dosage of drug given. Unfortunately, many of the studies of the biologic properties of the cytostatic drugs are derived from animal models, and the relevance of these to human marrow is, in some cases, uncertain.

Competitive inhibition of specific enzymatic activity is the basis of action of the synthetic metabolic analogues. These agents tend to be cycle-active, and therefore have a greater effect on more differentiated cells than upon their precursors. For the most part, they inhibit enzymes involved in nucleic acid synthesis, very often resulting in imbalanced DNA-RNA synthesis and megaloblastic changes. In general, they depress erythroid and myeloid elements more than platelet precursors. These drugs include the folic acid antagonist methotrexate, which, through inhibition of dihydrofolate reductase, leads to macrocytosis and megaloblastosis of red cells; bone marrow aplasia usually occurs only after large doses.[41] Depression of T-lymphocyte function and cellular depletion of lymphoid tissue also may occur after large doses of methotrexate or after chronic exposure to this agent.[9,46] Similar effects are seen with the purine analogues 6-mercaptopurine, thioguanine, and azothiaprine, which inhibit the de novo synthesis of adenine and guanine, and with the pyrimidine analogues 5-fluorouracil and floxuridine, which presumably inhibit thymidylate synthetase. Cytosine arabinoside, also a pyrimidine analogue, probably inhibits DNA polymerase.[49] Hydroxyurea inhibits the reductive conversion of ribonucleotides to deoxyribonucleotides and thereby also inhibits DNA synthesis.

Alkylating agents are compounds which form covalent linkages with a variety of biomolecules, resulting in the alkylation of electron-donating atoms such as nitrogen, sulfur, or oxygen, in proteins or nucleic acids. This may lead to single alkylations, cross-linkage, depurination, or single- or double-stranded breakage of the DNA molecule.[33] Alkylating agents may affect both resting and dividing cells, although the cytotoxicity of these agents is more evident when cells containing alkylated DNA are stimulated to divide.[43] Nitrogen mustard is the prototype of the alkylating agents, and a single injection of this drug will lead to combined reticulocytopenia, leukopenia, and thrombocytopenia; the effect occurs at both the differentiating cell level and at the multipotential stem cell. Cyclophosphamide also seems to act at the stem cell level in humans,[43] but it produces less depression of the megakaryocytes than of the erythroid and white cell precursors.[96] Busulfan demonstrates myelotoxic action primarily against granulocytic and thrombopoietic cells, and suppresses resting cells far more than dividing cells. The linkage of phenylalanine to nitrogen mustard results in a compound, melphalan, that penetrates cells active in protein synthesis.[43] Melphalan affects stem cells and differentiating cells similarly, and has a predilection for plasma cells. Chlorambucil and bischloroethylnitrosourea (BCNU) are also alkylating agents.

The vinca alkaloids, vinblastine and vincristine, impair the synthesis of microtubules, and hence inhibit mitosis.[32,33,49] These agents inhibit actively dividing cells because of the importance of the microtubles to spindle formation. White cells are the cells most severely affected[65] by the vinca alkaloids. Erythroid suppression is usually mild and transient with vinblastine, and even less marked with vincristine; thrombopoiesis may even be stimulated by certain dosages of these drugs.[96,144]

Of the antibiotics tested in cancer chemotherapy, actinomycin D, daunorubucin, and Adriamycin are the most frequently used. Each binds to DNA, causing inhibition of template function.[43,131] Actinomycin D is particularly toxic to erythroid cells, and may cause a specific blockade of erythropoietin-induced stem-cell differentiation.[139] Although actinomycin D is not cycle-dependent, cells in active proliferation are very vulnerable to it. Daunorubicin and Adriamycin have severe stem-cell suppressive effects; Adriamycin tends to produce more severe leukopenia than thrombocytopenia.[96] Another antibiotic, bleomycin, causes very little hematopoietic suppression.[43]

In addition to the hypoplasia and depression of the marrow elements and the megaloblastic changes described above, additional morphologic changes are often seen in the marrows of patients treated with the cytostatic agents, particularly when the cancer being treated is a hematopoietic neoplasm involving the bone marrow. Necrosis of the bone marrow has been reported in patients receiving cancer chemotherapy. In an autopsy study of 66 cases, Brown[16] felt that chemotherapy with cytostatic agents was a contributing factor to the presence of necrosis in 8 patients, 5 of whom, however, had underlying bone-marrow malignancy. Others have also reported bone-marrow necrosis following intensive chemotherapy for lymphoma[108] and leukemia.[82,185] However, this finding is probably a very uncommon sequel to chemotherapy, and since necrosis demonstrated in antemortem material is most frequently associated with a malignancy involving the bone marrow, a careful search for malignant tissue should be made before attributing the necrosis to cytostatic agents. Osteonecrosis and necrosis of adjacent bone marrow have also been reported following glucocorticoid therapy in conjunction with chemotherapy.[166]

Exudation of fibrin without an accompanying cellular infiltrate, referred to as "fibrinous myelitis" (Fig. 5-3), has been reported as a common finding in the marrows of patients given chemotherapy for cancer.[151,161] Wittels,[185] however, was unable to confirm that the exuded substance was fibrin. In a sequential study of 15 patients with leukemia, he

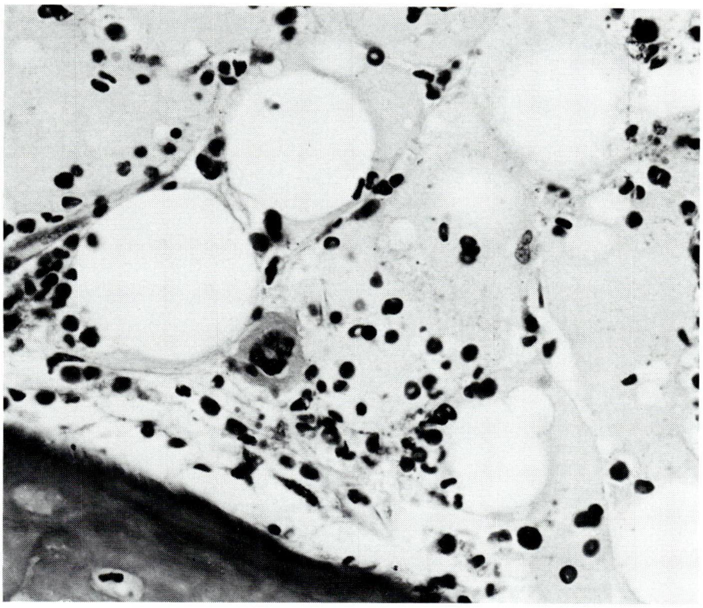

Fig. 5-3. Chemotherapy-induced fibrinous myelitis. The fat cells are separated and the marrow is hypocellular and replaced by edema and fibrin. H & E, × 440.

found that the changes occurring after chemotherapy could be demarcated into a phase of cellular depletion, usually lasting 2 to 4 weeks after the initiation of therapy, during which time there was a progressive emptying of the marrow with accentuation of the underlying reticulin stroma and dilatation of fibrin-filled sinusoids. A second phase of marrow reconstitution appeared during the next 5 to 10 weeks, during which time the intertrabecular spaces were refilled by a proliferation of hematopoietic cells and a generation of fat cells, collagen, and bone. However, although Wittels and others[151, 161] described scarring and fibrosis as possible sequelae to chemotherapy, it should again be emphasized that the underlying disease may produce similar changes, and that scarring and fibrosis should only be cautiously attributed to chemotherapy. In a patient with malignant lymphoma or carcinoma, areas of fibrosis in the marrow are an indication for the taking of multiple, deeper sections to rule out the presence of tumor.

Stromal hemorrhage, serous atrophy of the fat, and a plasmacytosis and lymphocytosis[10, 185] may also occur following cancer chemotherapy. Although there is some variation according to which drug is used, a marrow that is regenerating after chemotherapy will show erythroid replacement first, followed by granulocytic and megakaryocytic activity (Fig. 5-4).

Malignant hematopoietic neoplasms, particularly acute nonlymphocytic leukemia, may be a complication developing after the use of cytostatic agents.

Hemolytic Anemia

Drug-induced hemolytic anemias may be grouped into two distinct categories on the basis of their pathogenesis. In one group, an underlying, genetically determined biochemical abnormality predisposes the red cells to the hemolytic action of drugs or their metabolites. The most common defect in this group is a hereditary enzymopathy, such as G-6-PD deficiency, which results in hemolysis when a G-6-PD-deficient cell is exposed to a variety of oxidant drugs. Aminoquinolones, sulfones, sulfonamides, nitrofurans, and analgesics such as aspirin, phenacetin, and acetanilid are the

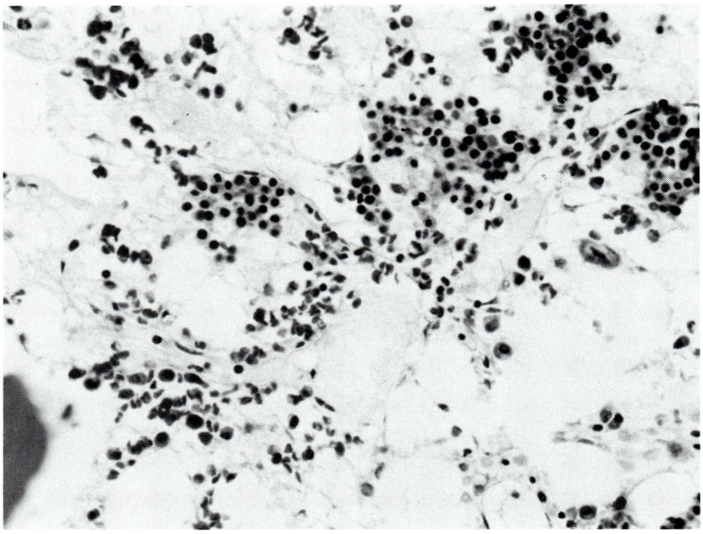

Fig. 5-4. Regenerating bone marrow after cytotoxic chemotherapy. Clones of erythroid precursors are the best evidence of regeneration. Fibrinous myelitis is still present in the hypocellular areas. H & E, × 265.

most frequent offenders. In the second large group of hemolytic anemias due to drugs, the pathogenesis is immune in nature. Within this subdivision, a variety of fundamental mechanisms exist, as already outlined in this chapter. Drugs producing immune hemolytic anemia include para-aminosalicylic acid, isoniazid, rifampicin, quinidine, quinine, phenacetin, pyramidon, dipyrone, sulfonamides, penicillin, cephalosporin, methyldopa, mefenamic acid, insulin, and stibophen.

Generally, there is erythroid hyperplasia in the bone marrow of patients with drug-induced hemolytic anemia, and often increased megakaryocytic and granulocytic precusors as well. If hemolysis is intravascular, there is hemosiderinuria with depletion of iron stores; whereas if hemolysis is extravascular, the bone marrow will show an increase in hemosiderin content. Details of the drug-induced hemolytic anemias, as well as more complete lists of drugs inducing hemolysis, can be found in standard texts.

Hyperplasia

Hyperplasia of the hematopoietic elements may be seen as a response to drug-induced peripheral destruction of circulating blood cells. Thus, in drug-induced thrombocytopenia due to circulating antibodies, megakaryocytic hyperplasia may be found, and in drug-related hemolytic anemias, erythroid hyperplasia may be seen. In addition, during the recovery phase of marrow hypoplasia, one or more hyperplastic cell lines may be found. However, some drugs may stimulate blood cell production, with a resulting hyperplasia of specific cells. This effect is, for these drugs, not a toxic action, but one from which the pharmacologic benefit of the drug may be derived.

Lithium is known to produce granulocytosis and granulocytic hyperplasia in the bone marrow.[55, 61, 63, 97, 172] The site of action of lithium is probably on the CFU-S,[97] although an enhancement of colony-stimulating factor (CSF) has also been demonstrated.[61, 64] This property of lithium is useful in the attenuation of myelosuppression due to drug therapy.[20, 55, 172]

The effects of some hormones are also stimulating to hematopoiesis. Androgens lead to increased erythroid activity, although granulopoiesis and, to a lesser extent, thrombopoiesis may be stimulated as well.[77] Androgens may exert their action on the erythroid elements by increasing erythropoietin levels,[3, 47] as well as by triggering hematopoietic stem cells into the cell cycle, and increasing the number of stem cells undergoing erythroid differentiation.[117, 159] There is some data to the effect that androgens may also increase endogenous CSF production, but other factors may also be operative here.[45] Glucocorticoids enhance granulopoietic activity, but prolonged doses may well suppress both erythroid and megakaryocytic proliferation.[36, 143] Evidence exists that the beneficial effect of glucocorticoids sometimes seen in patients with hypoplastic states may be due to inhibition of corticol-sensitive T-lymphocytes capable of suppressing granulopoiesis.[5]

A group of patients with persistent pancytopenia but with hyperplastic bone marrows has been described[156]; in some of these the abnormality was attributed to drug therapy. Chloramphenicol, sulfonamides, phenylbutazone, meprobamate, phenacetin, dipyrone, streptomycin, librium, penicillin, and codeine were among the drugs implicated. These patients exhibited hyperplasia of both the myeloid and erythroid series, with "shifts to the left" in each series; however, whether these patients' hematologic disorders were truly drug-related, or whether they represented a broader group of myeloproliferative disorders is unclear. Panhyperplasia with sideroblastic changes has been described with pyrazinoic acid amide therapy,[106] and sideroblastic anemias with hyperplastic bone marrows have been reported with other antituberculous drugs as well.[176]

The panhyperplasia associated with evolving, acute nonlymphocytic leukemia secondary to cytostatic drug therapy is described in the section on neoplasia.

Cytologic Atypia

The most common drug-induced cytologic abnormality is probably megaloblastic change. Megaloblastosis is the morphologic result of relatively slow DNA synthesis in relation to relatively normal RNA synthesis. Any drug that can inhibit DNA synthesis may cause megaloblastosis; Table 5-2 shows the most common of these. Caution should be used, however, before ascribing all megaloblastic changes to the drug therapy in patients receiving medications that may cause this abnormality. For example, triamterene, a diuretic, may cause megaloblastic changes because it is a dihydrofolate reductase inhibitor; in practice, however, it rarely causes megaloblastosis unless the patient already has, or is predisposed to, low folate stores.[163]

Table 5-2. Drugs That May Induce Megaloblastic Changes

Alcohol	6-Mercaptopurine
Aminopterin	Metformin
Azathioprine	Methotrexate
Barbiturates	Neomycin
	Nitrofurantoin
Colchicine	Nitrous oxide
Contraceptive agents	
Cycloserine	Pentamidine
Cytosine arabinoside	Primidone
	Pyrimethamine
Diphenylhydantoin	
	Thioguanine
5-Fluorodeoxyuridine	Triamterene
5-Fluorouracil	Trimethoprim
Hydroxyurea	

The mechanisms responsible for drug-induced megaloblastic changes are varied. Many medications interfere with folate metabolism. Within this group, the mechanism of action of the dihydrofolate reductase inhibitors is best understood. These agents include methotrexate, pyrimethamine, triamterene, and trimethoprim.[163, 164] Less well understood is how the anticonvulsants, including the phenytoins, phenobarbital, and primidone result in megaloblastic change, which is an uncommon side effect of therapy with these medications. It is probable that these medications inhibit the intestinal absorption of folate,[164] although stimulation of microsomal enzyme activity has also been suggested.[111] Low serum folate has been found in 58 percent of patients taking diphenylhydantoin, but megaloblastic anemia actually occurs in only 0.15 to 0.75 percent of patients exposed to this drug.[85] However, macrocytosis occurs much more commonly.[54] The occasional megaloblastic anemia associated with oral contraceptive agents is probably also related to impaired folate metabolism, as are the megaloblastic anemias associated with cycloserine, metformin, isoniazid, tetracycline, nitrofurantoin, and glutethemide.[164]

A second group of drugs leading to megaloblastic change are those agents that interfere with vitamin B_{12}, usually by inhibiting its absorption. Para-aminosalicylic acid, colchicine, neomycin, metformin, phenformin, and slow-release potassium chloride preparations have been reported to have such effects.[163,164]

Drugs that interfere with purine and pyrimidine synthesis also lead to impaired DNA-RNA synthetic rates. Chief among these drugs are the cytostatic agents discussed earlier: 6-mercaptopurine, thioguanine, azathioprine, 5-fluorouracil, hydroxyurea, and cytosine arabinoside. Compounds that produce megaloblastosis through unknown mechanisms include nitrous oxide,[92,93] azulphidine, and L-asparaginase.[164]

Vacuolization of cells is another common morphologic change following toxic injury by drugs[119] (Fig. 5-5). Although chloramphenicol and alcohol are the best known examples of drugs having this effect, primaquine, colchicine, vinblastine, nitrous oxide, and pyrazinoic acid also may lead to abnormal vacuolization within the nuclei and cytoplasm of erythroid and granulocytic cells.[92] This vacuole formation is nonspecific; the vacuoles are PAS- and Sudan red-negative.[187] Injury to the plasma membrane, with internalization by endocytosis, is a possible mechanism for the production of these vacuoles.

A cytologic change commonly observed in leukemias being treated with chemotherapy is the so-called "treated blast" alteration; often, blasts or neoplastic cells in the bone marrow or peripheral blood develop a more smudged chromatin and more irregular, often pyknotic, nuclei. This is illustrated in Figure 5-6.

A variety of other drug-induced, cellular morphologic abnormalities have been described, such as the occurrence of Döhle bodies after cyclophosphamide, busulfan, chlorambucil, and nitrogen mustard treatment[174]; acquired Pelger-Huet nuclei after sulfasoxazole[80]; toxic granulation of neutro-

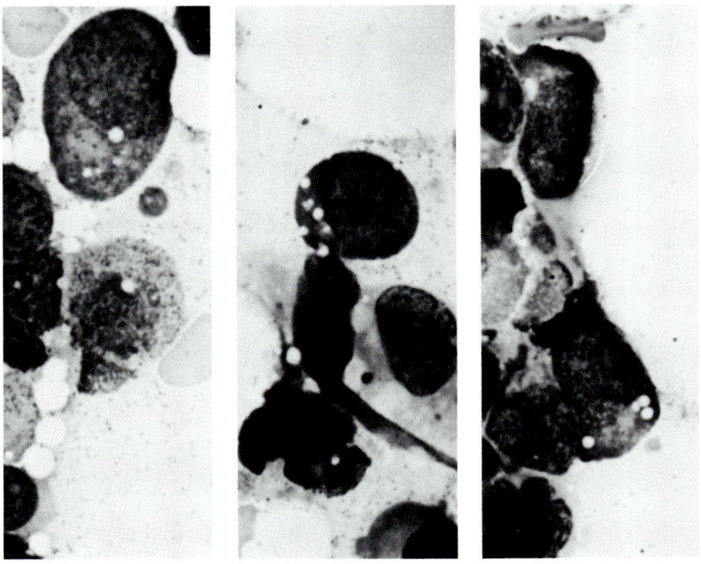

Fig. 5-5. Chloramphemicol effect is manifested by the vacuolation of the cytoplasm in the myeloid (left, right) and erythroid (center) precursors in the bone marrow aspirate composite. Wright-Giemsa, × 950.

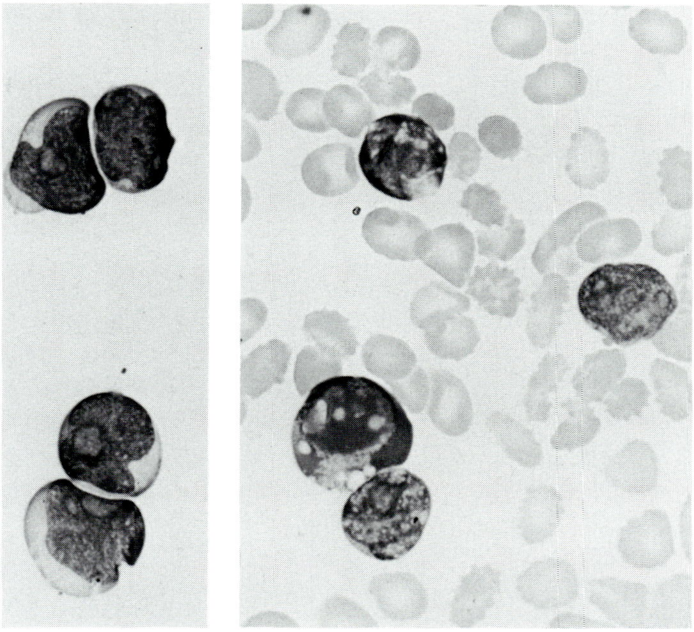

Fig. 5-6. (Left) Myeloblasts in the cerebrospinal fluid. The cells show immature nuclear chromatin and large nucleoli. (Right) After methotrexate, blasts from a repeat specimen show variable degrees of smudged nuclear chromatin and vacuolated cytoplasm. The cells are degenerating. Cytospin preparation of the cerebrospinal fluid. Wright-Giemsa, × 1,000.

phils after chloroquine; and spherocytosis of red cells after vinblastine.[75] For the most part, these changes are nonspecific and, although their occurrence may indicate serious physiologic alterations, their true significance is unknown.

Therapy-related Leukemia and Dysmyelopoietic Syndromes

The use of chemotherapy and radiotherapy for the malignant diseases has been complicated by the development of therapy-related neoplastic hematopoietic disorders, mainly acute nonlymphocytic leukemia (ANLL), as a terminal event. Treatment-related leukemias most frequently follow the use of radiotherapy or alkylating-agent chemotherapy, used singly or in combination, although potent immunosuppressive agents, such as azothioprine, have also been implicated.[159] This condition has been observed to occur in patients treated for Hodgkin's disease,[17,79,147] non-Hodgkin's lymphoma,[79] ovarian cancer,[79] breast cancer,[79] lung cancer,[79] myeloma,[8,53] and following immunosuppressive therapy in rheumatoid arthritis,[79] Sjogren's syndrome,[66] and renal transplant patients.[160]

ANLL may develop from 1.5 to 15.0 years after therapy has begun.[11,17,44,53,79,146] The relative role of the chemotherapeutic agents, radiation, and drug- or disease-related immunosuppression in this condition is not yet known. However, the finding of nonrandom chromosome abnormalities in the leukemic cells of over 95 percent of the patients developing this condition suggests that radiotherapy and chemotherapy can greatly alter the biochemical integrity of the DNA molecule.[79,149]

We had the opportunity to study serially the bone marrow aspirates, biopsies, and peripheral blood specimens of 10 patients who developed ANLL after treatment for Hodgkin's disease and non-Hodgkin's lymphoma.[175] A preleukemic period occurred in 6 of these 10 patients. This preleukemia phase was characterized by nucleated red cells, macrocytosis, marked anisopoikilocytosis of red cells, dysplastic neutrophils, basophilia, occasional myelocytes, promyelocytes, and a few blasts in the peripheral blood (Fig. 5-7). Erythroid hyperplasia with megaloblastoid features, a mild to moderate shift toward

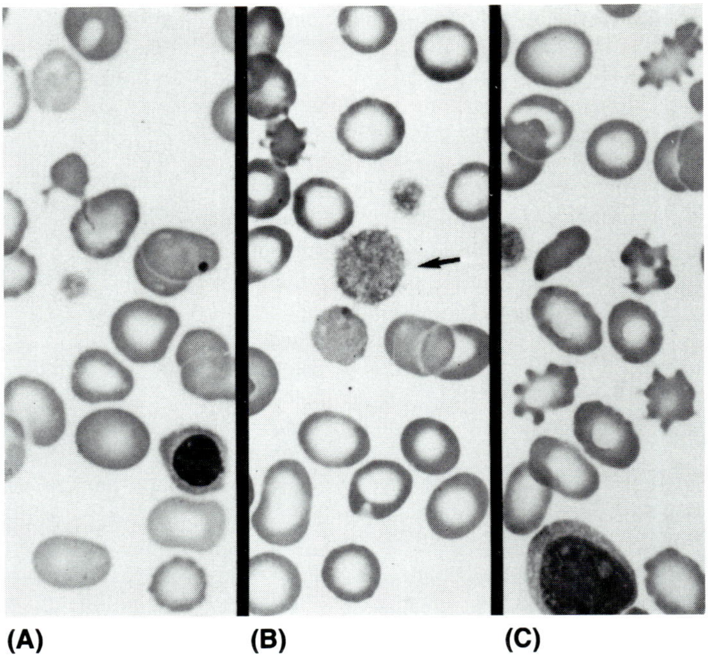

Fig. 5-7. Peripheral blood from patient treated with cytotoxic agents for Hodgkin's disease, who then developed a preleukemic phase, characterized by (A) nucleated red cells, (B) giant platelets, and (C) immature myeloid precursors. Wright-Giemsa, × 1,000. (Vardiman, J. W., Golomb, H. M., Rowley, J. D., et al.: Acute nonlymphocytic leukemia in malignant lymphoma. A morphologic study. Cancer 42:229, 1978.)

granulocytic immaturity, increased numbers of megakaryocytes with cytologic abnormalities, and increased amounts of reticulin were found in the marrow (Fig. 5-8). As overt leukemia evolved, serial marrow studies in 5 of the 6 patients showed a gradual increase in numbers of blasts and in the amount of reticulin, a decrease in the numbers of megakaryocytes, and a decrease in numbers of erythroid precursors; the sixth patient developed erythroleukemia. Two of our 10 patients had no apparent preleukemic phase, and information on 2 others was insufficient for a determination of whether there was a preleukemic period.

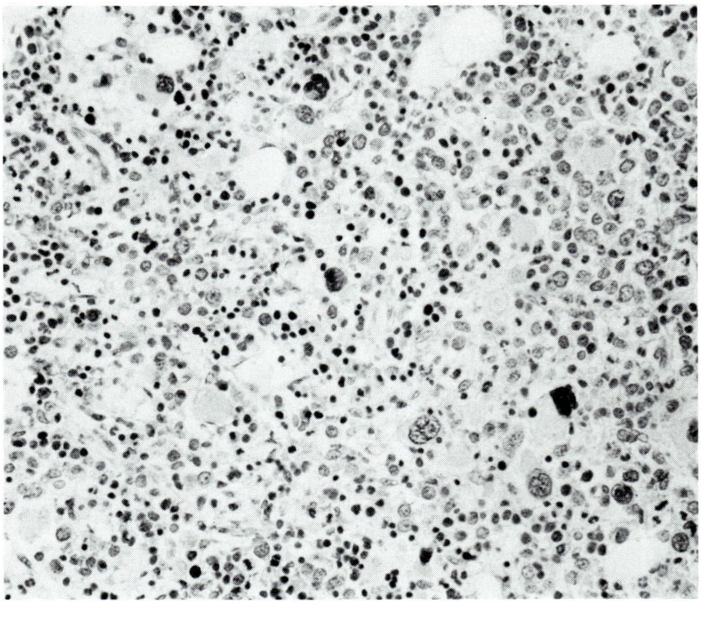

Fig. 5-8. Bone core biopsy from a patient in a preleukemic phase after therapy for non-Hodgkin's lymphoma. There is an increase in overall cellularity, with increased numbers of immature myeloid cells and megakaryocytes. The picture is that of a myeloproliferative process. H & E, × 500. (Vardiman, J. W., Golomb, H. M., Rowley, J. D., et al.: Acute nonlymphocytic leukemia in malignant lymphoma. A morphologic study. Cancer 42:229, 1978.)

The nonlymphocytic nature of the leukemic cells was confirmed by cytochemistry.

We have since expanded the number of patients studied to 21, and have made identical observations in this larger group; others have reported very similar changes.[17, 44, 79] Ringed sideroblasts have been described by some,[44] but were not a common finding in any of our patients. The bone-marrow morphologic picture described above, which, at points in the development of the leukemia, is a panmyelosis with severe dysplasia in all cell lines, appears to be a distinctive dysmyelopoietic syndrome occurring not only after therapy for lymphoma, but following therapy for other nonhematopoietic malignancies as well. Twenty of our 21 patients have had abnormal chromosomes, with a tendancy toward hypodiploidy. A loss of chromosome No. 5 and of chromosome No. 7 has been the most frequent finding.[149]

Although therapy-related leukemia occurs most frequently following treatment with cytotoxic drugs and irradiation, it may also occur after other types of therapy. Phenylbutazone, chloramphenicol, amidopyrine, sulfonamides, and phenothiazines are among the drugs implicated.[123] In some of these cases, leukemia has developed following aplastic anemia induced by the drug. Some investigators have postulated that marrow aplasia and depression of the bone marrow induced by any toxic agent may be an important event in the development of leukemia.[27, 34]

Inflammatory Lesions

Necrosis of bone marrow and hematopoietic cells has already been discussed in conjunction with the cytostatic agents used for cancer therapy, but we again urge caution before ascribing marrow necrosis to drugs. When necrosis is present, multiple sections may be necessary to rule out the presence of metastatic tumor or a primary hematopoietic malignancy. Glucocorticoid therapy has been implicated in bone necrosis[166] and in bony lytic lesions, probably due to the stimulation of fatty growth in the marrow cavity.[182] Alcohol may also be associated with marrow necrosis.[124]

Granulomata have been described with a variety of medications; diphenylhydantoin,[186] procainamide,[142] chlorpropamide,[141] and allopurinol[151] are among the drugs implicated. The granulomata have been poorly circumscribed, noncaseating, associated with few to many eosinophils, and may be the result of a localized antigen-antibody reaction. These drug-induced granulomata appear to differ from the lesion described as an eosinophilic fibrohistiocytic lesion by Rywlin et al.[152] The eosinophilic fibrohistiocytic lesion is also thought to be due to drug hypersensitivity, but consists of collections of cells characterized by regular, oval- to spindle-shaped nuclei with an indistinct, amphophilic cytoplasm. Many eosinophils are found with these cells, often forming eosinophilic abscesses. In some instances, these are associated with lymphoid nodules (type I), are perivascular (type II), or are perisinusoidal (type III). Ampicillin, allopurinol, and procainamide were responsible for the reported cases.

It is important not to confuse granulomata and the eosinophilic fibrohistiocytic reaction with the lesion of angioimmunoblastic lymphadenopathy (AILD) in the bone marrow. In some cases, it has been suspected that AILD represents a drug hypersensitivity reaction. In the marrow, AILD appears as an ill-defined, space-occupying lesion with increased numbers of lymphocytes, plasma cells, immunoblasts, histiocytes, and eosinophils, in a fibrovascular background[126] (Fig. 5-9).

EFFECT OF ALCOHOL ON THE HEMATOPOIETIC SYSTEM

Alcohol is such a commonly abused drug, with such diverse effects on the hematopoietic system, that a separate section is warranted for the description of ethanol toxicity. The mechanisms by which alcohol induces hematopoietic disease are multiple, and vary from

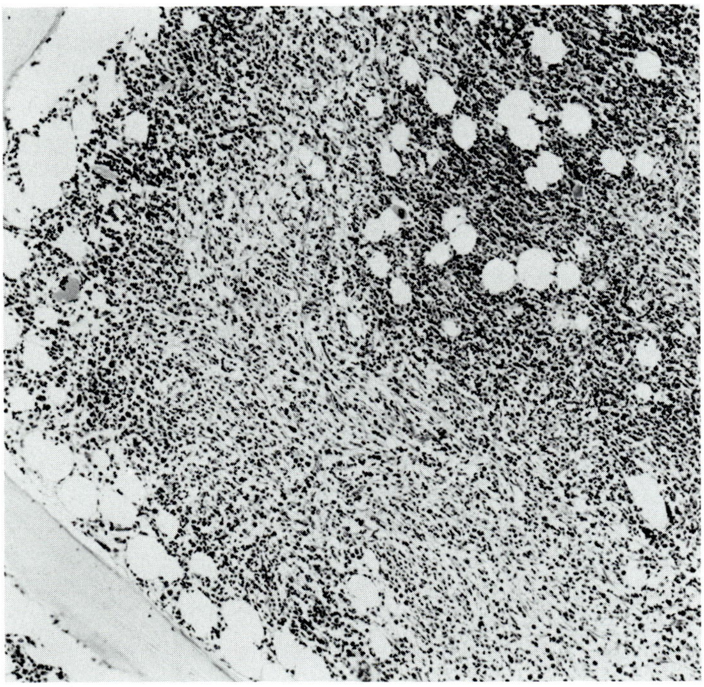

(A)

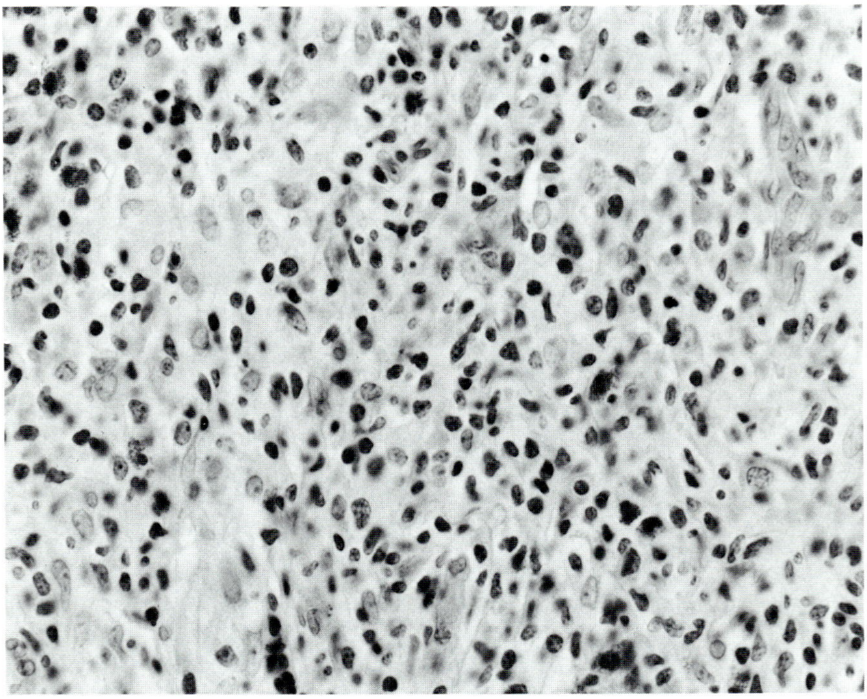

(B)

Fig. 5-9. (A) Bone core biopsy from a patient with angioimmunoblastic lymphoadenopathy. The biopsy shows an area of fibrosis and focal obliteration of normal bone marrow architecture, with a proliferation of lymphocytes, histiocytes, immunoblasts, and eosinophils. H & E, × 100. (B) Higher power showing a polymorphic infiltrate consisting of lymphocytes, histiocytes, immunoblasts, and eosinophils. H & E, × 500.

patient to patient, depending upon the quantity and duration of alcohol intake, the supplemental dietary habits of the patient, and the status of the liver. In addition to the direct toxic effects of ethanol and its metabolites on blood cells, the complicating effects of altered folate metabolism, altered plasma lipids and protein concentrations, loss of iron from hemorrhage, development of sideroblastic anemia, splenic enlargement with blood cell sequestration, the hemodilution of cirrhosis, and chronic infections contribute to the final morphology observed in the bone marrow and peripheral blood. At times, one of these factors may mask the influence of another, so that unraveling the complex nature of a hematopoietic disturbance in an individual patient may be difficult.

Anemia is probably the most common hematologic finding in the alcoholic patient. Its cause depends, to some extent, upon the acuteness of the situation. The sequence of events in acute alcoholism has been described[28, 40] as being initiated by a phase of rapidly declining serum folic acid levels, which is greater than would be expected from dietary deficiency alone, followed by megaloblastic conversion of the marrow within a week of onset of the alcoholic binge. Shortly after the megaloblastosis develops, ringed sideroblasts may be observed, perhaps due either to pyridoxine deficiency or to an intracellular enzyme defect. If the drinking stops and the patient recovers dietary intake, the megaloblastosis will disappear, and a phase of erythroid hyperplasia with reticulocytosis will develop. McCurdy et al.[113, 114] were the first to describe the vacuolation of erythroid precursors, most pronounced in the pronormoblast, that occurs with acute alcohol ingestion. Although similar to the vacuolation seen after chloramphenicol toxicity, the vacuolation present in ethanol ingestion differs from the former in being associated with the presence of continuing stages of red cell maturation, whereas that with chloramphenicol is usually associated with a maturation arrest in the erythroid series. The vacuoles usually disappear within 1 week after ethanol intake has stopped. The presence of macrocytosis without corresponding megaloblastic change is also a well known feature in alcoholic patients, but its nature has not been adequately explained.

Chronic alcoholic patients develop anemia for a variety of reasons. If there is liver disease, then blood loss, hemolysis, diminished red cell production, or a combination of these factors may contribute to the lowered red cell mass. Cooper[29] details three separate hemolytic syndromes occurring in alcoholic patients who have developed chronic liver disease. One is a mild, chronic hemolysis associated with peripheral blood spherocytes and target cells, probably resulting from congestive splenomegaly. The second is a more acute process, associated with hypertriglyceridemia and a fatty liver (Zieve's syndrome), probably associated with acute splenic congestion and splenic hemolysis. Severe hemolysis associated with spur cells (bizarrely spiculated red cells) is the third syndrome, and is due to an abnormality of red cell membrane cholesterol content resulting from abnormal plasma lipoprotein metabolism.

Diminished red cell production is common in both acute and chronic alcoholism. It may be due to impairment of folic acid metabolism, but may also be due to decreased iron stores if the patient has been bleeding. The presence of both of these factors simultaneously may obscure the typical morphologic features that would be seen if either folic acid deficiency or iron deficiency existed alone. Frequently, in the chronic alcoholic patient, the bone marrow is hypoplastic. Although protein deprivation may play a role in this hypoproliferative state, the exact mechanism by which it comes about is unknown.[28] Marrow necrosis has also been described,[124] but may be due to complicating factors, such as infection.

Granulocytopenia may occur in up to 10 percent of patients with acute alcoholism, and may occur in chronic alcoholism as well.[103] The finding of decreased granulocytes in the marrow of alcoholic patients, as well as the observation that in vitro exposure of human bone marrow cells to alcohol suppresses the growth of granulocyte colonies, suggest that ethanol may inhibit granulocytic production.[103] Of course, the complicating factors of folate deficiency, infection, and splenomegaly may also influence granulocyte production. The effect of alcohol on the survival of neutrophils in the vascular compartment is unknown.

Lymphopenia is present in most alcoholic patients with leukopenia[103]; the thymus-derived lymphocytes may be the most severely affected lymphocytes.[105] Alcohol suppresses the blastogenic transformation of lymphocytes.[173]

Inhibitory effects of alcohol on platelet production, survival, function, and structure have also been demonstrated.[32] It is probable that ethanol leads directly to ineffective thrombopoiesis, whether the alcoholic patient is folic-acid-depleted or not. Megakaryocyte numbers are not usually decreased in alcoholic patients—in fact, the total megakaryocytic mass may be increased.[30]

THE REACTION OF THE LYMPHOID SYSTEM TO DRUGS

Drug toxicity affecting the cells of the immune system is less well studied than the adverse effects of drugs on other blood cells. This is probably because aplastic anemia, agranulocytosis, thrombocytopenia, and hemolytic anemias are so dramatic in their presentation as life-threatening events, and because of the relative ease with which they may be studied. That less is known about the reaction of the lymphoid system to drugs is ironic, since many of the mechanisms whereby drugs injure hematopoietic tissue are immune-mediated. With the advent of recent techniques to separate and study subsets of lymphocytes, such as T and B cells, knowledge about drug-lymphocytic interactions will accumulate rapidly.

Perhaps the best known drug interaction with the lymphoid system is the effect of the glucocorticoids on lymphocyte numbers and function. The responses of lymphocytes to steroids are believed to be mediated by specific receptor molecules in the cytoplasm and nucleus of these cells.[155,184] Exposure of certain classes of lymphocytes to steroids leads to lysis of the lymphocytes, with a reduction in the amount of lymphoid tissue and in the lymphocyte count. T lymphocytes appear more susceptible to steroid lysis than do B cells; it is the T-zone area of peripheral lymphoid tissue that is most depleted following steroid therapy.[31] Within the human T-cell population, at least two subsets of cells exist with respect to their surface receptors.[60] One group comprises the Tμ cells, which have surface receptors for IgM, and which perform helper activities for the differentiation of B-lymphocytes into immunoglobulin-secreting plasma cells. T cells in the second group have surface receptors for IgG, are known as Ty cells, and appear to inhibit B-cell differentiation. Tμ cells appear more resistant to steroid-induced lysis and other effects than do Ty cells.[59]

B cells appear less susceptible than T cells to the effects of glucocorticoids, although suppression of immunoglobulin production may occur after steroid treatment. The latter effect may occur because induction of cells into the B-differentiation pathway is susceptible to steroid interference.[31] Mature, immunoglobulin-secreting cells are relatively resistant to steroids.[23] The earliest progenitor cells of the T- and B-cell system are evidently resistant to the glucocorticoids, since restoration of the lymphocyte areas occurs within a short time after steroid withdrawal.

Aspirin has been shown to inhibit lymphocyte transformation at the therapeutic levels commonly achieved with this drug.[35] This interference with lymphocyte function may well be one mechanism by which aspirin exerts its beneficial anti-inflammatory effects.

In general, chemotherapeutic agents used for the treatment of cancer lead to depressed lymphocyte function and an apparent alteration in lymphocyte numbers and distribution. Lymphopenia accompanies almost any stressful situation, and follows almost all varieties of chemotherapy.[78] Whether this lymphopenia is a result of a decrease in lymphocyte production or an increase in lymphocyte destruction, or is merely the result of a redistribution in tissue, is not really known. However, because of the inhibition of cell proliferation, it would be expected that immune responses requiring mitotic division of lymphocytes would be impaired, and since some cell proliferation is probably required in most immune responses, chemotherapy seriously suppresses the patient's immune-response capacity.

Diminished lymphoid tissue in the lymph nodes and spleen following cytostatic agent therapy would be expected, and in general this is true. Slavin and associates[161] detailed the changes in the lymph node and spleen following cyclophosphamide therapy. Moderately severe lymphoid depletion was present within the first 3 to 10 days after the therapy was begun; the splenic follicles also showed lymphoid depletion. Erythrophagocytosis, focal hemorrhages, and fibrin deposition were evident. This is the usual morphologic pattern seen in most chemotherapeutic regimens for malignancies. On the other hand, Irey[72] reports a case of a patient receiving methotrexate for exfoliative dermatitis who developed generalized lymphadenopathy with marked lymphoid hyperplasia.

Another drug that has been demonstrated to affect lymphoid cells is diphenylhydantoin, but there are conflicting reports concerning the mechanism of its action in this respect. An inverse correlation between serum drug levels and absolute lymphocyte counts has been observed in patients treated with diphenylhydantoin, and inhibition of DNA synthesis in lymphocytes from patients with a known hypersensitivity to this drug has been reported,[107] but opposite effects of diphenylhydantoin have been observed by others.[133] Whether one class of lymphocytes is selectively involved is not known. Abnormalities in immunoglobulin synthesis, particularly IgA synthesis, have been described in patients receiving long-term diphenylhydantoin therapy.[58]

Drug-induced Lymphadenopathy

Lymph node enlargement as a reaction to drugs is relatively common, and as a manifestation of idiosyncratic hypersensitivity reactions, is often associated with fever, urticaria or skin rashes, and atypical lymphocytes and eosinophilia in the peripheral blood. Nevertheless, since lymph node biopsies are not done in most cases of drug-induced lymphadenopathy, the histologic changes induced by many drugs are unknown. Some drugs, however, cause such severe reactions in selected patients that the clinical picture of malignant lymphoma is simulated, and biopsies in these patients have led to the description of well-defined clinicopathologic entities. The lymph node changes seen in patients receiving anticonvulsant therapy are the best known, although similar changes may be seen after sulfonamide and antibiotic therapy, phenylbutazone, indomethacin, and acetaminophen.[18, 168]

Dilantin-induced lymphadenopathy is characterized histologically by varying degrees of effacement of the normal lymph node architecture and by a pleomorphic cellular reaction consisting of immunoblasts, lymphocytes in varying stages of transformation, plasma cells, eosinophils, and neutrophils (Fig. 5-10). Foci of necrosis are common, and mitotic figures may be quite prominent; fibrosis is not a prominent feature. Diffuse hypergammaglobulinemia may be present; some patients may show hypogammaglobulinemia. Often the bone marrow shows a lymphoplasmacytic infiltrate and numerous eosinophils[26, 154] (Fig. 5-11). These effects of diphenylhydantoin are usually reversible when the drug is withdrawn.

However, diphenylhydantoin is also among the drugs implicated in the development of another abnormal immune response, angioimmunoblastic lymphadenopathy (AILD). This syndrome, characterized by generalized lymphadenopathy, hepatosplenomegaly, skin rash, Coomb's-positive hemolytic anemia, and polyclonal hypergammaglobulinemia,

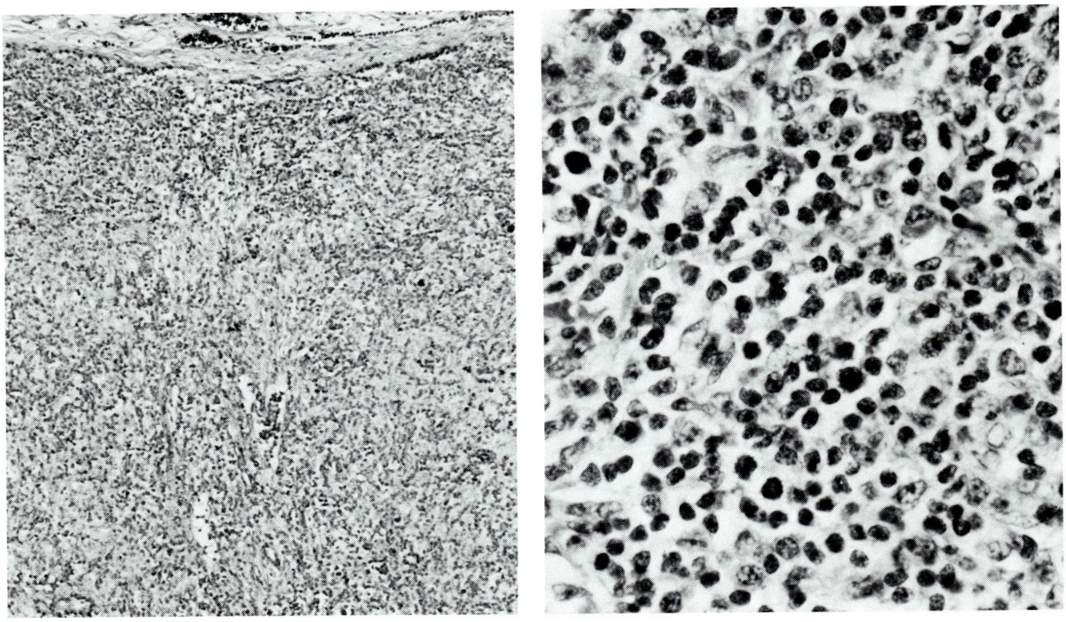

(A) **(B)**

Fig. 5-10. (A) Lymph node biopsy from diphenylhydantoin-induced lymphoadenopathy shows partially obliterated architecture without capsular infiltrate. H & E, × 100. (B) Higher magnification of the diphenylhydantoin-affected lymph node shows a diffuse proliferation of lymphocytes, immunoblasts, plasma cells, and histiocytes. H & E, × 500.

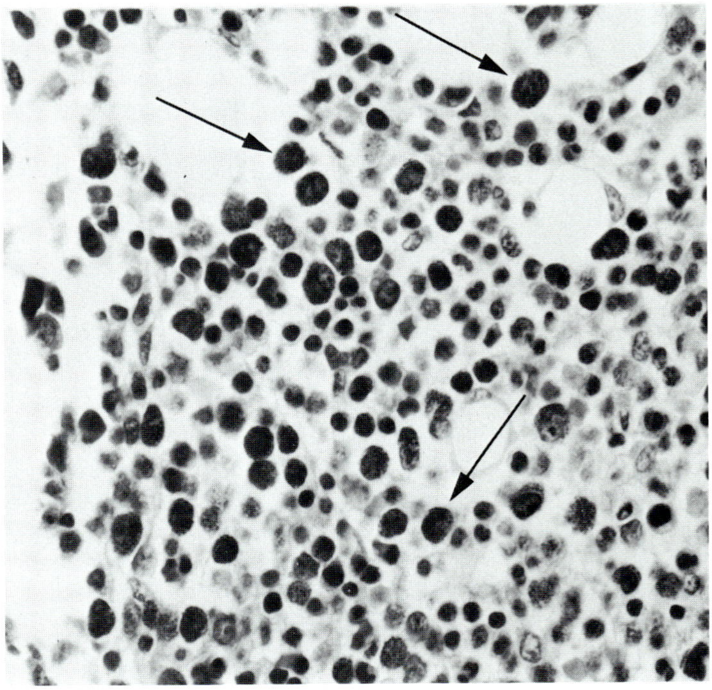

Fig. 5-11. Bone core biopsy from diphenylhydantoin-treated patient with lymphadenopathy. The most striking features are an increased number of eosinophils (arrows) and a lymphoplasmacytic infiltrate. H & E, × 500.

has gained widespread attention in recent years.[48,104,116,138] Histologically, the disease leads to obliteration of the normal lymph node architecture by a proliferation of small vessels, with a cellular infiltration of small lymphocytes, plasma cells, and numerous immunoblasts. Eosinophils and histiocytes may be present in varying numbers. An amorphous, eosinophilic, PAS-positive interstitial material is often present. Germinal centers are usually lacking or are represented as "burned out" follicles, often replaced by collections of epithelioid histiocytes (Fig. 5-12). The disorder is systemic, and the spleen and bone marrow are frequently involved. The exact nature of AILD is uncertain, but it probably represents an unregulated immune reaction to a variety of stimuli, among which may be some medications. Penicillins, sulfonamides, aspirin, halothane,[48] griseofulvin, diphenylhydantoin,[104] methyldopa,[180] and barbiturates[110,116] are among the drugs ingested by some patients prior to development of the disease. The findings of a lack of suppressor cell activity in some of these patients may indicate a specific susceptibility of certain classes of lymphocytes to the toxic action of these drugs.[12]

A variety of foreign substances used for diagnostic and therapeutic procedures, but which are not usually thought of as "drugs," may lead to lymphadenopathy. Perhaps the best recognized lymphadenopathic changes are those occurring after lymphangiography, in which the oily base of the contrast medium causes a granulomatous reaction that is most intense in the sinusoidal areas. Macrophages with ingested lipid, giant cells often surrounding large globules of oil, and eosinophils are the characteristic cells of the lymphangiogram effect. Neutrophils may be present for the first several days after the diagnostic procedure.[39]

Silicone is used in a variety of surgical techniques, and the silicone fluid may be absorbed and carried in the lymph to regional lymph nodes, where a marked histiocytic and granulomatous reaction may develop in the sinusoids and paracortical areas of the nodes. The silicone particles are highly refractile, do not polarize, and may be found surrounded by the inflammatory reaction or ingested by the histiocytic cells.[22,83]

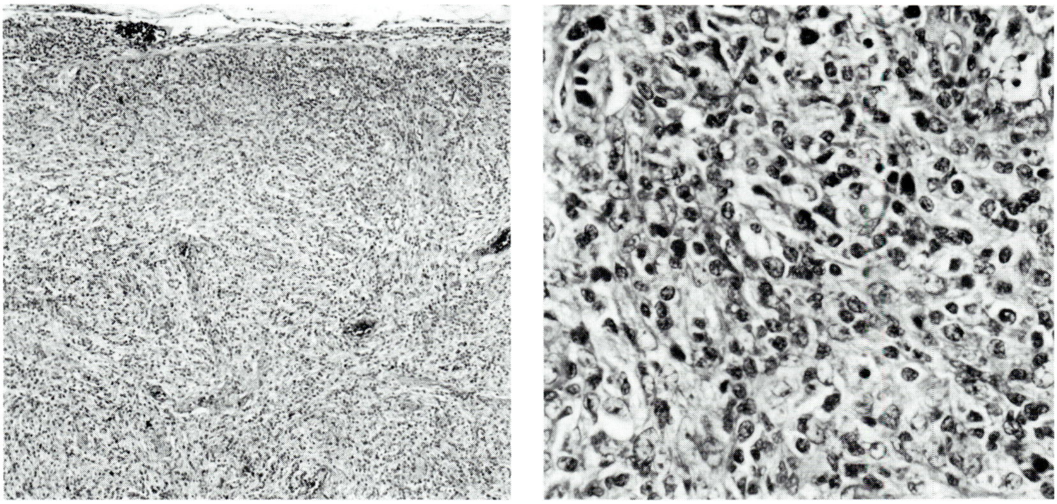

(A) **(B)**

Fig. 5-12. (A) Lymph node biopsy from a patient with angioimmunoblastic lymphadenopathy. The nodal architecture is effaced, showing a proliferation of blood vessels. H & E, × 75. (B) Higher power view of (A) shows a polymorphic proliferation of lymphocytes, many immunoblasts, some plasma cells, and eosinophils. H & E, × 365.

Drug-induced Changes in the Spleen

Very little information is available concerning histologic changes in the spleen following drug therapy. The changes seen after cancer chemotherapy have been mentioned in an earlier section; these consist primarily of loss of the lymphoid tissue of the spleen. After cyclophosphamide therapy, for example, lymphoid depletion is complete by 3 weeks, and transient myelopoiesis is sometimes observed in the depleted white pulp area of the spleen.[161] Hemorrhages, erythrophagocytosis, hemosiderin-laden histiocytes, and leukophagocytosis are commonly observed in the red pulp areas after cytostatic drug therapy.

Depletion of lymphoid tissue also occurs in the spleen following glucocorticoid therapy,[36] and lipid-laden histiocytes may also be encountered after such therapy.[72]

The lymphoid component of the spleen may react in exactly the same manner as described for other lymphatic organs when exposed to a variety of medications, such as diphenylhydantoin. Angioimmunoblastic lymphadenopathy frequently leads to an enlarged spleen,[48] and may represent one example of the type of response possible by the splenic white pulp.

Drugs that induce thrombocytopenia or hemolytic anemia through immune mechanisms may lead to secondary changes in the red pulp of the spleen, since the removal of antibody-coated red cells and platelets occurs by the splenic macrophages.

Malignant Lymphoma Following Drug Therapy

It is well-known that the incidence of malignancy is increased in patients who are being treated with agents that suppress the immune system; lymphoproliferative tumors show the greatest increase[68, 109, 129] in this group of patients.

Outside of the immunosuppressive and cytostatic agents, few other drugs have been implicated in the development of lymphoma with, of course, the exception of diphenylhydantoin. In some patients who exhibit diphenylhydantoin-induced lymphadenitis, there appears to develop a more malignant process. At present, the older literature concerning this development is probably not totally relevant, since the histologic picture of angioimmunoblastic lymphadenopathy, which may also be diphenylhydantoin-induced, may have been confused with Hodgkin's disease or other malignant lymphomas. (On the other hand, if the instances of immunoblastic sarcoma evolving in patients with AILD related to drug therapy are considered, the incidence of therapy-related lymphoma may be even greater.) Li and associates[100] considered the problem of diphenylhydantoin-induced lymphoma from a slightly different prespective, and found that of 516 patients with Hodgkin's disease or non-Hodgkin's lymphoma, 8 (1.6 percent) had a history of prolonged diphenylhydantoin ingestion, as compared with 3 (0.6 percent) of 516 patients with other cancers, and 2 (0.4 percent) of 516 tumor-free individuals. Their data suggests a small excess risk of lymphoma after prolonged diphenylhydantoin therapy. Non-Hodgkin's lymphoma is reported with greater frequency than Hodgkin's disease following diphenylhydantoin therapy.[71, 100]

EFFECTS OF IRRADIATION ON THE HEMATOPOIETIC SYSTEM

Ionizing irradiation has a profound effect on the hematopoietic and lymphoid systems, resulting in the destruction of lymphocytes and in suppression of blood cell development.

Much of the current information in the literature regarding the effects of irradiation on the bone marrow has been derived from animal studies or from clinical studies of patients being treated for various malignancies. Since animal models do not always translate into meaningful data for human beings, and since variability in dose, duration of exposure, and ports of delivery may vary from clinical study to clinical study, there is a surprising lack of detailed knowledge of what pathology to expect with therapeutic dosages of irradiation.

In classic studies by Knospe et al.[87, 88, 89] x-irradiation to a rat femur led to destruction of hematopoietic activity within 4 days, but at 2 weeks, hematopoiesis was restored because of "seeding" by hematopoietic stem cells from nonirradiated areas. Two months later, however, the marrow was again aplastic, evidently because of loss of the microcirculation due to the delayed death of vascular elements. Destruction of the microcirculation does not permit repopulation of the bone marrow. With 2,000 rads of irradiation, the rat femur showed dilatation of sinusoids, extravasation of erythrocytes, and pigment-laden macrophages. Restoration of hematopoietic activity began at 7 days, but disappeared again at 2 months; at 1 year, hematopoiesis was present but sparse. Similar but more severe changes were seen after 4,000 rads and, at 1 year, only rare foci of hematopoiesis were found. Although there was some increase in reticulin, diffuse fibrosis was not present. Massive amounts of fibrous tissue, interspersed with areas of fat, occurred only with very large doses of irradiation—such as 10,000 rads—to the rat femur.

Similar effects are found in human patients following therapeutic irradiation. The normal cellular elements are replaced by loose, edematous connective tissue, in which scattered islands of hematopoiesis are observed. Normoblasts tend to be reduced earlier than granulocytic precursors, although both are equally affected by 1 week.[95] The sinusoids became dilated and prominent, and moderate eosinophilia or plasma cell infiltration may be seen. Hemosiderin deposits may be heavy.[178] In our experience, fibrosis does not occur with the usual dosages of radiation used for therapeutic purposes. The presence of fibrosis in a marrow biopsy from a patient who has received radiotherapy for a malignancy should be suspected as being due to infiltrating tumor rather than to the irradiation.

Although initial peripheral blood counts may reflect the marrow damage, routine peripheral counts are unreliable in assessing the true status of bone marrow reserve following radiotherapy; there is no correlation between the return of the peripheral blood counts to normal and the return or repopulation of bone marrow to a functional status after radiation-induced suppression.[150] The length of time required for the marrow to return to normal, if ever, depends upon the total number of rads given and the amount of marrow exposed; the age of the patient is also important—the younger the patient the better the regeneration.[153] There is evidence of partial to complete return of function by 1 year in 50 percent of patients receiving radiation at dose levels of 4,000 rads, with this figure increasing to 80 percent at 2 to 3 years.[128, 150, 153]

Lymphoid tissue appears to be even more susceptible to radiation injury than the hematopoietic cells of the bone marrow. Early degeneration of the germinal centers is seen within hours after the irradiation of lymph nodes in animals. Swelling of the node, with congestion and edema, occurs, and lymphocyte pyknosis and destruction is progressive over the next several days; similar changes occur in the spleen.[178] The long-term effects of radiation on lymphoid tissue depend upon many factors, primarily the dose and duration of treatment. Irradiated nodes may be repopulated if the dose is small, but atrophy and fibrosis occur at higher doses. Hoppe and associates found that after regional irradiation, absolute lymphopenia, with suppression of both T and B cells, occurred and persisted in many patients 3 years or more following the completion of radiotherapy. On the other hand, total nodal irradiation was followed by an initial lymphopenia, with a persistent T-lymphopenia and B-lymphocytosis.[69] $T\mu$ cells are more sensitive than Ty cells to irradiation.[59]

The occurrence of nonlymphocytic leukemia following exposure to ongoing radiation and after combination radiotherapy and chemotherapy has been well described, and has been discussed in another section of this chapter. It is apparent that non-Hodgkin's lymphomas may also develop, probably as a consequence of therapy, in patients who have received both irradiation and chemotherapy for other malignancies; the relative role of the radiotherapy in these patients is not known at this time.[91] Although there are conflicting reports, a recent, well-controlled study[102] found no statistically significant increase in the development of leukemia with the radiation doses commonly used for diagnostic tests.

REFERENCES

1. Ackroyd, J. F.: The pathogenesis of thrombocytopenia purpura due to hypersensitivity with Sedormid. Clin. Sci. 7:249, 1949.
2. Aku, Y., & Yunis, A.: Antithyroid therapy and leukocytes. In: Dimitrov, N., & Nodine, J. eds.: Drugs and Hematologic Reactions. p. 249. Grune & Stratton, New York, 1974.
3. Alexanian, R., Vaughn, W. K., & Reichelman, M. W.: Erythropoietin excretion in man following androgens. J. Lab. Clin. Med. 70: 777, 1967.
4. Alter, B. P., Potter, N., & Li, F.: Classification and aetiology of the aplastic anemias. Clin. Haematol. 7:431, 1978.
5. Bagby, G. C., Goodnight, S. H., Mooney, W. M., et al.: Prednisone-responsive aplastic anemia. A mechanism of glucocorticoid action. Blood 54:322, 1979.
6. Barret, A. J., Waller, E., Rosengurt, N., et al.: Amidopyrine agranulocytosis. Drug inhibition of granulocyte colonies in the presence of patient's serum. Br. Med. J. 2:541, 1975.
7. Becker, A. J., McCulloch, E. A., Siminovitch, L., et al.: The effect of differing demands for blood cell production on DNA synthesis by hematopoietic colony-forming cells of mice. Blood 26:296, 1965.
8. Bergsagel, E. D., Barley, A. J., Langley, G. R., et al.: The chemotherapy of plasma-cell myeloma and the incidence of acute leukemia. N. Engl. J. Med. 301:743, 1979.
9. Bleyer, W. A.: Clinical pharmacology of methotrexate. New applications of an old drug. Cancer 41:36, 1978.
10. Block, M.: Text-Atlas of Hematology. Lea & Febiger, Philadelphia, 1976.
11. Bloomfield, C. D., & Brunning, R. D.: Acute leukemia as a terminal event in nonleukemic hematopoietic disorders. Semin. Oncol. 3:297, 1976.
12. Bluming, A. Z., Cohen, H. G., & Saxon, A.: Angioimmunoblastic lymphadenopathy with dysproteinemia. A pathogenetic link between physiologic lymphoid proliferation and malignant lymphoma. Am. J. Med. 67:421, 1979.
13. Böttiger, L. E., Furhoff, A. K., & Holmberg, L.: Drug-induced blood dyscrasias. A ten-year material from the Swedish Adverse Drug Reaction Committee. Acta Med. Scand. 205:457, 1979.
14. Böttiger, L. E., & Westerholm, B.: Drug-induced blood dyscrasias in Sweden. Br. Med. J. 3:339, 1973.
15. Brauer, M. J., & Dameshek, W.: Hypoplastic anemia and myeloblastic leukemia following chloramphenicol therapy. Report of three cases. N. Engl. J. Med. 277:1003, 1967.
16. Brown, C. H.: Bone marrow necrosis. A study of seventy cases. Johns Hopkins Med. J. 131:189, 1972.
17. Cadman, E. C., Capizzi, R. L., & Bertino, J. R.: Acute nonlymphocytic leukemia. A delayed complication of Hodgkin's disease therapy. Analysis of 109 cases. Cancer 40:1280, 1977.
18. Castleman, B., Scully, R. E., & McNeely, B. U., eds: Case records of the Massachusetts General Hospital. Weekly clinicopathological exercises—Case 33—1972. N. Engl. J. Med. 287:349, 1972.
19. Catalano, P. M.: Dapsone agranulocytosis. Arch. Dermatol. 104:675, 1971.
20. Catane, R., Kaufman, J., Mittelman, A., et al.: Attenuation of myelosuppression with lithium. N. Engl. J. Med. 297:452, 1977.
21. Chernevich, P. M., & Bogg, D. R.: In vitro growth of granulocytic and mononuclear cell colonies from blood of normal individuals. Blood 37:131, 1971.
22. Christie, A. J., Weinberger, K. A., & Dietrich, M.: Silicone lymphadenopathy and synovitis. J.A.M.A. 237:1463, 1977.
23. Claman, H. N.: Corticosteroids and lymphoid cells. N. Engl. J. Med. 287:388, 1972.
24. Clarke, B. J., & Houseman, D.: Characterization of an erythroid precusor cell of high proliferative capacity in normal human peripheral blood. Proc. Natl. Acad. Sci. U.S.A. 74:1105, 1977.
25. Cline, M. J., & Golde, D. W.: A review and reevaluation of the histiocytic disorders. Am. J. Med. 55:49, 1973.

26. Recant, L., & Hartcroft, W. S., eds.: Clinicopathologic conference. Lymphoma or drug reaction occuring during hydantoin therapy for epilepsy. Am. J. Med. 32:286, 1962.
27. Cohen, T., & Greger, W. P.: Acute myeloid leukemia following seven years of aplastic anemia induced by chloramphenicol. Am. J. Med. 43:762, 1967.
28. Conrad, M. E., & Baron, J. C.: Anemia and iron kinetics in alcoholism. Semin. Hematol. 17:149, 1980.
29. Cooper, R. A.: Hemolytic syndromes and red cell membrane abnormalities in liver disease. Semin. Hematol. 17:103, 1980.
30. Cowan, D. H.: Effect of alcoholism on hemostasis. Semin. Hematol. 17:137, 1980.
31. Craddock, C. G., Longmire, R. L., & McMillan, R.: Production and distribution of lymphocytes and plasma cells. In: Williams, W., Beutler, E., Erslev, A., & Rundles, R. W., eds.: Hematology. p. 903. McGraw-Hill, New York, 1977.
32. Creasey, W. A.: Vinca alkaloids and colchicine. In: Sartorelli, A. C. & Johns, D. G., eds.: Anti-neoplastic and Immunosuppressive Agents II. p. 670. Springer-Verlag, Berlin, 1975.
33. Creasey, W. A., Withers, H. R., & Casarett, G.: Basic Mechanisms. Cancer (Suppl.) 37:999, 1976.
34. Cronkite, E. P.: Evidence for radiation and chemicals as leukemogenic agents. Arch. Environ. Health 3:297, 1961.
35. Crout, J. E., Hepburn, B., & Ritts, R. E.: Suppression of lymphocyte transformation after aspirin ingestion. N. Engl. J. Med. 292:221, 1975.
36. David, D. S., Grieco, M. H., & Cushman, P.: Adrenal glucocorticoids after twenty years. A review of their clinically relevant consequences. J. Chron. Dis. 22:637, 1970.
37. de Gruchy, G. C.: Drug-induced Blood Disorders. Blackwell Scientific Publications, Oxford, 1975.
38. Dimitrov, N. V., Faix, J. D., & Ellegaard, J.: Leukocytes and phenylbutazone. In: Dimitrov, N. & Nodine, J., eds.: Drugs and Hematologic Reactions. p. 223. Grune & Stratton, New York, 1974.
39. Dominok, G. W.: Die histologischen Veränderungen menschlicher Lymphknoten nach Lymphographien. Virchows Arch. Pathol. Anat. 338:143, 1964.
40. Eichner, E. R., & Hellman, R. S.: The evolution of anemia in alcoholic patients. Am. J. Med. 50:218, 1971.
41. Ernest, D., & Kellmann, S. A.: Perturbation of generation cycle of human leukemic myeloblasts in vivo by methotrexate. Blood 38:689, 1971.
42. Erslev, A.: Pathophysiology of aplastic anemia. In: Dimitrov, N. & Nodine, J., eds.: Drugs and Hematologic Reactions. p. 65. Grune & Stratton, New York, 1974.
43. Erslev, A.: Chemotherapy and erythropoiesis. In: Brodsky, K., Kahn, S., & Conroy, J., eds.: Cancer Chemotherapy III. p. 287. Grune & Stratton, New York, 1978.
44. Foucar, K., McKenna, R. W., Bloomfield, C. D., et al.: Therapy-related leukemia. A panmyelosis. Cancer 43:1285, 1979.
45. Francis, G. E., Berney, J. J., Batemen, S. M., et al.: The effect of androstanes on granulopoiesis in vitro and in vivo. Br. J. Haematol. 36:501, 1977.
46. Freeman-Narrod, M., & Narrod, S. A.: Chronic toxicity of methotrexate in mice. J. Natl. Cancer Inst. 58:735, 1977.
47. Fried, W., & Gurney, C. W.: The erythropoietic stimulating effects of androgens. Ann. NY. Acad. Sci. 149:356, 1968.
48. Frizzera, G., Moran, E. M., & Rappaport, H.: Angio-immunoblastic lymphadenopathy. Diagnosis and clinical course. Am. J. Med. 59:803, 1975.
49. Furth, J., & Cohen, S. S.: Inhibition of mamalian DNA polymerase by the 5′-triphosphate of 1-beta-d-arabinofuranosylcytosine and the 5′-triphosphate of 9-beta-d-arabinofuranoxyladenine. Cancer Res. 28:2061, 1968.
50. Gerdwood, P. H.: The effects of drugs on the blood. In: Hanson, G. C., ed.: Adverse Effects of Drugs. p. 79. Beecham Research Laboratories, London, 1971.
51. Golde, D. W., Burgaleta, C., Sparkes, R. S., et al.: The Philadelphia chromosome in human macrophages. Blood 49:367, 1977.
52. Golde, D. W., Finley, T. N., & Cline, M. J.: Production of colony-stimulating factor by human macrophages. Lancet 2:1397, 1972.
53. Gonzalez, F., Trujillo, J. M., & Alexanian, R.: Acute leukemia in multiple myeloma. Ann. Intern. Med. 86:440, 1977.
54. Gordon, R. L., & Kahn, S. B.: Hematologic effects of anti-convulsant drugs. In Dimitrov, N. & Nodine, J., eds.: Drugs and Hematologic

Reactions. p. 155. Grune & Stratton, New York, 1974.
55. Greco, F. A., Brereton, H. D., & Pomeroy, T.: Lithium carbonate alteration of neutropenia from cancer chemotherapy. Proc Am. Ass. Chemotherapy Radiotherapy—Am. Soc. Clin. Oncologists 17:256, 1976.
56. Greenberg, M. S., & Zambrano, S. S.: Aplastic agranulocytosis after allopurinol therapy. Arthritis Rheum. 15:413, 1972.
57. Gregory, C., & Eaves, A. C.: Human marrow cells capable of erythropoietic differentiation in vitro. Definition of three erythroid colony responses. Blood 49:855, 1977.
58. Grob, P. J., & Herold, G. E.: Immunological abnormalities and hydantoins. Br. Med. J. 2:561, 1972.
59. Gupta, S., & Good, R. A.: Subpopulations of human T lymphocytes. II. Effects of thymopoietin, corticosteroids, and irradiation. Cell. Immunol. 34:10, 1977.
60. Gupta, S., & Good, R. A.: Markers of human lymphocyte subpopulations in primary immunodeficiency and lymphoproliferative disorders. Semin. Hematol. 17:1, 1980.
61. Gupta, S. C., Robinson, W. A., & Kurnick, J. E.: Felty's syndrome. Effect Felty's syndrome. Effect of lithium on granulopoiesis. Am. J. Med. 61:29, 1976.
62. Gussoff, B. D.: Chloramphenicol-induced hematopoietic depression. A controlled comparison with tetracycline. Am. J. Med. Sci. 251:8, 1966.
63. Gynn, T. N., Messmore, H. L., & Friedman, I. A. Drug-induced thrombocytopenia. Med. Clin. North Am. 56:65, 1972.
64. Harker, W. G., Rothatein, G., & Clarkson, D.: Enhancement of colony stimulating activity production by lithium. Blood 49:263, 1977.
65. Harrington, W. J.: Iatrogenic disorders from cancer treatment. Adv. Intern. Med. 24:141, 1979.
66. Hochberg, M. C., & Shulman, L. E.: Acute leukemia following cyclophosphamide therapy for Sjogren's syndrome. Johns Hopkins Med. J. 142:211, 1978.
67. Hoffman, R., Zanjani, E. S., Lutton, J. D., et al.: Suppression of erythroid-colony formation by lymphocytes from patients with aplastic anemia. N. Engl. J. Med. 296:10, 1977.
68. Hoover, R., & Fraumeni, J. F.: Risk of cancer in renal transplant recipients. Lancet 2:55, 1973.
69. Hoppe, R. T., Fuks, Z. Y., Strober, S., et al.: Long term effects of radiation on T and B lymphocytes in the peripheral blood after regional irradiation. Cancer 40:2071, 1977.
70. Howell, A., Andrews, T. M., & Watts, R. W.: Bone-marrow cells resistant to chloramphenicol in chloramphenicol-induced aplastic anaemia. Lancet 1:65, 1975.
71. Hyman, G. A., & Sommers, S. C.: Development of Hodgkin's disease and lymphoma during anticonvulsant therapy. Blood 28:416, 1966.
72. Irey, N. S.: Adverse reactions to cytostatic agents. Recent Results Cancer Res. 52:36, 1975.
73. Iscove, N., & Sieber, F.: Erythroid progenitors in mouse bone marrow detected by macroscopic colony formation in culture. Exp. Hematol. 3:32, 1975.
74. Iscove, N., Sieber, F., & Winterhalter, K. M.: Erythroid colony formation in cultures of mouse and human bone marrow. Analysis of the requirement for erythropoietin by gel filtation and affinity chromatography on agarose-Conervalin A. J. Cell. Physiol. 83:309, 1974.
75. Jacob, H., Amsden, T., & White, J.: Membrane microfilaments of erythrocytes. Alteration in intact cells reproduces the heriditary spherocytosis syndrome. Proc. Natl. Acad. Sci. U.S.A. 69:471, 1972.
76. Jepson, J. H.: Hypoplastic anemia. Pathophysiology and therapy. Med. Clin. North Am. 57:1079, 1973.
77. Jiji, R. M., Gangarosa, E. J., & DeLaMacorra, F.: Chloramphenicol and its sulfamoye analogue. Report of reversible erythropoietic toxicity in healthy volunteers. Arch. Intern. Med. 111:70, 1963.
78. Joyce, R. & Boggs, D.: Chemotherapy and leukokinetics. In: Brodsky, I., Kahn, S., & Conroy, J., eds.: Cancer Chemotherapy III. p. 297. Grune & Stratton, New York, 1978.
79. Kapadia, S. B., Krause, J. R., Ellis, L. D., et al.: Induced acute nonlymphocytic leukemia following long-term chemotherapy. A study of 20 cases. Cancer 45:1315, 1980.
80. Kaplan, J. M., & Barrett, O.: Reversible pseudo Pelger-Huet anomaly related to sulfisoxazole therapy. N. Engl. J. Med. 277:421, 1967.

81. Kelton, J. C., Mold, N. & Huang, A.: Quinidine-associated pancytopenia and marrow aplasia as demonstrated in marrow culture. Blood (Suppl.) 50:229, 1978.
82. Kiraly, J. F., & Wheby, M. S.: Bone marrow necrosis. Am. J. Med. 60:361, 1976.
83. Kircher, T.: Silicone lymphadenopathy. Hum. Pathol. 11:240, 1980.
84. Kirtland, H. H., Mohler, D. N., & Horwitz, D. A.: Methyldopa inhibition of suppressor-lymphocyte function. A proposed cause of autoimmune hemolytic anemia. N. Engl. J. Med. 302:825, 1980.
85. Klipstein, F. A.: Subnormal serum folate and macrocytosis associated with anti-convulsant drug therapy. Blood 23:68, 1964.
86. Klotz, S. A., & Kay, B. F.: Cimetidine and agranulocytosis. Ann. Intern. Med. 88:579, 1978.
87. Knospe, W. H., Blom, J., & Crosby, W. H.: Regeneration of locally irradiated bone marrow. I. Dose dependent, long-term changes in the rate, with particular emphasis upon vascular and stromal reaction. Blood 28:398, 1966.
88. Knospe, W. H., Blom, J., & Crosby, W. H.: Aplastic anemia. Dependence of function on structure in the bone marrow. Blood 30:851, 1967.
89. Knospe, W. H., Blom, J., & Crosby, W. H.: Regeneration of locally irradiated bone marrow. II. Induction of regeneration in permanently aplastic medullary cavities. Blood 31:400, 1968.
90. Knospe, W. H., & Crosby, W. H.: Aplastic anemia. A disorder of the bone-marrow sinusoidal microcirculation rather than stem-cell failure? Lancet 1:20, 1971.
91. Krikorian, J. G., Burke, J. S., Rosenber, S. A., et al.: Occurrence of non-Hodgkins lymphoma after therapy for Hodgkins disease. N. Engl. J. Med. 300:452, 1979.
92. Kripke, B. J., Talarico, L., Shah, N. K., et al.: Hematologic reaction to prolonged exposure to nitrous oxide. Anesthesiology 47:342, 1977.
93. Lancet. Nitrous oxide and the bone-marrow. Lancet 2:613, 1978.
94. LeBien, T. W., Hozier, J., Minowada, J., et al.: Origin of chronic myelocytic leukemia in a precursor of pre-B lymphocytes. N. Engl. J. Med. 301:144, 1979.
95. Lehar, T. J., Kiely, J. M., Pease, G. L., et al.: Effect of local irradiation on human bone marrow. Am. J. Roentgenol. 96:183, 1966.
96. Levin, J.: Chemotherapy and thrombopoiesis. In: Brodsky, K., Kahn, S., & Conroy, J., eds.: p. 313. Cancer Chemotherapy III. Grune & Stratton, New York, 1978.
97. Levitt, L. J., & Quesenberry, P. J.: The effect of lithium on murine hematopoiesis in a liquid culture system. N. Engl. J. Med. 302:713, 1980.
98. Lewis, S. M.: Abnormal erythropoiesis. In Hoffbrand, A. V., & Lewis, S. M., eds.: Haematology. p. 92. Heinemann, London, 1972.
99. Li, F. P., Alter, B. P., & Nathan, D. G.: The mortality of acquired aplastic anemia in children. Blood 40:153, 1972.
100. Li, F. P., Willard, D. R., Goodman, R., et al.: Malignant lymphoma after diphenylhydantoin (Dilantin) therapy. Cancer 36:1359, 1975.
101. Lind, D. E., Levi, J. A., & Vincent, P. C.: Amodiaquine-induced agranulocytosis. Toxic effect of amodiaquine in bone marrow cultures in vitro. Br. Med. J. 1:458, 1973.
102. Linos, A., Gray, J. E., Orvis, A. L., et al.: Low-dose radiation and leukemia. N. Engl. J. Med. 302:1101, 1980.
103. Liu, Y. K.: Effects of alcohol on granulocytes and lymphocytes. Semin. Hematol. 17:130, 1980.
104. Lukes, R. J., & Tindle, B. H.: Immunoblastic lymphadenopathy. A hyperimmune entity resembling Hodgkins disease. N. Engl. J. Med. 292:1, 1975.
105. Lundy, J., Raaf, J. H., Deakins, S., et al.: The acute and chronic effects of alcohol on the human immune system. Surg. Gynecol. Obstet. 141:212, 1975.
106. MacCurdy, R. K., & Simon, E. R.: Thrombocytopenia and sideroblastic anemia with pyrazinoic acid amide (Pyrazinamide) therapy. Chest 57:378, 1970.
107. MacKinney, A. A., & Booker, H. E.: Diphenylhydantoin effects on human lymphocytes in vitro and in vivo. Arch. Intern. Med. 129:988, 1972.
108. Mason, B. A., Klug, P. P., & Cohen, P.: Bone marrow necrosis during chemotherapy for lymphoma. J.A.M.A. 239:1158, 1978.
109. Matas, A. J., Hertel, B. F., Rosai, J., et al.: Post-transplant malignant lymphoma. Dis-

tinctive morphologic features related to its pathogenesis. Am. J. Med. 61:716, 1976.

110. Matz, L. R., Papadimitriou, J. M., Carroll, J. R., et al.: Angioimmunoblastic lymphadenopathy with dysproteinemia. Cancer 40:2152, 1977.

111. Maxwell, J. D., Hunter, S., Stewart, D. A., et al: Folate deficiency after anti-convulsant drugs. An effect of hepatic enzyme induction? Br. Med. J. 1:297, 1972.

112. McCulloch, E. A., Siminovitch, L., & Till, J. E.: Spleen-colony fomation in anemic mice of genotype WW^v. Science 144:844, 1964.

113. McCurdy, P. R., Pierce, L. E., & Rath, C. E.: Abnormal bone-marrow morphology in acute alcoholism. N. Engl. J. Med. 266:505, 1962.

114. McCurdy, P. R., & Roth, C. E.: Vacuolated nucleated bone marrow cells in alcoholism. Semin. Hematol. 17:100, 1980.

115. Metcalf, D.: In vitro cloning techniques for hemapoietic cells. Clinical applications. Ann. Intern. Med. 87:483, 1977.

116. Moore, S. B., Harrison, E. G., & Weiland, L. H.: Angioimmunoblastic lymphadenopathy. Mayo Clin. Proc. 51:273, 1976.

117. Moreyama, J., & Fisher, J. W.: Effects of testosterone and erythropoietin on erythroid colony formation in rabbit bone marrow culture. Life Sci. 15:1181, 1974.

118. Morley, A., Trainor, K., & Remes, J.: Residual marrow damage. Possible explanation for idiosyncrasy to chloramphenicol. Br. J. Haematol. 32:525, 1976.

119. Mullick, F. G., Drake, R. M., & Irey, N. S.: Morphologic changes in adverse drug reactions in infants and children. Hum. Pathol. 8:361, 1977.

120. Nagoa, T., & Mauer, A. M.: Concordance for drug-induced aplastic anemia in identical twins. N. Engl. J. Med. 281:7, 1969.

121. Nathan, D. G., Chess, R., Hellerman, D. G., et al.: Human erythroid burst-forming unit (BFU-E). T-cell requirement for proliferation in vitro. J. Exp. Med. 147:324, 1978.

122. Nawabi, I. U., & Ritz, N. D.: Agranulocytosis due to propranolol. J.A.M.A. 223:1376, 1973.

123. Nieweg, H. O.: Drug-induced diseases as seen by a haematologist. In Meyler, L. & Peck, P., eds.: Drug Induced Disease, Vol. 4. p. 325. Excerpta Medica Foundation, Amsterdam, 1972.

124. Norgard, M. J., Carpenter, J. T., & Conrad, M. E.: Bone marrow necrosis and degeneration. Arch. Intern. Med. 139:905, 1979.

125. Ognibene, A. J.: Agranulocytosis due to dapsone. Ann. Intern. Med. 72:521, 1970.

126. Pangalis, G. A., Moran, E. M., & Rappaport, H.: Blood and bone marrow findings in angioimmunoblastic lymphadenopathy. Blood 51:71, 1978.

127. Parkman, R.: The immunopathology of marrow failure. Clin. Haematol. 7:475, 1978.

128. Parker, R. G., & Berry, H. C.: Late effects of therapeutic irradiation on the skeleton and bone marrow. Cancer 7:1162, 1976.

129. Penn, I.: The incidence of malignancies in transplant recipients. Transplant Proc. 7:323, 1975.

130. Perry, S.: Appraisal of myelopoiesis. N. Engl. J. Med. 4:214, 1971.

131. Pigram, W. J., Fuller, W., & Hamilton, L. D.: Stereochemistry of intercalation. Interaction of daunocycin with DNA. Nature 235:17, 1972.

132. Pisciotta, A.: The effect of chlorpromazine on peripheral leukocytes. In Dimitrov, N. & Nodine, J., eds.: Drugs and Hematologic Reactions. p. 233. Grune & Stratton, New York, 1974.

133. Pruzanki, W.: Lymphadenopathy associated with dysgammaglobulinemia. Semin. Hematol. 17:44, 1980.

134. Quagliana, J. M., Cartwright, G. E., & Wintrobe, M. M.: Paroxysmal nocturnal hemoglobinuria following drug-induced aplastic anemia. Ann. Intern. Med. 61:1045, 1964.

135. Quesenberry, P., & Levitt, L.: Hematopoietic stem cells (First of three parts). N. Engl. J. Med. 14:755, 1979.

136. Quesenberry, P., & Levitt, L.: Hematopoietic stem cells (Second of three parts). N. Engl. J. Med. 15:819, 1979.

137. Quesenberry, P., & Levitt, L.: Hematopoietic stem cells (Third of three parts). N. Engl. J. Med. 16:868, 1979.

138. Radaszkiewicz, T., & Lennert, K.: Lymphogranulomatosis X. Kliniscnes bild, therapie und prognose. Dtsch. Med. Wochenschr. 100:1157, 1975.

139. Reissmann, K. R., & Ito, K.: Selective eradication of erythropoiesis by actinocycin D as the result of interference with hormonally controlled effector pathway of cell differentiation. Blood 28:201, 1966.

140. Richman, C. M., Chess, L., & Yankee,

R. A.: Purification and characterization of granulocytic progenitor cells (CFU-C) from human peripheral blood using immunologic surface markers. Blood 51:1, 1978.
141. Rigberg, L. A., Robinson, M. J., & Espiritu, C. R.: Chlorpropamide-induced granulomas. A probable hypersensitivity reaction in liver and bone marrow. J.A.M.A. 235:409, 1976.
142. Riker, J., Baker, J., & Swanson, M.: Bone marrow granulomas and neutropenia associated with procainamide. Report of a case. Arch. Intern. Med. 138:1731, 1978.
143. Robbin, G. P., Cooper, J. A., & Alt, H. L.: Effect of corticotropin on cellularity and mitosis in rate bone marrow, spleen, and thymus. Endocrinology 56:161, 1955.
144. Robertson, J. H., Crozier, E. H., & Woodend, B. E.: Vincristine-induced thrombocytosis studied with ^{75}Si selenomethionine. Acta. Haematol. 47:356, 1972.
145. Rosenszajn, L. A., Shoham, D., & Kalechmar, I.: Clonal proliferation of DNA stimulated lymphocytes in soft agar culture. Immunology 29:1041, 1975.
146. Rosner, F., & Grunwald, H.: Hodgkins disease and acute leukemia. Report of eight cases and review of the literature. Am. J. Med. 58:339, 1975.
147. Rosse, W.: Paroxysmal nocturnal hemoglobinuria in aplastic anemia. Clin. Haematol. 7:541, 1978.
148. Rowley, J. D.: A new consistent chromosomal abnormality in chronic myelogenous leukemia identified by quinacrine fluorescence and Giemsa staining. Nature 243:290, 1973.
149. Rowley, J. D., Golomb, H. M., & Vardiman, J.: Nonrandom chromosomal abnormalities in acute nonlymphocytic leukemia in patients treated for Hodgkin disease and non-Hodgkin lymphomas. Blood 50:759, 1977.
150. Rubin, P., Landman, S., Mayer, E., et al.: Bone marrow regeneration and extension after extended field irradiation in Hodgkins disease. Cancer 32:699, 1973.
151. Rywlin, A.: Histopathology of the Bone Marrow. Little, Brown & Co., Boston, 1976.
152. Rywlin, A. M., Hoffman, E. P., & Ortega, R. S.: Eosinophilic fibrohistiocytic lesion of bone marrow. A distinctive new morphologic finding, probably related to drug hypersensitivity. Blood 40:464, 1972.
153. Sacks, E. L., Goris, M. L., Glatstein, E., et al.: Bone marrow regeneration following large field radiation. Cancer 42:1057, 1978.
154. Saltzstein, S. L., & Ackerman, L. V.: Lymphadenopathy induced by anticonvulsant drugs and mimicking clinically and pathologically malignant lymphomas. Cancer 12:164, 1959.
155. Schaumberg, B. D., & Bojeson, E.: Specificity and thermodynamic properties of the corticosteroid binding to a receptor on rate thymocytes in vitro. Biochim. Biophys. Acta. 170:172, 1968.
156. Schiller, M., Rachmilewitz, E. A., & Izak, G.: Panytopenia with hypercellular hemopoietic tissue. Isr. J. Med. Sci. 5:69, 1969.
157. Schulman, N. R.: A mechanism of cell-destruction in individuals sensitized to foreign antigen and its implications in auto-immunity. Ann. Intern. Med. 60:506, 1964.
158. Schulman, N. R.: Immunologic reactions to drugs. N. Engl. J. Med. 287:400, 1972.
159. Shadhidi, N. T.: Androgens and erythropoiesis. N. Engl. J. Med. 289:72, 1973.
160. Silvergleid, A. J., & Schrier, S. L.: Acute myelogenous leukemia in two patients treated with azathioprine for nonmalignant disease. Am. J. Med. 57:885, 1974.
161. Slavin, R. E., Milan, J. C., & Mullins, G. M.: Pathology of high dose intermittent cyclophosphamide therapy. Hum. Pathol. 6:693, 1975.
162. Slichter, S. J., & Harker, L. A.: Thrombocytopenia. Mechanisms and management of defects in platelet production. Clin. Haematol. 7:523, 1978.
163. Stebbins, R., & Bertino, J. R.: Megaloblastic anemia produced by drugs. Clin. Haematol. 5:619, 1976.
164. Stebbins, R., Scott, J., & Herbert, V.: Drug-induced megaloblastic anemia. Semin. Hematol. 10:235, 1973.
165. Stephenson, J. R., Axelrad, A. A., McLeod, D. L., et al.: Induction of colonies of hemoglobin-synthesizing cells by erythropoietin in vitro. Proc. Natl. Acad. Sci. U.S.A. 68:1542, 1971.
166. Sweet, D. L., Roth, D. G., Desser, R. K., et al.: Avascular necrosis of the femoral head with combination therapy. Ann. Intern. Med. 85:67, 1976.
167. Swisher, S., & Burke, E.: Drug reactions involving antibodies reacting with erythrocytes. In: Williams, W., Beutler, E., Erslev, A., &

Rundles, R. W., eds.: Hematology. p. 607. McGraw-Hill, New York, 1977.

168. Symmers, W. St. C.: The lymphoreticular system. In: Symmers, W. S. C., ed.: Systemic Pathology, 2nd Ed. p. 701. Churchill-Livingstone, New York, 1978.
169. Taetle, R., Lane, T. A., & Mendelsohn, J.: Drug-induced agranulocytosis. In vitro evidence for immune suppression of granulopoiesis and a cross-reacting lymphocyte antibody. Blood 54:501, 1979.
170. Tepperman, A. D., Curtis, J. E., & McCulloch, E. A.: Erthropoietic colonies in culture of human marrow. Blood 44:659, 1974.
171. TeVelde, H., & Haak, H. L.: Aplastic anaemia. Histological investigation of methacrylate embedded bone marrow biopsy specimens; correlation with survival after conventional treatment in 15 adult patients. Br. J. Med. 35:61, 1977.
172. Tisman, G.: Lithium carbonate protection against drug-induced leukopenia in lymphosarcoma patients. Histology 2:509, 1974.
173. Tisman, G., & Herbert, V.: In vitro myelosuppression and immunosuppression by ethanol. J. Clin. Invest. 52:1410, 1973.
174. Trowbridge, A. A., & Linman, J. W.: Drug-induced morphologic changes in leukocytes. In: Dimitrov, N. & Nodine, J., eds.: Drug and Hematologic Reactions. p. 199. Grune & Stratton, New York, 1974.
175. Vardiman, J. W., Golomb, H. M., Rowley, J. D., et al.: Acute nonlymphocytic leukemia in malignant lymphoma. A morphologic study. Cancer 42:229, 1978.
176. Verwilghen, R., Reybrouch, G., Collins, L., et al.: Anti-tuberculous drugs and sideroblastic anemia. Br. J. Haematol. 11:92, 1965.
177. Vogler, L. B., Crist, W. M., Vinson, P. C., et al.: Philadelphia-chromosome-positive pre-B-cell leukemia presenting as blast crisis of chronic myelogenous leukemia. Blood 54:1164, 1979.
178. Warren, S.: Effects of radiation on normal tissues. III. Effects of radiation on the blood and the hemopoietic tissues, including the spleen, the thymus and the lymph nodes. Arch. Pathol. 34:562, 1942.
179. Weisberger, A. S.: Mechanism of action of chloramphenicol. J.A.M.A. 209:97, 1969.
180. Weisenburger, D. D.: Immunoblastic lymphadenopathy associated with methyldopa therapy. A case report. Cancer 42:2322, 1978.
181. Wi, A. M., Till, J. E., Siminovitch, L., et al.: A cytological study of the capacity for differentiation of normal hematopoietic colony-forming cells. J. Cell. Physiol. 69:177, 1967.
182. Wilkenfeld, M. J., & Sliwinski, A. J.: Fatty lesions of both humeri in a patient on corticosteroids and cyclophosphamide. Arthritis Rheum. 22:199, 1979.
183. Williams, D. M., Lynch, R. E., & Cartwright, G. E.: Prognostic factors in aplastic anemia. Clin. Heamtol. 7:467, 1978.
184. Wira, C., & Muncle, A.: Specific glucocorticoid receptors in thymus cells. Localization in the nucleus and extraction of the corticol receptor complex. J. Biol. Chem. 245:3436, 1970.
185. Wittles, B.: Bone marrow biopsy changes following chemotherapy for acute leukemia. Am. J. Surg. Pathol. 4:135, 1980.
186. Wu, H. V., & Kosmin, M.: Bone-marrow granulomata and phenytoin. Ann. Intern. Med. 86:663, 1977.
187. Yeung, K. Y., Klug, P. P., Brewer, M., et al.: Mechanism of alcohol-induced vacuolization in human bone-marrow cells. Blood 42:998, 1973.
188. Yunis, A. A.: Chloramphenicol-induced bone marrow suppression. Semin. Hematol. 10:225, 1973.
189. Yunis, A. A., Arimura, G. K., Lutcher, C. L., et al.: Biochemical lesion in Dilantin-induced erythroid aplasia. J. Clin. Invest. 44:1114, 1965.
190. Yunis, A. A., Arimura, G. K., Lutcher, C. L., et al: Biochemical lesion in Dilantin-induced erythroid aplasia. Blood 30:587, 1967.

6

The Skin

Maria Medenica

INTRODUCTION

Untoward reactions to drugs are an important medical problem. However, although drug reaction may involve any organ system, cutaneous eruptions—which may result from a drug administered by any route—are recognized more often than effects in other areas because of their visibility. Untoward cutaneous drug reactions[108] can result from immunologic or nonimmunologic mechanisms. Those drug reactions that occur through nonimmunologic mechanisms may be due to activation of cell injury effector pathways, overdosage, cumulative toxicity, idiosyncratic metabolism, interactions of drugs, and drug-related ecologic disturbances. Immunologic mechanisms depend on several factors and their interaction, which may influence the capacity of a drug to elicit an immunologic response. These factors include the molecular characteristics of the drug, the host effect, and environmental influences.

The molecular characteristics of allergenic drugs are an important factor in the induction of allergic drug reactions. Most drugs are small molecules having molecular weights below 1,000, and are thus unable to elicit antibody formation. It is necessary for such small molecules (haptens) to combine with tissue macromolecules in order to induce drug-specific antibodies. But because most drugs are stable molecules, they do not easily form covalent bonds with tissue components. However, minor contaminants or reactive metabolic products of the drug may form a compound that will be able to evoke an immune response. Large molecular size and the complexity of a drug are associated with increased immunogenicity; macromolecular drugs, including proteins and carbohydrates, are antigenic without metabolic alteration or degradation. Antigenic cross-reactivity among therapeutic agents is another structural characteristic contributing to drug allergy. Host effects, including the route of administration and immunogenic load of a therapeutic agent, will influence its immunogenicity. The immunogenic load may depend on the quantity and length of drug exposure, and the individual's ability to absorb and metabolize the drug. In inbred animals, immune responses to various antigens are genetically controlled. In the human population little is known about the genetic control of immune responses, but it is likely that such control plays a role in immune drug reactions. Age may also be a contributing factor; allergic drug reactions are less common in infants and old people, probably owing to an immature or involuting immune system, respectively. Environmental factors, such as sunlight, may directly affect the host's response to a drug, or may alter the drug in such a way that it becomes an effective immunogen. Immunochemical mechanisms underlying immune drug reactions include IgE-mediated drug reactions, immune-complex-mediated drug reactions, cytotoxic drug reactions, and cell-mediated drug reactions.

There are numerous clinical forms of drug eruption, mimicking many skin diseases. Each of these eruptions can be caused by numerous pharmacologic agents, and the same drug may produce a variety of reaction patterns on the skin. In this chapter, cutaneous drug reactions are classified mainly according to their clinical appearance.

Histologic changes are usually the same in the skin diseases whether a disease appears in its idiopathic form or is drug induced. However, some histologic features are suggestive of a drug eruption; these will be described.

The following conditions will be discussed:

1. Acneiform eruptions.
2. Alopecias.
3. Pigmentary disorders induced by drugs without preceding inflammation.
4. Exanthematous-morbiliform eruptions.
5. Exfoliative dermatitis.
6. Eczematous eruptions.
7. Photosensitivity reactions.
8. Lichenoid reactions.
9. Fixed drug eruptions.
10. Urticaria.
11. Leukocytoclastic angiitis.
12. Thrombocytopenic purpura.
13. Lupus erythematousus-like eruptions.
14. Erythema nodosum.
15. Pseudolymphoma syndrome.
16. Erythema multiform and Stevens-Johnson syndrome.
17. Toxic epidermal necrolysis.
18. Pemphigus foliaceus and vulgaris.
19. Porphyria cutanea tarda.
20. Bullous lesions in comatose states.
21. Halogenodermas.
22. Coumarin-induced necrosis of the skin.
23. Skin changes induced by local pentazocine injections.
24. Skin changes induced by systemically and locally administered corticosteroids.

ACNEIFORM DRUG REACTIONS

The primary lesion of acne vulgaris is the comedo, which consists of a widened channel of follicular infundibulum which is packed with cornified cells, while the epithelium has become thinned. The pustular lesion is characterized by collections of neutrophils within the follicular infundibulum and around it. Identical lesions may be seen in women given androgenic hormones,[23] and more rarely with progesterones. Antiepileptic drugs[57] (hydantoin and trimethadione) and antituberculous drugs[33] (isoniazid, ethambutol, and ethionamide) may either aggravate existing acne or induce it; patients who are "slow inactivators" of isoniazid are predisposed to acneiform eruptions. Halogens (bromides and iodides) and lithium[77] carbonate will cause inflammation of the pilosebaceous unit. Lithium causes enlargement of the total circulating neutrophil mass, and accelerates neutrophil production without impairing neutrophil migration into skin lesions; it may even enhance neutrophil migration.[90]

Corticotropin (ACTH) and corticosteroids induce acne-like eruptions after puberty.[102] The lesions in these eruptions are usually all, synchronously, in the same stage of development, and consist of small pustules and red papules. Similar lesions are seen after prolonged application of topical corticosteroids to the face. The histopathology of steroid acne is a focal folliculitis and perifolliculitis without prominent hyperkeratinization initially.

ALOPECIAS

Drug-induced alopecia mainly affects scalp hair.[61] The growth of hair is cyclic, consisting of three phases[1]: (1) the growing phase (anagen); (2) the involuting phase (catagen); and (3) the resting phase (telogen). Hairs of the scalp, beard, and sexual regions have follicles that extend into the subcutaneous tissue (Fig. 6-1). The roots of smaller hairs are in different levels of the dermis. The hair follicle is divided into three segments (Fig. 6-2): (1) the infundibulum, which is the part of the follicle extending from the follicular orifices above to the entrance of the sebaceous gland below. (2) The isthmus, which lies between the entrance of the sebaceous gland above and the insertion of the hair erector muscle below; this area also represents the lower border of the permanent part of the hair follicle. (3) The inferior segment of the hair follicle, which represents one-half of the entire follicle. The inferior segment extends from the insertion of the hair erector muscle to the base of the follicle, and disintegrates during the catagen phase and

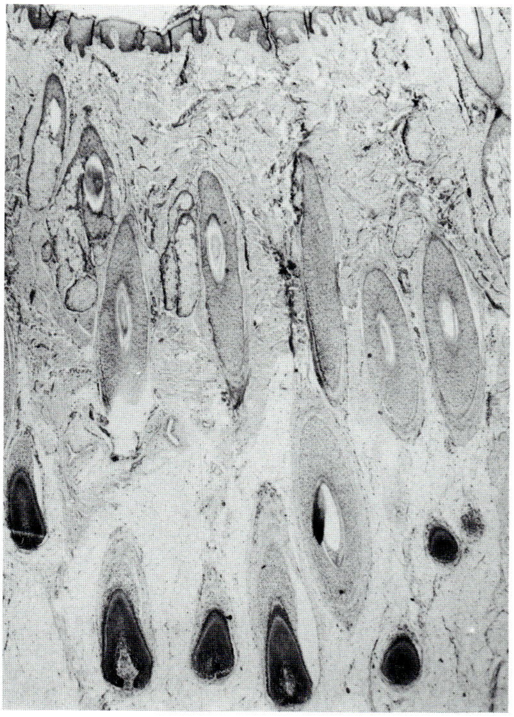

Fig. 6-1. Normal scalp hair with numerous hair follicles and their bulbs in the subcutaneous tissue. × 23.

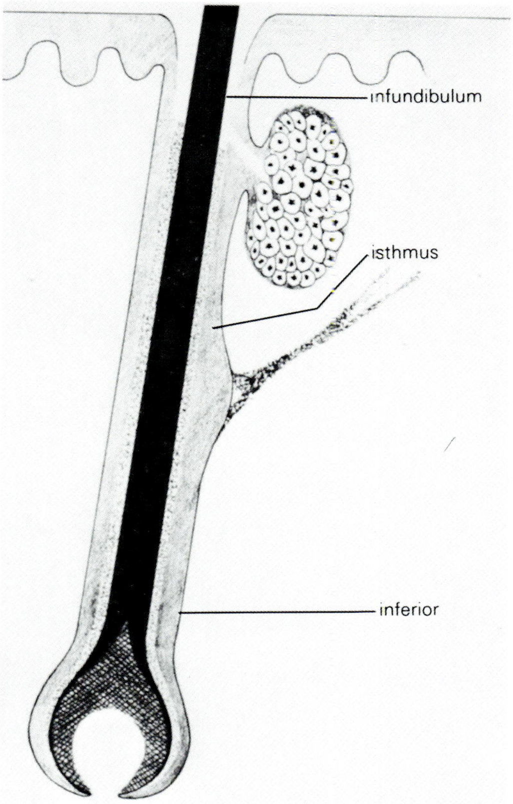

Fig. 6-2. Three segments of follicular structure: infundibulum, isthmus and inferior segment. (Ackerman, B.: Histologic Diagnosis of Inflammatory Skin Diseases. Lea and Febiger, Philadelphia, 1978.)

disappears during the telogen phase. The hair bulb, which is part of the inferior segment, encloses a small amount of vascular connective tissue called the papilla. At its distal portion, the papilla connects and becomes contiguous with the fibrous hair sheath which surrounds the entire follicle.

The hair follicle consists of the external root sheath, a continuation of the epidermis that encloses the hair itself and its internal root sheath. Between the external root sheath and the fibrous hair sheath is the glassy basement membrane of the hair follicle. In the anagen phase (Fig. 6-3) of hair growth, the follicle contains all three of the segments noted above—the infundibulum, the isthmus, and the inferior segment. During the catagen phase (Fig. 6-4), the melanocytic activity in the hair bulb ceases, and the entire inferior segment of the hair follicle becomes a narrow cord of epithelial cells. The glassy basement membrane becomes thicker, while the external root sheath retracts into a cornifying epithelial sac around the bulbous lower end of the hair shaft, creating a club hair. During the telogen phase of hair growth (Fig. 6-5), the epithelial cord becomes a small collection of undifferentiated cells, just below the epithelial sac of the club hair. The length of the hair follicle during this phase is about one-half of the length of the follicle in the anagen phase.

The anagen phase of epilated hair (Fig. 6-6A) is characterized by the presence of an external root sheath and an expanded lower portion of the hair. The telogen phase of epilated hair (Fig. 6-6B) shows the absence of

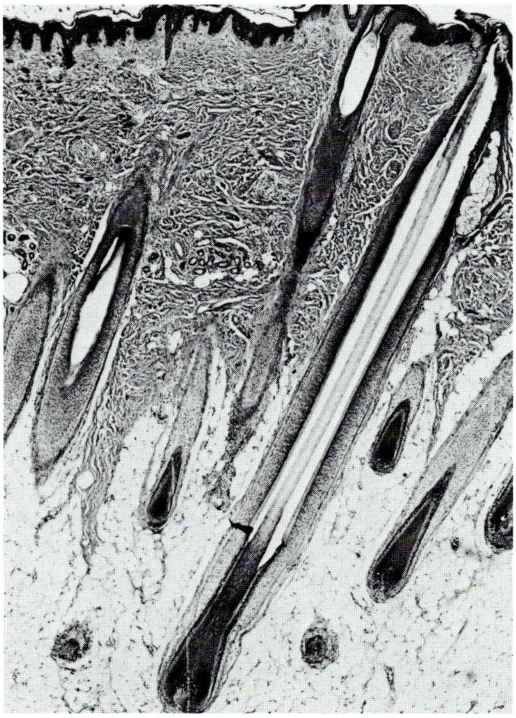

Fig. 6-3. Mature anagen hair follicle containing all three segments. × 23.

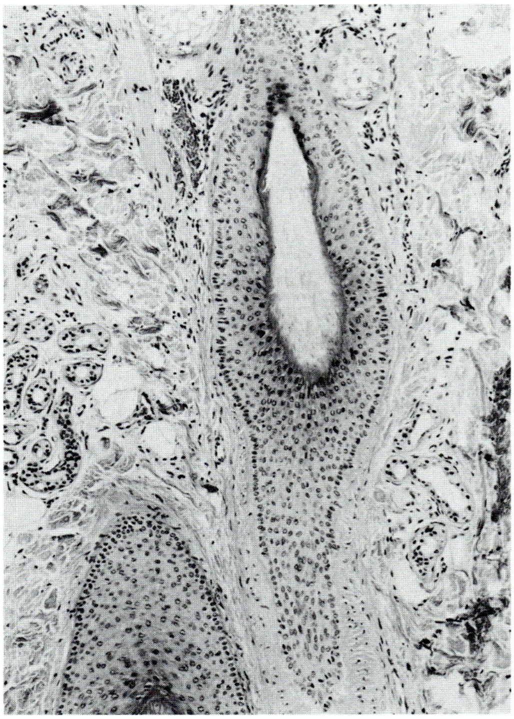

Fig. 6-4. Catagen hair follicle showing a thin cord of epithelial cells representing the remnants of its inferior segment. × 65.

the external root sheath and a rounded lower part of the hair.

There are different types of drug-induced hair losses. Anagen effluvium (the loss of hair while it is growing) consists of a sudden cessation of hair growth during the anagen phase. Small doses of drugs, or injuries of short duration, may produce this condition by temporarily impairing mitosis, decreasing the size of the hair bulb, and leading to a thin and weak area of hair shaft that breaks readily. The epilated hair follicles or a biopsy of the involved skin show a normal anagen:telogen ratio. Anagen alopecia begins 1 to 2 weeks after a drug treatment is instituted, and is reversible if the treatment is discontinued; antimitotic agents are among the drugs that cause this type of alopecia. These include alkylating agents (cyclophosphamide), antimetabilites (methotrexate), vinca alkaloids (vincristine), and miscellaneous agents (colchicine and hydroxyurea). Telogen effluvium consists of a prematurely induced resting phase in the hair follicles, caused by drugs. The scalp hair is mainly affected, but the eyebrows, axillary, and pubic regions may also be involved. The drugs implicated in this type of reaction are anticoagulants, mainly coumarins and heparin. The hair loss is maximal 3 months after initial administration of the drug. In the condition, the percentage of telogen hairs can increase to as much as 50. After the cessation of drug administration there is recovery of hair growth.

Oral contraceptives are incriminated as an occasional cause of diffuse hair loss.[49,61] This hair loss has been observed in some women while they were taking contraceptive pills; more commonly, the hair loss has been noticed 3 months following discontinuation of the pills. The mechanism of the hair loss is unknown; it is speculated that in the cases of hair loss that follow discontinuation of a con-

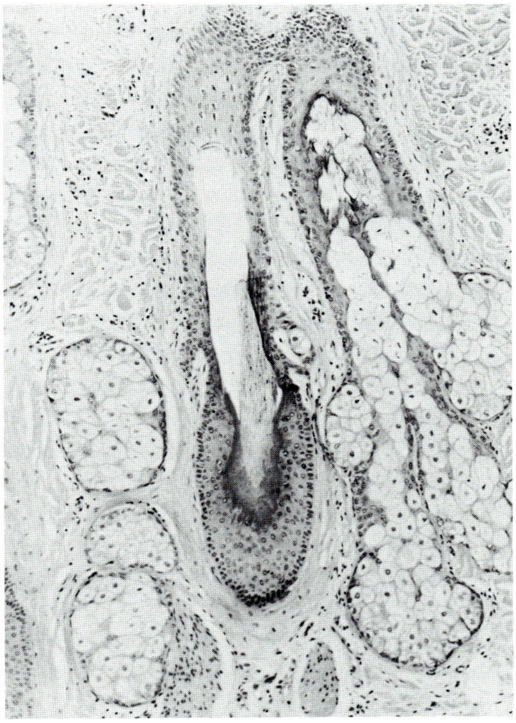

Fig. 6-5. Telogen hair follicle showing a club hair. × 70.

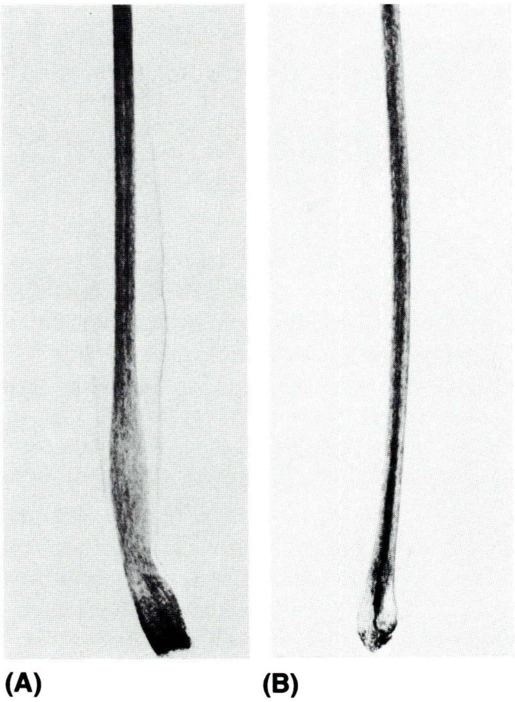

Fig. 6-6. (A) Epilated anagen hair. × 33. (B) Epilated catagen hair. × 31.

traceptive drug, the process resembles the telogen effluvium seen after parturition. In pattern alopecia (Fig. 6-7)—which is induced by androgens—the terminal hair becomes vellus hair. Vellus hairs have very short follicles; hair that is produced is of small diameter. This type of alopecia is permanent. Some other drugs, such as the antithyroid drugs carbimazole and thiouracil, anticonvulsants such as trimethadione, hypervitaminosis A, and ingestion of boric acid[100] may induce a hair loss that is reversible if the offending drug is discontinued.

Hirsutism is the excessive growth of body hair, with a male distribution, induced by androgens from any source in women and children.[43] The ordinarily fine, light-colored vellus hair becomes terminal hair that is longer, coarser, and darker. This type of hair growth is permanent.

Hypertrichosis is an excessive growth of vellus hair that can be either generalized or localized. Some drugs may induce a hypertrichosis[74] that is reversible within a year of discontinuation of the drug. Phenytoin, systemic steroids, minoxidil, and diazoxide have been reported to produce hair growth on the face, neck, and limbs. Penicillamine and systemic methoxypsoralens may also increase hair growth.

PIGMENTARY DISORDERS INDUCED BY DRUGS WITHOUT PRECEDING INFLAMMATION

The color of normal skin depends on oxyhemoglobin, reduced hemoglobin, melanin, and carotene. Drug-produced changes in skin color have different mechanisms. The drug itself may be responsible, or it may induce an alteration of melanin pigmentation, or both. The nature of the formed pigment that alters the skin color is sometimes unknown. The pigment disorders may be widespread or localized.

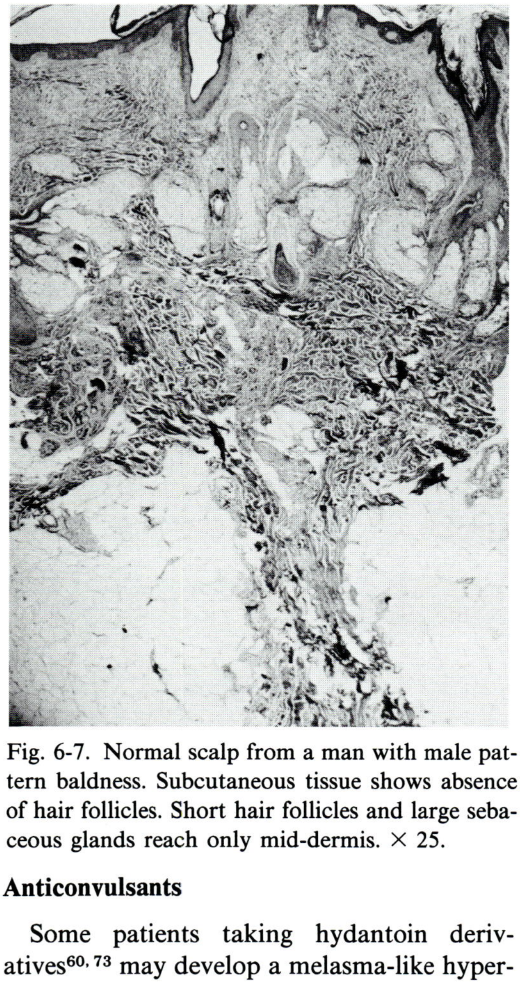

Fig. 6-7. Normal scalp from a man with male pattern baldness. Subcutaneous tissue shows absence of hair follicles. Short hair follicles and large sebaceous glands reach only mid-dermis. × 25.

Anticonvulsants

Some patients taking hydantoin derivatives[60, 73] may develop a melasma-like hyperpigmentation, which takes the form of symmetric macules, on sun-exposed areas of the face. Histologically, there is increased melanin pigment in the melanocytes and keratinocytes in the basal layer of the epidermis; there is also an increased production of melanosomes and an increased percentage of single melanosomes in keratinocytes. The pigmentation usually appears 1 year after administration of the drug. Nitrofurantoin is chemically closely related to the hydantoin derivatives, and may cause a similar type of pigmentation after prolonged use.

Antimalarials

Pigmentary changes may develop in patients receiving any of the antimalarial drugs for more than 3 to 4 months.[60, 73] Quinacrine and amodiaquine less frequently cause a diffuse yellowish discoloration of the skin. This discoloration is due to the drug itself, and disappears after the drug is discontinued. Squamous cell carcinoma of the palmar surface has been described[15] as a late sequel of quinacrine intake.

Quinine may produce a generalized hyperpigmentation of the skin, owing to melanocyte stimulation.[104] A localized blue-black pigmentation may affect the pretibial areas, face, hard palate, and subungal regions. However, such pigmentary changes are most frequently caused by chloroquine. Tuffanelli et al.[104] observed pigmentary changes in patients with lupus erythematosus receiving antimalarial drugs, with chloroquine being the drug most frequently used. The pigmentary change took several months following the cessation of drug administration to decrease in intensity. Histologically, the pigmented lesions showed yellowish to dark brown pigment granules intra- and extracellularly in the dermis, predominantly in the deeper areas of the dermis. Stains for melanin and hemosiderin were both positive. The hemosiderin was seen around capillaries and small blood vessels, while the melanin was present in deeper dermis. Chloroquine has an affinity for cutaneous and ocular melanin, and is not readily released from the pigmented tissue. The most important side effect of this drug is retinopathy, which is irreversible and dose related. Corneal deposits may also occur but are reversible (see Chapter 16).

Cystostatic Drugs

Busulfan, 5-fluorouracil, cyclophosphamide, and topical nitrogen mustard induce a diffuse brown hyperpigmentation of the skin.[73] Bleomycin may cause a linear hyperpigmentation on the back and chest.[68] Doxorubicin hydrochloride has been reported to cause longitudinal, pigmented bands on the fingernails.[86] Histologically, all of these conditions are marked by an increase in melanin in the epidermis. It is postulated[73] that the cause of the hyperpigmentation is secondary to depressed keratinocyte proliferation and to a prolonged contact between melanocytes and keratinocytes which become overloaded with melanosomes. With topical nitrogen mustard, the increased number of single melanosomes, is seen within keratinocytes.[42]

Tranquilizers

Chlorpromazine and related phenothiazines following prolonged use in large doses, will cause a slate-grey, progressive pigmentation in exposed areas of the skin.[112] Mild pigmentation of the cornea may also occur. Corneal and lens opacity and retinopathy are more serious complications; chlorpromazine is the drug most frequently implicated. The skin pigmentation is caused by the deposition of melanin pigment in the dermis. Light microscopic examination with H&E reveals dark brown pigment in the upper dermis extracellularly and in the melanophages in the same area; electron microscopic examination shows an increase in melanosomes in the epidermal cells. An increase in lysosomes in dermal phagocytes has also been found.[52] Light and EM examination of both[111] normal and pigmented skin from these patients, and analysis of the extracts and residues of their skin following chlorpromazine extraction, suggest that the pigment represents a combination of both drug and melanin, rather than melanin alone.

Antibiotics

Long-term treatment with methacycline[38] occasionally induces a dark-grey pigmentation of light-exposed skin and conjunctivae. Patients affected with this condition were treated daily, over a period of 2 to 7 years, with 600 mg of methacycline. Histopathologic examination of the skin reveals increased melanin pigment in the basal layer and elastotic degeneration of connective tissue, with increased melanophages among elastotic fibers. There is also extracellular depositon of granular pigment in the area of degenerated elastotic fibers. It was speculated that in the condition, a methacycline-melanin complex becomes bound to degenerated connective tissue.

Metals

Arsenic. The chronic ingestion of inorganic arsenic[60] may, after 1 to 20 years, result in a diffuse macular pigmentation, most pronounced on the trunk. In the past, arsenic was an ingredient in some tonics; it is also the main ingredient in Fowler's solution, which is still occasionally used. Histopathologic examination[72] reveals a focal increase in melanin pigment in the basal layer of the epidermis, with increased production of melanosomes and melanophages in the upper dermis. There is also absolute hyperkeratosis and atrophy of the remainder of the epidermis. The basal cells show pyknosis of nuclei: arsenic is not refractile under darkfield microscopic examination. Bowenoid keratosis, Bowen's disease, and basal and squamous cell carcinoma may appear in the skin and squamous cell carcinomas may appear in the viscera as late sequelae of chronic arsenic intake.

Silver. At present, silver is used only locally. The continued application of silver salts to mucous membrane may, if these salts are sufficiently absorbed, result in a slate blue-gray pigmentation of light-exposed areas of the skin, oral mucosa, conjunctiva, and fingernails. The pigmentation is permanent. Histopathologically,[72] there is an increase in melanin pigment in the epidermis, with an increased production of melanosomes[73] and dermal melanophages; additionally, small granules of silver can be seen in the lamina propria of sweat glands (Fig. 6-8A). The granules are best demonstrated by darkfield examination, in which they appear as uniform, small refractile granules around hair follicles, sebaceous glands, and sweat glands (Fig. 6-8B and F). The granules are scattered throughout the

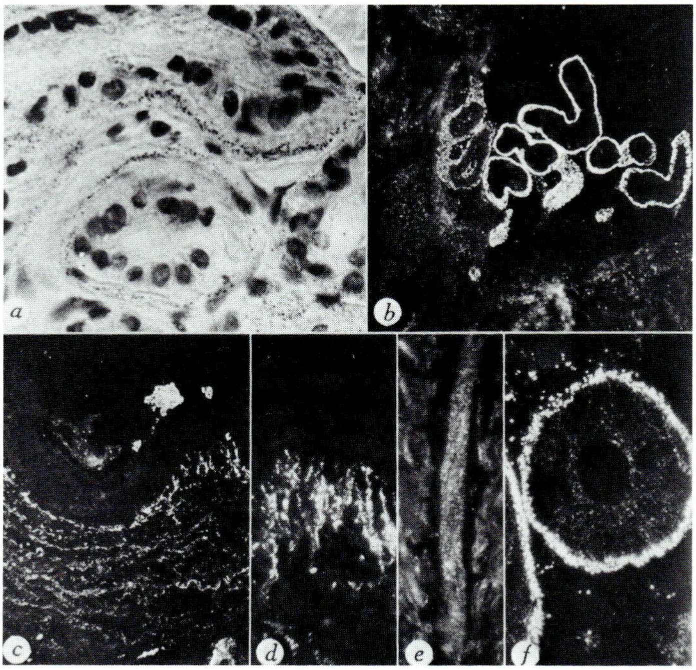

Fig. 6-8. Argyria. (A) Silver particles in the lamina propria of sweat glands. H & E, × 665. Darkfield illumination shows refractile silver particles in (B) lamina propria of sweat glands, × 140; (C) on elastic fibers in the dermis, × 150; (D) on elastic fibers in the papillary dermis, × 360; (E) on arrectores pilorum muscle, × 240; and (F) in lamina propria of sweat glands, × 665. (Montgomery, H.: Dermatopathology. Harper and Row Publishers, New York, 1967.)

dermis, and have a special affinity for elastic fibers (Fig. 6-8C and D). The granules of mercury and gold are also refractile but are much coarser than those of silver, and vary in size.

Gold is used systemically in the treatment of rheumatoid arthritis and some dermatologic diseases.[60] After prolonged administration it may produce a permanent, diffuse blue-grey pigmentation, especially on light-exposed areas of the skin. Histopathologic[72] examination reveals increased melanin in the epidermis, with an increased number of melanosomes[73] and of melanophages in the upper dermis. Gold is deposited in the dermis and is also found in histiocytes; it is especially deposited on elastic fibers, but is absent around sweat glands. In darkfield examination the gold granules, like silver granules, are refractile, but are larger than silver granules.

Bismuth will produce generalized blue-grey pigmentation of the skin and a characteristic blue-black "bismuth line" on the gingival margins.[60] However, bismuth is no longer used clinically.

Mercury. Repeated application of mercury-containing creams may induce a grey-brown pigmentation of the skin.[30, 60] As in the pigmentation produced by gold this is also due to an increase of melanin pigment in the basal layer of the epidermis, with increased melanosome production and melanophages in the upper dermis, and the deposition of mercurial granules in histiocytes and in elastic fibers; it is therefore indistinguishable from the changes induced by gold. For the accurate identification of heavy metals without a proper history of intake, more precise methods are required, such as neutron activation analysis. Specific-localization electron-microprobe analysis may also be used.

Hormones

Adrenocorticotrophic hormone (ACTH) and melanocyte stimulating hormone (MSH) may produce a diffuse, brownish, Addisonian type of pigmentation in the skin. The pigmentation is reversed through reduction of the dose of ACTH. Histopathologic examination reveals an increase in melanin pigment in the epidermis, caused by the increased production of melanosomes.

Oral contraceptives will produce a circumscribed, chloasma-like hyperpigmentation that is symmetric.[60, 73] This condition affects mainly the upper lip, forehead, the malar eminences, and the lower part of the cheeks. It fades more slowly than the chloasma of pregnancy. Histopathologically there is an increase in melanin pigmentation in the basal layer of the epidermis, with increased melanosome size and an increased number of single melanosomes in the keratinocytes.

LOSS OF HAIR COLOR

From 2 to 3 months after the initiation of treatment with chloroquine, the hair in some individuals with blond, red, and light brown hair becomes bleached[60]; dark brown and black hair are not affected. It has been claimed that hydroxychloroquine does not have an effect on hair color. It appears that chloroquine interferes with the formation of pheomelanin but not of melanin. The loss of color is reversible after withdrawal of the drug. Mephenesin has been reported to cause depigmentation of human hair.[99]

EXANTHEMATOUS—MORBILIFORM ERUPTIONS

Exanthematous-morbiliform eruptions are the most common type of drug-induced reactions.[24, 108] The eruptions may occur any time between the first day and 3 weeks after the beginning of administration of the drug. Reactions appearing within the first 2 to 3 days usually occur in patients already sensitized to the drug; in nonsensitized patients, the peak of reaction is commonly on the ninth day. Fever is frequent in these exanthematous types of reactions. Often, the eruptions appear as symmetric macules and papules, with a tendency to confluence. Histopathologically (Fig. 6-9), these lesions show a slight vacuolization of basal cells, and a sparse to moderately dense lymphohistiocytic infiltrate along the epi-

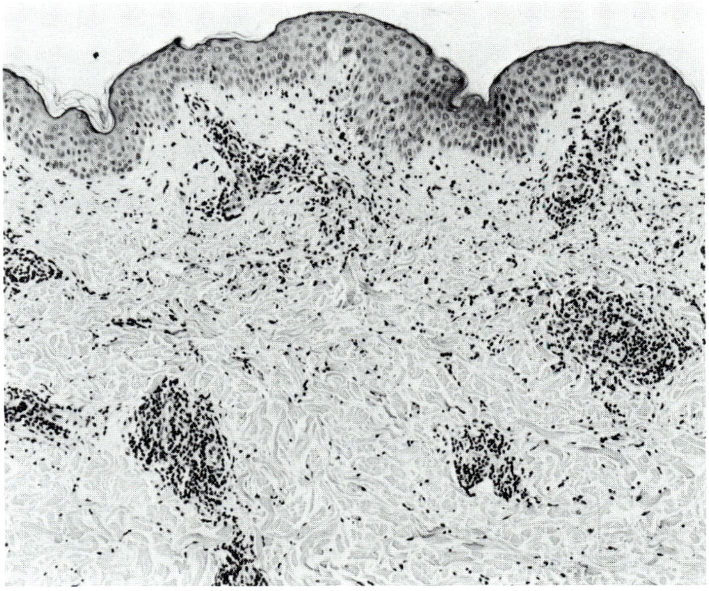

Fig. 6-9. Morbiliform drug eruption shows an unremarkable epidermis except for some mild edema of basal cells and a dense lymphohistiocytic perivascular infiltrate in the dermis. × 130.

dermo-dermal interface and superficial dermal blood vessels. These changes can also be seen in morbiliform viral eruptions. Although a multitude of drugs can cause exanthematous-morbiliform eruptions, the most common are penicillin and related antibiotics, sulphonamides, tetracycline, streptomycin, pyrazalone derivatives, barbiturates, nitrofurantoin, hydantoin derivatives, isoniazid, chloramphenicol, erythromycin, benzodiazepines, phenothiazines, carbamazepine, allopurinol, and gold salts. In the case of allopurinol, in particular, some patients present with an exanthematous eruption, fever, eosinophilia, hepatitis, and renal insufficiency. One patient with these symptoms also had granular IgM deposits at the epidermo-dermal junction, and circulating immune complexes were demonstrated at the height of the drug reaction by use of the Raji cell technique.[106]

The mechanism for drug-induced exanthematous-morbiliform eruptions is not known, but some investigators feel that they are mediated by cellular immunity.

EXFOLIATIVE DERMATITIS CAUSED BY DRUGS

This type of eruption begins a few weeks or longer after the administration of a causative drug.[76] The eruption is characterized clinically by an erythema which starts on the face and spreads over the entire body, and is followed by desquamation. Because of extensive erythema there is disturbance of temperature regulation. Healing of the eruption is slow, with 4 to 6 weeks required for the eruption to clear even if the causative drug is discontinued. The histopathology[63] of skin lesions in drug-induced exfoliative dermatitis is nonspecific, consisting of parakeratosis, inter- and intracellular edema, acanthosis with elongation of rete ridges, edema of the papillary dermis, and a mixed perivascular infiltrate consisting of lymphocytes, histiocytes, plasma cells, and eosinophils. The drugs most frequently implicated as being causative of the condition are pyrazolone derivatives carbamazepine, phenindione, hydantoin derivatives, nitrofurantoin, isoniazid, gold salts, streptomycin, and *p*-aminosalicylic acid.

URTICARIA

Drug-induced urticarial lesions are second in frequency of occurrence to drug-induced exanthematous reactions.[27,98,108] The drugs most commonly inducing urticaria are penicillin and related antibiotics, acetyl-salicylic acid, sulphonamides, opiates, indomethacin, acetaminophen (paracetamol), x-ray contrast media, and enzymes. Allergic urticarial lesions may occur from within minutes of administration of the drug up to 12 to 36 hours later. These reactions are mediated by IgE antibodies. Urticaria in the serum sickness syndrome develops from 7 to 10 days after the administration of a causative drug. The pathogenesis of the urticaria in this instance is not completely understood; it is possible that immune complexes are formed, with activation of the complement system and anaphylatoxin formation, which induces mast cell degranulation; however, IgE antibodies may also contribute to this response. In nonimmunologic urticaria the causative drug induces the urticaria by acting as a direct liberator of histamine from mast cells. Finally, some drugs inhibit the formation of prostaglandin from arachidonic acid by inhibiting cyclooxygenase.

The individual lesions of urticaria last less than 24 hours. Histologically, the lesions show (Fig. 6-10A and B) unremarkable epidermis, perivascular edema, and a sparse infiltrate of lymphocytes, neutrophils, and a few eosinophils in the upper dermis. Vessels are dilated, and there is an edema of the reticular dermis. In urticarial-like eruptions, the individual urticarial lesion lasts longer than 24 hours. Histologically, (Fig. 6-11A and B) such lesions are characterized by an unremarkable epidermis, edema of the papillary dermis, and a moderately dense perivascular infiltrate consisting of neutrophils, lymphocytes, histiocytes, eosi-

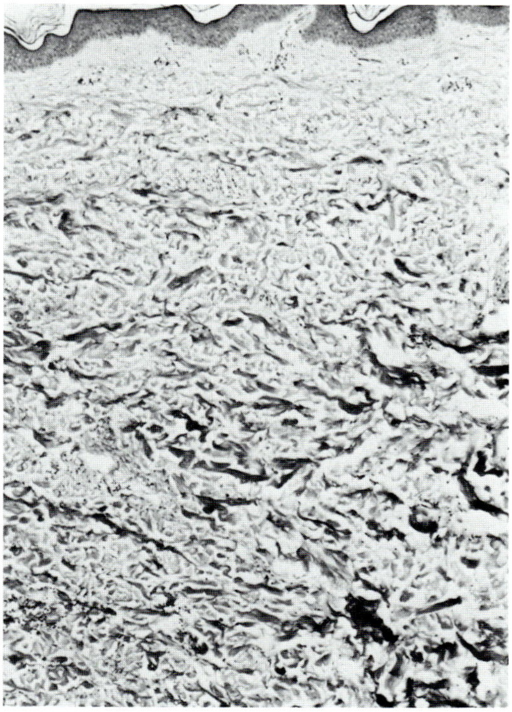

(A)

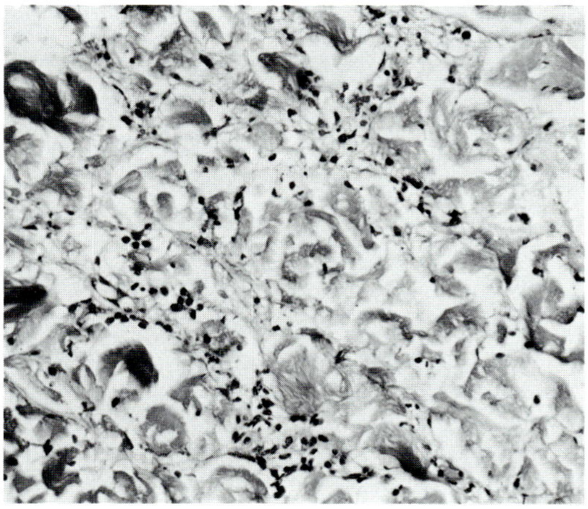

(B)

Fig. 6-10. Urticaria. (A) An unremarkable epidermis and some edema of reticular dermis × 35. (B) A sparse perivascular mixed-cell infiltrate in the dermis. × 170.

nophils, and mast cells. These infiltrates may be either superficial or both superficial and deep.

ECZEMATOUS-TYPE ERUPTIONS

These eruptions are often seen in patients already sensitized by external exposure to a drug, since some of the causative drugs are used externally and internally.[25, 34, 97] In addition, some individuals, such as medical personnel, are exposed to these drugs by handling them. Drugs commonly causing these reactions are the penicillins, streptomycin, neomycin, gentamycin, kananycin, sulphonamides, chlorpromazine and related phenothiazene compounds, meprobamate, promethazine, chlorothiazide and related compounds, mercurial diuretics, tolbutamide, chlorpropamide, iodide, procaine and other anesthetics, quinine, and quinidine. Cross-sensitivity is also one of the causes of eczematous eruptions; the para-amino group which is present in sulphonamides, local anesthetics, tolbutamide, and chlorpropamide is also found in numerous locally applied chemicals. Skin eruptions of the eczematous type usually appear within 1 to 2 days after administration of the drug. Clinically the eruption presents as an eczematous process similar to contact dermatitis. Histopathologic changes are the same as in eczematous contact dermatitis, consisting of spongiosis in the epidermis and a perivascular lymphohistiocytic infiltrate in the dermis, with or without eosinophils.[65]

PHOTOSENSITIVITY REACTIONS

All photosensitivity reactions result from the absorption of radiation of specific wavebands by specific molecules.[26, 79] Photosensitivity reactions are divided into phototoxic and photoallergic types. Phototoxic reactions are the most common, and are dose dependent for both the amount of drug and the amount of radiation. Ultraviolet radiation is said to "activate" the drug, damaging the cell, although the mechanisms by which affected cells are damaged are not understood. When a skin eruption is produced by a phototoxic agent taken systemically, the eruption is called a

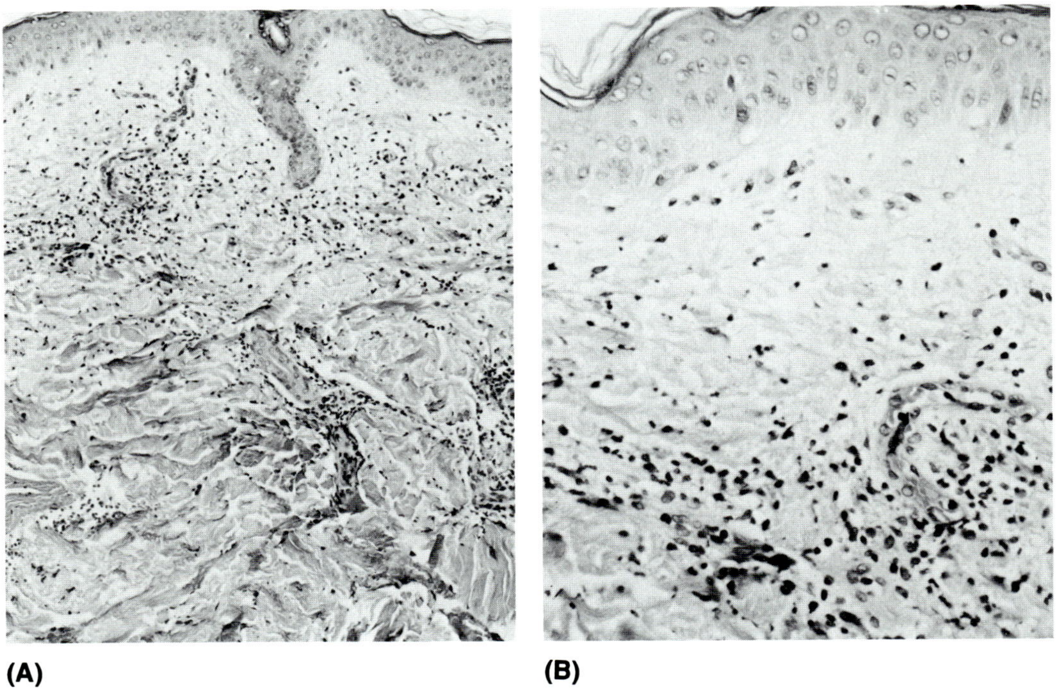

Fig. 6-11. Urticaria-like eruption. (A) There is an unremarkable epidermis and a moderately dense perivascular mixed cell infiltrate in the dermis. × 100. (B) Higher magnification of (A). × 250.

"phototoxic" dermatitis; if it is produced by external application of the phototoxic agent it is called a phototoxic contact dermatitis.[2]

The wavelengths producing these reactions are often in the long-wave spectrum of ultraviolet light. The long wavelength range between 320 and 400 nm, is called the ultraviolet A (UVA) region, while the wavelength range between 290 and 320 nm is called the ultraviolet B (UVB) region and is also referred to as the sunburn or erythema spectrum.

Clinically, phototoxic reactions appear as an intensified sunburn reaction, hours after sun exposure, over the tops of the ears, malar areas, lateral and posterior surfaces of neck, and dorsal aspects of the forearms and hands. Histologically (Fig. 6-12), the epidermis shows a normal stratum corneum, with necrosis of superficial epidermal cells. The basal cell layer shows some vacuolization, and the dermis a modest superficial perivascular lymphohistiocytic infiltrate. Some drugs often causing phototoxic reactions are tetracycline—with demeclocycline having a higher incidence—sulphonamides, psoralens, chlorpromazine, nalidixic acid, and quinidine; other drugs causing phototoxic contact dermatitis are coal tar and coal tar derivatives, psoralens, phenothiazines, halogenated salicylanilide compounds, and sulphonamides and related compounds. The last three groups of compounds may also be photoallergens.

In photoallergic reactions, the light reacts with the chemical or a metabolite of the chemical to produce a hapten, the hapten then combines with tissue protein to form a complete antigen. There is no evidence of dose dependency, and once sensitization is achieved, small doses of the responsible chemicals are sufficient to evoke the photosensitivity. These reactions have a delay from the first exposure to the chemical to the onset of eruption that is similar to that in other allergies. When the offending agent is applied externally, the reaction is called a photoallergic contact dermatitis; when the drug is introduced systemically, the reaction is called a photoallergic dermatitis.[2]

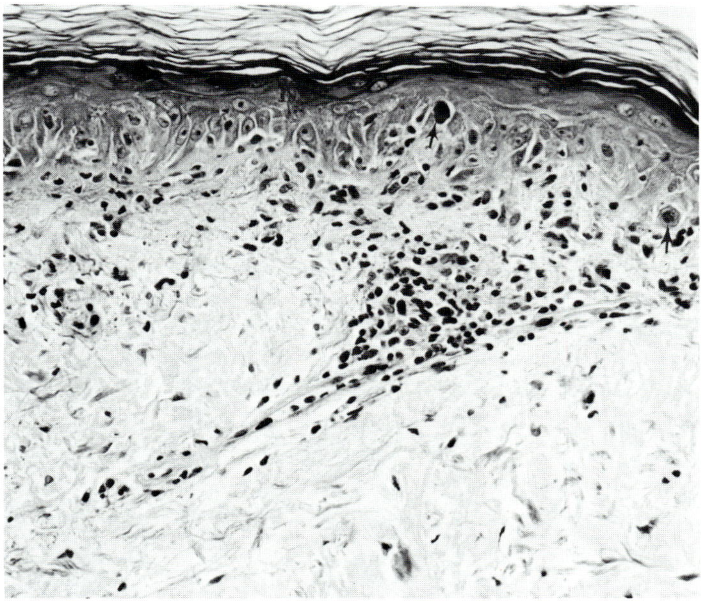

Fig. 6-12. Phototoxic eruption reveals a normal stratum corneum, few necrotic keratinocytes in the epidermis (arrows), some vacuolization of basal cells, and modest superficial perivascular lymphohistiocytic infiltrate in the dermis. × 225.

Most photosensitivity reactions due to systemically administered drugs are phototoxic reactions. Photoallergic contact dermatitis is commonly caused by sulfonamides, halogenated salicylanilides, and chlorpromazine. Clinically, photoallergic reactions appear as eczematous dermatitis on sun-exposed areas. Histologically they are characterized by spongiosis and acanthosis in the epidermis, edema in the papillary dermis, and superficial lymphohistiocytic perivasculitis with or without eosinophils.

In addition to the foregoing conditions, lichenoid photodermatitis[3] has been described following the administration of such systemic medications as chlorothiazides. Clinically, this condition is characterized by erythematous, edematous papules on sun-exposed areas of the skin. Histopathologically there is focal parakeratosis, moderate acanthosis, dyskeratotic cells, and vacuolar alteration of basal cells in the epidermis, together with a dense, band-like infiltrate in the papillary dermis; a superficial and deep perivascular, predominantly lymphocytic infiltrate is also seen.

Bullous eruptions occur after the ingestion of nalidixic acid[20] in association with considerable sun exposure. Bullae are present on exposed areas and especially on the legs and feet. Histopathologic examination reveals subepidermal bullae and a sparse, perivascular lymphohistiocytic infiltrate in the dermis. The lesions clear with avoidance of sun exposure.

Photosensitization due to psoralens[79] is activated by ultraviolet A (320 to 400 nm) waves and is designated by the acronym PUVA. Maximal photosensitization occurs when the UVA exposure takes place 2 hours after psoralen ingestion. The cutaneous changes following PUVA are similar to those in sunburn, including erythema, pigmentation, epidermal damage, and dermal changes. The difference is that the onset of erythema in PUVA is slower and of longer duration, and the pigmentation is greater and persists longer than in sunburn. PUVA inhibits epidermal cell DNA synthesis, probably by the covalent binding of photoactive psoralens to the DNA of epidermal cells. PUVA also increases the number of active melanocytes, the production of melanosomes, and the transfer of melanosomes to keratinocytes.

Currently, PUVA is used for the treatment of several skin diseases. There is considerable concern about the possible long-term side effects of this type of therapy. Repeated phototoxic reactions over long periods of time may produce irreversible changes in the epidermal cells, dermal cellular elements, blood vessels and connective tissue of the skin, leading to prematurely aged skin. The possibility of a carcinogenic effect should also be considered, although for the last 25 years PUVA has been used in the treatment of vitiligo, and no increased incidence of skin cancer has been observed in treated patients. However, in a recent 2.1-year study[101] of 1,373 patients who received PUVA therapy, it was found that the incidence of cutaneous squamous cell carcinoma was 2.6 times higher than that expected in a similar population matched for age, sex, and geography. Careful long-term followup is needed for patients who are treated with PUVA.

Besides its other effects, UVA penetrates the cornea and is absorbed by the lens, and may be a factor in the development of cataracts. Psoralen-related cataracts have been reported in animals. The first report of such a cataract found in humans[81] was in a patient who received photochemotherapy for vitiligo. It is therefore advisable to use protective, wrap-around sunglasses during daylight hours for the duration of psoralen ingestion throughout the entire treatment period, and for at least 1 week after the last treatment. Frequent eye examinations are also recommended.

LUPUS ERYTHEMATOSUS-LIKE ERUPTION

Hydralazine and procainamide are drugs that induce a lupus erythematosus-like syndrome in a significant number of patients[19,50,51,105,107,109,110]; isoniazid, hydantoin, trimethadione, penicillamine, methyldopa, sulfonamides, and oral contraceptives have also been implicated. Hydralazine- and isoniazid-induced lupus erythematosus is known to occur mainly in "slow acetylators"[110]; in procainamide-induced lupus erythematosus,[110] the syndrome appears earlier in "slow acetylators" than in "rapid acetylators." All three of these drugs contain a primary amine or hydrazine moiety that is acetylated by the hepatic n-acetyltransferase system; the patients called "slow acetylators" are deficient in this n-acetyltransferase enzyme, and it is postulated that a nonacetylated compound of these drugs, or their metabolites, binds to DNA or nucleoprotein, producing an antigenic complex; the acetylation serves as a probable pathway for reducing the amount of drug or its metabolite available to induce the immunologic reaction[110] that results in the lupus-like syndrome. Skin eruptions appear less frequently in the drug-induced lupus than in systemic lupus erythematosus and are variable, but frequently have the clinical and histologic features of typical lupus erythematosus. The epidermis shows liquefaction, degeneration of the basal layer, and thinning. The upper dermis shows edema, and there is lymphohistiocytic infiltrate through the entire thickness of the dermis. Among six patients included in four reports,[50,105,107,109] immunoglobulin deposition was found at the epidermo-dermal junction in five, and in the kidneys of two.

LEUKOCYTOCLASTIC ANGITIS

Drug-induced leukocytoclastic angitis[32,41] involves small blood vessels of the skin or internal organs, or both. Clinically, it appears as a palpable purpura, with urticarial papules that sometimes progress to nodules, vesicles, bullae, and ulcers. Histopathologic examination (Fig. 6-13) reveals numerous neutrophils, fragmented neutrophilic nuclei, and fibrin accumulation around and within the upper dermal blood vessels. Eosinophils, lymphocytes, mast cells, and histiocytes are also present. The epidermis is often unremarkable in the papular lesions, is separated in vesiculo-bullous lesions, or is necrotic in ulcerated lesions. Histologically these changes are identical to those seen in an Arthus reaction. It is postulated that the drug, which is a hapten, combines with a macromolecular carrier to form an antigen that initiates the formation of antibody. Subsequently, antigen will bind to the

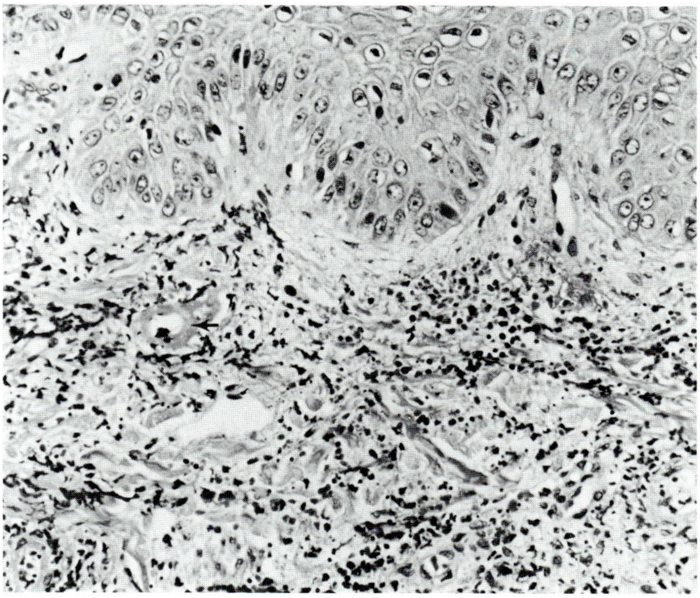

Fig. 6-13. Leucocytoclastic angiitis. Epidermis is unremarkable. Dermis shows a perivascular infiltrate consisting predominantly of neutrophils and nuclear dust, and invading blood vessel walls. Few vessel walls show fibrinoid degeneration (arrow). × 220.

antibody that is formed. Antigen-antibody complexes that are formed in antigen excess are soluble, circulate freely, and if not cleared by the reticuloendothelial system are deposited in blood vessel walls. After these antigen-antibody complexes are deposited, they combine with complement and induce the release of chemotactic factors for neutrophils. These cells then infiltrate the vessel walls and release their lysosomes, which damage the vessel walls and surrounding connective tissue. Direct immunofluorescence studies of skin lesions in leukocytoclastic angiitis[91,96] show wall-vessel deposits of IgG, IgM and C3. IgM and C3 appear to be the most common deposits. The biopsy should be taken from uninvolved skin next to the lesion.

Braverman and Yen[22] induced the skin lesions of leukocytoclastic angiitis by histamine injection in uninvolved skin in patients with active vasculitis. They studied spontaneous lesions, histamine induced lesions, and nonmanipulated uninvolved skin using direct immunofluorescence and electron microscopy, and concluded that immune complexes are first deposited and then followed by cellular infiltration. They also observed that the involved vessels are always postcapillary venules. In these reports,[22,96] only a few patients had leukocytoclastic angiitis secondary to drugs.

Drugs causing leukocytoclastic angiitic reactions include allopurinol, gold, phenothiazine, hydantoin, and sulfonamides. When the drug is discontinued, the leukocytoclastic vasculitis clears. Polyarteritis nodosa is a type of leukocytoclastic angiitis involving medium-sized arteries; the whole or only part of the vessel circumference may be involved. Fibrin, neutrophils, fragmented neutrophilic nuclei, eosinophils, plasma cells, and macrophages are present within the vessel wall. There is no extravascular involvement. Necrosis of the arterial wall may lead to formation of aneurysms that may rupture. Clinically, the lesions appear as subcutaneous nodules. The sulphonamides[87] occasionally cause this type of reaction.

THROMBOCYTOPENIC PURPURA

Thrombocytopenic purpura can be due to toxic or allergic reactions;[28,69] a purpura[28,69] usually does not occur unless the platelet count is less than 20,000/mm³. In toxic reactions, other blood elements besides platelets are involved. Drugs causing toxic thrombocytopenic purpura include most of the cancer chemotherapeutic agents; inducers of folate malabsorption such as hydantoins; estrogens; and birth control pills. In allergic reactions the drug acts as a hapten and combines with platelets, which then become autoantigenic and induce the production of antiplatelet antibodies. These antibodies agglutinate the platelets, and cause them to undergo lysis in the presence of complement. Drugs proven to cause immunologic platelet destruction include sulfathiazole, quinidine, hydroxychloroquine, methyldopa, and phenytoin. The skin lesions in both toxic and allergic thromocytopenic purpura are identical clinically and histologically, and appear as nonblanching red macules. Histologically, in the upper dermis, only extravasated red blood cells are seen. This is further discussed in Chapter 5.

COUMARIN

Coumarin-induced necrosis of the skin is a rare type of drug reaction[29,75]; usually it occurs in the first week of anticoagulant therapy and is described for all coumarin derivatives. It is not dose related. Obese women are especially susceptible, and sites of predilection are the breast (see Chapters 10 and 14), buttock, and thighs. Histologically,[64] thrombi are seen within capillaries in the dermis; capillaries are surrounded by numerous extravasated red blood cells and a few polymorphonuclear leukocytes. Subepidermal blister formation and necrosis of the epidermis are also present. The lesions may subside and heal by granulation and fibrosis, although surgical intervention is sometimes needed. Once the eruption has appeared, its course is not significantly changed by the continuation of therapy.

ERYTHEMA NODOSUM-LIKE LESIONS

Erythema nodosum-like lesions[37,48] are caused by oral contraceptives,[14] sulphonamides, salicylates, bromides, iodides, penicillin, and codeine. The lesions tend to occur in women, being manifest clinically by painful subcutaneous nodules on the lower extremities. Histologically, these lesions are indistinguishable from those in erythema nodosum of other causes; they are characterized by a moderately dense, mixed inflammatory infiltrate around blood vessels in the septa of subcutaneous tissues. This infiltrate consists of neutrophils, lymphocytes, and histiocytes.

PORPHYRIA CUTANEA TARDA

Estrogens, ethyl alcohol, and toxic chemicals such as hexachlorobenzene and chlorinated phenols are all known to induce porphyria cutanea tarda; indeed, every individual exposed to hexachlorbenzene will develop this condition, while alcohol and estrogens will induce prophyria cutanea tarda[17] in a genetically susceptible person. The condition usually first develops in the third or fourth decade. The biochemical enzymatic defect is a deficiency of uroporphyrinogen decarboxylase in the liver and red blood cells. All patients have increased urinary uroporphyrin and increased coproporphyrin in their urine and feces. Other associated conditions are diabetes mellitus, which is present in about 25 percent of patients, and, rarely, hepatic tumors. Increased liver iron stores and increased serum iron are also found (see Chapter 17).

The skin of patients with porphyria cutanea tarda has a purplish red color involving the periorbital area, hypertrichosis of fine lanugo hair on the temporal areas, hypermelanosis, sclerodermoid changes in the skin, and blisters on the hands and other areas exposed to trauma[17]; histologically,[66] the blisters are (Fig. 6-14A) subepidermal. There is preservation of papillae and absence of inflammation in the dermis. Basophilic degeneration of collagen is found and, sometimes, deposition of a homogenous eosinophilic material around the superficial blood vessels. This eosinophilic material is PAS positive before and after diastase digestion. Scleroderma-like changes (Fig. 6-14B) are characterized[83] by the sparing of sub-

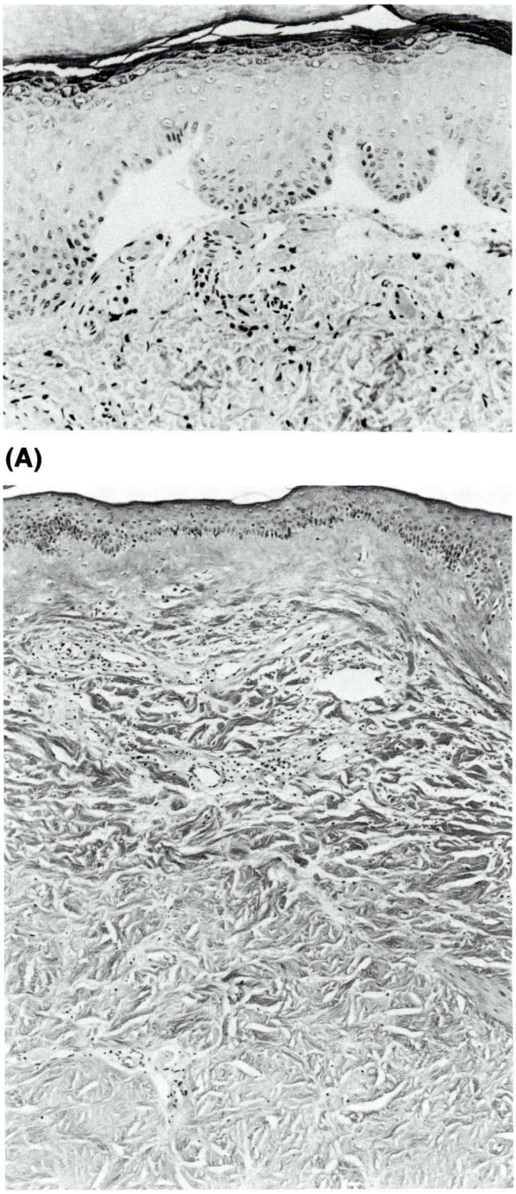

(B)

Fig. 6-14. Porphyria cutanea tarda. (A) Blister. There is a subepidermal separation with preservation of papillae and paucity of inflammatory infiltrate in the dermis × 50. (B) Sclerodermoid changes. Mid and lower dermis show thickening of collagen fibers with decreased spaces between them, and decreased cellularity. There is also some homogenization of papillary dermis. × 75.

cutaneous tissue, and solar elastosis in the upper dermis. The remainder of the dermis shows thickening of collagen fibers, decreased cellularity, and decreased spaces between collagen fibers.

LICHENOID ERUPTIONS

Drugs frequently inducing lichenoid reactions[12] are gold salts,[82] antimalarials, thiazides, chlordiazepoxide, and *p*-aminosalicylic acid. Clinically, the eruption resembles lichen planus and is characterized by small, violaceous lichenoid papules. In addition to these lesions there are also present moderately large, scaly, violaceous patches which are not usually seen with lichen planus. A predilection for flexor involvement and mucosal lesions—which is seen in lichen planus—is not usually seen in lichenoid drug eruptions. The drug-induced eruption starts several months after the beginning of treatment, but the pathogenic mechanism is not known. As in lichen planus, hyperpigmentation is considerable and fades slowly after the causative drug is discontinued. Histologically (Fig. 6-15), the epidermis shows parakeratosis, sawtoothing acanthosis, and liquefaction degeneration of basal cells.[4,82] The upper dermis contains a dense infiltrate which includes lymphocytes, histiocytes, melanophages, plasma cells, and eosinophils. Parakeratosis, plasma cells, and eosinophils are features that differentiate drug-induced lichenoid reactions from lichen planus.

FIXED DRUG ERUPTIONS

Drugs associated with fixed drug eruptions[36,58,80,92] include phenolphthalein, barbiturates, birth control pills, meprobamate, phenylbutazone, sulfonamides, salicylates, and tetracyclines. There is also evidence for a cross-sensitivity[79] between different sulphonamides, phenylbutazone and oxyphenbutazone, and between tetracycline and demethylchlortetracycline in fixed drug eruptions. The lesions in this eruption have an

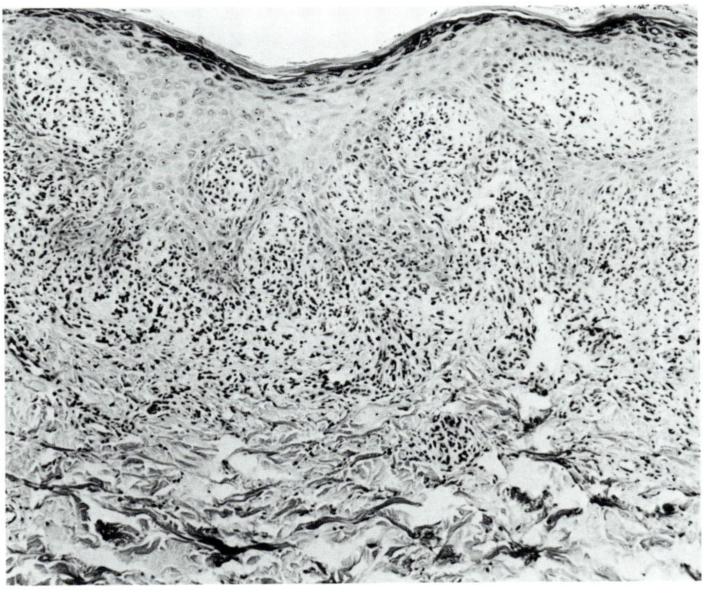

Fig. 6-15. Lichenoid eruption. There is sawtoothing acanthosis and a band-like infiltrate in the papillary dermis. These changes are indistinguishable from lichen planus. × 90.

acute and a late stage. The acute stage consists of a lesion that recurs in precisely the same site with each administration of the offending agent. It appears as a well circumscribed, red, edematous lesion with or without bullae. In the late stage the lesion appears as a macular hyperpigmented patch that remains for months or years. Occasionally the lesion may be urticarial[36] or eczematous. The lesions in a fixed drug eruption can be solitary or multiple, and may occur at any site on the skin, but the palms, soles, lips, and glans penis are favored places. Histologically,[5] in the acute stage (Fig. 6-16A) the epidermis shows necrotic keratinocytes, liquefaction degeneration of the basal layer, and sometimes subepidermal blister formation. Intracellular edema is also seen, which may progress to intraepidermal blister formation. The papillary dermis shows considerable edema. Moderately dense perivascular superficial and deep infiltrates are also observed; these consist of neutrophils, eosinophils, lymphocytes, and histiocytes.

In the late stage (Fig. 6-16B) of the eruption, liquefaction degeneration of the basal layer is minimal. The upper dermis shows a lymphohistiocytic infiltrate and numerous melanophages. Fixed drug eruptions sometimes have lichenoid features[70] (Fig. 6-16C) both clinically and histologically. The mechanism of this eruption is not known. Sometimes also, mouth lesions are present, and may progress to superficial erosions.

ERYTHEMA MULTIFORME AND STEVENS-JOHNSON SYNDROME

Drugs often responsible for this type of eruption[16,39] are the sulphonamides, hydantoin, penicillin, barbiturates, phenothiazines, sulfonamides, and thiazides. The pathogenesis of this reaction pattern is unknown, but an immunologic basis is postulated. Recently,[59] the deposition of IgM, complement, and fibrin has been found around superficial blood vessels by direct immunofluorescence in erythema multiforme.

Clinically, erythema multiforme is characterized by the appearance of erythematous macules and urticarial papules which are sometimes hemorrhagic, and by bullae. Stevens-Johnson syndrome is a more severe disease, with many bullous lesions and mucous membrane involvement, especially of the mucosa of the eyes and mouth. In addition, fever

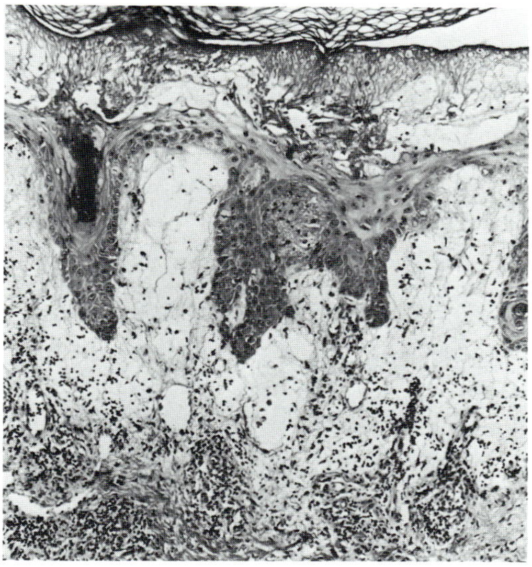

(A)

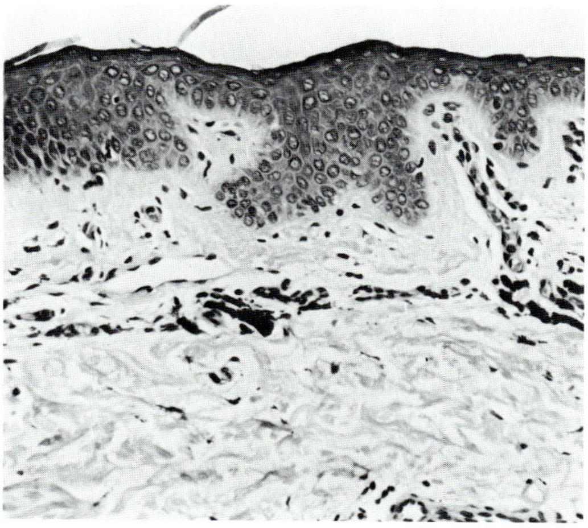

(B)

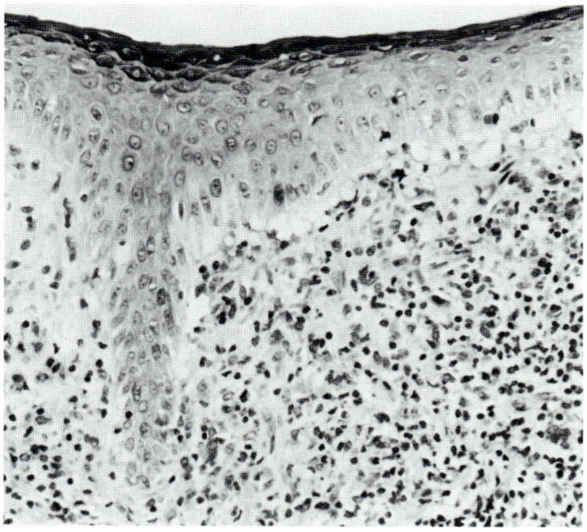

(C)

Fig. 6-16. Acute stage of fixed drug eruption. (A) There are intraepidermal vesicles and necrosis in the upper layers of epidermis. In the lower layers, scattered necrotic keratinocytes are seen. Considerable edema of the papillary dermis is present, together with a moderately dense mixed-cell perivascular infiltrate. × 100. (B) Inactive chronic stage of fixed drug eruption reveals a slight acanthosis of epidermis and a sparse lymphohistiocytic infiltrate with melanophages in the dermis. × 170. (C) Lichenoid type of fixed drug eruption. There is edema of the epidermal basal cells and a dense band like lymphohistiocytic infiltrate in the papillary dermis. × 170.

is present and the patient is acutely ill. The duration of the disease is about 2 to 3 weeks. In the early lesion,[6] histologic examination (Fig. 6-17A) reveals vacuolar degeneration of basal cells, numerous necrotic keratinocytes in all layers of the epidermis, and intercellular edema. The papillary dermis is edematous. A modest lymphohistiocytic infiltrate is seen around blood vessels in the upper dermis. The late lesion[6] (Fig. 6-17B) shows confluent necrosis of the epidermis and marked vacuolar degeneration of the basal layer.

TOXIC EPIDERMAL NECROLYSIS

The drugs most often implicated in inducing toxic epidermal necrolysis[45] are hydantoins, barbiturates, allopurinol, phenylbutazone, penicillin, sulfonamides, antituberculous drugs, and tetracycline. The disease is an acute one; it begins with skin tenderness which is followed by an erythema involving the face and extremities, with vesicles and bullae which rupture, leaving denuded areas. Mucous membranes are also involved, and fever and leukocytosis is also present. Electrolyte imbalance and renal failure may occur and are associated

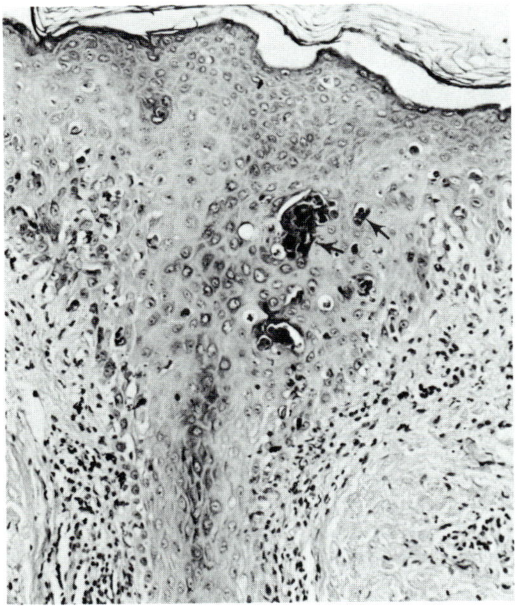

(A)

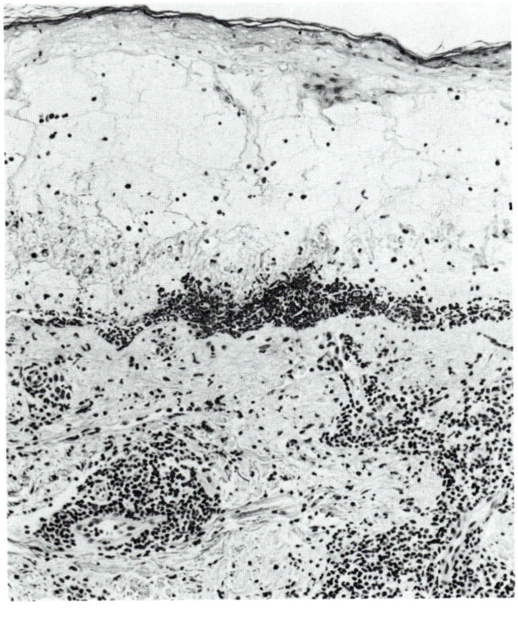

(B)

Fig. 6-17. Erythema multiforme. (A) Early lesion shows edema of the epidermal basal cells and necrotic keratinocytes (arrows) throughout the epidermis, with lymphohistiocytic perivascular infiltrate in the upper dermis. × 150. (B) Late lesion shows an epidermal-dermal separation with confluent epidermal necrosis and a dense dermal perivascular lymphohistiocytic infiltrate. × 100.

with a high mortality rate. After the acute episode, the lesions of toxic epidermal necrolysis heal without scars in 2 to 3 weeks. Histologically, there is vacuolization of the basal cells in the epidermis, with subepidermal separation and necrosis of all epidermal cells.[7] There is a paucity of infiltrate in the dermis and some swelling of the capillary endothelium.

The paucity of dermal infiltrate, the minimal papillary edema, and the marked necrosis of the epidermis (Fig. 6-18) differentiate toxic epidermal necrolysis from erythema multiforme, in which pronounced edema of the papillary dermis, a moderately dense perivascular inflammatory infiltrate in the upper dermis, and less pronounced changes in the epidermis are seen. Differentiation from the staphylococcal scalded skin syndrome[40] is made in the level of epidermal separation, which in the staphylococcal scalded skin syndrome is at the level of the granular layer. The prognosis in this condition is good. In toxic epidermal necrolysis, ultrastructural study[21] shows extensive cell damage of the basal and lower spinous layers.

PSEUDOLYMPHOMA SYNDROME

The clinical and histopathologic picture of a sudden illness resembling malignant lymphoma[53] can occur in patients taking anticonvulsants. Most of the hydantoins and hydantoin-type drugs have been implicated, in causing this condition, especially phenytoin and mephenytoin. Phenobarbital and mephobarbital may also produce this type of reaction. The skin lesions are most frequently exanthematous, but may be vesicular or hemorrhagic. Associated findings are fever, malaise, arthralgia, lymphodenopathy, and hepatosplenomegaly. Histopathologic examination of the skin usually reveals lymphohistiocytic pervasculitis in the dermis, with or without eosinophils. Occasionally, the infiltrate simulates Pautrier microabscesses,[95] while the appearance of the lymph nodes may

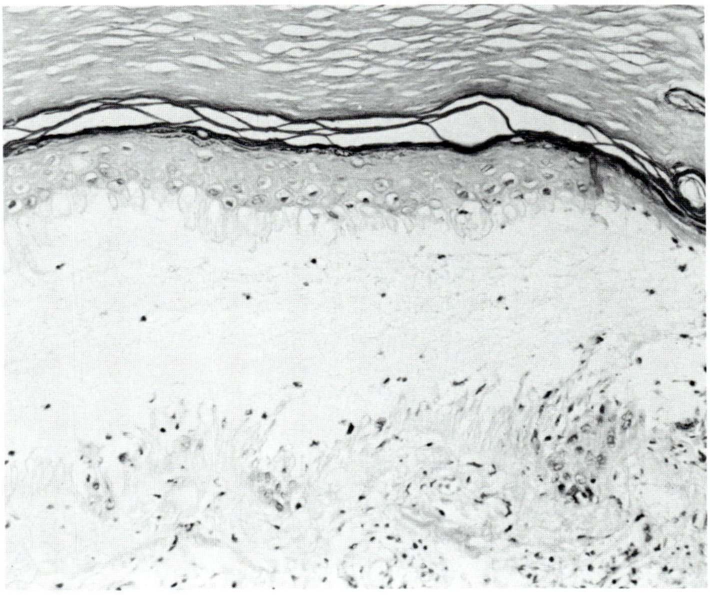

Fig. 6-18. Toxic epidermal necrolysis shows subepidermal blister with a necrotic epidermis and sparse dermal infiltrate. × 185.

mimic that in lymphoma. The liver may show changes similar to those seen in toxic cholangiolitis. All abnormalities in the pseudolymphoma syndrome usually resolve spontaneously within 3 to 4 weeks of discontinuation of the offending drug.

HALOGENODERMAS

Cutaneous lesions may occur as a result of the long-term ingestion of halogen-containing drugs or other substances.[18, 89, 103] Bromide and iodide preparations are the most common cause of halogenodermas. The lesions may be either single or multiple, appearing as fungating nodules, annular lesions with pustules at the periphery, and acneiform pustules. Iododermas sometimes appear as bullous lesions. Recently, papulonodular eruption secondary to fluoride ingestion[18] was described in two patients who had applied fluoride gel preparations to their teeth for the prophylaxis of postirradiation dental caries.

Histologically, bromodermas and iododermas show pseudoepitheliomatous hyperplasia, with intraepidermal abscesses and follicular involvement.[11, 62] Fluorodermas exhibit less epidermal hyperplasia and more surface erosions. In all halogenodermas the dermis shows a dense infiltrate of neutrophils, eosinophils, lymphocytes, plasma cells, and histiocytes (Fig. 6-19). Some early lesions of iododermas and bromodermas have minimal epidermal hyperplasia[10] and a dense infiltrate consisting of neutrophils and eosinophils; atypical mononuclear cells may be present. The bullous lesions in iododermas consist of subepidermal bullae and an infiltrate of neutrophils and eosinophils. As mentioned previously, iodides and bromides may induce acneiform lesions; erythema nodosum, and sometimes purpuric lesions with the histologic picture of leukocytoclastic angiitis, may also be seen.

PEMPHIGUS FOLIACEUS AND VULGARIS

The drugs implicated in causing these conditions are butazolidin,[31] rifampin,[47] and penicillamine.[35, 46, 54, 55] Histologically, there is acantholysis as well as a positive direct and indirect immunofluorescence reaction against intercellular antigens. In some cases, both the

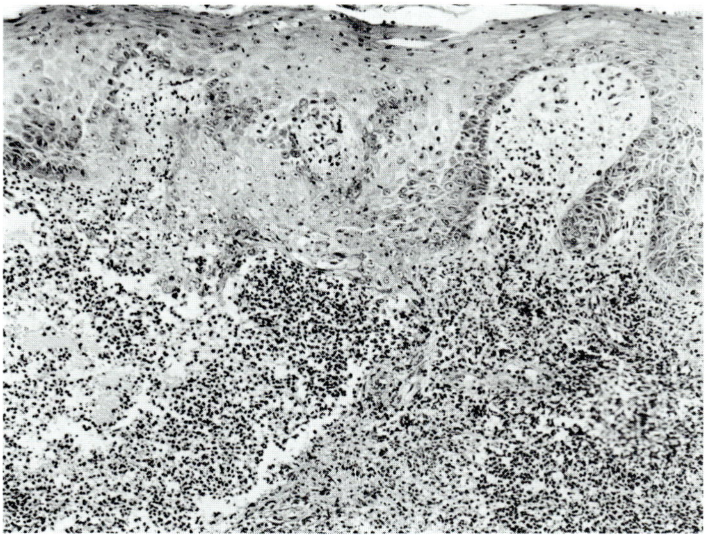

Fig. 6-19. Iododerma. There is considerable hyperplasia of the epidermis and a dense, mixed-cell infiltrate with predominance of neutrophils in the dermis. × 100.

lesions and intercellular antibodies disappear after withdrawal of the drug,[35,47,55] while in others maintenance therapy with steroids is required.[46] In nine cases of penicillamine-induced pemphigus reported by Hewitt et al.,[54] some cleared after penicillamine was stopped and others continued to have the usual course of the disease.

DERMATITIS HERPETIFORMIS

Ackerman described a patient on several drugs who developed a bullous drug eruption which resembled dermatitis herpetiformis only histologically. It was characterized by subepidermal blistering, basophilic necrosis of collagen, and a dense infiltrate of neutrophils.[8] Furthermore, in this case, numerous contiguous papillae were involved, while in true dermatitis herpetiformis fewer contiguous or only individual papillae are affected.

BULLOUS LESIONS IN COMOTOSE STATES

Bullous lesions appear on areas of long-standing local pressure in comatose patients.[13] The coma is usually drug-induced, especially by central nervous system depressants—usually barbiturates. However, CO intoxication and central nervous system diseases have also been implicated. Regardless of the etiologic factors, the bulla (Fig. 20A) is subepidermal,[9,13,84] with a necrotic epidermis. The dermal infiltrate is sparse, consisting of lymphocytes, histiocytes, and neutrophils. There is also necrosis of all epidermal appendages (Fig. 6-20B). It is postulated that the cutaneous lesions are the result of pressure-induced ischemia and anoxia during the comatose state, and are not related to toxic effects of any specific medication.

SKIN CHANGES INDUCED BY LOCAL PENTAZOCINE INJECTIONS

Repeated local injections of pentazocine may cause tissue damage at the site of the injection.[78,93,94] Clinically, the damage consists of a tense, woody fibrosis of the skin that extends beyond the site of injection, irregular deep ulcers, and a halo of hyperpigmentation about the ulcers. Histologically there is necrosis and fibrosis in the dermis and in the septa of subcutaneous tissues, with areas of acute and chronic inflammation. Some of the vessels

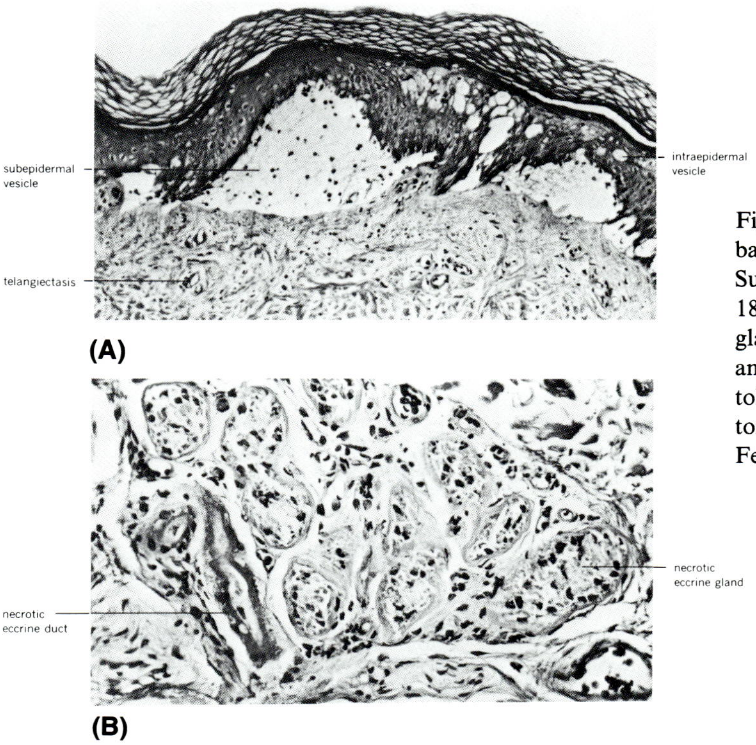

Fig. 6-20. Bulla secondary to barbiturate intoxication. (A) Subepidermal separation. × 180. (B) Necrosis of sweat glands. × 4,000. (Figs. 6-20 A and B from Ackerman, B.: Histologic Diagnosis of Inflammatory Skin Diseases. Lea and Febiger, Philadelphia, 1978.)

are occluded. Studies[78] in animals suggest that the primary insult is a vasoconstriction of vessels caused directly by pentazocine, with subsequent infarction of the dermis and epidermis, followed by fibrosis.

SKIN CHANGES INDUCED BY SYSTEMICALLY AND LOCALLY ADMINISTERED CORTICOSTEROIDS

Patients receiving long-term corticotropin and corticosteroids systemically often show cushinoid features.[44] The skin generally becomes atrophic, with a thin epidermis and a thin and loose dermis with the formation of striae. The skin becomes easily damaged and heals slowly; dermal vessels are fragile, leading to echymosis from slight trauma. Acne-like lesions and excessive growth of fine vellus hair are also present, mainly on the face. After discontinuation of the causative steroid, the skin changes, except for the striae, slowly fade. Local application of highly potent steroids[44] may produce local atrophy of the skin and telangiectasia; striae may also be seen in this condition, and adolescents are more prone to develop them than adults.

Histologically,[56] atrophic skin shows flattening of rete ridges in the epidermis, thinning of the epidermis, and a decrease in the size of the epidermal cells. The dermis displays collagen bundles which are thin and sometimes fragmented. Elastic fibers are thin and sparse in the upper dermis, while in the lower dermis they are more compact and dense than in normal skin. Sometimes the upper dermis shows large, compact bundles of fragmented elastic fibers. The number of fibrocytes may be decreased; the vessels are telangiectatic. Fresh striae (Fig. 6-21B) exhibit actual breakage and fragmentation of the elastic and collagen fibers in the reticular dermis and also edema.[85] Older striae (Fig. 6-22) show new formation of thin elastic fibers and fibrillar collagen in the upper dermis, which are parallel to the epidermis. Eventually loss of hair

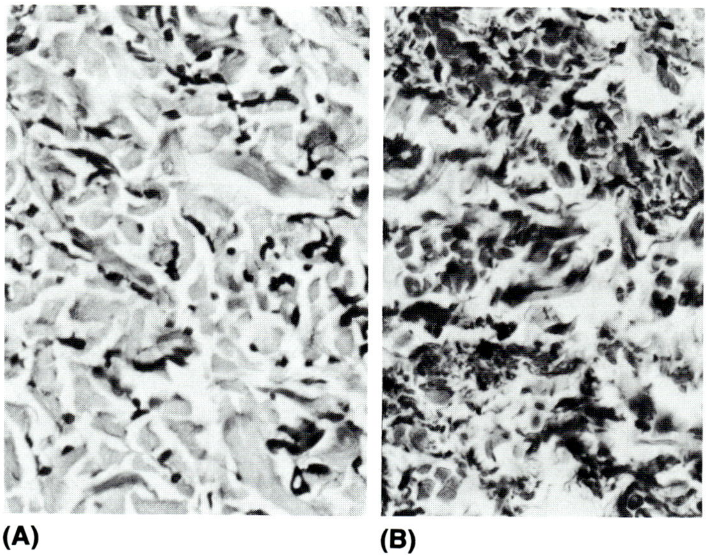

Fig. 6-21. (A) Normal elastic tissue. (B) Fresh striae distensae secondary to systemic corticosteroids reveal in the dermis fragmented elastic fibers, collagen fibers, and edema. Elastic tissue stain. (A) and (B) × 300.

follicles and most of the dermal appendages occurs.[71]

Although the striae in steroid-induced atrophy are permanent, the atrophy itself disappears within 6 months after steroids are discontinued. When very potent steroids are applied to the face for more than several weeks, a rosacea-like[67] eruption may occur. After withdrawal of steroids the skin eruption initially may become worse, but over a period of several months it gradually improves. Histologically there is a dense lymphocytic infiltrate around blood vessels. Hair follicles show disruption of the follicle wall and are surrounded by a lymphohistiocytic infiltrate and giant cells.

After sudden discontinuation of systemic corticosteroids, in patients who have been given systemic corticosteroids in large doses for long periods of time, panniculitis[88] may develop. When corticosteroids are reinstituted, the panniculitis gradually heals. Histo-

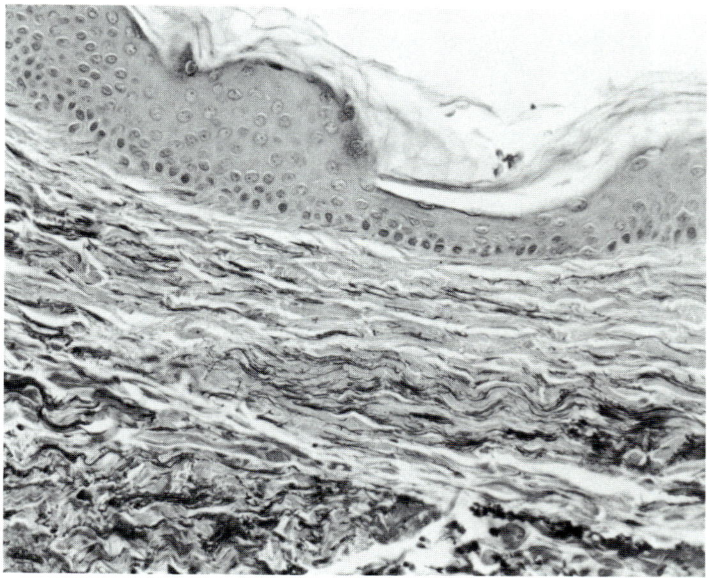

Fig. 6-22. Old striae distensae shows, in the dermis, newly formed thin elastic fibers and fibrillar collagen arranged parallel to the epidermis. Elastic tissue stain. × 230.

logically, the lesions in this condition are indistinguishable from subcutaneous fat necrosis of the newborn.

REFERENCES

1. Ackerman, B.: Hair follicle. In: Histologic Diagnosis of Inflammatory Skin Diseases. p. 50. Lea and Febiger, Philadelphia, 1978.
2. Ackerman, B.: Photoallergic contact dermatitis and photoallergic dermatitis. In: Histologic Diagnosis of Inflammatory Skin Diseases. p. 322. Lea and Febiger, Philadelphia, 1978.
3. Ackerman, B.: Lichenoid photodermatitis. In: Histologic Diagnosis of Inflammatory Skin Diseases. p. 322. Lea and Febiger, Philadelphia, 1978.
4. Ackerman, B.: Lichen planus like drug eruptions. In: Histologic Diagnosis of Inflammatory Skin Diseases. p. 210. Lea and Febiger, Philadelphia, 1978.
5. Ackerman, B.: Fixed drug eruption. In: Histologic Diagnosis of Inflammatory Skin Diseases. p. 516. Lea and Febiger, Philadelphia, 1978.
6. Ackerman, B.: Erythema multiforme. In: Histologic Diagnosis of Inflammatory Skin Diseases. p. 188. Lea and Febiger, Philadelphia, 1978.
7. Ackerman, B.: Toxic epidermal necrolysis (Lyell). In: Histologic Diagnosis of Inflammatory Skin Diseases. p. 605. Lea and Febiger, Philadelphia, 1978.
8. Ackerman, B.: Dermatitis herpetiformis-like drug eruption. In: Histologic Diagnosis of Inflammatory Skin Diseases. p. 626. Lea and Febiger; Philadelphia, 1978.
9. Ackerman, B.: Blisters secondary to hypoxemia and local pressure. In: Histologic Diagnosis of Inflammatory Skin Diseases. p. 595. Lea and Febiger, Philadelphia, 1978.
10. Ackerman, B.: Halogenodermas. In: Histologic Diagnosis of Inflammatory Skin Diseases. p. 463. Lea and Febiger, Philadelphia, 1978.
11. Alarcon-Segovia, D.: The necrotizing vasculitides. A new pathogenetic classification. Med. Clin. North Am. 61:24, 1977.
12. Almeyda, J., & Levantine, A.: Lichenoid drug eruptions. Br. J. Derm., 85:604, 1971.
13. Arndt, K. A., Mihm, H. C., & Parrish, J. A.: Bullae: A cutaneous sign of a variety of neurologic diseases. J. Invest. Dermatol. 60: 312, 1973.
14. Baden, H. P., & Holcomb, F. D.: Erythema nodosum from oral contraceptives. Arch. Dermatol. 98:634, 1968.
15. Bauer, F.: Late sequelae of atabrine dermatitis—A new pre-malignant entity. Aust. J. Dermatol. 19:9, 1978.
16. Biachine, J. R., Macaraeg, P. V. J., Lasagna, I. et al.: Drugs as etiologic factors in Stevens-Johnson syndrome. Am. J. Med. 44:390, 1968.
17. Bickers, D., Pathak, M. A., & Magnus, I. A.: The porphyrias, p. 1072. In: Fitzpatrick, T. B., et al., Eds.: Dermatology in General Medicine. 2nd Ed. McGraw-Hill Book Co., New York, 1979.
18. Blasik, L. G., & Spenser, S. K.: Fluoroderma. Arch. Dermatol. 115:1334, 1979.
19. Blomgren, S., Condemi, J., Vaughan, J. et al.: Procainamide-induced lupus erythematosus. Am. J. Med. 52:338, 1972.
20. Branner, G.: Bullous photoreaction to nalidixic acid. Am. J. Med. 58:576, 1975.
21. Braun Falco, O., & Woeff, H. H.: Zur ultrastruktur der epidermis beim Lyell-syndrome. Arch. Klin. Exp. Dermatol. 236:83, 1969.
22. Braverman, I. M., Yen, A.: Demonstration of immune complexes in spontaneous and histamine induced lesions and in normal skin of patients with leucoclastic angiitis. J. Invest. Dermatol. 64:105, 1975.
23. Bruinsma, W.: Acne. In: Guide to Drug Eruptions. Vol. 2. p. 17. The File of Adverse Reactions to the Skin, Department of Dermatology, Free University, distributed by DeZwaluw. Oosthuizem, The Netherlands, 1977.
24. Bruinsma, W.: Exanthematous eruptions. In: Guide to Drug Eruptions. p. 31. The File of Adverse Reactions to the Skin, Department of Dermatology, Free University, distributed by DeZwaluw. Oosthuizem, The Netherlands, 1977.
25. Bruinsma, W.: Eczematous type of eruptions. In: Guide to Drug Eruptions. p. 41. The File of Adverse Reactions to the Skin, Department of Dermatology, Free University, distributed by DeZwaluw. Oosthuizem, The Netherlands, 1977.
26. Bruinsma, W.: Photosensitivity. In: Guide to Drug Eruptions. The File of Adverse Reactions to the Skin. p. 43. Department of Derma-

tology, Free University, distributed by DeZwaluw. Oosthuizem, The Netherlands, 1977.
27. Bruinsma, W.: Urticaria. In: Guide to Drug Eruptions. p. 39. The File of Adverse Reactions to the Skin, Department of Dermatology, Free University, distributed by DeZwaluw. Oosthuizem, The Netherlands, 1977.
28. Bruinsma, W.: Purpura. In: Guide to Drug Eruptions. p. 53. The File of Adverse Reactions to the Skin, Department of Dermatology, Free University, distributed by DeZwaluw. Oosthuizem, The Netherlands, 1977.
29. Bruinsma, W.: Vascular reactions. In: Guide to Drug Eruptions. p. 49. The File of Adverse Reactions to the Skin, Department of Dermatology, Free University, distributed by DeZwaluw. Oosthuizem, The Netherlands, 1977.
30. Burger, L., & Winkelmann R.: Mercury pigmentation. Arch. Dermatol. 102:51, 1970.
31. Chorzelski, T., Jablonska, S., & Blaszczyk, M.: Autoantibodies in pemphigus. Acta Dermatol. Venereol. (Suppl.) 46:26, 1966.
32. Christian, C., & Sergent, J.: Vasculitis syndromes: Clinical and experimental models. Am. J. Med. 61:385, 1976.
33. Cohen, L. K., George, W., & Smith, R.: Isoniazid-induced acne and pellagra. Arch. Dermatol. 109:377, 1974.
34. Cronin, E.: Ekzematöse reactionen bei innerlecher aufnahme Von Kontact allergenen. Hautarzt 26:68, 1975.
35. Davis, M. G., and Holt, P.: Pemphigus in a patient treated with penicillamine for generalized morphea. Arch. Dermatol. 112:1308, 1976.
36. Delany, T. Y.: Tetracycline induced fixed drug eruptions. Br. J. Dermatol. 83:570, 1970.
37. de Moragas, J.: Panniculitis. In: Fitzpatrick, T. B. et al., Eds.: Dermatology in General Medicine. 2nd Ed. p. 784. McGraw-Hill Book Co., New York, 1979.
38. Dyster, A.: Pigment deposits in eyes and light exposed skin during long term methacycline therapy. Acta Derm. Venereol. 54:209, 1974.
39. Elias, P., & Fritsch, P.: Erythema multiforme. In: Fitzpatrick, T. B. et al., Eds.: Dermatology in General Medicine. 2nd Ed. p. 295. McGraw-Hill Book Co., New York, 1979.
40. Elias, P. M., Fritsch, P., & Epstein, E. Staphylococcal scalded skin syndrome. Arch. Dermatol. 113:207, 1977.
41. Fauci, A.: The spectrum of vasculitis. Clinical, pathologic, immunologic and therapeutic considerations. Ann. Intern. Med. 89:660, 1978.
42. Flaxman, B. A., Sosis, A. C., & Vanscott, E. J.: Changes in melanosomes distribution in causasoid skin following topical application of nitrogen mustard. J. Invest. Dermatol. 60:321, 1973.
43. Forbes, A.: Hirsutism. In: Fitzpatrick, T. B. et al., Eds.: Dermatology in General Medicine. 2nd Ed. P. 1266. McGraw-Hill Book Co., New York, 1979.
44. Freinkel, R., & Freinkel, N.: Dermatologic manifestations of endocrine disorders. In: Fitzpatrick, T. B. et al., Eds.: Dermatology in General Medicine. p. 1247. McGraw-Hill Book Co., New York, 1979.
45. Fritsch, P., & Elias, P.: Toxic epidermal necrolysis. In: Fitzpatrick, T. B. et al., Eds.: Dermatology in General Medicine. 2nd Ed. p. 303. McGraw-Hill Book Co., New York, 1979.
46. From, E., & Frederksen, P.: Pemphigus vulgaris following D penicillamine. Dermatologia 152:358, 1976.
47. Gauge, R. W., Rhodes, E. L., Edwa, R. D. S. et al.: Pemphigus induced by rifampicin. Br. J. Dermatol. 95:445, 1976.
48. Gordon, H.: Erythema nodosum review of 115 cases. Br. J. Dermatol. 73:393, 1961.
49. Griffits, W. A. D.: Diffuse hair loss and oral contraceptives. Br. J. Dermatol. 88:31, 1973.
50. Günther, R., Asamer, H., and Dittrich, P.: Das reversible procainamide-induzierte Lupus Erythematodes Syndrom. Dtsch. Med. Wochenschr. 94:2338, 1969.
51. Hahn, B. H., Sharp, G. C., Irwin, W. S. et al.: Immune responses to hydralazine and nuclear antigen in hydralazine-induced lupus erythematosus. Ann. Intern. Med. 76:365, 1972.
52. Hashimato, K., Wiener, W., Albert, J. et al.: An electron microscopic study of chlorpromazine pigmentation. J. Invest. Dermatol. 47:296, 1966.
53. Haymes, H. H., & Van Scott, E. J.: Lymphomas. In: Fitzpatrick, T. B. et al., Eds.: Dermatology in General Medicine. 2nd Ed. p. 749. McGraw-Hill Book Co., New York, 1979.
54. Hewitt, J., Beneviste, M., & Lessaner-Leibow-

itch, M.: Pemphigus induced by penicillamine and experimental pemphigus. Br. J. Dermatol. (Suppl.) 11:12, 1975.
55. Hewitt, J., Lessaner-Leibowitch, M., Beneviste, M. et al.: Un cas de pemphigus induit par la D penicillamine. Le pemphigus iatrogene exist-il. Ann. Med. Interne 122:1003, 1971.
56. Jablonska, S., Groniowska, M., & Dabroswki, J.: Comparative evaluation of skin atrophy in man induced by topical corticoids. Br. J. Dermatol. 100:193, 1979.
57. Jenkins, R. B., & Rattner, A. C.: Diphenylhydantoin and acne. N. Engl. J. Med. 287:148, 1972.
58. Jolly, H. W., Jr., Sherman, I. J., Jr., Carpenter, C. L., Jr. et al.: Fixed drug eruptions to tetracylcines. Arch. Dermatol. 114:1484, 1978.
59. Kazmierowski, J., & Wuepper, K. D.: Erythema multiforme, immune-complex vasculitis of the superficial cutaneous microvasculature. Clin. Res. 25:282a, 1977.
60. Levantine, A., & Almeyda, J.: Drug induced changes in pigmentation. Br. J. Dermatol. 89:105, 1973.
61. Levantine, A., & Almeyda, J.: Drug induced alopecia. Br. J. Dermatol. 89:549, 1973.
62. Lever, W., & Schaumburg-Lever, G.: Eruptions due to drugs. In: Histopathology of the Skin. p. 239. J. B. Lippincott Co., Philadelphia, 1975.
63. Lever, W., & Schaumburg-Lever, G. Dermatitis (eczema). In: Histopathology of the Skin. p. 96. J. B. Lippincott Co., Philadelphia, 1975.
64. Lever, W., & Schaumburg-Lever, G.: Noninflammatory purpuras. In: Histopathology of the Skin. p. 157. J. B. Lippincott Co., Philadelphia, 1975.
65. Lever, W., & Schaumburg-Lever, G.: Dermatitis (eczema). In: Histopathology of the Skin. p. 96. J. B. Lippincott Co., Philadelphia, 1975.
66. Lever, W., & Schaumburg-Lever, G.: Porphyria. In: Histopathology of the Skin. p. 397. J. B. Lippincott Co., Philadelphia, 1975.
67. Leyden, J. J., Thew, M., & Kligman, A. M.: Steroid rosacea. Arch. Dermatol. 110:619, 1974.
68. Lowitz, B. B.: Streaking with bleomycin. N. Engl. J. Med., 292:1300, 1975.
69. Lynch, P., & Boyer, J.: Clotting disorders and the skin (purpura). In: Fitzpatrick, T. B. et al., Eds.: Dermatology in General Medicine. 2nd Ed. p. 1168. McGraw-Hill Book Co., New York, 1979.
70. Montgomery, H.: Fixed drug eruptions. In: Dermatopathology. p. 261. Harper and Row Publishers, New York, 1967.
71. Montgomery, H.: Striae cutis distense. In: Dermatopathology. p. 776. Harper and Row Publishers, New York, 1967.
72. Montgomery, H.: Pigmentary disorders. In: Dermatopathology. p. 267. Harper and Row Publishers, New York, 1967.
73. Mosher, D., Fitzpatrick, T. B., & Ortonne, J. P.: Abnormalities of pigmentation. In: Fitzpatrick, T. B. et al., Eds.: Dermatology in General Medicine. p. 568. McGraw-Hill, Book Co., New York, 1979.
74. Munro, D. D., & Darley, C. R.: Hair. In: Fitzpatrick, T. B. et al., Eds.: Dermatology in General Medicine. 2nd Ed. p. 395. McGraw-Hill Book Co., New York, 1979.
75. Nalbandion, R. M.: Skin necrosis induced by coumarin congeners. J.A.M.A. 211:1699, 1970.
76. Nicholis, G. D., & Helwig, E. B.: Exfoliative dermatitis. Arch. Dermatol. 108:788, 1973.
77. Okrasinski, H.: Lithium acne. Dermatologica 154:251, 1977.
78. Parks, D. L.: Cutaneous complications of pentazocine injections. Arch. Dermatol. 104:231, 1971.
79. Parrish, J., White, H. A. D., & Pathak, M. A.: Photomedicine. In: Fitzpatrick, T. B. et al., Eds.: Dermatology in General Medicine. 2nd Ed. p. 942. McGraw-Hill Book Co., New York, 1979.
80. Pasricha, J. S.: Drugs causing fixed eruption. Br. J. Dermatol. 100:183, 1979.
81. Peduis-Leftick, A., Cyrlin, M. N., & Solomon, J. M.: Cataract in a patient with vitiligo who received photochemotherapy. Arch. Dermatol. 115:1253, 1979.
82. Penneys, N. S. et al.: Gold dermatitis, a clinical and histopathological study. Arch. Dermatol. 109:372, 1972.
83. Pinkus, H., & Mehregan, A. H.: Scleroderma. In: A Guide to Dermatohistopathology. 2nd Ed. p. 359. Appleton-Century Crofts, New York, 1976.
84. Pinkus, H., & Mehregan, A. H.: Unusual bullous lesions. In: A Guide to Dermatohistopa-

thology. 2nd Ed. p. 182. Appleton-Century-Crofts, New York, 1976.
85. Pinkus, H., & Mehregan, A. H. Striae distensae. In: A Guide to Dermatohistopathology. 2nd Ed. p. 386. Appleton-Century-Crofts, New York, 1976.
86. Priestman, T. J., & James, K. W.: Adriamycin and longitudinal pigmented banding of fingernails. Lancet 1:1337, 1975.
87. Rich, A. R.: Role of hypersensitivity in periarteritis nodosa as indicated by 7 cases developing during serum sickness and sulfonamide therapy. Bull. Johns Hopkins Hosp. 71:123, 1942.
88. Roenigk, H. H. et al.: Poststeroid panniculitis. Arch. Dermatol., 90:387, 1964.
89. Rosenberg, E. R., Einbinder, J., Wahzer, R. H., et al.: Vegetating iododerma. Arch. Dermatol. 105:900, 1972.
90. Rothstein, G., Clarkson, D. R., Larsen, W., & Grosser, B. I.: Effect of lithium on neutrophis mass and production. N. Engl. J. Med. 298:178, 1978.
91. Sams, W. M. et al.: Human necrotizing vasculitis immunoglobulins and complement in vessel walls of lesions and normal skin. J. Invest. Dermatol. 64:441, 1975.
92. Savin, J. A.: Current causes of fixed drug eruptions. Br. J. Dermatol. 83:546, 1970.
93. Schiff, B. L., & Kern, H. B.: Unusual cutaneous manifestations of pentazocine addiction. J.A.M.A. 238:1542, 1977.
94. Schlicher, J., Zucheke, R. L., Lynch, P. J. et al.: Local changes at the site of pentazocine injection. Arch. Dermatol. 104:90, 1971.
95. Schreiber, M. M., & McGregor, J. G.: Pseudolymphoma syndrome. Arch. Dermatol. 97:296, 1968.
96. Schroefer, A. L. et al.: Immunofluorescence of cutaneous vasculitis associated with systemic diseases. Arch Dermatol. 104:254, 1974.
97. Soter, N., & Fitzpatrick, T. B.: Introduction and classification. Cutaneous changes in disorders of altered reactivity: Eczematous dermatitis. In: Fritzpatrick, T. B. et al., Eds.: Dermatology in General Practice. 2nd Ed. p. 507. McGraw-Hill Book Co., New York, 1979.
98. Soter, W., & Wasserman, S.: IgE dependent urticaria, angioedema and anaphylaxis. In: Fitzpatrick, T. B. et al., Eds.: Dermatology in General Medicine. 2nd Ed. p. 532. McGraw-Hill Book Co., New York, 1979.
99. Spillane, J. D.: Brunette to blonde: Depigmentation of human hair during oral treatment with mephenesin. Br. Med. J. 1:997, 1963.
100. Stein, K. M., Odone, R. B., & Justice, G.: Toxic alopecia from ingestion of boric acid. Arch. Dermatol. 108:95, 1973.
101. Stern, L. S., Thibooleau, L. A., Kleinerman, R. A. et al.: Cutaneous carcinoma after PUVA treatment of psoriasis. N. Engl. J. Med. 300:809, 1979.
102. Strauss, J.: Sebaceous glands. In: Fitzpatrick, T. B. et al., Eds.: Dermatology in General Medicine. 2nd Ed. p. 437. McGraw-Hill Book Co., New York, 1979.
103. Teller, H.: Bromoderma and iododerma tuberosum. Dermatol. Wochenschr. 143:273, 1961.
104. Tuffanelli, D., Abraham, R. K., & Dubois, E.: Pigmentation from antimalarial therapy. Arch. Dermatol. 88:113, 1963.
105. Ullman, S., Wiik, A., Kobayasi, T. et al.: Drug induced lupus erythematosus syndrome. Acta Dermato. Venereol. 54:387, 1974.
106. Utsinger, P. D., & Yount, W. J.: Allopurinol hypersensitivity: Granular deposition of IgM at the dermal-epidermal junction. Am. J. Med. 61:287, 1976.
107. Whitle, T., Jr., & Ainsworth, S. K.: Procainamide-induced systemic lupus erythematosus. Arch. Pathol. Lab. Med. 100:469, 1976.
108. Wintroub, B., Shiffman, N. J., & Arndt, K.: Adverse cutaneous reactions to drugs. In: Fitzpatrick, T. B. et al., Eds.: Dermatology in General Medicine. 2nd Ed. p. 555. McGraw-Hill Book Co., New York, 1979.
109. Wittingham, S., & Mackay, I. R.: Systemic lupus erythematosus induced by procainamide. Aust. Am. Med. 4:358, 1970.
110. Woosley, R. L., Drayer, D. E., Reidenberg, M. M. et al.: Effect of acetylator phenotype on the rate at which procainamide induces antinuclear antibodies and the lupus syndrome. N. Engl. J. Med. 298:1157, 1978.
111. Zelickson, A.: Skin changes and chlorpromazine. J.A.M.A. 198:341, 1966.
112. Zelickson, A. S., & Zeller, H.: A new and unusual reaction to chlorpromazine. J.A.M.A. 188:394, 1964.

7

The Oral Cavity

Robert A. Goepp

The oral cavity may be affected by a variety of toxic events occurring through different mechanisms. The appearence of toxic disease may be consequent to direct surface contact by matter toxic to oral tissues; disease may follow the ingestion of a toxic substance that is then carried parenterally to oral sites; or diseases may present as lasting formative alterations in the teeth if exposure to a toxic substance occurred during the time of development of the teeth by either direct or parenteral route. The term oral toxicosis as used herein is restricted to toxic exposure causing necrosis or disabling alterations in the functions of oral tissues.

CONTACT TOXICOSIS

The opportunity for oral toxic disease precipitated by direct contact seems limitless because of the great variety of materials—including foods—that are put into the oral cavity. In addition, the mouth has a profound relationship to personality—a relationship that is apparently the basis for oral habits which are ubiquitous and worldwide. Beyond this, the tongue and taste are commonly used to explore unknown materials.

Yet, although many oral habits involve the use of potentially toxic materials, contact toxic disease of the oral cavity is relatively rare. The resistance to contact toxic disease is probably due to the highly protective surfaces of the oral tissues. The outer surface of the teeth is covered by dental enamal, an extremely hard, impervious, highly mineralized tissue composed of calcium hydroxyapatite crystals in a highly organized spatial arrangement. The remainder of the oral cavity surface is composed of stratified squamous epithelium, highly specialized in the mucosa of the tongue and keratinized in the common contact areas of the tongue, palate, and gingivae. Moreover, the oral surfaces are generously and constantly bathed in saliva containing a large amount of mucus, which provides both lubrication and a chemical barrier. The infrequent loss of adequate saliva through aging or specific disease processes results in the rapid destruction of dental enamel and the presence of mucositis, both of which are caused by contact toxic phenomena.

Exposure over a period of time to markedly unfavorable environments containing relatively high concentrations of acids may decalcify the teeth. While acid exposure may be found in some industrial environments,[14] decalcification is also possible through habitual sucking on citrus fruits. The fruit is usually pressed against the incisor teeth, with decalcification being seen only on the labial surfaces of these teeth. Strong alkalis put into the mouth produce a very rapid necrosis and sloughing of the oral mucosa. A variety of industrial chemicals may cause staining of the oral mucosa and teeth, although in most cases the staining of teeth is not intrinsic, but is rather a staining of debris adherent to tooth surfaces.[15] The effect of corrosives is considered in greater detail in Chapter 18.

Chemotherapy

The cytotoxic medications often used in the management of hematologic neoplasms may cause ulceration of the oral mucosa. Most often, the site of oral mucosal breakdown is that of a pre-existing inflammatory disease, such as marked gingivitis or periodontal disease. Occasionally, ulcerations can occur in areas where there is no prior chronic dental inflammatory disease, such as the palate; however, while this may seem to be the result of a singular effect of chemotherapy, it must be remembered that the oral mucosa is frequently subject to pressures and minor, usually unnoticed, lacerations from eating foods, such as crackers, which break into pieces with sharp edges. Such an event might be the nidus, under the influence of chemotherapy, for an oral ulceration. There appears to be no propensity for any of the different groups of chemotherapeutic medications to cause oral ulcerations; rather, oral toxicosis is related directly to the dose or length of time of treatment or to both.

Initial oral complaints during chemotherapy are a burning sensation in the mucosa and a soreness of the tongue, which may be erythematous. Atrophy of the lingual filiform papillae makes the fungiform papillae appear prominent. Necrotic lesions may appear about 2 weeks after chemotherapy is begun, as irregular, yellowish-gray areas. Secondary infection is common and causes the ulceration to become painful and to have an erythematous halo at its perimeter. An associated thrombocytopenia may allow hemmorrhage from the ulceration. Ulcerations occuring in such less well lubricated areas of the oral mucosa as the lips may demonstrate cracking or fissuring through the ulceration.

Microscopically, chemotherapeutic agents may cause nonspecific ulceration, with possibly little inflammatory infiltrate especially if leukopenia is present. Secondary infection of the ulcer is frequent.

Heavy Metals

The ingestion of or exposure to metals that are protoplasmic poisons can cause oral disease. Arsenic causes erythematous streaks in the oral mucosa. Petechial hemorrhages are consequent to the necrosis of small vessel walls. Such hemorrhages may coalesce and form vesicle-like subepithelial accumulations of blood.[15]

Bismuth or cadmium ingestion or contact produces a mild, uniform mucositis with pain probably caused by the considerable subepithelial edema. Bismuth can combine with sulfide in preexisting gingivitis, resulting in a bismuth sulfide precipitate that produces a blue discoloration of the gingiva.[8] Cadmium can cause intrinsic yellow staining of the teeth.[12]

The oral effects of lead ingestion appear to be restricted to a bluish discoloration of the gingiva in areas of gingivitis (Fig. 7-1).[4] If lead ingestion is during dental formative times, lead will be incorporated into hard dental tissues and, as such, teeth can be used to assess prior lead exposure.[1] The pathogenesis of lead precipation in the gingiva is, like that of other metals, combined with the deposition of sulfides in extracellular locations, and also seen in macrophages.

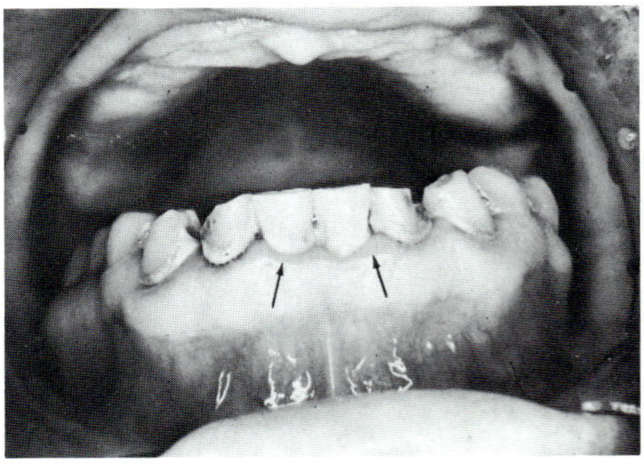

Fig. 7-1. Lead-line in gingiva. The metal is accumulated in sites of chronic inflammation, in this case causing a linear festooning, indicated by arrows, in the gingiva immediately adjacent to the teeth. (From Goepp, R. A.: Physical, chemical and radiation changes in the oral cavity. In: Tiecke, R. W., Ed.: Oral Pathology, p. 725. Copyright © 1965 McGraw-Hill. Used with the permission of McGraw-Hill Book Company, New York.)

Mercury ingestion or contact causes marked edema of the oral mucosa, most noticeable in the lips. The initial complaint is burning and soreness in the oral mucosa. Necrotic lesions that coalesce to form large patches are found in a chronic mercury poisoning. It is commonly reported that hypersalivation with drooling is a hallmark of mercury poisoning; however, the hypersalivation is probably not the direct result of mercury stimulation of salivary function, but is rather provoked by a gustatory stimulation which is in turn caused by the presence of large necrotic areas of oral mucosa. Mercury salts can also deposit in the mucosa, causing a bluish-gray discoloration. A unique exposure to mercury, occuring in infants and young children, has been termed acrodynia or pink disease.[17] The source of the causative mercury is an infant teething powder, the effects of exposure to which may last for several years, and are characterized by a red, raw dermatitis. The oral findings are gingival ulceration, hypersalivation, pain, and loose teeth which may be prematurely shed.

Aspirin

Among the more common oral sites for painful symptoms are the teeth, and the use of aspirin is almost as common as toothaches. Yet there are individuals who do not understand that aspirin is to be ingested, and instead put aspirin tablets directly on the apparent site of pain, usually between the cheek and the gingiva. Such application quickly causes a white, convoluted elevation of the oral mucosa. (Fig. 7-2). Microscopic examination reveals that the mucosal change is due to pronounced intra- and intercellular edema in the Malpighian layers of the stratified squamous epithelium. If exposure is continued, the epithelium disintegrates and the underlying basal cell layer is easily lost, resulting in frank ulceration.

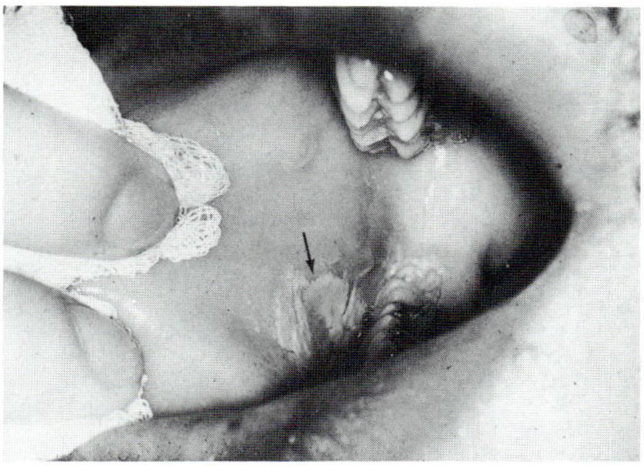

Fig. 7-2. Toxicity of aspirin applied locally to oral mucosa. The mucosa area in the cheek displays a raised white irregular area indicated by an arrow.

Gasoline

The oral siphoning of gasoline may, by miscalculation, cause gasoline to fill the mouth. While such an event has not been reported for decades, gasoline-induced mucositis has recently been reported.[7] The contact exposure of the oral mucosa to gasoline causes swelling, erythema, vesicles, and punctate ulcerations.

PARENTERAL-ROUTE ORAL TOXICOSIS

Radium

Among the more notable forms of parenteral-route oral toxicity was the radioactive poisoning discovered in 1923 among workers who painted watch dials, numbers, and hands with radium or thorium to make the watch faces visible in the dark.[2,10] The event was notable because it directed popular interest to the possible toxic effects of ionizing radiation, and served as the stimulus for an organized, public interest in occupational safety which in turn resulted in pioneering legislation for occupational protection.

The watch-dial painters ingested radioactive materials by pointing their small paint brushes with their lips. Since the ingested radioactive salts followed the same metabolic pathways as calcium, they became concentrated in the bone—first in the marrow, followed by a slower recycling to the bone cortices.

The deposition of ingested radium in the bone is not uniform; rather, there are random focal "hot spots." The necrosis of osteocytes interrupts the canalicular circulation in the bone, with consequent distal infarction and necrosis—in this case osteoradionecrosis of calcified bone matrix. Additionally, the presence of radioactive salts near the trabecular surfaces provokes sclerotic bone deposition, compromising the marrow space and vascular distribution, and again causing bone infarction and necrosis. While in most bones a degree of aseptic infarction and necrosis would not compromise function, the jawbones are particularly liable to infection as a consequence of these effects because of the prevalence of inflammatory dental disease, both dental caries and periodontal diseases, which can result in the access of bacteria into bone. Once established in bone in which the circulatory distribution has been interrupted, infection can persist and spread, because neither innate defensive mechanisms nor additive medical treatment are effective against it; the continuing bone necrosis persists until the entire bone is destroyed. The mandible is the bone most often affected; the maxilla, probably because of its more rich vascular distribution, is rarely affected.

The earliest sign of osteoradionecrosis of the mandible is a severe, constant pain in the bone[11]; the pain may continue for weeks before physical signs appear. Cortical sequestration results in loss of the soft tissue covering over the affected bone, and a denuded area of necrotic bone is commonly the first physical evidence of osteoradionecrosis of the jawbones. The radiologic findings of sequestration are seen only in an advanced state (Fig. 7-3). In very advanced cases, subperiosteal abscesses, with draining facial fistulas, can be found.

The effect of radium ingestion on the teeth is a generalized, multifocal external and internal resorption of the roots (Fig 7-4). There are a number of reasons, consequent to dental disease, why a tooth root may undergo internal or external resorption, or both; however, a generalized multifocal internal and external resorption of the roots is a specific sign of parenteral route toxicosis.[6,13]

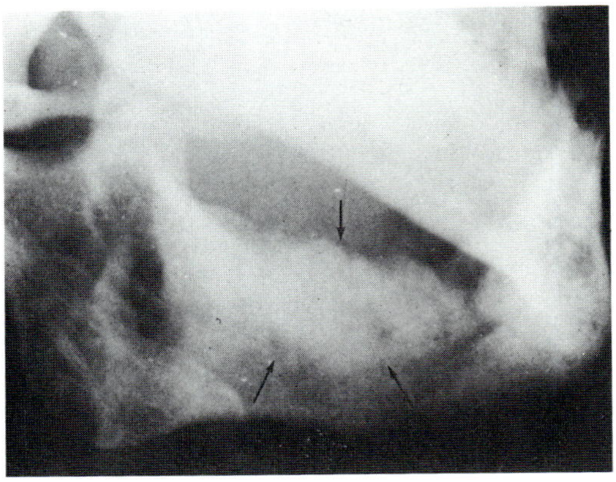

Fig. 7-3. Osteoradionecrosis. The lateral-jaw x-ray examination reveals a large sequestrum, outlined by arrows, in the edentulous left mandible.

Phosphorus

The term phossy jaw is used to describe a fulminating osteomyelitis of the jaws with extensive necrosis, usually of the mandible, cuased by the ingestion of white phosphorus.[9] Exposure to white phorphorus was mainly an occupational hazard in the latter half of the nineteenth century; in fact, the condition became so widespread that industrial safety pro-

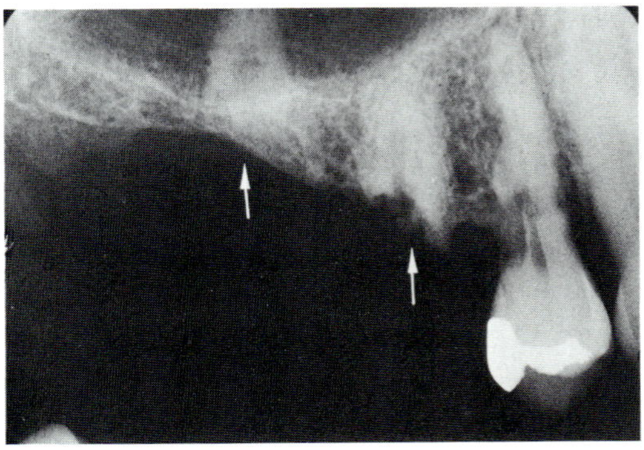

Fig. 7-4. Radium ingestion. The x-ray examination of the dental area reveals resorption of biscupid tooth root. Remaining roots of other teeth, indicated by arrows, can be seen in the bone.

cedures were established in the last decade of the nineteenth century. Presently, phossy jaw is a rare occurrence.

Dilantin

Dilantin (sodium diphenylhydantoin) is a medication that has been used for many decades to control seizures.[5] However, in the past decade, Dilantin has also been used to manage a wider variety of neurologic and neuromuscular difficulties. The increased indicated use of Dilantin has important consequences for oral toxicity. The parenteral use of Dilantin causes two changes in the gingiva: a basal cell hyperplasia of the squamous epithelium and a hypertrophy of submucosal collagen. The gingiva becomes enlarged immediately around (particularly between) teeth, causing the formation, between the teeth and gingiva, of a cul-de-sac that acts as an entrapment for oral debris, in turn causing a more severe inflammatory gingivitis (Fig. 7-5). The appositional epithelial surface usually becomes ulcerated, producing a Dilantin-induced toxicosis in conjunction with the banal gingivitis. In fact, Dilantin-induced change in the gingiva depends upon pre-existing gingivitis; in the absence of gingivitis, Dilantin causes little or no change in the gingiva. If Dilantin treatment is discontinued, the gingiva may revert to its original anatomy. However, if Dilantin treatment lasts many months (six or more) the gingiva probably will not resolve from its enlarged anatomy. The enlarged gingival anatomy is usually not self-cleaning and a progressive, destructive periodontitis would be expected (Fig. 7-5A). The gingival hypertrophy associated with long-term Dilantin treatment may even dislocate and spread teeth apart (Fig. 7-5B). Furthermore, Dilantin-related mucosal changes can occur in other areas of the oral mucosa besides the gingiva; such changes can be seen in edentulous jaws and in the palate when an ill-fitting artificial appliance causes low grade, chronic irritation, the same prerequisite as gingivitis, needed for the much more common gingival change.

FORMATIVE TOXICOSIS

Prenatal Icterus

Pigments consequent to blood cell destruction in the fetus may be incorporated into the mineralizing tissues of the teeth. Such prenatal

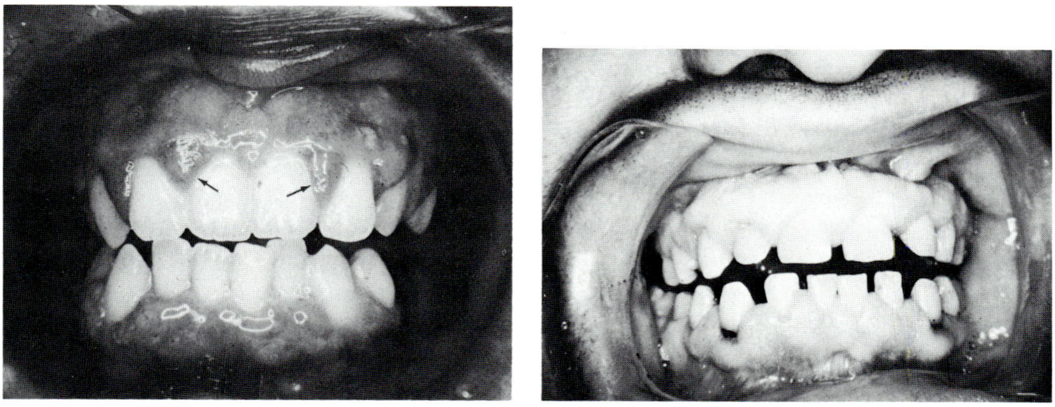

(A) **(B)**

Fig. 7-5. (A) Moderate Dilantin change. The gingiva displays a bulbous enlargement mainly in the interdental papillae. (B) Severe Dilantin change. The gingival displays a generalized bulbous enlargement with displacement of teeth.

pigmentation of the teeth is most commonly a consequence of Rh factor incompatability between parents; in such cases the primary, deciduous, teeth will incorporate pigment and be stained a reddish brown color. Necrosis or functional impairment occurs in the form of hypoplastic defects in the coronal anatomy, particularly involving the cusp tips or incisal edges of the teeth (Fig. 7-6). If a blood-cell destruction episode occurs in the latter part of the third trimester of pregnancy, certain secondary, permanent central incisors and first molars may be affected by hypoplasia in the areas of the cusp tips and incisal edges.[12] The incorporation of blood-cell products into calcifying tissues has an obvious pathogenesis; however, the hypoplastic defects of the teeth consequent upon blood-cell destruction are not precisely clear in their pathogenesis. It may be that focal hypoxia is responsible for the formative defects such as those seen in Figure 7.6.

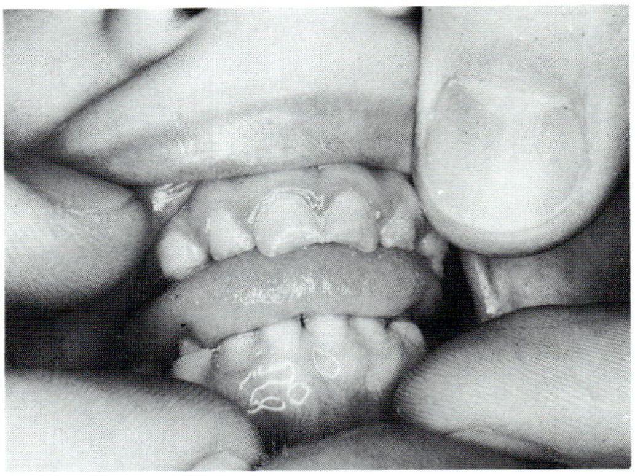

Fig. 7-6. Prenatal icterus. These teeth contain an intrinsic deep yellow discoloration. Formative defects are seen at the incisal edges of the incisor teeth and cuspid tips in the primary teeth. (From Goepp, R. A.: Physical, chemical and radiation changes in the oral cavity. In: Tiecke, R. W., Ed.: Oral Pathology, p. 725. Copyright © 1965 McGraw-Hill. Used with the permission of McGraw-Hill Book Company, New York.)

Nonspecific Dental Hypoplasia

Hypoplasia of an entire or major portion of a tooth is relatively rare; such a finding is almost always associated with radiation therapy. Additionally, uniquely small teeth may be found in a normal-size dentition; these are believed to result from genetic or programmed alterations. Such teeth are referred to as microdonts.

Focal hypoplasia is a somewhat horizontal linear defect in the surfaces of crowns of teeth. The borders and depth of the defect are irregular, giving the appearance of a line or collection of pits. Focal hypoplasia may involve single, isolated teeth or the entire dentition.

The pattern of generalized focal hypoplasia of the teeth follows the chronology of dental development; that is, the linear hypoplastic line will be located at different levels in different teeth, the levels being a mark of the degree of development achieved at the time of exposure to the causes of the hypoplasia (Fig. 7-7). The width of the linear hypoplastic line is roughly proportional to the length of exposure, in time, to the causative factor of the hypoplasia. This relationship is necessarily approximate because teeth do not form at a constant rate; rather, there are periods of active

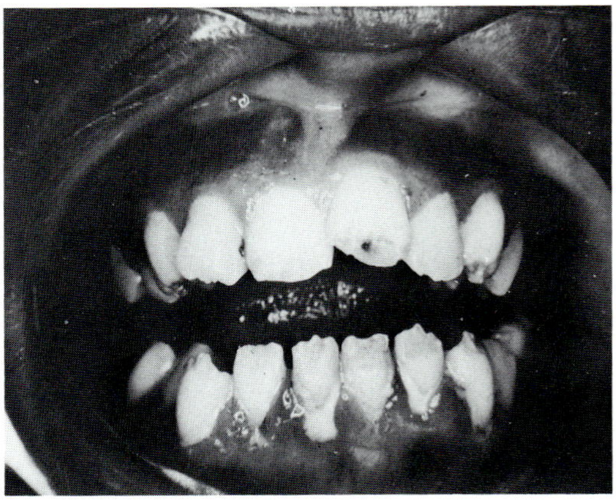

Fig. 7-7. Dental hypoplasia. The generalized focal dental hypoplasia exhibits a chronologic pattern ranging from a major part of the incisal thirds of the incisor crowns to the cusp tips of the cuspid teeth. This indicates a generalized interference with dental development during the first two years of life.

development alternating with periods of developmental rest.

The causes of focal dental hypoplasia may be toxic, nutritional, or physical. While the pathogenesis may involve an interference with matrix production, linear hypoplasia is more often believed to be associated with interference with mineralization of the matrix.

Focal linear hypoplasia of single teeth, called "Turner's teeth," is usually caused by localized inflammatory disease consequent to the presence of microorganisms. Carious destruction of a primary tooth, with bacterial toxic penetration into the subjacent bone crypt of the developing secondary tooth, may cause single focal hypoplasia.

Fluorine

The use of fluorine as a public health measure against dental caries has received wide attention, and has achieved remarkable results in the mass reduction of caries. Fluorine, in the form of fluoride, is usually used for this purpose through introduction into the water supply. The amount of fluoride in the water supply is critical; about 1 ppm has been found to be effective for caries prevention when available during the formation of teeth. Higher concentrations of fluoride are applied topically to erupted tooth surfaces, with a beneficial anticaries effect. However, the ingestion of larger amounts than 1 ppm of fluoride may have marked toxic effects during the tooth formative process.[3]

The toxic effect of excessive fluoride exposure on tooth formation is called fluorosis or mottled enamel. The exposure to excessive fluoride in such cases usually occurs through water supplies in which fluoride is naturally present at 3 or more ppm. The severity of formative defects is directly related to the amount of fluoride ingested. Considerable variation in the degree of dental fluorosis can be found in populations exposed to excessive levels of fluoride in the water supply; this variation is thought to reflect individual variation in the amount of water ingested related to alternate periods of active development and developmental rest.

The dental effects of excessive fluoride exposure during tooth formation are mottled enamel and hypoplastic defects. Mottled enamel may range in appearance from chalky white spots to more severe brown discolorations (Fig. 7-8). However, small chalky white spots incorporated in the tooth surfaces may have a variety of causes and are not pathognomonic of fluoride ingestion. Hypoplastic defects are in themselves nonspecific for fluorosis; they appear as irregularly sized pits or depressions in the tooth surface. The floors of the pits or depressions are also irregular as contrasted to the usually smooth tooth surfaces. In non-fluorosis cases, the white spots and hypoplastic defects are restricted to subtotal areas of one or a few teeth. The white spots, brown discoloration and hypoplastic defects of fluorosis are most often generalized for the complete surfaces of all teeth. If the exposure to excessive fluoride was of less time than the duration of dental development, the fluorosis effect would be seen only on the parts of those teeth formed during exposure. In severe cases of fluorosis the degree of hypoplasia

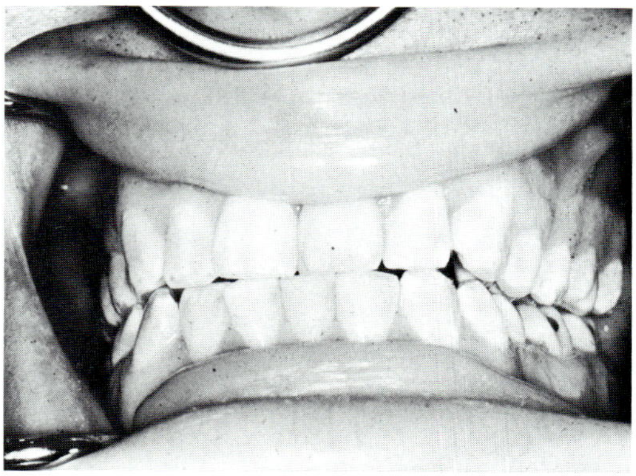

Fig. 7-8. Dental fluorosis. These teeth have a mottled appearance consisting of irregular tan and chalky white patches on the surface. The biting surfaces of the teeth have irregular rough surfaces due to flaking of brittle enamel also found in dental fluorosis. This case was due to naturally occurring excessive fluoride in the drinking water during formative years.

may so radically alter the surface anatomy of a tooth that the unique identification of the tooth can be done only through its location in the jaw. Teeth exhibiting fluorosis are rather brittle and tend to fracture more easily than teeth not involved by this condition.

Tetracycline

The prolonged administration of tetracycline during tooth formation will result in its incorporation into the tooth structure during calcification. This produces bright yellow rings or bands in the teeth. However, as the stained area—such as the tooth crown—is exposed to light after tooth eruption, the yellow-stained areas become progressively brown to dark brown.[16] Tetracycline incorporation into the teeth does not produce necrosis or anatomic abnormality. However, white teeth generally have considerable esthetic value, and darkly stained teeth may be considered a decrement in esthetic function. Hence, tetracycline incorporation into the teeth is considered here to be a toxicosis.

REFERENCES

1. Altshuller, L. F., Halak, D. B., Landing, B. H., and Kehoe, R. H.: Deciduous teeth as an index of body burden of lead. J. Pediatr. 60:224, 1962.
2. Blum, T.: Osteomyelitis of the mandible. J. Am. Dent. Assoc. 11:396, 1924.
3. Churchill, H. V.: Occurances of fluorides in some waters of the United States. Ind. Eng. Chem. 23:966, 1931.
4. Dreesen, W. C.: Health of lead exposed storage battery workers. Toxicology 25:60, 1943.
5. Glickman, I., and Levitus, M. P.: Hyperplasia of the gingiva associated with Dilantin. J. Am. Dent. Assoc. 28:199, 1941.
6. Goepp, R. A.: Physical, chemical and radiation changes in the oral cavity. In: Tiecke, R. W., Ed.: Oral Pathology. p. 725. McGraw-Hill, New York, 1965.
7. Hoffman, D. L., Swanson, B. Z., and Lutins, N. D.: Gasoline induced mucositis. J. Am. Dent. Assoc. 100:217, 1980.
8. Hunter, O.: The Diseases of Occupations. University Press, London, 1955.
9. Kennon, R., and Hallam, J. W.: Modern phosphorus caries and necrosis. Br. Dent. J. 76:321, 1944.
10. Martland, H. S.: Occupational poisoning in the manufacture of luminous watch dials. J.A.M.A. 92:466, 522, 1929.
11. Meyer, I.: Osteoradionecrosis of the Jaws. Year Book Publishers, Chicago, 1958.
12. Potter, E. L.: Pathology of the Fetus and Infant. 2 ed., Chapter 18. Year Book Publishers, Chicago, 1961.
13. Rowland, R. E.: Radium in human teeth. Arch. Oral Biol. 7:13, 1963.
14. Schour, I., and Sarnat, B. G.: Oral manifestations of occupational origin. J.A.M.A. 120:1197, 1942.
15. Schwartz, L., Tulipan, L., and Birmingham, D. J.: Occupational Diseases of the Skin, 3rd ed. Lea & Febiger, Philadelphia, 1957.
16. Wallman, I. S., and Hilton, H. B.: Teeth pigmented by tetracycline. Lancet 1:827, 1962.
17. Warkany, J., and Hubbard, D. M.: Acrodynia and mercury. J. Pediatr. 42:365, 1953.

8

The Inner Ear

Raul Hinojosa, John R. Lindsay, Gregory J. Matz, and Ralph F. Naunton

INTRODUCTION

Drug-induced inner ear damage is by now a well recognized hazard accompanying the use of a considerable and increasing number of medications. Among early examples of medications carrying this hazard (and therefore described as "ototoxic drugs") were arsenic, used in the treatment of syphilis; in this instance, however, as in some others, the inner ear effects of the disease itself may well have been confused with and mistaken for drug-induced changes in the inner ear. The salicylates and quinine have also been recognized for many years as ototoxic drugs.

The therapeutic problem of ototoxicity became a major issue—demanding and receiving the concerted attention of clinicians, histopathologists, and neurophysiologists—only as the first aminoglycoside antibiotics were introduced into clinical practice. The resulting studies led to the recognition that aminoglycosides may damage the cochlear system or the vestibular system or both, that the damage may develop and progress only while the drug is being taken or that it may start late and continue after discontinuing drug administration, and that the ototoxic effects are usually but not always irreversible. Newer aminoglycoside antibiotics have been developed since, all of them ototoxic to varying degrees.

Ototoxic changes have also been recognized in association with other types of drugs such as the "loop" diuretics and some of the antimetabolites. Thalidomide, a mild sedative, achieved notoriety because of its tragic tendency to induce amelia and phocomelia in the fetuses of pregnant women; one of its other, less-recognized dangers is that it may arrest inner ear formation during the early weeks of fetal development, thus leading to aplasia of the inner ear. Other, still less familiar instances of ototoxicity include those accompanying the use of radium, in the treatment of schizophrenia or as a "tonic," and ototoxicity in the anaphylactic reaction to penicillin.

SALICYLATES

Salicylates can lead to sensorineural hearing impairment which is usually completely reversible on discontinuation of the medication.[21] Commonly, patients with arthritis, taking more than eight 5-grain aspirin tablets daily (2,700 mg) will report a hearing impairment that proves to be sensorineural in nature; discontinuation of the drug is usually followed by complete recovery of hearing. We recently encountered the case of a young adult male who swallowed "a whole bottle" of aspirin tablets in an apparent suicide attempt; much of the drug was lost from vomiting, and emergency care saved the patient's life; there was no demonstrable permanent hearing loss, but apparently severe tinnitus persisted to the time the patient was lost to follow-up (over 1 year). Jarvis[9] reports a case of permanent hearing impairment following aspirin ingestion; the significance of this case, however, remains uncertain since the impairment was unilateral.

Crifo[3] administered salicylates to guinea pigs intraperitoneally in a study of the effects of these drugs upon hearing. He found that single doses of salicylates produced a high-tone hearing impairment that resolved completely by 72 hours following drug administration. Chronic drug administration to the animals over periods of 10 or 20 days resulted in apparently permanent hearing damage; however, no corresponding histopathologic changes could be seen in the cochlear ducts.

ETHACRYNIC ACID

Ethacrynic acid, a loop diuretic structurally related to salicylic acid, may lead to cellular damage in the stria vascularis, spiral limbus, and cochlear and vestibular hair cells of laboratory animals. Moreover, it is believed that ethacrynic acid may augment the electrophysiologic and histopathologic manifestations of the cochlear toxicity of aminoglycosides in guinea pigs.[15] Ethacrynic acid has also been incriminated in the causation of cochlear and vestibular damage in humans, especially when given in association with aminoglycosides. Most of the reported cases have been of patients in renal failure treated with moderate doses of ethacrynic acid which resulted in the rapid onset of bilateral transient hearing loss.[20] Histopathologic studies of the inner ears of clinical cases with permanent hearing loss have shown cochlear hair cell loss along with damage to the stria vascularis. Figure 8-1 shows the organ of Corti, from the basal turn, of a patient who received a single 50-mg dose of ethacrynic acid intravenously during a terminal illness. In this particular example there are no clear signs of strial damage, the changes being limited to outer hair cell damage.[16] Figure 8-2, of an experimental animal (cat) that received ethacrynic acid, shows the more characteristic strial changes: enlargement of the intercellular spaces between the marginal and intermediate cells.[17]

Furosemide, a loop diuretic with pharmacologic properties similar to those of ethacrynic acid, has replaced the latter in many medical centers. Transient hearing loss has been reported occasionally following the intravenous administration of 1,000 mg of furosemide, or if the infusion rate exceeds 25 mg/minute.[13] Cases of permanent deafness have also been reported.[22] At very high doses, furosemide potentiates the toxic effects of aminoglycosides on the guinea pig cochlea, but there is no evidence of a similar potentiation in humans with the usual clinical dosages of furosemide. The clinician should, however, use extreme caution when prescribing aminoglycoside antibiotics along with loop diuretics.

QUININE AND CHLOROQUINE

Quinine is the major medicinally important alkaloid obtained from the dried bark of the cinchona tree. It has also been synthesized, but its synthetic production on a large scale has proved to be economically unfeasible. Quinine, which has long been used in the treatment of all forms of malaria, was recognized

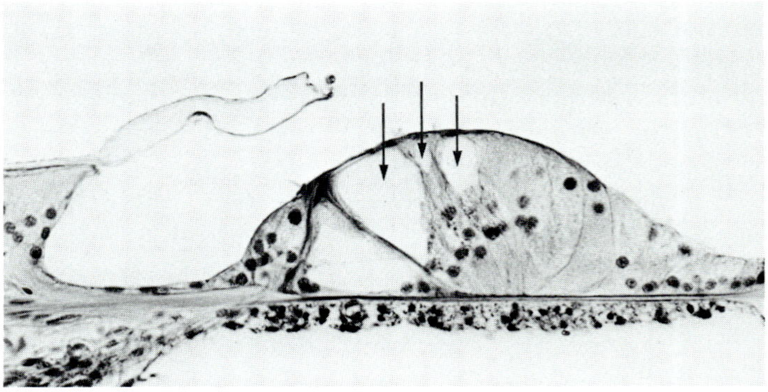

Fig. 8-1. Photomicrograph of the organ of Corti from the basal turn of the cochlea. This patient received one 50-mg dose of ethacrynic acid. The outer hair cells are absent (arrows); the inner hair cells and supporting cells are normal. (From Matz, G. J., Beal, D. D., and Krames, L.: Ototoxicity of ethacrynic acid—demonstrated in a human temporal bone. Arch. Otolaryngol. 90:152-155, 1969. Copyright 1969, American Medical Association.)

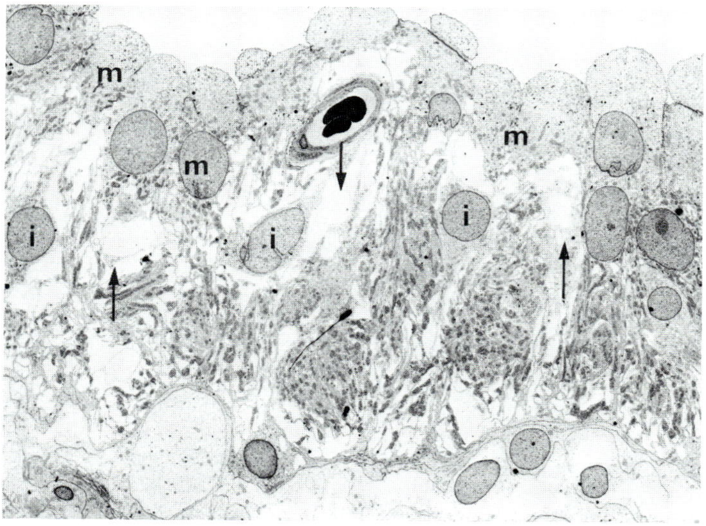

Fig. 8-2. Ethacrynic acid. Electron micrograph of the stria vascularis of the cat showing enlargement of intercellular spaces (arrows) between marginal (m) and intermediate cells (i). (From Matz, G. J., and Hinojosa, R.: Histopathology following use of ethacrynic acid. Surg. Forum. 24:488-489, 1973.)

by Taylor in 1934[23] as a cause of congenital deafness when taken during pregnancy; he reported severe sensorineural loss in the newborn following even as little as a single dose of quinine to the mother.

Chloroquine phosphate was developed in the United States during World War II for use as an antimalarial agent because of the shortage of natural quinine; it has more recently been used for the treatment of collagen diseases. Because chloroquine is chemically related to quinine, it has been suspected of being ototoxic. Dwivedi and Mehra reported in 1978[4] the case of a patient who suffered bilateral hearing damage after receiving only four doses of chloroquine for the treatment of malaria; the hearing impairment had not resolved after a 6-month follow-up.

A case reported by Matz and Naunton[18] in 1968 concerned one of two siblings who had profound congenital sensorineural hearing impairment and whose mother had taken chloroquine during her pregnancies; the reported case involved a 7-year old male who died from an epithelial ependymoma of the right cerebellum. The boy's mother had taken chloroquine phosphate, 250 mg twice daily, during the first trimester of pregnancy for the treatment of systemic lupus erythematosus; the pregnancy and birth were otherwise entirely normal. Hearing impairment was suspected in the infant, and a hearing evaluation done at 19 months showed a profound bilateral sensorineural hearing impairment; vestibular examination revealed a marked bilateral vestibular paresis.

The mother of this particular child had six pregnancies, during three of which she took chloroquine orally; the boy in the reported case was the result of the first of those three pregnancies; the second of the three resulted in a deaf child, and the third ended in a miscarriage. The other pregnancies, during which chloroquine was not taken, resulted in normal children with normal hearing.

Following the death of the boy at age 7, the right temporal bone was processed in the usual fashion, imbedded in celloidin, and stained with hematoxylin and eosin. The middle ear, tympanic membrane, and oval and round windows showed no abnormality; however, there was complete absence of the inner and outer hair cells throughout all of the turns of the cochlea. The organ of Corti and peripheral axons in the osseous spiral lamina were completely absent throughout most of the basal, second, and third turns. The ganglion cells were reduced in number, and in most areas the supporting cells of Hensen, Claudius, and Deiters were also missing except for a few supporting cell elements seen in the midmodiolar sections. The stria vascularis, with

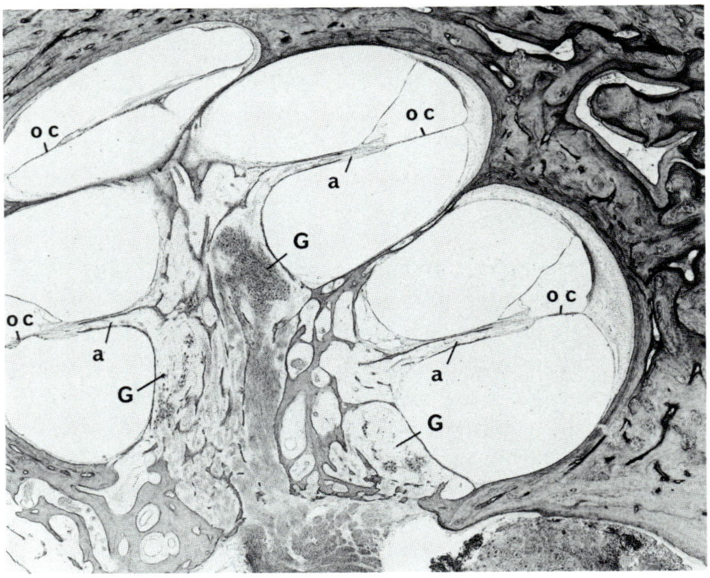

Fig. 8-3. Chloroquine ototoxicity. Photomicrograph of mid-modiolar section of the cochlea showing complete absence of the organ of Corti (oc) and peripheral axons in the osseous spiral lamina (a) in all turns. Ganglion cells (G) are reduced in number (From Matz, G. J., and Naunton, R. F.: Ototoxicity of chloroquine. Arch. Otolaryngol. 88:370-372, 1968. Copyright 1968, American Medical Association.)

the exception of some slight degenerative changes, was within normal limits throughout. The tectorial and Reissner's membranes were normal. There was no evidence of cochlear hydrops, and the semicircular canals and the maculae of the saccule and utricle were within normal limits (Figs. 8-3 and 8-4). In summary, the right inner ear of this case showed severe neuroepithelial cochlear degeneration.

AMINOGLYCOSIDE ANTIBIOTICS

The aminoglycoside antibiotics are employed in the treatment of serious infections with Gram-negative bacilli. As with any toxic drug, the indications for treatment with an aminoglycoside antibiotic should be continually reassessed with each patient so that ad-

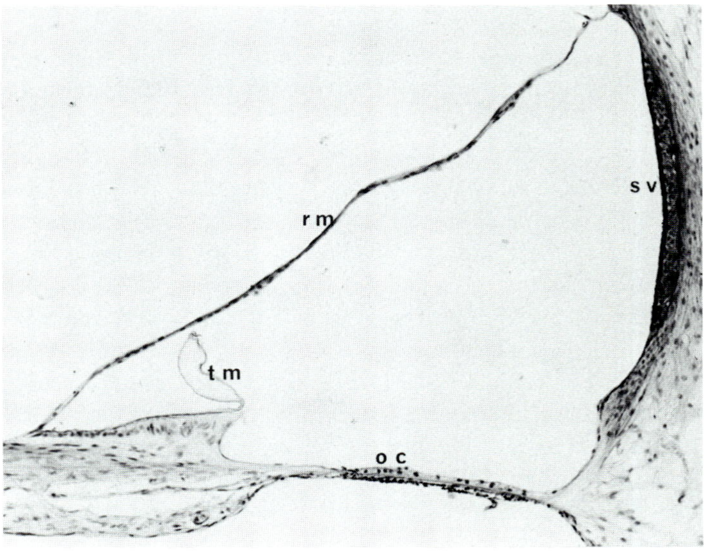

Fig. 8-4. Chloroquine ototoxicity. Photomicrograph of cochlear duct at higher magnification showing absence of organ of Corti (oc). The tectorial membrane (tm), Reissner's membrane (rm) and stria vascularis (sv) are normal (From Matz, G. J., and Naunton, R. F.: Ototoxicity of chloroquine. Arch. Otolaryngol. 88:370-372, 1968. Copyright 1968, American Medical Association.)

ministration can be stopped if it is no longer needed.

Since the introduction of streptomycin, ototoxicity has been recognized as a side effect of every aminoglycoside antibiotic. Impairment of cochlear function may manifest itself through the symptoms of decreased hearing, tinnitus, aural fullness or stuffiness, or dysacusis, and should be confirmed by audiometric testing. Impairment of vestibular function may result in vertigo, nausea, instability of gait, and problems with occular fixation; vestibular dysfunction may be confirmed by caloric testing. Each of the aminoglycosides has been considered to affect primarily either the auditory or vestibular system; thus, kanamycin has been considered cochleotoxic[5] and gentamicin primarily vestibulotoxic.[8] Our experience, however, suggests that gentamicin may cause auditory as well as vestibular changes, and that amikacin, a semisynthetic derivative of kanamycin, produces vestibular as well as auditory effects. It may well be that if kanamycin were subjected to careful prospective study in humans, its vestibulotoxic potential would be revealed. Each new aminoglycoside antibiotic should therefore be examined for effects on both the auditory and vestibular systems.

Cochlear hair cell damage has been observed by light-microscopy of temporal bones from patients who developed symptoms or signs of ototoxicity associated with aminoglycoside treatment.[11,19] The reports of this damage show that hair cells of the basal turn were more susceptible to aminoglycoside toxicity than were hair cells located nearer to the apical end of the cochlea. Nevertheless the outer hair cells at any level of the cochlea seem more susceptible than the inner hair cells. Neither the vestibular system nor the ganglion cells of the cochlea have been examined in detail. In most other reported cases of aminoglycoside toxicity, the patients either received an inordinately large dose of the drug, or there was renal impairment that delayed excretion of the drug. The patients were not studied prospectively in anticipation of possible clinical ototoxicity that could be correlated with histopathologic changes.

Figure 8-5 shows the organ of Corti of a

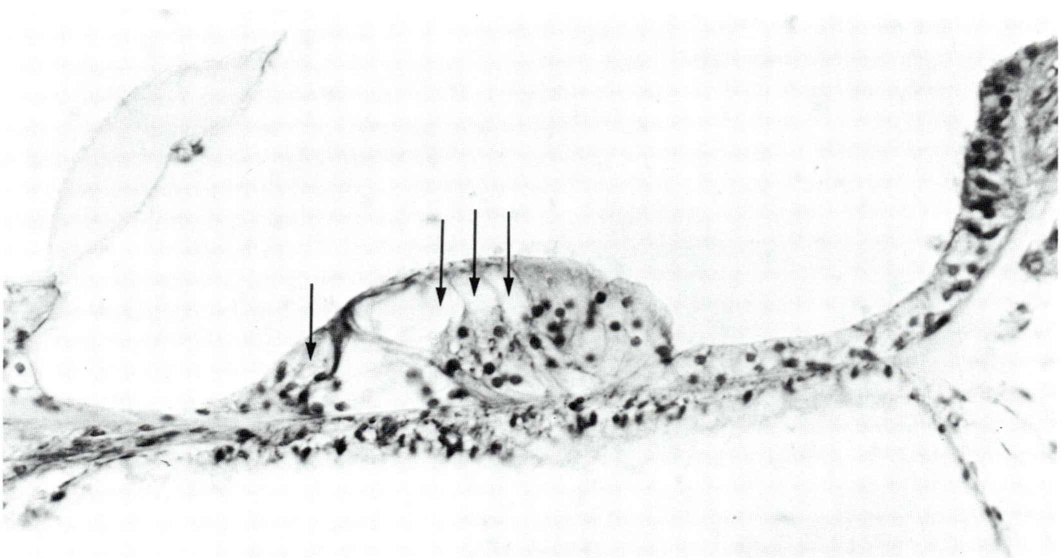

Fig. 8-5. Neomycin ototoxicity. Organ of Corti at high magnification. The inner and outer hair cells (arrows) are absent. The supporting cells are well preserved. (From Lowry, M. D., May, M., and Pastore, P.: Acute histopathologic inner ear changes in deafness due to neomycin: A case report. Ann. Otol. Rhinol. Laryngol. 82:876-880, 1973.)

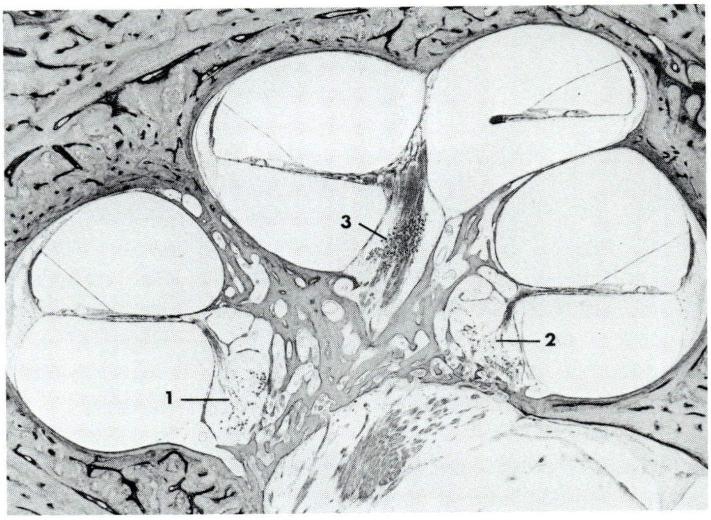

Fig. 8-6. Gentamicin ototoxicity. Mid-modiolar section of the cochlea. The ganglion cells are reduced by about 32 percent in the basal turn (1) and by about 45 percent in the second (2) and third (3) turns of the cochlea. The stria vascularis is normal in all turns.

patient treated with neomycin; the inner and outer hair cells are absent, but the supporting cells remain intact.[14] Figures 8-6 and 8-7 are sections of the inner ear of a patient who received gentamicin; the changes seen are not characteristic of those commonly seen in the experimental animal, in that the ganglion cells show marked reduction, while the stria vascularis and the organ of Corti are normal.

Experiments designed to examine the histopathology of aminoglycoside ototoxicity have been done with guinea pigs, cats, chinchillas, and monkeys.[7,24,25] In most of these investigations large doses of an aminoglycoside were administered daily, and the cochleas were examined at various times by conventional celloidin light-microscopy of horizontal sections or by phase-contrast microscopy of surface preparations. In these experimental animals, destruction of hair cells of the cochlea is the primary manifestation of aminoglycoside auditory toxicity; hair cells toward the basal turn are generally more susceptible. At any level of the cochlea, the temporal sequence of destruction suggests that the second and third rows of outer hair cells and the inner hair cells are the first to show histologic signs of damage. The earliest vestibular abnormality found in animal studies of cellular damage is to the type I hair cells of the ampulla of the semicircular canals.[26] Changes in the maculae of the utricle and saccule have not been well described, since this requires scanning electron microscopic techniques, which until recently have not been applied to the inner ear.

There is experimental evidence that aminoglycoside antibiotics may act synergistically

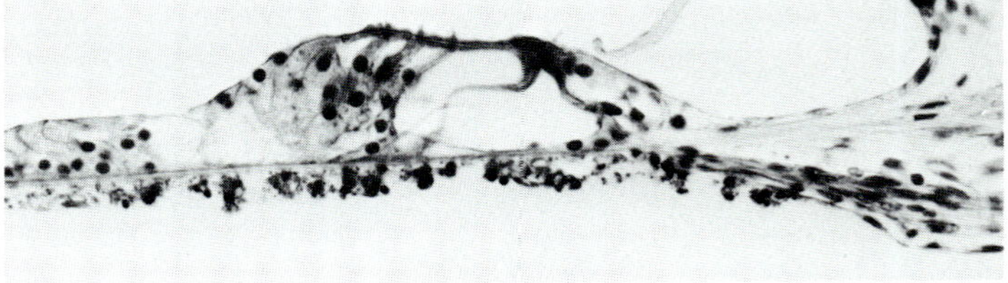

Fig. 8-7. Cochlear duct of the same case of gentamicin ototoxicity at higher magnification, showing normal organ of Corti.

with high-intensity noise in producing inner ear damage. Brown et al.[2] found marked interaction, leading to increased damage, when neomycin was given to guinea pigs exposed to 115 dB of noise. Loss in cochlear sensitivity was noted at all frequencies, with close to 100 percent hair-cell loss. Gannon et al.[6] studied guinea pigs who were given a low "safe" dose of kanamycin and, in some cases, were exposed to noise. None of the animals receiving kanamycin alone showed hair cell damage, but in those also exposed to noise the drug appeared to increase the susceptibility of the hair cells to damage—an effect that could persist more than 20 days after discontinuing the drug.

THALIDOMIDE

The histopathologic changes in a case of thalidomide-induced inner ear aplasia have been described by Jorgensen et al.[10] In this case, a female infant was born with severe deformity of the external ears, facial nerve palsy, and severe heart disease (atrioseptal defect). The mother had taken two Lulamin tablets, corresponding to 100 to 200 mg of thalidomide, about 25 days after conception. Polytomography of the inner ear showed a large, smooth-walled cavity in place of and apparently comprising the right inner ear, and only a tympanic cavity and epitympanic recess on the left. The external auditory canals were narrow. No auditory or vestibular responses were detected. The infant died at 4 months of age.

At autopsy, the left middle ear of the infant was slit-shaped, with a normally developed drum, malleus, incus, and incudostapedial articulation; but there was no oval window or stapes footplate. The inner ear was a smooth-walled cavity with a membranous labyrinth and the distinct primordia of sense organs corresponding to the utricle and canals, but no evidence of statoacoustic or facial nerves. On the right side there was a slit-shaped middle ear and a normal malleus and incus but no stapes. There was total aplasia of the inner ear and otic capsule (Fig. 8-8). The statoacoustic and facial nerves were also absent.

The authors of the case relate the mother's ingestion of thalidomide to the time at which the fetal otocyst was forming as an ingrowth from the ectoderm. They indicate that the aplasia of the seventh and eighth nerves could not be related to the labyrinthine aplasia, since the otocyst has been shown experimentally to have the capacity to differentiate independently of contact with the eighth cranial nerve. The middle and external ear dysplasia seems to have no causal relationship to the inner

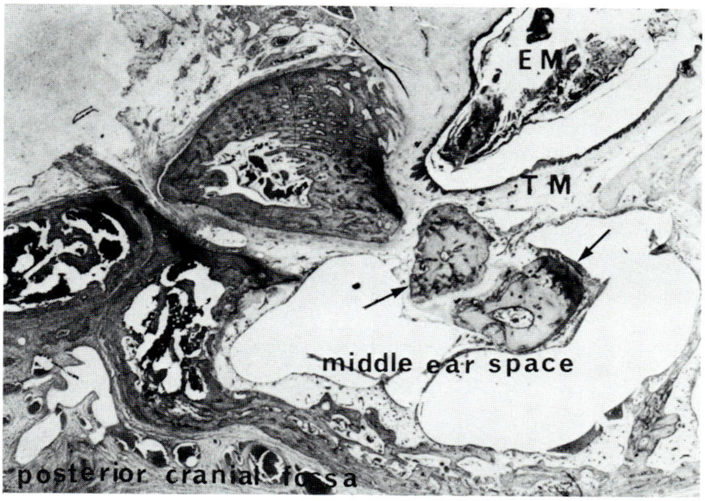

Fig. 8-8. Thalidomide. The external auditory meatus (EM) and the tympanic membrane (TM) are seen in the upper right corner. The malleus and incus (arrows) are in the middle ear space. There is total aplasia of the inner ear. (From Jorgensen, M. B., Kristensen, H. K., and Buch, N. H.: Thalidomide-induced aplasia of the inner ear. J. Laryngol. Otol. 80:318-320, 1966; reproduced by permission.)

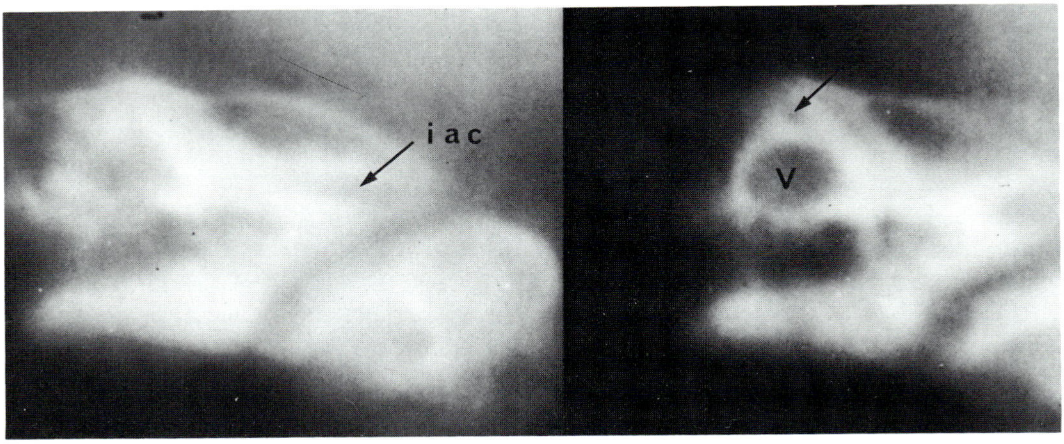

Fig. 8-9. Laminograms of the right inner ear of a 6-year-old child whose mother had taken thalidomide during pregnancy. The vestibule (V) is strikingly enlarged; the superior semicircular canal (arrow) appears to be normal; the internal auditory canal is narrowed (iac).

ear aplasia, since these two structures have independent embryonic origins.

We have encountered a case similar to that reported by Jorgensen et al.—that of a 6-year-old, totally deaf female whose mother had taken a "few thalidomide tablets" before pregnancy was recognized. Audiometry showed an unusually profound hearing impairment, there being no sound recognition in either ear at any audiometric frequency at maximum audiometer output. There was no other detectable physical abnormality. Laminograms of the ears (Fig. 8-9) showed no abnormality of the external and middle ears; the abnormalities seen in the inner ear were similar on the two sides, there being striking enlargement of the vestibule and anterior limb of the horizontal semicircular canal, with total absence of the cochlea but with a normal-appearing superior semicircular canal. The posterior semicircular canal and crus commune could not be identified. The internal auditory canal was approximately 1.0 mm in diameter at its widest point.

RADIUM

Carcinoma of the mastoid is infrequent in the general population, but in the selected population of radium-dial painters and patients treated during the third and fourth decades of this century with oral or intravenous radium solutions (who may or may not have known that they received this type of medication), the incidence of this cancer is markedly increased.[1] In these patients, radioactive elements have been found bound into the bone, and the chronic bombardment of closely approximated cells by radioactive particles has been considered a likely explanation for the tendency to develop neoplasms. Preceding the development of tumors, destructive changes in the bone, referred to as osteoradionecrosis (Fig. 8-10) or radiation osteitis, frequently develop. Radiation osteitis is characterized by the loss of normal bone structure, with disappearance of the osteocytes in the lacunae, widening and coalescence of the Haversian canals, and the replacement of resorbed bone by fibrous tissue. These defects in the bone appear as radiolucent areas on x-rays, and often increase the difficulty of making a diagnosis of malignancy.

Figure 8-11 shows a portion of the temporal bone of a female who, many years before her death, had been employed as a radium-dial painter; during her employment she absorbed a measurable quantity of radium. The apical

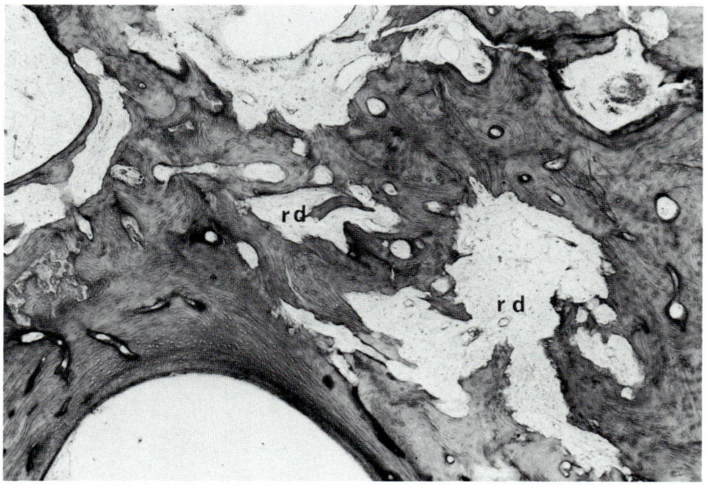

Fig. 8-10. Radium poisoning. Portion of the otic capsule showing osteoradionecrosis. In large areas (rd) the reabsorbed bone has been replaced by fibrous connective tissue.

portion of the petrous part of the temporal bone is invaded by squamous celled carcinoma, but the otic capsule is tumor-free.

INNER EAR DAMAGE RESULTING FROM ANAPHYLACTIC REACTION TO PENICILLIN

The patient reported here was a 66-year-old male who, 9 months before death, had had an operation for repair of an inguinal hernia.[12] Postoperatively, because he developed "a cold," the patient was given an injection of penicillin; within seconds of receiving the penicillin, his eyes swelled shut from edema of the eyelids and he lost consciousness. An eczematous rash was also noted at this time. Unconsciousness lasted for 2 to 3 weeks; following recovery of consciousness the patient was unable to move any of his extremities and complained of hearing difficulty and blurred vision; no vestibular symptoms were reported.

The extremities regained their strength slowly during the next 8 months, but the hearing impairment persisted. An air- and bone-conduction audiogram, taken 8 months after

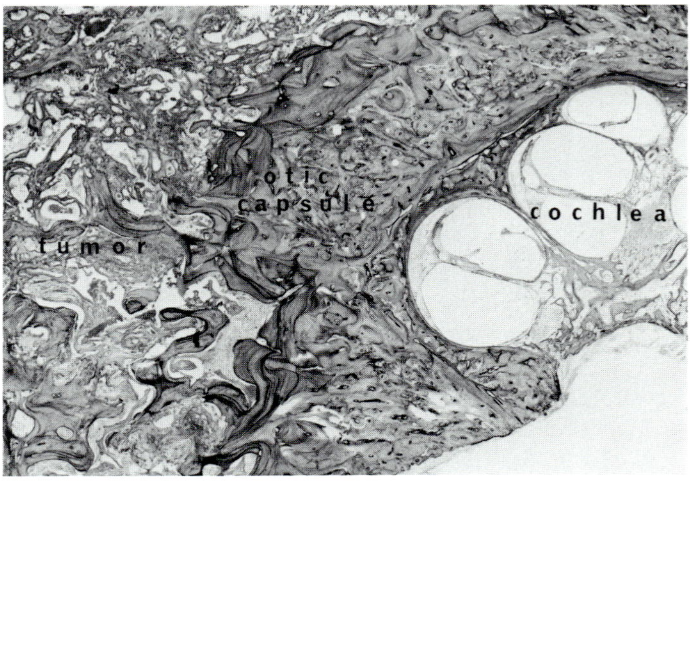

Fig. 8-11. Radium-dial painter. Portion of the temporal bone of a patient who had been a radium-dial painter, showing the cochlea and normal otic capsule. The apical region of the temporal bone has been invaded by tumor, but the otic capsule is tumor-free.

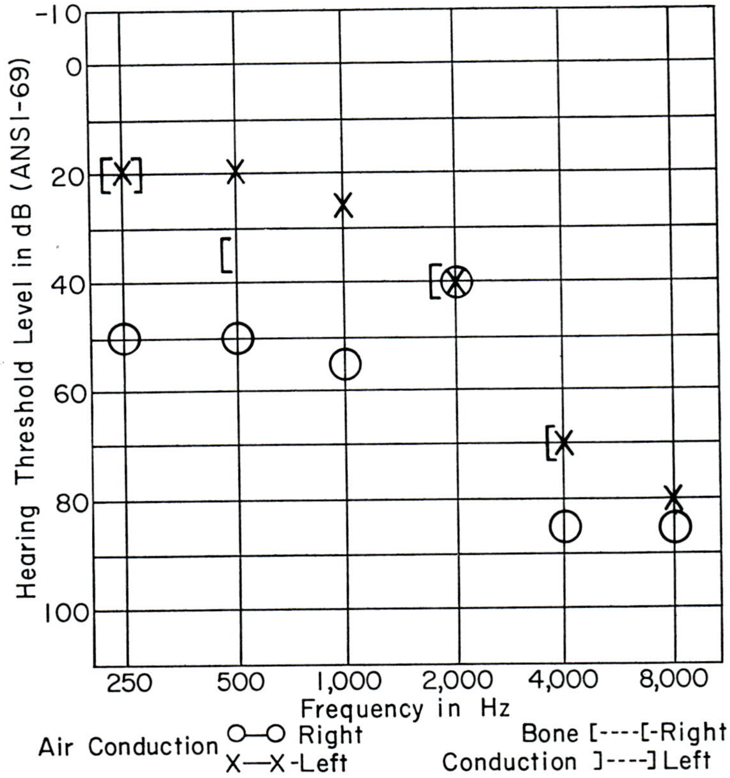

Fig. 8-12. Reaction to penicillin. Audiogram of a case of sensitivity reaction to penicillin taken 8 months after the event (Modified from Lindsay, J. R., & Schulthess, G. v.: An unusual case of labyrinthine hydrops. Acta Otolaryngol. 49: 315-324, 1958.) (The original audiogram was taken in 1955 using an audiometer whose air conduction system was calibrated according to ASA 1951 values and whose bone conduction system was calibrated in house on real ears. In order to provide closer correspondence to the current ANSI 1969 standard of reference, the air conduction figures have been corrected by 10 dB; the bone conduction values have not been changed.)

the penicillin-related episode, revealed a bilateral high-tone sensorineural impairment and a moderate low-tone impairment, worse on the right side than the left (Fig. 8-12). Neurologic opinion at the same time was that the patient had suffered multiple cerebral thromboses, possibly the result of an episode of cerebral anoxia. The patient expired 9 months after the original hernia operation and episode of consciousness loss, from a ruptured abdominal aortic aneurism.

At microscopic examination, the inner ear

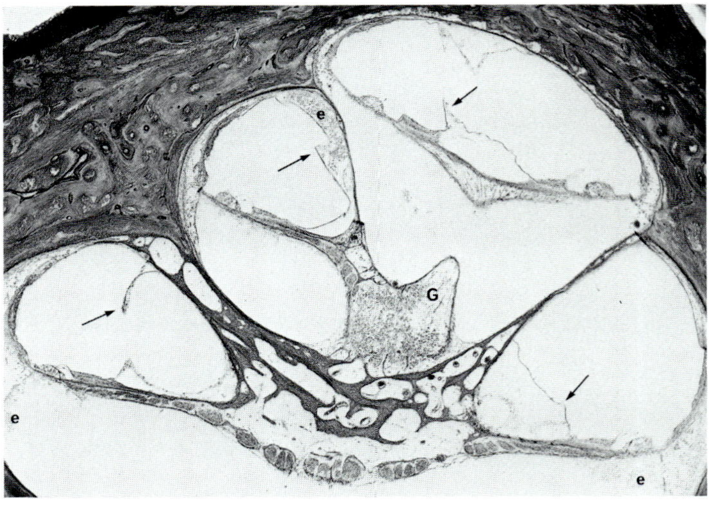

Fig. 8-13. Reaction to penicillin. The cochlea of the right ear, showing endolymphatic hydrops. The perilymphatic space contains an exudate (e). Notice the irregular contour of Reissner's membrane in all turns (arrows). The ganglion cells (G) and peripheral nerve fibers of the apical turn are reduced in number. (From Lindsay, J. R., & Schulthess, G. v.: An unusual case of labyrinthine hydrops. Acta Otolaryngol. 49:315-324, 1958.)

of the patient in the foregoing case showed endolymphatic hydrops, and the case was originally reported otologically as an unusual type of labyrinthine hydrops.[12] However, in the light of further information regarding "hydrops," and particularly in view of the history of extensive injury to the central nervous system, the case has been reviewed and reclassified as one of secondary hydrops limited to irregular dilatation of the cochlear duct. The most striking histopathologic features shown (Fig. 8-13) are an atypical endolymphatic hydrops (Reissner's membrane displaying a markedly irregular contour in all turns), reduction of the number of ganglion cells and nerve fibers at the apical turn, and the presence of an amorphous exudate most prominent in the perilymphatic space of all turns. It is now felt that the case was one of severe injury to the central nervous system, resulting from a sensitivity reaction to penicillin injection.

REFERENCES

1. Beal, D. D., Lindsay, J. R., & Ward, P. H.: Radiation-induced carcinoma of the mastoid. Arch. Otolaryngol. 81:9-16, 1965.
2. Brown, J. J., Brummett, R. E., Meikle, M. B., & Vernon, J.: Combined effects of noise and neomycin. Acta Otolaryngol. 86:394-400, 1978.
3. Crifo, S. Aspirin ototoxicity in the guinea pig. ORL, 37:27-34, 1975.
4. Dwivedi, G. S., & Mehra, Y. N.: Ototoxicity of chloroquine phosphate. A case report. J. Laryngol. Otol. 92:701-703, 1978.
5. Finegold, S.: Toxicity of kanamycin in adults. Ann. N.Y. Acad. Sci. 132, 942-956, 1966.
6. Gannon, R. P., Tso, S. S., & Chung, D. Y.: Interaction of kanamycin and noise exposure. J. Laryngol. Otol. 93:341-347, 1979.
7. Igarashi, M., Lundquist, P. G., Alford, B. R., & Miyata, H.: Experimental ototoxicity of gentamicin in squirrel monkeys. J. Infect. Dis. 124(Suppl.):S130-S137, 1971.
8. Jackson, G. G., & Arcieri, G.: Ototoxicity of gentamicin in man. A survey and controlled analysis of clinical experience in the United States. J. Infect. Dis. 124(Suppl.):S130-S137, 1971.
9. Jarvis, J. F.: A case of unilateral permanent deafness following acetylsalicylic acid. J. Laryngol. Otol. 80:318-320, 1966.
10. Jorgensen, M. B., Kristensen, H. K., & Buch, N. H.: Thalidomide-induced aplasia of the inner ear. J. Laryngol. 78:1095-1101, 1964.
11. Lindsay, J. R., Proctor, L. R., & Work, W. P.: Histopathologic inner ear changes in deafness due to neomycin in a human. Laryngoscope 70:382-392, 1960.
12. Lindsay, J. R., & Schulthess, G. v.: An unusual case of labyrinthine hydrops. Acta Otolaryngol. 49:315-324, 1958.
13. Lloyd-Mostyn, R. H., & Lord, I. J.: Ototoxicity of intravenous furosemide. Lancet 2:1156-1159, 1971.
14. Lowry, M. D., May, M., & Pastore, P.: Acute histopathologic inner ear changes in deafness due to neomycin: A case report. Ann. Otol. Rhinol. Laryngol. 82:876-880, 1973.
15. Matz, G. J.: Ototoxic effects of ethacrynic acid in man and animals. Laryngoscope 86:1065-1086, 1976.
16. Matz, G. J., Beal, D. D., & Krames, L.: Ototoxicity of ethacrynic acid—demonstrated in a human temporal bone. Arch. Otolaryngol. 90:152-155, 1969.
17. Matz, G. J., & Hinojosa, R.: Histopathology following use of ethacrynic acid. Surg. Forum 24:488-489, 1973.
18. Matz, G. J., & Naunton, R. F.: Ototoxicity of chloroquine. Arch. Otolaryngol. 88:370-372, 1968.
19. Matz, G. J., Wallace, T. H., & Ward, P. H.: The ototoxicity of kanamycin. A comparative histopathologic study. Laryngoscope 75:1690-1698, 1965.
20. Meriwether, W. D., Mange, R. J., & Serpick, A. A.: Deafness following standard intravenous dose of ethacrynic acid. J.A.M.A. 216:795-798, 1971.
21. Myers, E. N., Bernstein, J. M., & Fostiropolous, G.: Salicylate ototoxicity; a clinical study. N. Engl. J. Med. 273:587, 1965.
22. Quick, C. A., & Hoppe, W.: Permanent deafness associated with furosemide administration. Ann. Otol. Rhinol. Laryngol. 84:94-101, 1975.
23. Taylor, H. M.: Pre-natal medication as possible etiologic factor of deafness in newborn. Arch. Otolaryngol. 20:790-803, 1934.

24. Waitz, J. A., Moss, E. L., & Weinstein, M. J.: Aspects of the chronic toxicity of gentamicin sulfate in cats. J. Infect. Dis. 124(Suppl.):S125-S129, 1971.
25. Ward, P. H., & Fernandez, C.: The ototoxicity of kanamycin in guinea pigs. Ann. Otol. Rhinol. Laryngol. 70:132-150, 1961.
26. Wersäll, J., Björkroth, B., Flock, A., & Lundquist, P. G.: Sensory hair fusion in vestibular sensory cells after gentamicin exposure. Arch. Klin. Exp. Ohren Nasen Kehlkopfheilkd: 200, 1-14, 1971.

9

The Lung

W. F. Whimster and Wanda de Poitiers

INTRODUCTION

Drug-induced lung disease has become a popular topic for reviews.[28, 49, 57, 87, 93, 137, 175a, 176, 177, 198a, 202, 227a, 234] However, as a result of attempts to make such reviews comprehensive for clinicians, their practical value to pathologists has often been small. Pathologists faced with an urgent lung biopsy from a patient in respiratory distress, or with postmortem lungs, must consider several possibilities. The lungs may have been affected by the disease for which the patient is being treated; by one or more microorganisms; by therapy, including drugs, radiotherapy, and oxygen; by aspiration of vomit; or by some unrelated condition. Because most of these possibilities do not have pathognomonic structural macroscopic or microscopic features, the interpretation of the lung tissue findings may be controversial.

Over 40 therapeutic agents, and various toxic substances, have been reported in association with changes in the lung; for only a proportion of these, however, have there been reports of morphologic effects, and for only a very few has there been published evidence from experimental exposure of animals that the association between the agent and the structural changes is causal. This chapter will discuss the differential diagnoses to be considered by the tissue pathologist, the types of damage produced by drugs, and what to do with lung biopsies and postmortem lungs; these will be followed by a discussion of the agents for which tissue pathology is available. The latter are discussed individually, in alphabetical order. For each, an attempt has been made to describe the damage caused, the smallest doses reported to have caused the damage, and the shortest and longest times between the first exposure and the onset of pulmonary trouble.

Tissue pathologists depend very much upon published black-and-white photomicrographs, although these are highly selected and of variable quality. We believe that in a review, it is better to direct the reader to the many photomicrographs available rather than to reproduce many more. In the references at the end of this chapter, we have therefore drawn attention to relevant illustrations according to the following convention: macro: macroscopic pictures; LM: light microscopic pictures; EM: electron microscopic pictures; SEM: scanning electron microscopic pictures. References without this information contain none of these but may contain radiographs.

DIFFERENTIAL DIAGNOSIS

If a patient with a disease for which treatment has been prescribed develops symptoms, signs, or radiologic abnormalities referable to the respiratory system, and either a biopsy or a postmortem is done, the pathologist entrusted with interpreting the morphologic abnormalities in tissue specimens taken from the case must consider the following check-list of possibilities:

1. The disease being treated.
2. Infections.
3. Aspiration pneumonia.
4. Shock.
5. Disseminated intravascular coagulation (DIC).
6. Uremia.
7. Any of the therapeutic agents used.
8. Unrelated diseases.

Careful consideration of the patient's history, supplemented if possible by discussion with the patient him- or herself, and particularly of the patient's respiratory, smoking, and occupational history, with all of the clinical and laboratory findings, often rules out many of the possibilities in the preceding list. Nevertheless, distinguishing between the morphologic changes attributable to the remaining conditions and those attributable to therapy, and, indeed, distinguishing between conditions attributable to more than one therapeutic agent, must depend on the pathologist's knowledge not only of the effects of individual drugs, but also of the other conditions in the differential diagnosis, some of which call for mention here.

The Disease Being Treated

The appearance of a disease may be reasonably specific, as in carcinomatous involvement; less specific, as with lymphomatous involvement; or nonspecific, as with involvement by, for example, collagen diseases. The morphologic features of most diseases that can affect the respiratory tract are described by Spencer.[203]

Infections

Most accounts of drug-induced lung damage emphasize that the presence of all conceivable microorganisms had been excluded by every microbiologic technique available. Nevertheless, the presence of infectious microorganisms does not exclude drug-induced lung damage, and the infection may have been imposed on it. Generally, because drugs do not produce acute inflammatory infiltrations with neutrophilic polymorphonuclear leukocytes, bacterial, actinomycotic, nocardial, and some fungal infections should not present difficulties in differential diagnosis.

Legionnaire's disease is at present entering the differential diagnosis of lung biopsies. The disease is primarily a bronchopneumonia (which may be unilateral) with intra-alveolar exudation of fibrinous fluid, polymorphonuclear leucocytes, and macrophages, which may undergo extensive and striking lysis (Fig. 9-1); there is also interstitial edema and cellular infiltration, and abscesses may form.[27] Diffuse alveolar damage with hyaline membranes may be seen in areas without intra-alveolar exudate,[237] and may be the only feature in a biopsy.[119] The small irregular rods (400 nm to 2.5 μm) of the Legionnaire's bacillus can be revealed by the Dieterle stain and identified electron microscopically.[119]

Many microorganisms may be identified in association with granulomatous reactions including tuberculosis, histoplasmosis, and coccidioidomycosis. Granulomata attributable to

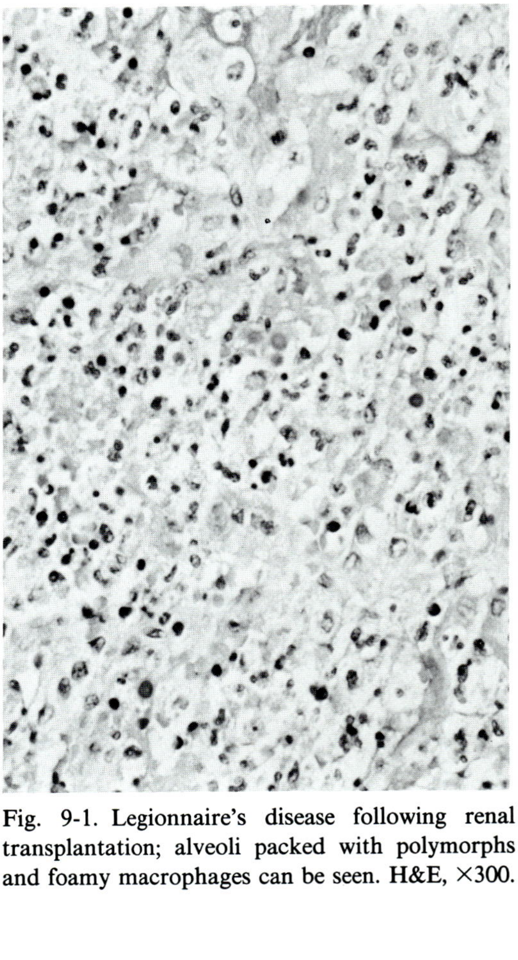

Fig. 9-1. Legionnaire's disease following renal transplantation; alveoli packed with polymorphs and foamy macrophages can be seen. H&E, ×300.

drugs and toxic substances are discussed in a later section.

It may be difficult to distinguish drug-induced from virus-induced diffuse alveolar damage. Unlike drugs, viruses have a tendency to damage bronchial and bronchiolar epithelium (which also lays the airways open to bacterial infection), to produce focal alveolar necrosis, to form inclusion bodies in the nuclei or cytoplasm of epithelial cells, and to have antigens detectable by fluorescein-conjugated antibodies upon fluorescence microscopy. Spencer[204] describes, illustrates, and gives references to the original descriptions of the pulmonary changes seen in viral infections, as shown in Table 9-1.

Intranuclear inclusions have been detected by sputum cytology in infections with adenoviruses, herpes hominis virus, and varicella.[46]

Like the viruses, *Coxiella burneti,* the causative organism of rickettsial pneumonia, also produces diffuse alveolar damage with bronchial inflammation,[205] while the *Bedsonia* (chlamydial) group of organisms, which cause psittacosis, produce a hemorrhagic consolidation and intra-alveolar exudation with only mild interstitial infiltration.[206] Intracytoplasmic (Levinthal) inclusions—small coccoid bodies just visible by light microscopy—may be demonstrated by prolonged Giemsa staining.[206]

Table 9-1. Virus Infections*

Adenoviruses	Note "smudge" cells and intranuclear inclusions
Coxsackie virus	Nonspecific morphology, isolate virus
Cytomegalovirus	Large intranuclear Feulgen-negative inclusions
Herpes hominis virus	Focal alveolar necrosis, intranuclear inclusions
Influenza virus	Intracytoplasmic inclusions, epithelial cell necrosis and regeneration, hyaline membranes
Measles	Multinucleate epithelial cells with intracytoplasmic inclusions
Respiratory syncytical virus	Bronchiolar epithelial damage, intracytoplasmic inclusions
Vaccinia	Interstitial infiltration, focal necrosis
Variola	Late appearance of calcified nodules
Varicella	Interstitial infiltration, focal necrosis which may calcify, intranuclear inclusions

* Adapted from refs. 204, 46, and 241.

In *Mycoplasma pneumoniae* infection, the lesions are nonspecific, with an intra-alveolar exudate containing red cells, macrophages, and sometimes hyaline membranes, together with interstitial lymphocyte infiltration. During recovery, the proliferating type II cells may become stratified, and there may be some interstitial fibrosis. The bronchioles also show lymphocytic infiltration. The organisms can be demonstrated with specific fluorescein-conjugated antisera.[241, 207]

In infections with *Pneumocystis carinii,* the lesions consist of a patchy consolidation that may be extensive or, less commonly, localized, without pleural involvement. Microscopically there is interstitial infiltration with lymphocytes, plasma cells, macrophages and, sometimes, many eosinophils. Pneumocystic pneumonia may possibly go on to interstitial fibrosis.[232] The alveolar spaces contain a foamy exudate in which the parasite can be demonstrated by the traditional PAS or Grocott stains; more rapid techniques, using a rapid methenamine silver technique[144] or toluidine blue O, have also been devised, and may be used on suspension smears of the exudate.[32] It is important to use control sections known to contain pneumocystis cysts in order to avoid missing the diagnosis through inadequate staining.[60] The exudate also contains macrophages and desquamated cells; these appear together with hyaline membranes in infants, but with neutrophilic polymorphonuclear leukocytes in adults (sometimes with minimal interstitial involvement). The exudate can plug the small bronchioles, but there is no true bronchiolitis.

Aspiration Pneumonia

Aspiration pneumonia due to the inhalation of oropharyngeal or gastrointestinal contents may complicate the clinical picture in unconscious or debilitated patients. Experimentally, the inhalation of acidic materials (less than pH 2.5) produces loss of bronchial epithelium, pulmonary edema and hemorrhages very quickly, with polymorphonuclear leukocyte infiltration and consolidation within 4 hours. Within 48 hours, hyaline membranes are seen, and by 72 hours resolution begins; this may leave some scarring, bronchiolitis obliterans, or a typical regeneration of epithelial cells. Large particles of food may, of course, obstruct large airways, but small, nonobstructive particles produce extensive hemorrhagic pneumonia within 6 hours and a granulomatous response within 48 hours. Oropharyngeal organisms can produce putrefactive necrosis of pulmonary tissue, and secondary infection by aerobic bacteria is always possible.[239] Apparent aspiration, owing to the passive displacement of gastric contents after death, may also denude the bronchial epithelium, but this is confined to the larger airways and there is no inflammatory reaction.

Shock

"Shock lung," in which progressive respiratory failure develops after severe hemorrhagic shock, was first recognized in 1965.[96] The pathologic features of this condition—heavy lungs, often more than 1,000 grams each, which are firm on slicing with little free edema fluid, and which microscopically have extensive interstitial edema with focal hemorrhages, microthrombi, and collapsed alveolar spaces containing desquamated cells and hyaline membranes—were subsequently found to be indistinguishable from those seen after severe trauma, shock of any cause, viral pneumonia, and near-drowning. The term "adult respiratory distress syndrome"[9] then came into use, and is still of value to clinicians,[168] although its subdivisions must be recognized in order for further progress to be made in the pathology and differential diagnosis of these conditions.[160] Whether or not shock—that is, hypotension—alone can cause pulmonary damage is open to question; it seems likely that thromboplastic substances are also necessary, and that disseminated intravascular coagulation is an essential part of shock lung pathology.[95]

Disseminated Intravascular Coagulation

Disseminated intravascular coagulation (DIC) is a process that may complicate many conditions, possibly including diffuse alveolar damage and certainly the various forms of shock.[193] It is associated with fibrin thrombi, particularly in the kidneys, lungs, and skin. Robboy et al.[173] have described four patterns of pathology in the lungs in DIC: emboli from venous catheters; tiny thrombi in arterioles, capillaries, and venules; hyaline membranes; and diffuse pulmonary hemorrhage. Saldeen[184] regarded the thrombi as microemboli, and described focal interstitial and alveolar edema, hemorrhages, and lymphatic stasis, together with occasional hyaline membranes in experimental animals into which thrombin had been injected. Microemboli may also be introduced by blood transfusion without adequate filtration, and this has been shown to damage alveolar epithelial and endothelial cells.[61] Extra megakaryocytes (more than 25 per square centimeter) may also be found in the pulmonary capillaries in DIC.[1] The tissue pathologist must therefore look for fibrin thrombi/microemboli, and correlate the findings with the clinical and hematologic findings in diagnosing DIC. Some of the difficulties facing the tissue pathologist are illustrated by case 13-1978 demonstrated at the Massachusetts General Hospital.[40]

Uremia

In fatal cases of uremia the lungs show an intra-alveolar exudate which is often organized into buds of young connective tissue.[63] There is little interstitial change. The same appearances, although tending to be more severe, may be seen as a result of treatment with hexamethonium, mecamylamine, and pentolinium. Perry et al.[167] studied 67 postmortems on uremic hypertensive patients not treated with hexamethonium, 27 treated with this drug, and 39 with mitral stenosis. Intra-alveolar fibrin masses were found in 34 percent, 59 percent, and 18 percent of the cases, respectively; hyaline membranes were found in 16 percent, 41 percent, and 6 percent; an organized exudate was found in 18 percent, 52 percent, and 6 percent. Thus, although differing in frequency, the same pulmonary changes were seen in association with uremia alone, with hexamethonium alone, and with chronic venous back-pressure from mitral stenosis. These changes cannot, therefore, be regarded as specific, and must be considered by the tissue pathologist in the light of the patient's renal function, drug therapy, and pulmonary venous state.

DIFFUSE ALVEOLAR DAMAGE

Diffuse alveolar damage is damage to the alveolar lining cells, especially the more easily damaged type I pneumocytes, and to the capillary endothelial cells; it can be caused by many therapeutic and toxic agents that reach the lung by inhalation or in the pulmonary blood. Mild alveolar pneumocyte damage without damage to the basement membrane may lead merely to type II cell proliferation, with subsequent differentiation into type I cells to cover the ulcerated area.[71] Mild endothelial cell damage may lead to a mild increase in capillary wall permeability, with transient interstitial edema. A transient increase in alveolar macrophage activity and number may be needed to remove the debris of cells and exuded proteins. Such mild damage probably occurs focally in everyday life, to be repaired and disappear without trace or notice. More severe damage, which breaches the alveolar basement membrane or produces cellular or fluid exudation through the capillary wall, or both, sets up an inflammatory reaction that attracts lymphocytes, and possibly plasma cells, neutrophils, eosinophils, and basophils to the site, and may lead to more longlasting intra-alveolar or interstitial changes. Thus the alveolar spaces may fill with shed pneumocytes or macrophages, or proteinaceous debris. This is plastered on the alveolar surface during inspiration, and takes on the microscopic appearance of hyaline membrane. Both protein-rich edema fluid and hyaline membranes may be invaded by interstitial fibroblasts and converted into collagen. This in turn may be covered over by alveolar pneumocytes and basement membrane so that it becomes enclosed within the interstitial compartment of the alveolar wall (Figs. 9-2 and 9-3).

The interstitial exudate of fluid and cells may also stimulate interstitial macrophages

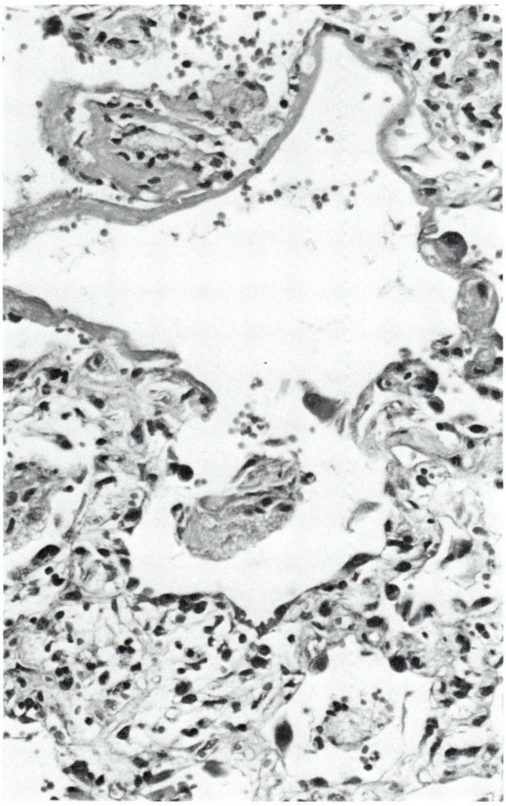

Fig. 9-2. Diffuse alveolar damage following multiple drug chemotherapy; hyaline membranes and interstitial pneumonia can be seen. H&E, ×250.

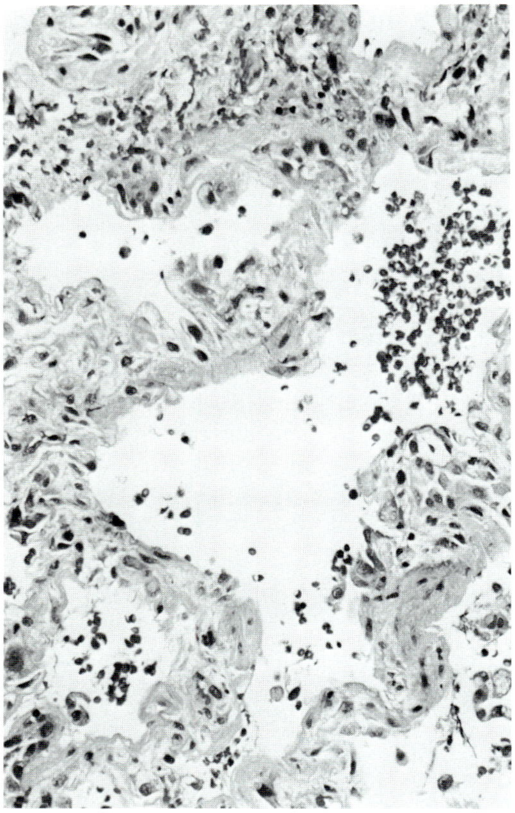

Fig. 9-3. Late stage of diffuse alveolar damage in which the membranes have become organized and incorporated into the thickened alveolar walls. H&E, ×200.

and fibroblasts so that collagen is laid down in this compartment. The formation of granulomata is, rightly or wrongly, not thought of as part of diffuse alveolar damage.

Finally, collagen itself is not a static substance. It may be removable, and it tends to contract and to be remodeled by fibroblasts, which may also add extra elastic fibers to the interstitial mixture, especially in lung adjacent to the pleura. Such fibrosis leads eventually to the loss of the normal three-dimensional structure of the acinus, leaving distorted air spaces lined by cuboidal type II pneumocytes. Eventually the process can reach an "end-stage" in which bronchiolectasis and scar emphysema contribute to the appearance known, inappropriately, as honeycomb lung.

In trying to comprehend the microscopic appearance of pulmonary histologic elements in a biopsy or postmortem specimen, one must remember that many different agents may cause diffuse alveolar damage. These agents may be applied to the lung in varying concentrations for different lengths of time, continuously or intermittently, and singly or in combination. They may be unevenly distributed within the lung as a result of variations in perfusion or ventilation which they, themselves, may bring about. The alveolar walls may react differently in different areas and in different subjects.

Furthermore, the pathologist has a major sampling problem—a glance at a slice of an affected, inflated whole lung shows that the changes have not affected all parts of the lung evenly; "diffuse" alveolar damage is an approximate description of something between "focal" and truly diffuse damage and would probably be better expressed as "patchy." Thus it is not surprising that biopsies or blocks taken for histology may show different features of the damaged alveolar condition: more or less normal, more or less cellular, more or less fibrotic, and with or without hyaline membranes; nor is it surprising that none of the resulting pictures can be attributed to specific agents, unless they can be identified within the tissue. Even the bizarre alveolar and bronchiolar cells sometimes associated with certain cytotoxic agents are not specific. Moreover, most of the drugs to be discussed produce pulmonary side effects in very few of the patients taking them.

It therefore behoves the pathologist once again to seek as much clinical information as possible, to search for all of the recognizable, possibly causative agents of the condition being investigated, to describe very carefully what is seen, and to be very cautious in interpreting the observations. Review of the literature shows that clinicians and radiologists are ready to attribute diffuse alveolar damage to drugs without the examination of lung tissue or experimental confirmation, and to read too much into macroscopic and microscopic find-

Table 9-2. Therapeutic Agents Associated with Diffuse Alveolar Damage

Amitriptyline overdose
Azathioprine
BCNU*
Bleomycin*
Busulphan
Chlorambucil
Cyclophosphamide*
Gold salts
Hexamethonium
Mecamylamine
Melphalan
Methotrexate
6-Mercaptopurine
Mitomycin
Nitrofurantoin
Oxygen*
Penicillamine
Pentolinium
Pindolol
Practolol
Radiotherapy
Sulfasalazine

* Also produced in experimental animals

ings. Nevertheless, diffuse alveolar damage has been attributed to the therapeutic agents listed in Table 9-2.

One must reiterate, however, that diffuse alveolar damage can also be caused by microorganisms, inhaled vomit, carbon dioxide, ozone, oxides of nitrogen, hot metal fumes, uremia, disseminated intra-vascular coagulation, and lymphangiography contrast media.[183, 195a, 231] Furthermore, the exact relationships between diffuse alveolar damage and the interstitial pneumonias[134] and idiopathic pulmonary fibrosis[54] have still largely to be worked out.

HYPERSENSITIVITY PNEUMONITIS

By this term we refer to the association between certain drugs and the appearance of pulmonary infiltrates in a chest x-ray—with or without a concomitant increase in circulating eosinophils—and which disappear when the drug is withdrawn.[87] The discussion of hypersensitivity pneumonitis is here not intended to include granulomatous disease or extrinsic allergic alveolitis, nor is there the intention to enter into arguments about immunology.

Table 9-3 lists the drugs associated with the syndrome of hypersensitivity pneumonitis (sometimes called Loeffler's syndrome (see ref. 135)). Part B of Table 9-3 shows the few instances in which the pathology of the infiltrates has been established by biopsy or postmortem examination.

Hypersensitivity pneumonitis also occurs in asthma (including that due to aspergillosis) and in parasitic infections. It was described by Liebow and Carrington[135] as "eosinophilic pneumonia" in which the principal features were alveolar spaces filled with eosinophils and large mononuclear cells, some having eosinophilic granules in their cytoplasm; an interstitial infiltration with inflammatory cells including eosinophils; occasional, poorly formed granulomas; and, rarely, necrotizing angiitis. Some degree of interstitial fibrosis may be seen. None of Liebow and Carrington's 16 cases was attributed to drugs, but the same

Table 9-3. Drugs Associated with Hypersensitivity Pneumonitis

A. Radiologic changes without Histologic Confirmation	
	Antitetanus serum[93]
	Aurothioglucose[84]
	Chlorpropamide[17]
	Disodium cromoglycate[139]
	Imipramine[235]
	Isoniazid[115]
	Mephenesin[175]
	Nitrofurantoin[159]
	Para-aminosalicylic acid[55, 219]
	Penicillin[172, 86]
	Sulphanilamide[123]
	Sulphasalazine[113, 214, 220, 51]
	Tetracycline[101]
B. Histologic confirmation (see also individual drugs)	
	Methotrexate[201]
	Nitrofurantoin[212]
	Sulphadimethoxine[75]
	Sulphonamide[82]
	Procarbazine[140, 62, 73]

features have been reported in association with procarbazine therapy[73] and sulphadimethoxine use.[75] Nitrofurantoin has been associated with both hypersensitivity pneumonitis[212] and diffuse alveolar damage,[107] while sulphasalazine is also associated with hypersensitivity pneumonitis (but without tissue confirmation), as well as with diffuse alveolar damage. Similarly diffuse alveolar damage due to methotrexate may be associated with eosinophil infiltration (see p. 184).

GRANULOMATOUS REACTIONS

From the tissue pathologist's viewpoint, it is a pity that more of the drug-induced pulmonary lesions are not granulomata, since these are easier to identify and analyze than are diffuse alveolar damage and hypersensitivity reactions. Macrophages collect in septal or bronchovascular connective tissue or alveolar walls into more or less well-defined granulomata with multinucleate forms, some fibrosis, and lymphocytic infiltration when they are presented with material that they cannot rapidly ingest, dissolve, and remove. One would not expect drugs to come into the category of such granuloma-inducing substances, although inhaled or injected substances might.

Nevertheless, granulomata have been seen in association with methotrexate[44, 201] and with nitrofurantoin.[212] Granulomata have also been described after long periods of inhalation of extracts of porcine and bovine pituitary gland, or "pituitary snuff,"[145] and this reaction is regarded as a form of extrinsic allergic alveolitis. Eosinophilia may also be present.

Granulomatous reactions occur in response to inhaled food particles (see aspiration pneumonia, p. 169), to oil such as liquid paraffin,[185] in which multinucleate giant cells are seen in relation to the oil globules, and also in response to vaporized vaseline and light oils in "black fat tobacco disease."[153]

Granulomata may also be caused by the inhalation, injection, or pleural instillation of talc. The inhalation of this substance may be occupational[152, 158] or domestic,[228] and with its massive aspiration in childhood, death may precede granuloma formation.[157] Talc granulomata associated with pulmonary arterioles are seen in the lungs of drug addicts who inject suspensions of tablets intravenously; these may lead to pulmonary hypertension.[8, 133] Factor[72] reported granulomatous consolidation of the lung at postmortem in a patient who had had bilateral recurrent pleural effusions treated with intrapleural instillation of quinacrine hydrochloride and talcum powder.

Talc particles can usually be detected in multinucleate or mononucleate macrophages by polarized light microscopy. Their nature may be confirmed by x-ray diffraction patterns on ashed tissue or on the residue of tissue dissolved in domestic bleach, or by electron probe analysis on paraffin sections. Sometimes the particles are too small to be seen with the light microscope but can be found with the electron microscope.[152] Cornstarch and cotton fiber granulomata have also been reported, and other unidentified refractile and nonrefractile particles have been observed in drug addicts.[195]

Pulmonary granulomatosis has recently been described in a patient whose malignant melanoma was treated intralesionally with the methanol-extracted residue (MER) of BCG, and has also been seen in animals given this substance.[222]

Drugs and toxic substances are, of course, among the less common of the many causes of pulmonary granulomata, all of which may have to be considered before finally making a diagnosis.

MISCELLANEOUS RESPONSES

Apart from the pulmonary reactions already mentioned, various other toxic reactions of the lungs have been reported. Of these, pleural reactions, systemic lupus erythematosus-like reactions, pulmonary edema, pulmonary hypertension, pulmonary hemorrhage, and pulmonary calcification are recognizable by the tissue pathologist and will be considered here.

The relationships between pulmonary disease (including chronic bronchitis, emphysema, and lung cancer) and cigarette smoking would require a separate review. Furthermore, much more work is still needed to identify which of the three hundred-odd components of cigarette smoke are, in fact, toxic. At present, the tissue pathologist can do no more than record the patient's cigarette consumption, the presence of bronchial gland hypertrophy, the type and extent of emphysema, and the type of lung cancer for future correlation. Similarly, the association between carcinogenesis and certain drugs and toxins is so far from proved that—with the exception of mesothelioma and asbestos—this association will not be considered here. We also exclude reactions such as bronchospasm and respiratory muscle paralysis, attributable to certain drugs, which cannot be recognized through tissue pathology.

PLEURAL REACTIONS

Serous pleural effusions, pleural fibrosis, and malignant pleural mesothelioma have been attributed to drugs and inhaled substances.

Serous pleural effusions are either transudates or exudates, distinguishable on protein estimation and cytology. Those caused by drugs are presumably inflammatory exudates produced by the action of the drug on the pleura. Unfortunately, there are no reports about the protein content or cytology of drug-induced pleural effusions, except for those drugs that produce pleural effusions as part of systemic lupus erythematosus-like reactions, in which LE cells may sometimes be seen (hydralazine, procainamide, see p. 176). However, even if their protein and cell content were known, pleural effusions are too nonspecific for the cytologist or pathologist to attribute, in individual cases, to drugs or toxic substances. Nevertheless, pleural effusions have been associated with isoniazid,[240] methotrexate,[225] methysergide,[100a] mephenytoin and diphenylhydantoin,[170] nitrofurantoin,[106] practolol,[94] tetracycline,[101] radiation,[11] and asbestos.[83]

Pleural fibrosis is also a nonspecific reaction that can be conceived to be the result of chronic inflammation, even when it is very hyaline and hypocellular. It has been associated with methysergide[100a] oxprenolol,[166] practolol,[94] and asbestos.[151] The latter can cause: (1) a widespread parietal and visceral exudative pleural reaction that may obliterate the pleural space; or (2) localized hyaline and sometimes calcified—plaques, usually on the parietal pleural surface.[14] The latter type of plaques, particularly in the protuberant form, are almost always associated with exposure to asbestos. Furthermore, pleural fibrosis (pleurodesis) is sometimes deliberately induced in order to prevent recurrent pneumothoraces, and many substances have been used for this, including iodized talc and silver nitrate. Mepacrin has been used to prevent recurrent malignant pleural effusion.

Many reports have supported a close association between malignant pleural mesothelioma and asbestos inhalation (see Becklake's[14] Table 6). Of the four histologic patterns of malignant pleural mesothelioma described,[233] the mixed type appears to be more commonly associated with asbestos exposure.[143] Malignant mesothelioma has been seen in close association with pleural plaques,[132] but whether there is any pathogenetic relationship between these two types of lesion is not known. That asbestos can cause malignant mesotheliomas is supported by the production of these lesions in rats after the instillation of asbestos fibers into the pleural cavities[223]; however, other fibers can also produce mesothelioma in rats.[224] Indeed, the instillation of asbestos and glass fibers into the pericardium (to improve collateral coronary circulation) has been reported to produce malignant mesothelioma in a human.[42] Nevertheless, patients not exposed to any sort of fiber (as far as can be ascertained) also develop malignant mesotheliomata, with the effect that, although this diagnosis should provoke enquiry into possible exposure, it cannot be assumed that the inhalation of toxic fibers was the cause; nor is the finding of "asbestos bodies" or fibers in the lung or in a tumor proof that these bodies caused a mesothelioma.

Parenthetically, industrial exposure to asbestos is also believed to cause diffuse alveolar damage and pulmonary fibrosis—"asbestosis"[14]—but the pneumoconioses are not under consideration in this chapter. Industrial exposure to asbestos is also epidemiologically associated with carcinoma of the bronchus and with other human malignant tumors[14]; but while a complete occupational history should be obtained, in every case of lung disease, individual carcinomas cannot be attributed to exposure to asbestos.

SYSTEMIC LUPUS ERYTHEMATOSUS-LIKE REACTIONS

Many drugs have been associated with the development of systemic lupus erythematosus (SLE), on the basis of the presence of LE cells or high antinuclear factor titers in patients who recover when the suspected drug has been stopped[5,129,176]; however, the respiratory organs are rarely involved in this condition. Moreover, the pulmonary manifestations of SLE—pleurisy, pleural effusion, and atelectasis—are not usually specific, although LE cells in the pleural fluid must be regarded as diagnostic. These have been reported in association with hydralazine[226] and procainamide.[33,117] Pleural effusions have also been described in association with mephenytoin and diphenylhydantoin[170] and isoniazid.[240] Additionally, three patients developed reversible radiologic pulmonary infiltrates and high antinuclear factor titers in association with nitrofurantoin therapy.[190]

PULMONARY EDEMA

Although it can easily be recognized by the tissue pathologist, pulmonary edema is so common, particularly terminally, that it cannot reliably be attributed by the pathologist to any drug or toxin. The mechanisms of edema production and the value of measuring the pulmonary capillary wedge pressure during life are discussed by Gillett and Ford,[87] who have also tabulated and referenced the drugs involved in causing pulmonary edema.

PULMONARY HYPERTENSION

Drugs and toxins may cause pulmonary hypertension directly, as aminorex has been reported to do in humans[80] but not in animals.[121] or as the alkaloids of bush teas have been shown to do in animals.[200] Pulmonary hypertension may also be caused indirectly by drugs in three ways: oral contraceptives cause thromboemboli,[69] and hence pulmonary hypertension; the injection of talc by drug addicts produces granulomata in the pulmonary vasculature, which can lead to pulmonary hypertension (see p. 174); chronic diffuse fibrosing alveolar damage also leads to pulmonary hypertension, which means that any drug causing diffuse alveolar damage may indirectly cause pulmonary hypertension.

Patients coming to lung biopsy or postmortem may not have had their pulmonary pressures measured during life and the question of the existence of pulmonary hypertension may therefore have to be deduced from the clinical signs, the radiographs, and examination of the right ventricle[127] and pulmonary arterial system.[6] Conversely, any patient with "idiopathic" pulmonary hypertension should be closely questioned about any drugs they may have taken, although the results of such questioning may be confusing.[146]

PULMONARY HEMORRHAGE

Significant pulmonary hemorrhage caused by drugs or toxins is uncommon. Massive pulmonary hemorrhage in neonates is thought by some to be related to intensive oxygen therapy (see p. 186). Microscopic hemorrhage is a feature of paraquat poisoning (see p. 187) and of bleomycin caused lung damage (see p. 180). Intrapulmonary hemorrhage can certainly complicate drug or toxin-induced thrombocytopenia. Pulmonary hemorrhage is a feature of Goodpasture's syndrome, and the latter has been described as a complication of penicillamine therapy (p. 188).

Finley et al.[77] described a syndrome of occult pulmonary hemorrhage (dyspnea, unexplained acute anemia, and alveolar infiltrates on x-rays, hemoptysis) in three patients receiving oral anticoagulants. The authors gave a method of scoring hemosiderin in alveolar macrophages obtained by bronchopulmonary lavage, in order to help diagnosis of the condition. Simon et al.[196] described a fatal case of hemothorax in a patient receiving anticoagulants.

PULMONARY CALCIFICATION

Pulmonary calcification caused by therapeutic agents is uncommon. Cooke and Hyland[52] described a patient with Crohn's disease, who was given large doses of calcium salts and vitamin D for tetany, and whose lungs at autopsy "had the consistency of pumice stone," with extensive calcification in the alveolar walls; there was no calcification elsewhere. This is in contrast to cases of excessive milk and alkali intake in which alveolar wall calcification was part of a more widespread, metastatic calcification[229] (Fig. 9-4).

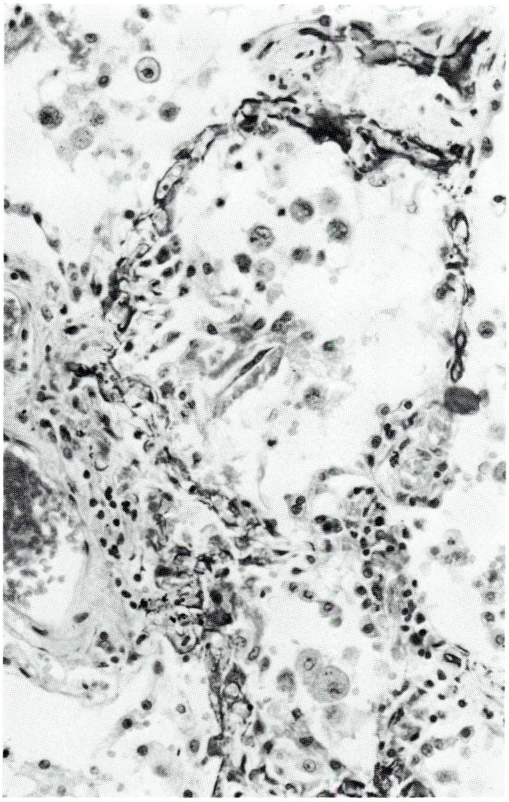

Fig. 9-4. Metastatic calcification that was diffuse throughout the alveoli. H&E, ×250.

LUNG BIOPSY

The pathologist may receive lung biopsies obtained transbronchially through a fiberoptic bronchoscope, or transpleurally by open thoracotomy or percutaneous needle biopsy. Several fiberoptic or needle biopsy samples may be taken for light microscopy, electron microscopy, microbiologic examination or chemical analysis[183] although nothing can be done to maintain the anatomic relationships of the elements of such a specimen. However, open lung biopsies for light- or electron microscopy should be taken from between two clamps and dropped immediately into fixative; this keeps some air in the alveolar spaces and retains the normal anatomy of the specimen. With this approach Carrington and Gaensler[34] identified 43 different pathologic entities in 490 biopsies, although none was attributed to drugs.

To cover the possibilities listed in the differential diagnosis, the clinician should discuss the case—including the precise details of therapy (timing and dosage)—with the tissue pathologist and the microbiologist before the biopsy is done, so that appropriate microbiologic, microscopic, and chemical analyses can be arranged. If the microbiologic work reveals no significant organism, and no organisms are seen in tissue sections stained for bacteria (gram stain), Legionnaire's organism (Dieterle stain), mycobacteria (Ziehl-Nielsen stain), fungi and protozoa (methenamine silver stain), or viral inclusions (phloxine tartrazine stain), then the pathologist can consider—for a possibly toxic etiology—the morphologic changes seen with hematoxylin and eosin (H&E) staining (also viewed with polarized light for birefringent particles) and those seen in sections stained for collagen and elastic fibers (elastic-van Giesen stain), reticulin fibers (Gordon & Sweets stain), and fibrin (Martius scarlet-blue stain). Lesions due to drugs or toxins may be present even if microorganisms are found, but their elucidation is more difficult.

With regard to restoring the function of the lung, fluid and cellular exudation and cellular proliferation in the alveolar spaces or alveolar walls are more easily reversible than fiber deposition; each of these components should therefore be mentioned in the report, as should the presence or absence of birefringent particles and asbestos bodies (identified with Perl's stain), although there may be further argument about the significance of these findings in each individual case. The organization of a comprehensively planned approach to a lung biopsy is well described by Weisenberger.[227]

Tissue samples may also be collected and fixed for electron microscopy, although at present this technique seldom contributes to routine diagnosis. Extra samples can be collected and deep frozen or fixed in formalin for chemical or particle analysis. The latter may be done by digesting the tissue in domestic bleach and examining the residue by electron microscopy and x-ray diffraction. In the end, however, the pathologist in each individual case can usually say only that the drug or toxin to which the patient had been exposed could or could not, given our present state of knowledge, have produced the damage seen, and whether that drug is the only agent in the patient's history likely to have produced the particular pattern of damage seen.

POSTMORTEM LUNGS

By the time death has occurred, the various pathologic changes in the lungs that have called for diagnosis earlier in the course of the illness have often had terminal changes added to them. The latter may include changes caused by terminal infection, oxygen therapy, inhalation of vomit, uremia, hypotension, disseminated intravascular coagulation, emboli, and heart failure. Microbiologic investigation, electron microscopy, and immunofluorescent detection of viruses may be precluded, particularly if the postmortem is delayed.

Attributing pathologic changes in the lung to one or another of the drugs the patient has had can therefore be difficult, but is not impossible (see Chapter 1). However, as already noted, it is not always convincingly done in published reports, particularly of individual cases.

Nevertheless, if the pathologist is satisfied with the documentation of all the factors bearing on the pulmonary changes, he or she has the advantage at postmortem of having the entire respiratory system to study. In infants, it is appropriate to remove the thoracic organs intact, to cut off the right lung at the main bronchus distal to a clamp, and then to pour 10 percent formalin, via the trachea, into the left lung, thus fixing it in inflation. The uninflated right lung may be sliced saggitally and the lateral half given, without fixation, to the microbiologist for bacterial and viral isolation. The whole medial half may then be fixed for 24 hours in formalin, processed, and embedded in wax; whole lung sections can then be cut from the cut surface and mounted on large glass slides for staining. The inflated left lung may also be sliced saggitally after fixation for 24 hours, and the medial half treated in the same way as that of the right lung. The whole, uninflated right lung section gives a good view of the pathologic lesions and their distribution, while the whole inflated left lung section shows the anatomy well, although the formalin flow sometimes distorts the pathology. Bronchopulmonary dysplasia caused by oxygen therapy, congenital lobar emphysema, and infections caused by *Aspergillus* species and *Serratia marcescens,* for example, have been among the conditions recently elucidated by this approach in our laboratory.

The same system is largely applicable to adult lungs. The right and left main bronchi should be severed at their origin from the trachea, and both lungs should be weighed. The left lung, with the longer main bronchus, should be inflated with 10 percent formalin via the bronchus until the pleura is fully distended; it should then be clamped and allowed to float in formalin for 24 hours before slicing. In the right lung, first the bronchi and then the arteries should be opened and examined before the entire lung is sliced saggitally and a portion of the lateral half given to the microbiologist for appropriate microbiologic examination. Although whole-lung slices can be cut from either lung for macroscopic examination, it is not practicable to cut, mount, and stain whole adult lung sections for transmitted light microscopy—although whole-lung sections can be rapidly mounted on paper[230] to show the distribution of lesions. For light microscopic appearances, one is thus thrown back on processing as many small samples as is judged necessary, although these can often be bigger than those obtained at open lung biopsy, and can include samples from larger airways. The histologic stains used for these autopsy specimens, have been described for biopsies (p. 177).

By the foregoing means, it is usually possible to judge reasonably accurately the final extent of an original disease, the extent of pneumonia and of pulmonary edema, and the extent of any radiation-induced in the lung changes (which are usually localized to the area irradiated (see p. 189)). Interpretation of any further diffuse alveolar damage may be somewhat more subjective, but reference to the timing and dosage for each drug under consideration, and the type of lesion previously reported in association with each drug, together with any experimental data, may enable the pathologist to reach moderately firm conclusions as to the contribution of any drug or toxin to the lesions found.

DRUGS

Amitriptyline

Damage. Diffuse alveolar damage has been reported at autopsy, both without[210] and with intra-alveolar fibrosis and hyaline membranes.[136] Hyaline membranes alone have been also reported.[148]

Experimental Data. None.

Dose and Time Relationships. The minimum recorded dose causing damage was 750 mg (an overdose of 30 tablets[136]), with pulmonary changes apparent from day 3 (the patient died on day 12). Marshall and Moore's case[148] was a child of 15 months who ingested at least 1,000 mg, had generalized seizures and laryngeal stridor, and died on day 3.

Azathioprine

This drug is a derivative of 6-mercaptopurine, which is metabolized to 6-mercaptopurine.

Damage. Diffuse alveolar damage has been seen on biopsy[227]; the damage cleared radiologically when azathioprine was stopped.

Experimental Data. None.

Dose and Time Relationships. The dose of this drug causing damage was 150 mg per day for 2 years.[227] The case of Rubin et al.[180] had 100 mg per day for 6 weeks, and cleared when the drug was stopped, but no tissue was examined.

BIS-Chloroethylnitrosourea (BCNU)

Damage. Fatal diffuse alveolar damage has been reported by Holoye et al.[102] in a man of 19, and by Bailey et al.[12] in a girl of 22 months. Durant et al.[65] reviewed 10 patients with pulmonary fibrosis, of whom 7 died and 8 had biopsy or autopsy lung tissue examined. In Holoye's case, apart from diffuse alveolar damage particularly affecting the lower lobes, there was fibrous thickening of the pleura. In Bailey's case the pleura was normal but there was severe subpleural fibrosis of the upper lobe parenchyma. There were also areas of pneumonia, hyaline membranes, alveolar hemorrhages, and intra-alveolar fibrin.

Experimental Data. Animal experiments have produced pleural effusions and pulmonary edema in beagles, plus pneumonitis in rhesus monkeys.[35]

Dose and Time Relationships. In Holoye's case, 100 mg per square meter of BCNU was given intravenously every 3 to 4 weeks for 36 months, to a total of 3,330 mg. The first respiratory symptoms developed 34 months after starting the drug, and the patient died 7 months after the drug was stopped. Bailey's case was given vincristine, dexamethazone, and radiotherapy before starting BCNU 50 mg intravenously at 6-week intervals, to a total of 775 mg over 2 years. The patient developed pulmonary symptoms 2 months after the drug was stopped, and died 1 month later. All but one of Durant et al.'s 10 cases had combination chemotherapy with BCNU, cyclophosphamide, vincristine, prednisone, and procarbazine. (NB: cyclophosphamide (p. 182) and procarbazine (p. 189) can also cause pulmonary damage). The one patient who was given no other chemotherapy had a total dose of BCNU of 800 mg per square meter, and 12 months elapsed between the start of chemotherapy and the onset of pulmonary symptoms.

Bleomycin

Damage. Diffuse alveolar damage. Luna et al.[141] described lesions, particularly subpleurally and in the lower lobes, in 12 of 37 patients given bleomycin intravenously. Intra-alveolar proteinaceous material was the most consistent feature of the lesions. Proliferation of alveolar and bronchiolar epithelium, with squamous metaplasia and even dysplasia is described,[59] with basal honeycombing in advanced cases. Jones[111] found no particular distribution of damage, but emphasized intra-alveolar hemorrhage. Electron microscopic appearances of the effects caused by bleomycin[16] include intra-alveolar collagen. The differential diagnosis of bleomycin-induced lung damage has been helpfully discussed.[38]

Experimental Data. The effects of intravenous bleomycin on the lung have been studied in dogs[79, 187] and pheasants.[15] The dogs developed subpleural lesions and mesothelial hyperplasia which turned into fibrous plaques, while the pheasants developed confluent interstitial pneumonia. Diffuse alveolar damage occurs after the intratracheal injection of bleomycin in hamsters[208] and in rats.[215] Thrall et al.[215] also found that after a single intratracheal dose of 1.5 units of bleomycin, daily injections of indomethacin (2 mg per kilogram per day) prevented the fibrosis. Electron microscopic changes have been reported after intraperitoneal injections of bleomycin in mice[10, 112] and after tritiated thymidine labeling.[2] These studies suggest that both endothelial and epithelial damage can result from bleomycin therapy.

Dose and Time Relationships. There is confusion about the dosage of bleomycin required to produce pulmonary damage because some authors use units and others milligrams. Fatal pulmonary involvement has been described after a dose as low as 75 mg per square meter[21]; however, pulmonary damage associated with low doses can be completely reversible in humans[164] and in baboons.[142] High doses (up to 1,215 mg), on the other hand, may produce only a small mortality, possibly enhanced by radiotherapy.[186] De Lena et al.[59] gave parenteral doses ranging from 115 mg to 800 mg, but did not report any time intervals. Blum et al.[19] noted a 5 percent incidence of lung involvement if the total dose of bleomycin was less than 500 mg, rising to 17 percent when the 500 mg figure was exceeded.

The shortest time of onset of pulmonary toxicity after the onset of bleomycin therapy in 67 patients reported by De Lena et al.[59] was 28 days. This was produced by 15 mg per square meter given twice weekly—that is, a total dose of 120 mg per square meter—in 7 out of 26 patients given this dosage. Ten milligrams per square meter given twice weekly for 4 weeks, and repeated after a 1 month interval, produced no pulmonary symptoms. Rudders and Hensley[182] reported pulmonary involvement by bleomycin in a case of Kaposi's sarcoma only 3 days after starting a course of intravenous injections (9 mg per day).

Busulphan

Damage. Busulphan has produced diffuse alveolar damage with interstitial and intra-alveolar fibrosis.[138] Striking enlargement of alveolar and bronchial epithelial cells and the nuclei of some of these cells has been reported histologically and cytologically in the sputum, even 6 months after stopping busulphan[125] (Fig. 9-5). Multinucleate cells have been reported,[30] and these atypical cells have been thought to be premalignant,[154] although the exact relationship between 5 years of busulphan therapy for chronic myeloid leukemia and honeycomb lung and adenocarcinoma was not clear. "Busulphan lung" does not appear to have been reported except in patients with chronic myeloid leukemia. Kirschner and Esterly[122] compared 40 patients with chronic myeloid leukemia treated with busulphan with 41 not treated. All the changes attributed to busulphan were found in both groups except the atypical "busulphan cells" (see also ref. 36).

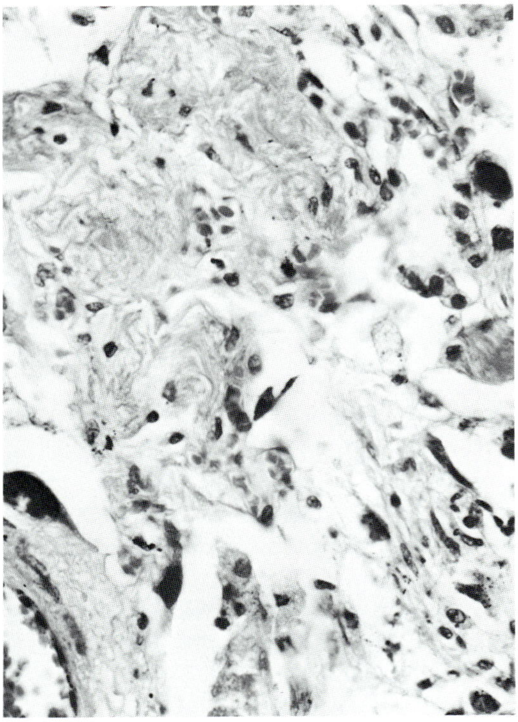

Fig. 9-5. "Busulphan" lung with interstitial fibrosis and many large atypical alveolar cells. H&E, ×360.

Experimental Data. None.

Dose and Time Relationships. Pulmonary changes have been reported with busulphan as early as 3 months after beginning therapy with to 4 to 6 mg per day,[156] and as long as 13 years[126] after starting continuous busulphan therapy (this patient also had diffuse pulmonary ossification). The pulmonary changes are thus unlikely to be dose-related.

Chlorambucil

Damage. Chlorambucil produces diffuse alveolar damage. The only significant report of such damage[50] refers to a 73-year-old woman given chlorambucil for polycythemia rubra vera for 21 months before developing cough and breathlessness. Lung biopsy revealed patchy interstitial fibrosis with lymphocytic and histiocytic infiltration, some intra-alveolar cells, and marked alveolar cell hyperplasia and atypia. Electron microscopy revealed no epithelial damage. The symptoms regressed within 2 weeks of stopping the drug. Rubio[181] refers to four patients who died of severe interstitial fibrosis, two of whom were biopsied on the suspicion of *Pneumocystis carinii,* but in whom fibrosis was found instead.

Experimental Data. None.

Dose and Time Relationships. The patient of Cole et al.[50] developed pulmonary symptoms after a total dose of 4,120 mg of busulphan in the 21-month period. Rubio[181] gives no relevant data.

Colchicine

A postmortem on a woman of 80 who died 36 hours after taking 150 mg of commercial grade colchicine in tea revealed interstitial and airspace edema and interstitial polymorphs, but no hyaline membranes.[100] How much of the pulmonary pathology was due to colchicine is not clear.

Cyclophosphamide

Damage. Cyclophosphamide produces diffuse alveolar damage. There have been three clinical reports of this. Rodin et al.[174] described a child of 3 years with a rhabdomyosarcoma of the bladder who received cyclophosphamide (30 to 40 mg per kilogram per week) for 22 weeks, then prednisone and vincristine for 8 weeks, and radiotherapy (2,000 r). The child had a *Klebsiella* infection for a week and 2 days in an oxygen tent before he died. A woman of 66 was described at a clinicopathologic conference[37] who had carcinoma of the breast treated with radiotherapy, vincristine, prednisone, and cyclophosphamide. After 8 weeks on the cyclophosphamide she became breathless and died after another 9 days, during which she was given streptomycin, isoniazid, pyridoxine, 5-fluorouracil, and oxygen. The alveolar lining cells of her lungs were hyperplastic, and there was squamous metaplasia. Topilow et al.[218] described a 33-year-old woman with Hodgkin's disease treated initially with nitrogen mustard and radiotherapy. A year later, cyclophosphamide was started and continued for 27 months in doses of 50 to 300 mg/day. The cyclophosphamide was stopped when the woman developed chest pain and a cough. Vinblastine and isoniazid were then given. After 6 months she was admitted for breathlessness and given oxygen, prednisone, hydroxystilbamidine, pyramethamine, and sulphadiazine, but died.

Thus cyclophosphamide was not the only possible cause of the diffuse alveolar damage in any of these cases.

Experimental Data. Dogs given cyclophosphamide in an injection of 500 mg/kg developed hemorrhagic myocarditis and pulmonary edema, and died within 6 hours.[163] Rats given a single dose (20 mg/100 mg body weight) intraperitoneally developed interstitial and intra-alveolar hemorrhages within 2 days, hyaline membranes within 4 days, proliferating alveolar cells within 1 week and, later, interstitial fibrosis and atypical alveolar cells. Electron microscopy confirmed initial endothelial and type I cell pneumocyte damage.[89]

Dose and Time Relationships. There is little information on this (see above). Eight weeks (with no dose specified) appears to be the shortest time on cyclophosphamide before respiratory involvement has been noted.[37]

Gold Salts

Damage. Gold salts produce diffuse alveolar damage. Interstitial fibrosis, lymphocytes, and plasma cells, but no granulomas or vasculitis, were described in two open-lung biopsies by Winterbauer et al.[238]; Since one patient relapsed when gold injections were resumed, and the other had osteoarthritis, the gold damage was convincingly distinguished from rheumatoid lung damage. Miyachi[155] reported the same findings in an open biopsy from a patient given 1,080 mg of gold thioglucose for bronchial asthma. Geddes and Brostoff[85] added a case in which lymphoblastic transformation to gold was positive. Gould et al.[88] added the case of a patient who died and additionally had hyaline membranes. James et al.[108] reported a case of gold-induced alveolar cell hyperplasia so florid as to suggest adenocarcinoma; intra-alveolar cells and fibrosis were generally inconspicuous. Sepuya et al.[191] report a further example in a patient with seropositive rheumatoid arthritis which showed 80 percent resolution radiologically 4 months after gold salts had been stopped.

Pulmonary eosinophilia has been reported after aurothioglucose,[84] but no pulmonary tissue was examined (see p. 173).

Experimental Data. None.

Dose and Time Relationships. The lowest initiating dose of gold salts reported for lung damage was 50 mg.[191] Gould et al.[88] give a table of their own cases and three others in which the smallest dose was 325 mg and the shortest time for development of effects was 5 weeks. In one of the cases the onset was delayed for 16 weeks. Scharf et al.[188] describe a case of seronegative rheumatoid arthritis in which respiratory disease developed after only 175 mg of sodium aurothiomalate, but no pulmonary tissue was examined.

Hexamethonium

Hexamethonium, mecamylamine, and pentolinium were once popular ganglion blocking agents for hypertension. They produce striking pulmonary damage similar to that seen in uremia (p. 170).

Damage. Hexamethonium produces intra-alveolar fibrosis, together with some interstitial fibrosis, affecting the central portion of the lungs (case 2) or periphery (case 3).[64] Case 3 was described again after the patient had lived much longer and died of uremia[45, 97]; intra-alveolar fibrosis was no longer seen, but there was interstitial fibrosis and bronchiolectasis, plus partial degeneration of elastic fibers with adherent, laminated PAS- and Perl-positive conchoidal bodies. Perry et al.[167] reviewed three groups of cases: malignant hypertension not treated with hexamethonium; malignant hypertension treated with hexamethonium; and mitral stenosis. Hyaline membranes, intra-alveolar fibrin, and intra-alveolar fibrosis were found in all three groups, but more frequently in those treated with hexamethonium and at lower blood urea levels. The lung tissue appearances found in uremia[103] are indistinguishable from those in hexamethonium-induced damage, but in uremia the perihilar radiologic shadows may be associated with only minor breathlessness. Neither the pathogenesis of uremic lung damage nor of that due to ganglion blocking drugs is known—one may potentiate the other. With mecamylamine, similar interstitial and intra-alveolar fibrosis is also seen,[179] as it is with pentolinium as well.[99]

Experimental Data. None.

Dose and Time Relationships. Pulmonary lesions have been reported as early as 7 months after beginning treatment with hexamethonium at 50 mg tds[64]; with mecamylamine 2.5 mg increased to 5 mg bd[179]; and after 15 months on pentolinium at 80 mg qds.[99] Doniach's third case[45, 97] was given hexamethonium at 70 mg b.i.d., increasing this to 240 mg b.i.d. for several months before shadows were noted with chest x-ray. Hexamethonium was stopped for a month and then restarted, but the shadows continued to diminish. For the next 6 years the patient received hexamethonium at night and pentolinium by day. He was changed to pempidine for 2 years before he eventually died of uremia. It is hard to know the parts that hexamethonium, pentolinium, and uremia each played in this case.

Mecamylamine

See hexamethonium.

Melphalan

Damage. Melphalan causes diffuse alveolar damage. There are only two case reports—both postmortems in elderly men being treated for multiple myelomatosis with melphalan and prednisone. Codling and Chakera[48] found solid lungs with foci of honeycomb change, an intra-alveolar fibrinous exudate undergoing organization, interstitial fibrosis, and proliferation of alveolar lining cells. Taetle et al.[211] found marked atypical epithelial proliferation with widespread fibrosis. They reviewed tissues from 10 other patients with myeloma treated with melphalan, and found atypical epithelial proliferation in 5 others and fibrosis in 1. In 11 myeloma patients not treated with melphalan, and in 11 age- and sex-matched controls, no atypical epithelial proliferation or fibrosis was found.

Experimental Data. None.

Dose and Time Relationships. Both Codling and Chakera's[48] and Taetle et al.'s[211] patients received 2 mg of melphalan b.i.d., but this was reduced to 2 mg on alternate days in Taetle's case, in which the patient died after 2 months. Codling and Chakera's patient[48] developed widespread consolidation after 3 months and died 1 month later.

6-Mercaptopurine

There are three reports (quoted by Sostman et al.[202]) of pulmonary damage caused by this drug, but all are unsatisfactory because other drugs were involved. Sostman et al. also reported a 2-year-old child whose lung biopsy showed "exuberant epithelial proliferation and round cell infiltration with no evidence of fibrosis," and who recovered. No dose or time relationships were given.

Since azathioprine (p. 179) is metabolized to 6-mercaptopurine and appears to cause pulmonary damage, it is perhaps surprising that 6-mercaptopurine has not been reported to do so more often.

Methotrexate

Damage. Sostman et al.[201] reviewed 29 cases of pulmonary damage due to methotrexate, and added 7 of their own. There was a wide range of appearances. Generally, diffuse alveolar damage was present with prominent, often atypical epithelial cells, and intra-alveolar cells and hyaline membranes together with interstitial infiltration. Some cases, however, had eosinophils in the infiltrate and peripheral blood eosinophilia (see p. 174); others showed granulomatous reactions, with multinucleate giant cells (see p. 174). Fibrosis was unusual. Pulmonary involvement occurred whether the patient was being treated for cancer, skin disease, or connective tissue disease, or whether they were already receiving corticosteroids or not. There was clinical recovery after stopping the drug in most cases, but some patients died.

Experimental Data. None.

Dose and Time Relationships. The dose of methotrexate received in all cases exceeded 20 mg per week, and the total dosage ranged from 40 mg to 41 grams given over periods ranging from 12 days to 5 years.

Methysergide

Damage. Reversible pleural fibrosis has been reported by Graham,[91] in an anecdotal account of 2 cases of his own and 10 others reported to him; one of these latter 10 cases had both retroperitoneal and "pleuropulmonary" fibrosis. Another case of methysergide-induced pulmonary damage referred to by Graham et al.[92] had fibrosis around vessels and terminal bronchioles on lung biopsy. Hindle et al.[100a] report dense hyaline fibrous tissue on pleural biopsy.

Experimental Data. None.

Dose and Time Relationships. Both of Graham's cases had been taking methysergide for 2 years, but no doses are given. Hindle's case had had 1 mg t.i.d. for 6 months.

Mitomycin

Damage. Diffuse alveolar damage from mitomycin has been reported by Orwoll et al.[165] in three cases; there was interstitial edema, infiltration with plasma and mononuclear cells, and some fibrosis, together with mild alveolar epithelial proliferation, but no intra-alveolar fluid or hyaline membranes. Fielding et al.[76] have described a case in which transbronchial biopsies showed interstitial fibrosis and proliferation of alveolar lining cells. At postmortem there was diffuse and focal interstitial fibrosis with no intra-alveolar fibrosis. This patient and one of Orwoll's had also had 5-fluorouracil, but there is no record of lung damage due to 5-fluorouracil.

Experimental data. None.

Dose and Time Relationships. The minimum time for mitomycin-induced lung damage appears to be 6 months,[165] and the minimum dose seems to have been 60 mg over a period of 6 months.[165]

Nitrofurantoin

Nitrofurantoin has produced a wide range of reactions including hypersensitivity reactions (see p. 174), granulomatous reactions (see p. 174), pleural reactions (see p. 175), systemic lupus erythematosus-like reactions (see p. 176), and diffuse alveolar damage. The nitrofurantoin reactions are sometimes classified as acute, subacute, and chronic. There are few reports of tissue examination in the acute and subacute reactions apart from that of Taskinen et al.[212]

Chronic reactions refer to diffuse alveolar damage. Five cases with lung biopsies were described by Rosenow et al.,[178] although the one death seems only tenuously related to nitrofurantoin. There are three other reports with histology.[39, 22, 137] All cases improved clinically and radiologically after stopping the drug.

Experimental data. None.

Dose and Time Relationships. The duration of exposure to nitrofurantoin before symptoms of diffuse alveolar damage have appeared has varied from 1 year to 6 years.[178] It is impossible to work out the dose relationships.

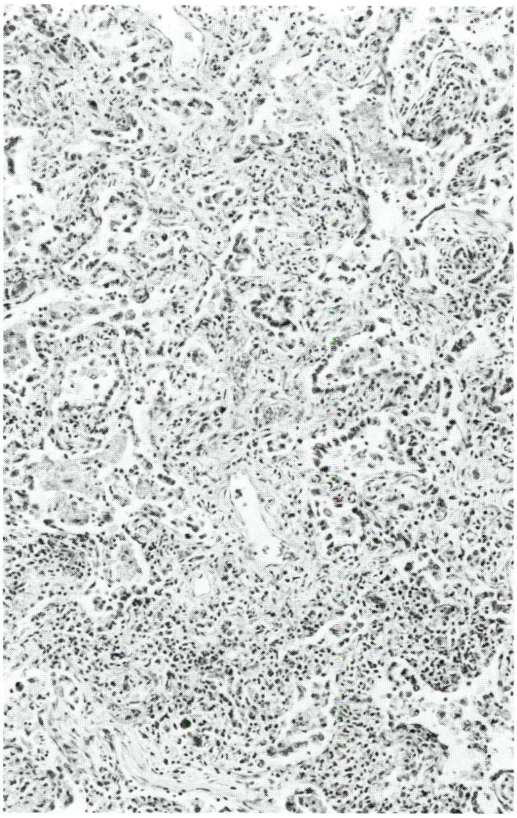

Fig. 9-6. Patient who died following a head injury and 4 weeks on a respirator during which time the pO_2 had to be gradually raised. Note the marked interstitial fibrosis and prominent type II proliferation. H&E, ×100.

Oxygen

The complex subject of oxygen toxicity has recently been well reviewed by Frank and Massaro[81, 81a] and Deneke and Fanburg.[60a]

Diffuse Alveolar Damage in Adults. By 1976, 90 cases had been reported, but in 80 of these the use of oxygen had followed one or more of the conditions which can, in themselves, cause diffuse alveolar damage, and 7 more had underlying pulmonary disorders.[120] Nevertheless, Katzenstein et al.[120] carefully correlated the concentrations and duration of exposure to oxygen with histology in 16 further patients in previous good health and without pulmonary disease who required oxygen before their deaths. All 16 had been treated with 80 to 100 percent oxygen via a respirator for from 22 hours to 32 days (see Fig. 9-6). All of those exposed for less than 3 days had congestion and focal intra-alveolar edema, and some had fibrin thrombi in small vessels (see disseminated intravascular coagulation, p. 170). Hyaline membranes were present in all cases exposed for 7 days or less. Interstitial edema was seen after 3 days, and there was a striking interstitial infiltrate of lymphocytes, plasma cells, and mononuclear cells, most evident in those dying within less than a week. Focal type II cell proliferation could be seen as early as 3 days after treatment began, but was marked in all cases after a week. Sometimes the cells were atypical, with large bizarre nuclei and nucleoli. Small foci of interstitial fibrosis could be seen after 3 days, and this was extensive in all cases after 8 days and by 14 days looked surprisingly chronic. Sevitt[192] noted that patients inhaling 25 to 40 percent oxygen had either no lesions or subclinical focal lesions at postmortem. With the electron microscope, Gould et al.[90] showed swollen membranous pneumocytes and endothelial cells after only 14 hours exposure to 70 percent oxygen.

Although many patients who develop oxygen toxicity die, Hyde and Rawson[104] reported three patients on respirators for muscular weakness who were given 83 percent or more oxygen and developed oxygen pneumonitis radiologically which regressed when the oxygen intake was lowered; the chest x-rays in these cases took 42 to 50 days to clear. Frank and Massaro[81] comment on the great individual variation in susceptibility/resistance to oxygen toxicity.

"Broncho-pulmonary Dysplasia" in Infants. The term "bronchopulmonary dysplasia" has been given to the radiologic and pathologic features produced by prolonged, high concentrations of oxygen given to neonates with respiratory distress.[162] The pathology includes airway epithelial hyperplasia and squamous metaplasia, fibroblast proliferation around bronchioles and muscle hypertrophy, and interstitial fibroblast proliferation (resembling premature interstitium), with type II cells lining the alveoli. This pathology is well illustrated by Banerjee et al.,[13] who found changes as early as 55 hours, and hyaline membranes present up to 8 days; and by Anderson et al.,[7] who also found endothelial and epithelial cell damage ultrastructurally. Edwards et al.[68] reviewed 299 babies ventilated for respiratory distress, and found that those who survived to be given 80 to 100 percent oxygen for more than 6 days developed bronchopulmonary dysplasia, as did those given 40 to 70 percent oxygen for more than 18 days, or 22 to 30 percent oxygen for more than 53 days. There is some individual variation in susceptibility, and mechanical ventilation may play some part. None of the babies reviewed by Edwards et al. survived, but Shepard et al.[194] described 19 patients who survived after requiring mechanical assistance for hyaline membrane disease; 6 had radiologic evidence of pulmonary fibrosis or overexpansion of the lung, or both, and biopsy revealed pulmonary fibrosis in 2.

Massive Pulmonary Hemorrhage in Neonates. This fatal condition (also called hemorrhagic pulmonary edema by Adamson et al.[4]), defined by Boothby and de Sa[24] as confluent hemorrhage, either alveolar or interstitial and involving two or more lobes of the lung in the absence of infection, has been associated with intensive oxygen therapy, particularly in premature babies.[24, 74] Although it has been noted[128] that the data are at present too limited to allow the assumption of a single cause for this condition, oxygen exposure should be considered and recorded in each case.

Experimental Data. Much work has been done on oxygen toxicity,[81, 43] revealing considerable differences in susceptibility between species; for example, frogs survive well but dogs do not. In general, laboratory animals (mice, rats) and primates react similarly to humans, although oxygen concentrations of other than 100 percent have rarely been used.

In adult mice, Bowden et al.[26] showed focal endothelial cell damage, caused by 90 percent oxygen at 7 days, to be the earliest lesion, and also[25] that mice who recover after oxygen toxicity have only minor focal residual damage. Newborn mice can survive continuous 100 percent oxygen treatment for up to 6 weeks[23]; the damage in these animals falls particularly on the airway epithelium. There is marked type II cell proliferation by 2 weeks, cellular infiltration of alveolar walls by 3 weeks, and the alveolar spaces are filled with undifferentiated cells, polymorphs, and collagen by 4 weeks. By 6 weeks there are many thrombi in various stages of organization in alveolar capillaries. Lung growth is considerably inhibited.

Monkeys breathing 100 percent oxygen have their alveolar pneumocytes almost totally destroyed within 4 days,[118,116] but these cells are replaced by type II pneumocytes in 7 days. There are inconspicuous changes at the intercellular junctions of the endothelial cells in 2 days and a 50 percent loss of endothelial cell volume by 7 days, with interstitial hemorrhage. Weaning back to room air after 8 days of exposure produced clinical and functional recovery within 2 to 3 months, but pathologically there was residual interstitial fibrosis.

Paraquat

Paraquat is a herbicide whose worldwide economic value far outstrips in importance the fact that it is toxic and has caused accidental, homicidal, and suicidal deaths. It is sold for agricultural purposes as a 20 percent solution, and to domestic gardeners in granules that give a 5 percent paraquat solution when dissolved in water according to the instructions.[47] A rapid immunoassay method for measuring plasma paraquat concentrations is now available.[131]

Damage. Paraquat causes diffuse alveolar damage. Of 188 cases reported to the London Centre of the British National Poisons Information Service from 1974 to 1976, 57 died acutely within 7 days, and only 12 died later with evidence of pulmonary fibrosis (see Fig. 9-7). The remaining 119 survived without ill effects; 111 of these had taken the granular form of paraquat.[98] Sequential reports were not common (a resected lung at 8 days and a postmortem lung at 20 days[150]; a biopsy at 7 days and a postmortem at 17 days[217]), and findings in patients at different times were therefore required. Rebello and Mason[171] reported a persistent but patchy hemorrhage occurring within 16 hours; intra-alveolar edema with strands of fibrin and phagocytes; hyaline membranes (PAS and picro-Mallory positive) after 6 days; and early septal thickening with hemorrhage and fibrin; but fibroblastic activity from 6 days onwards. They saw little intra-alveolar fibrosis except in one case. Our own experience is that both the interstitial and intra-alveolar fibrosis are patchy and are seen in different parts of the same lung; the former is more peripheral, the latter more central in whole-lung slices. This same effect was shown by Thurlbeck and Thurlbeck,[216] who also observed the cystic dilatation of air spaces or "honeycombing" described by Rebello and Mason[171] as early as 1 day after the ingestion of paraquat. Our cases have shown this to be a bronchiolectasis, often containing mucopurulent secretions.

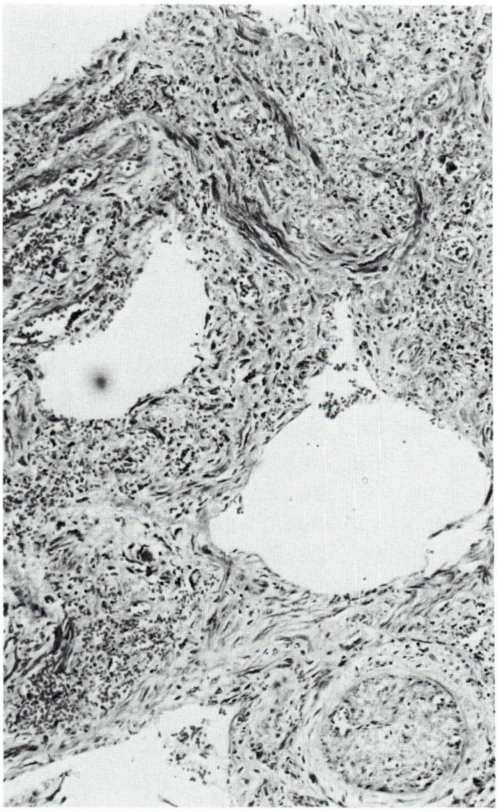

Fig. 9-7. Paraquat lung from a male who had ingested the herbicide approximately 2 weeks prior to death. There is tremendous interstitial fibrosis with cystic spaces (honeycombing). H&E, ×100.

Toner et al.[217] viewed their 7-day biopsy, taken before oxygen was given, and studied electron microscopically, and found alveolar walls varying from normal to markedly disturbed. In places the pneumocytes had disappeared, leaving bare basement membrane; in others there was endothelial swelling and interstitial edema with swollen fibroblasts. There was massive intra-alveolar and interstitial fibrosis at autopsy 10 days later, and there was also proliferation of the terminal bronchiolar epithelium. Electron microscopy of a lung biopsy taken 22 days after the ingestion of paraquat[58] showed collapsed alveolar spaces lined by type II pneumocytes and filled with proteinaceous fluid containing a variety of cells, including "profibroblasts." The interstitial areas were greatly expanded, endothelial cells were abnormal, and there was patchy disruption of the capillary basement membrane.

A fatal case reported after the percutaneous absorption of 2.8 percent paraquat solution 17 days previously also showed medial hypertrophy of pulmonary arterioles. Biopsies from fellow workers who survived also had these features, plus organizing thrombi,[130] and this picture was reproduced in rats.[130] Smith and Heath[199] have also noticed vascular changes characteristic of chronic hypoxia, which paraquat poisoning may have rapidly brought about.

There have been some discussions as to whether oxygen therapy may not potentiate paraquat damage.[47, 53]

Experimental Data. Similar diffuse alveolar damage has been produced by parenteral paraquat in rats,[221, 78] mice,[29] and hamsters, with a lesser effect produced and protection given by ACTH and Freund's adjuvant[31]; in rabbits, alveolar damage has been produced with a paraquat aerosol.[189]

Penicillamine

"Diffuse Alveolitis." This has been reported in one case[67] after 450 mg per day of penicillamine given for a year to a patient with severe rheumatoid arthritis. The symptoms and x-ray changes thought to be characteristic of alveolitis improved within a week of stopping the drug, and disappeared at 1 month. No tissue was examined.

Goodpasture's Syndrome. This was reported[209] in three fatal cases given penicillamine at 1 to 3.5 grams/day for Wilson's disease for 2 to 3½ years. In the case described in detail, however, immunofluorescence microscopy revealed only patchy deposition of IgG and C3 in the kidneys, and no deposits in the lungs, although the pulmonary hemorrhage was convincing. No reports of other drugs causing Goodpasture's syndrome are known.

Pentolinium

See hexamethonium (p. 183).

Pindolol

Damage. Pindolol produces diffuse alveolar damage. There is one report[161] referring to a patient who had an open lung biopsy after taking pindolol (no dose given) for 7 years for essential hypertension. The biopsy from the left upper lobe showed desquamated cells in the alveoli and small airways, patchy interstitial fibrosis and infiltration with mononuclear cells, patchy type II cell hyperplasia and atypia, mild thickening of the pulmonary arterioles, and prominent type II cells on electron microscopy. The authors note that pindolol and practolol have a stereochemical configuration similar to methysergide.

Practolol

This drug was introduced into clinical practice in 1970 but was withdrawn in 1976.

Polyserositis. First recognized in the peritoneum, sclerosing peritonitis in patients given practolol was subsequently associated at postmortem with fine tacky adhesions between the visceral and parietal pleura and the pericardium,[236, 66] and at thoracotomy with a dense fibrosis up to 2 cm thick.[94]

Interstitial Pulmonary Fibrosis. This has

been reported in one patient on biopsy.[70] Marshall et al.[147] followed 6 patients successfully treated for practolol-induced sclerosing peritonitis, and showed parenchymal changes (including "honeycomb" appearances) in addition to bilateral pleural thickening radiologically, but no tissue was examined.

Experimental Data. None.

Dose and Time Relationships. The case of Windsor et al.[236] had had 100 mg of practolol three times a day for about 2 years; Dyer and Varley's[66] case 100 mg given 3 times a day for 3 years; Hall et al.'s[94] case had 300 mg a day for 17 months, sclerosing peritonitis after 24 months, and progressive dyspnea and pleural biopsy after that, although the treatment had been stopped. Erwteman's case[70] had 150 mg of practolol given 3 times a day for 18 months, a laparotomy for peritonitis, and interstitial fibrosis with cough and dyspnea after a further 6 months.

Procarbazine

This drug is usually used as part of a quadruple chemotherapeutic regimen for malignant disease, in conjunction with nitrogen mustard, vincristine, and prednisone, none of which are reported to cause pulmonary reactions.

Damage. Procarbazine causes a pulmonary hypersensitivity reaction. Interstitial infiltration with mononuclear cells appears to predominate, and to include eosinophils,[62,73] although a fibrotic element is also reported.[140] In Farney's[73] second case, poorly circumscribed granulomas were described. No hyaline membranes have been reported. Although blood eosinophilia has not been described, the eosinophils in the infiltrate have suggested a hypersensitivity reaction, and a rapid reaction to procarbazine challenge supports this.[114] Procarbazine is a hydrazine derivative, as is isoniazid, but Lokich's[140] patient did not react to isoniazid when this was given subsequently to procarbazine.

Experimental Data. None.

Dose and Time Relationships. Quadruple chemotherapy is given in courses with intervals. Farney et al.[73] gave three courses, with unspecified intervals, which included 100 mg procarbazine daily for 14 days each, before pulmonary symptoms developed in one case, and 75 mg given similarly for six courses in the other case. Dohner's[62] case had 2.5 mg/kg/day in the first course of therapy, and developed dyspnea during the second course.

Radiotherapy

Damage. Radiotherapy produces diffuse alveolar damage to the lungs. Documentation of the morphologic changes in this condition is surprisingly poor. Clinically, a phase of coughing and dyspnea appears in some patients from 4 to 6 months after irradiation, but this usually disappears spontaneously, although Smith[198] reported a fatal case. Progressive respiratory impairment may develop several years after irradiation.[197] These phases have been called acute and chronic[137] and also early and late,[197] although these terms appear to have no pathologic counterparts. The most comprehensive account of postmortem pulmonary changes induced by radiotherapy is that of Jennings and Arden,[110] who studied 173 cases selected retrospectively; all had had less than 500 to more than 6,000 rads, and had died from less than 30 days to more than 5 years after irradiation. Eight percent showed no pulmonary changes. A fibrin-rich, intra-alveolar exudation, often with hyaline membranes, was seen in 41 percent that had had all doses and intervals of therapy, but the exudation was more frequent with dosages of more than 2,000 rads and more than 6 months after irradiation. Fibrillar deposits and thickening of alveolar walls was seen in 27 percent, of Jennings and Arden's cases usually after less than 3,000 rads and less than 6 months after irradiation, but one case was seen after less than 500 rads and less than 5 months after irradiation. There was increased interstitial cellularity in only 16 percent, mostly after more than 2,000 rads and more than 6 months after irradiation. In 42 percent there was interstitial fibrosis, which could occur in less than 30 days. Obliterative endoarteriolitis was seen in 14 percent; the occlusion of arterioles with subintimal collections of lipid-laden macrophages has been regarded as pathognomonic of radiation damage.[18] Bachman and Macken found bilateral radiation damage in 7 of 72 postmortems on patients with symptoms starting 3 to 7 weeks after 4,000 to 5,000 rad dosages of radiation were given for lung cancer. Pleural effusions have been attributed to radiation,[11] but pleural fibrosis does not appear to have been.

There has been discussion about the mechanism of radiation-induced damage to the lung, particularly with regard to bilateral damage in cases of unilateral irradiation,[198] and hypersensitivity,[137] and the possibility that the withdrawal of steroids could activate latent radiation injury[41] has been put forward. None of these proposals are convincing, and it seems likely that the usual mechanisms of diffuse alveolar damage (see p. 171) apply when the lung is irradiated. The difficulties in the differential diagnosis of lung damage due to radiation were highlighted in a clinicopathological conference in 1972.[37]

Experimental Data. This is also poorly reported. Jennings and Arden[109] gave 3,000 rads fractionated in three different ways to rats. With each mode they found congestion after 2 days, interstitial edema after 6 days, intra-alveolar edema after 12 days, and fibrillar material expanding the alveolar walls after 17 days. This material progressed to fibrosis; there were no hyaline membranes. Smith[197] gave one dose of 3,000 rads to rats, with much the same results, although he emphasized the macroscopic atrophy and hyalinization of the lung that followed, as well as hyalinization of the alveolar walls with fragmentation and phagocytosis of elastic fibers. The ultrastructure of affected lung tissue has been examined by Adamson et al.[3] in mice and rats in which the earliest injury was the vacuolation and destruction of capillary endothelial cells followed by necrosis of type I pneumocytes. Fibrosis was seen before the expected time of immunologic recovery, and these authors concluded that radiation-induced pulmonary fibrosis was a direct result of vascular injury, rather than a delayed immunologic response.

Masse et al.[149] have explored the interesting side issue of the effects of inhaling alpha-emitting particles, and have shown that such alpha emitters produce diffuse alveolar damage in both rats and monkeys, but that dogs are less sensitive.

Steroids

Damage. Mediastinal fat deposition, of which 15 cases have been reported. Koerner and Sun[124] described three asthma cases, in which the mediastinal widening seen radiologically was shown to be due to mediastinal lipomatosis at thoracotomy in two cases, and at postmortem in the third. Bodman and Condemi[20] reviewed Koerner and Sun's[124] second case, and added one that came to postmortem (see color picture of open thorax in reference 20). Price and Rigler[169] reported seven examples of mediastinal lipomatosis in renal transplant cases, one of which came to postmortem, a patient in whom Cushing's syndrome was due to a pituitary tumor, and another receiving treatment for systemic lupus erythematosus. Teates[213] added yet another example.

Experimental Data. None.

Dose and Time Relationships. Koerner and Sun's[124] first case developed mediastinal widening after 5 years on 7.5 mg prednisone per day; their second case developed this after 20 mg prednisone per day for 23 months, with the widening in this case regressing when the dose was reduced to 15 mg per day, but reappearing (with other Cushingoid features) when the dose was put back to 20 mg per day. Teates'[213] case showed mediastinal widening after 7 months on 30 mg prednisone per day; this persisted but did not increase over the next 4 years, and regressed when prednisone was then stopped.

Sulphasalazine

Diffuse Alveolar Damage. There are two reports of diffuse alveolar damage from sulphasalazine: Davies and MacFarlane[56] describe a case of ulcerative colitis treated with sulphasalazine for 15 months, in which the patient died. At postmortem there was fibrosing alveolitis, with honeycombing particularly of the lower lobes which was tentatively attributed to the sulphasalazine. Isenberg et al.[105] described a patient with ulcerative colitis treated with sulphasalazine not quite continuously for 15 years, who was then admitted for total colectomy. The patient was found to have infiltrates upon the chest x-ray; an open lung biopsy showed interstitial fibrosis and arteritis, with fibrinoid necrosis and eosinophil infiltration. After total colectomy (and stopping the drug) the lung fields cleared radiologically within 5 weeks. Ulcerative colitis itself does not appear to be associated with pulmonary lesions.

Hypersensitivity Reactions. There are four case reports of hypersensitivity reactions in patients treated with sulphasalazine for ulcerative colitis: three associated with blood eosinophilia.[113] There is no morphologic data on this reaction (see hypersensitivity pneumonitis, p. 173).

Experimental Data. None.

Dose and Time Relationships. Davies and MacFarlane's[56] case had between 6 and 8 grams of sulphasalazine per day for 15 months before developing symptoms. Isenberg's[105] case had between 2 and 4 grams per day over the 15 year period.

CONCLUSIONS

Reviewing the evidence for the association of drugs and toxic substances with pulmonary damage reminded us that the respiratory tract can respond to attack in only a few ways. Furthermore, the constellations of changes identified as diffuse alveolar damage, hypersensitivity pneumonitis, granulomata, and so on are not mutually exclusive. Therefore it is not surprising that it is seldom possible to incriminate a particular toxic substance purely on the basis of morphologic changes in the lung tissues.

We were also impressed by how far short the published evidence often falls in definitely establishing an association between a substance and a pulmonary reaction, let alone establishing cause and effect. It seems that an initial case report may be followed by further case reports until the alleged association becomes "common knowledge," and is then accepted uncritically and not tested further.

Only in the cases of BCNU, bleomycin, cyclophosphamide, and oxygen have therapeutic agents apparently been tested to see whether, in appropriate doses for appropriate times, each can produce lesions in healthy lung tissue in healthy animals. We tested this assumption by writing to the manufacturers of all of the drugs under consideration, on the possibility that we had not looked hard enough for damage reports, but little more published experimental data was forthcoming, although there may be unpublished data in the files.

We therefore conclude that physicians should be encouraged to continue publishing case reports, with full therapeutic and clinical details, when histology is available, and that someone—perhaps the drug regulatory agencies—should ensure that the necessary experimental work on toxic pulmonary damage is not only done but also published.

REFERENCES

Notations in parentheses indicate the number of illustrations included. Abbreviations are: Macro—macroscopic pictures; LM—light microscopic pictures; EM—transmission electron micrographs; SEM—scanning electron micrographs.

1. Aabo, K., & Hansen, K. B.: Megakaryocytes in pulmonary blood vessels. 1. Incidence at autopsy, clinicopathological relations especially to disseminated intravascular coagulation. Acta Pathol. Microbiol. Scand. (A) 86:285, 1978. (LM 2).

2. Adamson, I. Y. R., & Bowden, D. H.: Origin of alveolar epithelial cells in bleomycin-induced lung injury. Am. J. Pathol. 87:569, 1977. (EM 10).
3. Adamson, I. Y. R., Bowden, D. H., & Wyatt, J. P.: A pathway to pulmonary fibrosis: an ultrastructural study of mouse and rat following radiation to the whole body and hemithorax. Am. J. Pathol. 58:481, 1970. (EM 1).
4. Adamson, T. M., Boyd, R. D. H., Normand, I. C. S. et al.: Haemorrhagic pulmonary oedema (massive pulmonary haemorrhage) in the newborn. Lancet 1:494, 1969.
5. Alarcon-Segovia, D.: Drug-induced lupus syndromes. Mayo Clin. Proc. 44:664, 1969.
6. Anderson, E. G., Simon, G., & Reid, L.: Primary and thrombo-embolic pulmonary hypertension: a quantitative pathological study. J. Pathol. 110:273, 1973. (LM 2).
7. Anderson, W. R., Strickland, M. B., Tsai, S. H. et al.: Light microscopic and ultrastructural study of the adverse effects of oxygen therapy on the neonate lung. Am. J. Pathol. 73:327, 1973. (LM 8, EM 4).
8. Arnett, E. N., Battle, W., Russo, J. V. et al.: Intravenous injection of talc-containing drugs intended for oral use. Am. J. Med. 60:711, 1976. (LM 12.)
9. Ashbaugh, D. G., Bigelow, D. B., Petty, T. L. et al.: Acute respiratory distress in adults. Lancet 2:319, 1967. (LM 3).
10. Aso, Y., Yoneda, K., & Kikkawa, Y.: Morphologic and biochemical study of pulmonary changes induced by bleomycin in mice. Lab. Invest. 35:558, 1976. (LM 4, EM 8).
11. Bachman, A. L., & Macken, K.: Pleural effusions following super voltage radiation for breast carcinoma. Radiology 72:699, 1959.
12. Bailey, C. C., Marsden, H. B., & Jones, P. H. M.: Fatal pulmonary fibrosis following 1,3-bis(2-chloroethyl)-1-nitrosourea (BCNU) therapy. Cancer 42:74, 1978.
13. Banerjee, C. K., Girling, D. J., & Wigglesworth, J. S.: Pulmonary fibroplasia in newborn babies treated with oxygen and artificial ventilation. Arch. Dis. Child. 47:509, 1972. (LM 8).
14. Becklake, M. R.: Asbestos-related diseases of the lung and other organs: their epidemiology and implications for clinical practice. Am. Rev. Resp. Dis. 114:187, 1976.
15. Bedrossian, C. W. M., Greenberg, S. D., Yawn, D. H. et al.: Experimentally induced bleomycin sulphate pulmonary toxicity: histopathological and ultrastructural study in the pheasant. Arch. Pathol. Lab. Med. 101:248, 1977. (LM 3, EM 5).
16. Bedrossian, C. W. M., Luna, M. A., Mackay, B., et al.: Ultrastructure of pulmonary bleomycin toxicity. Cancer 32:44, 1973. (EM 5).
17. Bell, R. J. M.: Pulmonary infiltration with eosinophils caused by chlorpropamide. Lancet 1:1249, 1964.
18. Bennett, D. E., Million, R. R., & Ackerman, L. V.: Bilateral radiation pneumonitis, a complication of the radiotherapy of bronchogenic carcinoma. Cancer 23:1001, 1969. (Macro 1, LM 7).
19. Blum, R. H., Carter, S. K., & Agre, K.: A clinical review of bleomycin—a new antineoplastic agent. Cancer 31:903, 1973.
20. Bodman, S. F., & Condemi, J. J.: Mediastinal widening in iatrogenic Cushing's syndrome. Ann. Intern. Med. 67:399, 1967. (Macro 1).
21. Bonadonna, G., De Luna, M., Monfardini, S., et al.: Clinical trials with bleomycin in lymphomas and in solid tumors. Eur. J. Cancer 8:205, 1972.
22. Bone, R. C., Wolfe, J., Sobonya, R. E. et al.: Desquamative interstitial pneumonia following long-term nitrofurantoin therapy. Am. J. Med. 60:697, 1976. (LM 2, EM 2).
23. Bonikos, D. S., Bensch, K. G., & Northway, W. H.: Oxygen toxicity in the newborn. The effect of chronic continuous 100 percent oxygen exposure on the lungs of newborn mice. Am. J. Pathol. 85:623, 1976. (Macro 1, LM 1, EM 12).
24. Boothby, C. B., & De Sa, D. J.: Massive pulmonary haemorrhage in the newborn. A changing pattern. Arch. Dis. Child. 48:21, 1973. (LM 10).
25. Bowden, D. H., & Adamson, I. Y. R.: Reparative changes following pulmonary cell injury. Ultrastructural, cytodynamic and surfactant studies after oxygen exposure. Arch. Pathol. 92:279, 1971. (EM 4).
26. Bowden, D. H., Adamson, I. Y. R., & Wyatt, J. P.: Reaction of the lung cells to a high concentration of oxygen. Arch. Pathol. 86:671, 1968. (LM 1, EM 2).
27. Brettman, L. R., Goldstein, E. J. C., Holzman, R. S. et al.: Legionnaire's disease: cause of severe abscess pneumonia. Am. J. Med. 67:339, 1979.
28. Brettner, A., Heitzman, R. E., & Woodin,

W. G.: Pulmonary complications of drug therapy. Radiology 96:31, 1970.

29. Brooks, R. E.: Ultrastructure of lung lesions produced by ingested chemicals: 1. Effect of the herbicide paraquat on mouse lung. Lab. Invest. 25:536, 1971. (LM 4, EM 7).
30. Burns, W. A., McFarland, W., & Matthews, M. J.: Busulfan-induced pulmonary disease: report of a case and review of the literature. Am. Rev. Respir. Dis. 101:408, 1970. (LM 4).
31. Butler, C.: Pulmonary interstitial fibrosis from paraquat in the hamster. Arch. Pathol. 99:503, 1975. (LM 2).
32. Cameron, R. B., Watts, J. C. & Kasten, B. L.: Pneumocystis carinii pneumonia: an approach to rapid laboratory diagnosis. Am. J. Clin. Pathol. 72:90, 1979. (LM 2).
33. Carel, R. S., Shapiro, M. S., Shoham, D. et al.: Lupus erythematosus cells in pleural effusion: The initial manifestation of procainamide-induced lupus erythematosus. Chest 72:670, 1977. (LM 1).
34. Carrington, C. B., & Gaensler, E. A.: Clinical-pathologic approach to diffuse infiltrative lung disease. In: Thurlbeck, W. M., & Abell, M. R., Eds.: The Lung. p. 58. Williams and Wilkins Co., Baltimore, 1978. (LM 12).
35. Carter, S. K., & Newman, J. W.: Nitrosoureas 1,3-bis(2-chloroethyl)-1-nitrosourea (NSC-409962; BCNU) and 1-(2-chloroethyl)-3-cyclohexyl-1-nitrosourea (NSC 79037; CCNU). Clinical brochure. Cancer Chemother. Rep. 1:115, 1968.
36. Case records of the Massachusetts General Hospital: weekly clinicopathological exercises: (Case 40-1971). N. Engl. J. Med. 285:847, 1971. (LM 5).
37. Case records of the Massachusetts General Hospital: (Case 26-1972). N. Engl. J. Med. 286:1405, 1972. (LM 3).
38. Case records of the Massachusetts General Hospital: (Case 6-1974). N. Engl. J. Med. 290:390, 1974. (LM 3).
39. Case records of the Massachusetts General Hospital: (Case 22-1974). N. Engl. J. Med. 290:1309, 1974. (LM 2).
40. Case records of the Massachusetts General Hospital: (Case 13-1978). N. Engl. J. Med. 298:786, 1978.
41. Castellino, R. A., Glatstein, E., Turbow, M. M., et al.: Latent radiation injury of lungs or heart activated by steroid withdrawal. Ann. Intern. Med. 80:593, 1974.
42. Churg, A., Warnock, M. L., & Bensch, K. G.: Malignant mesothelioma arising after direct application of asbestos and fiberglass to the pericardium. Am. Rev. Respir. Dis. 118:419, 1978. (Macro 1, LM 3).
43. Clark, J. M., & Lambertsen, C. J.: Pulmonary oxygen toxicity. Pharmacol. Rev. 23:37, 1971.
44. Clarysse, A. M., Cathay, W. J., Cartwright, G. E., et al.: Pulmonary disease complicating intermittent therapy with methotrexate. J.A.M.A. 209:1861, 1969. (LM 2).
45. Clinicopathological Conference: A case of malignant hypertension. Br. Med. J. 1:569, 1961. (LM 1).
46. Clinicopathological Conference: Adult respiratory distress syndrome. Am. J. Med. 50:521, 1971. (LM 1).
47. Clinicopathological Conference: Paraquat poisoning. Scott. Med. J. 16:407, 1971. (Macro 2, LM 5).
48. Codling, B. W., & Chakera, T. M. H.: Pulmonary fibrosis following therapy with melphalan for multiple myeloma. J. Clin. Pathol. 25:668, 1972. (LM 5).
49. Cole, P.: Drug-induced lung disease. Drugs 13:422, 1977.
50. Cole, S. R., Myers, T. J., & Klatsky, A. U.: Pulmonary disease with chlorambucil therapy. Cancer 41:455, 1978. (LM 2, EM 2).
51. Constantinidis, K. A.: Eosinophilic pneumonia: an unusual side effect of therapy with salicylazosulfapyridine (sulphasalazine). Chest 70:315, 1976.
52. Cooke, C. R., & Hyland, J. W.: Pathological calcification of the lungs following intravenous administration of calcium. Am. J. Med. 29:363, 1960. (Macro 1, LM 2).
53. Copland, G. M., Kolin, A., & Shulman, H. S.: Fatal pulmonary intraalveolar fibrosis after paraquat ingestion. N. Engl. J. Med. 291:290, 1974. (LM 4).
54. Crystal, R. G., Fulmer, J. D., Roberts, W. C., et al.: Idiopathic pulmonary fibrosis. Clinical, histologic, radiographic, physiologic, scintigraphic, cytologic and biochemical aspects. Ann. Intern. Med. 85:769, 1976. (LM 18).
55. Cuthbert, R. J.: Löffler's syndrome occurring during streptomycin and PAS therapy. Br. Med. J. 2:398, 1954.
56. Davies, D., & MacFarlane, A.: Fibrosing alveolitis and treatment with sulphasalazine. Gut 15:185, 1974. (Macro 1, LM 3).

57. Davies, P. D. B.: Drug-induced lung disease. Br. J. Dis. Chest 63:57, 1969.
58. Dearden, L. C., Fairshter, R. D., McRae, D. M. et al.: Pulmonary ultrastructure of the late aspects of human paraquat poisoning. Am. J. Pathol. 93:667, 1978. (LM 2, EM 11).
59. De Lena, M., Guzzon, A., Monfardini, S. et al.: Clinical, radiologic and histopathologic studies on pulmonary toxicity induced by treatment with bleomycin (NSC-125066). Cancer Chemother. Rep. 56:343, 1972. (LM 4).
60. Demicco, W. A., Stein, A., Urbanetti, J. S. et al.: False negative biopsy in pneumocystis carinii pneumonia. Chest 75:389, 1979. (LM 1).
60a. Deneke, S. M., & Fanburg, B. L.: Normobaric oxygen toxicity of the lung. N. Engl. J. Med. 303:76, 1980.
61. Dhurandhar, H. N., Brown, C., Barrett, J. et al.: Pulmonary structural changes following microembolism and blood transfusion. Arch. Pathol. Lab. Med. 103:335, 1979. (LM 4, EM 4).
62. Dohner, V. A., Ward, H. P., & Standord, R. E.: Alveolitis during procarbazine, vincristine and cyclophosphamide therapy. Chest 62:636, 1972. (LM 2).
63. Doniach, I.: Uraemic edema of the lungs. Am. J. Roentgenol. 58:620, 1947. (LM 2).
64. Doniach, I., Morrison, B., & Steiner, R. E.: Lung changes during hexamethonium therapy for hypertension. Br. Heart J. 16:101, 1954. (LM 6).
65. Durant, J. R., Norgard, M. J., Murad, T. M. et al.: Pulmonary toxicity associated with bischloroethylnitrosourea (BCNU). Ann. Intern. Med. 90:191, 1979.
66. Dyer, N. H., & Varley, C. C.: Practolol-induced pleurisy and constrictive pericarditis. Br. Med. J. 2:443, 1975.
67. Eastmond, C. J.: Diffuse alveolitis as complication of penicillamine treatment for rheumatoid arthritis. Br. Med. J. 1:1506, 1976.
68. Edwards, D. K., Dyer, W. M., & Northway, W. H.: Twelve years' experience with bronchopulmonary dysplasia. Pediatrics 59:839, 1977.
69. Elgee, N. J.: Medical aspects of oral contraceptives. Ann. Intern. Med. 72:409, 1970.
70. Erwteman, T. M., Braat, M. C. P., & Van Aken, W. G.: Interstitial pulmonary fibrosis: a new side effect of practolol. Br. Med. J. 2:297, 1977. (LM 1).
71. Evans, M. J., Cabral, L. J., Stephens, R. J. et al.: Renewal of alveolar epithelium in the rat following exposure to NO_2. Am. J. Pathol. 70:175, 1973. (LM 7, EM 11).
72. Factor, S. M.: Granulomatous pneumonitis. A result of intrapleural instillation of quinacrine and talcum powder. Arch. Pathol. Lab. Med. 99:499, 1975. (LM 4).
73. Farney, R. J., Morris, A. H., Armstrong, J. D. et al.: Diffuse pulmonary disease after therapy with nitrogen mustard, vincristine, procarbazine and prednisone. Am. Rev. Respir. Dis. 115:135, 1977. (LM 4).
74. Fekete, M., Horvath, M., Bardosi, L. et al.: Oxygen therapy and massive pulmonary haemorrhage in newborn infants. Acta Paediatr. Acad. Sci. Hung. 18:53, 1977.
75. Fiegenberg, D. S., Weiss, H., & Kirshman, H.: Migratory pneumonia with eosinophilia. Arch. Intern. Med. 120:85, 1967. (LM 2).
76. Fielding, J. W. L., Stockley, R. A., & Brookes, V. S.: Interstitial lung disease in a patient treated with 5-fluorouracil and mitomycin C. Br. Med. J. 2:62, 1978. (LM 1).
77. Finley, T. N., Aronow, A., Cosentino, A. M. et al.: Occult pulmonary haemorrhage in anticoagulated patients. Am. Rev. Respir. Dis. 112:23, 1975.
78. Fisher, H. K., Clements, J. A., & Wright, R. R.: Enhancement of oxygen toxicity by the herbicide paraquat. Am. Rev. Respir. Dis. 107:246, 1973. (LM 4).
79. Fleischman, R. W., Baker, J. R., Thompson, G. R., et al.: Bleomycin-induced interstitial pneumonia in dogs. Thorax 26:675, 1971. (Macro 1, LM 12).
80. Follath, F., Burkart, F., & Schweizer, W.: Drug-induced pulmonary hypertension? Br. Med. J. 1:265, 1971.
81. Frank, L., & Massaro, D.: The lung and oxygen toxicity. Arch. Intern. Med. 139:347, 1979.
81a. Frank, L., & Massaro, D.: Oxygen toxicity. Am. J. Med. 69:117, 1980.
82. French, A. J.: Hypersensitivity in pathogenesis of histopathologic changes associated with sulphonamide chemotherapy. Am. J. Pathol. 22:679, 1946.
83. Gaensler, E. A., & Kaplan, A. I.: Asbestos pleural effusion. Ann. Intern. Med. 74:178, 1971. (LM 9).

84. Garrell, M.: Löffler's syndrome. Report of a case associated with the administration of aurothioglucose (solganal). Arch. Intern. Med. 106:874, 1960.
85. Geddes, D. M., & Brostoff, J.: Pulmonary fibrosis associated with hypersensitivity to gold salts. Br. Med. J. 1:1444, 1976.
86. Geller, M., Kriz, R. J., Zimmerman, S. W., et al.: Penicillin-associated pulmonary hypersensitivity reaction and interstitial nephritis. Ann. Allergy 37:183, 1976.
87. Gillett, D. G., & Ford, G. T.: Drug-induced lung disease. In: Thurlbeck, W. M. & Abell, M. R., Eds.: The Lung: Structure, Function and Disease. p. 21. The Williams & Wilkins Co., Baltimore, 1978. (LM 16).
88. Gould, P. W., McCormack, P. L., & Palmer, D. G.: Pulmonary damage associated with sodium aurothiomalate therapy. J. Rheumatol. 2:252, 1977. (LM 1).
89. Gould, V. E., & Miller, J.: Sclerosing alveolitis induced by cyclophosphamide. Ultrastructural observations on alveolar injury and repair. Am. J. Pathol. 81:513, 1975. (LM 4, EM 10).
90. Gould, V. E., Tosco, R., Wheelis, R. F. et al.: Oxygen pneumonitis in man. Ultrastructural observations on the development of alveolar lesions. Lab. Invest., 26:499, 1972. (EM 12).
91. Graham, J. R.: Cardiac and pulmonary fibrosis during methysergide therapy for headache. Am. J. Med. Sci. 254:1, 1967. (LM 1).
92. Graham. J. R., Suby, H. I., Lecompte, P. R., et al.: Fibrotic disorders associated with methysergide therapy for headache. N. Engl. J. Med. 274:359, 1966.
93. Van Haeringen, J. R., Hilvering, C., & Sluiter, H. J.: Diseases of the respiratory tract due to drugs. In: Meyler, L. & Peck, H. M., Eds.: Drug-Induced Diseases. Vol. 4. p. 498. Excerpta Medica Foundation, Amsterdam, 1972.
94. Hall, D. R., Morrison, J. B., & Edwards, F. R.: Pleural fibrosis after practolol therapy. Thorax 33:822, 1978.
95. Hardaway, R. M.: Acute respiratory distress syndrome and disseminated intravascular coagulation. South. Med. J. 71:596, 1978.
96. Hardaway, R. M., James, P. M., Anderson, R. W., et al.: Intensive study and treatment of shock in man. J.A.M.A. 199:779, 1967.
97. Heard, B. E.: Fibrous healing of old iatrogenic pulmonary oedema ("hexamethonium lung"). J. Pathol. Bacteriol. 83:159, 1962. (Macro 3, LM 4).
98. Higenbottam, T., Crone, P., Parkinson, C., et. al.: Further clinical observations on the pulmonary effects of paraquat ingestion. Thorax 34:161, 1979.
99. Hilden, T., Krogsgaard, A. R., & Vimtrup, B.: Fatal pulmonary changes during the medical treatment of malignant hypertension. Lancet 2:830, 1958. (LM 3).
100. Hill, R. N., Spragg, R. G., Wedel, M. K., et al.: Adult respiratory distress syndrome associated with colchicine intoxication. Ann. Intern. Med. 83:523, 1975.
100a. Hindle, W., Posner, E., Sweetnam, M. T., et al.: Pleural effusion and fibrosis during treatment with methysergide. Br. Med. J. 1:605, 1970.
101. Ho, D., Tashkin, D. P., Bein, M. E., et al.: Pulmonary infiltrates with eosinophilia associated with tetracycline. Chest 76:33, 1979.
102. Holoye, P. Y., Jenkins, D. E., & Greenberg, S. D.: Pulmonary toxicity in long term administration of BCNU. Cancer Treat. Rep. 60:1691, 1976. (LM 1).
103. Hopps, H. C., & Wissler, R. W.: Uremic pneumonitis. Am. J. Pathol. 31:261, 1955. (LM 4).
104. Hyde, R. W., & Rawson, A. J.: Unintentional iatrogenic oxygen pneumonitis—response to therapy. Ann. Intern. Med. 71:517, 1969. (LM 2).
105. Isenberg, J. I., Goldstein, H., Korn, A. R., et al.: Pulmonary vasculitis—an uncommon complication of ulcerative colitis. N. Engl. J. Med. 297:1376, 1969. (LM 1).
106. Israel, H. L., & Diamond, P.: Recurrent pulmonary infiltration and pleural effusion due to nitrofurantoin sensitivity. N. Engl. J. Med. 266:1024, 1962.
107. Israel, K. S., Brashear, R. E., Sharma, H. M., et al.: Pulmonary fibrosis and nitrofurantoin. Am. Rev. Respir. Dis. 108:353, 1973.
108. James, D. W., Whimster, W. F., & Hamilton, E. B. D.: Gold Lung. Br. Med. J. 1:1523, 1978. (LM 1).
109. Jennings, F. L., & Arden, A.: Development of experimental radiation pneumonitis. Arch. Pathol. 71:437, 1961. (LM 14).
110. Jennings, F. L., & Arden, A.: Development of radiation pneumonitis. Arch. Pathol. 74:351, 1962. (LM 17).

111. Jones, A. W.: Bleomycin lung damage: the pathology and nature of the lesion. Br. J. Dis. Chest 72:321, 1978. (LM 3, EM 1).
112. Jones, A. W., & Reeve, N. L.: Ultrastructure of bleomycin-induced pulmonary changes in mice. J. Pathol. 124:227, 1978. (LM 5, EM 9).
113. Jones, G. R., & Malone, D. N. S.: Sulphasalazine induced lung disease. Thorax 27:713, 1972.
114. Jones, S. E., Moore, M., Blank, N., et al.: Hypersensitivity to procarbazine (Matulane) manifested by fever and pleuropulmonary reaction. Cancer 29:498, 1972.
115. Kalinowski, S. Z., Lloyd, T. W., & Moyes, E. N.: Complications in the chemotherapy of tuberculosis. Am. Rev. Respir. Dis. 83:359, 1961.
116. Kapanci, Y., Weibel, E. R., Kaplan, H. P., et al.: Pathogenesis and reversibility of the pulmonary lesions of oxygen toxicity in monkeys. II. Ultrastructural and morphometric studies. Lab. Invest. 20:101, 1969. (LM 2, EM 20).
117. Kaplan, A. I., Zakher, F., & Sabin, S.: Drug-induced lupus erythematosus with in vivo lupus erythematosus cells in pleural fluid. Chest 73:875, 1978. (LM 1).
118. Kaplan, H. P., Robinson, F. R., Kapanci, Y., et al.: Pathogenesis and reversibility of pulmonary lesions of oxygen toxicity in monkeys. I. Clinical and light microscopic studies. Lab. Invest. 20:94, 1969. (LM 10).
119. Katz, S. M., Brodsky, I., & Kahn, S. B.: Legionnaire's disease: ultrastructural appearance of the agent in a lung biopsy specimen. Arch. Pathol. Lab. Med. 103:261, 1979. (LM 2, EM 3).
120. Katzenstein, A. A., Bloor, C. M., & Liebow, A. A.: Diffuse alveolar damage—the role of oxygen, shock, and related factors. A review. Am. J. Pathol. 85:210, 1976. (LM 16).
121. Kay, J. M., Smith, P., & Heath, D.: Aminorex and the pulmonary circulation. Thorax 26:262, 1971. (LM 4).
122. Kirschner, R. H., & Esterly, J. R.: Pulmonary lesions associated with busulfan therapy of chronic myelogenous leukemia. Cancer 27:1074, 1971. (LM 8).
123. Klinghoffer, J. F.: Löffler's syndrome following use of a vaginal cream. Ann. Intern. Med. 40:343, 1954.
124. Koerner, H. J., & Sun, D. I. C.: Mediastinal lipomatosis secondary to steroid therapy. Am. J. Roentgen. 98:461, 1966.
125. Koss, L. G., Melamed, M. R., & Mayer, K.: The effect of busulfan on human epithelia. Am. J. Clin. Pathol. 44:385, 1965. (LM 21).
126. Kuplic, J. B., Higley, C. S., & Niewoehner, D. E.: Pulmonary ossification associated with long-term busulfan therapy in chronic myeloid leukemia: case report. Am. Rev. Respir. Dis. 106:759, 1972. (Macro 1, LM 1).
127. Lamb, D.: Heart weight and assessment of ventricular hypertrophy. In: Dyke, S. C., Ed.: Recent Advances in Clinical Pathology. p. 133. Churchill Livingstone, Edinburgh, 1973.
128. Leading Article: Massive pulmonary haemorrhage in the newborn. Br. Med. J. 3:553, 1973.
129. Lee, S. L., Rivero, I., & Siegel, M.: Activation of systemic lupus erythematosus by drugs. Arch. Intern. Med. 117:620, 1966.
130. Levin, P. J., Klaff, L. J., Rose, A. G., et al.: Pulmonary effects of contact exposure to paraquat: a clinical and experimental study. Thorax 34:150, 1979. (LM 13).
131. Levitt, T.: Radioimmunoassay for paraquat. Lancet 2:358, 1977.
132. Lewinsohn, H. C.: Early malignant changes in pleural plaques due to asbestos exposure: a case report. Br. J. Dis. Chest 68:121, 1974. (Macro 1, LM 4).
133. Lewman, L. V.: Fatal pulmonary hypertension from intravenous injection of methylphenidate (Ritalin) tablets. Hum. Pathol. 3:67, 1972. (LM 3).
134. Liebow, A. A.: Definition and classification of interstitial pneumonias in human pathology. In: Basset, F. & Georges, R., Eds.: Progress in Respiration Research. Vol. 8. Alveolar Interstitium of the Lung: Pathological and Physiological Aspects. p. 1. Karger, New York, 1975. (Macro 2, LM 26).
135. Liebow, A. A., & Carrington, C. B.: The eosinophilic pneumonias. Medicine 48:251, 1969. (LM 22, EM 1).
136. Lindström, F. D., Flodmark, O., & Gustafsson, B.: Respiratory distress syndrome and thrombotic, non-bacterial endocarditis after amitriptyline overdose. Acta Med. Scand. 202:203, 1977. (LM 4).
137. Lippmann, M.: Pulmonary reactions to drugs. Med. Clin. North Am. Symposium on pulmonary disease. 61(6):1353, 1977.

138. Littler, W. A., Kay, J. M., Hasleton, P. S., et al.: Busulphan lung. Thorax 24:639, 1969. (Macro 3, LM 5, EM 7).
139. Löbel, H., Machtey, I., & Eldror, M. Y.: Pulmonary infiltrates with eosinophilia in an asthmatic patient treated with disodium cromoglycate. Lancet 2:1032, 1972.
140. Lokich, J. J., & Moloney, W. C.: Allergic reaction to procarbazine. Clin. Pharmacol. Ther. 13:573, 1972.
141. Luna, M. A., Bedrossian, C. W. M., Lichtiger, B., et al.: Interstitial pneumonitis associated with bleomycin therapy. Am. J. Clin. Pathol. 58:501, 1972. (Macro 1, LM 7).
142. McCullough, B., Collins, J. F., Johanson, W. G., et al.: Bleomycin-induced diffuse interstitial pulmonary fibrosis in baboons. J. Clin. Invest. 61:79, 1978. (LM 5).
143. Magner, D., & McDonald, A. D.: Malignant mesothelial tumours: histologic type and asbestos exposure. N. Engl. J. Med. 287:570, 1972.
144. Mahan, C. T., & Sale, G. E.: Rapid methenamine silver stain for pneumocystis and fungi. Arch. Pathol. Lab. Med. 102:351, 1979. (LM 2).
145. Mahon, W. E., Scott, D. J., Ansell, G. et al.: Hypersensitivity to pituitary snuff with miliary shadowing in the lungs. Thorax 22:13, 1967. (LM 3).
146. Malmquist, J., Trell, E., Torp, A., et al.: A case of drug induced (?) pulmonary hypertension. Acta Med. Scand. 188:265, 1970. (LM 2).
147. Marshall, A. J., Barritt, D. W., Griffiths, D. A., et al.: Respiratory disease associated with practolol therapy. Lancet 2:1254, 1977.
148. Marshall, A., & Moore, K.: Pulmonary disease after amitriptyline overdosage. Br. Med. J. 1:716, 1973.
149. Masse, R., Nolibe, D., Fritsch, P., et al.: Chronic interstitial pneumonitis induced by internal α-irradiation of the lung. In: Basset, F. & Georges, R., Eds.: Progress in Respiration Research. Vol. 8. Alveolar Interstitium of the Lung: Pathological and Physiological Aspects. p. 74. Karger, New York, 1975.
150. Matthew, H., Logan, A., Woodruff, M. F. A., et al.: Paraquat poisoning—lung transplantation. Br. Med. J. 3:759, 1968. (Macro 6, LM 10).
151. Mattson, S. B., & Ringqvist, T.: Pleural plaques and exposure to asbestos. Scand. J. Respir. Dis. (Suppl.) 75:3-41, 1970.
152. Miller, A., Teirstein, A. S., Bader, M. E., et al.: Talc pneumoconiosis: significance of sublight microscopic mineral particles. Am. J. Med. 50:395, 1971. (LM 4).
153. Miller, G. J., Ashcroft, M. T., Beadnell, H. M. S. G., et al.: The lipoid pneumonia of blackfat tobacco smokers in Guyana. Q. J. Med. (N.S.) 40:457, 1971. (LM 4).
154. Min, K. W., & Gyorkey, F.: Interstitial pulmonary fibrosis, atypical epithelial changes and bronchiolar cell carcinoma following busulfan therapy. Cancer 22:1027, 1968. (Macro 2, LM 4).
155. Miyachi, S.: Pulmonary reaction to chrysotherapy. N. Engl. J. Med. 295:506, 1976.
156. Miyashita, T., Ojima, A., Tuji, T. et al.: Varied pulmonary lesions with intra-alveolar large lamella bodies in an autopsy case with busulfan therapy. Acta Pathol. Jpn. 27:239, 1977. (Macro 1, LM 10, EM 3).
157. Molnar, J. J., Nathenson, G., & Edberg, S.: Fatal aspiration of talcum powder by a child. N. Engl. J. Med. 266:36, 1962.
158. Moskowitz, R. L.: Talc pneumoconiosis: a treated case. Chest 58:37, 1970. (LM 3).
159. Muir, D. C. F., & Stanton, J. A.: Allergic pulmonary infiltration due to nitrofurantoin. Br. Med. J. 1:1072, 1963.
160. Murray, J. F.: The adult respiratory distress syndrome (may it rest in peace). Am. Rev. Respir. Dis. 111:716, 1975.
161. Musk, A. W., & Pollard, J. A.: Pindolol and pulmonary fibrosis. Br. Med. J. 2:581, 1979.
162. Northway, W. H., Rosan, R. C., & Porter, D. Y.: Pulmonary disease following respirator therapy of hyaline-membrane disease. Bronchopulmonary dysplasia. N. Engl. J. Med. 276:357, 1967. (Macro 1, LM 4).
163. O'Connell, T. X., & Berenbaum, M. C.: Cardiac and pulmonary effects of high doses of cyclophosphamide and isophosphamide. Cancer Res. 34:1586, 1974. (LM 1).
164. O'Neill, T. J., Kardinal, C. G., & Tierney, L. M.: Reversible interstitial pneumonitis associated with low dose bleomycin. Chest 68:265, 1975.
165. Orwoll, E. S., Kiessling, P. J., & Patterson, J. R.: Interstitial pneumonia from mitomycin. Ann. Intern. Med. 89:352, 1978. (LM 3).
166. Page, R. L.: Progressive pleural thickening

during oxprenolol therapy. Br. J. Dis. Chest 73:195, 1979.
167. Perry, H. M., O'Neal, R. M., & Thomas, W. A.: Pulmonary disease following chronic chemical ganglionic blockade. Am. J. Med. 22:37, 1957. (LM 4).
168. Petty, T. L.: The adult respiratory distress syndrome (confessions of a "lumper"). Am. Rev. Respir. Dis. 111:713, 1975.
169. Price, J. E., & Rigler, L. G.: Widening of the mediastinum resulting from fat accumulation. Radiology 96:497, 1970.
170. Rallison, M. L., Carlisle, J. W., Lee, R. E., et al.: Lupus erythematosus and Stevens-Johnson syndrome: occurrence as reactions to anticonvulsant medication. Am. J. Dis. Child. 101:725, 1961.
171. Rebello, G., & Mason, J. K.: Pulmonary histological appearances in fatal paraquat poisoning. Histopathology 2:53, 1978. (LM 11).
172. Reichlin, S., Loveless, M. H., & Kane, E. G.: Loeffler's syndrome following penicillin therapy. Ann. Intern. Med. 38:113, 1953.
173. Robboy, S. J., Colman, R. W., & Minna, J. D.: Pathology of disseminated intravascular coagulation (DIC). Analysis of 26 cases. Hum. Pathol. 3:327, 1972. (LM 1).
174. Rodin, A. E., Haggard, M. E., & Travis, L. B.: Lung changes and chemotherapeutic agents in childhood. Report of a case associated with cyclophosphamide therapy. Am. J. Dis. Child. 120:337, 1970. (LM 3).
175. Rodman, T., Fraimow, W., & Myerson, R. M.: Löffler's syndrome: report of a case associated with administration of mephenesin carbarmate (Tolseran). Ann. Intern. Med. 48:668, 1958.
175a. Rohlfing, B. M., & Stauffer, J. L.: Drug induced pulmonary disease. In: Preger, L., Ed.: Induced Disease. pp. 45–76. Grune & Stratton, New York, 1980.
176. Rosenow, E. C.: The spectrum of drug-induced pulmonary disease. Ann. Intern. Med. 77:977, 1972.
177. Rosenow, E. C.: Drugs that may induce pulmonary disease. Geriatrics 33:64, 1978.
178. Rosenow, E. C., de Remee, R. A., & Dines, D. E.: Chronic nitrofurantoin pulmonary reaction. Report of five cases. N. Engl. J. Med. 279:1258, 1968.
179. Rosketh, P., & Storstein, O.: Pulmonary complications during mecamylamine therapy. Acta Med. Scand. 167:23, 1960. (LM 2).
180. Rubin, G., Baume, P., & Vanderburg, R.: Azathioprine and acute restrictive lung disease. Aust. N. Z. J. Med. 3:272, 1972.
181. Rubio, F. A.: Possible pulmonary effects of alkylating agents. N. Engl. J. Med. 287:1150, 1972.
182. Rudders, R. A., & Hensley, G. T.: Bleomycin pulmonary toxicity. Chest 63:626, 1973. (LM 3).
183. Rüttner, J. R., Spycher, M. A., & Sticher, H.: Detection of etiologic agents in interstitial pulmonary fibrosis. Hum. Pathol. 4:497, 1973. (LM 3, EM 2).
184. Saldeen, T.: The microembolism syndrome: Forensic Sci. 1:179, 1972.
185. Salm, R., & Hughes, E. W.: A case of chronic paraffin pneumonitis. Thorax 25:762, 1970. (Macro 1, LM 4).
186. Samuels, M. L., Johnson, D. E., Holoye, P. Y., et al.: Large-dose bleomycin therapy and pulmonary toxicity. A possible role of prior radiotherapy. J.A.M.A., 235:1117, 1976.
187. Schaeppi, U., Phelan, R., Stadnicki, S. W., et al.: Pulmonary fibrosis following multiple treatment with bleomycin (NSC-125066) in dogs. Cancer Chemother. Rep. 58:301, 1974.
188. Scharf, J., Nahir, M., Kleinhaus, U., et al.: Diffuse pulmonary injury associated with gold therapy. J.A.M.A. 237:2412, 1977.
189. Seidenfeld, J. J., Wycoff, D., Zavala, D. C. et al.: Paraquat lung injury in rabbits. Br. J. Ind. Med. 35:245, 1978. (Macro 1, LM 8, SEM 1).
190. Selroos, O., & Edgren, J.: Lupus-like syndrome associated with pulmonary reaction to nitrofurantoin: report of three cases. Acta Med. Scand. 197:125, 1975.
191. Sepuya, S. M., Grzybowski, S., Burton, J. D., et al.: Diffuse lung changes associated with gold therapy. Can. Med. Assoc. J. 118:816, 1978. (LM 1).
192. Sevitt, S.: Diffuse and focal oxygen pneumonitis. A preliminary report on the threshold of pulmonary oxygen toxicity in man. J. Clin. Pathol. 27:21, 1974. (LM 9).
193. Sharp, A. A.: Diagnosis and management of disseminated intravascular coagulation. Br. Med. Bull. 33:265, 1977.
194. Shepard, F. M., Johnston, R. B., Klatte, E. C., et al.: Residual pulmonary findings in clinical hyaline-membrane disease. N. Engl. J. Med. 279:1063, 1969. (LM 1).
195. Siegel, H.: Human pulmonary pathology asso-

ciated with narcotic and other addictive drugs. Hum. Pathol. 3:55, 1972. (Macro 3, LM 10).

195a. Silvestri, R. C., Huseby, J. S., Rughani, I., et al.: Respiratory distress syndrome from lymphography contrast media. Am. Rev. Respir. Dis. 122:543, 1980.

196. Simon, H. B., Daggett, W. H., & Desanctis, R. W.: Haemothorax as a complication of anticoagulant therapy in the presence of pulmonary infarction. J.A.M.A. 208:1830, 1969.

197. Smith, J. C.: Experimental radiation pneumonitis. Am. Rev. Respir. Dis. 87:656, 1963. (Macro 3, LM 4).

198. Smith, J. C.: Radiation pneumonitis: case report of bilateral reaction after unilateral irradiation. Am. Rev. Respir. Dis. 89:264, 1964. (Macro 1, LM 2).

198a. Smith, L. H., Ed.: Respiratory manifestations. In: Clinical Problems with Drugs. Vol. 5, Major Problems in Internal Medicine. p. 142. W. B. Saunders Co., Philadelphia, 1975.

199. Smith, P., & Heath, D.: Paraquat lung: a reappraisal. Thorax 29:643, 1974. (LM 12).

200. Smith, P., Kay, J. M., & Heath, D.: Hypertensive pulmonary vascular disease in rats after prolonged feeding with *Crotalaria spectabilis* seeds. J. Pathol. 102:97, 1970. (LM 14).

201. Sostman, H. D., Matthay, R. A., Putman, C. E., et al.: Methotrexate-induced pneumonitis. Medicine 55:371, 1976. (LM 4).

202. Sostman, H. D., Matthay, R. A., & Putman, C. E.: Cytotoxic drug-induced lung disease. Am. J. Med. 62:608, 1977.

203. Spencer, H.: Pathology of the Lung. 3rd Ed. Vol. 1. Pergamon Press, Oxford, 1977.

204. Spencer, H.: Pathology of the Lung. 3rd Ed. Vol. 1. p. 139 et seq. Pergamon Press, Oxford, 1977.

205. Spencer, H.: Pathology of the Lung. 3rd Ed. Vol. 1. p. 195. Pergamon Press, Oxford, 1977.

206. Spencer, H.: Pathology of the Lung. 3rd Ed. Vol. 1. p. 198. Pergamon Press, Oxford, 1977.

207. Spencer, H.: Pathology of the Lung. 3rd Ed. Vol. 1. p. 229. Pergamon Press, Oxford, 1977.

208. Starcher, B. C., Kuhn, C., & Overton, J. E.: Increased elastin and collagen content in the lungs of hamsters receiving an intratracheal injection of bleomycin. Am. Rev. Respir. Dis. 117:299, 1978. (LM 5).

209. Sternlieb, I., Bennett, B., & Scheinberg, I. H.: D-penicillamine induced Goodpastures syndrome in Wilson's disease. Ann. Intern. Med. 82:673, 1975.

210. Sunshine, P., & Yaffe, S. J.: Amitriptyline poisoning: clinical and pathological findings in a fatal case. Am. J. Dis. Child. 106:501, 1963.

211. Taetle, R., Dickman, P. S., & Feldman, P. S.: Pulmonary histopathologic changes associated with melphalan therapy. Cancer 42:1239, 1978. (LM 3).

212. Taskinen, E., Tukiainen, P., & Sovijärvi, A. R. A.: Nitrofurantoin-induced alterations in pulmonary tissue. A report on five patients with acute or subacute reactions. Acta Pathol. Microbiol. Scand. (A) 85:713, 1977.

213. Teates, C. D.: Steroid-induced mediastinal lipomatosis. Radiology 96:501, 1970.

214. Thomas, P., Seaton, A., & Edwards, J.: Respiratory disease due to sulphasalazine. Clin. Allergy 4:41, 1974.

215. Thrall, R. S., McCormick, J. R., Jack, R. M., et al.: Bleomycin-induced pulmonary fibrosis in the rat: inhibition by indomethacin. Am. J. Pathol. 95:117, 1979. (LM 4).

216. Thurlbeck, W. M., & Thurlbeck, S. M.: Pulmonary effects of paraquat poisoning. Chest 69 (Suppl. 2) 276-280, 1976. (Macro 1, LM 4, EM 1).

217. Toner, P. G., Vetters, J. M., Spilg, W. G. S., et al.: Fine structure of the lung lesion in a case of paraquat poisoning. J. Pathol. 102:182, 1970. (LM 4, EM 2).

218. Topilow, A. A., Rothenberg, S. P., & Cottrell, T. S.: Interstitial pneumonia after prolonged treatment with cyclophosphamide. Am. Rev. Respir. Dis. 108:114, 1973. (LM 2).

219. Tuchman, H.: Löffler's reaction to paraaminosalicylic acid. Am. Rev. Tuberc. 70:171, 1954.

220. Tydd, T. F., & Dyer, N. H.: Sulphasalazine lung. Med. J. Aust. 1:570, 1976.

221. Vijeyaratnam, G. S., & Corrin, B.: Experimental paraquat poisoning: a histological and electron-optical study of the changes in the lung. J. Pathol. 103:123, 1971. (LM 5, EM 18).

222. Voith, M. A., Lichtenfeld, K. M., Schimpff, S. C., et al.: Systemic complication of MER immunotherapy of cancer. Pulmonary granulomatosis and rash. Cancer 43:500, 1979. (LM 1).

223. Wagner, J. C.: Experimental production of mesothelial tumours of the pleura by implantation of dusts in laboratory animals. Nature 196:180, 1962.

224. Wagner, J. C., Berry, G., & Timbrell, V.: Mesotheliomata in rats after inoculation with asbestos and other materials. Br. J. Cancer 28:173, 1973.
225. Walden, P. A. M., Mitchell-Heggs, P. F., Coppin, C. C., et al.: Pleurisy and methotrexate treatment. Br. Med. J. 2:867, 1977.
226. Weinstein, J.: Hypocomplementemia in hydralazine-associated systemic lupus erythematosis. Am. J. Med. 65:553, 1978.
227. Weisenberger, D. D.: Interstitial pneumonitis associated with azathioprine therapy. Am. J. Clin. Pathol. 69:181, 1978. (LM 4).
227a. Weiss, R. B., & Muggia, F. M.: Cytotoxic drug-induced pulmonary disease: Update 1980. Am. J. Med. 68:259, 1980.
228. Wells, I. P., Dubbins, P. A., & Whimster, W. F.: Pulmonary disease caused by the inhalation of cosmetic talcum powder. Br. J. Radiol. 52:586, 1979. (LM 1).
229. Wermer, P., Kuschner, M., & Riley, E. A.: Reversible metastatic calcification associated with excessive milk and alkali intake. Am. J. Med. 14:108, 1953. (LM 1).
230. Whimster, W. F.: Rapid giant paper sections of lungs. Thorax 24:737, 1969. (Macro 3).
231. Whimster, W. F.: Interstitial lung disease. Proc. R. Soc. Med. 70:300, 1977.
232. Whitcombe, M. E., Schwarz, M. I., Charles, M. A., et al.: Interstitial fibrosis after pneumocystis carinii pneumonia. Ann. Intern. Med. 73:761, 1970. (LM 4).
233. Whitwell, F., & Rawcliffe, R. M.: Diffuse malignant pleural mesothelioma and asbestos exposure. Thorax 26:6, 1971. (LM 13).
234. Willson, J. K. V.: Pulmonary toxicity of antineoplastic drugs. Cancer Treat. Rep. 62:2003, 1978.
235. Wilson, I. C., Gambill, J. M., & Sandifer, M. G.: Loeffler's syndrome occurring during imipramine therapy. Am. J. Psychiatry 119:892, 1963.
236. Windsor, W. O., Kurrein, F., & Dyer, N. H.: Fibrinous peritonitis: a complication of practolol therapy. Br. Med. J. 2:68, 1975.
237. Winn, W. C., Glavin, F. L., Perl, D. P., et al.: The pathology of Legionnaire's disease. Arch. Pathol. Lab. Med. 102:344, 1979. (Macro 5, LM 11).
238. Winterbauer, R. H., Wilske, K. R., & Wheelis, R. F.: Diffuse pulmonary injury associated with gold treatment. N. Engl. J. Med. 294:919, 1976. (LM 1).
239. Wynne, J. W., & Modell, J. H.: Respiratory aspiration of stomach contents. Ann. Intern. Med. 87:466, 1977.
240. Zingale, S. B., Minzer, L., Rosenberg, B., et al.: Drug induced lupus-like syndrome. Arch. Intern. Med. 112:63, 1963.
241. Zinserling, A.: Peculiarities of lesions in viral and mycoplasma infections of the respiratory tract. Virchows Arch. [Pathol. Anat.] 356:259, 1972. (LM 28).

10

The Cardiovascular System

Hugh A. McAllister, Jr., and Florabel G. Mullick

Although many drugs adversely affect the cardiovascular system, the patterns of injury they produce may be morphologically similar. The major morphologic changes in the heart include hypersensitivity myocarditis, toxic myocarditis, cardiomyopathy, myocardial infarction, endocardial and valvular fibrosis, drug-associated infective endocarditis, pericarditis, and pericardial hemorrhage. The major morphologic changes that drugs produce in the blood vessels include hypersensitivity vasculitis, toxic vasculitis, intimal proliferation, accelerated artherosclerosis, arterial calcification, thrombosis and thromboembolism, and drug-associated infective vasculitis.

HYPERSENSITIVITY MYOCARDITIS

Hypersensitivity myocarditis is characterized by an inflammatory cell infiltrate consisting of prominent numbers of eosinophils, lymphocytes, and plasma cells. Numerous foci of myocytolysis are common, but there is minimal, if any, muscle cell necrosis.[32] The inflammatory cell infiltrate is prominent in the interstitium, and is also present in small intramural coronary arteries, arterioles, and venules, resulting in a bland-appearing vasculitis that is similar to the hypersensitivity vasculitis associated with the use of some therapeutic drugs (Fig. 10-1). Necrotizing vascular lesions, such as those present in patients with Wegener's granulomatosis, systemic lupus erythematosus, and panarteritis (polyarteritis) nodosa (P.A.N.) are not a feature of hypersensitivity myocarditis.[68a] Aggregates of the inflammatory cells characteristic of the myocarditis are often present adjacent to intramyocardial blood vessels, simulating Aschoff bodies; however, there is no fibrinoid necrosis, and Anitschkoff cells are not prominent. There is no myocardial fibrosis unless this process has been caused by a pre-existing myocardial disease. There is a uniform appearance of the inflammatory process throughout the heart and, although the myocardial involvement is focal and patchy, it affects both the ventricles and the atria without apparent predilection for either side of the heart.[32] Frequently, foci of hypersensitivity myocarditis are more prominent in the subendocardial myocardium, and occasionally may involve the endocardium proper, with or without superimposed thrombus. The inflammatory cell infiltrates may also involve the pericardium, especially the visceral pericardium, but characteristically the cardiac valves are spared. The precise pathogenesis of hypersensitivity myocarditis remains unclear, but appears to be immunologically mediated, perhaps as a delayed hypersensitivity reaction.[56a]

Other forms of myocarditis in which eosinophils are prominent, such as parasitic infections of the heart and Loeffler's endomyocardial fibrosis, can usually be distinguished from hypersensitivity myocarditis by the presence of focal myocardial necrosis and myocardial scarring. Eosinophils have also been described as part of the inflammatory cell infiltrate in isolated and granulomatous myocarditis. However, in both of these entities,

The opinions or assertions contained herein are the private views of the authors and are not to be construed as being official or as reflecting the views of the Department of the Army or the Department of Defense.

This study was supported in part by the Food and Drug Administration (under contract FDA 224-77-3001), Department of Health and Human Services.

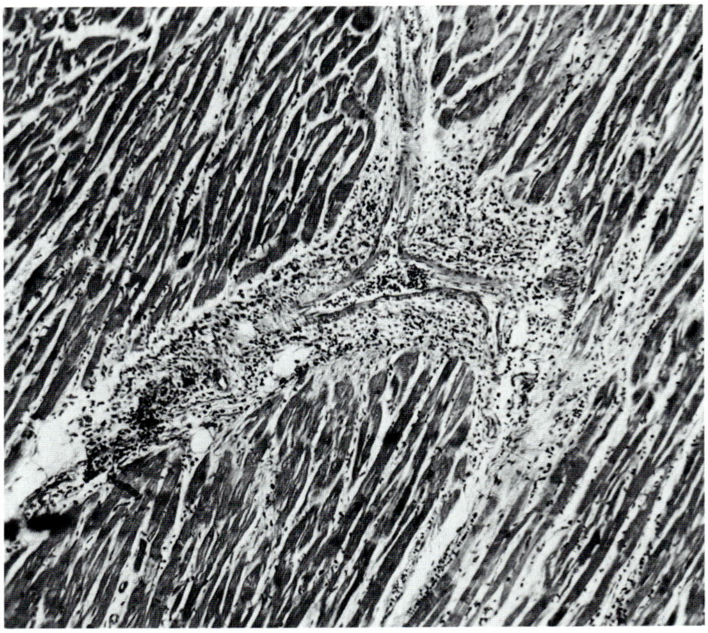

Fig. 10-1. Section of myocardium from a 39-year-old-male who had been taking methyl-DOPA for 18 days showing a prominent interstitial infiltrate involving a small intramural coronary artery. H & E, × 80.

Table 10-1. Drugs Associated with Hypersensitivity Myocarditis

Methyldopa	Phenindione
Hydrochlorothiazide	Phenylbutazone
Sulfadiazine	Oxyphenbutazone
Sulfisoxazole	Tetracycline
Sulfonylureas	Diphenylhydantoin
Chloramphenicol	Acetazolamide
Paraminosalicylic acid (PAS)	Ampicillin
Amitriptyline	Chlorthalidone
Carbamazepine	Spironolactone
Indomethacin	Streptomycin
Pencillin	

myocardial cell necrosis or fibrosis is usually present, distinguishing them from hypersensitivity myocarditis.[32]

The drugs that have been associated with hypersensitivity myocarditis in humans are listed in Table 10-1. It should be noted that many of these drugs have also been associated with hypersensitivity vasculitis.

TOXIC MYOCARDITIS

In acute toxic myocarditis there is interstitial edema, necrosis of myocardial cells with contraction bands (myofibrillar damage leading to myocytolysis), and a mixed inflammatory cell infiltrate consisting of lymphocytes, plasma cells, and polymorphonuclear leukocytes (Fig. 10-2). Although eosinophils may be present, they are usually not prominent. There is endothelial damage, but no true vasculitis. Prolonged therapy with a drug that is causing acute toxic myocarditis can allow progression of the condition to a chronic stage in which there are the gross and microscopic findings of dilated cardiomyopathy, with scattered foci of myocytolysis and myocardial fibrosis, as well as focal endocardial thickening and mural thrombi (Fig. 10-3). The progression of acute toxic myocarditis to cardiomyopathy can occur even after a causative drug (such as Adriamycin or daunomycin) has been discontinued.

Many highly specific biochemical and pharmacologic mechanisms can mediate the cardiac cellular damage produced by toxic drugs and chemical agents; however, the time course of these changes presents a complex variable. Even specific, localized disturbances of the equilibrium of cell functions can lead rapidly to the morphologic pattern of generalized cell

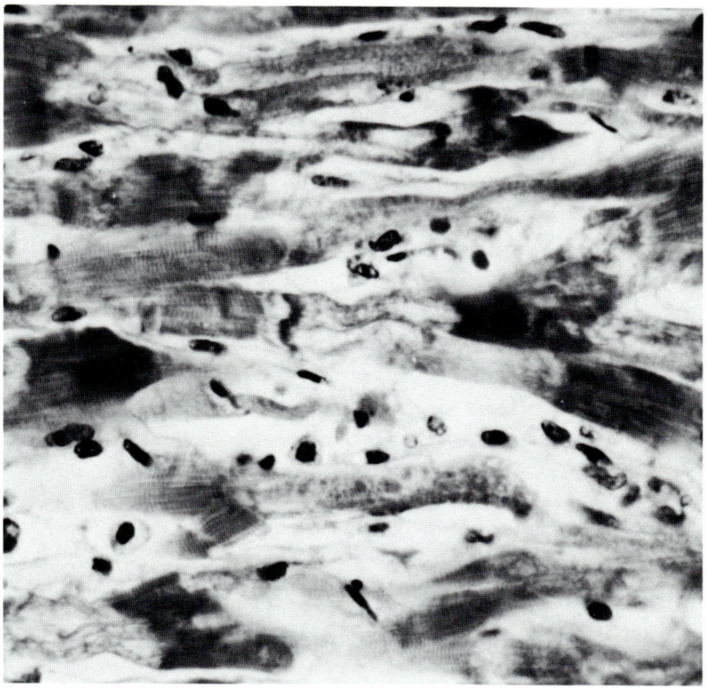

Fig. 10-2. Section of myocardium from a 22-year-old man who died 18 hours after eating food contaminated with arsenic. It shows focal contraction band necrosis, myocytolysis and minimal inflammation. H & E, × 440.

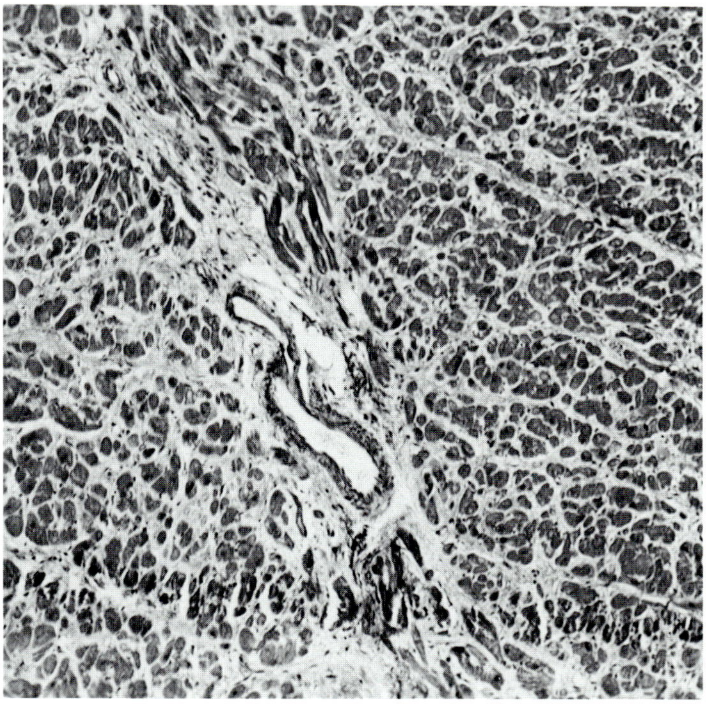

Fig. 10-3. Section of myocardium with interstitial fibrosis from a 43-year-old woman who had been treated with daunorubicin for 3 months. Masson, × 80.

Table 10-2. Drugs Associated with Toxic Myocarditis

Adriamycin	Cyclophosphamide
Daunomycin	Arsenicals
Fluorouracil	Lithium carbonate
Emetine hydrochloride	Phenothiazines
Antimony compounds	Mitomycin C
Amphetamines	Catecholamines

damage or cell necrosis.[34] Among toxic agents that produce specific damage to various subcellular organelles of cardiac muscle cells are: (1) Compounds that interfere with mitochondrial enzymes (cyanide,[112] thyroid hormone[88]), uncouple oxidative phosphorylation (dinitrophenol, emetine[88]), or bind to mitochondrial DNA (acriflavine[62]). These substances can produce a number of alterations in mitochondrial morphology. (2) Compounds that induce intracellular calcification, usually localized within the mitochondria (dehydrotachysterol,[91] sodium phosphate[85]). (3) Compounds that primarily cause myofibrillar lesions (sympathomimetic amines,[35-37,100] plasmocid,[9] diuretics, or other agents that lead to potassium deficiency[104]). (4) Drugs that cause accumulations of electron-dense lamellae (chloroquine[96]). (5) Drugs that produce nuclear or nucleolar lesions (anthracyclines[33]); and (6) Agents that produce massive dilatation of the sarcoplasmic reticulum (anthracyclines[33]). These changes, together with alterations in the permeability of plasma membranes, determine whether or not cellular injury progresses to the point of irreversibility, so resulting in cellular necrosis. The increasing number of drugs that can cause acute as well as chronic toxic myocarditis is listed in Table 10-2.

ISCHEMIC NECROSIS

Cardiac muscle cell damage secondary to capillary endothelial damage, and microthrombosis with structural alterations similar to those in ischemic necrosis, may also occur with the use of certain drugs (cyclophosphamide, catecholamines, selenium-vitamin E deficiency).[34] The damaged areas are usually microscopic and patchy.

MYOCARDIAL INFARCTION

Macroscopic myocardial infarction may occur when the extramural coronary arteries are involved by drug-induced arteritis, as from amphetamines, by intimal proliferation, as from oral contraceptives, by embolization from drug-associated endocarditis or, in patients with normal coronary arteries, following exposure to toxic levels of carbon monoxide, nitrates, thyroid preparation, methysergide, or ergot derivatives.[21]

ENDOCARDIAL FIBROSIS

Endocardial fibrosis may occur adjacent to subendocardial areas of hypersensitivity myocarditis or toxic myocarditis with or without mural thrombus. An identical form of endocardial thickening is commonly located adjacent to areas of myocardial ischemia; microscopically, this consists of collagen as well as elastic fibers, smooth muscle cells, and variable amounts of acid mucopolysaccharide. When the lesions are induced by drug hypersensitivity or toxicity alone, without antecedent valvular disease, the cardiac valves are seldom involved. In contrast, another form of drug-induced endocardial fibrosis commonly involves the cardiac valves; this latter form is most commonly associated with methysergide therapy, although ergotamine tartrate has also been implicated in the induction of the fibrotic lesions.[5,42,75] The cardiac valves most commonly involved are the mitral and aortic; however, involvement of the tricuspid valve has also been reported.[75] The valves are thickened and distorted secondary to a dense layer of fibrous tissue that is devoid of elastic fibers and is superimposed over the normal valve. Microscopically, this lesion is identical to that seen with valvular involvement in the carcinoid syndrome, containing fibroblasts, myofibroblasts, and smooth muscle cells embedded in a stroma rich in collagen and proteoglycans but lacking in elastic fibers (Fig. 10-4). When the atrioventricular valves are involved, the fibrous thickening not uncommonly involves the chordae tendineae and tips of the papillary muscles. The chordae tendineae may be thickened and fused. The endocardium may contain similar lesions, with or without contiguity with the valvular lesions. Occasionally, extensive endocardial fibrosis may be associated with adjacent intramyocardial fibrosis as well.[75]

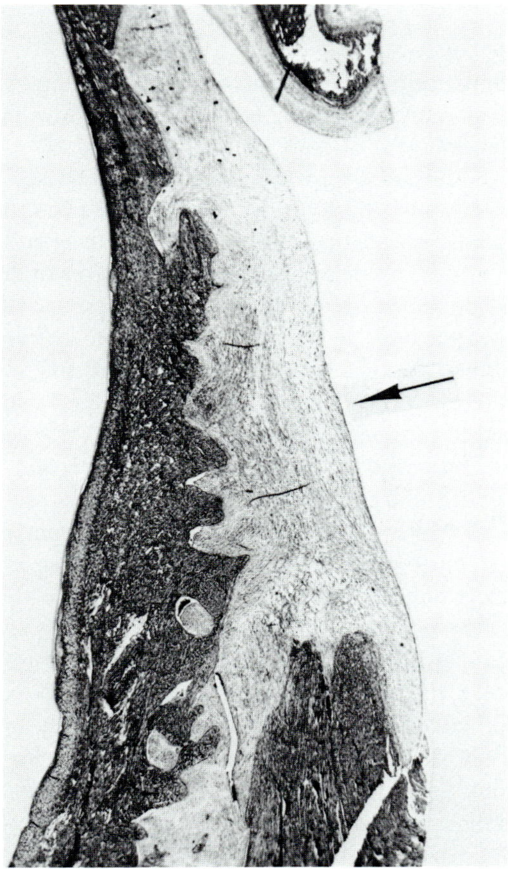

Fig. 10-4. Section of atrial septum with extensive fibrosis of the left atrial endocardium. The lesion is devoid of elastic fibers (arrow). Movat, × 5.

INFECTIVE ENDOCARDITIS

Infective endocarditis is one of several serious complications of parenteral narcotic abuse. Although the incidence of this infection in the addict population has not been precisely determined, it may be conservatively estimated at 1.5 to 2 cases per thousand at risk per year. Since the number of daily narcotic users in the United States is believed to be between 400,000 and 600,000, almost 1,000 cases of narcotic-associated infective endocarditis can be anticipated annually.[108] A history of prior heart disease can be elicited from only 20 percent of patients with narcotic-associated infective endocarditis; in contrast, 60 percent of nonaddicts with infective endocarditis have valvular, congenital, or degenerative heart disease.[108]

Also in contrast to the nonaddict population, the tricuspid valve is frequently involved in narcotic-associated infective endocarditis. Indeed, in one large study 50 percent of the patients with narcotic-associated infective endocarditis had primary tricuspid valve infection.[108]

Nonbacterial thrombotic endocarditis (NBTE) may also affect the cardiac valves in patients with drug-induced disseminated intravascular coagulation (DIC). NBTE differs morphologically from infective endocarditis in that no organisms are present in the lesions, and there is no significant destruction of the cardiac valve. The valves most commonly involved are the mitral and aortic.

The organisms isolated from blood cultures grown from patients with narcotic-associated infective endocarditis differ significantly from those in the nonaddict population. Furthermore, in the addict population in the United States, the clustering of infection with particular microorganisms has been noted in different geographic areas. *Staphylococcus aureus* has been the most common microorganism in Washington D.C., Chicago, New York City, and Cincinnati, whereas *Pseudomonas aeruginosa* appears to be predominant in Detroit;

Serratia marcescens in San Francisco; and *Enterococcus* in Cleveland. In Washington D.C. the prevalence of *Staphylococcus aureus* infection was correlated with skin carriage rates of this organism.[108] Generally, it has not been possible to account for the prevalence of particular infecting microorganisms by contamination of the drug supply or the equipment used for the intravenous injection of drugs. Fungal endocarditis and endocarditis caused by Gram-negative organisms are much more common in the addict than in the nonaddict population. The fungi most commonly isolated in patients with this complication are *Candida* species.

Table 10-3. Drugs that Induce a Lupus-Like Syndrome

Hydralazine	Tetracycline
Procainamide	Propylthiouracil
Isoniazid	Methylthiouracil
Aminosalicylic acid	Alphamethyldopa
Diphenylhydantoin	Barbiturates
Methylphenylethylhydantoin	Griseofulvin
Mephenytoin	Streptomycin
Primidone	Quinidine
Trimethadione	Phenylbutazone
Ethosuximide	Chlorpromazine
Methsuximide	Methotrimeprazine
Trimethadione	Perphenazine
Penicillin	Promazine
Penicillamine	Reserpine
Sulfonamides	

PERICARDITIS

Pericarditis with or without effusion has been reported in patients with drug-induced systemic lupus erythematosus (SLE). It is rare, however, for patients with drug-induced SLE to present with pericarditis as the major initial manifestation, and cardiac tamponade is exceptional.[69] When the offending drug is discontinued, the signs and symptoms of pericarditis disappear, but may recur promptly upon readministration of the drug. There has been a steady accumulation of reports describing the induction of lupus-like syndromes by various drugs[99]; the list of drugs implicated in this manner continues to grow and is itemized in Table 10-3. In many of these reports, the evidence linking drugs to disease is often highly circumstantial, and in some cases symptoms suggestive of SLE have antedated the use of the drug in question. Lupus-like syndromes with pericarditis usually occur only after prolonged treatment with large doses of a causative drug, and affect only a small group of the patients exposed to the drug. As in spontaneously occurring SLE, women are affected more commonly than men.[99] The syndromes that have been most extensively investigated, and most firmly established, have been those that have followed the use of hydralazine and procainamide. Administration of procainamide, methysergide, or practolol has also been associated with the development of constrictive pericarditis.

Some patients with active drug-induced SLE precipitated by hydralazine have been found to have ciruclating antibodies to the drug and evidence of a delayed hypersensitivity reaction (lymphocyte transformation upon exposure to hydralazine), as well as antibodies to native human deoxyribonucleic acid.[45] In patients receiving procainamide for an appreciable length of time, antinuclear antibodies develop in 75 percent[79]; however, only a small percentage of these patients develop a lupus-like reaction. Nevertheless, procainamide is currently the most commonly recognized offender in drug-induced SLE.

Those drugs that cause hypersensitivity myocarditis or toxic myocarditis may also involve the contiguous pericardium, especially the visceral pericardium, resulting acutely in a fibrinous pericarditis with or without effusion. In toxic myocarditis, the pericardium is most commonly affected in patients receiving cyclophosphamide, anthracyclines, or arsenic.

Patients receiving immunosuppressive drugs may develop an infective pericarditis with opportunistic organisms. Virus infections may result in a fibrinous pericarditis, whereas bacteria and fungi commonly cause a purulent pericarditis which may occasionally be accompanied by myocardial abscesses. Either fibrinous or purulent pericarditis may result in cardiac tamponade or may evolve into chronic constrictive pericarditis. The rare occurrence of tuberculous pericarditis in patients immunologically compromised through the administration of immunosuppressive drugs must also be considered in the differential diagnosis.

The organisms responsible for nontuberculous infective pericarditis have changed considerably since the introduction of antibiotics and immunosuppression.[65] In the preantibiotic and preimmunosuppressive era, gram-positive bacteria were responsible for 80 percent of these cases and gram-negative bacteria for 4 percent; in a recent study of patients with purulent pericarditis, gram-positive bacteria were responsible for 42 percent of the cases of this condition, gram-negative bacteria for 39 percent, and fungi for 19 percent. Additionally, the types of gram-positive bacteria causing infective pericarditis have changed considerably. *Streptococcus* and the pneumococcus were the most common causative gram-positive organisms in the preantibiotic era, but these have been replaced by *Staphylococcus* in the more recent antibiotic era. Fungal pericarditis has significantly increased in frequency with the use of immunosuppressive agents[112]; furthermore, although usually granulomatous, fungal pericarditis may be purulent. While many different fungi have been implicated as being causative of pericarditis, the most common are *Candida* species, in patients with leukemia who are receiving immunosuppressive drugs.

PERICARDIAL HEMORRHAGE

Pericardial hemorrhage most commonly occurs in patients receiving anticoagulants; it may exist in the form of focal extravasations contained within the pericardium, or may result in hemorrhage into the pericardial sac, occasionally resulting in cardiac tamponade. The latter is especially the case with uremic patients receiving heparin in conjunction with hemodialysis.[69] If the pericardium is not damaged, the presence of blood within the pericardial sac leaves no residuum. However, in these patients with pericarditis, hemorrhagic effusion frequently results in pericardial adhesions that are initially fibrinous. If minimal, this fibrinous pericarditis may resolve completely; if the fibrinous pericarditis is more extensive, the exudate becomes organized and is replaced by fibrous tissue. If the exudate is abundant, the visceral and parietal layers of the pericardium may become bound together by adhesions, or the pericardial cavity may become virtually obliterated by fibrous adhesions. In cases of extensive fibrous adhesions, chronic constrictive pericarditis may develop, and has been reported to occur as early as 6 weeks and as late as 11 months following acute hemorrhagic pericarditis.

HYPERSENSITIVITY VASCULITIS

Hypersensitivity vasculitis related to therapeutic drugs most commonly involves the arterioles, capillaries, and venules; small veins and occasionally small arteries may also be affected, but the muscular and elastic arteries and the large veins are spared. In hypersensitivity vasculitis an inflammatory cell infiltrate is present in all three layers of the involved vessel wall, there is no evidence of necrotizing vascular lesions or of fibrinoid necrosis[83]; therefore, the media is not weakened, and in contrast to the situation in panarteritis nodosa, aneurysm formation is not a feature of hypersensitivity vasculitis. The inflammatory cell infiltrate in hypersensitivity vasculitis consists primarily of mononuclear cells—mainly lymphocytes, and prominent numbers of eosinophils (Fig. 10-5). There is usually also an extensive perivascular infiltrate consisting of the same population of inflammatory cells; the inflammatory process appears to spread from the affected blood vessels to the adjacent

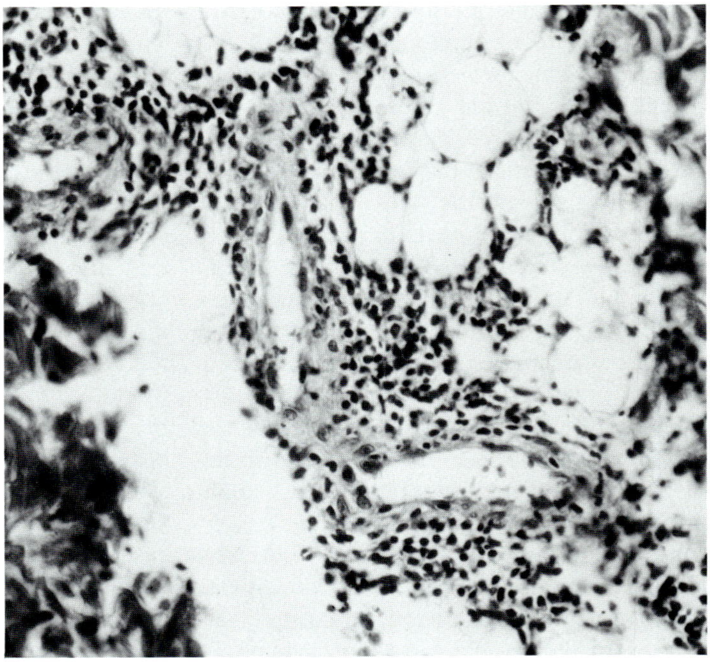

Fig. 10-5. Section of skin from a 24-year-old male who had been taking diazepam daily for 8 weeks, illustrating arterioles with infiltration of their wall by lymphocytes and a few eosinophils. H & E, × 440.

structures.[82] The perivascular infiltrate alone is insufficient evidence upon which to base a diagnosis of hypersensitivity vasculitis. The endothelial lining of the involved blood vessels appears intact, and thrombosis is not a feature of this disease process.

Drug hypersensitivity reactions are presumed to be the result of antigen-antibody interactions. Numerous attempts, however, to define the immunologic mechanisms of hypersensitivity angiitis have been unsuccessful.[83] The interval between the first administration of a drug and the development of vasculitis is extremely variable; the history that a patient has been taking the drug for months or years without side effects does not exclude that drug as a possible etiologic agent of vasculitis. Nor is hypersensitivity dose or time dependent; it may occur at any time while a drug is being administered; however, the temporal relationship of drug administration to the onset of symptoms is an important clinical-pathological correlation in possible drug hypersensitivity reactions.[83] Furthermore, it is possible for lesions to occur from 1 day to 1 week after a medication has been discontinued. Therefore, in considering the diagnosis of drug-related vasculitis, a complete drug history, including current medications as well as discontinued medications, and the temporal relationship of drug administration to the onset of symptoms, is imperative.

The growing list of drugs that have been associated with hypersensitivity vasculitis is itemized in Table 10-4.

Table 10-4. Drugs Associated with Hypersensitivity Vasculitis

Allopurinol	Indocin
Ampicillin	Isoniazid
Bromide	Levamisole
Carbamazepine	Methylthiouracil
Chloramphenicol	Oxyphenbutazone
Chlorpropamide	Phenylbutazone
Chlortetracycline	Potassium iodide
Chlorthalidone	Procainamide
Cromolyn sodium	Propylthiouracil
Colchicine	Quinidine
Dextran	Spironolactone
Diazepam	Sulfonamides
Diphenylhydantoin	Tetracycline
Diphenhydramine	Trimethadione
Griseofulvin	

TOXIC VASCULITIS

Toxic vasculitis is usually necrotizing, with morphologic similarities to panarteritis nodosa. The blood vessels most frequently involved are the medium-sized and small arteries; however, in contrast to classic panarteritis nodosa, capillaries, arterioles, and veins may also be affected by the inflammatory process in toxic vasculitis. The lesions tend to be segmental, with a predilection for the bifurcations of arteries. Grossly, they appear as nodules 2 to 4 mm in diameter; microscopically, the lesions consist of a segmental necrosis and inflammation of all layers of the arterial wall as well as of the contiguous connective tissue. The inflammatory cell population is mixed, but in the active lesion, polymorphonuclear leukocytes are the most common inflammatory cells. Fibrinoid necrosis is usually present in the intima and inner third of the media, and a superimposed thrombus is frequently encountered (Fig. 10-6); an aneurysm may form in the weakened arterial wall. The lesions in toxic vasculitis are usually present in varying stages of evolution and devolution, and the arterial lumen may be occluded by fresh thrombus or by granulation tissue, fibrosis, and recanalization, in varying combinations (Fig. 10-7).

The etiology of toxic vasculitis appears to vary, depending upon the nature of the offending agent as well as the host response. Serum sickness in its classic form results from the injection into a human of a foreign heterologous serum and is the human counterpart of the classic immune complex-mediated experimental serum sickness.[23] Similar reactions resulting in a necrotizing vasculitis—and which are essentially indistinguishable from classic serum sickness—can occur after the administration of nonprotein drugs. The offender is often penicillin, although other drugs have been clearly implicated. In many of these necrotizing vasculitides, especially those associated with sulfonamide administration, precipitated drug or foreign material may occasionally be present in the blood vessel wall, especially in areas of necrosis.[83]

Patients who abuse drugs intravenously may also develop arterial lesions. Disseminated lesions morphologically identical to those in panarteritis nodosa are not uncommonly seen in patients who inject amphetamines intravenously.[22] Although the etiology of this necrotizing vasculitis in drug abusers

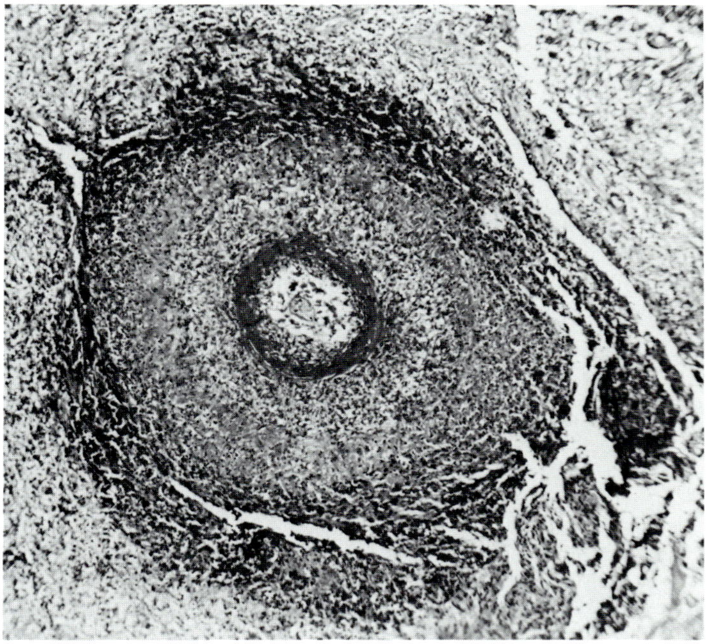

Fig. 10-6. Medium-sized artery from a 25-year-old woman with a 3-year history of drug abuse, showing fibrinoid necrosis and inflammation of all layers of the vessel wall and contiguous connective tissue. H & E, × 80.

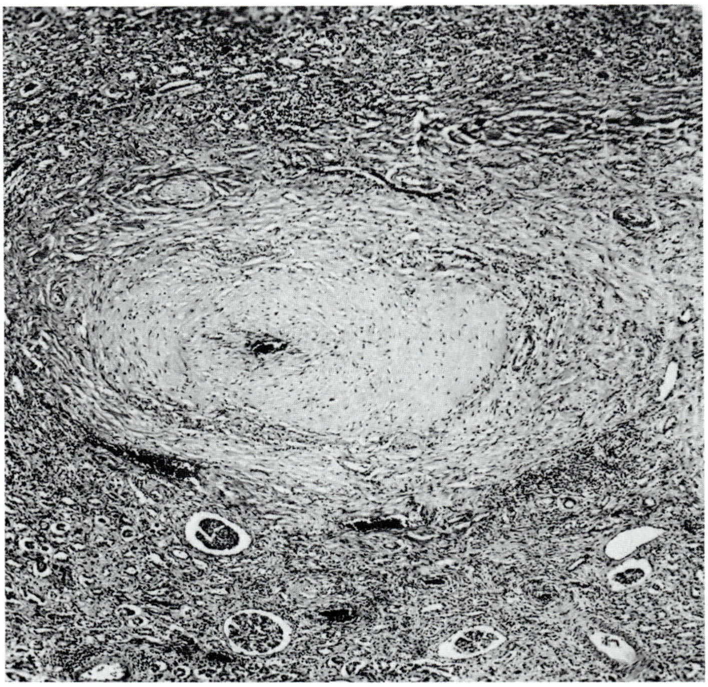

Fig. 10-7. Section of kidney illustrating an arcuate artery with fibrosis of all layers of the arterial wall resulting in marked luminal compromise. H & E, × 80.

is unclear, it has been speculated that it may be secondary to the transmission of hepatitis B antigen from contaminated needles, resulting in antigen exposure and subsequent abnormal immunologic reactivity.[39] Indeed, the hepatitis B antigen has been demonstrated in the wall of an artery containing a lesion identical to that in panarteritis nodosa.[4] This association suggests the possibility that the immune complex deposition of viral antigen and antibodies may be a mechanism of the vascular damage in some patients with necrotizing vasculitis.

Drugs that have been associated with toxic vasculitis are listed in Table 10-5.

Table 10-5. Drugs Associated with Toxic Vasculitis

Organic arsenicals
Gold salts
Mercurials
Bismuth
Amphetamine
Methamphetamine
DDT
Serum
Sulfonamides

INTIMAL PROLIFERATION

Intimal proliferation with and without associated thrombosis has been found in women taking oral contraceptives, in pregnant and postpartum women, and in a few men with severe liver disease.[51] These lesions may occur in any of the branches of the pulmonic, portal, or systemic arteries. Microscopically, the focal areas of intimal thickening are usually eccentric and consist mainly of smooth muscle cells and collagen, with variable amounts of acid mucopolysaccharide (Fig. 10-8). The internal elastic membrane is intact, but in areas of intimal thickening, it is usually thickened and replicated into the intima. The arterial media is usually of normal thickness; however, there may be focal areas of apparent decrease in the expected number of smooth muscle cells, with an increased amount of stainable acid mucopolysaccharide in these areas. The adventitia appears normal. Frequently, there is an occlusive thrombus which appears loosely attached to the intimal proliferative lesion, without intimal ulceration or inflammation. Indeed, the presence of inflammatory cells in intimal proliferative lesions is rare, and there

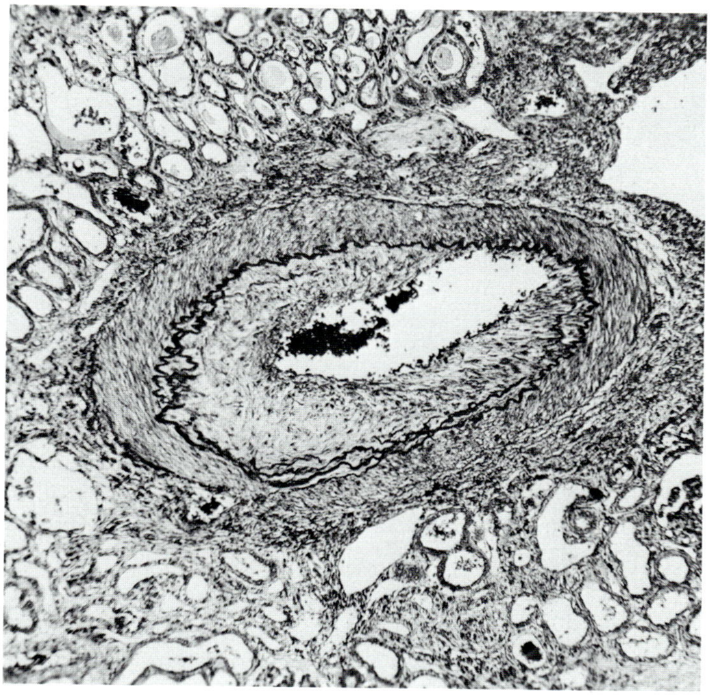

Fig. 10-8. Section of kidney illustrating an arcuate artery with eccentric fibromuscular intimal thickening from a 21 year old woman who had been taking oral contraceptives. The internal elastic membrane is intact but is replicated into the thickened intima. The media and adventitia are unaffected. H & E, × 80.

is no evidence of a necrotizing arteritis or of fibrinoid necrosis in this condition.[50-52]

The arterial lesions induced by ergotamine are those of intimal proliferation and hyalinization, with medial hypertrophy resulting in compromise of the arterial lumen. Superimposed thrombosis frequently completes the occlusion, and gangrene results (Fig. 10-9). The arteries most commonly involved are the tibial, radial, and ulnar arteries, or small tributaries of these, down to arterioles.[41,116,117] Methysergide maleate also may produce spasm and occlusive lesions of the arteries.[92,106] Rarely, the intimal proliferation may be so extensive that distal ischemia persists after withdrawal of the drug (Fig. 10-10).

The pulmonary arterioles may be occluded by an intimal proliferation containing talc or magnesium silicate—both fillers used in the manufacture of certain drugs—in persons who inject these drugs intravenously[66,107]; in those individuals with extensive intimal proliferation of the pulmonary arterioles, pulmonary hypertension and cor pulmonale result. Usually, granulomas containing foreign body giant cells are present in the pulmonary parenchyma adjacent to the intimal lesions, and the talc or magnesium silicate in the lesions can be identified with the polarizing lens of the light microscope (Fig. 10-11). Extravasation of this filler material frequently occurs at the injection site, permitting the diagnosis to be confirmed by skin biopsy. Some of the polarizable material in drug-induced arteriolar intimal proliferation passes through the pulmonary circulation and may be identified in reticuloendothelial tissues of the body, especially in portal histiocytes and Kupffer cells of the liver. The drugs most commonly implicated in this pulmonary arteriopathy are methylphenidate, propoxyphene, and "blue velvet" (paregoric and tripelennamine).[66]

ACCELERATED ATHEROSCLEROSIS

Although scientific proof is lacking, epidemiologic studies have associated the chronic intake of certain drugs, including oral contraceptives and oral hypoglycemic agents, with accelerated atherosclerosis[57]; oral contraceptives have also been associated with intimal

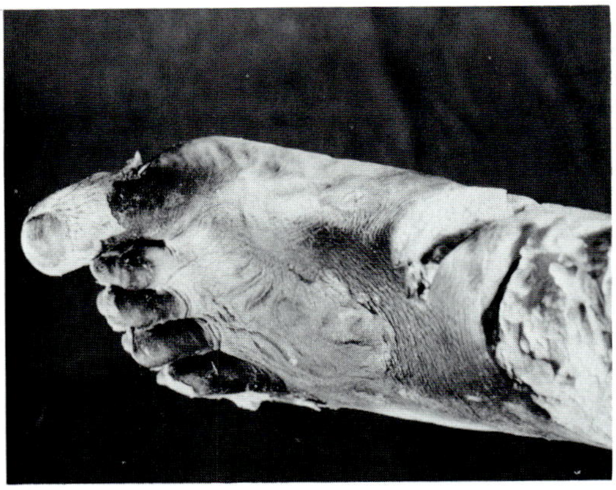

(A)

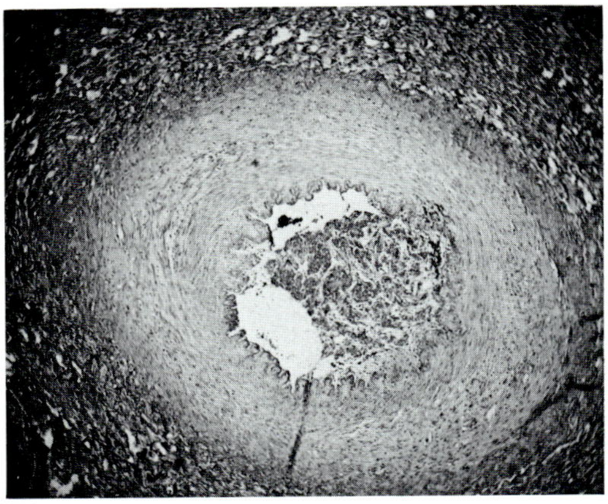

(B)

Fig. 10-9. (A) Amputated foot with gangrenous toes from a 21-year-old woman who was treated with ergot suppositories. (B) Section of posterior tibial artery from the same patient illustrating medial hypertrophy and a superimposed thrombus resulting in marked luminal compromise. H & E, × 25.

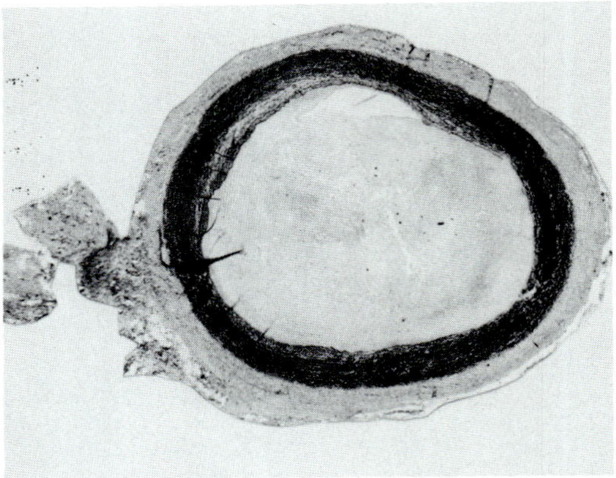

Fig. 10-10. Section of common carotid artery from a 45-year-old man who had been treated with methysergide, illustrating marked intimal proliferation. The media and adventitia appear normal. Movat, × 3.

proliferative lesions.[52] The proliferating cell in the arterial intima appears morphologically identical, by light and electron microscopy, to the proliferating cell in early atherosclerosis. Therefore, the chronic consumption of oral contraceptives and oral hypoglycemic agents by patients with known atherogenic risk factors such as cigarette smoking, hypertension, or hyperlipidemia, could predispose these individuals to increased lipid accumulation in the thickened intima.

Epidemiologic studies have shown that the plasma high-density lipoprotein (HDL) concentration is negatively correlated with the risk of developing ischemic heart disease.[45a] Therefore, HDL seems to retard the process of atherogenesis and to protect against ischemic heart disease. With regard to this, women taking oral contraceptives containing more estrogen have higher levels of HDL, while those taking contraceptives mainly containing progestins have lower serum HDL levels[13]; low plasma HDL levels have also been reported in patients taking oral hypoglycemic agents,[18] and in those being treated concurrently with hydrochlorathiazide and propranolol.[46]

Drug-induced calcification of the arterial wall is a process distinct from atherosclerosis. Calcification of the internal elastic membrane and the adjacent media may occur in vitamin D intoxication or hypersensitivity.[69] The medial calcification in these disorders is similar to that seen in hyperparathyroidism, pseudoxanthoma elasticum, and juvenile intimal sclerosis (idiopathic arterial calcification of infancy) in that there is an associated fibromuscular hyperplasia of the intima resulting in significant luminal compromise. The calcification is not associated with any inflammatory reaction, and the adventitia is largely unaffected. In contrast, the medial calcification in

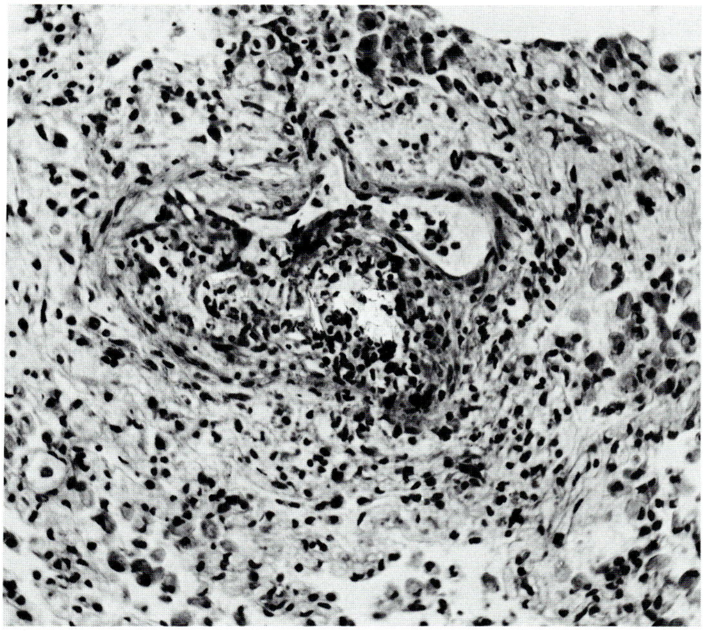

Fig. 10-11. Section of lung from a 26-year-old known drug abuser who died following an overdose of methadone, showing a pulmonary arteriole with marked intimal proliferation. Talc is present within the intimal proliferative lesion. H & E, × 195, with partial polarization.

the pure, uncomplicated form of Monckeberg's sclerosis is not associated with intimal thickening.

THROMBOSIS AND THROMBOEMBOLISM

Thrombosis with or without subsequent thromboembolism may occur in both the arteries and veins. Venous thrombosis may result from damage to the veins at an injection site from the toxic effects of a drug, diluent, or excipient; from hypersensitivity to the metals contained in an injection needle; or from infection. Drugs that increase coagulation, damage the endothelium, cause spasm, or stimulate intimal proliferation may result in localized or diffuse thrombosis.

Arterial thrombosis is less common than venous thrombosis, but usually more catastrophic. Arterial thrombosis may occur from inadvertent injections that produce an intimal flap or a perivascular hematoma, or from a perivascular injection, false aneurysm, infective arteritis with or without mycotic aneurysm, vasopasm, excipient injection with particulate embolism, or idiosyncratic reaction.

Drugs administrated nonarterially may also result in arterial thrombosis. The majority of these drugs are associated with intimal proliferation (oral contraceptives), or with arterial spasm acutely and with intimal proliferation chronically (ergotamine, methysergide maleate). Arterial thrombosis has been associated with the conjunctive use of human chorionic gonadotrophin and human menopausal gonadotrophins (menotropins), although the precise mechanism of the responsible reaction has not yet been defined.[49]

DRUG-RELATED INFECTIVE VASCULITIS

Drug-related infective vasculitis occurs almost exclusively in patients receiving intravenously administered drugs. The infection may remain localized to the injection site as a phlebitis, or the organisms may become disseminated, resulting in an infective endocarditis or infective arteritis. The inflammatory reaction to an infection of an artery depends upon the infecting organism and the ability of the arterial wall to react to injury. Some organisms excite little or no inflammatory response, whereas others may completely destroy the arterial wall. The inflammatory response in an artery also varies greatly according to the type of artery involved, the mode of involvement, and the stage of reaction. The inflammatory lesions may be relatively diffuse or localized. In addition to the routine histologic examination, cultures for bacteria and fungi, as well as serologic studies for viruses, are frequently necessary in order to identify the infectious agent. The use of special histochemical stains for organisms and immunofluorescence techniques are usually helpful diagnostic aids.[70]

ANTICOAGULANTS

Hypersensitivity reactions to heparin are well known, but fortunately are rare. The most dramatic cardiovascular effect of heparin hypersensitivity is a vasospastic reaction.[67] Vasospasm may develop independent of the route of heparin administration. These reactions usually occur from 6 to 10 days after initiation of injections of the drug, and last for 4 to 6 hours. Women are affected more commonly than men. The affected limb is painful, ischemic, and cyanosed.[115] If heparin treatment is not discontinued, similar but progressively more severe reactions will occur following each injection. In addition, there may be signs of generalized vasospasm. These vasospastic reactions appear to be induced by a heparin-protein complex in which heparin acts as a hapten, and which induces antibody production, followed by an antigen-antibody reaction with histamine liberation.[24] Protamine sulfate treatment has no marked therapeutic effect on the vasospastic condition. Generally, the prognosis in heparin-induced vasospasm is good, although ischemic necrosis has been reported.[38]

The observations of "spontaneous" arterial emboli following subcutaneous injections of heparin have not been confirmed pathologically; vasospastic reactions in acute hypersensitivity reactions to heparin may have been misinterpreted clinically as arterial embolization.[67] Disseminated intravascular coagulation (DIC), with or without cardiogenic shock, may rarely occur following heparin injection. In such cases, the DIC may partly be due to antibodies against heparin.[67] There is evidence that the neutralization of heparin with protamine in vivo induces a hypercoagulable state associated with an increased risk of thromboembolism; this may be caused by the activation of factor VII or factor XII, or both, by heparin-protamine, as evidenced by a marked shortening of the Thrombotest in vitro.[40] Metastatic arterial calcification in patients with chronic renal failure undergoing hemodialysis may be enhanced by the action of heparin, since the intravenous injection of large doses of heparin induces the mobilization of calcium and inorganic phosphate. The widespread use of intermittent hemodialysis in uremic patients appears to have increased the incidence of pericardial tamponade and fibrinohemorrhagic pericarditis, perhaps influenced by heparinization.[69] Additionally, heparin activates liproprotein lipase, thereby inducing an increase in circulating nonesterified fatty acids; this effect may be associated with arrhythmias and death in patients with myocardial infarction.[60]

Patients receiving coumarin derivatives may rarely develop skin necrosis secondary to vascular damage.[67] It has been suggested that coumarin congeners exert a toxic effect at the site of the dermovascular loop near the junction of the capillary and the percapillary arterioles, which may lead to hemorrhage into the skin, particularly in the presence of preexisting cutaneous lesions or following minor trauma.[84] In cases of coumarin-induced vascular damage with skin necrosis, petechiae appear in the skin secondary to ruptured capillaries and often become confluent within 24 hours. During the next 24 hours, thrombotic occlusion of the veins causes infarction, with necrosis of skin and subcutaneous fat. These lesions have a predilection for sites rich in adipose tissue, such as the breast, abdomen, buttocks, thighs, and calves; however, other sites of the body may occasionally be involved. Obese, elderly women account for the vast majority of the cases of coumarin-induced vascular necrosis with skin damage.[67]

Hemorrhagic skin necrosis has been described as occurring with all coumarin derivatives and during combined therapy with heparin and phenindione; in the latter situation the necrosis may be unusually extensive.[29] Hemopericardium with or without cardiac rupture is distinctly more frequent in cardiac patients treated with anticoagulants as compared with patients not treated with these drugs[1]; less commonly, cases of "spontaneous" hemopericardium in patients receiving long term anticoagulant treatment have been reported.[31] Overdosage or virus infection have been suspected as precipitating causes in some of these patients with spontaneous or idiopathic pericardial effusion.[77] Anticoagulants may also intensify the postmyocardial-infarction syndrome. Although one study concluded that the frequency of hemorrhage into atherosclerotic plaques was no different in patients receiving anticoagulants than in untreated patients, additional investigation of this potential problem is needed.[56]

The indandione derivatives do not differ from the coumarin derivatives with respect to their anti-vitamin K activity, bleeding complications, or liability to produce skin necrosis, but their use, unlike that of the coumarins, involves the hazard of hypersensitivity, including hypersensitivity myocarditis[59]; it is conceivable that the benzene ring in the indandione molecule is significant in the pathogenesis of this hypersensitivity reaction.

Although a causal relationship has not been proven, there is suggestive evidence that antifibrinolytic agents may be capable of inducing a thrombotic microangiopathy. In some patients with carcinomatosis—most probably associated with DIC—acute heart failure[55] and renal failure due to glomerular capillary thrombosis[19] have occurred during treatment with epsilon-aminocaproic acid.

ORAL CONTRACEPTIVES

Women receiving oral contraceptives have an increased incidence of: (1) superficial venous thrombosis; (2) thrombosis of deep veins; (3) pulmonary embolism; (4) cerebral ischemia and thrombosis; (5) hypertension; (6) intimal proliferation with or without associated thrombosis; and (7) accelerated atherosclerosis. Both retrospective and prospective studies indicate that the risk of deep vein thrombophlebitis and pulmonary embolism is fivefold greater, and that the risk of stroke is tenfold greater in women taking oral contraceptives than in age-matched controls.[61,105] The risk of oral contraceptive-associated thromboembolic disease is greatest in women under 35 years of age, and does not appear to correlate with smoking[54]; the duration of the use of oral contraceptives apparently does not affect the risk.

The effect of contraceptive steroids on the clotting mechanism is complex. Platelet aggregation is increased, and the platelet count may fall slightly.[76] There is an increase in platelet factor 3.[95] Some women demonstrate a slightly increased intravascular coagulation activity, and in some women blood viscosity is increased.[3] In many patients, soluble fibrin increases up to 97 percent. Sequential oral contraceptive administration apparently causes more pronounced changes in clotting factors than the usual combined administration of these drugs.[78]

Retrospective epidemiologic studies have suggested an association between the use of oral contraceptives and myocardial infarction in premenopausal women.[54,73] These studies indicate that the risk of myocardial infarction is increased fivefold in oral contraceptive users; the risk is greatest in women with preexisting medical conditions, especially diabetes mellitus, hypertension, or a previous history of ischemic heart disease. Intimal proliferation may be present in the extramural as well as the intramural coronary arteries. The intimal proliferation may be extensive, resulting in marked luminal compromise, and occasionally, there may be a superimposed occlusive thrombus.[52] Other women dying with myocardial infarction may have classic atherosclerotic lesions in the extramural coronary arteries. Oral contraceptives are also associated with multiple risk factors known to accelerate atherosclerosis. These risk factors include the induction or exacerbation of hypertension in some patients, increased platelet aggregation and altered coagulation, an increase in serum cholestrol with an occasional decrease in the HDL fraction, an increase in triglyceride as well as phospholipid and fatty acid levels, and altered carbohydrate metabolism with a decrease in glucose tolerance and increased plasma insulin levels. Additionally, women taking the contraceptive pill have significantly lower blood levels of vitamin B_6 than do other women.[44] Vitamin B_6 is necessary for the clearing of homocystine from the blood, and experimental studies in baboons indicate that homocystine is a potent inducer of atherosclerosis.[44] These alterations induced by the contraceptive pill, when combined with other risk factors such as cigarette smoking, may well accelerate atherogenesis.

Besides their other effects, oral contraceptives may induce hypertension or exacerbate preexisting hypertension through alterations of the renin-angiotensin system.[8,68] Estrogen causes a marked elevation of plasma angiotensin (renin substrate); renin acts on this substrate to produce angiotensin I, which is hydrolized to produce angiotensin II, an active pressor substance. Angiotensin II stimulates the adrenal cortex to produce aldosterone, which causes water and sodium retention. This, along with such variables as blood volume and increased arterial tone, may produce hypertension, especially if there is increased cardiac output and a compensatory failure of sodium and water excretion. The estrogen component of oral contraceptives appears to be the main agent responsible for hypertension in users of these drugs, but the progestin component has not been completely absolved.[25] However, it is not possible to allocate the elevation of blood pressure in oral contraceptive users to the renin-angiotensin system alone; plasma renin substrate and plasma renin activity are increased in both hypertensive and normotensive patients taking oral contraceptives. When hypertension occurs with oral contraceptive use, it usually occurs within the first 6 months of such use. Both the diastolic and systolic pressure levels may be elevated, and although the hypertension is usually mild, there are rare reports of hypertensive crisis and renal failure in patients receiving contraceptive steroids.[113] Usually, blood pressure levels return to normal within 3 to 6 months after the cessation of oral contraceptive therapy.[25]

A rare but catastrophic complication associated with the use of oral contraceptives is hepatic vein thrombosis (Budd-Chiari Syndrome).[28] Additionally, hereditary hemorrhagic telangiectasia is aggravated by oral contraceptives.[102]

CORTICOSTEROIDS

Long-term treatment with corticosteroids may be accompanied by an arteritis involving small and medium-sized arteries. In most cases it is not clear whether the arteritis is caused by the disease which the corticosteroids are being used to treat, or is causally related to the steroid treatment itself; most of the available evidence points to the first possibility.[27] Corticosteroids also alter carbohydrate metabolism, inducing abnormal glucose tolerance, especially in patients with a family history indicating a predisposition to diabetes mellitus.[72] Additionally treatment with steroids predisposes to an increased incidence of thromboembolic complications in both adults and children.[27] Although the evidence is not conclusive, it has been suggested that corticosteroids may induce, in the arteries and veins of susceptible individuals, an intimal proliferation similar to that seen in patients receiving oral contraceptives. The combination of damage to the arterial wall with arteritis, an increased tendency to thrombosis, alteration of carbohydrate metabolism, and possible intimal proliferation suggests that the long-term administration of corticosteroids may accelerate atherosclerosis. Steroid-induced hypertension must also be considered as an additional risk factor in accelerating atherogenesis.

Focal myocardial necrosis has been induced in experimental animals receiving large doses of corticosteroids, but the induction of these lesions in humans has not been documented.[58] Some patients who die while receiving large doses of corticosteroids will have myocytes with cytoplasmic vacuoles, similar to the monocytes seen in patients with Cushing's syndrome or hypokalemia. Patients with cardiac sarcoidosis treated with steroids have an increased incidence of ventricular aneurysm.[98] Additionally, the immunosuppressive effect of corticosteroids predisposes patients receiving these drugs to infection of the heart and blood vessels by opportunistic organisms.

IMMUNOSUPPRESSANTS

The immunosuppressant drugs most commonly associated with cardiotoxicity are the anthracycline antibiotics (daunomycin and its analogues, especially Adriamycin) and cyclophosphamide. Although the anthracycline antibiotics can produce acute and subacute cardiac toxicity, these agents are more notoriously known for the chronic congestive cardiomyopathy that they produce in humans and experimental animals. The cardiotoxic effects of Adriamycin are dose related, and an accumulative dose below 500 mg per square meter yields a low incidence of cardiomyopathy; however, approximately 30 percent of the patients receiving a larger dose will develop cardiomyopathy.[64]

The pathogenesis of Adriamycin-induced cardiomyopathy remains uncertain; however, a number of possible mechanisms have been proposed, including damage to DNA in cardiac muscle cells, and peroxidative damage to cell membranes, mitochondrial membranes, and membranes of the sarcoplasmic reticulum.[34] Mural thrombi are frequently present in both ventricles. Microscopically, the lesions are both focal and disseminated. The earliest lesions are most common in the subendocardium. In these early lesions, single, isolated myocytes with degenerative changes are often disbursed in an otherwise morphologically intact myocardium.[10]

The cardiac degeneration induced by anthracyclines is manifested microscopically by myofibrillar loss and cytoplasmic vacuolization.[11, 16, 53] The latter is a prominent but focal finding that involves individual cells rather than large, confluent areas of myocardium, and is caused by massive dilatation of tubules of the sarcoplasmic reticulum; some dilatation of T-tubules also occurs. This vacuolar degeneration can occur with apparent preservation of the nucleus and mitochondria of affected cells. The two types of degeneration may occur concomitantly in the same cell or in separate cells. There does not appear to be a relationship between the two types of injury and the severity or course of the cardiotoxicity.[10]

The cellular lesions in anthracycline-induced cardiomyopathy eventually progress to the death of the myocyte, at which time the nuclei become pyknotic and disintegrate, and the mitochondria swell and develop myelin figures. When the myocardial cells die, they are replaced by fibrous tissue, resulting in patchy stellate scars throughout the myocardium. Although the microscopic and ultrastructural changes of anthracycline cardiotoxicity are characteristic, these changes are not specific, and can be seen in cardiomyopathies due to other conditions. The severity of the cardiac morphologic changes induced by anthracyclines has been evaluated by myocardial biopsies, and these have been found to be useful in determining whether or not patients suspected of developing anthracycline-induced cardiomyopathy can receive additional amounts of the drug.[10] In addition to the myocardial degnerative lesions described above, which characteristically are not accompanied by an inflammatory cell infiltrate, patients receiving anthracycline antibiotics may develop an acute myopericarditis which is thought to be reversible.

Like the anthracycline antibiotics, cyclophosphamide, an alkylating agent used in the treatment of cancer, is also associated with a high incidence of cardiac toxicity, especially when administered in high-dose combination chemotherapy.[14,20] Cyclophosphamide-induced cardiotoxicity usually has an acute onset, within hours or days after the beginning of treatment. Morphologically, there may be numerous large foci of hemorrhagic necrosis in the myocardium, in association with an extensive capillary microthrombosis, erythrocytes and fibrin in the interstitum, and necrotic myocytes.[15] Subpericardial and subendocardial ecchymosis, with an acute inflammatory infiltrate, may also be present. Additionally, treatment with cyclophosphamide may result in an acute myopericarditis with or without hemorrhagic necrosis of the myocardium.[10] Electron microscopic examination of the myocardial lesions reveals capillary endothelial damage and the unraveling of nuclear chromatin in both myocytes and endothelial cell nuclei, producing prominent thick, thin, and intermediate filaments.[15]

Antineoplastic drugs may indirectly cause damage to the cardiovascular system by their immunosuppressive effect, resulting in infectious vasculitis, endocarditis, myocarditis, or pericarditis caused by opportunistic organisms.

ANTIMICROBIAL AGENTS

Most of the morphologic changes in the heart and blood vessels associated with antibiotic therapy result from hypersensitivity myocarditis, hypersensitivity vasculitis, or both. Those antibiotics that have been associated with hypersensitivity myocarditis in humans are included in Table 10-1. The antibiotics that have been associated with hypersensitivity vasculitis in humans are included in Table 10-3. Less commonly, antimicrobials may be associated with toxic myocarditis (emetine, antineoplastic antibiotics), or toxic vasculitis (penicillin, sulfonamides).

Occlusion and thrombosis following the arterial injection of penicillin is rare; however, the consequences of such complications may be catastrophic; most often, the injection of depot-penicillin preparations into the gluteal area is involved, and the superior gluteal artery has been accidentally entered.[47] Ischemic reactions followed by gangrene have been described not only following the injection of depot-penicillin preparations, but also after the injection of water-soluble penicillin solutions.[48] The high pressure used for the injection of viscous fluids may produce a retrograde flow of the drug into the larger arteries such as the common iliac, abdominal aorta, renal, and spinal cord arteries. The resulting ischemia may therefore involve not only the region of the inferior branch of the superior gluteal artery, but may also result in intestinal and renal hemorrhage, necrosis of the entire lower extremity, or paraplegia from spinal cord damage.[47] Although benzathine penicillin crystals have been identified in an artery following arterial embolization, it is not certain whether the distal ischemia that follows the injection of the drug results from a direct vascular toxic effect of the drug on the endothelium, inducing thrombosis, or from the induction of an arterial spasm resulting in secondary thrombosis.[110] In rare cases, a thrombotic vascular occlusion, with propagation of the thrombus, embolization, or both, may result from the trauma of arterial puncture alone. The accidental intravenous injection of penicillin compounds may also occur, resulting in venous thrombosis and occasionally pulmonary embolization.

The Jarisch-Herxheimer reaction may occur in some patients with syphilis treated with penicillin, resulting in sudden aneurysmal dilatation of the arch of the aorta[30] or acute coronary occlusion producing myocardial infarction.[17] The Herxheimer reaction has also been documented in patients with typhoid fever or with sepsis caused by *Salmonella, E.*

coli, or *Proteus* treated with chloramphenicol. Isoniazid may produce a lupus-like syndrome with pericarditis; antinuclear antibodies and LE cells can be uniformly demonstrated in this condition.[81] The discontinuation of isoniazid usually causes complete disappearance of the symptoms, but occasionally it may take many months for the LE cells and the antibodies to disappear. Spontaneous recurrences of the syndrome have been described.[81]

Although thrombophlebitis may be associated with the intravenous administration of any antimicrobial agent, it most commonly occurs with the intravenous administration of vancomycin or amphotericin B. Purpura-like vasculitis has been described rarely in patients receiving ethambutol.[81]

Other antimicrobial agents, and especially the antihelminthic drugs, may be associated with electrocardiographic changes; however, the histologic changes in the heart that occur with the use of these drugs have not been fully described. Because of the rapid onset of the electrocardiographic changes following the administration of the drug, and the usual disappearance of these changes following the cessation of therapy, the mechanism of the cardiac damage appears to be a toxic effect. Sinus tachycardia and nonspecific electrocardiographic changes have been described following the injection of streptomycin.[74] Stibocaptate has been associated with myocardial enzyme changes, together with T-wave changes on the electrocardiogram and chest pain.[63] Electrocardiographic changes—primarily a T-wave inversion that disappeared after the completion of treatment—have been described in patients receiving piperazine.[63] T-wave flattening and inversion have been observed in patients receiving hycanthone and niridazole.[63] The electrocardiographic changes associated with the administration of niridazole have been reversed with atropine.[63]

DIURETICS

Those diuretics associated with hypersensitivity myocarditis and hypersensitivity vasculitis are summarized in Tables 10-1 and 10-3. Additionally, necrotizing vasculitis of the skin has been reported in patients taking benzothiazides or chlorthalidone,[12] and Henoch-Schonlein purpura has been described in patients taking ethacrynic acid or chlorothiazide.[6,94] Carbonic anhydrase inhibitors (acetazolamide) may induce allergic reactions that demonstrate a cross antigenicity with sulfonamides.[26] Sudden death of presumed cardiac origin has followed the intravenous injection of furosemide and the intravenous administration of mercurial diuretics.[26,71] Clorexolone, quinethazone, metolazone, and mefruside have metabolic effects similar to those of the benzothiazine diuretics; these include hypokalemia, hyperuricemia, and hyperglycemia. Primarily because of their potassium depleting effect, the incidence of adverse reactions to digitalis is two to three times higher in patients taking one of these diuretics than in those not doing so.[26] There are no available data indicating that the hyperglycemia and hyperuricemia caused by clorexolone, quinethazone, metolazone, and mefruside accelerates atherosclerosis in patients receiving them for the treatment of hypertension. However, further investigation of this potential complication is necessary in light of the recent report that concurrent treatment with hydrochlorothiazide and propranolol may lower the high-density lipoprotein (HDL) cholesterol.[46] In contrast to the hypokalemic effects of the diuretics just discussed, spironolactone, triamterene, or amiloride cause retention of potassium, which may result in the disturbances of cardiac rhythm attendant to hyperkalemia. Drugs often used in conjunction with diuretics in the treatment of hypertension may also cause hypersensitivity myocarditis; this is especially true of methyldopa.[82]

ANALGESICS

Most of the cardiovascular effects of aspirin are hoped to be beneficial, in that aspirin is a potent inhibitor of platelet aggregation, which is instrumental in the progression of atherosclerosis. Whether or not the long-term ingestion of small amounts of aspirin will indeed inhibit atherogenesis in humans, however, has yet to be proven. There is preliminary evidence that large doses of aspirin may actually increase endothelial permeability, allowing the influx of lipids into an atherosclerotic plaque. Some patients with aspirin sensitivity may develop a hemorrhagic vasculitis when exposed to the drug.[89] The precise mechanisms involved in aspirin sensitivity are unknown. An immunologic basis is suspected, but a specific allergic response has yet to be related to clinical sensitivity to the drug. Probably the most damaging effect of aspirin on the cardiovascular system is mediated by the effects of hypertension secondary to analgesic nephropathy. Analgesic nephropathy has been reported in patients who have consumed large amounts of aspirin, and also in patients taking phenacetin.[89] Aspirin is teratogenic and embryotoxic in animals, and there is some evidence that it may cause human congenital malformations, including congenital heart defects.[89]

Paracetamol (acetaminophen) when taken in overdosage may result in myocardial damage with subendocardial hemorrhage and focal muscle necrosis.[103] Indomethacin has been associated with hypersensitivity vasculitis, and experimentally reduces systemic blood pressure and myocardial blood flow when given intravenously to anesthetized cats, suggesting that indomethacin may aggreviate angina pectoris and predispose toward myocardial infarction.[90] Phenylbutazone has been associated with both hypersensitivity myocarditis and the induction of a lupus-like syndrome.[90] Allopurinol and colchicine, drugs used in the treatment of gout, have both been associated with hypersensitivity vasculitis, whereas gold, when used in the treatment of rheumatoid arthritis, has been associated with necrotizing vasculitis.[90]

Methysergide, and less frequently ergotamine, may induce cardiac valvular lesions microscopically identical to those present in the carcinoid syndrome; the endocardium may contain similar lesions with or without contiguity with the valvular lesions.[5] Ergotamine and methysergide can both induce marked arterial spasm with resulting ischemia[41,92]; when the coronary arteries are involved, angina pectoris or myocardial infarction may be precipitated.[21] With prolonged administration of these drugs, intimal proliferation, hyalinization, and medial hypertrophy may occur, resulting in structural compromise of the arterial lumen. Arterial thrombosis may result either during the period of intense spasm or superimposed upon an intimal proliferative lesion. Tolazoline has been implicated as a precipitating factor in myocardial infarction, and may occasionally produce hypertension.[97]

The cardiovascular complications of opiate dependence (generally heroin dependence) are usually of two types: (1)Those directly related to the drug (overdose syndrome, acute pulmonary edema); and (2) infection associated with nonsterile techniques of injection by addicts. Additionally, the pulmonary arterioles may be occluded by intimal proliferative lesions containing silicates or corn starch in those patients who inject certain drugs intravenously. Usually, granulomas containing foreign body giant cells are present in the pulmonary parenchyma adjacent to these lesions.[66,107]

Many of the mood-altering drugs are associated with adverse cardiovascular reactions, including hypersensitivity myocarditis (amitriptyline), hypersensitivity vasculitis (diazepam), toxic myocarditis (lithium carbonate, phenothiazines, amphetamines), and toxic vasculitis (amphetamines).

Malignant hyperthermia is an inherited disorder in which affected individuals may react adversely to certain anethestic agents and other stressful stimuli. The condition is inherited as an autosomal dominant trait with variable penetrance and expressivity. In susceptible individuals, potent inhalation agents or skeletal muscle relaxants may cause fever, skeletal muscle rigidity, cardiac arrythmias, and occasionally sudden death. Those patients who are malignant hyperthermia-susceptible may also develop myopathic disorders, including cardiomyopathy. The hearts of patients dying during an episode of malignant hyperthermia usually contain extensive contraction-band necrosis.

TOXINS

Ethyl Alcohol

The role of ethyl alcohol as an etiologic factor in heart disease has been debated over the years, and often attributed to coexistent malnutrition. The latter factor, however, has been dissociated from ethanol use in many patients with cardiomyopathy and heart failure. Major support for the role of ethanol as a toxic agent, when used in large amounts for a prolonged period, has been obtained in various species of animals, including subhuman primates. The cardiac abnormalities produced by ethanol include depression of ventricular function, and metabolic and morphologic changes that parallel the changes in humans with preclinical malfunction of the heart.[93] Although the mechanism of progression of the heart failure or arrythmias associated with alcohol use is not known, several factors may be related to this. These include the accumulative effects of ethanol alone or after intensified drinking episodes, simultaneous exposure to trace metals in excess, and occasional specific nutritional deficiency or superimposed infection.[93] The low prevalence of clinical malnutrition in patients with alcoholic cardiomyopathy, and the infrequency of heart disease in patients with cirrhosis or neuropathy support the view that the cardiac abnormality induced by ethanol is not commonly dependent on nutritional deficiency. Clinical data indicate that the cessation of alcohol intake may reverse the disease or interrupt its progress in many patients who become abstinent.[93]

The pathogenetic mechanisms of alcoholic cardiomyopathy remain uncertain, since such cardiomyopathy develops in only a small percentage of alcoholic patients, although a much higher percentage of these patients develop less obvious anatomic and functional cardiac abnormalities. Furthermore, the complete clinical picture of alcoholic cardiomyopathy seen in humans has not been reproduced in experimental animals by ethanol feeding, even though various morphologic and functional changes have been observed.[34] It appears likely that the toxic effect of ethanol on the myocardium is modified by other factors, and that alcoholic cardiomyopathy is a multifactorial disease.

No specific pathologic features have been described in alcoholic cardiomyopathy. Myocardial biopsies in patients with this condition have revealed a wide variety of nonspecific degenerative changes which tend to reflect the duration and severity of the disease.[34] Histochemical studies have demonstrated large amounts of triglyceride within the myocardial fibers, and the myocardial oxidative enzymes are usually reduced.[93] Myocardial fibrosis may be a prominent feature in those patients with a long-standing cardiomyopathy. Electron microscopic studies have shown mitochondrial swelling with disruption of the cristae, and lipid droplets and lipofuchsin granules are prominent, while intramitochondrial inclusions of cristal debris, as well as membrane-bound vesicles containing cell debris, are common. Myofibrillary disruption is also present. But although these changes can be interpreted as indicative of myocardial cell damage, they are not specific ultrastructural features of alcoholic cardiomyopathy.[34]

Cobalt

During 1965 and 1966, an outbreak of cardiomyopathy with sudden onset and rapid clinical course was observed in Quebec.[80] Epidemiologic studies revealed that the patients affected by the condition drank brands of beer to which cobalt had been added as an anti-frothing agent.[111] Subsequently, other cases of cardiomyopathy were recorded in beer drinkers exposed to cobalt-treated brands of beer in the United States and Europe.[43] Experimental proof of the direct toxic action of cobalt on the myocardium of animals has been documented; however, such other factors as alcohol intake and vitamin deficiency may potentiate the toxic effect of cobalt. Although there is widespread industrial exposure to cobalt, only isolated cases of cobalt-associated cardiomyopathy have been recorded in this area.

The gross and microscopic characteristics of cobalt-induced cardiomyopathy resemble those in other forms of dilated congestive cardiomyopathies. Grossly, the heart weight is usually increased, with proportionate hypertrophy and dilatation of the cardiac chambers. Mural thrombi are frequently present. Microscopically, diffuse lesions involving all parts of the myocardium are present and are characterized by variations in the staining properties and size of the muscle fibers, and by a decrease in the number of myofibrils, vacuolization, interstitial edema, focal fibrosis, and the virtual absence of an inflammatory reaction. Occasionally, scattered foci of mononuclear cells may be encountered. The vacuoles in the myocardial fibers contain both glycogen and neutral fats.[80] The foci of fibrosis are usually minimal and apparently result from myocytolysis with myofibrillar collapse, rather than from fibrous connective tissue proliferation. Many of the myocardial fibers seen in cobalt-induced cardiomyopathy contain an increased amount of lipochrome pigment. Empty sarcolemmal sheaths, occasionally with fatty replacement of the vanished myofibers, are scattered throughout the myocardium. The intramyocardial coronary arterioles may be edematous, with separation of the intimal and adventitial layers, giving rise to a double contour image. Thromboembolism involving any of the major arteries is frequently encountered in patients with cobalt-induced cardiomyopathy.

Arsenic

Chronic arsenical intoxication has been associated with intimal thickening in small and medium-sized arteries, occasionally with superimposed atherosclerosis; the arteries of the extremities, heart, gastrointestinal tract, liver, skin, and pancreas are most often involved. An endemic proliferative vascular disorder resulting in gangrene of the extremities, especially the feet (blackfoot disease), has been described in inhabitants of a limited area of Taiwan where there was a high level of arsenic in the water from artisian wells[114]; a report from Antofagasta, in northern Chile, also demonstrated vascular lesions in patients drinking water with a high arsenic content.[101] Two children in this latter series died from myocardial infarction at the age of 2 years. Exposure to arsine not only causes severe hemolysis, but also has a direct toxic effect on cardiac muscle; this effect is manifested by generalized gross and microscopic evidence of necrosis accompanied by striking abnormalities in the electrocardiogram. Indeed, the electrocardiogram may be the most sensitive indicator of arsine poisoning.[7] In addition to their deleterious effect on arteries and the myocardium, arsenic compounds can induce pericarditis.

Carbon Monoxide

The toxicity of carbon monoxide is directly related to its great affinity for hemoglobin and to the low disassociation rate of carbon methemoglobin.[7] The effect of carbon monoxide on the heart depends on the intensity and duration of the hypoxemia produced and on the state of the heart and the coronary arteries; objective evidence of myocardial injury by carbon monoxide may not be manifested until several days after the exposure to this gas, sometimes even in those who appear to be recovering from the intoxication.[7] A variety of electrocardiographic changes have been observed in carbon monoxide cardiomyopathy, the most common of which are abnormalities of the T-waves and S-T segments; other changes encountered include ventricular extrasystoles, atrial fibrillation, AV nodal rhythm, and bundle branch block.[7] In fatal carbon monoxide poisoning the heart contains focal areas of necrosis, most marked in the subendocardial region of the left ventricle and its papillary muscles. The histologic features resemble those produced by prolonged coronary insufficiency, even though the coronary arteries may not be occluded. The effect of aromatic nitro- and amino-compounds on the cardiovascular system is like that of carbon monoxide, related to the formation of methemoglobin, and is similar to that in carbon monoxide poisoning.[7]

Halogenated Hydrocarbons

Interest in the cardiovascular effects of halogenated hydrocarbons stems from the frequency of the arrythmias that follow exposure to many of the commonly used halogenated hydrocarbon compounds. Large doses of certain halogenated hydrocarbons can cause cardiac depression owing to their effect on heart muscle and vagal reflexes. When death ensues, it is usually ascribed to ventricular fibrillation and most often follows the use of halogenated hydrocarbon compounds as anesthetic agents[7]; such death usually immediately follows exposure to these compounds, so that morphologic changes in the heart are usually minimal and nonspecific. Fatal arrythmias with similar nonspecific morphologic change may also occur following exposure to concentrated doses of ozonized air.[7]

Viper Venom

Viper venom contains four major components that promote either direct or indirect effects on the cardiovascular system. The hemolysins and neurotoxins act indirectly while the cytolysins and hemorrhagins destroy, by direct action, the endothelial cells in small blood vessels and lymphatic spaces, causing widespread destruction of the capillaries in all the viscera. In the heart these destructive changes are most pronounced in the endocardium and pericardium.[7]

Paraquat

Patients who die with paraquat intoxication, especially if the paraquat has been ingested, may have a toxic myocarditis.[86] Grossly, the hearts of these persons are usually soft and flabby. Microscopically, there are focal areas of myocardial necrosis with varying numbers of polymorphonuclear leukocytes. Occasionally, there may be petechial hemorrhage of the epicardium. There may also be a moderate degree of right ventricular hypertrophy secondary to pulmonary hypertension induced by the extensive damage paraquat does to the lungs, including the pulmonary arteries and veins.[109]

REFERENCES

1. Aarseth, S., & Lange, H: The influence of anticoagulant therapy on the occurrence of cardiac rupture and haemopericardium following heart infarction. Am. Heart J. 56:250, 1958.
2. Applebaum, F. R., Strauchen, J. A., & Graw, R. G. Jr.: Acute lethal carditis caused by high dose combination chemotherapy. A unique clinical pathologic entity. Lancet 1:58, 1976.
3. Aronson, H. B., Magora, F., & Schewker, J. G.: Effect of oral contraceptives on blood viscosity. Am. J. Obstet. Gynecol. 110:997, 1971.
4. Baker, A. L., Marshall, M. K., Wendy, C. B., et al: Polyarteritis associated with Australian antigen-positive hepatitis. Gastroenterology 62:105, 1972.
5. Bana, D. S., McNeal, P. S., LeCompte, P. M., et al: Cardiac murmurs and endocar-

dial fibrosis associated with methysergide therapy. Am. Heart J. 88:640, 1975.
6. Bar-On, H., Eisenberg, S., & Eliakin, M.: Clinical experience with ethacrynic acid—with reference to a possible complication of the Schoenlein-Henoch type. Israel J. Med. Sci. 3:113, 1967.
7. Batsakis, J. C.: Degenerative lesions of the heart. In: Gould, S. E., Ed.: In pathology of the heart and blood vessels. 3rd Ed. p. 479. Charles C Thomas, Springfield, Illinois. 1968.
8. Beckerhoff, R., Luetscher, J. A., Wilkinson, R., et al.: Plasma renin concentration, activity and substrate in hypertension induced by oral contraceptives. J. Clin. Endocrinol. Metab. 34:1067, 1972.
9. Berger, J. M., & Bencosme, S. A.: Divergence in patterns of atrial and ventricular cardiocyte degeneration: studies with plasmacide. J. Mol. Cell. Cardiol. 2:41, 1971.
10. Billingham, M. E.: Some recent advances in cardiac pathology. Hum. Pathol. 10:367, 1979.
11. Billingham, M. E., Mason, J. W., Bistow, M. R., et al: Anthracycline cardiomyopathy monitored by morphologic changes. Cancer Treat. Rep. 62:865, 1978.
12. Bjomberg, A., & Gisslen, H.: Thiazides: a cause of necrotizing vasculitis? Lancet 2:982, 1965.
13. Bradley, D. D., Petitti, D. B., Wingerd, J., et al: Serum high-density-lipoprotein cholesterol in women using oral contraceptives, estrogens and progestins. N. Engl. J. Med. 299:17, 1978.
14. Buckner, C. D., Rudolf, R. H., Fefer, A., et al: High dose cyclophosphamide therapy for malignant disease. Cancer 29:357, 1972.
15. Buja, L. M., & Ferrans, V. J.: Myocardial injury produced by antineoplastic drugs. In: Fleckenstein A. and Rona G., Eds.: Recent Advances in Studies on Cardiac Structure and Metabolism. Vol. 6. p. 487. Baltimore University Park Press, 1975.
16. Buja, L. M., Ferrans, V. J., Mayer, R. J., et al: Cardiac ultrastructural changes induced by daunorubicin therapy. Cancer 32:771, 1973.
17. Butterly, J. M., & Fishman, L: Jarish Herxheimer reaction following penicillin therapy in case of syphilitic aortitis. J.A.M.A. 148:370, 1952.
18. Calvert, G. D., Mannik, T., Graham, J. J., et al: Effects of therapy on plasma-high-density-lipoprotein-cholesterol concentration in diabetes mellitus. Lancet 2:66, 1978.
19. Charitan, Ch., & Purtilo, D.: Glomerular capillary thrombosis and acute renal failure after epsilon amino caproic acid. N. Engl. J. Med. 280:1102, 1969.
20. Chatterjee, S. S., & Thakre, M. W.: Fiedler's myocarditis: report of a fatal cause following intramuscular injection of streptomycin. Tubercle 39:240, 1958.
21. Cheitlin, M. D., McAllister, H. A., & DeCastro, C. M.: Myocardial infarction without atherosclerosis. J.A.M.A. 231:951, 1975.
22. Citron, B. P., Halpern, M., McCarron, M., et al: Necrotizing angiitis associated with drug abuse. N. Engl. J. Med. 283:1003, 1970.
23. Clark, E., Kaplan, B. I.: Endocardial, arterial and other mesenchymal alterations associated with serum disease in man. Arch. Pathol. 24:458, 1937.
24. Coon, W. W., & Willis, P. W., III: Some side-effects of heparin heparinoids and their antagonists. Clin. Pharmacol. Ther. 7:379, 1966.
25. Crane, M. G., & Harris, J. J.: Plasma renin activity and aldosterone excretion rate in normal subjects. II. Effects of oral contraceptive agents. J. Clin. Endocrinol. Metab. 29:558, 1969.
26. Dargie, H. J., & Dollery, C. T.: Adverse reaction to diuretic drugs. In: Dukes, M. N. G., Ed.: Meyler's Side Effects of Drugs. Vol. 8. p. 483. American Elsevier Publishing Co., Inc., New York, 1975.
27. deLange, W. E., & Doorenbos, H.: Corticotrophins and corticosteroids. p. 812. In: Dukes, M. N. G., Ed.: Meyler's Side Effects of Drugs. Vol. 8. American Elsevier Publishing Co., Inc., New York, 1975.
28. deLange, W. E., & Doorenbos, H.: Sex hormones, anabolic agents and related drugs. p. 841. In: Dukes, M. N. G., Ed.: Meyler's Side Effects of Drugs. Vol. 8. American Elsevier Publishing Co., Inc., New York, 1975.
29. Desai, S. N.: Extensive skin necrosis following anticoagulant therapy. Br. J. Plast. Surg. 20:325, 1967.
30. Diefenbach, W. C. L.: Fatal Jarish-Herxheimer reaction with sudden aneurysmal dilatation and complete bronchial occlusion following penicillin therapy. N. Engl. J. Med. 241:95, 1949.
31. Fell, S. C., Rubin, I. L., Enselberg, Ch. D., et al: Anticoagulant-induced haemopericardium with tamponade; its occurrence in the

absence of myocardial infarction or pericarditis. N. Engl. J. Med. 272:670, 1965.
32. Fenoglio, J. J., McAllister, H. A., & Mullick, F. G.: Drug related myocarditis I. hypersensitivity myocarditis. Hum. Pathol. 12:900, 1981.
33. Ferrans, V. J.: Overview of cardiac pathology in relation to anthracycline cardiotoxicity. Cancer Treat. Rep. 62:977, 1978.
34. Ferrans, V. J.: Overview of morphologic reactions of the heart to toxic injury. In: T. Balazs, Ed.: Cardiac Toxicology. CRC Press, Cleveland, (in press).
35. Ferrans, V. J., Hibbs, R. G., Cipriano, P. R., & Buja, L. M.: Histochemical and electron-microscopic studies in norepinephrine-induced myocardial necrosis in rats. In: Rona, G., & Bajusz, E., Eds.: Recent Advances in Studies on Cardiac Structure and Metabolism. Vol. 1. University Park Press, Baltimore. 495, 1972.
36. Ferrans, V. J., Hibbs, R. G., Walsh, J. J., & Burch, G. E.: Histochemical and electron microscopical studies on the cardiac necroses produced by sympathomimetic agents. Ann. N.Y. Acad. Sci. 156:309, 1969.
37. Ferrans, V. J., Hibbs, R. G., Weily, H. S., Weilbaecher, D. G., Walsh, J. J., & Burch, G. E.: A histochemical and electron microscopic study of epinephrine-induced myocardial necrosis. J. Mol. Cell. Cardiol. 1:11, 1970.
38. Gayer, W.: Seltene Blobachtungen von Heparin-Unvertaglichkeit. Gynalcologia (Basel). 166:25, 1968.
39. Gocke, D. J., Hsu, K., Morgan, C., et al: Association between polyarteritis and Australian antigen. Lancet 2:1149, 1970.
40. Godal, H. C., & Gjengedal, G.: Activation of coagulation by heparine-protamine complexes as demonstrated by thrombotest. Scan. J. Haematol. 8:194, 1971.
41. Gould, S. E., Price, A. E., & Ginsberg, H. I.: Gangrene and death following ergotamine tartrate (Gynergen) therapy. J.A.M.A. 106:1631, 1936.
42. Grahan, J. R.: Cardiac and pulmonary fibrosis during methysergide therapy for headache. Am. J. Med. Sci. 254:1, 1967.
43. Grinvalsky, H. T., & Fitch, D. M.: Pathology of a myocardiopathy. Ann. N.Y. Acad. Sci. 156:544, 1969.
44. Gruberg, E. R., & Raymond, S. A.: Beyond cholesterol: A new theory on arteriosclerosis. Atlanta Monthly: 59, 1979.
45. Hahn, B. H., Shapp, G. C., Irvin, W. S., Kantor, O. S., et al: Immune responses to hydralazine and nuclear antigens in hydralazine-induced lupus erythematosis. Ann. Intern. Med. 76:365, 1972.
45a. H. D. L., C. H. D.: Editorial. Lancet 2:131, 1976.
46. Helgeland, A., Hjermann, I., & Leren, P.: High-density-lipoprotein cholesterol and antihypertensive drugs. The Oslo study. Br. Med. J. 2:403, 1978.
47. Hoigne, R.: Penicillins, cephalosporins and tetracyclines. In: Dukes, M. N. G., Ed.: Meyler's Side Effects of Drugs. Vol. 8. p. 551. American Elsevier Publishing Co., Inc., New York, 1975.
48. Hoigne, R.: Penicillins, cephalosporins and tetracyclines. In: Dukes, M. N. G., Ed.: Meyler's Side Effects of Drugs. Vol. 8. p. 554. American Elsevier Publishing Co., Inc., New York, 1975.
49. Humbert, G., Delaunay, P., Leroy, J., et al: Accidentvasculaire cerebral an cours d'un traitement par les gonadotiophins. Norw. Presse. Med. 2:28, 1973.
50. Irey, N. S., McAllister, H. A., & Henry, J. M.: Oral contraceptives and stroke in young women: A clinicopathologic correlation. Neurology 28:1216, 1978.
51. Irey, N. S., Manion, W. C., & Taylor, H. B.: Vascular lesions in women taking oral contraceptives. Arch. Pathol. 89:1, 1970.
52. Irey, N. S., & Norris, H. J.: Intimal vascular lesions associated with female reproductive steroids. Arch. Pathol. 96:227, 1973.
53. Jaenke, R. S., & Fajardo, L. F.: Adriamycin-induced myocardial lesions; report of a workshop. Am. J. Surg. Pathol. 1:55, 1977.
54. Jick, H., Dinan, B., Herman, R., et al: Myocardial infarction and other vascular diseases in young women: role of estrogen and other factors. J.A.M.A. 240:2548, 1978.
55. Johansson, S.: Acute right heart failure during treatment with epsilon amino caproic acid (EACA). Act. Med. Scand. 182:331, 1967.
56. Jorgensen, L., Chandler, A. B., & Borchgrevink, C. F.: Acute lesions of coronary arteries in anticoagulant-treated and in untreated patients. Atherosclerosis 13:21, 1971.
56a. Kalikshtein, D. B., Odinokova, V. A., Paleev, N. R., & Gurevich, M. A.: Hypersensitivity of delayed type manifested during the development of allergic lesions of the myocardium. Bull. Exp. Biol. Med. 77:89, 1975.

57. Kannel, W. B.: Editorial: Possible hazards of oral contraceptive use. Circulation 60:490, 1979.
58. Karstad, L., Tabel, H., & Gordon, D.: Myocardial necrosis and mineralization in normal and Aleutian disease in mink fed dexamethasone. Can. J. Comp. Med. 33:253, 1969.
59. Kerwin, A. J.: Fatal myocarditis due to sensitivity to phenindione. Can. Med. Assoc. J. 90:1418, 1964.
60. Kurien, V. A., Yates, P. A., & Oliver, M. F.: Free fatty acids, heparin and arrhythmias during experimental myocardial infarction. Lancet 2:185, 1969.
61. Kyser, F. A., Finsberg, H., & Gilbert, N. C.: The effect of certain drugs upon the cardiotoxic lesions of digitalis in the dog. Am. Heart J. 31:451, 1946.
62. Laguens, R., Meckert, P. C., & Segal, A.: Effect of acriflavin on the fine structure of the heart muscle cell mitochondria of normal and exercised rats. J. Mol. Cell. Cardiol. 4:185, 1972.
63. Langman, M. J. S.: Anthelminthic drugs. In: Dukes, M. N. G., Ed.: Meyler's Side Effects of Drugs. Vol. 8. p. 690. American Elsevier Publishing Co., Inc., New York, 1975.
64. Lefrak, E. A., Pitha, J., Rosenheim, S., et al: A clincopathologic anatomy of adriamycin cardiotoxicity. Cancer 32:302, 1973.
65. Lerner, P. I., & Weinstein, L.: Infective endocarditis in the antibiotic era. N. Engl. J. Med. 274:199, 1966.
66. Lewman, L. V.: Fatal pulmonary hypertension from intravenous injection of methylphenidate (Ritalin) tablets. Hum. Pathol. 3:67, 1972.
67. Loeliger, E. A.: Drug affecting blood clotting and fibrinolysis. In: Dukes, M. N. G., Ed.: Meyler's Side Effects of Drugs. Vol. 8. p. 764. American Elsevier Publishing Co., Inc., New York, 1975.
68. Low, J., & Oparil, S.: Oral contraceptive pill hypertension. J. Reprod. Med. 15:201, 1975.
68a. McAllister, H. A.: Collagen vascular diseases and the cardiovascular system. In Silver, M. D., Ed.: Cardiovascular Pathology. Churchill Livingstone, Inc., New York (in press).
69. McAllister, H. A.: Pathology of the cardiovascular system. In: Lowenthal, D. T., Pennock, R. L., Likoff, W., and Onesti, G., Eds.: Management of Cardiovascular Disease in Renal Failure. pp. 1–16. F. A. Davis, Philadelphia, 1981.
70. McAllister, H. A., & Ferrans, V. J.: The heart and blood vessels. In: Silverberg, J. S., Ed.: Principles and Practice of Surgical Pathology. John Wiley and Sons, New York (in press).
71. Machtely, I.: Sudden death after intramuscular furosemide. Lancet 2:1301, 1968.
72. McKiddie, M. T., Jasani, M. K., Buchanan, K. D., et al: The relationship between glucose tolerance, plasma insulin and corticosteroid therapy in patients with rheumatoid arthritis. Metabolism 17:730, 1968.
73. Mann, J. I., & Inman, W. H. W.: Oral contraceptives and death from myocardial infarction. Br. Med. J. 2:245, 1975.
74. Martin, P. D.: ECG change associated with streptomycin. Chest 65:478, 1974.
75. Mason, J. W., Billingham, M. E., & Friedman, J. P.: Methysergide-induced heart disease. A case of multivalvular and myocardial fibrosis. Circulation 56:889, 1977.
76. Mettler, Z., & Selchow, B. M.: Oral contraceptives and platelet function. Thromb. Diath. Haemorrh. (Stuttgart) 28:213, 1972.
77. Miller, R. L.: Haemopericardium with use of oral anticoagulant therapy. J.A.M.A. 209:1362, 1969.
78. Mink, I. B., Courey, N. G., Niswander, K. R., et al: Progestational agents and blood coagulation. V. Changes induced by sequential oral contraceptive therapy. Am. J. Obstet. Gynecol. 119:401, 1974.
79. Molina, J., Dubois, E., Bilitch, M., et al: Procainamide-induced serologic changes in asymptomatic patients. Arthritis Rheum. 12:608, 1969.
80. Morin, Y. L., Folley, A. R., Martineau, G., et al: Quebec "beer-drinkers cardiomyopathy": forty eight cases. Can. Med. Assoc. J. 15:881, 1967.
81. Mulder-DeJong, M. T., & Mulder, R. J.: Drugs used in the treatment of tuberculosis and leprosy. In: Dukes, M. N. G., Ed.: Meyler's Side Effects of Drugs. Vol. 8. p. 676. American Elsevier Publishing Co., Inc., New York, 1975.
82. Mullick, F. G., & McAllister, H. A.: Myocarditis associated with methyldopa J.A.M.A. 237:1699, 1977.
83. Mullick, F. G., McAllister, H. A. et al.: Drug related vasculitis: clinicopathologic correla-

tion in 30 patients. Hum. Pathol. 10:313, 1979.

84. Nalbandian, R. M., Mader, I. J., Barret, J. L., et al: Petechiae echymoses and necrosis of skin induced by coumarin congeners. J.A.M.A. 192:603, 1958.
85. Nienhand, H., Poche, R., & Reimold, E.: Elektrolytverschiebungen, histologische veranderungen der Organe und Ultrastruktur des Herzmuskels nach belastung mit Cortisol, Aldosteron und Primarem Natriumphosphat bei der Ratte. Virchows Arch. Pathol. Anat. 337:245, 1963.
86. Parkinson, C.: The changing pattern of paraquat poisoning in man. Histopathology 4:171, 1980.
87. Pileram, L. O., Ellison, J., Vomdern, & Bussche, G.: Oral contraceptives and increased formation of soluble fibrin. Br. Med. J. 3:556, 1974.
88. Poche, P.: Uber den einfluss von dinitrophenol und thyroxin auf die ultrastruktur des herzmuskels bei der ratte. Virchows Arch. Pathol. Anat. 335:282, 1962.
89. Prescott, L. F.: Antipyretic analgesics. In: Dukes, M. N. G., Ed.: Meyler's Side Effects of Drugs. Vol. 8. p. 154. American Elsevier Publishing Co., Inc., New York, 1975.
90. Prescott, L. F.: Anti-inflammatory analgesics and drugs used in the treatment of rheumatoid arthritis and gout. In: Dukes, M. N. G., Ed.: Meyler's Side Effects of Drugs. Vol. 8. p. 207. American Elsevier Publishing Co., Inc., New York, 1975.
91. Raute-Kreinsen, U., Berlet, H., Biihler, F., & Rixner, P.: Elektronenmikroskopische befunde am herzmuskel der ratte bei experimentell induzierten electrolytveranderrungen. Virchows Arch. Pathol. Anat. 275:331, 1977.
92. Regan, J. F., & Poletti, B. J.: Vascular adventitial fibrosis in a patient taking methysergide maleate. J.A.M.A. 203:1069, 1968.
93. Regan, T. J., Ettinger, P. O., Lyons, M. M., et al: Ethyl alcohol as a cardiac risk factor. Current problems in cardiology, Vol. 2. p. 7. Year Book Publishers, Chicago, 1977.
94. Reid, J. M., Stevenson, J. G., & Orr, M.: Nonthrombocytopenic purpura due to chlorothiazide. Scot. Med. J. 14:309, 1969.
95. Renaud, S., & Gautheron, P.: Role of platelet factor 3 in the hypercoagulability induced by pregnancy and oral contraceptives. Thromb. Diath. Haemorrh. (Stuttgart) 30:299, 1973.
96. Ridout, R. M., Decker, R. S., & Wildenthal, K.: Chloroquine-induced lysosomal abnormalities in cultured fetal mouse heart. J. Mol. Cell. Cardiol. 10:175, 1978.
97. Roberts, J. B., & Breckenridge, A. M.: Drugs affecting autonomic functions. In: Dukes, M. N. G., Ed.: Meyler's Side Effects of Drugs, Vol. 8. P. 304. American Elsevier Publishing Co., Inc., New York, 1975.
98. Roberts, W. C., McAllister, H. A., & Ferrans, V. J.: Sarcoidosis of the heart: a clinicopathologic study of 35 necropsy patients (group I) and review of 78 previously described necropsy patients (group II). Am. J. Med. 63:86, 1977.
99. Rodnan, G. P., McEwen, C., & Wallace, S. L. (Eds.): Primer on rheumatic diseases. J.A.M.A. 224(suppl.):705, 1973.
100. Rona, G., Hiitner, I., & Boutet, M.: Microcirculatory changes in myocardium with particular reference to catecholamine-induced cardiac muscle cell injury. In: Meesen, H., Ed.: Handbuch der allgemoiner Pathologie, Vol. III. Part 7. Mikrozirkulat Microcirculation. Springer-Verlag, Berlin, Heidelberg, 1977.
101. Rosenberg, H. G.: Systemic arterial disease and chronic arsenicism in infants, Arch. Pathol. 97:360, 1974.
102. Rowley, P. T., Kurnick, J., & Cheville, R.: Hereditary haemorrhagic telangiectasia, aggravation by oral contraceptives. Lancet 1:474, 1970.
103. Sanerkin, N. G.: Acute myocardial necrosis in paracetamol poisoning. Br. Med. J. 3:478, 1971.
104. Sarkar, K., & Levine, D. Z.: Repair of the myocardial lesion during potassium repletion of Kaliopenic rats: an ultrastructural study. J. Mol. Cell. Cardiol. 11:1165, 1979.
105. Sartwell, P. E., Masi, A. T., Arthes, F. G., et al: Thromboembolism and oral contraceptives: an epidemiologic case-control study. Am. J. Epidemiol. 90:365, 1969.
106. Schwarts, D. T.: Relation of superior mesenteric artery obstruction to renal hypertension. N. Engl. J. Med. 272:1318, 1965.
107. Siegel, H.: Human pulmonary pathology associated with narcotic and other addictive drugs. Hum. Pathol. 8:55, 1972.

108. Simherkoff, M. S.: Narcotic associated infective endocarditis. In: Kaplan, E. L., Taranta, A. V., Eds.: Infective Endocarditis: An American Heart Association Symposium. p. 46. American Heart Association Monograph, No. 42. American Heart Association, Inc., Dallas, 1977.
109. Smith, P., & Heath, D.: Paraquat. Crit. Rev. Toxicol. 4:411, 1976.
110. Stiehl, P., Weissbach, G., & Schroter, K.: Das nicolan-syndrom. Zur pathogenese and klinik arteriellembolischer penicillinzwischenfalle. Schweiz. Med. Wochenschr. 101:377, 1971.
111. Sullivan, J., Parker, M., & Carson, S. B.: Tissue cobalt content in beer-drinkers myocardiopathy. J. Lab. Clin. Med. 7:983, 1968.
112. Suzuki, T.: Ultrastructural changes of heart muscle in cyanide poisoning. Tohoku J. Exp. Med. 95:271, 1968.
113. Tobon, H.: Malignant hypertension, uremia and hemolytic anemia in a patient on oral contraceptives. Obstet. Gynecol. 40:681, 1972.
114. Tseng, W. P., Chu, H. M., How, W. S., et al: Prevalence of skin cancer in an endemic area of chronic arsenicism in Taiwan. J. Nat. Cancer Inst. 40: 453, 1968.
115. Turcotte, J. G., Kraft, R. O., & Fry, W. J.: Heparin reactions in patients with vascular disease, Arch. Surg. 90:375, 1965.
116. Yater, W. M., & Cahill, J. A.: Bilateral gangrene of feet due to ergotamine tartrate used for pruritus and jaundice. J.A.M.A. 106:1625, 1936.
117. Young, J. R., & Humphries, A. W.: Severe arteriospasm after use of ergotamine tartrate suppositories. J.A.M.A. 175:1141, 1961.

11

The Kidney and Urinary Tract

Wellington Jao

Our day-to-day exposure to drugs and chemicals has put increasing demands on numerous organs of the body. Within these organs, the response of any given cell or tissue to an insult caused by a drug or chemical, or its metabolites is determined by the interplay of many factors. Because the urinary system is involved in eliminating toxic and waste substances, both drugs and chemicals may either generally or selectively damage the system as filtration, secretion, and excretion occur. Exposure of the renal pelvis, ureter, and urinary bladder to a drug or chemical after its filtration may put these organs in almost equal jeopardy.

Although subtle, transient functional or structural changes, or both, may follow exposure of the kidney to some of these substances, these effects may be sufficiently short-lived to go clinically undetected. However, overt nephropathy secondary to drug or chemical exposure occurs frequently and accounts for approximately 5 percent of all nephrology consultations[226] and 20 to 30 percent of all cases of acute renal failure.[34, 254, 338] For example, in Australia and certain Scandinavian countries, analgesic nephropathy alone is responsible for 20 percent of dialysis and transplantation cases,[89] and approximately 8 percent of carcinomas of the renal pelvis are attributable to the abuse of phenacetin alone.[260]

It is important to recognize the potential renal toxicity of such drugs, because the adverse effects of these agents may be preventable by their elimination, modification, or substitution, or adjustments in their dosage, especially in patients with pre-existing renal disease. It is equally important to know that most of the adverse, toxic reactions of the kidney to drugs and chemicals are reversible when the offending agent is discontinued; an understanding of these processes will prevent the unnecessary, invasive, corrective procedures that are potentially more harmful to the patient than is such discontinuation itself.

Toxic nephropathy has been defined as "adverse functional and/or structural changes in the kidney caused by chemical or biologic products that are inhaled, ingested, injected, absorbed, or yield metabolites with an identifiable toxic effect on the kidney."[310] A number of considerations underlie the vulnerability of the kidney to the adverse effects of drugs and chemicals[225]:

1. The kidneys constitute 0.4 percent of the total body weight, and normally receive from 20 to 25 percent of the resting cardiac output. Because of this extremely rich vascular perfusion, the kidney is maximally exposed to any circulating nephrotoxic drugs or toxic solutes.

2. Hypertonicity in the renal medulla, generated by the countercurrent filtration mechanism, enhances the concentration of drugs and their toxic metabolites in the interstitium.

3. The processes of glomerular filtration, tubular resorption, and secretion progressively concentrate nephrotoxic agents within the tubular lumen, thus exposing the tubular epithelial lining cells to high concentrations of such agents.

4. The complexity of metabolic functions of the renal tubular cells, particularly when the reactions within these cells depend upon enzymes containing sulfhydryl groups, makes the kidney susceptible to enzyme inhibitors.

5. The kidney has a high rate of oxygen consumption, making it vulnerable to agents producing cellular anoxia.

6. The changes in the urinary pH will favor

the intraluminal precipitation of certain excreted compounds.

7. The kidney has the largest endothelial cell surface area by weight, making it especially susceptible to damage by immune-complex deposition.

In order to gain a measurable appreciation of the toxic effects of various drugs and chemicals and their manifestations at cellular and tissue levels, within the kidney, both the renal functional changes produced by these insulting agents, and the associated pathologic lesions, should be studied. Functional changes may occur before the morphologic indications of damage are seen; however, histologic data derived from biopsy material frequently provides more useful information than can be gained from a battery of functional tests. It is important to correlate both the physiologic and morphologic data to arrive at the most appropriate diagnosis.

A number of toxic agents of current concern will be discussed in this chapter, using prototype drugs and chemicals as examples. It is, however, beyond the scope of the chapter to discuss the detailed effects of individual nephrotoxic agents, since virtually every drug or chemical has at one time or another been implicated as a cause of renal lesions.

MECHANISMS

Many drugs, chemicals, and metals in common use today are potentially nephrotoxic. Among the best studied drugs are antibiotics of the aminoglycoside group, such as gentamicin, kanamycin, and neomycin; the fungicides, such as amphotericin B; and chemicals such as glycols, carbon tetrachloride, and tetrachloroethylene. Among the best known nephrotoxic heavy metals are mercury, gold, lead, bismuth, and cadmium.

Because the kidney can respond to injury in only a limited number of ways, similar underlying morphologic derangements and clinical manifestations are repeatedly seen in the toxic nephropathies induced by different etiologic agents. An appreciation of the preferential affinity of certain drugs, chemicals, and metals for a particular segment of the nephron may permit the pathologic lesions these substances may produce to be predicted (Fig. 11-1).

The adverse effects of nephrotoxic agents on the kidney may be caused by one or more pathogenetic mechanisms. One mechanism is the direct action of the nephrotoxic agent at the cytoplasmic level, in which direct damage is done to the tubular epithelial cell when a toxic concentration of the agent is reached within the tubular lumen. In addition, some drugs have a preferential affinity for a certain segment of the nephron, such as mercury for the proximal tubular epithelium. Another mechanism is that of hypersensitivity resulting in the formation of antigen-antibody complexes. The endothelial surfaces of the glomerular capillaries, arterioles, and arteries are favorite entrance sites of immune-complexes, and such complexes can be deposited in the renal interstitium. Thus, the deposition of gamma globulin and complement has been demonstrated in the glomeruli of patients with the penicillamine-induced nephrotic syndrome.[213] Inhalation of hydrocarbons may cause dissolution of basement membranes and the induction of antiglomerular basement-membrane antibodies, with the development of extracapillary proliferative or crescentic glomerulonephritis.[28, 202] Hypersensitivity to methicillin can result in the formation of antitubular basement-membrane antibodies and the induction of an acute interstitial nephritis.[45] In some instances, toxic tubular necrosis results in the release of tubular epithelial antigen, which can elicit autoantibody formation and lead to immune complex injury to glomeruli and the renal interstitium. Another indirect mechanism is that caused by such therapeutic agents as potassium-depleting diuretics, which predispose to the development of pyelonephritis and other types of secondary renal damage.

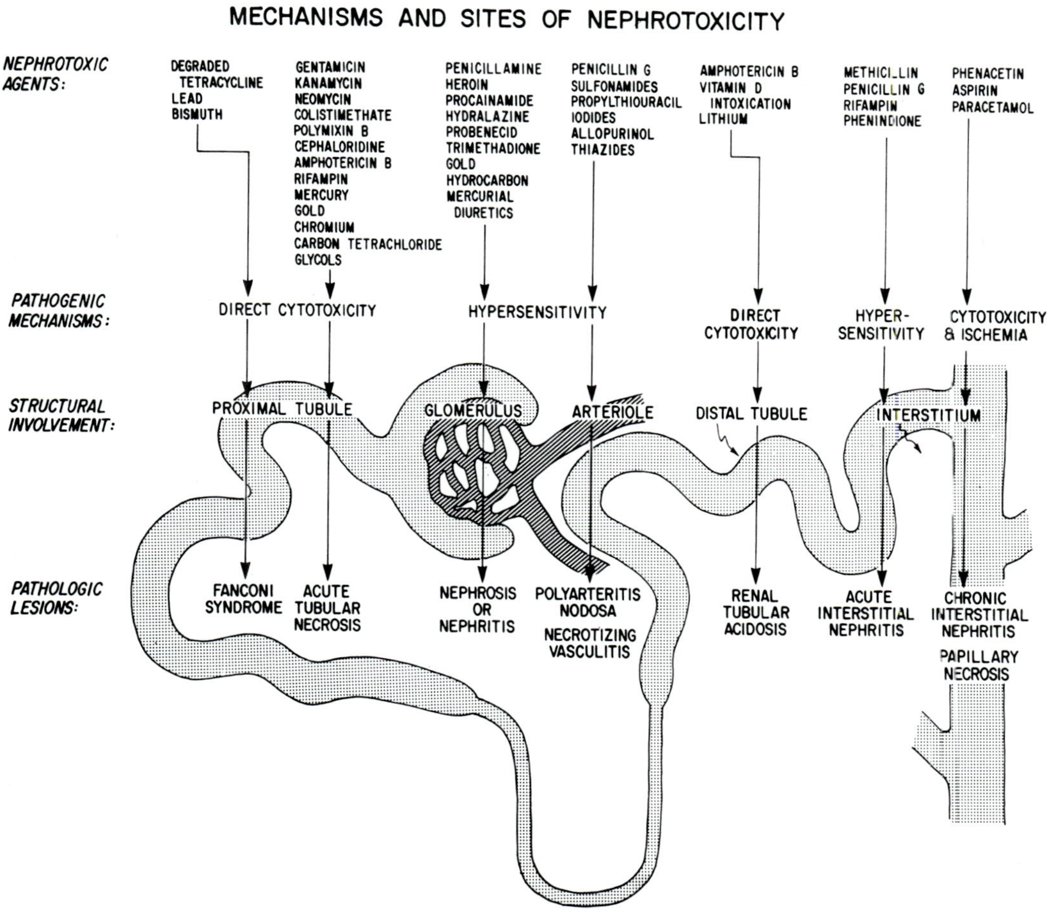

Fig. 11-1. Mechanisms and sites of nephrotoxicity.

Hypersensitivity to drugs may produce a wide spectrum of glomerular lesions, such as minimal change disease (probenecid), membranous glomerulonephropathy (D-penicillamine, gold, trimethadione),[22] acute proliferative glomerulonephritis (hydralazine, procainamide, heroin), and focal glomerulosclerosis (heroin). Such tubular lesions as acute tubular necrosis frequently result from direct toxic damage to the tubular epithelial cells, which is induced mainly by an antibiotic of the aminoglycoside group, heavy metals (particularly mercury and bismuth), or chemicals (especially carbon tetrachloride and ethylene glycol). Chronic diuretic abuse may trigger the development of massive vacuolar lesions in the tubular epithelial cells. Renal tubular obstruction can be produced by the deposition of oxalate crystals derived from methoxyflurane.[15,113] Interstitial diseases such as acute interstitial nephritis—frequently a manifestation of hypersensitivity—are sometimes precipitated by methicillin therapy. Chronic interstitial nephritis can result from the prolonged, excessive ingestion of analgesics, from chronic lead poisoning, or from renal radiation. Vascular complications involving the kidney, such as generalized polyarteritis or hypersensitivity angiitis, may complicate therapy with iodides,[296] propylthiouracil,[240] and the thiazides.[40] Drug-induced uricosuria may lead to the formation of uric acid calculi, with eventual ureteric obstruction; and obstructive uropathy may result from methysergide-induced retroperitoneal fibrosis

A number of drugs and chemical compounds have been identified as causes of malignant tumors in the urinary tract. With most of these, the carcinogenic effects are mediated through metabolites of the drugs or chemical compounds rather than by the parent agent. *N*-hydroxylated metabolites of phenacetin are both nephrotoxic and carcinogenic, and are responsible for the increased incidence of transitional cell carcinoma of the renal pelvis. Beta naphthylamine, a byproduct of many industries, is a potent carcinogen, inducing bladder cancer.

THE KIDNEY

The kidney can conveniently be divided into four major compartments: the glomerular, tubular, interstitial, and vascular. Most nephrotoxic agents interact preferentially in these structural compartments within the kidney to produce a spectrum of renal diseases.

GLOMERULAR DISEASES

A number of drugs, heavy metals, and environmental chemicals have been implicated as the cause of glomerulonephropathy. The diagnosis of this condition frequently depends upon a sequential relationship between the administration of the agent and the onset of renal manifestations. The renal symptoms and glomerular lesions of toxic glomerulonephropathy are usually reversible when the nephrotoxic agent is discontinued[4, 156]; however, a progressive deterioration of renal function ending in renal failure does occur in some cases.[103, 313, 366] Nephrotic syndrome, characterized by edema, massive proteinuria, hypoalbuminemia, and hyperlipidemia has frequently been found in drug-induced glomerulonephropathy[4, 22, 58, 97, 105, 146, 213, 309, 370]; additionally, hematuria and acute renal failure secondary to acute proliferative glomerulonephritis have been associated with exposure to toxins and drugs.[239, 334]

Drug- and chemical-induced glomerulonephropathy encompasses a variety of pathologic changes in the glomerulus (Table 11-1). The nephrotic syndrome associated with probenecid therapy for gout is usually accompanied by minimal changes in the glomeruli[160]; membranous glomerulonephropathy has been found in patients receiving gold therapy for rheumatoid arthritis,[188, 217, 319] and focal glomerulonephritis, with a lupus-like syndrome, has been described in patients taking procainamide.[65, 368] Conversely, a wide spectrum of glomerular histopathology can be induced by a single drug. The glomerular histologic findings in D-penicillamine nephropathy have not been uniform; membranous glomerulonephropathy is the most common lesion,[88, 179, 213] but acute proliferative glomerulonephritis with crescent formation,[239, 334] minimal change disease,[103] and focal glomerulonephritis[98, 158] have also been reported with this drug. Renal biopsies on heroin addicts with the nephrotic syndrome have shown focal and segmental glomerulosclerosis[230]; however, a spectrum of glomerular lesions (such as minimal change disease,[330, 345] membranous glomerulonephropathy,[97, 243] focal membranoproliferative glomerulonephritis,[343, 345] and renal amyloidosis[309]) have also been found. Heroin addicts, may develop an immune-complex glomerulonephritis additionally caused by multiple antigens associated with nonsterile, intravenous narcotic injections.

The exact pathogenic mechanism for most drug- and chemical-induced glomerulonephropathy is not known. In some patients, hypersensitivity to the responsible drug may result in the formation of antigen-antibody complexes. The demonstration of gamma globulin and complement deposited in the glomeruli,[88, 213] and the identification of antibodies to penicillamine,[6] have indicated that the glomerular damage in drug-induced glomerulonephropathy is of the immune-complex type, secondary to sensitization to the drug.

Table 11-1. Histopathologic Findings in the Glomerulus in Drug-associated Glomerulonephritis

Minimal change glomerulonephritis	Membranoproliferative glomerulonephritis
Probenecid[160]	Sulfadiazine silver[275]
D-Penicillamine[103]	Heroin[146, 343, 345]
Heroin[146, 242, 243, 330, 345]	
Mercurial diuretics[298]	Focal glomerulosclerosis
Gold[370]	Heroin[146, 230, 242, 269, 331, 345]
Practolol[105]	Renal amyloidosis
	Heroin[309]
Membranous glomerulonephropathy	
Gold[217, 319, 337, 344]	
D-Penicillamine[88, 179, 213, 326]	
Heroin[97, 243]	
Mercurial diuretics[58]	
Trimethadione[22]	
Focal glomerulonephritis with or without lupus-like syndrome	
Procainamide[65, 147, 367, 368]	
Hydralazine[5, 366]	
D-Penicillamine[98, 158]	
Proliferative glomerulonephritis with crescent formation	
D-Penicillamine[239, 334]	

Certain metallic compounds can act as haptens, combining with a protein to become antigenic and eliciting an antibody response in a susceptible individual. The nephrotoxic effect of mercuric chloride may cause tubular necrosis with focal dissolution of the tubular basement membrane; this results in autoantibody formation against the released tubular antigens, with antigen-antibody complexes depositing in the glomeruli.

Penicillamine-induced Nephropathy

Penicillamine (B,B-dimethylcysteine), a drug of broad pharmacologic activity, has been used to treat a variety of diseases. Its efficacy as a chelating agent has been convincingly demonstrated in the treatment of hepatolenticular degeneration (Wilson's disease),[335] lead poisoning,[132] cystinuria,[60] and rheumatoid arthritis.[178] However, the clinical usefulness of penicillamine has been somewhat compromised by its toxic properties. Renal complications are among the most serious of the adverse effects of this drug,[17, 155, 213, 216, 334] with the incidence of penicillamine-induced nephropathy varying from 0 to 17 percent.[38, 257]

Penicillamine-induced nephropathy has been associated with a variety of renal lesions. Although almost all of the nephrotoxic effects of penicillamine have as a rule been reversed when the drug has been discontinued, a more serious type of renal lesion, characterized by crescentic proliferative glomerulonephritis and leading to uremia and death, has been reported.[239, 334] There have been reports of a total of 34 cases of penicillamine-induced nephropathy, confirmed by studies of renal tissue.[88, 98, 158, 179, 213, 239, 326, 334] Light, electron, immunofluorescence microscopic studies have shown the histopathologic type of the nephropathy to be membranous glomerulonephropathy[88, 179, 213, 326] in 22 patients (65 percent), focal glomerulonephropathy in 7 patients (21 percent),[98, 158] crescentic proliferative glomerulonephritis in 4 patients (12 percent),[239, 334] and minimal change glomerulonephritis in 1 patient (2 percent).[103]

In penicillamine-induced membranous glomerulonephropathy[88, 179, 213, 326] the glomeruli are normocellular and the appearance of the capillary walls ranges from normal to having a slight diffuse thickening (Fig. 11-2). No subepithelial "spike" was evident with the silver methenamine stain. However, electron microscopic examination showed numerous

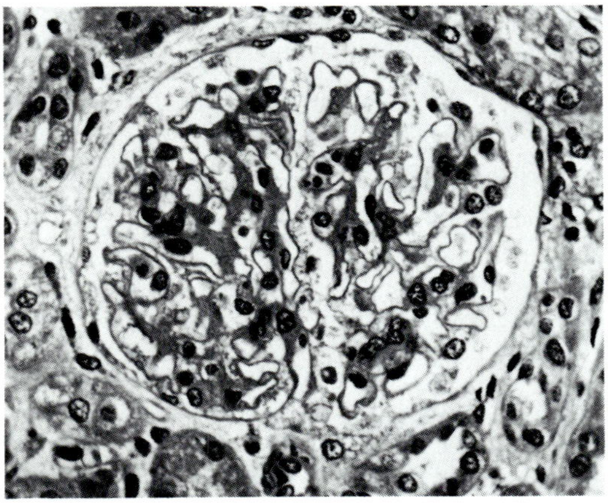

Fig. 11-2. Early or mild membranous glomerulonephropathy from a 20-year-old patient who developed nephrotic syndrome while receiving D-penicillamine therapy for Wilson's disease. H & E, × 400. (Courtesy of Dr. J. R. Manaligod.)

electron-dense granular deposits situated on the epithelial side of the basement membrane (Fig. 11-3), with projections of basement membranes observed between these deposits. Immunofluorescence microscopy demonstrated the presence of finely granular deposits

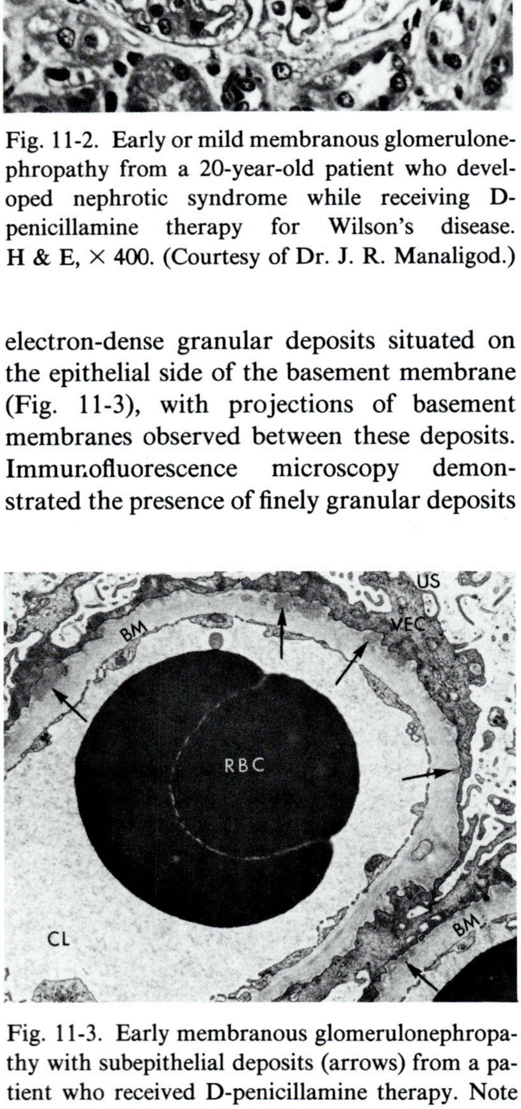

Fig. 11-3. Early membranous glomerulonephropathy with subepithelial deposits (arrows) from a patient who received D-penicillamine therapy. Note the fusion of foot processes of visceral epithelial cells (VEC). BM = basement membrane; RBC = red blood cell; US = urinary space; CL = capillary lumen. Electron micrograph, × 7,300.

of IgG and complement along the peripheral capillary walls.[360]

Heyslett et al.[158] presented three patients with penicillamine-induced nephropathy having histologic features of focal glomerulonephritis. The most profound change was a focal, necrotizing glomerular lesion with a segmental cellular increase. The capillary lumina were obliterated by the proliferation of endothelial cells, and occasionally by the exudation of polymorphonuclear leukocytes. Expansion of the subendothelial spaces and the presence of electron-dense deposits in the subepithelial region were seen electron microscopically.

Sternlieh et al.[334] presented three patients with penicillamine-induced Goodpasture's syndrome. The histologic sections of the patients' kidneys showed proliferation of the parietal and visceral epithelial cells of the glomeruli, with epithelial crescent formation. A granular, interrupted (rather than continuous) staining for IgG and C3 complement was observed along the capillary walls by immunofluorescence microscopy.

The histopathologic features of penicillamine-induced nephropathy resemble the changes that develop in immunologically induced glomerulonephritis produced by the deposition of circulating antigen-antibody complexes.[90] The demonstration of circulating antibodies to penicillamine supports the impression that penicillamine-induced nephropathy is caused by a hypersensitivity reaction, with immune-complex deposition.

Heroin-associated Nephropathy

Numerous reports during the last 10 years have described the clinical and pathologic findings in renal diseases associated with heroin abuse.[146, 331] More than 70 percent of the patients reported experienced a typical nephrotic syndrome, with heavy proteinuria, edema, hypoalbuminemia, and hyperlipidemia; the syndrome was frequently associated with varying degrees of renal insufficiency.[146] Patients were generally unresponsive to corticosteroid, immunosuppressive or anticoagulant therapy,[119,230] and the renal insufficiency was frequently rapidly progressive, terminanting in end-stage renal failure in less than 1 year.[119] A small number of patients experienced mild, acute glomerulonephritis characterized by mild to moderate proteinuria and microscopic hematuria.[331, 343]

A variety of diagnostic terminologies have been used to describe the histologic findings in 152 patients with heroin-associated nephropathy reported in the literature; among the many diagnoses that appear to represent similar lesions, the most commonly described histologic pattern (100 patients) was focal and segmental glomerulosclerosis, with or without proliferative features.[146, 230, 242, 269, 331, 345] With regard to the remaining 52 patients, focal membranoproliferative glomerulonephritis was found in 19 patients,[146, 343, 345] minimal change disease was found in 15,[146, 242, 243, 330, 345] lobular glomerulonephritis was found in 6 patients,[242, 345] renal amyloidosis was found in 4,[309] end-stage kidney disease was found in 5,[16] and membranous glomerulonephropathy was found in 3.[97, 243] Immunofluorescent studies showed granular deposits of IgM, $B1_c$, and $C1_q$ in the glomeruli,[230, 345] principally in the mesangium, but also in the capillary basement membrane in some patients. Electron microscopic examinations revealed changes in patients with the nephrotic syndrome; these included extensive "fusion" of the foot processes of visceral epithelial cells, focal glomerular basement-membrane thickening, mesangial matrix expansion with or without associated cellular increase, and, in approximately 50 percent of the patients, varying amounts of electron-dense deposits, which were most frequently seen in a mesangial position and occasionally in the subendothelial space.[119, 146, 269, 345] Typical subepithelial "humps" were observed in some patients with septicemia; however, these were usually associated with bacterial endocarditis.[345] In renal amyloidosis, characteristic amyloid fibrils were deposited in the mesangial region and on either side of the basement membrane. In

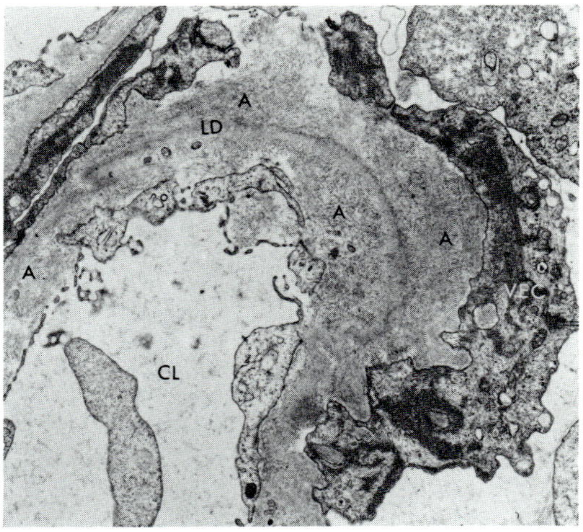

Fig. 11-4. Randomly oriented amyloid fibrils (A) on both sides of lamina densa (LD), causing focal cytoplasmic invagination of the visceral epithelial cells (VEC) in a 48-year-old heroin addict. Electron micrograph, × 6,000.

some capillary loops, the fibrils traversed the ill-defined lamina densa and streamed out into the urinary space (Fig. 11-4).[309]

Evidence suggests that the renal lesions in heroin addicts are of multifactorial etiology and share several of the characteristics of an immune-complex glomerulonephritis.[331] The drug or its associated contaminants may behave as haptens, attaching to a protein to become antigenic and elicit an antibody response.

Probenecid-induced Nephropathy

Both proteinuria and the nephrotic syndrome occur as complications of probenecid (Benemid) therapy for patients with gout[160, 313]; the proteinuria usually recedes when the drug is discontinued.[160] In one study, light microscopic examination of renal biopsy specimens from four patients revealed glomeruli of normal histologic appearance. The diagnosis of minimal change glomerulonephritis was supported by immunofluorescent and electron microscopic examinations of renal tis-

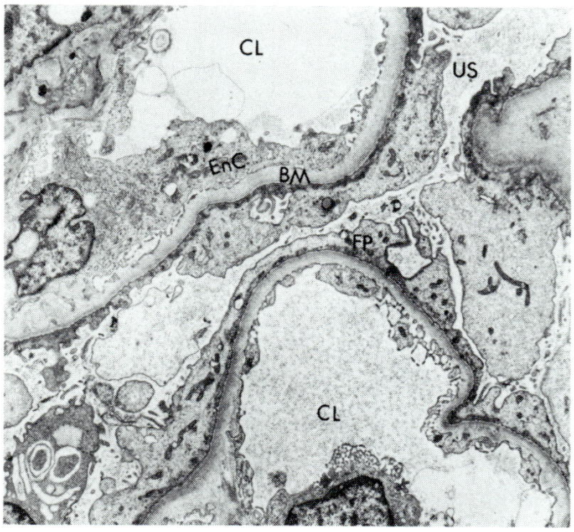

Fig. 11-5. Extensive foot-process fusion (FP) in minimal change glomerulonephritis from a patient who developed nephrotic syndrome while receiving probenecid treatment for gout. BM = basement membrane; CL = capillary lumen; EnC = endothelial cell; US = urinary space. Electron micrograph, × 1,600.

sue from one patient[160]; the examinations showed the complete absence of staining for IgG, IgA, IgM, and complement in the glomeruli. The only abnormality seen by electron microscopy was the fusion of foot processes of visceral epithelial cells (Fig. 11-5).

Lupus Glomerulonephritis

Many drugs have been associated with the induction of a lupus erythematosus-like syndrome[4, 156, 194, 288, 315]; these drugs differ significantly in their chemical structure and pharmacologic action. Their lupus-inducing potential can be activated either through their peculiar pharmacologic properties, or provoked by their elicitation of an allergic reaction, which in turn precipitates the preexisting lupus diathesis.[4] The lupus-like syndrome generally develops only after prolonged administration of the causative drug in high doses[4, 5, 92, 218]; the clinical and laboratory manifestations usually subside when the drug is discontinued.[4, 5, 92, 218]

Drug-induced lupus rarely causes renal disease; when the latter does occur, it is less severe than the renal involvement in the spontaneously occuring systemic lupus erythematosus, and is usually reversible with stoppage of the drug.[4, 92, 218] Among the growing list of drugs considered capable of evoking a lupus-like syndrome, significant renal involvement has been reported to occur with hydralazine,[5, 366] procainamide,[65, 147, 218, 303, 367, 368] trimethadione,[27] quinidine,[377] and D-penicillamine.[156]

Procainamide-induced Lupus Glomerulonephritis. Procainamide, an antiarrhythmic drug, is one of the drugs most commonly implicated as the cause of a lupus erythematosus-like syndrome. Since this association was first described by Ladd in 1962,[214] an increasing number of cases have been reported.[43, 92, 303]

The incidence of a lupus-like syndrome in patients receiving procainamide is estimated to be from 5 to 9 percent[171]; antinuclear antibodies occur regularly in the condition.[145] However, although antibodies to single-stranded DNA may be present, antinative (double-stranded) DNA antibody is not found.[145] On the other hand, hypocomplementemia,[350] circulating anticoagulant,[29] and cryoglobulins[244] have all been reported to occur in procainamide-induced lupus.

The clinical manifestations of procainamide-induced lupus are similar to those of idiopathic systemic lupus erythematosus,[92, 214] but renal involvement is rare compared to the frequency of renal involvement in the latter.[92, 318] Dubois[92] found no clinical renal involvement in 61 patients with a procainamide-induced lupus-like syndrome, and to date, only 6 patients with clinically significant lupus nephritis induced by procainamide have been described.[65, 147, 218, 303, 367, 368] Renal tissues from 4 of these patients were available for histopathologic evaluation,[65, 147, 367, 368] and all showed focal glomerulonephritis.

Light microscopic studies of the glomeruli of the four patients referred to above showed a mild, segmental proliferation of mesangial cells, and an expansion of the mesangial matrix without associated necrosis.[65, 368] Proteinaceous basophilic material, reminiscent of a hematoxylin body, was seen plugging a glomerular capillary.[368] There was focal tubular atrophy and interstitial fibrosis. Electron microscopic examination showed electron-dense, immune-complex deposits in the subendothelial region of the basement membrane and mesangium.[368] Immunofluorescence microscopic examination showed abundant granular deposits of IgG, IgM, and complement, located predominantly in the mesangial regions of the glomeruli[147, 367, 368]; deposits of IgA, IgE, and fibrinogen were also observed.[368]

Hydralazine-induced Lupus Glomerulonephritis. A lupus-like syndrome was reported in 1953 in hypertensive patients receiving hydralazine therapy.[190] Hydralazine is now well recognized as being capable of inducing systemic lupus erythematosus,[4, 5] and an estimated 8 to 13 percent of hypertensive patients receiving this drug develop a lupus-like syndrome[4, 256, 280]; in most instances, the lupus-like syndrome occurs after prolonged therapy with high doses of the drug.[5] The clinical manifestations have been reversed when the drug was discontinued.[4, 5]

Renal involvement, although rare, is more frequent in hydralazine-induced lupus erythematosus than in procainamide-induced lupus erythematosus; Alarcon-Segovia et al.[5] described renal involvement in 10 of 50 patients with the hydralazine-induced lupus-like syndrome. Proteinuria occurred in 8 of these patients; 7 patients had microscopic hematuria. Histologic studies of the kidneys were done on 2 patients; 1 of these showed the extensive changes of diabetic glomerulosclerosis, with wire-loop formations; the other patient had a mild, membranous glomerulonephritis.

Although renal manifestations have usually abated when hydralazine has been discontinued, fatal renal failure, despite stoppage of the drug, was reported in two patients.[366] Unfortunately, no histologic studies of the kidneys were available from these patients.

Hydrocarbon-induced Extracapillary Proliferative Glomerulonephritis

There have been scattered case reports of an association between an exposure to hydrocarbons and the development of extracapillary proliferative glomerulonephritis with crescent formation.[28, 202, 308, 378] Klavis and Dommer,[202] in 1970, described a 26-year-old painter who, within 2 months after a heavy exposure to a gasoline-based paint spray, developed pulmonary hemorrhage and rapidly progressive glomerulonephritis. The two authors were also able to induce similar pulmonary and renal lesions in rats by chronic exposure to gasoline vapors. In 1972, Beirne and Brennan[28] cited 6 of 8 patients with Goodpasture's syndrome who had a previous history of exposure to various hydrocarbon solvents. They postulated that the antibodies to glomerular basement membrane found in these patients could be considered as a secondary response to chemical injury to the pulmonary or renal basement membranes. Scheele et al.[308] cited a 59-year-old man who developed a nephrotic syndrome 40 days after hydrocarbon exposure. Renal biopsy showed a proliferative glomerulonephritis. The renal disease improved with immunosuppressive therapy.

In hydrocarbon-induced extracapillary proliferative glomerulonephritis, a light-microscopic examination of renal tissue shows proliferation of parietal epithelial cells, leading to the formation of an epithelial crescent (Fig. 11-6). The glomerular tuft is compressed and there is collapse of the capillary loops. The tubular lumina occasionally contain aggregates of red blood cells.

In patients with Goodpasture's syndrome, electron microscopic examination reveals a characteristic linear, homogeneously dense deposit along the glomerular capillary basement membranes. Immunofluorescent microscopy shows a diffuse, linear deposit of IgG along the glomerular capillary walls; similar, but weaker and focal linear deposits of IgG are present in Bowman's capsules and the tubular basement membranes.

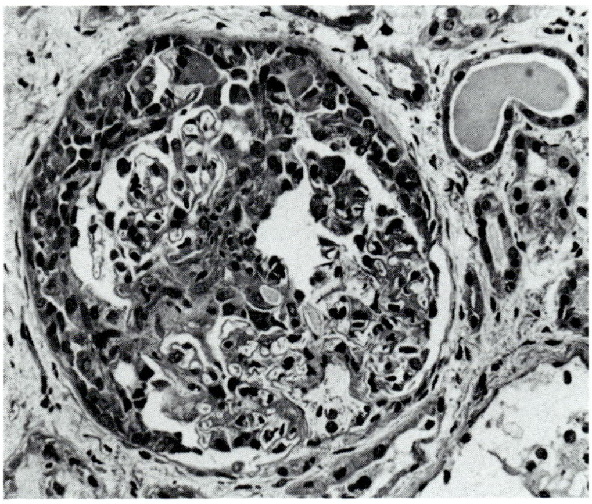

Fig. 11-6. Glomerulus with epithelial crescent formation in a patient with severe oliguria after heavy exposure to hydrocarbon solvent for several months. H & E, × 200.

Gold Nephropathy

Several reports describe membranous glomerulonephropathy in patients receiving gold injections for rheumatoid arthritis (Fig. 11-7).[188, 217, 319, 337] Stunk and Zift[337] described two patients with no apparent glomerular changes evidenced by light microscopy; upon electron microscopy, however, dense granular deposits were observed on the epithelial side of the glomerular basement membrane.

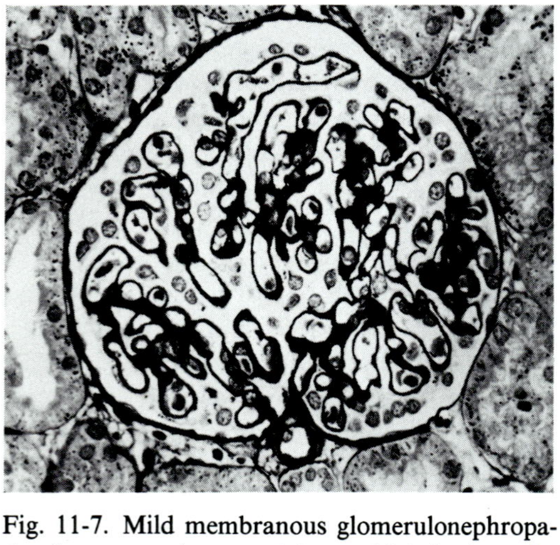

Fig. 11-7. Mild membranous glomerulonephropathy from a patient receiving gold injections for rheumatoid arthritis. Methenamine-silver stain, × 400.

Clusters of gold deposits are observed in proximal tubular cells in experimental studies of gold-induced nephropathy,[375] and are also seen in the human disease.[319] However, the extent of these deposits does not differ in patients with or without the nephrotic syndrome. Immunofluorescence studies demonstrate the presence of granular deposits of IgG and complement fractions along the capillary walls of the glomeruli,[344] suggesting an immune-complex basis for gold-induced glomerulonephritis; similar glomerular lesions have been observed following the therapeutic administration of mercury. The mechanism by which these two metallic compounds induce membranous lesions is unknown; however, attempts have been made to explain the mechanism on the basis of the formation of an immune complex. One possibility is that the metallic compound acts as a hapten, attaching itself to a protein to become antigenic, and then eliciting an antibody response. A second possibility is that the membranous lesions reflect an autologous immune-complex disease, in which substances such as mercuric chloride (and occasionally gold) induce focal dissolution of the tubular basement membrane. This process results in autoantibody formation against released tubular antigens, creating antigen-antibody complexes which are then deposited in the glomeruli.

TUBULAR DISEASES

A variety of nephrotoxic agents or their metabolites have been implicated as causes of functional and structural damage specifically to the renal tubules. Most of these agents effect a direct cytoplasmic poisoning of the tubular cells, chiefly of the proximal convoluted tubules; the results are manifested as an acute tubular necrosis. Other agents induce renal tubular injury indirectly, by provoking water and electrolyte imbalance.

Tubular blockage can be caused by the precipitation of Tamm-Horsfall protein in the tubular lumen, brought about by the combined effects of dehydration and hypertonic contrast media[35]; however, only the commonly offending nephrotoxic agents will be discussed in this section.

Acute Tubular Necrosis

There are numerous causes of tubular necrosis, probably implying that no single factor is all-important in the production of the associated morphologic lesions. The causes of tubular necrosis can be divided into two major groups: nephrotoxic and ischemic, although the absolute distinction between these two groups is not constant. Oliver,[268] using microdissection, demonstrated complete necrosis of the tubular epithelial lining cells, with basement membrane disruption, in ischemic-induced, acute tubular necrosis. In contrast, he also found tubular necrosis with intact basement membranes in nephrotoxin-induced acute oliguria, which leads to the belief that, in nephrotoxin-induced acute tubular necrosis, the preservation of the integrity of basement membranes was a major factor in the orderly growth and regeneration of tubular epithelial cells.

Acute tubular necrosis is by far one of the most common pathologic lesions responsible for the clinical manifestations of acute renal failure secondary to nephrotoxic agents. A growing list of drugs, metals, and chemicals are primarily and potentially toxic to tubular epithelial cells (Table 11-2). The site of the tubular injury may vary, depending on the etiologic agent. Thus, for example, the proximal third of the tubule is affected on potassium chromate poisoning, while the terminal third of the tubule is involved in mercuric chloride and ethylene glycol poisoning.

The probability of nephrotoxicity with some antibiotics, particularly aminoglycosides, appears to be dose related. On the basis of experimental studies,[82] the mechanism of tubular injury with these drugs appears to be an interference, by the drugs, in the energy-producing and oxidative metabolism of mitochondria in the proximal tubular cells. Many heavy metals (such as mercury, lead, bismuth, and cadmium) may be concentrated in the tubular cells, thus interfering with cellular enzymatic activity.[53] Proximal renal tubular cells are particularly vulnerable to acute injury by organic solvents such as carbon tetrachloride[264] and trichlorethylene.[149]

Table 11-2. Nephrotoxic Agents That Cause Acute Tubular Necrosis

Antibiotics	Metals
Aminoglycosides	Mercury
Gentamicin	Lead
Kanamycin	Chromium
Neomycin	Bismuth
Amikacin	Cadmium
Tobramycin	Arsenic
Streptomycin	Uranium
Polymixin B	Silver
Colistimethate	Iron
Cephaloridine	Antimony
Amphotericin B	Copper
Tetracycline	Others
Bacitracin	Sulfonamides
Rifampin	Methoxyflurane
Viomycin	Radioiodinated contrast agents
Organic solvents	Hexadimethrine bromide
Ethylene glycol	Carbamazepine
Carbon tetrachloride	Potassium chloride
Trichloroethylene	

Antibiotic Nephrotoxicity

Nephrotoxicity is a well-known side effect of some antibiotics, particularly in patients with pre-existing renal disease or impaired renal function. There is considerable variation in the frequency and severity of nephrotoxicity arising from the administration of different antibiotics. Among the aminoglycoside antibiotics, neomycin is considered the most toxic to the kidney; kanamycin, gentamicin, and streptomycin are of decreasing toxicity, in that order.[104] On the other hand, among the most commonly used aminoglycoside antibiotics, gentamicin appears to be a "prototype" with regard to nephrotoxicity, in that it has been the most widely studied; the other drugs are known to produce somewhat similar functional and morphologic alterations in the kidney.

Gentamicin Nephrotoxicity. Gentamicin, an effective and widely used aminoglycoside antibiotic, is potentially nephrotoxic. The degree of renal injury with this drug has been variable, ranging from a decrease in the glomerular filtration rate, with mild elevations in serum urea nitrogen and creatinine concentrations or abnormalities in urinary sediments[12, 104] to severe renal insufficiency.[127, 369] Renal functional abnormalities and renal lesions were reversible in most patients when gentamicin therapy was discontinued.[369]

The incidence of gentamicin nephrotoxicity varies from 2 to 14 percent,[12, 57, 161] depending upon the criteria used to assess renal damage. The probability of nephrotoxicity is related to both the dose and duration of gentamicin therapy, and the risk of renal damage is enhanced in the presence of pre-existing renal disease,[362] metabolic acidosis,[174] sodium depletion,[33] and concomitant administration of methoxyflurane[24] or diuretics.[33]

Pathologic changes in the kidney secondary to gentamicin toxicity have been described.[24, 32, 172, 209, 362] The kidney appears enlarged, with edematous cut surfaces. The cortex is pale, with congestion of the medulla. Light-microscopic examination of the glomeruli shows no significant changes, an observation confirmed by electron microscopy. The most profound histologic changes occur in the proximal tubules and are characterized by granular or vacuolar degeneration and necrosis of the proximal tubular epithelial cells.[24] Desquamation of necrotic epithelial cells, with amorphous eosinophilic material, is frequently found in the tubular lumina bordered by intact basement membranes[24] (Fig. 11-8). Scattered foci of dilated proximal tubules lined by flattened epithelium, which frequently shows increased basophilia of the cytoplasm, can be demonstrated. Mitotic figures may sometimes be present, thus indicating focal tubular regeneration. Edema in the interstitial tissue is evidenced by an undue separation of the tubules from each other.

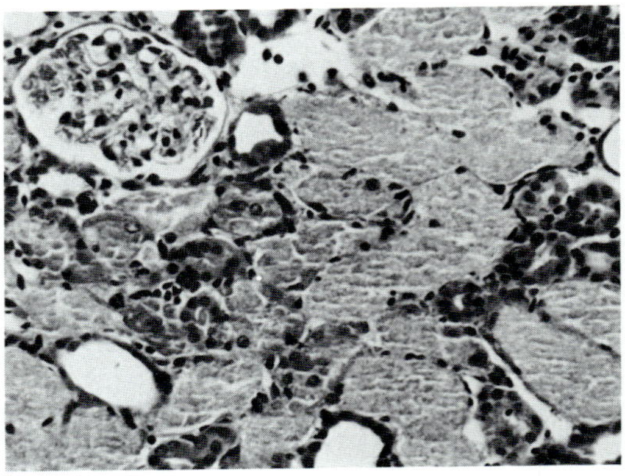

Fig. 11-8. Gentamicin-induced necrosis of the proximal tubular epithelium. H & E, × 190.

Upon electron microscopic examination, most of the proximal tubular epithelial cells in cases of gentamicin nephrotoxicity contain increased numbers of large, irregular lysosomal cytosegresomes, many of which contain prominent myeloid bodies[32, 172, 209] (Fig. 11-9). The mitochondria are swollen, with fragmented cristae, and the cisternae of the rough endoplasmic reticulum are distended. In severely damaged tubules, disintegrated cells,

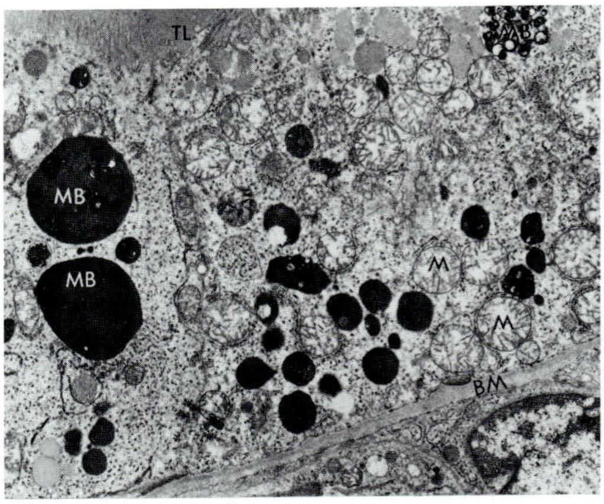

Fig. 11-9. Portion of proximal tubule exhibiting numerous lysosomal cytosegresomes with myeloid bodies (MB) from gentamicin-induced acute renal failure. There is swelling of the mitochondria (M). TL = tubular lumen; BM = basement membrane. Electron micrograph, × 5,500.

with disorganized and degenerated organelles, are seen. The tubular basement membrane remains intact in most instances.

The increased numbers of large lysosomal cytosegresomes in the proximal tubular epithelial cells may in cases of gentamicin nephrotoxicity indicate that gentamicin-induced focal cytoplasmic injury results in an increased rate of autophagic activity[172]; the pathologic significance and the origin of the intralysosomal myeloid bodies is not known. Hruban et al.[173] speculated that myeloid bodies represent a delay in the degradation of membrane material, primarily smooth endoplasmic reticulum, in autophagic vacuoles. Others have suggested that myeloid bodies may indicate the lysosomal isolation of gentamicin-bound cytoplasmic structures as a cellular mechanism for degrading toxic substances[172]; these bodies have been observed in the cells of many tissues of experimental animals following the administration of various drugs.[142, 173] Currently, myeloid bodies are believed to be histologic markers of drug administration and cellular uptake.[34, 321] The demonstration of myeloid bodies in the urine of patients with acute renal failure who are receiving gentamicin may suggest the diagnosis of gentamicin-induced nephrotoxicity.[189]

Kanamycin Nephrotoxicity. Renal tubular toxicity occurs in from 10 to 20 percent of patients receiving kanamycin at a dose of 25 to 50 mg/kg/day[376]; the toxicity is usually manifested clinically by proteinuria, microscopic hematuria, cylindruria, and transient azotemia. Acute renal insufficiency caused by kanamycin is reversible in most instances when the drug is discontinued, and renal function returns to normal within 6 weeks. However, an occasional acute renal failure secondary to extensive tubular necrosis has been reported.[310] Kanamycin nephrotoxicity occurs more frequently in elderly patients or those with underlying renal disease.[37] Increased kanamycin nephrotoxicity has been found in patients receiving prior therapy with streptomycin or viomycin,[310] and in patients with sodium depletion.[169]

Neomycin Nephrotoxicity. Neomycin, an aminoglycoside antibiotic that is used primarily as a topical antibiotic, can be extremely nephrotoxic when given orally. In patients with renal dysfunction, high oral doses of neomycin may induce audiotoxicity and nephrotoxicity.[144] Patients who are inadvertently given neomycin parenterally develop cylindruria, proteinuria, and azotemia, which progress to acute renal failure.[84, 99]

Neomycin causes vacuolar degeneration and necrosis of the proximal tubular epithelium, and exfoliated cellular casts in the lumina; additionally, the peritubular basement membranes may become thickened.[99]

Tobramycin Nephrotoxicity. Tobramycin, another aminoglycoside antibiotic, is excreted almost entirely by the kidneys. A dose adjustment should be made if there is renal impairment. Tobramycin renal toxicity is characterized by cylindruria, proteinuria, and progressive azotemia.

Administration of tobramycin to animals has produced pathologic changes in the proximal tubules identical to those seen with gentamicin. The incidence of tobramycin nephrotoxicity is low; it occurs in only 1 to 2 percent of patients treated with the drug.[263]

Polymyxin B and Colistimethate Nephrotoxicity. The nephrotoxicity of polymyxin B is characterized by proteinuria, cylindruria, cellular casts, and a loss of urine-concentrating ability[12, 251]; at a polymyxin B dose level of 3 mg/kg/day, azotemia and decrement of the glomerular filtration rate occur in patients with previously normal renal function.[180] The toxicity is dose related, and polymyxin B accumulates if renal function is impaired.[180, 276] Degeneration and necrosis of the tubular epithelial cells may occur at a dose of 5 mg/kg.[251] The renal lesions are usually reversible when therapy is discontinued, but renal function may be impaired permanently.[12]

Colistimethate, a sulfomethyl derivative of polymyxin E, has become popular as an alternative to polymyxin B. The incidence of colistimethate nephrotoxicity is estimated at 20 percent[207]; the nephrotoxicity, manifested by proteinuria, hematuria, cylindruria, and azotemia is more likely to occur in patients with pre-existing renal diseases[207] and in those receiving a cephalosporin concurrently than in others. As a rule, renal damage is reversible when the drug is discontinued[12, 289]; however, acute renal failure[48] and death[304] have been reported. Gross examination of the kidneys reveals cortical pallor and medullary congestion. Histologic examination reveals irregular dilatation of tubules, cellular casts, and necrosis of the tubular epithelial cells.[286, 289, 304]

Cephalosporin Nephrotoxicity. The excretion of cephalosporins predominantly involves a renal tubular mechanism. Cephaloridine is the most nephrotoxic of this group of drugs in common clinical use,[46]; its nephrotoxicity is thought to be secondary to the high concentration of cephloridine in the proximal tubular fluid and in tubular cells in patients treated with this antibiotic.[347] Dose-related tubular injury occurs frequently with cephaloridine, although renal toxicity from cephalothin occurs only after a high dose of this drug, or occurs in patients with a pre-existing renal disease.[106]

Cephalosporin nephrotoxicity is typically manifested by proteinuria, hematuria, cylindruria, and azotemia; the damage is usually reversible when the drug is discontinued.[277] Reports have claimed a synergistic effect in the renal toxicity of cephalothin in combination with other nephrotoxic antibiotics, notably gentamicin,[203] and tobramycin.[201] However, a combination of cephalothin and gentamicin, given to experimental animals, failed to show a potentiation of renal toxicity clinically or greater tubular damage histologically than was apparent in those animals given gentamicin alone.[157]

Histologic examination of cephalosporin-damaged renal tissue revealed cytoplasmic swelling, vacuolization, and necrosis of proximal tubular epithelial cells. Interstitial edema was associated with a variable, mononuclear cellular infiltrate.[205] The glomeruli and vessels were normal.[203, 277]

The results of electron microscopic studies of cephaloridine-induced renal damage are available from published experimental work. These show an abnormality in the proximal tubular brush border within 1 hour following cephaloridine administration; this was followed by the loss of microvilli, a disorganization of lateral membrane interdigitations, mitochondrial swelling, and necrosis.[320] The middle segment of the proximal tubules of the outer renal cortex was the most damaged area; however, the tubular basement membrane was preserved.[14]

Amphotericin B Nephrotoxicity. Amphotericin B is a polyene antifungal agent whose major adverse side effect is a nephrotoxicity that frequently requires the interruption of therapy. A large study in patients treated with amphotericin B documented dose-related renal abnormalities in 25 percent of patients receiving the drug.[56] Cylindruria frequently heralds amphotericin B-induced renal toxicity, and may be accompanied by hematuria, pyuria, mild proteinuria, and azotemia. The maximum concentrating capacity of the kidney is frequently reduced during therapy with the drug, but renal function can revert to normal when amphotericin treatment is discontinued[371]; however, progressive, irreversible renal failure with severe uremia has been reported.[339] Reversible but profound hypokalemia may occur because of excessive renal losses of potassium in patients receiving amphotericin,[237] and further damage to the renal tubules may result from the hypokalemia per se. Renal tubular acidosis, primarily of the distal type, is also well documented with amphotericin B.[241]

On histologic examination, the predominant changes in amphotericin B nephrotoxicity are those of tubular necrosis and degeneration involving both the proximal and distal renal tubules,[365] and deposition of calcium within the tubules and interstitium[56, 163, 365] (Fig. 11-10). The tubular lumina are frequently plugged with necrotic cellular debris, proteinaceous casts, and calcium material; the tubular basement membranes are frequently thickened.[361]

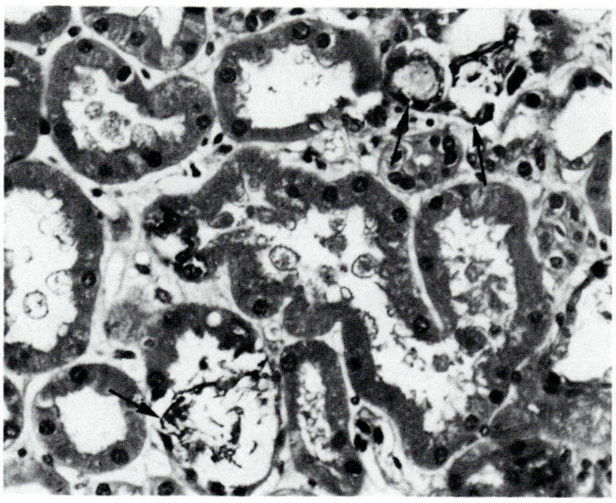

Fig. 11-10. Calcium deposits (arrows) in the tubular lumina from a patient receiving amphotericin B therapy for systemic fungal infection. H & E, × 200.

Tetracycline Nephrotoxicity. Tetracycline causes progressive azotemia, hyperphosphaturia, and acidosis[95] in patients with pre-existing renal disease. Ingestion of degraded tetracycline has been associated with the development of a reversible Fanconi syndrome[121,124,232] characterized by a proximal tubular defect leading to glycosuria, aminoaciduria, phosphaturia, hypercalciuria, hypokalemia, hypouricemia, acidosis, polyuria, and polydypsia. These effects are most likely to be caused by epianhydrotetracycline and anhydrotetracycline, which are produced by the degradation of tetracyclines when the outdated drug is exposed to heat, high humidity, and low pH.[121] The administration of nondegraded demethylchlortetracycline has led to nephrogenic diabetes insipidus.[64]

Histopathologic examination of biopsied renal tissues in cases of tetracycline nephrotoxicity has revealed vacuolization and hydropic degeneration of the proximal and distal convoluted tubular epithelium.[232] The glomeruli have shown segmental mesangial hypercellularity with irregular thickening of the capillary basement membranes.[124]

Bacitracin Nephrotoxicity. The apparent toxic effects of bacitracin on the renal tubules have limited the use of this drug to topical application.[247] Parenteral administration of the drug involves a high risk of nephrotoxicity resulting in the development of proteinuria, cylindruria, azotemia, and occasionally acute oliguria, which can cause death.[130] Histologic examination of the kidney in cases of bacitracin nephrotoxicity shows necrosis and degeneration of the cells of the proximal and distal convoluted tubules, with tubular obstruction by necrotic cellular debris.[12]

Rifampin Nephrotoxicity. Rifampin, an antituberculous agent, has been incriminated in the precipitation of acute oliguric renal failure in patients receiving intermittent therapy.[204,262] Most of the affected patients have oliguria, azotemia, hematuria, and cylindruria, and follow a typical course of reversible, acute renal failure with return of renal function to normal.[59,107]

Histopathologic examination of renal tissue from patients with rifampin nephrotoxicity reveals varying degrees of finely granular or vacuolar degeneration and necrosis of the proximal tubular epithelial cells, and interstitial edema with mononuclear cellular infiltrates. The glomeruli are normal. Immunofluorescent staining for IgG, IgA, IgM, Bl_c, and fibrinogen is negative[59,204]; however, rifampin-dependent antibodies have been demonstrated in the serum,[204] thus favoring a a hypersensitivity reaction as the mechanism for the nephrotoxicity produced by this drug.

Heavy Metals

Heavy metals tend to accumulate in the kidney and cause a variety of morphologic and functional alterations. Metals are excreted through the kidney in two ways: (1) metals filtered by the glomerulus may be reabsorbed and concentrated in the tubular cells; or (2) metals may be secreted directly into the tubular fluid by active transport across tubular epithelial cells from peritubular capillaries. These two processes enhance the vulnerability of tubular epithelial cells to the nephrotoxic effects of heavy metals.[135]

Mercury Nephrotoxicity. In general, inorganic compounds of mercury (mercury chloride) have a more toxic effect on parenchymal cells than do organic mercurials (methyl mercury chloride and methyl mercury dicyandiamide). Elementary mercury vapor is readily oxidized to ionic mercury after it is inhaled, and behaves biologically in a manner similar to mercury chloride.[135] Oral intake of mercury usually occurs in cases of suicide or as a result of the accidental contamination of food and drink.

The nephrotoxicity of mercury and its compounds has been well documented both clinically and experimentally.[126,310] Depending on the biochemical form of the metal and the mode of exposure to it, two major types of renal lesions can occur. The first type, in which there is massive damage to the proximal convoluted tubules resulting in acute renal failure, is characteristic in acute mercury poisoning; the kidneys are grossly enlarged, with a pale and swollen cortex and congested medulla (Fig. 11-11). By light microscopy, the proximal convoluted tubules show extensive cellular necrosis, with the lumina being filled with eosinophilic granular cytoplasmic debris (Fig. 11-12); the basement membranes of the tubules remain intact. Cellular casts are also seen in the ascending limbs, distal convoluted tubules, and collecting tubules. Focal calcification may occur in the proximal convoluted tubules, and interstitial edema is evident. The glomeruli appear normal.

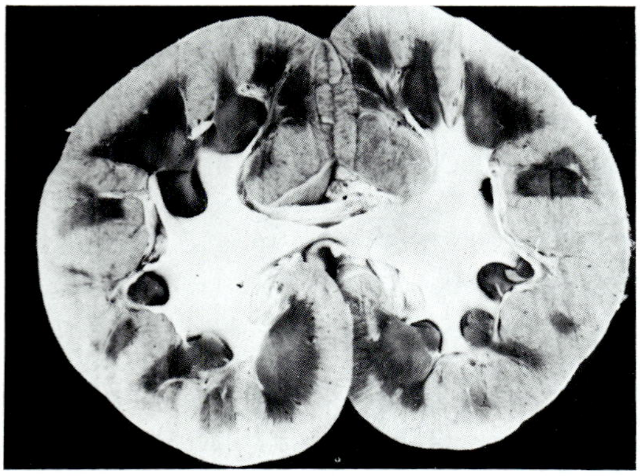

Fig. 11-11. Enlarged kidney from a patient with mercuric chloride poisoning accompanied by anuria. Note the pale, swollen cortex and dark, congested medulla.

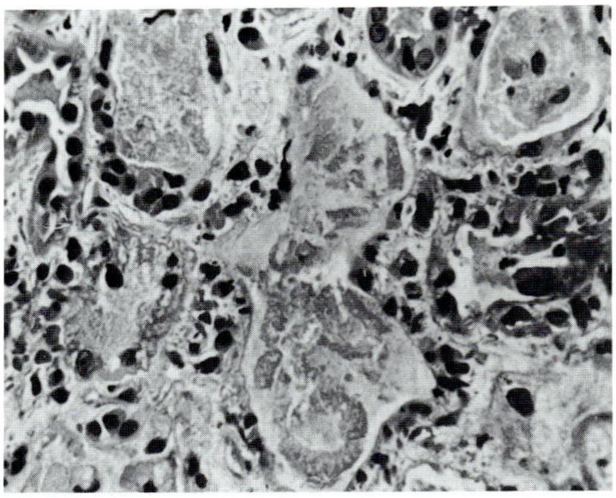

Fig. 11-12. Focal necrosis of the proximal tubules from mercuric chloride poisoning. Note that the basement membrane is intact. H & E, × 365.

Electron microscopic examination of the proximal tubular epithelium in cases of mercury poisoning shows changes ranging from complete cellular disintegration (Fig. 11-13) to cellular damage characterized by the loss of brush borders, fragmentation, disruption of plasma membranes, dispersion of ribosomes, vesiculation, disruption of the endoplasmic reticulum, and swelling of the mitochondria with dense granular deposits.

If the patient survives the period of acute

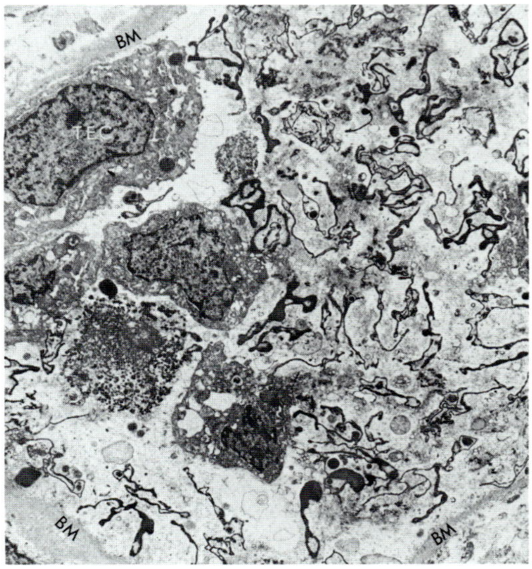

Fig. 11-13. Extensive disintegration of tubular epithelial cells in mercuric chloride poisoning. Electron micrograph, × 2,700.

renal failure, regeneration of the tubular epithelial cells occurs along the intact basement membrane.[310]

The second type of renal lesion induced by mercury and its compounds—characterized clinically by a nephrotic syndrome[298]—occurs frequently in persons chronically exposed to elemental mercury vapor.[192] The main lesion usually consists of a membranous glomerulonephropathy, with electron-dense deposits in the subepithelial region of the glomerular basement membranes.[58] The pathogenesis of this lesion is not well understood, but experimental studies suggest an immune-complex disease.[20]

Repeated administration of mercuric chloride to rats is followed by the development of antibodies directed against the tubular basement membrane and renal tubular epithelial antigen. This is followed by the formation of antigen-antibody complexes, with the subsequent deposition of these complexes in the glomerular basement membrane.[193]

Lead Nephropathy. Lead nephropathy is manifested clinically as tubular dysfunction with aminoaciduria, glycosuria, proteinuria, casts, and an increased excretion of lead, delta aminolevulinic acid, coproporphyrin, and urobilinogen in the urine.

Two distinct histopathologic patterns accompany lead nephropathy[135, 138]; the first pattern has been ascribed to an acute but reversible effect of lead toxicity. This pattern consists of morphologic alterations in the epithelial cells of the proximal convoluted tubules and loops of Henle. These alterations, including the formation of inclusion bodies, are found predominantly in the intranuclear region; but may occasionally be observed in the cytoplasm. The inclusion bodies are variable in size and shape, and are dense, eosinophilic, and acid fast.[41] Large inclusion bodies may fill the nucleus entirely, or may be surrounded by a "halo." Desquamated cells with intranuclear inclusion bodies may also be seen in the urinary sediment.[215] The protein that binds with the lead to form the inclusion bodies is thought to be nonhistone chromosomal protein that results from the degradation and restructuring of a pre-existing intranuclear protein.[136] It is also possible that the protein is synthesized in the cytoplasm, becomes bound to lead, and is transported to and polymerized in the nucleus.

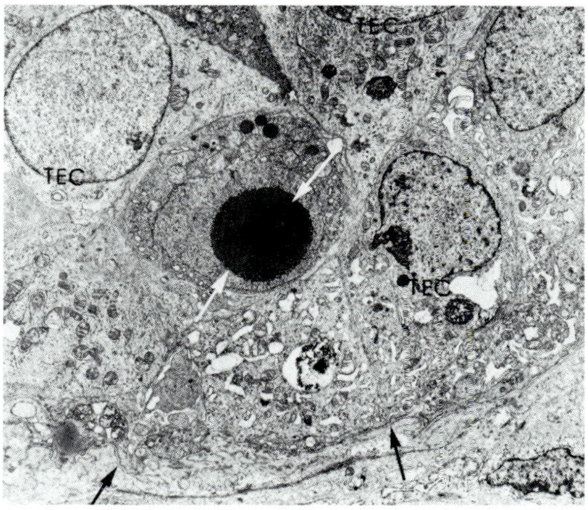

Fig. 11-14. Tubular epithelial cell with intranuclear inclusion body (white arrows) in lead nephropathy. The tubular basement membrane (black arrows) is intact. TEC = tubular epithelial cell. Electron micrograph, × 3,150.

Electron microscopy shows that the inclusion bodies in lead nephropathy consist of a dense central core, with a circumferential fibrillary meshwork that varies considerably in thickness (Fig. 11-14). The intranuclear inclusion bodies—which may be induced in cultured renal cells by exposure to lead[357]—may persist for a long period. The mitochondria in the proximal tubular epithelial cells show swelling with a severe distortion of cristae; multiple, large, irregular osmiophilic densities may be seen between the cristae. The mitochondria isolated from the kidneys of lead-intoxicated experimental animals have been shown to have impaired respiratory and phosphorylative functions.[137] The resultant impaired energy metabolism in proximal tubular epithelial cells may be responsible for the aminoaciduria, glycosuria, and phosphaturia found in acute lead nephropathy.

The second pattern of lead nephropathy is frequently observed in chronic lead exposure in humans; it is characterized by the histologic appearance of an interstitial nephritis. This type of lead nephropathy can be produced in experimental animals by feeding high doses of lead for more than a year[135]; it may also be found in humans who have had excessive lead exposure for more than 3 years. The interstitium shows proliferation of fibrous connective tissue accompanied by the infiltration of mononuclear leucocytes. The tubules show focal atrophy and dilatation. However, intranuclear inclusion bodies are rarely identified in chronic lead nephropathy.[135] The glomeruli may be normal or near normal, with focal and segmental mesangial accentuation and thickening of the capillary basement membrane. In end-stage kidney disease, the glomeruli are sclerotic.

Chromium Nephrotoxicity. Chromium is absorbed primarily through inhalation. Once absorbed, it is transported by the red blood cells[143] and accumulates primarily in highly vascularized organs such as the lungs, kidneys, liver, and spleen.[354] Chromium is excreted predominantly through the kidneys.[74]

Chromium is heavily used in the metal and galvanizing industries. Most acute chromium poisoning—usually among workers exposed to the metal—is accidental. Renal chromium toxicity is manifested clinically by acute renal failure; histologic study of biopsied renal tissue reveals focal degeneration and necrosis of the epithelial cells; other tubular cells have hyperchromatic nuclei and a basophilic cytoplasm indicative of regenerative changes. Mitoses are occasionally seen. The basement membranes of the tubules appear intact. There is mild interstitial edema associated with mononuclear cell infiltrates.[354]

Electron microscopic analysis of renal tissue in cases of chromium nephrotoxicity reveals focal swelling of proximal tubular epithelial cells, with blunting of the microvilli. There are unevenly swollen mitochondria and fragmentation of the mitochondrial cristae. Variably sized vacuoles, lysosomes, and autophagosomes are seen (Fig. 11-15). The cells in some tubules are completely disintegrated, with nuclear dissolution, and there is extrusion of degenerated cytoplasmic organelles into the tubular lumen. The interstitial tissue is edematous, with widely separated collagen fibers. No glomerular lesions are evident. Similar histopathologic changes are seen in tissues from experimental animals with chromium-induced acute tubular necrosis.[112]

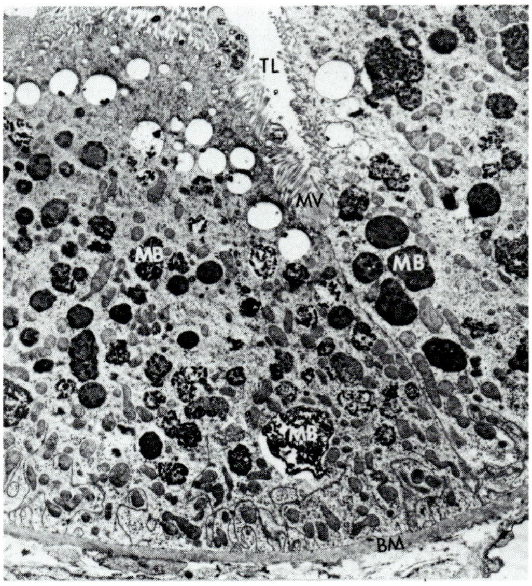

Fig. 11-15. Portion of proximal tubular epithelium from a 63-year-old man with renal failure from chromium poisoning. There are various-sized autophagosomes with myeloid bodies (MB). MV = microvilli; TL = tubular lumen; BM = basement membrane. Electron micrograph, × 4,140. (Courtesy of Dr. J. R. Manaligod.)

Bismuth Nephropathy. Bismuth has been used to treat a variety of ailments, including syphilis. Acute bismuth toxicity usually arises from accidental poisoning; the parenteral administration of bismuth compounds causes acute renal failure, while oral intake of this metal results in acute renal failure or the nephrotic syndrome.[349]

Bismuth nephropathy is usually manifested clinically as hyposthenuria, glycosuria, and proteinuria. Pathologically, degeneration and necrosis of the proximal tubular cells are seen in acute bismuth poisoning; intracytoplasmic and intranuclear inclusion bodies in the proximal tubular epithelial cells are seen in as many as 86 percent of patients with chronic bismuth ingestion.[25] These inclusion bodies are brownish-yellow and refractile, stain positively with the periodic acid Schiff or Ziehl-Neelson stains,[355] and are composed of a bismuth-protein complex. The bismuth content of the inclusion bodies has been confirmed by x-ray microanalysis of tissue sections.[110] Remarkably, bismuth inclusion bodies have been found at postmortem 30 years after a course of bismuth therapy.[26]

Cadmium Nephropathy. Cadmium can be extremely toxic because of its cumulative properties.[117] The biologic half life of this metal is long—more than 20 years; therefore, practically all cadmium ingested or inhaled is retained in the body. Exposure to cadmium is widespread because it is a contaminant in air and food.[117] The preferential accumulation of cadmium in the kidney is thought to be related to its affinity for metallothionein, a low-molecular-weight protein in the cytoplasm of renal tubular cells.[67] The cadmium-metallothionein complex in the extracellular compartment is thought to be the major nephrotoxin in cadmium-induced nephropathy.[68]

The incidence of proteinuria in chronic industrial exposure to cadmium is as high as 80 percent[116]; associated features are glycosuria, aminoaciduria, and impairment of the urinary concentrating ability.[116] The renal histopathology in chronic cadmium toxicity is inconsistent, ranging from indistinct renal lesions[115] to vacuolar degeneration with lipid droplets in the proximal tubular cells.[66]

Electron microscopic studies of experimental animals treated with cadmium reveal, on the luminal surface of the proximal tubular cells, blebs containing numerous vacuoles, swollen mitochondria, a focal proliferation of smooth endoplasmic reticulum, microbodies, and intranuclear inclusions. Flattening of the basal infolding is also seen in some proximal tubular cells.[66] Although disruption of cellular membranes, with the extrusion of degenerated organelles, is seen 24 hours after cadmium administration, the distal tubular cells remain intact; the lumina contain proteinaceous and cellular debris.[66, 68, 267]

Organic Solvents

Ethylene Glycol Nephrotoxicity. Ethylene glycol, a component of antifreeze, is one of the most widely known and most toxic glycols. It is rapidly metabolized to oxalic acid after ingestion. Nephrotoxicity is brought about by the direct cytotoxic effect of ethylene glycol on the tubular epithelial cells, causing tubular necrosis, and by the production and deposition of masses of birefrigent, sheaf-shaped calcium oxalate crystals in the renal tubules.[118] These effects result in a focal destruction of the tubular epithelial cells, dilatation of the tubules proximal to the site of obstruction, and a mononuclear cell response in the interstitium.

Carbon Tetrachloride Nephrotoxicity. Carbon tetrachloride is widely used as an industrial solvent and household cleaning agent; alcohol potentiates the nephrotoxic and hepatotoxic effects of carbon tetrachloride.[182] The clinical manifestations of renal involvement by carbon tetrachloride are usually insidious and accompanied by oliguria, proteinuria, hematuria, and crystalluria.

Carbon tetrachloride has a direct toxic effect on the proximal tubule.[183] Histologically, in the early stage of the nephrotoxicity, the proximal tubules contain sudanophilic droplets in the basal portion of the tubular epithelial cells. As the disease progresses, coagulation necrosis involving the proximal tubules and limbs of Henle's loop can be observed. Epithelial and red blood cell casts are also seen in the tubular lumina. Leucine, oxalate, and uric acid crystals are sometimes observed. The glomeruli, however, are normal.

Trichloroethylene Nephrotoxicity. Trichloroethylene, another nephrotoxic hydrocarbon, has been reported to cause acute renal failure and hepatic insufficiency following excessive sniffing of a spot remover.[18, 222] The nephrotoxicity is manifested by oliguria, proteinuria, and sometimes hematuria. Histologically, there is degeneration of the epithelial cells of the proximal convoluted tubules.

Other Tubulotoxins

A number of drugs and chemicals have caused acute tubular injury through an undetermined pathogenic mechanism. High doses of anticoagulant hexadimethrine bromide have been followed by acute tubular necrosis[153]; methotrexate administration has been associated with the development of azotemia and proximal tubular necrosis[76]; carbamazepine, an anticonvulsant, has occasionally caused acute renal failure[265]; uranium causes necrosis of the pars recta of the proximal tubules similar to that caused by mercury[42]; occupational exposure to arsine gas is frequently accompanied by acute tubular necrosis[255]; thioacetamide induces necrosis of the proximal tubular cells in rats[21]; lithium salts accumulate in the renal papilla, causing injury to the collecting ducts and distal tubules.[101]

Iodinated contrast media for radiographic study of the vasculature of the kidneys and gallbladder have been implicated in causing acute renal failure, especially in patients with dehydration, pre-existing renal disease, or both.[9, 332] The renal failure is secondary either to necrosis of both the proximal and distal tubules, with calcium oxalate crystals being deposited within the tubular lumina,[317] or to the intratubular precipitation of Tamm-Horsfall protein.[35] Sulfonamide- and methoxyflurane-induced nephropathy warrants a brief discussion.

Sulfonamide Nephropathy. A wide spectrum of renal lesions is induced by the sulfonamides. The most frequent of these is obstructive uropathy produced by the crystallization of sulfonamides in various parts of the urinary tract[284]; among the sulfonamide group of drugs, sulfapyridine, sulfathiazole, and sulfadiazine have been frequently implicated as causes of this form of renal damage.[91] The solubility of sulfonamides in the urine depends on the drug concentration, the state of dehydration, the urinary pH, renal function,[302] and the solubility properties of the particular drug and its acetylated derivatives.[91] Toxicity is manifested as hematuria, crystalluria, pyuria, cylindruria, azotemia and, occasionally, renal colic. Examination of the urinary sediment shows characteristic crystalline patterns for certain types of sulfonamides.[219] A histologic examination of the renal tissue reveals crystalline deposits in the distal tubules; these are accompanied by focal swelling, degeneration, and necrosis of the tubular epithelial cells. The interstitium frequently shows mononuclear cell infiltration.

Hypersensitivity reactions to the sulfonamides have allegedly induced renal lesions resembling acute interstitial nephritis,[299] focal granulomatous interstitial nephritis, periarteritis nodosa,[220] and focal glomerulonephritis with necrotizing features.[114] The nephrotic syndrome has also occurred after topical sulfonamide therapy.[275]

Methoxyflurane Nephropathy. Methoxyflurane (Penthrane) is a nonexplosive, volatile, fluorinated anesthetic agent. It has been incriminated as a cause of postoperative renal failure characterized by transient vasopressin-resistant polyuria and hyposthenuria.[80, 113] The syndrome of polyuric renal failure was observed in 16 percent of 274 patients anesthetized with methoxyflurane.[80, 281] Of a small number of patients dying from renal failure after surgery under methoxyflurane anesthesia, numerous calcium oxalate crystals were found in the renal parenchyma[154, 285]; in some of these patients the precipitation of the oxalate crystals in the kidney was extensive but, by itself, was not considered a sufficient morphologic alteration to account for the development of renal failure. The functional impairment of the kidney in methoxyfluorane nephropathy is probably mediated mainly by the acute, toxic effect of inorganic fluoride resulting from the metabolism of the anesthetic.[80, 340] A dose-related increase in plasma and urinary inorganic fluoride and oxalic acid, which are metabolites of methoxyflurane, correlates with the degree of renal functional and structural changes.[234]

The mechanism for the renal toxicity of inorganic fluoride is not clearly understood, but is probably related to its potent inhibitory effects on many enzyme systems, particularly those involved with cellular energy transfer mechanisms.[372] The inhibitory effect of inorganic fluoride on adenyl cyclase, which is an intermediary in the action of antidiuretic hormone,[271] may provide a partial explanation for the polyuria produced by methoxyflurane.

The gross appearance of the kidney in methoxyflurane nephropathy is usually normal, with a slight increase in renal weight. A light-microscopic examination of the kidney shows many sheaflike crystals of calcium oxalate in the lumina of the cortical tubules[15]; the crystals range from transparent and colorless to brown-tinged, and are primarily deposited in the proximal tubules, but occasionally also in Henle's loop. A foreign-body giant-cell reaction to the crystal is rarely demonstrated[113] (Fig. 11-16). The tubular epithelium generally appears well preserved, and degeneration or necrosis of epithelial cells is rarely encountered. Scattered foci of interstitial fibrosis are associated with a mild, chronic inflammatory cellular infiltrate. The glomeruli are normal and no arterial alteration can be seen.

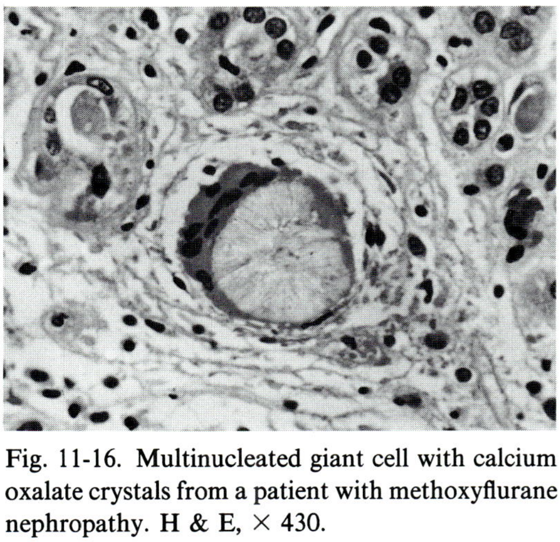

Fig. 11-16. Multinucleated giant cell with calcium oxalate crystals from a patient with methoxyflurane nephropathy. H & E, × 430.

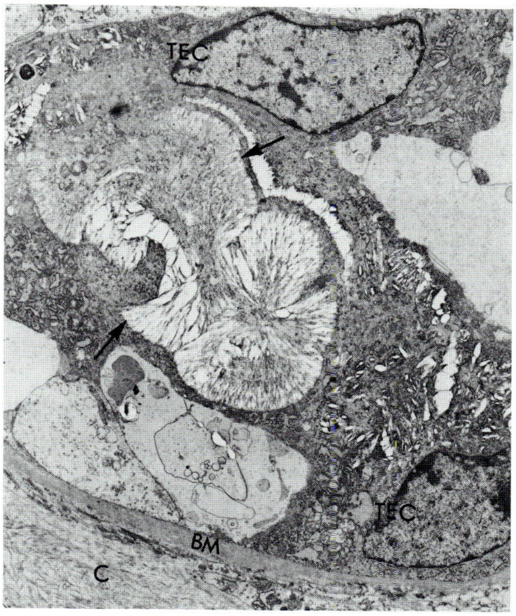

Fig. 11-17. Electron micrograph of calcium oxalate crystals (arrows) surrounded by tubular epithelial cells (TEC) in methoxyflurane nephropathy. BM = basement membrane; C = collagen. × 3,400.

An electron microscopic examination of the kidney in methoxyfluorane nephropathy shows mitochondrial swelling and disruption of cristae in the epithelial cells of the proximal tubules[208, 285]; similar but less severe changes are observed in some of the epithelial cells of the distal tubules. Intracytoplasmic lipid droplets are numerous. Calcium oxalate crystals are demonstrated in the tubular lumina (Fig. 11-17), and are frequently surrounded by intact or shed epithelial cells. The interstitial deposition of calcium oxalate crystals is rarely observed.

From a functional viewpoint, the polyuric renal insufficiency induced by methoxyflurane suggests a lesion in the distal or collecting tubules[235]; however, the anatomic alterations in this condition are usually found in the proximal tubules. Kosek et al.[208] proposed two possible explanations for this discrepancy: (1) damage to the distal or collecting tubules—or both—is insufficient to be demonstrable anatomically by the currently available methods; and (2) injury to the proximal convoluted tubules places an excessive load on, or otherwise impairs, the function of the more distal nephron.

Osmotic Nephrosis

The intravenous administration of substances such as sucrose, mannitol, or low-molecular-weight dextran will induce fine vacuolation or hydropic change in the cytoplasm of the tubular epithelial cells.[231, 312, 346] However, this type of histologic change may also be observed when there is no obvious etiology.

The finely and diffusely dispersed vacuolar changes induced by substances such as those named above are most pronounced in the epithelial cells of the pars convoluta and pars recta of the proximal tubules (Fig. 11-18). The brush borders of these cells frequently are preserved and prominent. The tubular lumen may be narrowed. Hydropic or vacuolar change may also be seen in the parietal epithelial cells and, rarely, in the visceral epithelial cells of the glomerulus. Histochemical staining for both lipid and glycogen is negative. Tubular vacuolarization also can be seen in diabetic nephropathy, the nephrotic syndrome, and phosphorus poisoning; however, the vacuoles in these conditions are of lipid origin, are not diffusely distributed throughout the proximal convoluted tubules, and are not evenly dispersed throughout the cytoplasm.

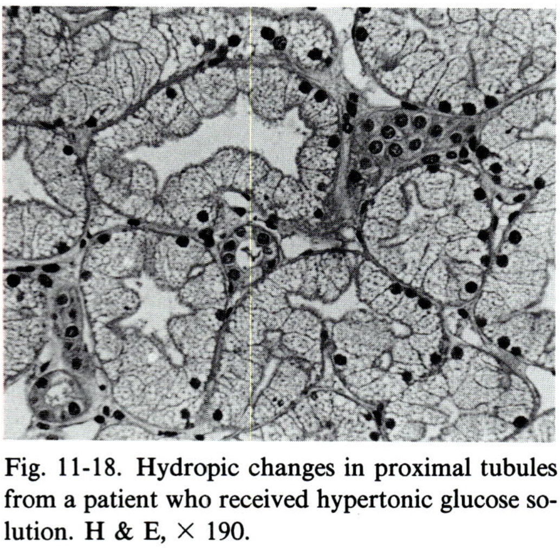

Fig. 11-18. Hydropic changes in proximal tubules from a patient who received hypertonic glucose solution. H & E, × 190.

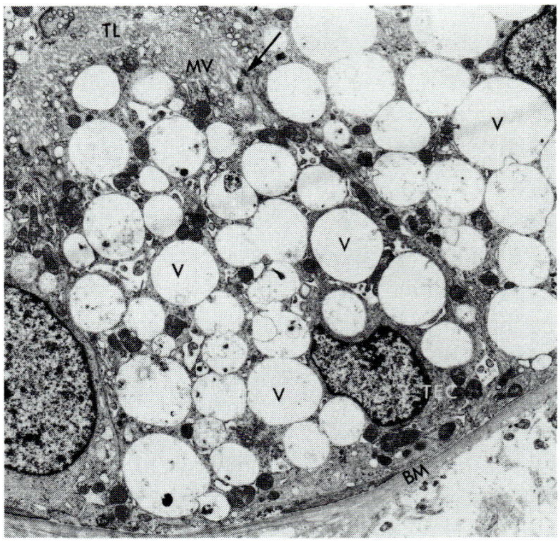

Fig. 11-19. Portion of proximal tubular epithelium with numerous, variably-sized vacuoles (V) from a 54-year-old man who received low-molecular-weight dextran. Tight junction is indicated by the arrow. BM = basement membrane, TEC = tubular epithelial cell, MV = microvilli; TL = tubular lumen. Electron micrograph, × 5,300.

Electron microscopic studies of the proximal tubules in rats administered hypertonic sucrose solutions showed variably sized vacuoles bounded by a single membrane[231, 346] (Fig. 11-19). Initially these vacuoles were small and situated beneath the brush border; with time, they moved basally and became larger.[231] Schwartz and Johnson,[312] using radioactively-labeled sucrose, concluded that the sucrose-induced proximal tubular vacuolation was a result of the incorporation of the sucrose into the phagolysosomal structures of the cells. As a rule, this type of tubular change is entirely reversible within 96 hours after the withdrawal of the offending agent, and the renal function remains normal.

Hypokalemic Nephropathy

The administration of diuretics of the thiazide group is one of the many potential causes of potassium depletion.[295] Prolonged potassium deficiency is manifested clinically by muscular weakness, polyuria, anorexia, and decreased reflexes. Pathologically, there is specific tubular vacuolation. Hypokalemia is frequently accompanied by faulty tubular concentrating mechanisms. These functional disturbances are caused by impaired resorption of sodium and chloride, with diminished back diffusion of water at the distal tubular sites.[168, 229] Both the functional change and the morphologic lesion can be resolved by potassium repletion.[168, 294] Potassium depletion may predispose the kidney to infection; however, the temporal relationship between the potassium depletion and pyelonephritis is not always clear.[168] Furthermore, conflicting evidence has been generated in numerous experimental animal studies.[61, 253]

Light-microscopic examination of the hypokalemic kidney shows that large, well-defined, clear vacuoles occupy the main part of the tubular epithelial cell, and that the nuclei of the cell are basally located; the vacuoles do not contain fat or glycogen. The vacuolar change is most pronounced in the proximal convoluted tubules, although the distal tubules also may be affected. The loops of Henle and the collecting tubules are generally not involved. The vacuolar swelling of the epithelial cells produces a considerable diminution of the tubular lumen.

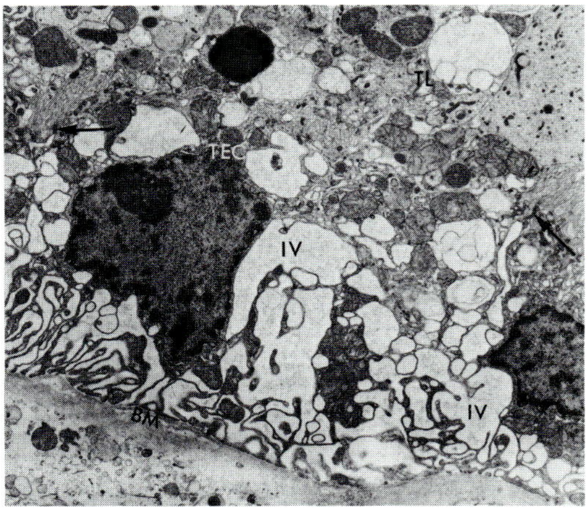

Fig. 11-20. Portion of proximal tubular epithelium with distention of intercellular spaces in hypokalemic nephrosis. Electron micrograph, × 5,400.

Biava et al.,[39] using electron microscopy, indicated that the vacuolation of the tubules in a patient with primary aldosteronism and hypokalemia was caused mainly by distention of the extracellular spaces, with separation of the basal plasma membranes (Fig. 11-20); the apical tight-junction of two adjacent cells remained intact. Intracytoplasmic vacuoles of variable sizes were also demonstrated.[325]

INTERSTITIAL DISEASES

A variety of nephrotoxic agents can elicit a primarily interstitial, inflammatory cellular response in the kidney. However, the recognition of the interstitium as the primary site of toxic injury may be difficult because interstitial damage is invariably accompanied by varying degrees of tubular lesions. From a histologic viewpoint, it is difficult to determine whether the interstitial inflammation is the primary event, or whether it is secondary to tubular damage. The term "tubulo-interstitial nephritis" appears to be more appropriate than "interstitial nephritis" because many interstitial nephrotoxic agents are potentially cytotoxic to the epithelial cells of the tubules.

At least two possible pathogenic mechanisms are responsible for toxic interstitial nephritis: (1) The hypersensitivity reaction to nephrotoxic agents may trigger an interstitial immunologic reaction; this mechanism is exemplified in the acute interstitial nephritis induced by such drugs as methicillin. (2) The counterpart multiplier system of the kidney may result in the concentration of nephrotoxic agents or their metabolites to toxic levels in the interstitium of the renal medulla, thus leading to interstitial damage; chronic analgesic nephropathy with papillary necrosis is an example of a condition mediated by such a mechanism.

Toxic interstitial nephritis may be divided into two groups: acute interstitial nephritis and chronic interstitial nephritis. The distinction between these two types of nephritis cannot be based solely on the type of cellular response, it also depends on the temporal relationship between the administration of the drug and the onset of the clinical renal symptoms. The inflammatory cellular response in many cases of acute interstitial nephritis may primarily comprise lymphocytes and plasma cells, with no polymorphonuclear leukocytes or eosinophils.

Acute Interstitial Nephritis

Acute interstitial nephritis associated with renal insufficiency has been increasingly recognized as a complication with a number of drugs. Sulfonamides were among the first drugs to be incriminated in this condition[114]; in recent years, the penicillins (penicillin G, methicillin, and ampicillin) have been the most commonly implicated agents.[19, 45, 75, 125, 233, 270] However, drugs as diversified as phenindione,[69] the thiazides,[123, 224] rifampin,[204] allopurinol,[128] azathioprine,[324] and diphenylhydantoin[159] have all been reported to cause acute interstitial nephritis.

Methicillin is by far the best studied and most common antibiotic implicated in drug-induced interstitial nephritis.[19, 45, 75, 233, 270] Prior exposure to the drug is the rule, with evidence of renal failure gradually appearing from 5 to 45 days after exposure. Symptoms included fever, skin rashes, macroscopic hematuria, mild proteinuria, and eosinophilia; the latter two findings are present in about 10 to 40 percent of patients with the syndrome.[206] The renal disease usually resolves when the offending drug is withdrawn, although permanent renal damage[233] and death[19] have been reported.

On gross examination, the kidney in drug-induced acute interstitial nephritis is usually slightly enlarged because of a generalized edema of the renal parenchyma. Light-microscopic examination of the renal tissue shows intense but focal inflammatory cell infiltrates in the interstitial tissues of both the cortex and medulla; the infiltrates consist primarily of lymphocytes, of plasma cells with a significant number of eosinophils,[19, 270] and occasionally of polymorphonuclear leukocytes. Aggregates of inflammatory cells are frequently seen in the periglomerular and peritubular regions, and are in close contact with the basement membranes of the tubules (Fig. 11-21). Interstitial granulomas with multinucleated giant cells are rarely seen.[225, 246] Interstitial edema and scattered foci of fibrosis are sometimes found. There is mild to moderate tubular atrophy associated with degenerative features. The distal tubules appear to be affected more severely than the proximal tubules. An interesting histologic feature of drug-induced interstitial nephritis is "tubulitis," which is characterized by the presence of chronic or acute inflammatory cells—or both—between the intact tubular epithelial cells[270] (Fig. 11-22). Focal and segmental thickening of the peritubular basement membranes is evident. The glomeruli are usually normal.

Electron microscopic examination of the

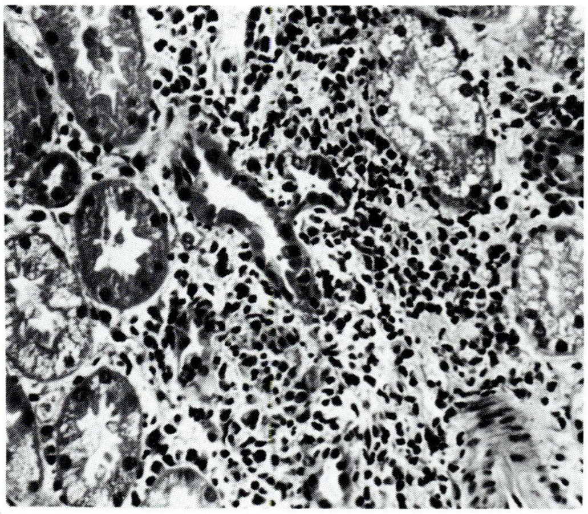

Fig. 11-21. Renal biopsy from a patient with methicillin-induced acute interstitial nephritis showing peritubular lymphocytic and neutrophilic infiltration. H & E, × 200.

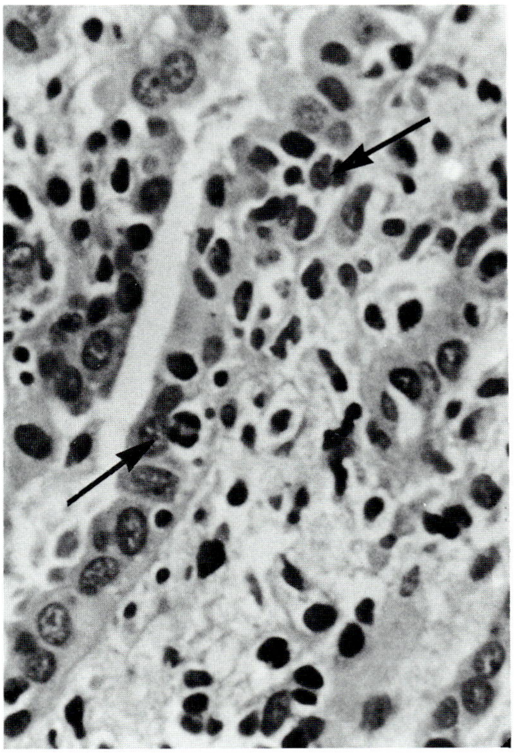

Fig. 11-22. Tubulitis with neutrophils and lymphocytes (arrows) interposed between tubular cells and basement membrane from a patient with methicillin-induced interstitial nephritis. H & E, × 865.

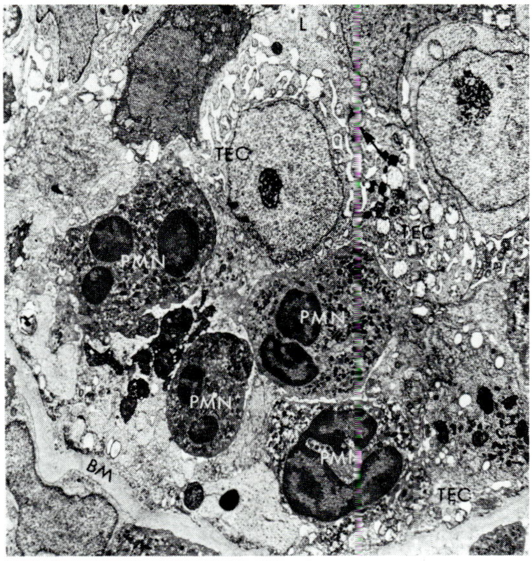

Fig. 11-23. Numerous polymorphonuclear leukocytes (PMN) are interposed between the tubular epithelial cells (TEC) from a patient with methicillin-induced interstitial nephritis. L = lumen; BM = basement membrane. Electron micrograph, × 3,900.

proximal and distal tubular epithelium in drug-induced interstitial nephritis reveals swelling of the mitochondria, with fragmentation of the cristae; giant mitochondria are found occasionally.[270] Myelin figures, frequently in close association with the swollen mitochondria, are seen in the cytoplasm of degenerated epithelial cells. Inflammatory cells, primarily lymphocytes and polymorphonuclear leukocytes, are seen interposed between the basement membrane and the tubular cells (Figs. 11-23 and 11-24). The distal tubules are more severely affected than the proximal tubules. Simplification and partial separation of the plasma membranes of two adjacent epithelial cells having intact, tight junctions are observed. The peritubular basement membranes are focally thickened and reduplicated, and small amounts of electron-

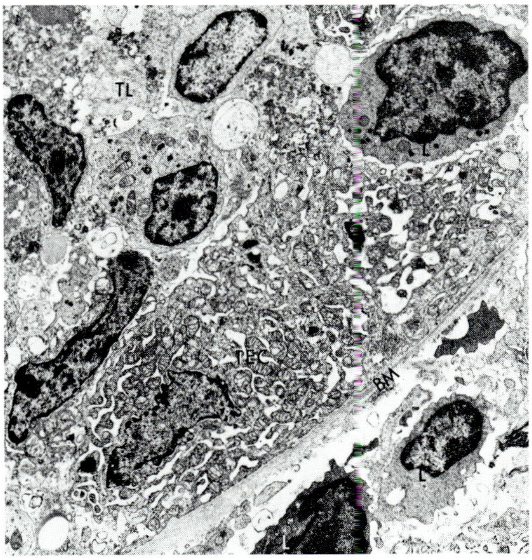

Fig. 11-24. Portion of distal tubular epithelium from a patient with methicillin-induced interstitial nephritis. Note that lymphocyte (L) is interposed between tubular cells (TEC). TL = tubular lumen; BM = basement membrane. Electron micrograph, × 6,660.

dense deposits and clusters of round bodies are seen occasionally in the basement membrane.[270] The interstitial inflammatory cells consist of lymphocytes, plasma cells, eosinophils, and polymorphonuclear leukocytes.

Immunofluorescence microscopy reveals an occasional deposition of $B1_c$ globulin along the tubular basement membrane, and patchy interstitial deposits of IgG and fibrinogen.[270] A dimethoxyphenyl penicilloyl (DPO) hapten and IgG deposits, in a linear pattern along the tubular basement membranes, have been detected by some investigators.[19,45]

Many clinical and pathologic features of drug-induced acute interstitial nephritis, especially that caused by methicillin, indicate an immunologic mechanism for the renal lesion. These features are as follows: the latent period before the onset of renal symptoms; the presence of eosinophilia and skin rashes; non-dose-related nephropathy; the elevation of serum IgE; the demonstration of immunoglobulins and complement in the interstitial tissues and along the tubular basement membranes; and the intense mononuclear cellular response.

The identification of antitubular basement membrane antibodies in methicillin-associated interstitial nephritis has led to the postulation that methicillin behaves as a hapten, combining with the tubular basement membrane to form a hapten-protein conjugate that may stimulate antibody formation.[45] Anti-tubular basement membrane antibody formation might also be initiated by the antigenic components of the tubular basement membrane released into the circulation from methicillin-damaged tubules.

Chronic Interstitial Nephritis

Chronic interstitial nephritis is characterized histologically by an increase of interstitial fibrous connective tissue, accompanied by an infiltration of chronic inflammatory cells, focal tubular atrophy, and periglomerular fibrosis. This pathologic lesion in this condition does not always indicate that the interstitium is the primary or initial site of injury, since damage to other structural components of the kidney can elicit the same type of interstitial response. Failure to appreciate the nonspecific nature of these parenchymal changes has led to an overdiagnosis of chronic pyelonephritis.

Nephrotoxic injury to the interstitium may result from vitamin D intoxication, which can cause nephrocalcinosis, or from analgesic abuse, which can result in papillary necrosis with cortical interstitial nephritis.

Analgesic Nephropathy

In 1953, Spühler and Zollinger[329] first drew attention to the high incidence of chronic interstitial nephritis and papillary necrosis in patients with a history of heavy consumption of analgesic agents containing phenacetin. Subsequently, many studies were done on the nature of this association, and on the possible pathogenic mechanisms and the morphogenesis of the pathologic lesions in it.

A causal relationship between prolonged, excessive ingestion of analgesics and renal damage is now well established. Several analgesics are considered as prime causative agents for such damage, including aspirin,[94] paracetamol,[211] phenylbutazone,[249] and phenacetin.[1,165] Analgesics are usually taken as compounds and mixtures, and there has been a tendency to single out phenacetin as being responsible for the production of renal papillary necrosis, a hallmark of analgesic nephropathy; however, a review of experimental work indicates that aspirin has a greater nephrotoxic effect than phenacetin, and produces papillary necrosis in a far more predictable manner, although there is less nephrotoxicity than when the two agents are combined.[248,305]

Analgesic nephropathy has been reported from most countries in the world; however, the incidence is alarmingly high in some countries.[198] For example, analgesic nephropathy with renal failure is the underlying cause in 20 percent of the patients requiring dialysis and transplantation in Australia,[89] compared to 7 percent in the United States,[259] 5.5 percent in Canada,[221] and 3.1 percent in Europe.[49]

Analgesic nephropathy is predominantly a female disease, with peak occurrence in the fourth and fifth decades of life.[260] The renal manifestations of this condition are characterized by an impaired concentrating and acidifying capacity, and a sodium-losing state[78, 212]; the nonrenal manifestations include peptic ulcer (35 percent), anemia (60 to 90 percent), hypertension (15 to 70 percent), and ischemic heart disease (35 percent).[260] There is usually a rapid improvement and stabilization of renal function when all analgesics are discontinued.[199]

On gross examination, both kidneys in cases of analgesic nephropathy are equally contracted, with much scarring of the subcapsular surface. A "linear bar" or "nodular ridge," representing normal tissue in the columns of Bertini, may be noted. The cut surface usually reveals a dark, thin cortex and brownish discoloration of the papillae. Necrosis of the papillae (usually at or near the tip of the pyramid) varies from minute to a total papillary necrosis. The necrotic papilla may slough off and lie loose in the renal pelvis.

According to Burry[54, 55] and Gloor,[131] three stages in the development of papillary necrosis can be recognized by light-microscopy: early, partial or intermediate, and total necrosis.

The papillary changes in early necrosis are confined to the inner medulla, and are characterized by homogeneous thickening of the basement membranes of the loops of Henle and of the capillaries. The interstitial matrix is increased and stains more intensely with periodic acid-Schiff than normal matrix does. Fine granules of calcium and lipid droplets may be detected. Some epithelial cells of the loops of Henle may show necrosis. The outer medulla and the cortex show no changes, except for the brownish pigment, which most likely represents lipofuscin granules in the tubular cells. Electron microscopic examination shows concentric thickening and reduplication of the basement membranes of the loops of Henle and, rarely, of the capillaries.

In partial or intermediate necrosis there is patchy necrosis of all elements in the inner medullary region except the collecting ducts and vasa recta; many tubules appear as "ghost" outlines (Fig. 11-25). Calcium deposits and lipid droplets may be prominent. There is no cellular reaction to the necrotic zone. At this stage, the outer medullary zone and the overlying cortex may show varying degrees of lymphocytic infiltration and fibroblastic proliferation.

In total necrosis there is total necrosis of the inner medulla (Fig. 11-26), with a line of demarcation between the necrotic zone and the viable renal tissue. One or two surviving collecting ducts may be seen. A band of fibrosis may be found parallel to the line of necrosis in the outer medulla. The overlying cortex shows progressively increasing tubular atrophy, lymphocytic infiltration (Fig. 11-27), and fibroblastic proliferation. Lipofuscin may be evident in the atrophic tubular cells.

Papillary necrosis is the primary and predominant histopathologic change in analgesic nephropathy; the chronic interstitial nephritis occurring in the renal cortex is a secondary event.[2, 54, 200] The pathogenic mechanism for the subsequent cortical damage is believed to involve an intrarenal tubular obstruction caused by fibrosis in the outer medulla.[248]

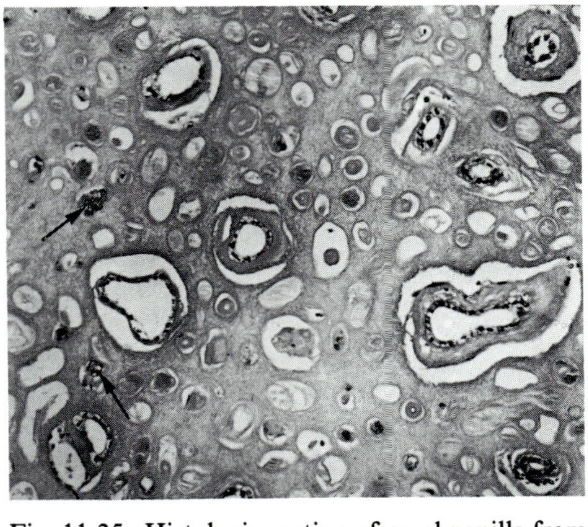

Fig. 11-25. Histologic section of renal papilla from a patient with analgesic abuse shows thickening of the peritubular basement membranes. Many tubules appear as "ghost" outlines. Calcium deposits are indicated by arrows. H & E, × 200.

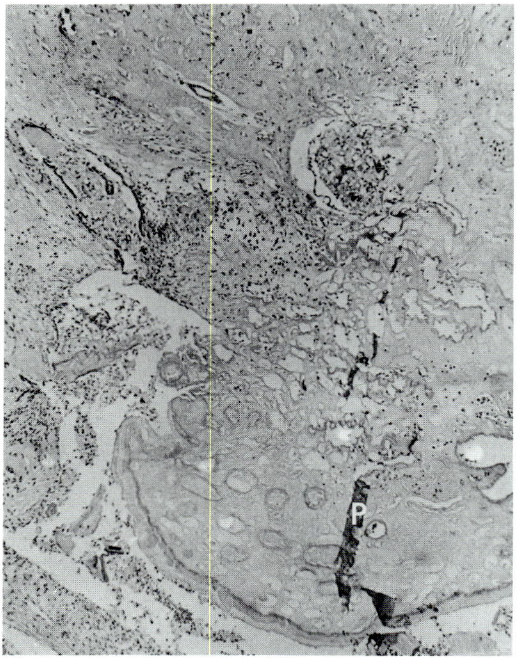

Fig. 11-26. Renal papillary necrosis (P) with focal calcification from a patient with analgesic nephropathy. H & E, × 70.

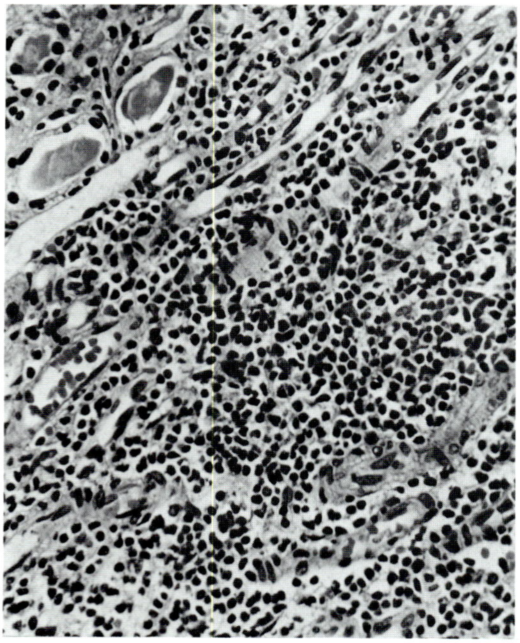

Fig. 11-27. Interstitial lymphocytic infiltration in chronic interstitial nephritis from a patient with analgesic nephropathy. H & E, × 250.

The pathogenesis of analgesic nephropathy is controversial. The evidence thus far from experimental studies suggests that the initiating event in the development of papillary necrosis is either a direct toxic effect of the analgesic metabolites on the tubular epithelial or interstitial cells,[44, 329] or an ischemic process.[200] Within the papillae, acetaminophen and aspirin reach a higher concentration in the tubular cells than in the interstitial or intratubular fluid[93]; this concentration gradient is accentuated by dehydration.[44] One potential toxic effect of acetaminophen is oxidative injury in the medulla. The renal cells normally protect against oxidative injury through the intracellular accumulation of reducing agents generated by the hexose monophosphate pathway; acetaminophen and aspirin inhibit this pathway.[133, 252]

However, Kincaid-Smith et al.[200] believed that the medullary damage in analgesic nephropathy was caused by ischemia. They demonstrated occlusive lesions in the vascular bundles of the outer medulla in rats given an APC mixture; other investigators have shown necrosis of endothelial cells of the efferent vasa recta.[248] The foregoing effects, coupled with the direct effect of aspirin's action as an inhibitor of prostaglandin PGE_2 synthesis,[351] cause a drastic reduction in medullary blood flow. Additionally, the interstitial cells—the source of arachidonic acid, which is the precursor of prostaglandins[266]—have been shown to be damaged. The early loss of medullary mucopolysaccharides in analgesic nephropathy may be related to interstitial cell damage. Possibly, all of the foregoing factors operate. The early papillary changes may be caused by ischemia secondary to inhibition of prostaglandin synthesis; and the late stage, leading to total papillary necrosis, may be caused by lesions in the vasa recta.[248]

Vitamin D-induced Nephrocalcinosis

Excessive intake of vitamin D is one of the many causes for the deposition of calcium salts in the kidneys.[176] Clinically, a patient with an overdose of vitamin D usually has polydipsia, polyuria, isosthenuria, weakness, gastrointestinal disturbances, and mild psychosis. Calcification in the kidneys, and osteoporosis, may be detected by radiologic examination.

Scarpelli,[306] in his study of vitamin D-induced nephrocalcinosis, found a sequence of cytochemical and morphologic alterations in the tubular epithelial cells that eventually led to calcium deposition. He demonstrated that hypervitaminosis D caused progressive uncoupling of oxidative phosphorylation, and decreased the calcium uptake by isolated renal tubular mitochondria. He postulated that in the vitamin D-induced hypercalcemic stage, there was an increased uptake of calcium by the tubular epithelial cells; as the intracellular calcium concentration rose, there was decreased active binding or impaired transport of calcium by mitochondria, eventually resulting in nephrocalcinosis. At the ultrastructural level, the earliest alterations Scarpelli saw were an increase in the number of cytoplasmic vacuoles and swelling of the mitochondria. This was followed by the appearance of calcium deposits in the cytoplasmic vacuoles, in the mitochondria, in the basilar infoldings of the plasma membrane, and in the basement membrane of the epithelial cells of the proximal convoluted tubules.

On gross examination, the kidneys in vitamin D-induced nephrocalcinosis are usually of normal size. Whitish granules of calcific deposits may be discernible on the cut surfaces. Light-microscopic examination of the kidney shows the deposition of calcium salts on the basement membranes of the tubules, in the interstitium, and in the tubular lumen, with destruction of the tubular epithelial cells. Foreign-body giant cells are sometimes seen. Occasionally, the walls of the arteries or arterioles are focally calcified. In the five cases of hypervitaminosis D reported by Fabre et al.[102] in 1968, there were diffuse glomerular lesions with proliferation of the epithelial cells and thickening of the capillary basement membranes.

Electron microscopic observations in vitamin D-induced nephrocalcinosis have been derived mainly from animal experiments. Dense granules of calcium salts can be observed in the cytoplasmic vacuoles and mitochondria of tubular cells. Multilamellar calcium deposits, consisting of closely packed, needle-shaped crystals, are present in the interstitium and basal laminae of the proximal, distal, and collecting tubules. Concentric layers of calcium crystals are also noted in the tubular lumina.

Pharmaceutical agents other than vitamin D can also cause the development of nephrocalcinosis. Acetazolamide induces a renal tubular acidosis with reduced citrate excretion; this causes nephrocalcinosis and calcium phosphate stone formation[279]; long-term therapy with dihydrotachysterol has caused hypercalcemia with metastatic calcification and nephrocalcinosis[87]; excessive ingestion of absorbable alkali and calcium is followed by the development of a milk-alkali syndrome characterized by systemic alkalosis, nephrocalcinosis, and uremia.[290] Nephrocalcinosis of varying etiology may sometimes be partially reversed when the hypercalcemic state is eliminated.[176,290]

VASCULAR DISEASES

Hypersensitivity Angiitis

Approximately 30 to 40 percent of cases of hypersensitivity angiitis have been associated with drug reactions.[122, 181, 238] Among the drugs implicated are penicillin, sulfonamides,[79] thiazides,[40] iodides,[296] phenylbutazone,[181] and propylthiouracil.[240]

The renal manifestations of hypersensitivity angiitis are the same as those of an acute glomerulonephritis, with microscopic hematuria, a variable degree of proteinuria, azotemia, and eosinophilia.

A light-microscopic examination of the kidney reveals lesions affecting interlobular arteries, arterioles, and venules.[238] These vascular lesions are characterized by transmural fibrinoid necrosis, and an inflammation comprising polymorphonuclear leukocytes, eosinophils, and lymphocytes. Intramural thrombosis is occasionally observed. The glomeruli show a focal and segmental proliferation of mesangial cells, with infiltration of polymorphonuclear leukocytes, and there are segmental areas of glomerular capillary thrombosis and necrosis.

The most consistent finding upon immunofluorescent microscopy in hypersensitivity angiitis has been fibrinogen in the vascular walls; additionally, variable amounts of granular deposits of IgG, IgA, IgM, and $B1_c$ have been demonstrated in the glomeruli.

Electron microscopic examination of the glomeruli shows proliferation of the mesangial cells, with expansion of the matrix. The capillary lumen is obliterated by swelling of the endothelial cells and exudation of polymorphonuclear leukocytes. Variable amounts of electron-dense granular deposits can be seen in the mesangial and intramembranous areas. The glomerular capillary basement membranes are segmentally wrinkled and laminated.

Acute Vascular Thrombosis

Drug-induced acute intravascular thrombosis unaccompanied by vasculitis is extremely rare; a thrombotic complication has been considered to result from the toxic effect of therapy with epsilon aminocaproic acid (EACA). Widespread glomerular capillary thrombosis with acute renal failure has been described in a patient with bleeding from disseminated intravascular coagulation who received EACA therapy.[141]

THE URETER

Intrinsic Obstruction of the Ureter

Obstruction of both ureters or the ureter of a single, functioning kidney can precipitate acute renal failure. Ureteric obstruction can follow impaction with sloughed renal papillae as a complication of analgesic nephropathy, or can be caused by occlusion with calculi or a blood clot.[300] Deposits of uric acid crystals in the renal tubules or ureters may follow successful treatment with radiation or chemotherapy for lymphoreticular diseases[227]; crystalluria also occurs with the less soluble sulfonamides, such as sulphadiazine, and can potentially be a cause of obstructive uropathy.

Additionally, unilateral obstruction of the ureter may be due to a primary urothelial tumor of the ureter. Johansson et al.[185] described four patients with transitional cell carcinoma of the ureter, and in three of these, associated renal papillary necrosis was found. All of these patients had a history of abuse of phenacetin-containing analgesics.

Extrinsic Obstruction of the Ureter

Methysergide-induced Retroperitoneal Fibrosis

In 1949, Ormond[272] described the formation of a dense, fibrous plaque in the retroperitoneum, causing bilateral ureteric obstruction. Numerous case reports and reviews followed, and retroperitoneal fibrosis is now an established clinical entity.[62, 191, 195, 196, 359]

Many theories have been proposed in an attempt to clarify the etiology and pathogenesis of methysergide-induced retroperitoneal fibrosis.[77, 150, 191] In one theory, the role of infection in the lower urinary tract has been stressed,[258] and there is also a theory suggesting that the fibrotic reaction represents an organization of a hematoma following trauma.[150] Others believe that the initial lesion may be an allergic vasculitis, with subsequent fibrous tissue reaction.[166]

Graham[139] first noted an association between retroperitoneal fibrosis and the administration of methysergide for the treatment of headache in 1964. Two years later, Graham et al.[140] reported on 27 patients who developed retroperitoneal fibrosis during methysergide therapy, and implicated other ergot derivatives as possible causative agents. A causal relationship between methysergide and the development of retroperitoneal fibrosis has been amply confirmed by subsequent reports.[62,195,359]

The clinical manifestations of methysergide-induced retroperitoneal fibrosis consist of loin pain, weight loss, fever, a high erythrocyte sedimentation rate, and acute or chronic renal failure. Intravenous or retrograde pyelography will demonstrate bilateral hydronephrosis, with the ureters drawn medially. In most of the reported cases, regression of the pathologic process, with amelioration of clinical symptoms, occurs as soon as methysergide is withdrawn[77,140,191]; occasionally, however, the disease progresses far enough that surgical ureterolysis or corticosteroid therapy become necessary.[311]

The gross pathologic appearance is that of an ill-defined, plaque-like fibrous mass, which is usually centered over the level of the third lumbar vertebra and extends to the promontory of the sacrum. The lesion extends laterally to the outer edge of the psoas muscle, and the fibrous process tends to pull the ureters toward the midline. Fibrosis may also encase the inferior vena cava and grow around the rectosigmoid colon,[129] in the scrotum, in the mediastinum, in the heart valves, and in the pleura.[164]

Light-microscopic examination of the plaque-like mass shows an active proliferation of fibroblasts, deposition of collagen fibers, and an infiltration of histiocytes, lymphocytes, plasma cells, and a few polymorphonuclear leukocytes. Aggregates of adipose cells may be surrounded by fibrous connective tissue. Arteriolitis may also be seen.[77] Dense, hyalinized collagenous tissue with a light lymphocytic infiltration can be seen in other areas.

In 1975, Iversen et al.[177] described retroperitoneal fibrosis in a patient taking methyldopa; it has been suggested that other drugs that induce autoimmune reactions and interfere with nervous transmission will also provoke a proliferation of fibrous connective tissue.[81] The mechanism of spontaneous or methysergide-induced retroperitoneal fibrosis is unknown.

THE URINARY BLADDER

Cyclophosphamide-induced Acute Hemorrhagic Cystitis

Cyclophosphamide is a cytotoxic alkylating agent used extensively as an effective chemotherapeutic agent against cancer. Recently it also has been used as an immunosuppressive drug in the treatment of nonneoplastic diseases, such as systemic lupus erythematosus and rheumatoid arthritis. The activation of cyclophosphamide to its cytotoxic alkylating metabolites is accomplished primarily in the liver.[72,322] Thereafter, there is a rapid, systemic distribution of the drug and its metabolites, and a prompt appearance of a significant amount of these metabolites in the urine.[47]

The urinary bladder complications associated with the use of cyclophosphamide are becoming common. These complications include acute hemorrhagic cystitis,[7,108,134,186,283,323,327,358,373] interstitial fibrosis,[7,186] telangiectasia,[186,323] eosinophilic cystitis,[108] and transitional cell carcinoma.[10,374] Acute hemorrhagic cystitis is the most common of these complications[373]; it has been reported from 2 to 40 percent of patients undergoing cylophosphamide therapy.[292,327]

Acute hemorrhagic cystitis may occur after either intravenous or oral administration of cyclophosphamide; the urinary symptoms of this condition generally appear earlier if the intravenous route is used. The usual clinical symptoms are burning on urination, urgency, and hematuria. The urine is sterile on culture. Acute hemorrhagic cystitis usually subsides if cyclophosphamide therapy is discontinued[7,358]; however, severe, protracted bleeding resulting in death has been reported.[283]

On gross examination, the mucosa of the urinary bladder is diffusely hemorrhagic, with focal areas of ulceration that are covered by necrotic debris and blood clots. Multiple, coarse, mucosal folds caused by hemorrhage and edema in the underlying lamina propria are prominent. The bladder wall is thickened and relatively inelastic in patients with interstitial fibrosis.

Histologic examination of the urinary bladder in cyclophosphamide-induced acute hemorrhagic cystitis reveals focal areas of complete desquamation of the urothelium; the residual epithelium may show a few atypical epithelial cells with enlarged vesicular nuclei. The most evident changes within the lamina propria are characterized by severe edema and hemorrhage (Fig. 11-28). Telangiectasia of the capillaries and venules is a dominant feature. Occasionally, vessels may show focal necrosis and transmural hemorrhage. Bizarre, atypical stromal cells containing enlarged hyperchromatic nuclei in association with abundant cytoplasm are observed (Fig. 11-29). Multinucleated stromal cells are frequently identified, and a few polymorphonuclear and mononuclear leukocytes are found. Interstitial fibrosis may be seen in chronic cases. Intranuclear and cytoplasmic inclusions characteristic of the cytomegalovirus within the endothelial cells have been reported.[134]

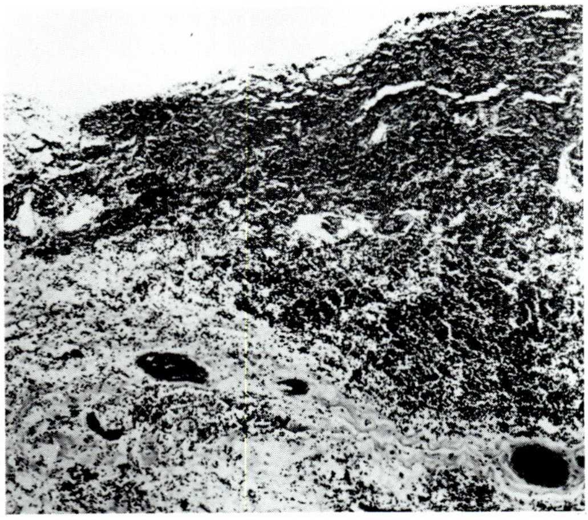

Fig. 11-28. Diffuse submucosal hemorrhage of urinary bladder from a patient receiving cyclophosphamide therapy for Hodgkin's disease. H & E, × 40.

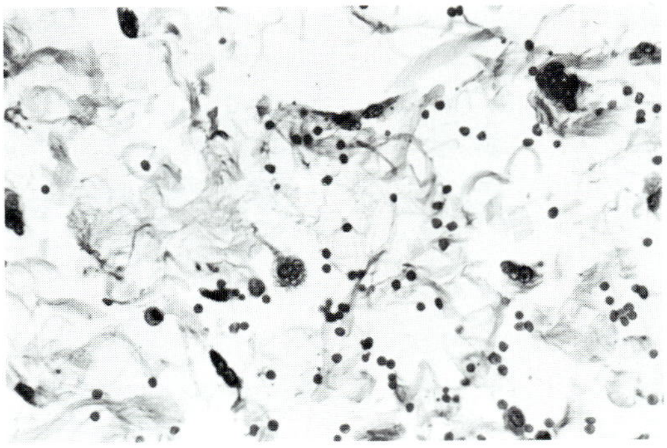

Fig. 11-29. Hyperchromatic and multinucleated atypical stromal cells are frequently found in the submucosa of urinary bladder in acute hemorrhagic cystitis due to cyclophosphamide therapy. H & E, × 275.

An experimental study has indicated that the cytotoxic effects of cyclophosphamide on the urinary bladder may be caused by its urinary metabolites rather than the parent drug[282]; urine from dogs given cyclophosphamide was instilled into the bladder of dogs not receiving the drug, and the characteristic lesions of acute hemorrhagic cystitis were induced. However, instillation of cyclophosphamide alone into the dogs' bladders caused no significant effect.[282] The relatively prolonged contact of the urinary bladder with the metabolites of cyclophosphamide could conceivably account for the selective toxicity to this organ.

DRUG- AND CHEMICAL-ASSOCIATED MALIGNANCIES OF THE KIDNEY AND LOWER URINARY TRACT

Various parts of the urinary tract—the renal pelvis, ureters, urinary bladder, and the major part of the urethra—are lined with a continuous, histologically identical layer of transitional epithelium (urothelium). Therefore, a single, common carcinogen is potentially capable of causing tumor formation in any one area; alternatively, several areas may be affected simultaneously. Thus, multifocal transitional cell carcinoma, which becomes apparent over a period of years, can occur; for example, a renal pelvic tumor may be followed by a bladder tumor. Although a single, common etiologic agent may be responsible for such malignancy, other factors, such as direct surface spread of the tumor by continuity, or implantation of tumor cells in the lower urinary tract from a lesion higher up, may also be the cause of the multicentricity of the tumors.

A number of drugs and chemical substances have been implicated as the cause of malignant tumors in the urinary tract. Among them are phenacetin-containing analgesics, cyclophosphamide, chlornaphazin, cyclamate, benzidine, alpha and beta naphthylamine, 4-aminodiphenyl, and 4-nitrodiphenyl.

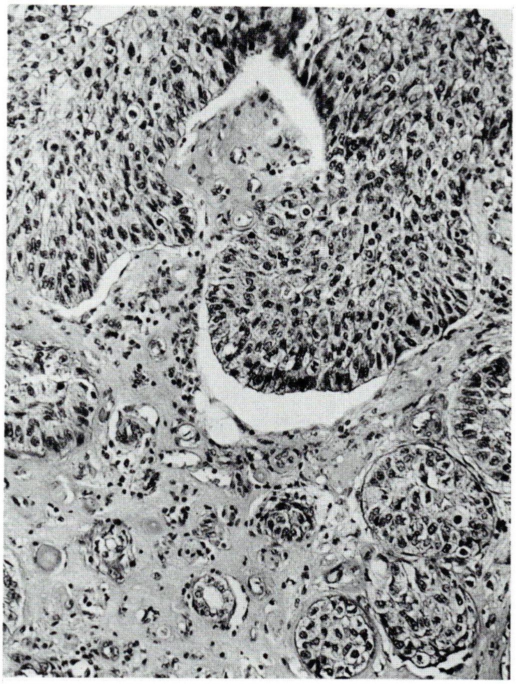

Fig. 11-30. Transitional cell carcinoma infiltrating the renal papilla in a patient with analgesic nephropathy. H & E, × 130.

Phenacetin-associated Carcinomas of the Renal Pelvis, Ureter, and Urinary Bladder

In 1965, Hutengren et al.[75] first drew attention to a possible causal relationship between the excessive use of phenacetin-containing analgesics and carcinoma of the renal pelvis. They described 6 patients with transitional cell carcinoma of the renal pelvis associated with papillary necrosis; 5 of these patients were known phenacetin abusers. In 1968, Bengtsson et al.[30] reported 9 instances of carcinoma of the renal pelvis and 2 instances of carcinoma of the urinary bladder in 104 patients with analgesic nephropathy. Subsequently, this type of association has been demonstrated in several studies, particularly in Sweden[8, 30, 184]; similar observations also have been reported from other countries.[3, 85, 167, 187, 223, 291]

Phenacetin is an aromatic amide with *N*-hydroxylated metabolites. Nery[261] found azoxy-4-ethoxybenzene, a condensation product of *N*-hydroxyphenacetin, in the urine of rats fed with phenacetin. The *N*-hydroxylated metabolites seem to be nephrotoxic and carcinogenic. Their excretion is enhanced by the simultaneous administration of caffeine, barbiturates, and phenozene.

There is an increasing incidence of transitional cell carcinomas in the renal pelvis (Fig. 11-30) and urinary tract in patients who abuse phenacetin. The sex ratio is 1 : 1,[185, 291] in contrast to the typical male preponderance in nonphenacetin-related bladder carcinomas[86]; this phenomenon apparently results from the fact that more women are phenacetin abusers than men.[260] The mean age of tumor occurrence is a decade younger in phenacetin abusers than in nonabusers.[291] Gross hematuria is the major clinical symptom, occurring in 95 percent of cases.[291]

In Sweden,[31] the incidence of bladder carcinoma is usually 15 times more common than renal pelvic carcinoma in the general population. However, in phenacetin abusers, renal pelvic carcinoma seems to be more frequent than bladder tumors,[261] and occurs in an estimated 8 percent of patients with analgesic nephropathy.[260] The induction time for bladder carcinoma is estimated to be 30 years; for renal pelvic carcinoma it is 22 years.[185]

Multicentric and bilateral tumors are common in the urinary tracts of patients having a history of phenacetin abuse[291]; 5 percent of the patients have had simultaneous, bilateral pelvic tumors, while an estimated 35 percent have had an earlier, simultaneous, or later development of urothelial carcinoma elsewhere in the urinary tract.[3, 31, 85, 167, 184, 187, 223, 291]

Carcinomas of the renal pelvis are usually located in the calyces or pelvic ampulla, carcinomas of the ureter are seen predominantly in the distal third, and carcinomas of the bladder are localized in the trigone area.[185] Most renal pelvic carcinomas, and to a lesser extent bladder carcinomas, are usually less differentiated in patients with analgesic abuse than in nonabusers; in 43 percent of the patients, distant metastases to lungs, liver, and the skeletal system occur.[31] The overall prognosis of renal pelvic tumor is not as good in analgesic abusers as in nonabusers.

Cyclophosphamide-associated Bladder Cancers

Cyclophosphamide (Cytoxan) is a chemotherapeutic agent used in the treatment of neoplastic diseases, and as an immunosuppressive agent.[228] In 1964, Forni et al.[109] reported their observation of large, atypical transitional cells with hyperchromatic nuclei in the urine sediment of patients receiving cyclophosphamide. In 1971, Worth[374] described the first case of transitional cell carcinoma of the urinary bladder with a temporal relationship to cyclophosphamide therapy. Since then, an additional 14 instances of bladder cancer following cyclophosphamide therapy have been reported[10, 83, 278, 297, 301, 316, 356, 364] (Table 11-3).

All of the reported patients with cyclophosphamide-associated bladder cancers have had underlying lymphoreticular or hematologic malignancies, except one woman who had carcinoma of the breast.[316] Multiple myeloma and Hodgkin's disease were the most common primary malignancies, the mean age was 54 years, and 13 of the 16 reported patients were males. Ten of these 16 patients had a diagnosis of hemorrhagic cystitis based on either clinical evaluation or cystoscopic examination. The most common histologic type of tumor was transitional cell carcinoma, occurring in 9 of the 16 patients; 4 patients had squamous cell carcinoma; adenocarcinoma, undifferentiated carcinoma, and fibrosarcoma occurred in 1 patient each. In some of these patients, the malignancies developed in areas of hemorrhagic cystitis.

Questions about whether cyclophosphamide has an etiologic role in the development of bladder cancer, and whether lymphoproliferative or hematologic diseases predispose to a second malignancy, are difficult to resolve. There have been reports of the frequent association of lymphoproliferative disease with other cancers,[148] especially skin cancers[36]; however, Stavraky et al.[333] conducted a retrospective study on 258 patients with chronic lymphocytic leukemia in an attempt to study the incidence of a second malignancy. They concluded that there was no statistically significant increase in the incidence of a second malignancy after the diagnosis of lymphoproliferative disease. Arseneau et al.[13] indicated that there was a definite, increasing risk of a secondary malignancy among patients who received both chemotherapy and radiotherapy; they pointed out a 29-fold increase in the incidence of a second malignancy among patients receiving intensive treatment with both modalities.

The carcinogenic effect of cyclophosphamide in experimental animal studies remains inconclusive and circumstantial. A single dose of cyclophosphamide given to rats fed with the carcinogen *N*-2-fluorenylacetamide and a vitamin B_6-deficient diet reduced the induction time of tumor development.[210]

Cyclophosphamide suppresses both the cell-mediated and humoral immune systems[111];

Table 11-3. Cyclophosphamide-associated Urinary Bladder Malignancies

Case	Authors	Age	Sex	Primary Disease	Hemorrhagic Cystitis	Bladder Malignancies
1	Worth[374]	49	M	Hodgkin's disease	Yes	Transitional cell carcinoma
2	Worth[374]	67	M	Lymphosarcoma	Yes	Transitional cell carcinoma
3	Rupprecht and Blessing[301]	12	M	Hodgkin's disease	—	Fibrosarcoma
4	Dale and Smith[83]	73	M	Multiple myeloma	Yes	Transitional cell carcinoma
5	Dale and Smith[83]	61	M	Macroglobulinemia	No	Transitional cell carcinoma
6	Weinstein et al.[364]	68	M	Multiple myeloma	No	Transitional cell carcinoma
7	Ansell and Castro[10]	50	F	Hodgkin's disease	Yes	Transitional cell carcinoma
8	Ansell and Castro[10]	61	F	Follicular lymphoma	Yes	Transitional cell carcinoma
9	Wall and Clausen[356]	47	M	Multiple myeloma	Yes	Squamous cell carcinoma
10	Wall and Clausen[356]	57	M	Multiple myeloma	Yes	Squamous cell carcinoma
11	Wall and Clausen[356]	27	M	Hodgkin's disease	Yes	Squamous cell carcinoma
12	Wall and Clausen[356]	60	M	Multiple myeloma	No	Undifferentiated carcinoma
13	Wall and Clausen[356]	63	M	Multiple myeloma	Yes	Squamous cell carcinoma
14	Seltzer et al.[316]	52	F	Breast carcinoma	Yes	Transitional cell carcinoma
15	Pearson and Soloway[278]	40	M	Malignant lymphoma	No	Adenocarcinoma
16	Richtsmeier[297]	65	M	Hodgkin's disease	No	Transitional cell carcinoma

there is a selective toxic effect of cyclophosphamide against B lymphocytes,[348] which interferes with the B-lymphocyte production of immunoglobulin G, an antibody that has been demonstrated to induce cell-mediated cytotoxicity against transitional cell carcinoma of the urinary bladder.[152, 274, 356]

Azathioprine-associated Bladder Carcinoma

Azathioprine (Imuran), a derivative of 6-mercaptopurine, has been widely used as an immunosuppressive agent in patients who have undergone organ transplantation, and to a lesser extent in those suffering from neoplastic or nonneoplastic diseases.

An increased incidence of malignant neoplasms (a high proportion of which are malignant lymphomas) occurs in azathioprine-treated patients with renal allografts or with underlying neoplastic disease; malignancy rarely occurs in patients receiving azathioprine therapy for other diseases. McAdam et al.[236] presented a 39-year-old woman with lupus nephritis in whom adenocarcinoma of the lung developed 4 years after she received azathioprine therapy. Recently, Scharf et al.[307] described two patients with transitional cell carcinoma of the urinary bladder that developed after they received long-term azathioprine therapy for ulcerative colitis. However, it is not known at this time if the appearance of bladder carcinoma and azathioprine therapy are associated or coincidental.

Chlornaphazin-induced Bladder Carcinoma

Chlornaphazin (Erysan) was introduced as a chemotherapeutic agent in 1949 because of its pronounced cytostatic effect on experimental tumors.[151] It was used primarily in Denmark and Italy for the treatment of polycythemia vera and Hodgkin's disease.

Chlornaphazin is a derivative of 2-naphthylamine and apparently is not carcinogenic per se; it is readily absorbed from the intestine. Hydroxylated chlornaphazin and conjugated compounds of the drug are excreted mainly in the urine. The high B-glucuronidase activity in the urinary bladder hydrolyzes the conjugates to form 2-naphthylhydroxylamine and 2-amino-1-naphthol, both of which are potent carcinogens.

In 1962, Chievitz and Thiede[70] described 2 patients with bladder carcinoma and 1 with renal cell carcinoma among 26 patients with polycythemia vera who had been treated with high doses of chlornaphazine: a daily dose of 300 mg or more for a 3-month period. In 1964 an additional 5 patients with bladder carcinoma associated with chlornaphazine therapy were reported.[341] In the same year, Videbaek[353] described 2 cases in patients with Hodgkin's disease. Chlornaphazine has been prohibited for clinical use in Denmark since 1963. A follow-up study in 1969 by Thiebe and Christensen[342] reported another 3 cases of bladder carcinoma among 27 surviving patients.

Nonnutritive Sweetener-associated Bladder Carcinoma

Considerable data have been generated regarding the carcinogenic potential of nonnutritive sweeteners in experimental animal studies.[50, 51, 52, 96, 273, 287] In 1970, Price et al.[287] provided evidence that extremely high doses of a cyclamate-saccharin mixture fed to rats were associated with a small, but significant, incidence of bladder cancer. Subsequent reports, using vesical implantation or oral feeding methods, confirmed the carcinogenic propensity of these substances in laboratory animals,[50, 51, 52, 96, 120, 162, 273] although others have failed to substantiate these findings.[100]

Findings in experimental animal studies are difficult to extrapolate to the etiology of human bladder cancer; there were some inconsistencies in these studies, and the histologic confirmation of the cancer was not always available. The doses used in experiments were frequently nonphysiologic, and invariably far exceeded the level of normal, human consumption.

There are relatively few human studies and epidemiologic surveys relating nonnutritive sweeteners and human bladder-cancer risk. In 1969, Stone et al.[336] found that cyclamates could adversely influence normal, human leukocytes by inducing chromosome breaks in vitro. Kessler,[197] in 1970, showed no increased incidence of bladder cancer in diabetics who consumed large amounts of nonnutritive sweeteners for many years. Morgan and Jain[250] also found no statistically significant increase in the risk of bladder cancer after the prolonged use of artificial sweeteners. However, a recent study reported an increase of bladder cancer in males taking saccharin as compared to a matched control population. In 1977, Barkin et al.[23] reported on three patients in whom the development of transitional cell carcinoma of the urinary bladder occurred after an unusually high intake of cyclamate for a long period.

Occupational or Industrial Carcinogens Causing Bladder Cancers

Human beings are exposed to a variety of occupational carcinogens. Unfortunately, our understanding of the full impact or hazards of these carcinogens and the means for their identification are rudimentary. Although certain, specific industries have been associated with an increased incidence of bladder cancer, there are a number of variables that make the identification of a specific carcinogen difficult. The amount of carcinogen necessary to induce a cancer is unknown; it is reasonable to assume that the critical exposure to carcinogens varies with the offending agent and the susceptibility of an individual. The time between the exposure to the carcinogen and the eventual development of the cancer is also unknown, although the latency period has been estimated to range from 18 to 40 years.[63, 170] Therefore, it is highly probable that a patient's current occupation may bear little relation to his or her tumor. A detailed investigation of the patient's occupational history is needed if the full impact of occupational exposure to carcinogens is to be meaningful.

Anthony and Thomas,[11] in 1970, reported that approximately 25 percent of male bladder cancer patients had a history of exposure to an occupational carcinogen. Veys,[352] in 1974, estimated that approximately 33 percent of men who died from bladder cancer in a highly industrialized area in England had a history of "potentially significant" occupational exposure. Cole et al.,[73] in 1972, identified five specific occupations associated with bladder cancers: work with dyestuffs, rubber, leather and leather products, paints, and organic chemicals. They estimated that, in a designated area in eastern Massachusetts, 18 percent of the bladder cancers in men and 6 percent in women were associated with these occupations.

At least four industrial-chemical carcinogens have been incriminated for the increased incidence of occupation-associated bladder cancer. Beta naphthylamine is a byproduct of many industries. In 1895, Rehn[293] first recognized an increased risk of bladder cancer among dyestuff workers; it is now well recognized that the risk of bladder cancer in this industry is associated with the naphthylamines and not with aniline, as was long suspected. Benzidine was first incriminated as a carcinogen in 1950 by Spitz et al.,[328] when they reported a relationship between benzidine exposure and the occurrence of human bladder cancer. This observation was confirmed by numerous case reports published subsequently.[63, 314] Wendel et al.,[363] in 1974, described 25 men engaged in the manufacture of benzidine, 13 of whom developed bladder cancers and 3 who developed renal pelvic cancers, one of which was bilateral. 4-Amino-diphenyl (xenylamine)[245] and 4-nitrodiphenyl[71] are byproducts of many industrial compounds, and have been shown to induce human bladder cancer. However, the exact impact of these agents on the incidence of urinary bladder cancer is unknown.

REFERENCES

1. Abel, J. A.: Analgesic nephropathy: A review of the literature 1967-70. Clin. Pharmacol. Ther. 12:583, 1971.
2. Abrahams, C., & Levin, N.W.: Experimentally induced analgesic nephropathy: Its pathogenesis. Med. Proc. 13:506, 1967.
3. Adam, W. R., Dawborn, J. K., Price, C. G., Ridell, J., & Story, H.: Anaplastic transitional cell carcinoma of the renal pelvis in association with analgesic abuse Med. J. Aust. 1:1108, 1970.
4. Alarcon-Segovia, D.: Drug-induced lupus syndromes. Mayo Clin. Proc. 44:664, 1969.
5. Alarcon-Segovia, D., Wakim, K. G., Worthington, J. W., and Ward, L. E.: Clinical and experimental studies on the hydralazine syndrome and its relationship to systemic lupus erythematosus. Medicine 46:1, 1967.
6. Amos, H.: Detection of antibodies in penicillamine sensitivity. Postgrad. Med. J. 44 (Suppl): 27, 1968.
7. Anderson, E. E., Cobb, O. E., & Glenn, J. F.: Cyclosphosphamide hemorrhagic cystitis. J. Urol. 97:857, 1967.
8. Angervall, L., Bengtsson, U., Zetterlund, C. G., & Zsigmond, M.: Renal pelvic carcinoma in a Swedish district with abuse of a phenacetin-containing drug. Br. J. Urol. 41:401, 1969.

9. Ansari, Z., & Baldwin, D. S.: Acute renal failure due to radio-contrast agents. Nephron 17:28, 1976.
10. Ansell, J. D., & Castro, J. E.: Carcinoma of the bladder complicating cyclophosphamide therapy. Br. J. Urol. 47:413, 1975.
11. Anthony, H. M., & Thomas, G. M.: Tumors of the urinary bladder: An analysis of the occupation of 1,030 patients in Leeds, England. J. Natl. Cancer Inst. 45:879, 1970.
12. Appel, G. B., & Neu, H. C.: The nephrotoxicity of antimicrobial agents. N. Engl. J. Med. 296:663, 722, 784, 1977.
13. Arseneau, J. C.: Non-lymphomatous malignant tumors complicating Hodgkin's disease. Possible association with intensive therapy. N. Engl. J. Med. 287:1119, 1972.
14. Atkinson, R. M., Currie, J. P., Davis, B., Pratt, D. A. H., Sharpe, H. M., & Tomich, E. G.: Acute toxicity of cephaloridine, an antobiotic derived from cephalosporin. Toxicol. Appl. Pharmacol. 8:398, 1966.
15. Aufderheide, A. C.: Renal tubular calcium oxalate crystal deposition. Its possible relation to methoxyflurane anesthesia. Arch. Pathol. 92:162, 1971.
16. Avram, M. M., Iancu, M., & Weiss, S.: Heroin usage nephropathy—Subclinical to end stage nephrotic syndrome. (Abstract). Am. Soc. Nephrol. 4th Annual Meeting, Washington, D.C., 1971.
17. Bacon, P. A., Tribe, C. R., Mackenzie, J. C., Verrier Jones, J., Cumming, R. H., & Amer, B.: Penicillamine nephropathy in rheumatoid arthritis. A clinical, pathological and immunological study. Q. J. Med., New Series XLV 661-684. 1976.
18. Baerg, R. D., & Kimberg, D. V.: Centrilobular hepatic necrosis and acute renal failure in solvent sniffers. Ann. Intern. Med. 73:713, 1970.
19. Baldwin, D. S., Levin, B. B., McCluskey, R. T., & Gallo, G.: Renal failure and interstitial nephritis due to penicillin and methicillin. N. Engl. J. Med 279:1245, 1968.
20. Bariety, J., Druet, P., Laliberte, F., & Sabin, C.: Glomerulonephritis with γ and Bl_c globulin deposits induced in rats by mercuric chloride. Am. J. Pathol. 65:293, 1971.
21. Barker, E. A., & Smuckler, E. A.: Nonhepatic thioacetamide injury. II. The morphologic features of proximal renal tubular injury. Am. J. Pathol. 74:575, 1974.
22. Bar-Khayim, Y., Teplitz, C., Garella, S., & Chazan, J. A.: Trimethadione (Tridione)-induced nephrotic syndrome. A report of a case with unique ultrastructural renal pathology. Am. J. Med. 54:272, 1973.
23. Barkin, M., Comisarow, R. H., Taranger, L. A., & Canada, A.: Three cases of human bladder cancer following high dose cyclamate ingestion. J. Urol. 118:258, 1977.
24. Barr, G. A., Mazze, R. I., Cousins, M. J., et al.: An animal model for combined methoxyflurane and gentamicin nephrotoxicity. Br. J. Anaesth. 45:306, 1973.
25. Beaver, D. L., & Burr, R. E.: Bismuth inclusions in the human kidney. A long term autopsy study. Arch. Pathol. 76:89, 1963.
26. Beaver, D. L., & Burr, R. E.: Electron microscopy of bismuth inclusions. Am. J. Pathol. 42:609, 1963.
27. Beernink, D. H., & Miller, J. J.: Anticonvulsant-induced antinuclear antibodies and lupus like disease in children. J. Pediatr. 82:113, 1973.
28. Beirne, G. J., & Brennan, J. T.: Glomerulonephritis associated with hydrocarbon solvents. Arch. Environ. Health 25:365, 1972.
29. Bell, W. R., Boss, G. R., & Wolfson, J. S.: Circulating coagulant in the procainamide-induced lupus syndrome. Arch. Intern. Med. 137:1471, 1977.
30. Bengtsson, U., Angervall, L., Ekman, H., & Lehmann, L.: Transitional cell tumors of the renal pelvis in analgesic abusers. Scand. J. Urol. Nephrol. 2:145, 1968.
31. Bengtsson, U., Johansson, S., & Angervall, L.: Malignancies of the urinary tract and their relation to analgesic abuse. Kidney Int. 13:107, 1978.
32. Bennett, W. M., Gilbert, D. N., Houghton, D., & Porter, G. A.: Gentamicin nephrotoxicity-morphologic and pharmacologic features. West. J. Med. 126:65, 1977.
33. Bennett, W. M., Hartnett, M. N., Gilbert, D., Houghton, D., & Porter, G. A.: Effect of sodium intake on gentamicin nephrotoxicity in the rat. Proc. Soc. Exp. Biol. Med. 151:736, 1976.
34. Bennett, W. M., Plamp, C., & Porter, G. A.: Drug-related syndromes in clinical nephrology. Ann. Intern. Med. 87:582, 1977.
35. Berdon, W. E., Schwartz, R. H., Becker, J., & Baker, D.: Tamm-Horsfall proteinuria: Its relationship to prolonged nephrogram in in-

fants and children and to renal failure following intravenous urography in adults with multiple myeloma. Radiology 92:714, 1969.
36. Berg, J. W.: The incidence of multiple primary cancers. I. Development of further cancer in patients with lymphomas, leukemias, and myelomas. J. Natl. Cancer Inst. 38:741, 1967.
37. Berman, L. B., & Katz, S.: Kanamycin nephrotoxicity. Ann. N.Y. Acad. Sci. 76:149, 1958.
38. Berry, H., Liyanage, S. P., Durance, R. A., Barnes, C. G., Berger, L. A., & Evans, S.: A controlled trial comparing azathioprine and penicillamine in the treatment of rheumatoid arthritis. Br. Med. J. 1:1052, 1976.
39. Biava, C. G., Dyrda, I., Genest, J., & Bencosme, S. A.: Kaliopenic nephropathy: A correlated light and electron microscopic study. Lab. Invest 12:443, 1963.
40. Bjornberg, A., & Gisslen, A.: Thiazides: A cause of necrotizing vasculitis. Lancet 2:982, 1965.
41. Blackman, S. S.: Intranuclear inclusion bodies in the kidney and liver caused by lead poisoning. Bull. Johns Hopkins Hosp. 58:384, 1936.
42. Blantz, R. C.: The mechanism of acute renal failure after uranyl nitrate. J. Clin. Invest. 55:621, 1975.
43. Blomgren, S. E., Condemi, J. J., & Vaughan, J. H.: Procainamide-induced lupus erythematosus. Am. J. Med. 52:338, 1972.
44. Bluemle, L. W., & Goldberg, M.: Renal accumulation of salicylate and phenacetin: Possible mechanisms in the nephropathy of analgesic abuse. J. Clin. Invest. 47:2507, 1968.
45. Border, W. A., Lehman, D. H., Egan, J. D., Sass, H. J., Glode, J. E., & Wilson, C. G.: Antitubular basement-membrane antibodies in methicillin-associated interstitial nephritis. N. Engl. J. Med. 291:381, 1974.
46. Boyd, J. F., Butcher, B. T., & Steward, G. T.: The nephrotoxic effect of cephaloridine and its polymers. Int. J. Clin. Pharmacol. 7:307, 1973.
47. Brock, N., Hohorst, H. J.: Metabolism of cyclophosphamide. Cancer 20:900, 1967.
48. Brown, J. M., Dorman, D. C., & Roy, L. P.: Acute renal failure due to overdosage of colistin. Med. J. Aust. 2:923, 1970.
49. Brunner, F. P., Giesecke, B., Gurland, H. J., Jacobs, C., Parsons, F. M., Scharer, K., Seyffat, G., Spies, G., & Wing, A. L.: Combined report on regular dialysis and transplantation in Europe. Proc. Eur. Dial. Transplant Assoc. 12:3, 1975.
50. Bryan, G. T., & Ertürk, E.: Production of mouse urinary bladder carcinomas by sodium cyclamate. Science 167:996, 1970.
51. Bryan, G. T., Ertürk, E., & Yoshida, O.: Production of urinary bladder carcinomas in mice by sodium saccharin. Science 168:1238, 1970.
52. Bryan, G. T., & Yoshida, O.: Artificial sweeteners as urinary bladder carcinogens. Arch. Environ., Health 23:6, 1971.
53. Bulger, R. E., & Siegel, F. L.: Alterations of the renal papilla during mercuric chloride-induced acute tubular necrosis. Lab. Invest. 33:712, 1975.
54. Burry, A. F.: The evolution of analgesic nephropathy. Nephron 5:185, 1968.
55. Burry, A. F.: Pathology of analgesic nephropathy: Australian experience. Kidney Int., 13:34, 1978.
56. Butler, W. T., Bennett, J. E., Alling, D. W., et al.: Nephrotoxicity of amphotericin B, early and later effects in 81 patients. Ann. Intern. Med. 61:175, 1964.
57. Bygbjerg, I. C., & Møller, R.: Genatmicin-induced nephropathy. Scand. J. Infect. Dis. 8:203, 1976.
58. Cameron, J. S., & Trounce, J. R.: Membranous glomerulonephritis and the nephrotic syndrome appearing during mersalyl therapy. Guy's Hosp. Rep. 114:101, 1965.
59. Campese, V. M., Marzullo, F., Schena, F. P., & Coratelli, P.: Acute renal failure during intermittent rifampicin therapy. Nephron 10:256, 1973.
60. Caranhall, J. C., Scowen, E. F., & Watts, R. W. E.: Effects of penicillamine in cystinuria. Br. Med. J. 1:588, 1963.
61. Carone, F. A., Kashgarian, M., & Epstein, F. H.: Effect of acute potassium deficiency on susceptibility of infection with particular reference to the kidney. Yale J. Biol. Med. 32:100, 1959.
62. Carr, R. J., & Biswas, B. K.: Methysergide and retroperitoneal fibrosis. Br. Med. J. 11:1116, 1966.
63. Case, R. A. M., Hosker, M. E., MacDonald, D. B., & Pearson, J. T.: Tumors of the urinary bladder in workmen engaged in the manufacture and use of certain dyestuff intermediates in the British chemical industry. I. The role of aniline, benzidine, alpha-naphthylamine

and beta-naphthylamine. Br. J. Industr. Med. 11:75, 1954.
64. Castell, D. O., & Sparks, H. A.: Nephrogenic diabetes insipidus due to demethylchlortetracycline hydrochloride. J.A.M.A. 193:237A, 1965.
65. Castleman, B., & McNeely, B. V.: Case records of Massachusetts General Hospital. N. Engl. J. Med. 278:1167, 1968.
66. Chang, L. W., & Sprecher, J. A.: pathological changes in the kidney after methyl cadmium intoxication. Environ. Res. 12:92, 1976.
67. Cherian, M. G., & Goyer, R. A.: Role of metallothioneins in disease. Ann. Clin. Lab. Sci. 8:91, 1978.
68. Cherian, M. G., Goyer, R. A., & Delaquerriere-Richardson, L.: Cadmium-metallothionein-induced nephropathy. Toxicol. Appl. Pharmacol. 38:399, 1976.
69. Chevet, D., Garre, M., Thomas, R., Ramée, M. P., Goasguen, J., & Alquier, P.: Nephropathies induites par la phényl-indanedione. Intérêt du test d'inhibition de migration des leucocytes. Nouv. Presse Med. 5:588, 1976.
70. Chievitz, E., & Thiede, T.: Complications and causes of death in polycythemia vera. Acta Med. Scand. 172:513, 1962.
71. Clayson, D. B., & Cooper, E. H.: Cancer of the urinary tract. In: Klein, G., Weinhouse, S., and Haddow, A., Eds: Advances in Cancer Research. Vol. 13. p. 271. Academic Press, London, 1970.
72. Cohen, J. L., & Jao, J. Y.: Enzymatic basis of cyclophosphamide activation by hepatic microsomes of the rat. J. Pharmacol. Exp. Ther. 174:206, 1970.
73. Cole, P., Hoover, R., & Friedell, G. H.: Occupation and cancer of the lower urinary tract. Cancer 29:1250, 1972.
74. Collins, R. J., Fromm, P. O., & Collings, W. D.: Chromium excretion in dog. Am. J. Physiol. 201:795, 1961.
75. Colvin, R. B., Burton, J. R., Hyslop, M. E., Jr., Spitz, L., & Lichtenstein, N. S.: Penicillin-associated interstitial nephritis. Ann. Intern. Med. 81:404, 1974.
76. Condit, P. T., Chanes, R. E., & Joel, W.: Renal toxicity of methotrexate. Cancer 23:126, 1969.
77. Cosbie Ross, J., & Goldsmith, H. J.: The combined surgical and medical treatment of retroperitoneal fibrosis. Br. J. Surg. 58:422, 1971.
78. Cove-Smith, J. R., & Knapp, M. S.: Sodium handling in analgesic nephropathy. Lancet 2:70, 1973.
79. Cox, J. N.: Fatal necrotizing angiitis after sulfa-dimethoxine therapy presenting as anaphylactoid purpura. Virchows Arch. [Pathol. Anat.] 359:97, 1973.
80. Crandell, W. B., Pappas, S. G., & Macdonald, A.: Nephrotoxicity associated with methoxyflurane anesthesia. Anesthesiology 27:591, 1966.
81. Croft, J. D., Swisher, S. N., Gilliland, B. C., Bakemeier, R. T., Leddy, J. P., & Weed, R. J.: Coombs'-Test positivity induced by drugs. Mechanisms of immunologic reactions and red cell destruction. Ann. Intern. Med. 68:176, 1968.
82. Cuppage, F. E., Setter, K., Sullivan, L. P., Reitzes, E. J., & Melnykovych, A. O.: Gentamicin nephrotoxicity. II. Physiological, biochemical and morphological effects of prolonged administration to rats. Virchows Arch. [Cell Pathol.], 24:121, 1977.
83. Dale, G. A., & Smith, R. B.: Transitional cell carcinoma of the bladder associated with cyclophosphamide. J. Urol. 112:603, 1974.
84. DeBeukelaer, M. M., Travis, L. B., Dodge, W. F., & Guerra, F. A.: Deafness and acute tubular necrosis following parenteral administration of neomycin. Am. J. Dis. Child. 121:250, 1971.
85. Deichgräber, E., & Johansson, S.: Urothelial renal pelvic tumors in phenacetin abusers. Acta. Radiol. 16:633, 1975.
86. Deming, C. L.: Tumors of the kidney, p. 895. In: Campbell, M. F., Ed.: Urology. Vol. 2. W. B. Saunders, Philadelphia, 1963.
87. Dinkel, L.: Nephrocalcinosis und dihychotachysterm-medikation. Dtsch. Med. Wochenschr. 90:1569, 1965.
88. Dische, F. E., Swinson, D. R., Hamilton, E. B. D., & Parsons, V.: Immunopathology of penicillamine-induced glomerular disease. J. Rheumatol. 3:145, 1976.
89. Disney, A. P. S., & Row, P. G.: A subcommittee of the Australia Kidney Foundation: Australia maintenance dialysis survey. Med. J. Aust. 2:651, 1974.
90. Dixon, F. J., Feldman, J. D., & Vazquez, J. J.: Experimental glomerulonephritis. The pathogenesis of a laboratory model resembling the spectrum of human glomerulonephritis. J. Exp. Med. 113:899, 1961.

91. Dowling, H. F., & Lepper, M. H.: Toxic reactions following therapy with sulfapyridine, sulfathiazole and sulfadiazine. J.A.M.A. 121:1190, 1943.
92. Dubois, E. L.: Procainamide induction of a systemic lupus erythematosus syndrome. Medicine 48:217, 1969.
93. Duggin, G., & Mudge, G.: Analgesic nephropathy: Renal distribution of acetaminophen and its conjugates. J. Pharmacol. Exp. Ther. 199:1, 1976.
94. Editorial: Analgesic nephropathy and aspirin. N. Z. Med. J. 79:1073, 1974.
95. Edwards, O. M., Huskisson, E. C., & Taylor, R. T.: Azotaemia aggravated by tetracycline. Br. Med. J. 1:26, 1970.
96. Egeberg, R. O., Steinfeld, J. L., Frantz, I., Griffith, G. C., Knowles, H., Jr., Rosenow, E., Serbrell, H., & Van Itallie, T.: Report to the secretary of HEW from the Medical Advisory Group on cyclamates. J.A.M.A. 221:1358, 1970.
97. Eknoyan, G., Gyorkey, F., Dichoso, C., Hyde, S., Gyorkey, P., Suki, W., & Martinez-Maldonado, M.: Renal involvement in drug abuse. Arch. Intern. Med. 132:801, 1973.
98. Elasa, L. J., Hayslett, J. P., & Spargo, B. H.: Wilson's Disease with reversible renal tubular dysfunction. Am. Intern. Med. 75:427, 1971.
99. Emmerson, B. T., & Pryse-Davies, J.: Studies on the nephrotoxic effect of neomycin. Aust. Ann. Med. 13:149, 1964.
100. Ershoff, B. H., & Bajwa, G. S.: Inhibitory effect of sodium cyclamate and sodium saccharin on tumor induction by 2-acetylaminofluorene in rats. Proc. Soc. Exp. Biol. Med. 145:1293, 1974.
101. Evan, A. P., & Ollerich, D. A.: The effect of lithium carbonate on the structures of the rat kidney. Am. J. Anat. 134:97, 1972.
102. Fabre, M. T., Fabre, J., Barthe, P. H., Yacoubi, B., & Regnier, C. L.: Etude ultrastructurale des modifications glomerularies dans l'hypervitaminose D. A propos de 5 observations. J. Urol. Nephrol. 74:982, 1968.
103. Falck, H. M., Tornroth, T., Kock, B., & Wegelius, O.: Fatal renal vasculitis and minimal change glomerulonephritis complicating treatment with penicillamine. Acta. Med. Scand. 205:133, 1979.
104. Falco, F. G., Smith, H. M., & Arcieri, G. M.: Nephrotoxicity of aminoglycosides and gentamicin. J. Infect. Dis. 119:406, 1969.
105. Farr, M. J., Wingate, J. P., & Shaw, J. N.: Practolol and the nephrotic syndrome. Br. Med. J. 2, 68, 1975.
106. Fillastre, J. P., & Kleinknecht, D.: Acute renal failure associated with cephalosporin therapy. Am. Heart. J. 89:809, 1975.
107. Flynn, C. T., Fainford, D. J., & Hope, E.: Acute renal failure and rifampicin: Danger of unsuspected intermittent dosage. Br. Med. J. 2:482, 1974.
108. Foad, B. S. I., & Hess, E. V.: Urinary bladder complications with cyclophosphamide therapy. Arch. Intern. Med. 136:616, 1976.
109. Forni, A. M., Koss, L. G., & Geller, W.: Cytologic study of the effect of cyclophosphamide on the epithelium of the urinary bladder in man. Cancer 17:1348, 1964.
110. Fowler, B. A., & Goyer, R. A.: Bismuth localization within nuclear inclusions by x-ray microanalysis. Effects of accelerating voltage. J. Histochem. Cytochem. 23:722, 1976.
111. Fox, M.: Suppression of tissue immunity by cyclophosphamide. Transplant 2:475, 1964.
112. Franchini, I., Mutti, A., Cavatorta, A., Corradi, A., Cosi, A., Olivetti, G., and Borghetti, A.: Nephrotoxicity of chromium. Remarks on an experimental and epidemiological investigation. Contrib. Nephrol. 10:98, 1978.
113. Frascino, J. A., Vanamee, P., & Rosen, P. P.: Renal oxalosis and azotemia after methoxyflurane anesthesia. N. Engl. J. Med. 283:676, 1970.
114. French, A. J.: Hypersensitivity in the pathogenesis of the histopathologic changes associated with sulfonamide chemotherapy. Am. J. Pathol. 22:679, 1946.
115. Frieberg, L.: Health hazards in the manufacture of alkaline accumulators with special reference to chronic cadmium poisoning: A clinical and experimental study. Acta Med. Scand. 138 (Suppl. 240): 1, 1950.
116. Frieberg, L.: Chronic cadmium poisoning. Arch. Ind. Health 20:401, 1959.
117. Frieberg, L., Piscator, M., Norberg, G., & Kjellstrom, T.: Cadmium in the Environment. 2nd Ed. CRC Press, Cleveland, 1974.
118. Friedman, E. A., Greenberg, J. D., Merrill, J. P., & Dammin, G. J.: Consequences of ethylene glycol poisoning: Report of 4 cases and

review of the literature. Am. J. Med 32:891, 1962.
119. Friedman, E. A., Sreepada Rao, T. K., & Nicastri, A. D.: Editorial. Heroin associated nephropathy. Nephron 13:421, 1974.
120. Friedman, L., Richardson, H. L., Richardson, M. E., Lethco, E. J., Wallace, W. C., & Sauro, F. M.: Toxic response of rats to cyclamates in chow and semi-synthetic diets. J. Natl. Cancer Inst. 49:751, 1972.
121. Frimpter, G. W., Timpanelli, A. E., Eisenmenger, W. J., Stein, H. S., & Ehrlich, L. I.: Reversible "Fanconi syndrome" caused by degraded tetracycline. J.A.M.A. 184:111, 1963.
122. Frohnert, P. P., & Sheps, S. G.: Long-term follow-up study of periarteritis nodosa. Am. J. Med. 43:8, 1967.
123. Fuller, T. J., Barcenas, C. G., & White, M. G.: Diuretic-induced interstitial nephritis. J.A.M.A. 235:1998, 1976.
124. Fulop, M., & Drapkin, A.: Potassium-depletion syndrome secondary to nephropathy apparently caused by "outdated tetracycline." N. Engl. J. Med. 272:986, 1965.
125. Galpin, J. E., Friedman, G. S., Shinaberger, J. H., Shapiro, D. J., Blumenkrantz, M. J., Stanley, T. M., Montgomerie, J. Z., Guze, L. B., & Coburn, J. W.: Acute interstitial nephritis due to methicillin and similar drugs. Kidney Int. 8:411A, 1975.
126. Ganota, C. E., Reimer, K. A., & Jennings, R. B.: Acute mercuric chloride nephrotoxicity. An electron microscopic and metabolic study. Lab. Invest. 31:633, 1974.
127. Gary, N. E., Buzzeo, L., Salaki, J., & Eisinger, R. P.: Gentamicin-associated acute renal failure. Arch. Intern. Med. 136:1101, 1976.
128. Gelbart, D. R., Weinstein, A. B., & Fajardo, L. F.: Allopurinol-induced interstitial nephritis. Ann. Intern. Med. 86:196, 1977.
129. Gelford, G. J., & Cromwell, D. K.: Methysergide retroperitoneal fibrosis and rectosigmoid stricture. Amer. J. Roentgenol. 104:566, 1968.
130. Genkins, G., Uhr, J. W., & Bryer, M. S.: Bacitracin nephropathy; Report of a case of acute renal failure and death. J.A.M.A. 155:894, 1954.
131. Gloor, F. J.: Changing concepts in pathogenesis and morphology of analgesic nephropathy as seen in Europe. Kidney Int., 13:27, 1978.
132. Goldberg, A., Smith, J. M., & Lockhead, A. C.: Treatment of lead poisoning with oral penicillamine. Br. Med. J. 1:1270, 1963.
133. Goldberg, M., Myers, C., English, P., & Peschel, W.: The mechanism of analgesic abuse nephropathy (abstr). J. Clin. Invest. 47:27a, 1971.
134. Goldman, R. L., & Warner, N. E.: Hemorrhagic cystitis and cytomegalic inclusions in the bladder associated with cyclophosphamide therapy. Cancer 25:7, 1970.
135. Goyer, R. A.: Effect of toxic, chemical, and environmental factors of the kidneys. In: Churg, J., Spargo, B. H., Mostofi, F. K., and Abell, M. R., Eds.: Kidney Disease: Present Status. pp. 202-217. Williams and Wilkins, Baltimore, 1979.
136. Goyer, R. A., May, P., Cates, M. M., & Krigman, M. R.: Lead and protein content of isolated intranuclear inclusion bodies from kidneys of lead poisoned rats. Lab. Invest. 22:245, 1970.
137. Goyer, R. A., & Krall, R.: Ultrastructural transformation in mitochondria isolated from kidneys of normal and lead-intoxicated rats. J. Cell Biol. 41:393, 1969.
138. Goyer, R. A., & Rhyne, B. C.: Pathological effects of lead. Int. Rev. Exp. Pathol. 12:1, 1973.
139. Graham, J. R.: Methysergide for prevention of headache: experience in five hundred patients over three years. N. Engl. J. Med 270:67, 1964.
140. Graham, J. R., Suby, H. I., LeCompte, P. R., & Sadowski, N. L.: Fibrotic disorders associated with methysergide therapy for headache. N. Engl. J. Med. 274:359, 1966.
141. Gralnick, H. R., & Greipp, P.: Thrombosis with epsilon aminocaproic acid therapy. Am. J. Clin. Pathol. 56:151, 1971.
142. Gray, J. E., Purmalis, A., Purmalis, B., & Mathews, J.: Ultrastructural studies of the hepatic changes brought about by clindamycin and erythromycin in animals. Toxicol. Appl. Pharmacol. 19:217, 1971.
143. Gray, S. J., & Sterling, K.: The tagging of red cells and plasma proteins with radioactive chromium. J. Clin. Invest. 29:1604, 1950.
144. Greenberg, L. H., & Mormary, H.: Audiotoxicity and nephrotoxicity due to orally administered neomycin. J.A.M.A. 195:827, 1965.
145. Griesemer, D. A., Muna, W., Osterman, Jr., F. A., Stevens, M. B., & Bell, W. R.: Procain-

amide-induced lupus. Johns Hopkins Med. J. 138:289, 1976.
146. Grishman, E., Churg, J., & Porush, J. G.: Glomerular morphology in nephrotic heroin addicts. Lab. Invest. 35:415, 1976.
147. Gunther, R., Asamer, H., & Dittrich, P.: DAS reversible procainamide-induzierte lupus-erythematodes syndrom. Dtsch. Med. Wochenschr. 94:2338, 1969.
148. Gunz, F. W., & Angus, H. B.: Leukemia and cancer in the same patient. Cancer 18:145, 1965.
149. Gutch, C. F. Tomhave, W. G., & Stevens, S. C.: Acute renal failure due to inhalation of trichlorethylene. Ann. Intern. Med. 63:128, 1965.
150. Hackett, E.: Idiopathic retroperitoneal fibrosis: A condition involving the ureters, the aorts, and the inferior vena cava. Br. J. Surg. 46:3, 1958.
151. Haddow, A., Kon, G. A. R., & Ross, W. C. Y.: Effects upon tumors of various haloalkylarylamines. Nature 162:824, 1948.
152. Hakala, T. R., Lange, P. H., Castro, A. E., et al.: Antibody induction of lymphocyte-mediated cytotoxicity against human transitional-cell carcinomas of the urinary tract. N. Engl. J. Med. 291:637, 1974.
153. Haller, J. A., Jr., Randell, H. T., Jr., Stowens, D., & Rubel, W. F.: Renal toxicity of polybrene in open heart surgery. J. Thorac. Cardiovasc. Surg. 44:486, 1962.
154. Halpren, B. A., Kempson, R. L., & Coplon, N. S.: Interstitial fibrosis and chronic renal failure following methoxyflurane anesthesia. J.A.M.A. 223:1239, 1973.
155. Hamilton, E. B.: Renal disease and penicillamine. In: Penicillamine Research in Rheumatoid Disease. Fabritius, Oslo, 1977 QV 354. p, 4043, 1976.
156. Harkcom, T. M., Conn, D. L., & Holley, K. E.: D-penicillamine and lupus erythematosus-like syndrome. Ann. Intern. Med., 89:1012, 1978.
157. Harrison, W. O., Silberblatt, F. J., & Turck, M.: Gentamicin nephrotoxicity. Failure of three cephalosporins to potentiate injury in rats. Antimicrob. Agts. Chemother., 8:209, 1975.
158. Hayslett, J. P., Bensch, K. G., Kashgarian, M., & Rosenberg, L. E.: Focal glomerulitis due to penicillamine. Lab. Invest. 19:376, 1968.
159. Heptinstall, R.: Pathology of the Kidney. 2nd Ed. Little, Brown, & Co., Boston, 1974.
160. Hertz, P., Yager, H., & Richardson, J. A.: Probenecid-induced nephrotic syndrome. Arch. Pathol. 94:241, 1972.
161. Hewitt, W. L: Gentamicin toxicity in perspective. Postgrad. Med. 50:(Supp.)7:55-59, 1974.
162. Hicks, R. M., Wakefield, J., & Chowaniec, J.: Evaluation of a new model to detect bladder carcinogens or co-carcinogens: Results obtained with saccharin, cyclamate and cyclophosphamide. Chem. Biol. Interact. 11:225, 1975.
163. Hill-II, G. J.: Amphotericin B toxicity, changes in renal morphology. Ann. Intern. Med. 61(Suppl):349-354, 1964.
164. Hindle, W., Posner, E., Sweetnam, M. T., & Tan, R. S. H.: Pleural effusion and fibrosis during treatment with methysergide. Br. Med. J. 1:605, 1970.
165. Hoffler, D.: Renal insufficiency due to phenacetin. Dtsch. Arztebl. 21:1447, 1976.
166. Hoffman, W. W., & Trippel, O. H.: Retroperitoneal fibrosis: Etiologic considerations. J. Urol 86:222, 1961.
167. Hojbye, G., & Nielsen, O. E.: Renal pelvic carcinoma in phenacetin abusers. Scand. J. Urol. Nephrol. 5:190, 1971.
168. Hollander, W., Jr., & Blythe, W. B.: Nephropathy of potassium depletion. In: Strauss, M. B., and Welt, L. G., Ed.: Diseases of the Kidney. 2nd Ed. p. 933. Little, Brown, & Co., Boston, 1971.
169. Hollenberg, N. K., Adams, D. F., Oken, D. E., Abrams, H. L., & Merrill, J. P.: Acute renal failure due to nephrotoxins. Renal hemodynamic and angiographic studies in man. N. Engl. J. Med. 282:1329, 1970.
170. Hoover, R., & Cole, P.: Population trends in cigarette smoking and bladder cancer. Am. J. Epidemiol. 94:409, 1971.
171. Hope, R. R., & Bater, L. A.: The frequency of procainamide-induced systemic lupus erythematosus. Med. J. Aust. 2:298, 1972.
172. Houghton, D. C., Hartnett, M., Campbell-Boswell, M., Porter, G., & Bennett, W.: A light and electron microscopic analysis of gentamicin nephrotoxicity in rats. Am. J. Pathol. 82:589, 1976.
173. Hruban, Z., Slesers, A. & Hopkins, E.: Drug-

induced and naturally occurring myeloid bodies. Lab. Invest. 27:62, 1972.

174. Hsu, C. H., Kurtz, T. W., Easterling, R. E., & Weller, J. M.: Potentiation of gentamicin nephrotoxicity by metabolic acidosis. Proc. Soc. Exp. Biol. Med. 146:894, 1974.
175. Hultengren, N., Lagergren, C., & Ljungqvist, A.: Carcinoma of the renal pelvis in renal papillary necrosis. Acta. Chir. Scand. 130:314, 1965.
176. Irnell, L.: Metastatic calcification of soft tissue on overdosage of vitamin D. Acta. Med. Scand. 185:147, 1969.
177. Iversen, B. M., Nordahl, E., Thunold, S., Jahannesen, J. W., Ofstad, J., & Willassen, Y.: Retroperitoneal fibrosis during treatment with methyldopa. Lancet 11:302, 1975.
178. Jaffe, I. A.: The effect of penicillamine on the laboratory parameters in rheumatoid arthritis. Arthritis Rheum. 8:1064, 1965.
179. Jaffe, I. A., Treser, G., Suzuki, K., & Ehrenreich, T.: Nephropathy induced by D-penicillamine. Ann. Intern. Med. 69:549, 1968.
180. Jawetz, E.: Polymyxin, colistin and bacitracin. Pediatr. Clin. North Am. 8:1057, 1961.
181. Jenis, E. H., & Lowenthal, D. T.: Kidney Biopsy Interpretation. pp. 190. F. A. Davis Co., Philadelphia, 1977.
182. Jennings, R. B.: Fatal fulminant acute carbon tetrachloride poisoning. Arch. Pathol. 59:269, 1955.
183. Jennings, R. W., & Kearns, W. M.: Necrotizing nephrosis in the rat following administration of carbon tetrachloride. Arch. Pathol. 56:348, 1953.
184. Johansson, S., Angervall, L., Bengtsson, U., & Wahlqvist, L.: Uroepithelial tumours of the renal pelvis associated with abuse of phenacetin-containing analgesics. Cancer 33:743, 1974.
185. Johansson, S., & Wahlqvist, L.: Tumors of urinary bladder and ureter associated with abuse of phenacetin-containing analgesics. Acta. Pathol. Microbiol. Scand., Sect. A 85:768, 1977.
186. Johnson, W. W., & Meadows, D. C.: Urinary-bladder fibrosis and telangiectasia associated with long-term cyclophosphamide therapy. N. Engl. J. Med. 284:290, 1971.
187. Junsela, H.: Carcinoma of the renal pelvis and its relationship to analgesic abuse. Ann. Chir. Gynaecol. Fenn. 62:386, 1973.
188. Katz, A., & Little, H. A.: Gold nephropathy; an immunopathologic study. Arch. Pathol. 96:133, 1973.
189. Katz, S. M., Sufian, S., & Matsumoto, T.: Urinary myelin figures in gentamicin nephrotoxicity. Am. J. Clin. Pathol. 72:621, 1979.
190. Kaufman, M.: Pancytopenia following use of hydralazine ("Apresoline"): Report of a case. J.A.M.A. 151:1488, 1953.
191. Kay, R. G.: Retroperitoneal vasculitis with perivascular fibrosis. Br. J. Urol. 35:284, 1963.
192. Kazantzis, G., Schiller, K. F. R., Asscher, A. W., & Drew, R. G.: Albuminuria and the nephrotic syndrome following exposure to mercury and its compounds. Q. J. Med. 31 (N.S.):403-418, 1962.
193. Kelchner, J., McIntosh, J. R., Boedecker, E., Guggenheim, S., & McIntosh, R. M.: Experimental autologous immune deposit nephritis in rats associated with mercuric chloride administration. Experientia 32:1204, 1976.
194. Kendall, M. J., & Hawkins, C. F.: Quinidine-induced systemic lupus erythematosus. Postgrad. Med. J., 46:729, 1970.
195. Kerbel, N. C.: Retroperitoneal fibrosis secondary to methysergide bimaleate. Can. Med. Assoc. J., 96:1420, 1967.
196. Kerr, W. S., Jr., Suby, H. I., Vickery, A., & Fraley, E.: Idiopathic retroperitoneal fibrosis: clinical experiences with 15 cases, 1956-1967. J. Urol. 99:575, 1968.
197. Kessler, I. I.: Non-nutritive sweetners and human bladder cancer: Preliminary findings. J. Urol. 115:143, 1976.
198. Kincaid-Smith, P.: Analgesic nephropathy, a common form of renal disease in Australia. Med. J. Aust. 2:1131, 1969.
199. Kincaid-Smith, P., Nanra, R. S., & Fairley, K. F.: Analgesic nephropathy: A recoverable form of chronic renal failure. In: Kincaid-Smith, P., & Fairley, K., Eds.: Renal Infection and Renal Scarring. p. 385 Mercedes Publishing Services, Melbourne 1971.
200. Kincaid-Smith, P., Saker, B. M., & McKenzie, I. F. C., & Muriden, K. D.: Lesions in the blood supply of the papilla in experimental analgesic nephropathy. Med. J. Aust. 1:203, 1968.
201. Klasterky, J., Hensgens, C., & Dubusscher, L.: Empiric therapy for cancer patients: Comparative study of ticarcillin-tobramycin, ticarcillin-cephalothin and cephalothin-tobramy-

cin. Antimicrob. Agents Chemother. 7:640, 1975.

202. Klavis, G., & Drommer, N.: Goodpasture syndrome und Benzineinwirkung. Arch. Toxikol. 26:40, 1970.
203. Kleinknecht, D., Ganeval, D., & Droz, D.: Acute renal failure after high doses of gentamicin and cephalothin. Lancet 1:1129, 1973.
204. Kleinknecht, D., Homberg, J. C., & Decroix, G.: Acute renal failure after rifampicin. Lancet 1:1238, 1972.
205. Kleinknecht, D., Jungers, P., & Fillastre, J. P.: Nephrotoxicity of cephaloridine. Ann. Intern. Med. 80:421, 1974.
206. Kleinknecht, D., Kanfer, A., Morel-Maroger, L., & Méry, J. Ph.: Immunologically mediated drug-induced acute renal failure. Contr. Nephrol. 10:42-52, 1978.
207. Koch-Weser, J., Sidel, V. W., Federman, E. B., et al.: Adverse effects of sodium colistimethate: Manifestations and specific reaction rates during 317 courses of therapy. Ann. Intern. Med. 72:857, 1970.
208. Kosek, J. C., Mazze, R. I., & Cousins, M. J.: The morphology and pathogenesis of nephrotoxicity following methoxyflurane (Penthrane) anesthesia. An experimental model in rats. Lab. Invest. 27:575, 1972.
209. Kosek, J. C., Mazze, R. I., & Cousins, M. J.: Nephrotoxicity of gentamicin. Lab. Invest. 30:48, 1974.
210. Koss, L. G., & Lavin, P.: Studies of experimental bladder carcinoma in Fischer 344 female rats. I. Induction of tumors with diet low in vitamin B_6 containing N-2 fluorenlyacetamide after single dose of cyclophosphamide. J. Natl. Cancer Inst. 46:585, 1971.
211. Krikler, D. M.: Paracetamol and the kidney. Br. Med. J. 2:615, 1967.
212. Krishnaswamy, S., Kuna, K., & Nanra, R. S.: Pattern of changes in renal function with analgesic abuse. Aust. N. Z. J. Med. 6:88, 1976.
213. Lachmann, P. J.: Nephrotic syndrome from penicillamine. Postgrad. Med. J. 44:23, 1968.
214. Ladd, A. T.: Procainamide-induced lupus erythematosus. New Engl. J. Med. 267:1357, 1962.
215. Landing, B. H., & Naki, H.: Histochemical properties of renal lead inclusion and their demonstration in urinary sediment. Am. J. Clin. Pathol. 31:499, 1959.
216. Lange, K.: Nephropathy induced by D-penicillamine. Contrib. Nephrol 10:63, 1978.
217. Lee, J. C., Dushkin, M., Eyring, E. J., Englemen, E. P., & Hopper, J., Jr.: Renal lesions associated with gold therapy. Light and electron microscopic studies. Arthritis Rheum. 8:1, 1965.
218. Lee, S. L., & Chase, H. P.: Drug-induced lupus. Seminars in Arthritis and Rheumatism 5:83, 1975.
219. Lehr, D., & Antropol, W.: Specific morphology of crystals appearing in the urine during administration of sulfonilamide derivatives. Am J. Clin. Pathol. 12:200, 1942.
220. Lichtenstein, L., & Fox, L. J.: Necrotizing arterial lesions resembling those of periarteritis nodosa and focal visceral necrosis following administration of sulfathiazole: Report of a case. Am. J. Pathol. 22:665, 1946.
221. Linton, A. L.: Renal disease due to analgesic. Can. Med. Assoc. J. 107:749, 1972.
222. Litt, I. F., & Cohen, M. I.: Danger-vapor harmful: Spot remover sniffing. N. Engl. J. Med. 281:543, 1969.
223. Liu, T., Smith, G. W., & Rankin, J. T.: Renal pelvic tumor associated with analgesic abuse. Can. Med. Assoc. J. 107:768, 1972.
224. Lyons, H., Pinn, V. W., Cortell, S., Cohen, J. J., & Harrington, J. T.: Allergic interstitial nephritis causing reversible renal failure in four patients with idiopathic nephrotic syndrome. N. Engl. J. Med. 288:124, 1973.
225. Maher, J. F.: Toxic nephropathy, p. 1355. In: Brenner, B. M., and Rector, F. C., Ed.: The Kidney. W. B. Saunders, Philadelphia, 1976.
226. Maher, J. F., Nolph, K. D., Bryan, C. W., & Grim, C. E.: Etiology and distribution of renal disease in central Missouri. Mo. Med. 69:799, 1972.
227. Maher, J. F., Raith, C. E., & Schreiner, G. E.: Hyperuricemia complicating leukemia. Treatment with allopurinol and dialysis. Arch. Intern. Med. 123:198, 1969.
228. Makinodan, T., Santos, G. W., & Quinn, R. P.: Immunosuppressive drugs. Pharmacol Rev. 22:189, 1970.
229. Manitius, A., Levitin, H., Beck, D., & Epstein, F. H.: On the mechanism of impairment of renal concentrating ability in potassium deficiency. J. Clin. Invest. 39:684, 1960.
230. Matalon, R., Katz, L., Gallo, G., Waldo, E., Cabaluna, C., & Eisinger, R.: Glomerular

sclerosis in adults with nephrotic syndrome. Ann. Interv. Med. 80:488, 1974.

231. Maunsbach, A. B., Madden, S. C., & Latta, H.: Light and electron microscopic changes in proximal tubules of rats after administration of glucose, mannitol, sucrose or dextran. Lab. Invest. 11:421, 1962.
232. Mavromatis, F.: Tetracycline nephropathy: Case report with renal biopsy. J.A.M.A. 193:191, 1965.
233. Mayaud, C., Kourilsky, O., Kanfer, A., & Sraer, J. D.: Interstitial nephritis after methicillin. N. Engl. J. Med. 292:1132, 1975.
234. Mazze, R. I., Cousins, M. J., & Kosek, J. C.: Dose related methoxyflurane nephrotoxicity in rats. Anesthesiology 36:571, 1973.
235. Mazze, R. I., Shue, G. L., & Jackson, S. H.: Renal dysfunction associated with methoxyflurane anesthesia. J.A.M.A. 216:27, 1971.
236. McAdam, L., Paulus, A. E., & Peter, B. J.: Adenocarcinoma of the lung during azathioprine therapy. Arthritis Rheum. 17:92, 1974.
237. McChesney, J. A., & Marquardt, J. F.: Hypokalemic paralysis induced by amphotericin B. J.A.M.A. 189:1029, 1964.
238. McCombs, R. P.: Systemic "allergic" vasculitis. Clinical and pathological relationships. J.A.M.A. 194:1059, 1965.
239. McCormick, J. N., Wood, P., & Bell, D.: Penicillamin-induced Goodpasture's syndrome. In: E. Munthe, Ed.: Penicillamine Research in Rheumatoid Disease. p. 268. Merck Sharp and Dohme, Symposium at Spatind, Norway, March, 1976.
240. McCormick, R. V.: Periarteritis occurring during propylthiouracil therapy. J.A.M.A. 144:1453, 1950.
241. McCurdy, D. K.: Distal tubule affected by amphotericin B. N. Engl. J. Med. 280:220, 1969.
242. McGinn, J. T., McGinn, T. G., Cherubin, C. E., & Hoffman, R. S.: Nephrotic Syndrome in drug addicts. N. Y. State J. Med. 74:92, 1974.
243. McGinn, J. T., McGinn, T. G., & Hoffman, R. S.: Nephrotic syndrome in heroin and cocaine addicts (abstract). Clin. Res. 18:699, 1970.
244. McLain, D. A., & Hahn, B. H.: Cryoglobulins in the procainamide-induced lupus syndrome. Arthritis Rheum. 22:305, 1979.
245. Melick, W. F., Escue, H. M., Naryka, J. J., Mezera, R. A., & Wheeler, E. P.: The first reported cases of human bladder tumors due to a new carcinogen: Xenylamine. J. Urol. 74:760, 1955.
246. Méry, J. Ph., & Morel-Maroger, L.: Acute interstitial nephritis. A hypersensitivity reaction to drugs. In: Giovannetti, Bonomini and D'Amico. Proceedings of the 6th International Congress on Nephrology, Florence, 1975. pp. 524-529. Karger, Basel, 1976.
247. Miller, J. M., MacConald, R. K., & Shock, N. W.: The effect of bacitracin on renal function. J. Clin. Invest. 29:389, 1950.
248. Molland, E. A.: Experimental renal papillary necrosis. Kidney Int. 13:5, 1978.
249. Morales, A., & Steyn, J.: Papillary necrosis following phenylbutazone ingestion. Arch. Surg. 103:420, 1971.
250. Morgan, R. W., & Jain, M. G.: Bladder cancer: Smoking, beverages, and artificial sweeteners. Can. Med. Assoc. J. 111:1067, 1974.
251. Moyer, J. H., Mills, E. C., & Yow, E. M.: Toxicity of polymyxin B. I. Animal studies with particular reference to evaluation of renal function. Arch. Intern. Med. 92:238, 1953.
252. Mudge, G.: Symposium on mechanisms of nephropathy: Analgesics. Proc. Am. Soc. Nephrol., 9th Annual Meeting, Washington, D.C., 1976.
253. Muehrcke, R. C.: Prolonged potassium deficiency and chronic pyelonephritis in man and animals, p. 581. In: Quinn, E. L., and Kass, E. H., Eds.: Henry Ford International Symposium on Biology of Pyelonephritis. Little, Brown, & Co., Boston, 1960.
254. Muehrcke, R. C.: Acute Renal Failure: Diagnosis and Management. C. V. Mosby Co., St. Louis, 1969.
255. Muehrcke, R. C., & Pirani, C. L.: Arsine induced anuria: A correlative clinicopathology study with electron microscopic observations. Ann. Intern. Med. 68:853, 1968.
256. Muller, J. C., Rast, C. I., Jr., Pryor, W. W., & Orgain, E. S.: Late systemic complications of hydralazine (Apresoline) therapy. J.A.M.A. 157:894, 1955.
257. Multicentric Trial Group: Controlled trial of D-penicillamine in severe rheumatoid arthritis. Lancet 1:275, 1973.
258. Mulvancy, W. P.: Periureteritis obliterans: A retroperitoneal inflammatory disease. J. Urol. 79:410,1958.

259. Murray, T., & Goldberg, M.: Chronic interstitial nephritis: Etiologic factors. Ann. Intern. Med. 82:453, 1975.
260. Nanra, R. S., Stuart-Taylor, J., DeLeon, A. H., & White, K. H.: Analgesic nephropathy: Etiology, clinical syndrome, and clinicopathologic correlations in Australia. Kidney Int. 13:79, 1978.
261. Nery, R.: The possible role of N-hydroxylation in the biological effects of phenacetin. Xenobiotica 1:339, 1971.
262. Nessi, R., Bonoldi, G. L., Redaelli, B., & DiFilippo, G.: Acute renal failure after rifampicin: a case report and survey of the literature. Nephron 16:148, 1976.
263. Neu, H. C.: Tobramycin: An overview. J. Infect. Dis. 134(Suppl.):S3-S19, 1976.
264. Neu, P. S., Lubash, G. D., Scherr, L., & Rubin, A. L.: Acute renal failure associated with carbon tetrachloride intoxication. J.A.M.A. 181:903, 1962.
265. Nicholls, D. P., Yasin, M.: Acute renal failure from carbamazepine. Br. Med. J. 4:490, 1972.
266. Nissen, H. M., & Bojesen, I.: On lipid droplets in renal interstitial cells: IV. Isolation and identification. Z. Zellforsch. Mikrosk. Anat. 97:274, 1969.
267. Nishizumi, M.: Electron microscopic study of cadmium nephrotoxicity in the rat. Arch. Environ. Health 24:215, 1972.
268. Oliver, J., MacDowell, M., & Tracy, A.: The pathogenesis of acute renal failure associated with traumatic and toxic injury. Renal ischemia, nephrotoxic damage and the ischaemuric episode. J. Clin. Invest. 30:1307, 1951.
269. Olivero, J., Bacque, F., Carlton, C. E., & Eknoyan, G.: Renal complications of drug addiction. Urology 8:526, 1976.
270. Ooi, B. S., Jao, W., First, M. R., Mancilla, R., & Pollak, V. E.: Acute interstitial nephritis. A clinical and pathologic study based on renal biopsies. Am. J. Med. 59:614, 1975.
271. Orloff, J., & Handler, J. S.: The cellular mode of action of antidiuretic hormone. Am. J. Med. 36:686, 1964.
272. Ormond, J. K.: Bilateral ureteral obstruction due to envelopment and compression by an inflammatory retroperitoneal process. J. Urol. 59:1072, 1948.
273. Oser, B. L., Carson, S., Cox, G. E., Vogin, E. E., & Sternberg, S. S.: Chronic toxicity study of cyclamate: Saccharin (10:1) in rats. Toxicology 4:315, 1975.
274. O'Toole, C.: Lymphocyte cytotoxicity in bladder cancer: No requirement for thymus-derived effector cells? Lancet 1:1085, 1973.
275. Owens, C. J., Yarbrough, D. R. III., & Brackett, N. C., Jr.: Nephrotic syndromes following topically applied sulfadiazine silver therapy. Arch. Intern. Med. 134:322, 1974.
276. Parker, R. H., & Hoeprich, P.: Toxicity associated with intravenous and intramuscular polymyxin B sulfate. Clin. Res. 12:244, 1964.
277. Pasternak, D. P., & Stephens, B. G.: Reversible nephrotoxicity associated with cephalothin therapy. Arch. Intern. Med. 135:599, 1975.
278. Pearson, R. M., & Soloway, M. S.: Does cyclophosphamide induce bladder cancer? Urol. XI:437, 1978.
279. Pepys, M. B.: Acetazolamide and renal stone formation. Lancet 2:837, 1970.
280. Perry, H. M., Jr., & Schroeder, H. A.: Syndrome simulating collagen disease caused by hydralazine (Apresoline). J.A.M.A. 154:670, 1954.
281. Pezzi, P. F., Frobese, A. S., & Greenberg, S. R.: Methoxyflurane and renal toxicity. Lancet 1:823, 1966.
282. Philips, F. S., Sternberg, S. S., Cronin, A. P., & Vidal, P. M.: Cyclophosphamide and urinary bladder toxicity. Cancer Res. 21:1577, 1961.
283. Phillip, G.: Haemorrhagic cystitis and cyclophosphamide. Lancet 2:942, 1963.
284. Plummer, N., & Wheeler, C.: Toxicity of sulfadiazine; Observations of 1357 cases. Am. J. Med. Sci. 207:175, 1944.
285. Powell, H. C., Garrett, R. S., Bernstein, L., & Mazze, R. I.: Methoxyflurane nephropathy. Human Pathol. 5:359, 1974.
286. Price, D. J. E., & Graham, D. I.: Effects of large doses of colistin sulphomethate sodium on renal function. Br. Med. J. 4:525, 1970.
287. Price, J. M., Biava, C. G., Oser, B. L., Vogin, E. E., Steinfeld, J., & Ley, H. L.: Bladder tumors in rats fed cyclohexylamine or high doses of a mixture of cyclamate and saccharin. Science 167:1131, 1970.
288. Raffery, E. B., & Denman, A. M.: Systemic lupus erythematosus syndrome induced by practolol. Br. Med. J. 2:452, 1973.
289. Randall, R. E., Jr., Bridi, G. S., et al.: Recov-

ery from colistimethate nephrotoxicity. Ann. Intern. Med. 73:491, 1970.

290. Randell, R. E., Strauss, M. B., & McNeely, W. F.: The milk-alkali syndrome. Arch. Intern. Med. 107:163, 1961.
291. Rathert, P., Melchior, H., & Lutzeyer, W.: Phenacetin: A carcinogen for the urinary tract. J. Urol. 113:653, 1975.
292. Reeve, T. S.: Treatment of malignant disease with an alkylating agent: Review of 100 patients treated with "Endoxan." Med. J. Aust. 48:686, 1961.
293. Rehn, L.: Über Blasengeschwulste bei Fuchsin-Arbeitern. Arch. Klin. Chir. 50:588, 1895.
294. Relman, A. S., & Schwartz, W. B.: The nephropathy of potassium depletion: A clinical and pathological entity. N. Engl. J. Med. 255;195, 1956.
295. Relman, A. S., & Schwartz, W. B.: The kidney in potassium depletion. Am. J. Med. 24:764, 1958.
296. Rich, A. R. L.: Hypersensitivity to iodine as a cause of periarteritis nodosa. Bull. Johns Hopkins Hosp. 77:43, 1945.
297. Richtsmeier, A. J.: Urinary bladder tumors after cyclophosphamide. N. Engl. J. Med. 293:1044, 1975.
298. Riddle, M., Gardner, F., Beswick, I., & Filshie, I.: The nephrotic syndrome complicating mercurial diuretic therapy. Br. Med. J., 1:1274, 1958.
299. Robson, M., Levi, J., Dolberg, L., & Rosenfeld, J. B.: Acute tubulo-interstitial nephritis following sulfadiazine therapy. Israel J. Med. Sci. 6:561, 1970.
300. Rosen, M.: Acute urinary suppression presumed due to bilateral ureteric obstruction by blood clot: an unusual feature of anticoagulant therapy. Med. J. Aust. 1:660, 1972.
301. Rupprecht, L., & Blessing, M. H.: Fibrosarcoma of the bladder after seven year chemotherapy of Hodgkin's disease in childhood. Dtsch. Med. Wochenschr. 98:1663, 1973.
302. Rutenburg, A. M.: The clinical use of sulfisomidine in urinary tract infections. Ann. N.Y. Acad. Sci. 69:389, 1957.
303. Rutherford, B. D.: Procainamide-induced systemic lupus erythematosus. N. Z. Med. J. 68:235, 1968.
304. Ryan, K. J., Schainuck, L. I., Hickman, R. O., et al.: Colistimethate toxicity: Report of a fatal case in a previously healthy child. J.A.M.A., 207:2099, 1969.
305. Saker, B. M., & Kincaid-Smith, P.: Papillary necrosis in experimental analgesic nephropathy. Br. Med. J. 1:161, 1969.
306. Scarpelli, D. G.: Experimental pathology of Vitamin-D induced nephrocalcinosis. In: Bajusz, E., and Jasmin, G., Eds: Methods and Achievements in Experimental Pathology. Vol 1. S. Karger, Basel/New York, 1966, p. 560-584.
307. Scharf, J., Nahir, M., Eidelman, S., Jacobs, R., & Levin, D.: Carcinoma of the bladder with azathioprine therapy. J.A.M.A. 237:152, 1977.
308. Scheele, C. V., Althoff, P., Kempi, V., & Schelin, U.: Nephrotic syndrome due to subacute glomerulonephritis—associated with hydrocarbon exposure? Acta Med. Scand. 200:427, 1976.
309. Scholes, J., Derosena, R., Appel, G. B., Jao, W., Boyd, M. T., & Pirani, C. L.: Amyloidosis in chronic heroin addicts with the nephrotic syndrome. Ann. Intern. Med. 91:26, 1979.
310. Schreiner, G. E., & Maher, J. F.: Toxic nephropathy. Am. J. Med. 38:409, 1965.
311. Schwartz, F. D., & Dunea, G.: Progression of retroperitoneal fibrosis despite cessation of treatment with methysergide. Lancet 1:955, 1966.
312. Schwartz, S. L., & Johnson, C. B. I.: Pinocytosis as the cause of sucrose nephrosis. Nephron 8:246, 1971.
313. Scott, J. T., & O'Brien, P. K.: Probenecid, nephrotic syndrome, and renal failure. Ann. Rheum. Dis. 27:249, 1968.
314. Scott, T. S.: The incidence of bladder tumours in a dyestuffs factory. Br. J. Indust. Med., 9:127, 1952.
315. Selroos, O., & Edgren, J.: Lupus-like syndrome associated with pulmonary reaction to nitrofurantoin. Acta Med. Scand. 197:125, 1975.
316. Seltzer, S. E., Benazzi, R. B., Kearney, G. P.: Cyclophosphamide and carcinoma of bladder. Urology 11:352, 1978.
317. Setter, J. G., Maher, J. F., & Schreiner, G. E.: Acute renal failure following cholecystography. J.A.M.A. 184:102, 1963.
318. Sheldon, P. J. H. S., & Williams, W. R.: Procainamide-induced systemic lupus erythematosus. Ann. Rheum. Dis. 29:236, 1970.
319. Silverberg, D. S., Kidd, E. G., & Shnitka, T. K.: Gold nephropathy: A clinical and pathologic study. Arthritis Rheum. 13:812, 1970.
320. Silverblatt, F., Turck, M.: & Bulger, R.:

Nephrotoxicity due to cephaloridine: A light and electron microscopic study in rabbits. J. Infect. Dis. 122:33, 1970.

321. Silverblatt, F. J., & Kuehn, C.: Autoradiography of gentamicin uptake by the rat proximal tubule cell. Kid. Int. 15:335, 1979.

322. Sladeck, N. E.: Metabolism of cyclophosphamide by rat hepatic microsomes. Cancer Res. 31:904, 1971.

323. Slavin, R. E., Millan, J. C., & Mullins, G. M.: Pathology of high dose intermittent cyclophosphamide therapy. Human Pathol. 6:693, 1975.

324. Sloth, K., & Thompsen, A. C.: Acute renal insufficiency during treatment with azathioprine. Acta Med. Scand. 189:145, 1971.

325. Spargo, B. H.: Renal changes with potassium depletion. In: Becker, E. L., Ed.: Structural Basis of Renal Disease. p. 565. Harper and Row, New York, 1968.

326. Sparrow, G. P.: Penicillamine pemphigus and the nephrotic syndrome occurring simultaneously. Br. J. Dermatol. 98:103, 1978.

327. Spiers, A. S.: Haemorrhagic cystitis and cyclophosphamide. Lancet 2:1282, 1963.

328. Spitz, S., Maguigan, W. H., & Dobriner, K.: The carcinogenic action of benzedine. Cancer 3:789, 1950.

329. Spühler, O., & Zollinger, H. U.: Die chronische interstitielle. Nephritis. Z. Klin. Med. 151:1, 1953.

330. Sreepada Rao, T. K., Niscastri, A. D., & Friedman, E. A.: Natural history of heroin associated nephrotic syndrome. N. Engl. J. Med. 290:19, 1974.

331. Sreepada Rao, T. K., Nicastri, A. D., & Friedman, E. A.: Renal consequences of narcotic abuse. Adv. Nephrol. 7:261, 1978.

332. Stark, F. R., & Coburn, J. W.: Renal failure following methylglucamine diatrizoate (Renografin) aortography. Report of a case with unilateral renal artery stenosis. J. Urol. 96:845, 1966.

333. Stavraky, K. M., Watson, T. A., White, D. F., & Miles, E. M.: Chronic lymphocytic leukemia and subsequent cancer in the same patient. Cancer 26:410, 1970.

334. Sternlieb, I., Bennett, B., & Scheinberg, I. H.: D-penicillamine induced Goodpasture's syndrome in Wilson's disease. Ann. Intern. Med. 82:673, 1975.

335. Sternlieb, I., & Scheinberg, I. L.: Penicillamine therapy for hepatolenticular degeneration. J.A.M.A. 189:748, 1964.

336. Stone, D., Lamson, E., Chang, Y. S., & Pickering, K. W.: Cytogenic effects of cyclamates on human cells in vitro. Science 164:568, 1969.

337. Strunk, S. W. & Ziff, M.: Ultra-structural studies of the passage of gold thiomalate across the renal glomerular capillary wall. Arthritis Rheum. 13:39, 1970.

338. Suki, W. N., Minuth, A. N., & Terrell, J. B.: Acute renal failure. A study of etiology, prognosis and the role of flurosemide. (abstract). Proc. West. Dialysis Transplant. Soc. 3:19, 1973.

339. Takacs, F. J., Tomkiewicz, Z. M., & Merrill, J. P.: Amphotericin B nephrotoxicity with irreversible renal failure. Ann. Intern. Med. 59:716, 1963.

340. Taves, D. R., Fry, B. W., Freeman, R. B., & Gillies, A.: Toxicity following methoxylfurane anesthesia. II. Fluoride concentrations in nephrotoxicity. J.A.M.A. 214:91, 1970.

341. Thiede, T., Chievitz, E., & Christensen, B. C.: Chlornaphazine as a bladder carcinogen. Acta Med. Scand. 175:721, 1964.

342. Thiede, T., & Christensen, B. C.: Bladder tumors induced by chlornaphazine: A five-year follow-up study of chlornaphazine-treated patients with polycythemia. Acta Med. Scand. 185:133, 1969.

343. Thompson, A. M., Antonovych, T., Lin, R., Wilson, R., Raposo, C., Venkatesan, R., Gula, A., Kramer, N., & Parrish, A. E.: Focal membranoproliferative glomerulonephritis (MPGN) in heroin users (Abstract). Am. Soc. Nephrol., 6th Annual Meeting, Washington, D.C., 1973.

344. Törnroth, T., & Skrifvars, B.: Gold nephropathy: prototype of membranous glomerulonephritis. Am. J. Pathol., 75:573, 1974.

345. Treser, G., Cherubin, C., Lonergan, E. T., Yoshizawa, N., Viswanathan, N., Tannenberg, A. M., Pompa, D., & Lange, K.: Renal lesions in narcotic addicts. Am. J. Med. 57:687, 1974.

346. Trump, B. F., & Janigan, D. T.: The pathogenesis of cytologic vacuolization in sucrose nephrosis: An electron microscopic and histochemical study. Lab. Invest. 11:395, 1962.

347. Tune, B. M., Fernholt, M., & Schwartz, A.: Mechanism of cephaloridine transport in the kidney. J. Pharmcol. Exp. Ther. 191:311, 1974.

348. Turk, J. L., & Poulter, L. W.: Selective deple-

tion of lymphoid tissue by cyclophosphamide. Clin. Exp. Immunol. 10:285, 1972.
349. Urizar, R., & Vernier, R. L.: Bismuth nephropathy. J.A.M.A. 198:187, 1966.
350. Utsinger, P. D., Zvaifler, N. J., & Bluestein, H. G.: Hypocomplementemia in procainamide-associated systemic lupus erythematosus. Ann. Intern. Med. 84:294, 1976.
351. Vane, J. R.: Inhibition of prostaglandin synthesis as a mechanism of action for aspirin-like drugs. Nature (New Biol.) 231:232, 1971.
352. Veys, C. A.: Bladder tumours and occupation: A coroner's notification scheme. Br. J. Indust. Med. 31:65, 1974.
353. Videbaek, A.: Chlornaphazin (Erysan) may induce cancer of the urinary bladder. Acta Med. Scand. 176:45, 1964.
354. Visek, W. J., Whitney, I. B., Kuhn, U. S. G., & Comar, C. L.: Metabolism of ^{51}Cr by animals is influenced by chemical state. Proc. Soc. Exp. Biol. Med. 24:610, 1953.
355. Wachstein, M.: Studies on inclusion bodies. I. Acid fastness of nuclear inclusion that are induced by ingestion of lead and bismuth. Am. J. Clin. Pathol. 19:608, 1949.
356. Wall, R. L., & Clausen, K. P.: Carcinoma of urinary bladder in patients receiving cyclophosphamide. N. Engl. J. Med. 293:271, 1975.
357. Walton, J. R.: Intranuclear inclusions in the lead-poisoned cultured kidney cell. J. Pathol. 112:213, 1974.
358. Watson, N. A., & Notley, R. G.: Urological complications of cyclophosphamide. Br. J. Urol. 45:606, 1973.
359. Watts, H. G.: Retroperitoneal fibrosis. N. Z. Med. J. 78:247, 1973.
360. Weiss, A. S., Markenson, J. A., Weiss, M. S., & Kammerer, W. H.: Toxicity of D-penicillamine in rheumatoid arthritis. A report of 63 patients including two with aplastic anemia and one with the nephrotic syndrome. Am. J. Med. 64:114, 1978.
361. Weldon, M. W., & Schultz, M. E.: Renal ultrastructure after amphotericin B. Pathology 6:191, 1974.
362. Wellwood, J. M., Simpson, P. M., Tighe, Jr., & Thompson, A. E.: Evidence of gentamicin nephrotoxicity in patients with renal allographs. Br. Med. J. 3:278, 1975.
363. Wendel, R. G., Hoegg, U. R., & Zaron, M. R.: Benzidine: a bladder carcinogen. J. Urol. 111:607, 1974.
364. Weinstein, S. H., Milleman, L. A., & Schmidt, J. D.: Cyclophosphamide. J. Urol. 114:157, 1975.
365. Wertlake, P. T., Butler, W. T., Hill, G. J., & Utz, J. P.: Nephrotoxic tubular damage and calcium deposition following amphotericin B therapy. Am. J. Pathol. 43:499, 1963.
366. White, A. B.: Hydralazine (apresoline) lupus with fatal renal failure. J. Am. Geriatr. Soc. 14:361, 1966.
367. Whittingham, S., & Mackay, I. R.: Systemic lupus erythematosus induced by procaine amide. Aust. Ann. Med. 19:358, 1970.
368. Whittle, T. S., Jr., & Ainsworth, S. K.: Procanamide-induced systemic lupus erythematosus. Renal involvement with deposition of immune complexes. Arch. Pathol. Lab. Med. 100:469, 1976.
369. Wilfert, J. N., Burke, J. P., Bloomer, H. A., & Smith, C. B.: Renal insufficiency associated with gentamicin therapy. J. Infect. Dis., 124 (Suppl): 148-153, 1971.
370. Wilkinson, R., & Eccleston, D. W.: Nephrotic syndrome induced by gold therapy. Br. Med. J. 2:772, 1970.
371. Winn, W. A.: Coccidiodomycosis and amphotericin B. Med. Clin. North Am. 47:1131, 1963.
372. Wiseman, A.: Effects of inorganic fluoride on enzymes, p. 48. In: Smith, F. A., Ed.: Handbook of Experimental Pharmacology of Fluoride. Springer-Verlag, New York, 1970.
373. Wiseman, J. C., & Hambly, C. K.: Cyclophosphamide and haemorrhagic cystitis. Med. J. Aust. 2:516, 1971.
374. Worth, P. H. L.: Cyclophosphamide and the bladder. Br. Med. J. 3:182, 1971.
375. Yarom, R., Stein, H., Peters, P. D., Slavin, S., & Hale, T. A.: Nephrotoxic effect of parenteral and intra-articular gold. Arch. Pathol. 99:36, 1975.
376. Yow, E. M., & Abu-Nassar, H.: Kanamycin: a re-evaluation after three years' experience. Antibiot. Chemother. 11:148, 1963.
377. Yudis, M., & Meehan, J. J.: Quinidine-induced lupus nephritis. J.A.M.A. 235:2000, 1976.
378. Zimmerman, S. W., Groehler, K., & Beirne, G. J.: Hydrocarbon exposure and chronic glomerulitis. Lancet 2:199, 1975.

12

The Testis

Francis H. Straus II

NORMAL TESTICULAR MORPHOLOGY AND TESTICULAR BIOPSY

Morphologic evaluations of the testes have always been rather vague. Organ weight is a quantitative record, but is obtainable only from experimental animal work or postmortem examination, and even here the presence of the epididymis and varying lengths of spermatic cord render testicular weights a more qualitative than quantitative measurement. Microscopic evaluation of testicular morphology usually centers on the diameter of the seminiferous tubules, the thickness of the tubular wall (tunica propria), the depth of the maturing germ-cell element within the tubular lumen, as well as the presence of all stages in the maturation process, from spermatogonia to morphologically mature spermatozoa. Finally, a rough evaluation of the quantity and quality of the Sertoli cell and Leydig cell populations is made. Quantitative measurements of morphologic abnormality are singularly lacking, and such modifiers as mild, moderate, or severe are often used to indicate a qualitative degree of severity to the morphologic observations. An advantage of the less precise, qualitative evaluation of the microscopic picture is that it allows the observer to discount the frequent artifactual changes that creep into histologic preparations of testes tissue even when these are obtained by careful surgeons, handled by serious pathologists, and prepared by a capable staff.

One pronounced defect of histologic preparations of the testes is the artifactual shrinkage commonly found in formalin-fixed testes tissue (Fig. 12-1), in which germ cells pull away from the basal lamina and from each other, leaving unnatural space between cells within the seminiferous tubule. This can be remedied by the use of Bouin's fixative, which hardens the abnormally soft testes, rendering it less likely to shrink (Fig. 12-2), and gives it more the consistency of liver, with which the microtomist can deal in a successful manner.

Two other frequent artifacts in histologic preparations of testes tissue and to which the observer should be alerted are mechanical, and again relate to the softness of the testicular tubular parenchyma and the fact that there are only delicate intercellular connections between the maturing germ-cell elements. The germ cells are gently held in place by engulfment in the Sertoli cell cytoplasm, and any squeezing or crushing of the soft tubule dislodges the maturing germ cells from this supporting cytoplasm, propelling them into the tubular lumen where—as a disorganized cell cluster—they are squeezed either retrograde or ahead, to a different segment of the tubule (Fig. 12-3). For this reason, sloughed intraluminal cell clusters should be disregarded in the interpretation of testicular morphology. The peripheral tubules in a biopsy fragment are often severely mechanically disrupted by cutting (Fig. 12-4), and should be given less importance than central tubular cross-sections.

In order to minimize tubular content distortion, we do not recommend, during testicular biopsy, a single incision through the tunica albuginea, with circumferential pressure causing the tubular parenchyma to squeeze up through the narrow slit, followed by slicing of the soft tubules at the base of the protruding mass leading to a badly distorted sample of seminiferous tubules. A better testicular biopsy technique cuts an ellipse in the tunica

(Text continues on p. 282.)

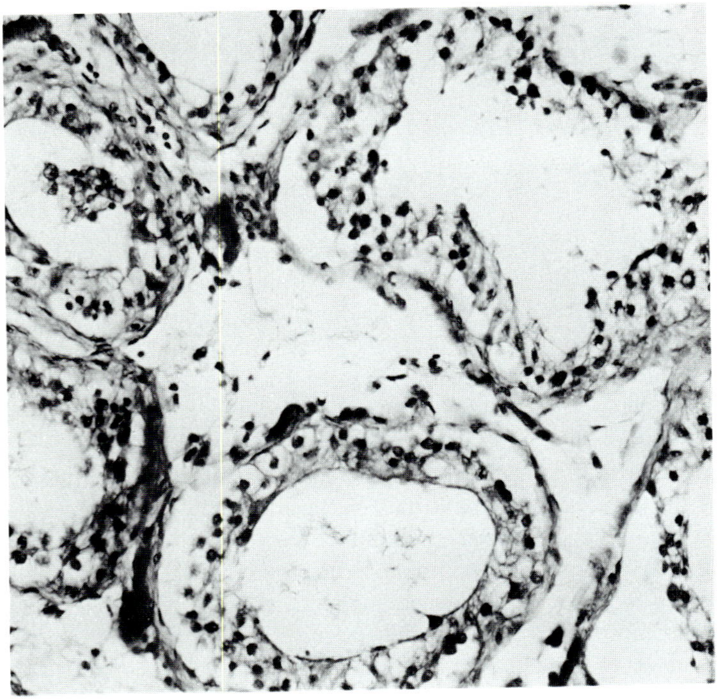

Fig. 12-1. Tubular disruption, cell vacuolization, and cell shrinkage typical of formalin fixation artifact of the testis. H&E, × 200.

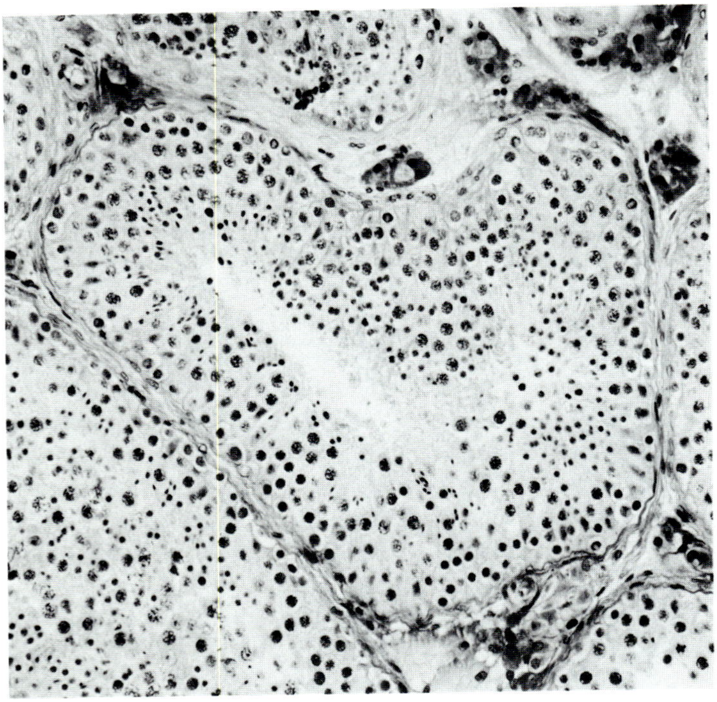

Fig. 12-2. Bouin's fixation normal seminiferous tubule with thin tunica propria (wall) and 10 cell layers of germinal epithelium with all maturation levels represented. H&E, × 200.

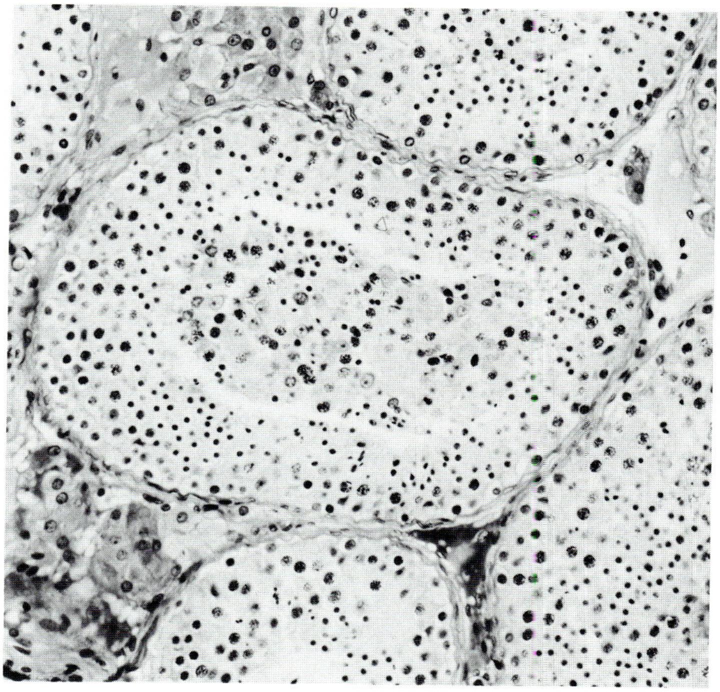

Fig. 12-3. Typical appearance of dislodged germinal epithelial cells occupying intraluminal position. H&E, × 200.

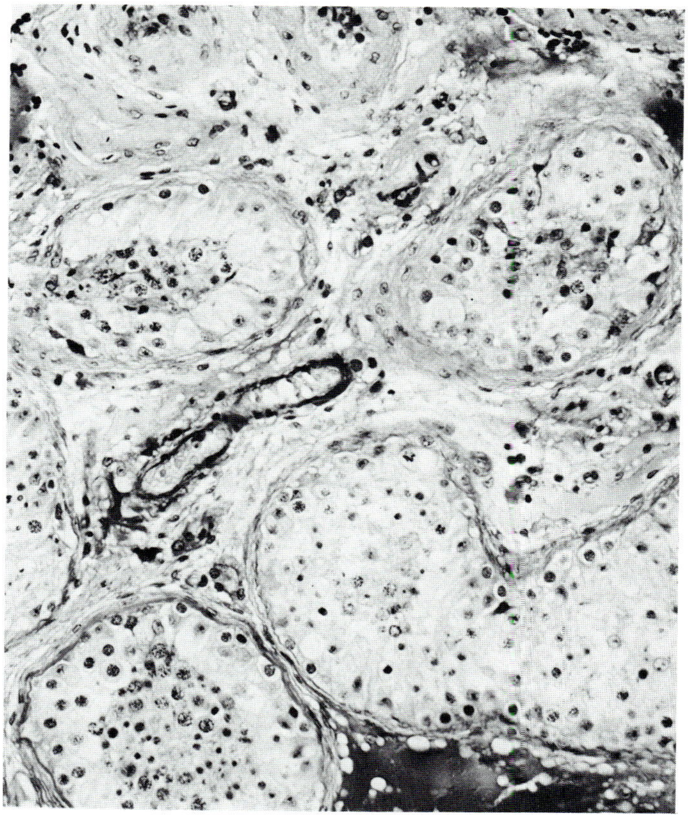

Fig. 12-4. Outside margin of biopsy fragment with severest mechanical distortion at top with small thick-walled empty seminiferous tubules. H&E, × 200.

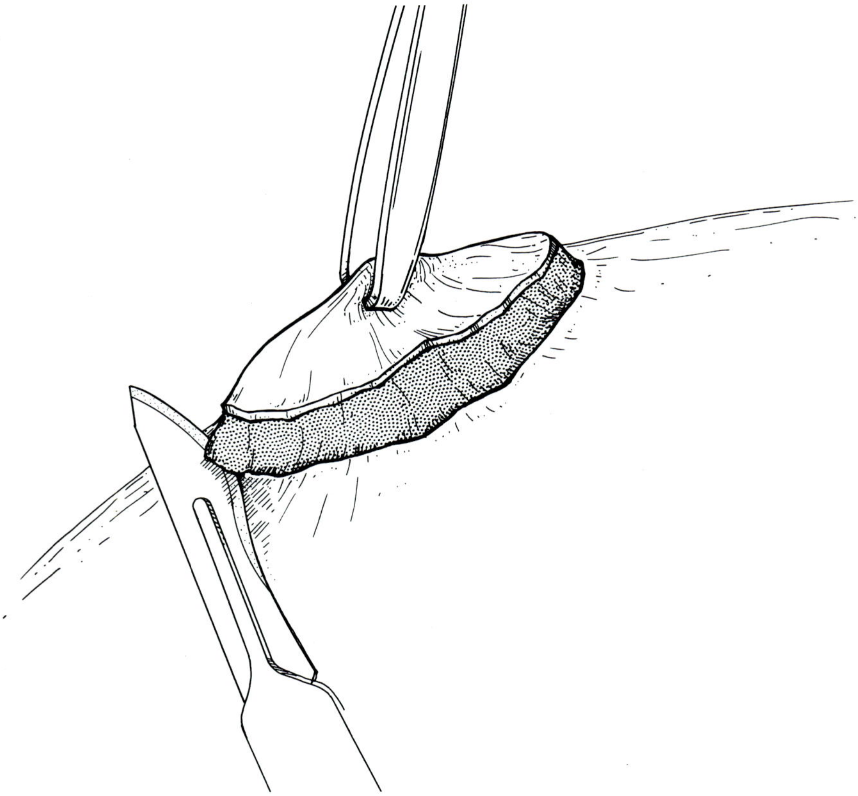

Fig. 12-5. Schematic view of separation of testicular biopsy fragment after elipse in tunica albuginea has been cut and tubular parenchyma extruded.

albuginea, and then raises this ellipse by gentle elevation with a forceps fastened to the tough tunica, followed by separation of the underlying adherent parenchyma from the rest of the testes parenchyma by scalpel slicing across the elliptical capsular defect in the same plane as the tunica albuginea. The specimen is always handled by the attached tunica, resulting in less distortion of the soft tubular contents (Fig. 12-5).

Attempts have been made to develop quantitative observations of testis morphology using histometric techniques. This is done by the statistically acceptable method of placing several random dots in the microscope eye piece and recording, in a number of random fields, whether the dots fall on the tubular lumen, tubular wall, Leydig cells, or interstitial connective tissue. Averages of the number of dots falling on any tissue compartment are then taken, and a more quantitative evaluation of the testicular morphology is made.[10] Difficulties arise when the evaluation points fall on margins or on artifactual configurations. Can the observer then disregard these points; or must they be included? This chapter will include only qualitative microscopic evaluations of the testicular parenchyma after various types of toxic damage. Some day, we may be able to replace these qualitative evaluations with quantitative observations.

Strangely, the rather intricate morphology of the adult human testes shows only a few avenues of morphologic change that express toxic damage. Generally, the least pronounced of these is maturation arrest (Fig. 12-6) (diminished-to-absent spermatozoa and spermatids toward the lumen of the seminiferous tubules), followed by the more severe change of hypospermatogenesis (Fig. 12-7) (propor-

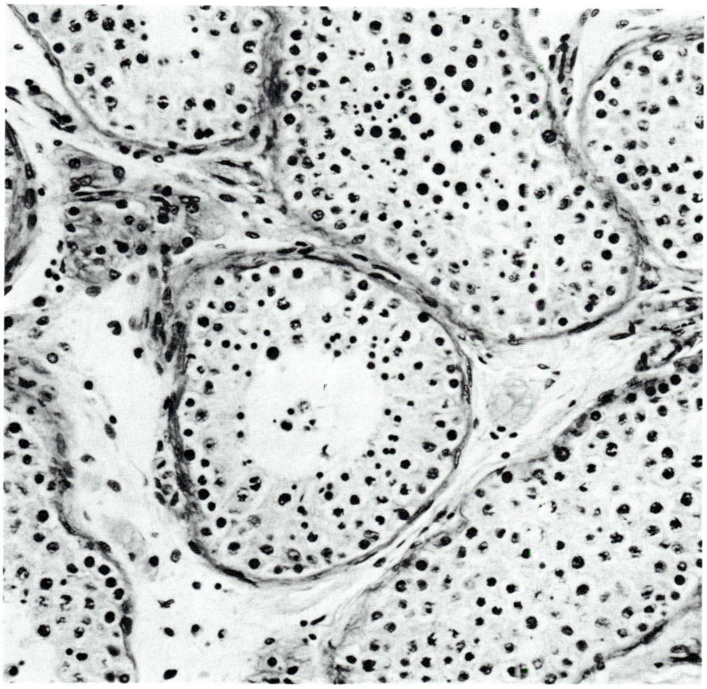

Fig. 12-6. Maturation arrest shows earlier stages of spermatogenesis are usual, but few or no mature spermatozoa are present. H&E, × 200.

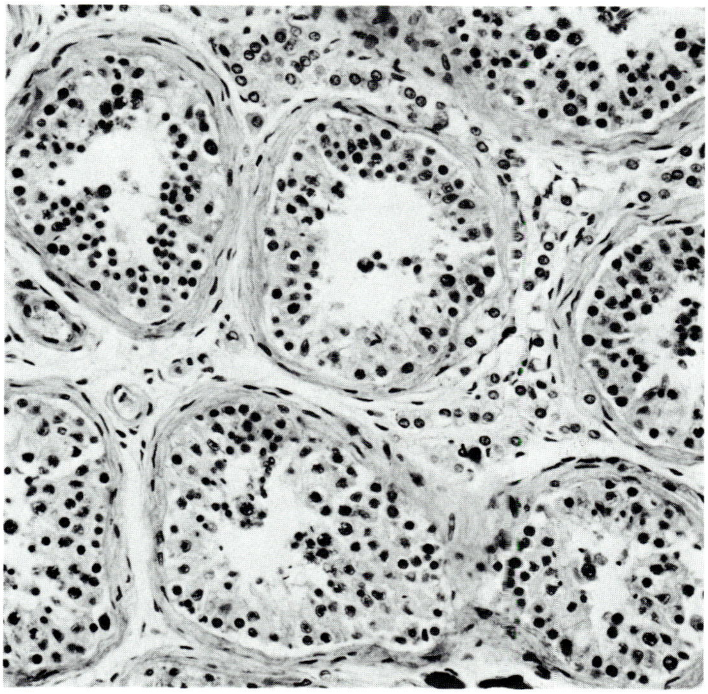

Fig. 12-7. Hypospermatogenesis with diminished population at all levels of spermatogenesis, diminished tubular diameter, and early apparent thickening of the tunica propria. H&E, × 200.

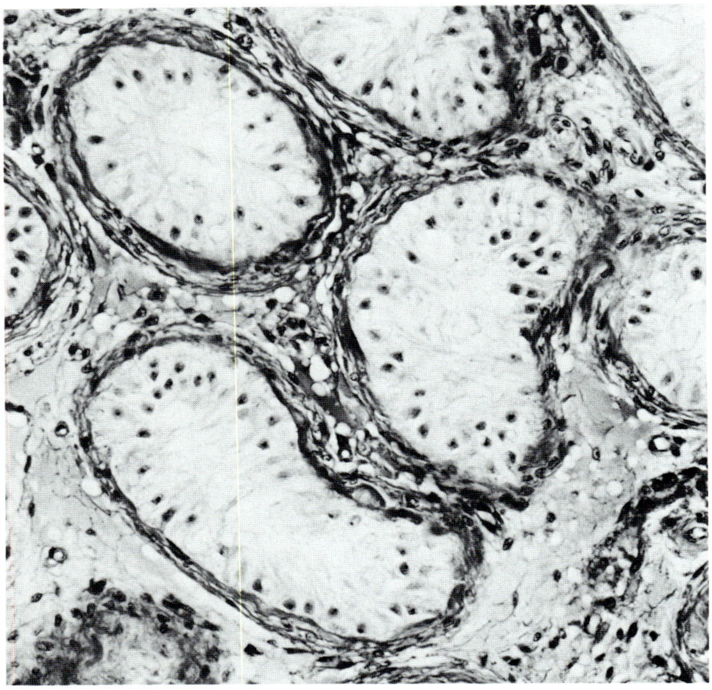

Fig. 12-8. Shrunken thick-walled tubules containing only Sertoli cells. H&E, × 200.

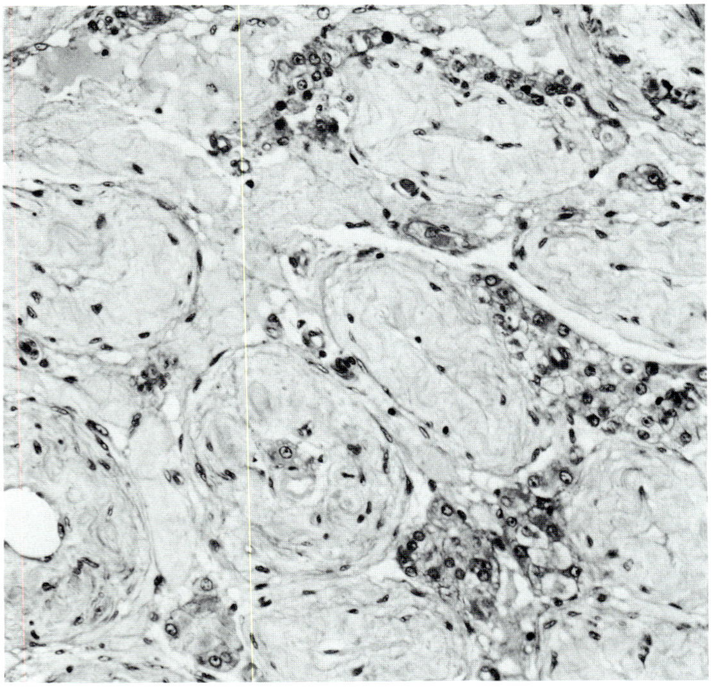

Fig. 12-9. Empty totally sclerosed seminiferous tubules with active interstitial Leydig cells.

tional hypoplasia of the maturing germ cell elements in the seminiferous tubule). The latter change leads to marked thinning of the maturing germ-cell layer, although representatives of each stage in the maturation process are still evident. More severe toxic effects lead to destruction of all germ-cell elements, including the stem germ cells—the spermatogonia—leaving only Sertoli cells within the shrinking seminiferous tubule (Fig. 12-8). Finally, with destruction of lumenal cells, the diminished lumenal volume will lead to diminished tubular diameter, progressive sclerosis of the tunica propria, and loss of lumenal Sertoli cells until the seminiferous tubules are entirely represented by a small, collagenous scar (Fig. 12-9). Sertoli cells and Leydig cells do respond sensitively to endocrine manipulations, and to some enzyme inhibitors.

Armed with the concept of a limited morphologic expression of testes injury, let us now proceed to identify four classes of drugs that damage the adult testes. A fifth class—which we shall call "other"—will identify some further known damaging agents and their effects on the testes.

DRUGS WITH HORMONAL ACTIONS

Sex Steroids

Certainly, small amounts of carefully administered testosterone given to a man with proven androgen deficiency may initiate more active spermatogenesis and improve fertility. But just as certainly, excessive administration of androgens or lesser exposure to natural or synthetic estrogens will reduce the secretion of hypothalamic gonadotropin-releasing substances (GRH), which in return will severely diminish follicle stimulating hormone (FSH) and lutenizing hormone (LH) production by the anterior pituitary. The first effect of this on the testes will be diminished prominence of the Leydig cells, with shrinking cytoplasmic volume and loss of the intense acidophilic character of their cytoplasm (Fig. 12-10 and

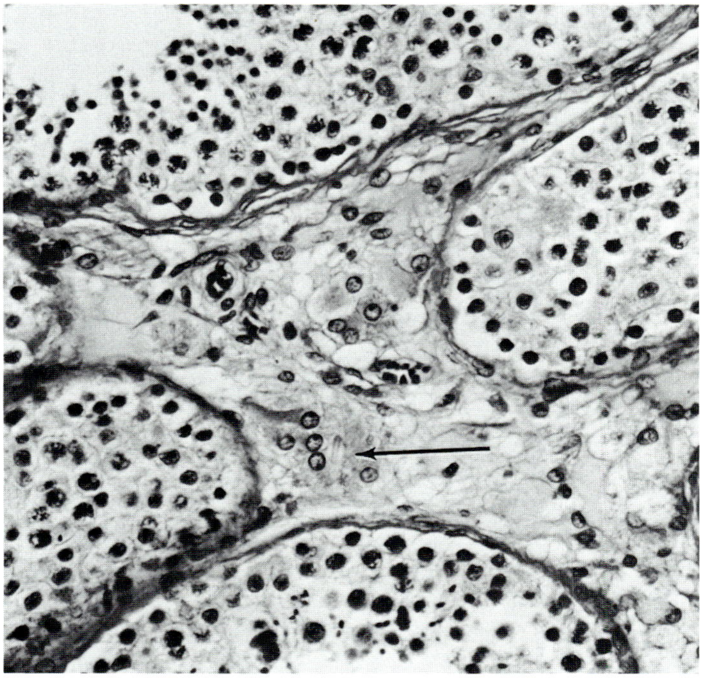

Fig. 12-10. Plump active Leydig cells with acidophilic cytoplasm (steroid-producing smooth-walled endoplasmic reticulum) and vacuolated cytoplasm (lipid storage, raw material for generating steroid hormones). Arrow localizes a crystalloid of Reinke (the normal protein crystalloid found in Leydig cells). H&E, × 300.

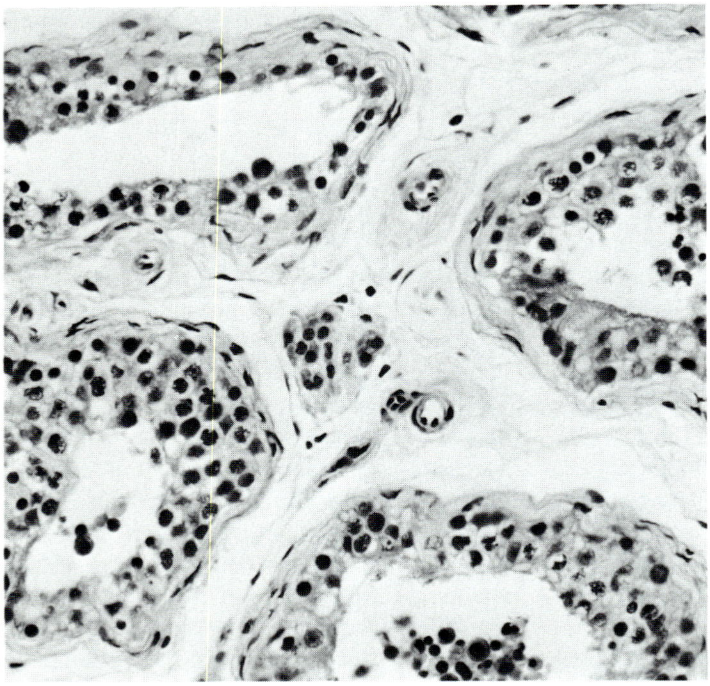

Fig. 12-11. Small atrophic Leydig cells filled with brown lipofuchsin pigment in a setting of severe hypospermatogenesis. H&E, × 300.

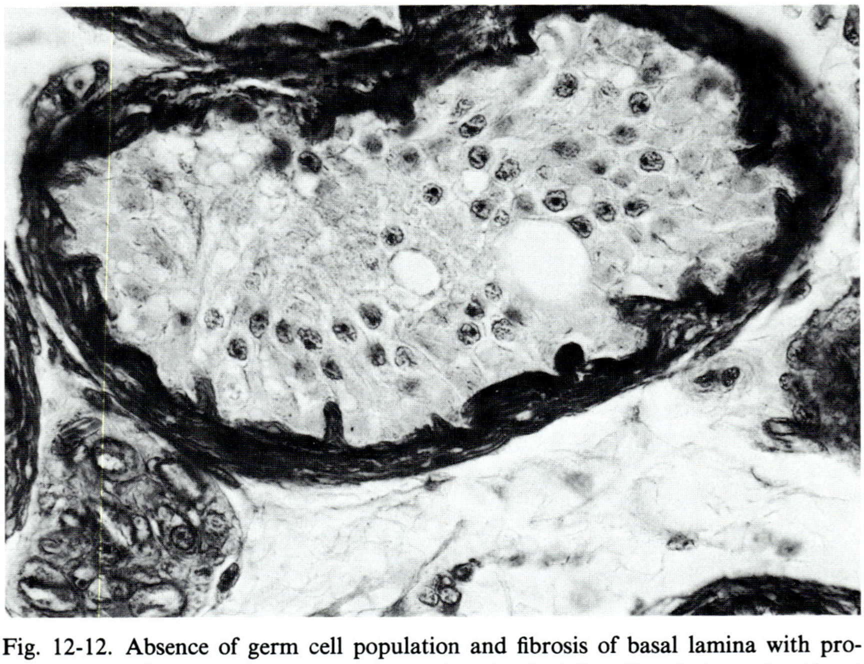

Fig. 12-12. Absence of germ cell population and fibrosis of basal lamina with projections of collagen up between remaining intraluminal Sertoli cells in an irradiated patient. Mallory trichrome, × 500.

12-11). The Leydig cells will appear small and lipid laden, and will exhibit increasing amounts of lipochrome pigment. Later, active spermatogenesis wanes, giving the picture of hypospermatogenesis. Finally, tubular atrophy is accompanied by increasing sclerosis of the tunica propria, with small projections of basal lamina and collagen between the peripheral Sertoli cells and spermatogonia (Fig. 12-12). When the tubular fibrosis is extensive enough, the seminiferous tubules are irreversibly damaged and the individual is rendered permanently infertile.

Cimetidine

Cimetidine is a nonsteroidal antiandrogen (a histamine H_2 receptor antagonist) which competes with androgen at cytosol receptor sites.[34] This partially accounts for the reported gynecomastia in human males treated with cimetidine, and the reported decrease in prostate and seminal vesicle weights in cimetidine-treated rats and dogs.

Van Thiel et al. reported endocrine studies on seven men before and after cimetidine therapy for peptic erosion and ulceration in the upper gastrointestinal tract.[32] All of these patients experienced reduction in the sperm count in ejaculate specimens, with a mean reduction of 43 percent; their seminal fluid volume remained the same before and after cimetidine treatment. The treatment did not alter basal FSH or LH levels, but did blunt the peak response of LH and LRF stimulation, thus giving testosterone levels 12 percent lower than normal in the cimetidine-treated patients. Clomifene stimulation also led to a blunted FSH response and a paradoxical decrease in the LH level. The testicular effects of cimetidine therefore appear to be secondary to alteration of pituitary gonadatropin secretion and androgen receptor site blockade, both of which could diminish testicular gamete production. A direct toxic effect of cimetidine on spermatogenesis has not yet been ruled out, nor have the antiandrogen effects of this drug on sperm transport or ejaculation been evaluated.

Prolactin

The effect of excess prolactin on testicular morphology is not at all clear. Jequier reported on three hyperprolactinemic men, all of whom showed varying degrees of impotence.[14] Testicular morphology revealed normal histology in two of these three cases, and severe maturation arrest with a thickened tunica propria in the third. All of the patients had low-normal testerone levels. After bromocriptine therapy the prolactin levels fell into the normal range, and the patients' impotence disappeared. Ejaculate examination revealed azoospermia in all three subjects, and therefore no improvement in fertility occurred. Excretory duct obstruction was assumed to be present in the two men with normal testicular histology; the azoospermia in the third patient followed inability of the testes to produce mature spermatozoa.

Another approach was used by Segal et al.[28] They studied 127 infertile men, finding elevated levels of prolactin in the group as a whole compared to 25 fertile men. Five of their patients showed markedly elevated prolactin levels, two with oligospermia, one with azoospermia, and one with hypogonadotropic hypogonadism; all five responded to bromocriptine therapy with reduction of their hyperprolactinemia into the normal range. Yet only one patient with oligospermia responded, demonstrating an improved sperm count up to 60 million/ml.

Both of the preceding reports tell us little about the gonadal effect of hyperprolactinemia because the patients seem to have had other, preexisting testicular and excretory duct pathologies. For this reason the report by Fang et al. on rats serving as hosts for a transplantable prolactin growth-hormone-secreting pituitary tumor is of interest.[12] At the height of tumor growth, these animals showed marked testicular atrophy, with gonads weighing half those of control animals. The secondary sex organs of the experimental animals weighed one-third those of controls. The animals' estrogen levels were elevated and their testerone levels were low. Testicular histology revealed reduction in seminiferous tubular diameter, totally arrested spermatogenesis (maturation between the spermatid and spermatozoon stages), and markedly reduced spermatogenesis (diminished meiotic divisions and maturation between resting spermatogonia and spermatozoa). Sertoli cells were relatively prominent in the depopulated tubular lumens, and Leydig cells were atrophic. Either prolactin excess has a strongly suppressive effect upon Leydig cell function and spermatogenesis in these animals, or the transplantable pituitary tumor in the animals was secreting another, as yet undescribed endocrine substance with such effects.[27]

ANTICANCER DRUGS

Alkylating agents (chlorambucil, cyclophosphamide, and thiotepa) cross-link DNA in the helix, or sever strands of DNA, primarily affecting rapidly multiplying cells. Alkylation probably also occurs in resting cells, but in slowly multiplying cell populations, DNA repair mechanisms correct the abnormality before the next cell division occurs. In the testes the most sensitive cell population comprises the immature germ cell elements, among which the spermatogonia and primary spermatocytes seem to be damaged first. Morphologically, this appears as diminished spermatogenesis (hypospermatogenesis), and finally, as more and more germ cells are damaged, there is total loss of all germ cell elements, with thickening of the tunica propria and narrowing of tubular diameters, rendering the patient irreversibly azoospermic and infertile (Fig. 12-13). Radiation leads to a similar change to that found after treatment with alkylating agents (Fig. 12-14). If treatment ceases before total germ-cell destruction, recovery may occur, but will extend over many months.[26] Rat germ-cell populations appear more resistant to the toxic effects of alkylating agents than do human immature germ cells.

The antimetabolite-folic acid analog drugs

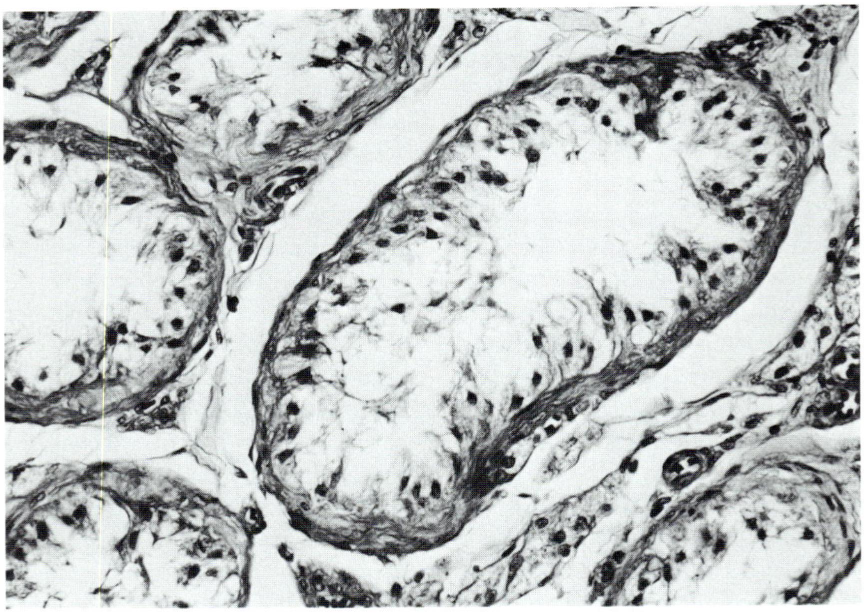

Fig. 12-13. Typical germ cell loss with thickened tunica propria Sertoli cells and Leydig cells remaining after destructive chemotherapy. H&E, × 200.

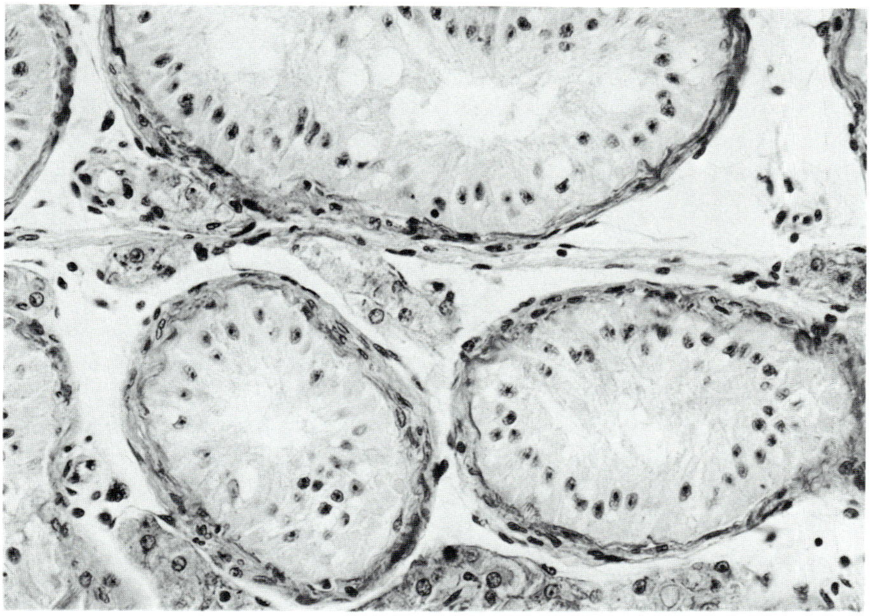

Fig. 12-14. Similar appearance to Figure 12-13 with better fixation in irradiated testes. H&E, × 200.

such as methotrexate function by blocking purine ring biosynthesis and do not show remarkable toxic effects on the testes. The antimetabolite pyrimidine analogs, 5-fluorouracil and cytosine arabinoside, inhibit pyrimidine synthesis and DNA polymerase; again there appears to be little toxic effect on the testes. The antimetabolite purine analogs, such as mercaptopurine, thioguanine, and azathioprine, inhibit purine synthesis and also do not show direct testicular toxic effects.

The vinca alkaloids inhibit microtubule function but do not alter the testes. The antibiotics actinomycin, daunorubicin, Adriamycin, and bleomycin tend to bind to the DNA and damage the helix, as well as inhibiting RNA synthesis. None of these drugs seem to affect the testes negatively.

HALOGENATED ORGANIC COMPOUNDS

A few reports on the effects of the toxic, halogenated organic compounds on the testes have been published. One describes the effects of the long-term respiratory exposure of 20 men to dibromochloropropane (DBCP) because of their employment in a pesticide factory. Three of the men had normal sperm counts and testes biopsies without diagnostic abnormality (they had worked only from 3 to 21 months in the factory). Five of the 20 men showed oligospermia and moderate to marked hypospermatogenesis, but their Leydig cells were unremarkable; these men had worked from 2 to 10 years in the factory. Finally, two men who had been exposed for more than 10 years were azoospermic; no germ cells remained in their testicular biopsies, and their Sertoli cells exhibited increased lipid and glycogen deposition. From these observations Biava et al.[4] suggest that spermatogonia are selectively sensitive to DBCP damage, with such damage first causing diminished spermatogenesis, and then loss of gamete production. Biava et al. also suggest that spermatogonia are preferentially affected because they are not protected by the blood-testes barrier provided more centrally within the tubule by the Sertoli cells.

Two rat experiments with polychlorinated

biphenyl (PCB) and dimethyl-2-dichlorovinyl phosphate (DDVP) produced varying effects, the most consistent of which were Leydig cell changes of hypertrophy, hyperplasia, increased acid phosphatase activity, and diminished androgen production. The last of these leads to diminished spermatogenesis, and in one report fragmentation and desquamation of maturing germ-cell elements within the seminiferous tubule occurred, until only spermatogonia and Sertoli cells remained.[18] The other report described no testicular weight change and no necrosis, but occasional sporadic chromosome breaks and exchange figures with bridging, in cytogenetic evaluations of the testes material.[8] Krause and Homla suggest that the organic halogen compounds adversely inhibit Leydig and Sertoli cell cholinesterase and nonspecific esterases, causing Sertoli cell fragmentation and diminished androgen production, with secondary LH stimulation leading to increased Leydig cell prominence.[18]

DDT (chlorophenothane), another hologenated organic compound widely studied in mammals, seems to have little effect on the testes. Tomatis et al.[29] reported that oral administration of DDT in doses varying from 2 to 250 ppm, given to CF-1 mice, did not impair fertility in these animals. There is a general statement in Goodman and Gilman saying that DDT has an estrogenic effect in mammals due to its inhibition of the hepatic metabolism of endogenous estrogens[13]; this, of course, might have an adverse effect on testicular function, but none has been specifically described.

A thorough study of the effect of the antispermatogenic compound bis-(dichloroacetyl)-diamine (Win 18446) has been reported by Reddy and Svoboda.[24] They describe the earliest changes as occurring in ultrastructural examinations of spermatids, which showed acrosomal abnormalities and dimorphic forms. Alterations in the disposition of axial filaments in the spermatid flagellum were also noted in the first few days of treatment, after which desquamation and degeneration of spermatids and spermatocytes occurred. Lysosomal bodies in Sertoli cells increased in number and contained fragments of organelles from the degenerating germ cells. By 3 weeks of steady treatment, numerous multinucleate giant cells (aggregated spermatids) were present along with the degenerating germ cells. At 4 weeks the seminiferous tubules were depopulated of maturing germ cells, leaving only Sertoli cells and spermatogonia; these two cell types appeared intact and viable. The Leydig cell mass underwent remarkable hyperplasia, increasing 100 percent by 8 weeks and showing active DNA synthesis. This Leydig cell hyperplasia was thought to occur in response to increased gonadotropin stimulation secondary to the diminished spermatogenesis.

HEAVY METALS

The toxic effects of several heavy metal salts on the rat testes have been described; no changes related to heavy-metal toxicity have yet been identified in human testes. The human male is a poorly conceived experimental animal because of attempts to protect him from known toxic exposures. There is also a strong desire by industry not to recognize toxic damage when it does occur, and an equally understandable reticence to document toxic testicular effects by parenchymal biopsy or orchiectomy.

It is very unlikely that the human species is totally protected from the toxic effects of heavy-metal accumulation, but so far documentation of this phenomenon is lacking. I have included here descriptions of such toxic effects in rodents, which may respond differently than humans, so that pathologists will be aware of the possibilities and may in the future document similar toxic effects in primates.

Cadmium

The adverse effects of cadmium salt administration on the testes were first described by Parizek and Zahor in 1956.[22] The acute toxic effects noted are capillary stasis, vessel damage, and hemorrhagic infarction within 24 to 48 hours of administration of cadmium, either intraperitoneally or intravenously. One month later revascularization occurs with Leydig cell regeneration and remasculinization. One year or more after cadmium administration there occurs an increased incidence of Leydig cell tumor formation in rats. Further investigations showed that cadmium toxicity of the testes appeared only in mammals with relatively exteriorized testes; frogs, fowl, lobsters, armadilloes, and opposums do not exhibit the toxic effects.[23] Why the oppossum testes is spared is at present unexplained.[1]

A more detailed description of the acute effects of a lethal dose of cadmium administrated to gerbils is reported by Berliner and Jones-Whittlers.[3] They describe capillary endothelial desmosome dissolution 3 hours after cadmium administration, leading to loss of vascular fluid into the interstitial compartment. This is later followed by extravasation of red blood corpuscles through the endothelial cell defects into the interstitial space. The authors suggest that the cadmium disrupts the calcium ion in the desmosomes, allowing the intercellular connections to break down. Similar observations were made by Aoki and Hoffer in the rat testes, showing extravasation of carbon particles and trypan blue from the capillary lumen into the interstitial space.[1] Aoki and Hoffer also describe clumps of adherent platelets piling up on the sites of endothelial cell detachment, and that these clumps attain sufficient bulk to obstruct the capillary channels, eventually leading to generalized organ ischemia and coagulative necrosis.[1] The desquamation and dissolution of germ cells within the seminiferous tubules is most likely an ischemic effect rather than a direct toxic effect of cadmium. The Aoki and Hoffer paper suggests that cadmium inhibits endothelial cell carbonic anhydrase, leading to rupture of desmosomal connections and increased capillary permeability.

The end-stage histologic appearance of the cadmium affected rat testes is of collagenized ghost forms of shrunken seminiferous tubules, some of which undergo dystrophic calcification. The interstitial space contains regenerated Leydig cells and is more fibrotic than usual. These testes are irreversibly infertile, but function as a source of androgens. In some rat and mouse experiments 80 percent of the animals showed multiple Leydig cell tumors when sacrificed 1 year after a single subcutaneous injection of cadmium chloride.[25] These tumors are indistinguishable from spontaneous Leydig cell tumors, and consist of closely packed, polyhedral acidophilic cells, with medium-sized vesicular nuclei usually containing a prominent central nucleolus.

Pre-exposure to a number of chemicals invokes a protective state in rats, blocking the toxic testicular damage that follows cadmium administration. Zinc salts, selenium, cobaltous chloride, thiols, cysteine, dimercaptopropanol, British anti-Lewisite (BAL), and low-dose preexposure to cadmium are all protective.[23]

Lead

The Russian literature contains sporadic reports of inorganic lead toxicity leading to male infertility in rats. Another paper, published in English, reports on the reproductive ability of 150 men occupationally exposed to lead fumes. This group as a whole showed decreased fertility, with asthenospermia (reduction in sperm vitality), hypospermia (reduction in numbers of sperm), and terato spermia (malformed sperm) found on examination of their ejaculate specimens. Because no abnormality of the pituitary-gonadal axis could be demonstrated, changes in spermatogenesis were thought to be due to the toxic effect of lead.[20] Tissue pathology that would document any morphologic abnormalities in lead-affected human testes is still lacking.

Mercury

There is no known human male gonadal toxicity due to inorganic mercury excess. There is some feeling that organomercury (alkymercury) compounds may damage gametes prior to fertilization.[17]

Aluminum

Aluminum sulfate given to rats in the concentration of 2.67 mmol/kg/day for 30 days led to testicular atrophy and "spermatogenic arrest"; no Leydig cell changes were noted.[15] In another study, Dixon et al. gave aluminum chloride to rats in the concentration of 4476 mg/liter for 90 days and found no abnormalities of the testes, no deviation of gonadatropin levels, and finally no loss in fertility in a post-experiment mating test.[9]

I am not aware of any reports of the effects of aluminum salts on human testes.

Boron

The toxic effects of boron have been known[6] since the mid-1960s, when boric acid delivered to rats in the concentrations of 25 mmol/kg was found to cause complete degeneration of the seminiferous epithelium of the testes. Adminsitration of borax at 140 mg/kg for 90 days to rats led to severe testicular atrophy and spermatogenic arrest.[33] Finally, experiments exposing rats to 2,000 ppm boron equivalent for 60 days led to testicular atrophy (testes one-third the weight of control testes), tubular atrophy (decreased tubular diameter), and extensive degeneration of germinal elements within the seminiferous tubules. Increased activity of premeiotic enzymes and decreases in postmeiotic enzyme activity after histochemical analysis were reported. FSH became elevated, and its increase was time- and dose-dependent; LH was less affected, and acid phosphatase was unchanged.[9] Again, no reports of toxic effects of boron salts on human testes are available.

OTHER

Alcohol

For years it has been said that excessive human ethanol intake leads to liver damage that inhibits the normal detoxification of natural estrogens. These estrogens then reduce the hypothalamic production of gonadatropin-releasing hormones and the pituitary production of FSH and LH, resulting in testicular atrophy. More recently it has been suggested that besides the mechanism outlined above, there is a direct toxic effect of ethanol on the testes, leading to diminished spermatogenesis, tubular atrophy, and tubular fibrosis; spermatogonia and Sertoli cells are relatively spared. These observations were made in male patients with chronic alcoholism, who had not developed severe liver damage, yet were azospermic or oligospermic.[5,11]

It is difficult to separate the endocrine effects of ethanol from its direct toxic effects in the testes. The state of preservation of the Leydig cell mass might be an important way of differentiating between the two proposed mechanisms of testicular atrophy in chronic alcoholism. If the atrophy were secondary to diminished hypophyseal stimulation, the Leydig cell mass would shrink, owing to diminished LH support, whereas if the atrophy were due to a direct toxic effect upon the spermatogenic elements within the seminiferous tubules, the stromal Leydig cells would be less directly affected. Unfortunately, separation of pituitary insufficiency from ethanol's direct toxic effect on the testes is further confused by Edmondson,[11] who described Leydig cell atrophy in 30 Los Angeles County alcoholics who did not have measurable liver disease.

Ethionine

When added to the diets of rats, *d,l*-ethionine (alpha-amino gamma-ethylmercaptobutyric acid), at a concentration of 0.5 percent, leads to early testicular degeneration at 10 days and severe uniform degeneration by 63 days.[16] There is early desquamation of spermatozoa and spermatids, with interstitial edema. Later, there are degenerative changes in spermatocytes, followed by multinucleate giant-cell formation among spermatocytes and spermatids. Finally, there is the loss of all maturing germ-cell elements, with only Sertoli cells and a few spermatogonia remaining. The tubular diameters steadily diminish, to less than one-third their original size, and the tunica propria is severely wrinkled. The secondary sex glands also become atrophic. The treated rats also showed pancreatitis and liver fibrosis.[16]

The recovery of test rats from *d,l*-ethionine administration in dosages of 25 mg/100 gm body weight, given daily by i.p. injection for 2 months, was marked by proliferation of the remaining spermatogonia, which formed laterally spreading clusters in the atrophic seminiferous tubules. After repopulation by the spermatogonia, primary spermatocytes began to appear, and in this way there was renewal of the entire germ-cell maturation process. Epididymal sperm granulomata were commonly found in the treated animals.[2] The authors suggest that ethionine is toxic to spermatocytes and some spermatogonia, but that the initial abnormality produced by this agent shows up later in the maturation process, leading to a "delayed lethal effect."

Monoamine Oxidase (MAO) Inhibitors

Administration of pargyline to young male rats leads to testicular weight loss, irregular sloughing of spermatozoa, spermatids, and spermatocytes, and to a final appearance of hypospermatogenesis and maturation arrest.[31]

Methadone

Study of a group of men in a methadone support group revealed widespread impotence, a decreased volume of ejaculate, increased sperm counts per cubic millimeter, and decreased motility of spermatozoa.[7] No testicular biopsies were performed. This group of men had fathered 53 children before being started on methadone, but since methadone therapy had begun, none had fathered any children. In contrast, individuals said to be using heroin remained fertile.

Nitrous Oxide

Because of the already observed effects of nitrous oxide exposure on rapidly proliferating cell populations, and because of the current concerns over chronic exposure to N_2O in operating theaters and in its long-term use for pain, Kripke et al. reported their findings in rats exposed to an atmosphere containing 20 percent N_2O for 35 days.[19] Focal loss of maturing germ cells was noted as early as the second day of exposure; by 14 days, all of the animals' testes showed weight loss, diminished seminiferous tubular diameters, and initial desquamation of spermatozoa and spermatids followed by later desquamation of spermatocytes. At 30 days exposure, virtually all tubular cross sections showed atrophic changes, with multinucleate giant-cell formation (spermatids in the syncytium); spermatogonia, Sertoli cells, Leydig cells, support cells, and vessels all remained unaffected. Rats returned to room air showed nearly complete recovery after 6 days. The toxic effect of nitrous oxide seems to directly affect meiotic cell division and its products, and is similar to the effect of some halogenated hydrocarbons. The mechanisms of action is not understood.

Sulphasalazine

Two reports characterizing anatomic and functional abnormalities in the spermatozoa of patients on long-term sulphasalazine therapy for ulcerative colitis have been published.[30,21] Both suggest that this antibiotic has a toxic effect directly on the spermatozoa, leading to diminished sperm counts, increased numbers of abnormal forms in the ejaculate specimen (the identification of 3 to 8 percent megalosperms with large, swollen sperm heads), and a generalized decrease in sperm motility. Testicular biopsy in one sulphasalazine-treated individual revealed no alteration from a normal configuration of seminiferous tubules with active spermatogenesis. The discontinuation of sulphasalazine treatment leads to rapid recovery (2 to 4 weeks) of semen abnormalities, and the wives of several patients became pregnant after discontinuation of the drug.[30]

REFERENCES

1. Aoki, A. & Hoffer, A.: Reexamination of the lesions in rat testes caused by cadmium. Biol. Reprod. 18(4:579–591) May 1978.
2. Benson, W. R., & Clark, F. S.: Regenerative changes and spermatocytic granulomas in the rat testes after treatment with DL Ethionine. Am. J. Pathol. 49:981–995, 1966.
3. Berliner, A. F., & Jones-Wittlers, P.: Early effects of a lethal casmium dose on gerbil testes. Biol. Reprod. 13:240–247, 1975.
4. Biava, C., Smuckler, E., & Whorton, D.: The testicular morphology of individuals exposed to dibromochloropropane. J. Exp. Mol. Pathol. 29:448–458, 1978.
5. Boiessen, P. T., Lindholm, J., Hagen, C. et al.: Histological changes in testicular biopsies from chronic alcoholics with and without liver disease. Acta Pathol. Microbiol. Scand. (Sect A) 87:139–142, 1979.
6. Bouissou, H., & Castagnol, R.: Action de l'acide borique sur le testicule du rat. Arch. Mal. Prof. 26:293, 1965.
7. Cicero, T. J., Bell, R. D., Wiest, W. G., et al.: Function of the male sex organs in heroin and methadone users. N. Engl. J. Med. 292:882–997, 1975.
8. Dikshith, T. S., Rockwood, W., & Coulston, F.: Effects of a polychlorinated biphenyl (Aroclor 254) on rat testes. J. Exp. Mol. Pathol. 22(3)376–385, 1975.
9. Dixon, R. L., Sherins, R. J., & Lee, I. P.: Assessment of environmental factors affecting male fertility. Environ. Health Perspect. 30:53–68, 1979.
10. Dykes, J. R. W.: Histometric assessment of human testicular biopsies. J. Pathol. 97:429–440, 1969.
11. Edmondson, A.: Pathology of alcoholism. Am. J. Clin. Pathol. 74(5):725–742, 1980.
12. Fang, V. S., Refetoff, S., & Rosenfield, R. L.: Hypogonadism induced by a transplantable prolactin producing tumor in male rats. Hormonal and morphologic studies. Endocrinology 95(4):991–998, 1974.
13. Harvey, S. C.: Antiseptics and disinfectants; fungicides; ectoparasiticides. In: Goodman, L., & Gilman, A. Eds.: The Pharmacological Basis of Therapeutics. 5th Ed. pp 1014. MacMillan, New York, 1975.
14. Jequier, A., Crich, J. C., & Ansell, I. D.: Clinical findings and testicular histology in three hyperprolactinemic infertile men. Fertil. Steril. 31(5):525–530, 1979.
15. Kamboj, V. P., & Kar, A. B.: Antitesticular effect of metallic and rare earth salts. J. Reprod. Fertil. 7:21–28, 1964.
16. Kaufman, N., Klavins, J. V., & Kinney, T. D.: Testicular damage following ethionine administration. Am. J. Pathol. 32(1):105–116, 1956.
17. Khera, K. S.: Reproductive capability of male rats and mice treated with methyl mercury. Toxicol. Appl. Pharmacol. 24:167–177, 1973.
18. Krause, W., & Homola, S.: Alteration of the seminiferous epithelium and the Leydig cells of the rat testes after IM application of Dichlorvos (DDVP). Bull. Environ. Contam. Toxicol. 2(5):429–433, 1974.
19. Krieke, B. J., Kelman, A. P., Shah, W. K., et al.: Testicular reaction to prolonged exposure to nitrous oxide. Anesthesiology 44(2):104–113, 1976.
20. Lancranjan, I., Popescu, H. I., Gavanescu, O., et al.: Reproductive ability of workmen occupationally exposed to lead. Arch. Environ. Health 30:396–401, 1975.
21. Levi, A. J., Fisher, A. M., Hughes, L., et al.: Male infertility due to sulphasalazine. Lancet 2(8137):276–278, 1979.
22. Parizek, J., & Zahor, Z.: Effect of cadmium salts on testicular tissue. Nature 177:1036, 1956.
23. Parizek, J., & Zahor, Z.: The destructive effect of cadmium ion on testicular tissue and its prevention by zinc. J. Endocrinol. 15:56, 1957.
24. Reddy, K., & Svoboda, D. J.: Alterations in rat testes due to an antispermatogenic agent: Light and electron microscopic study. Arch. Pathol. 84:376–392, 1967.

25. Reddy, J., Svoboda, D., Azarnoff, D., et al.: Cadmium induced Leydig cell tumors of rat testes: Morphologic and cytochemical study. J. Natl. Cancer Inst. 52:891–903, 1973.
26. Richter, P., Calamera, J. C., Morgenfeld, M. C., et al.: Effects of chlorambucil on spermatogenesis in the human with malignant lymphoma. Cancer 25:1026–1030, 1970.
27. Rosenfield, R. L.: Personal communication.
28. Segel, S., Polishuk, W. Z., & Ben-David, M.: Hyperprolactinemic male infertility. Fert. Steril. 27:1425–1427, 1976.
29. Tomatis, L., Turnsov, V., Day, N., et al.: The effect of long-term exposure to DDT on CF-1 mice. Int. J. Cancer 10:489–506, 1972.
30. Toth, A.: Reversible toxic effect of salicylasosulfapyridine on semen quality. Fert. Steril. 31(5):538–540, 1979.
31. Urry, R. L., Dougherty, K. A., & Cockett, A. J. K.: Age-related changes in male rat reproductive organ weights and plasma testosterone concentrations after administration of a monoamine oxidase inhibitor. Fert. Steril. 27:1326–1334, 1976.
32. Van Thiel, D. H., Gavaler, J. S., Smith, W. I., et al.: Hypothalamic-pituitary-gonadal dysfunction in men using cimetidine. N. Engl. J. Med. 300(18):1012–1015, 1979.
33. Weir, R. J., & Fisher, R. S.: Toxicological studies on borax and boric acid. Toxicol. Appl. Pharmacol. 23:351–364, 1972.
34. Winter, S. J., Banks, J. L., & Loriaux, D. L.: Cimetidine as an antiandrogen in the rat. Gastroenterology 76:504–508, 1979.

13

The Female Genital Tract

Barbara Winkler, Henry J. Norris, and Cecilia M. Fenoglio

The female genital tract contains diverse tissue components of germinal, epithelial, and mesenchymal origin whose hormonal sensitivity and biologic function in reproduction make the study of drug effects on female organs an interesting and complex subject. The normal physiologic changes at the time of menarche, menstruation, fertility, and menopause, the easy clinical availability of the vulva, vagina, and cervix, and the frequency of cytologic studies on women all serve to make drug effects more readily detectable in the female genital tract than in many other organ systems.

Hormonal influences are discussed in this chapter with respect to their effects on morphology, reproductive function, and contraception. The relationship between estrogen administration and the development of endometrial hyperplasia and adenocarcinoma is discussed and contrasted with the therapeutic use of progestins, antiestrogens, and androgens in the treatment of endometrial neoplasia and endometriosis. The effects of intrauterine exposure to diethylstilbestrol are discussed in the appendix to this chapter (see p. 325).

The transformation of normal physiologic processes into pathologic processes by pharmacologic intervention is illustrated by the development of ovarian hyperstimulation during the induction of ovulation, and by the development of corpus luteum hemorrhage during anticoagulant therapy.

Careful follow-up of patients undergoing immunosuppression and chemotherapy is emphasized because of the reported relationship between these modalities and the development of epithelial neoplasia of the vagina and cervix; this is of special importance in light of the increasing use of cytotoxic drugs in the treatment of both neoplastic and nonneoplastic conditions in which chronic maintenance doses of such drugs may be required over long periods. The ovarian ablative effects of these same drugs are also worthy of consideration because of their use in treating children and teenagers, whose subsequent reproductive function may be adversely affected. The use of alcohol and heroin are seen to have similar adverse ovarian effects.

In this chapter we will summarize the functional and pathologic alterations produced by agents that indirectly alter the hormonal environment, and the direct effects of steroid hormones, chemotherapy, immunosuppression, antibiotic therapy, and anticoagulation.

THE EFFECT OF STEROID HORMONES

Vagina

Vaginal epithelium undergoes a characteristic response and displays a distinct sensitivity to both estrogens and progesterone. Under the influence of estrogen the vaginal epithelium becomes thickened and the superficial cells mature. The epithelium becomes glycogenated, and with marked estrogenic effects, many of the superficial cells may become anucleated.[35] Progesterone, on the other hand, causes cell maturation only through the intermediate layer; therefore, a smear of the lateral vaginal wall will contain cells of the intermediate type, indicating incomplete maturation.

Estrogen-dominated oral contraceptives induce cornification of the vaginal surface epithelium, whereas in users of progestin-dominated oral contraceptives the incomplete cornification and consequent altered local carbohydrate metabolism[161] may predispose to monilial vaginitis.[61]

Cervix

The squamous epithelium of the exocervix is also altered by both estrogen and progesterone. However, the response of the cervical squamous epithelium to estrogen and progesterone is less than that seen in the squamous epithelium of the vagina. Estrogen promotes proliferation, maturation, and glycogenation of the squamous epithelium (Fig. 13-1); progesterone inhibits squamous maturation at the intermediate layer. The mucus-secreting columnar epithelium of the endocervix also responds to cyclic ovarian steroids; estrogen promotes endocervical epithelial cell growth and is responsible for the formation of moderate amounts of thin, alkaline, watery mucus. Under the influence of progesterone, cell height decreases and the endocervical mucus becomes thick, diminishes in amount, and is less alkaline.[35]

The major abnormal effect of oral contraceptive steroids (OCS) on the cervix is microglandular hyperplasia,[14, 169] which presents as a soft polyp, rarely larger than 1.5 cm. The polyp is usually asymptomatic but may cause postcoital or intermenstrual bleeding. Microscopically, the polyp is a racemose, cribriform agglomeration of glands lined by a single layer of flattened, cuboidal, or columnar mucinous cells (Fig. 13-2); these cells are generally uniform, but some may have hyperchromatic nuclei. Inflammatory cells and squamous metaplasia are common. With higher-dose progestins, the cervix may also show a decidual change (Fig. 13-3). Increased size of individual mucinous cells, increased mucus secretion, and hyperplasia of the mucinous epithelium of the endocervix occur. In oral contraceptive users, progesterone stimulation is apparently the cause of microglandular hyperplasia, which has not been seen in postmenopausal patients receiving estrogen except in a single report.[172] Microglandular hyperplasia is reversible once oral contraceptive therapy is discontinued.

There is no evidence that the OCS cause abnormal cervical cytology, dysplasia, carcinoma-in-situ, or carcinoma,[125] although one

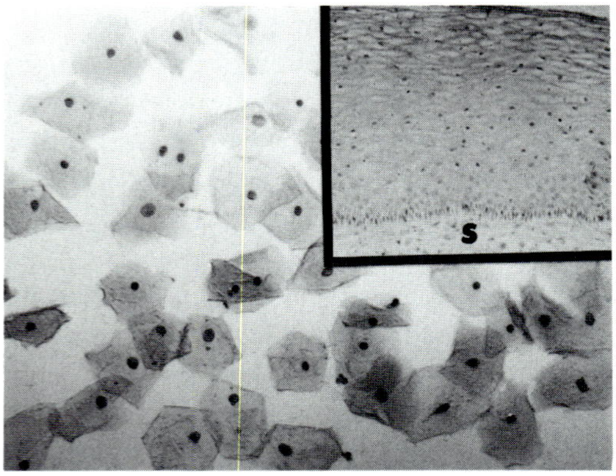

Fig. 13-1. Cytologic preparation demonstrating well-glycogenated, mature squamous epithelial cells. Insert shows normal maturation of squamous epithelium of the cervix. This epithelium is seen overlying the cervical stroma (s). × 175; insert × 50.

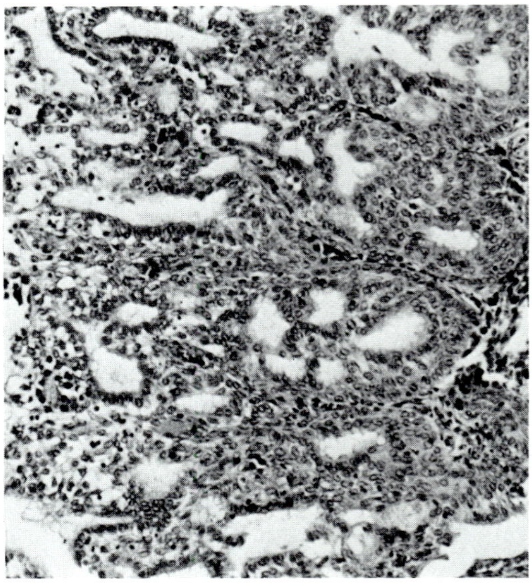

Fig. 13-2. Microglandular hyperplasia of the cervix in a patient taking an oral contraceptive. Note the squamous metaplasia (arrow) and inflammatory infiltrate. × 70. (Courtesy of Dr. C. Crum, Columbia-Presbyterian Medical Center, New York.)

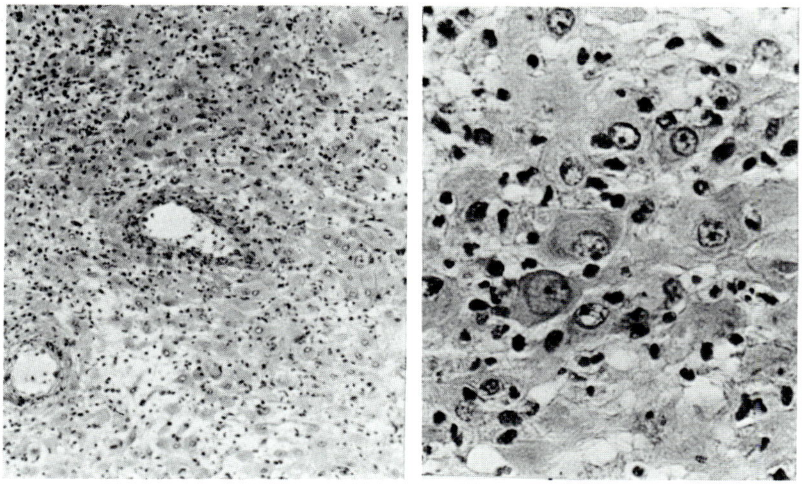

(A) **(B)**

Fig. 13-3. Progestin effect on the endocervix. (A) Low-power picture of an endocervix with extensive decidualization. (B) Decidualized cells at higher magnification. Note the large round cells with abundant cytoplasm. (A): × 95; (B): × 200.

report suggests that dysplasia may progress more rapidly in oral contraceptive users.[164]

Endometrium

Estrogen Effect. In order to understand the effects of exogenously administered steroid hormones on the female genital tract, it is necessary to understand physiologic cellular changes that occur in patients not taking steroids. The details of proliferative and secretory activity throughout the menstrual cycle, as seen by light microscopy, are provided in detail by Noyes, Hertig, and Rock[119, 120]; the corresponding ultrastructural changes that occur in both the glands and stroma during the menstrual cycle are summarized in detail by Cavazos[16] and Ferenczy.[31]

At the cellular level, estrogen, in physiologic doses, stimulates the endometrium by increasing mitotic activity, cell division, and the rate of glandular, vascular, and stromal growth. (Fig.13-4) Within the cell, estrogen is bound by protein receptors and is transported to the nucleus, where it binds to DNA, resulting in the production of a messenger RNA with specific information for the synthesis of certain enzymes. The uptake of nucleotide precursors of RNA and RNA polymerase increases. Estrogen induces estrogen-dependent pyridine nucleotide transhydrogenase

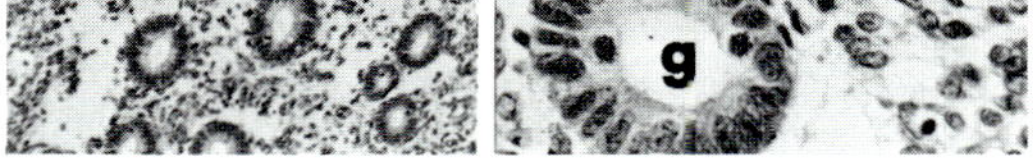

(A) **(B)**

Fig. 13-4. Normal proliferative endometrium. (A) Classical straight tubular endometrial glands separated by a loose stroma. (B) Mitotic figures in one of the glands (g) at higher magnification. (A): × 55; (B): × 210.

synthesis, and induces the production or release of the histamine needed for rapid production of endometrial edema and hyperemia.[119] The template activity of chromatin in the nucleus is increased, as is the rate of glycolysis and the uptake of water, electrolytes, and amino acids. A series of enzymatic activities are stimulated.[8, 120]

Progesterone Effect. Progesterone, elaborated by the corpus luteum, dominates the postovulatory pattern of the endometrium. This hormone induces secretory activity of the glands and decidual transformation of the stroma (Fig. 13-5); it also inhibits the endometrial response to estrogen by inhibiting DNA synthesis and mitotic activity, thus suppressing growth. Within the cell progesterone induces secretory differentiation, as reflected by a marked increase in the Golgi apparatus, increased protein synthesis, a marked increase in free ribosomes, and endoplasmic reticulum cisternae distended by a granular secretory product. (Fig. 13-6) Phagocytic activity of the cell increases, along with increases in lysosomes, lipid, and glycogen early in the secretory phase.[16, 51] The number of progesterone receptors in the endometrial glands varies during the menstrual cycle, and is regulated by the amount of estradiol. The synthesis of these receptors is stimulated by the binding of the estrogen receptor complex to nuclear DNA.

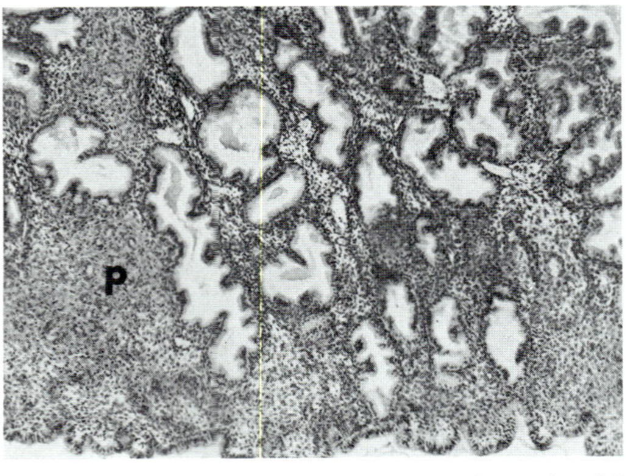

Fig. 13-5. Normal secretory endometrium, day 25 of the menstrual cycle. Note the tortuous endometrial glands and well developed predecidua around the spiral arterioles (d). × 45.

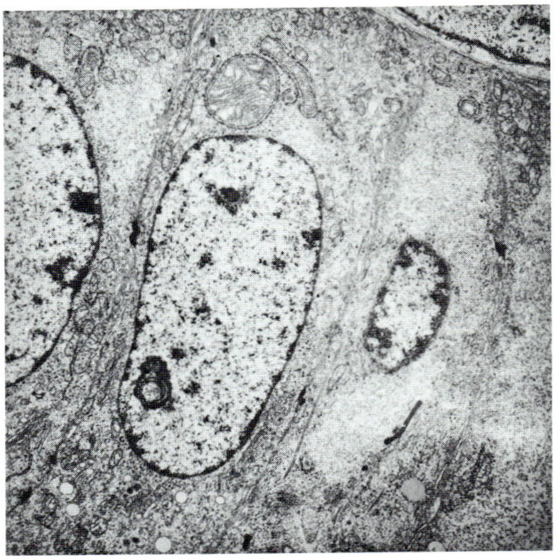

Fig. 13-6. Electron micrograph of the endometrial lining cells in day-20 secretory endometrium. Note the supranuclear and subnuclear glycogen accumulation. × 4,180.

Physiologic doses of progesterone, administered to produce augmentation of a deficient corpus luteum, results in endometrial biopsies having a correlation with the basal body temperature and subsequent menses.[65]

Effect of Contraceptive Steroids. The histologic alterations produced by exogenous estrogens and progestins on the endometrium depend upon: (1) whether these hormones are administered cyclically or continuously; (2) whether a hormone is given alone or in combination; (3) the dose and the duration of hormone use, and (4) the particular time of the cycle at which a tissue specimen was obtained for histologic study.[52, 122, 123] Most oral contraceptive regimens use ethinyl estradiol or its methyl ether, mestranol, in combination with a progestin—usually a 19-nortestosterone derivative.[5] Synthetic progestins fall into two groups; those derived from 17-α-acetoxyprogesterone and those derived from 19-nortestosterone. The 17-α-acetoxyprogesterone derivatives, when combined with estrogen, produce similar but less marked effects than the 19-nortestosterone derivatives.[72]

Two regimens have been developed for contraception: (1) the combined regimen, in which a synthetic progestin is combined with a synthetic estrogen into a single tablet; and (2) the sequential regimen, in which estrogen is taken for 14 to 16 days, followed by 5 to 6 days in which a tablet that contains both an estrogen and progestin is taken, as in the combined regimen. Only the combined regimen is available in the United States, although formerly the sequential regimen, still available in some countries outside of the United States, was used. In the combined regimen, the first pill is taken on day 5 of the cycle, and pills are then taken for 20 to 21 more days. Some packets contain 28 pills, of which the last 7 tablets are either inert or contain some form of iron. In the combined regimen, progestin dominates. The major effects of the combined regimen on the endometrium are summarized in Table 13-1.

A detailed description of the histologic effects of oral contraceptives can be found in the descriptions by Ober.[122, 123] In the combined regimen subnuclear vacuoles appear by day 10 of the cycle (after 5 days on the drug) and inhibition of glandular growth occurs.[72] The secretory changes develop slowly, if at all. The glands, being inhibited by the progestin in the regimen, remain small, and many gradually disappear. By day 20 of the cycle, there is an increased stroma-to-gland ratio (Fig. 13-7). Endometrial vessels may show an endothelial and intimal proliferation. Occasionally, fibrin thrombi occur in dilated vessels. The spiral arterioles do not develop.[72, 122, 123, 143] With lower-dose progestins, a decidual reaction may not be evident. On repeated cycles of the contraceptive regimen, the endometrium becomes thinner and less bleeding occurs.

Descriptions of the ultrastructure aspects seen with combined contraceptive regimens are also available. Cavazos,[16] in the most de-

Table 13-1. Effects of Oral Contraceptive Agents on the Endometrium

Combined Regimen	Day of Cycle	Sequential Regimen
Take pill no. 1	5	Take first of 14 estrogen pills
	6	
Little or no gland development	7	
	8	
	9	
Subnuclear vacuoles appear	10	
	11	
Glands gradually disappear	12	Glands slowly develop as usual
Large stroma/gland ratio	13	
	14	
Variable degree of supranuclear vacuoles	15	
	16	
	17	
	18	
	19	Begin Estrogen and Progestin Pill
Regression of secretory changes	20	
	21	Subnuclear vacuoles appear
	22	Atrophy or glands optional
	23	Stroma/gland ratio approximately normal
	24	
Stop pills	25	Stop pills
Decidual changes appear in Host (endometrium thin with repeated cycles)	26	Decidual change optional; secretory glands present
	27	
Bleeding starts (less than usual)	28	Bleeding starts (approximately normal)

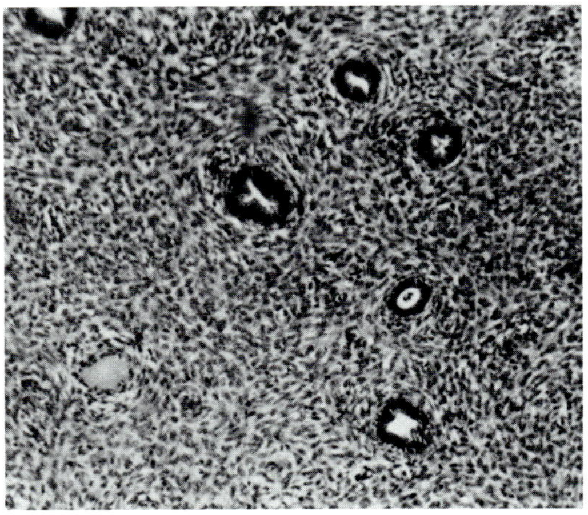

Fig. 13-7. Endometrium suppressed by an oral contraceptive regimen of 0.03 mg of ethinyl estradiol and 0.3 mg of norgestryl at day 20 of the cycle (day 15 of the contraceptive regimen). The stroma-to-gland ratio is high. × 80.

tailed ultrastructural study to date, found that under the influence of a combined regimen, the estrogen-dependent cell functions are depressed, and an intercellular progesterone milieu appears. The initial increase in glycogen, protein and carbohydrate synthesis, along with increased ribosomal activity and development of the Golgi apparatus, are evident in the early phase of the cycle, but these activities are depressed in the latter half as compared with the same parameters in the normal menstrual cycle. Large mitochondria, intranuclear canaliculi, and increased glycogen and rough endoplasmic reticulum characteristic of the secretory phase also appear, but are suppressed in the latter half of the cycle, and do not achieve the development found in the normal postovulatory phase.

The sequential regimen is important historically, because it was associated with an increased incidence of endometrial hyperplasia and carcinoma,[68, 99, 153, 154] and was therefore withdrawn from the market in the United States. The sequential regimen was characterized by 14 to 16 days of unopposed estrogen, leading, in some women, to a mild hyperplasia. The 4 to 6 days of progestin at the end of the cycle may not have been sufficient to inhibit the earlier-stimulated endometrium. The combination oral contraceptive regimen has not been associated with the development of endometrial hyperplasia or carcinoma, nor would it be expected to because it tends to inhibit glands and stroma by progestin domination.[52]

Progestins, when used alone and in small doses, cause the glands to mature irregularly, producing a histologic appearance that cannot be dated. Decidual change occurs, and there is glandular atrophy secondary to gland inhibition. (Fig. 13-8) A prominent pattern of dilated capillaries develops. In the continuous microdose progestins, the endometrium is similar to that seen in patients receiving combination oral contraceptives,[111, 112] but there is more of a decidual reaction. There may be an asynchronous endometrium with glandular atrophy and absent or focal stromal edema. Seventy-five percent of patients receiving the microdose progestins continue to ovulate,[111, 112, 124] adding variability to the histologic pattern of the endometrium. The effectiveness of these contraceptive steroids lies in the combination of an altered endometrium and the inhibition of sperm transport through the production of a scanty viscous

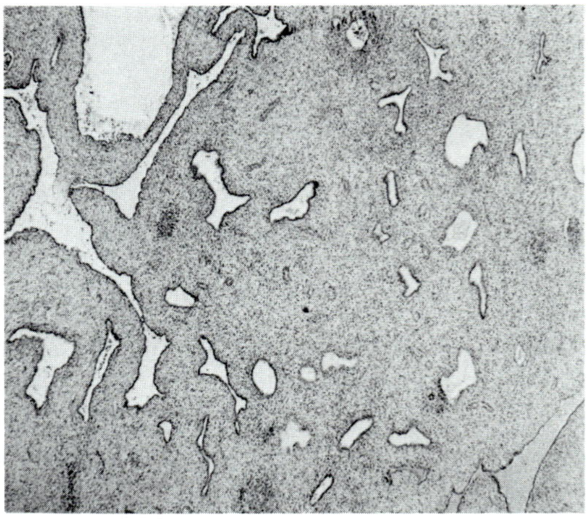

Fig. 13-8. Progestin effect on the endometrium. Note the irregular endometrial glands with atrophic lining and markedly decidualized stroma. × 20.

mucus of the cervix. The major disadvantages of the continuous progestin regimen are the occurrence of unpredictable bleeding and a greater failure rate in contraception compared to that with the combined preparations.[111]

Relationship of Estrogen to Endometrial Cancer and Hyperplasia. The incidence of endometrial cancer was stable in the United States until about 1970, when the rates—adjusted for the diminishing numbers of women with intact uteri—rose by about 10 percent per year in the few states with data available (Connecticut, New York, Hawaii, New Mexico, Oregon, Utah). Case control studies detected a four- to eightfold increase in the risk of endometrial cancer in estrogen users compared with nonusers.[41, 46, 56, 77, 106, 155] Little risk appears among those taking a dose of less than 1.25 mg for a period of less than 5 years. Few of the studies, however, have stated how the estrogen was given, with what safeguards, or whether it was given cyclically or continuously. In the United States, about 14 percent of women 45 years and older take estrogens. In one urban survey, 51 percent of menopausal women had used estrogen for at least 3 months; the median duration of use was over 10 years. During the period from 1963 to 1973, the use of conjugated estrogen quadrupled in menopausal women, and its use overall has doubled in the last 10 years.[77]

There are three reasons given for why there may be an association of exogenous estrogen with endometrial cancer: (1) estrogen probably promotes bleeding of the cancer in asymptomatic women, allowing for earlier detection; (2) recently, pathologists have been reporting carcinoma-in-situ of the endometrium (which is difficult to distinguish objectively from atypical hyperplasia) much more frequently than in the past; and (3) there is a cause-effect relationship.

The association of estrogen with endometrial carcinoma is strengthened by the recognition that young women with gonadal dysgenesis who use stilbestrol for a long time have an increased risk of developing endometrial cancer.[121] In a study of women who received stilbestrol as therapy for breast cancer, the subsequent incidence of endometrial cancer was about twice that expected. Endometrial carcinoma has occurred in from 3 to 38 percent of women with estrogen-secreting tumors of the ovary, and is more frequent than expected among patients with the Stein-Leventhal syndrome.[77] The increased conversion of androstenedione to the potent estrogen estrone, present in this syndrome, has been suggested as a factor in this increased frequency. Carcinoma rarely occurs in patients with Turner's syndrome unless they have taken estrogens. Few of the carcinomas associated with estrogen-secreting tumors and Stein-Leventhal syndrome have proved fatal. Invasive carcinomas of the endometrium have been infrequently associated with the use of exogenous estrogen, suggesting that overdiagnosis of hyperplasia as carcinoma may be common, or that if such tumors are induced by estrogens, they have a different biologic behavior than non-estrogen-induced tumors.

With respect to the relationship of oral contraceptive steroids and endometrial cancer, the combined regimen would be expected to inhibit, and the sequential preparation to promote, the development of endometrial cancer.[52, 72] This appears to be the case, because 11 of the first 13 patients found to have endometrial cancer while taking oral contraceptives had been taking the sequential regimen, instead of the 2 that would have been predicted on the basis of the low proportion of women taking this regimen.[153, 154] In contrast, the finding that users of combined oral contraceptives have only 50 percent of the incidence of endometrial carcinoma that nonusers have emphasizes the sensitivity of endometrial neoplasia to hormonal factors, and implies that combined contraceptive preparations may actually protect against the development of endometrial carcinoma.[190]

The unopposed action of estrogenic substances induces hyperplasia. (Fig. 13-9) A synthetic estrogen (tri-*p*-anisylchloroethylene),

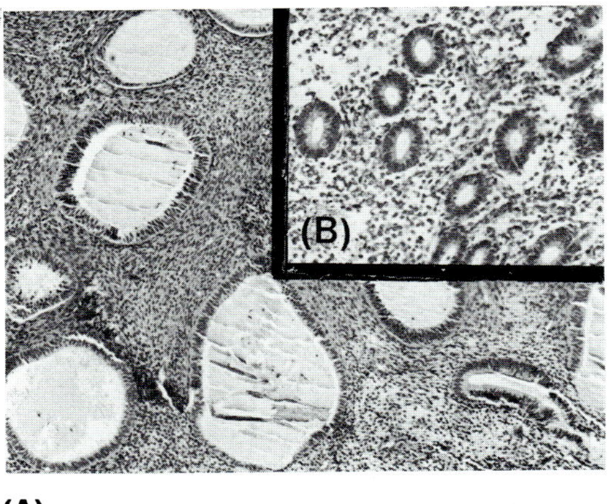

Fig. 13-9. (A) Endometrial biopsy from a postmenopausal woman on estrogen replacement therapy. Note the dilated, irregular endometrial glands with stratified nuclei and dense stroma. Contrast with (B) representing normal proliferative endometrium. (A): × 50; (B): × 70.

given for periods of from 45 to 100 days to 44 patients, induced hyperplasia in 34 percent and a more atypical lesion in 9 percent.[73] This illustrates the magnitude of the action of a potent estrogen.

Many women with endometrial carcinoma are obese, hypertensive, arthritic, and have a diabetic glucose tolerance test.[158] Obesity is related to endometrial carcinoma since it is well known that fat deposits convert adrenal precursors, including androstenedione, to estrone, a potent estrogen.[77] Ovarian stromal hyperplasia, adrenocortical hyperplasia, hyperplasia of cells of the anterior pituitary, sterility, fibrocystic disease of the breast, and persistence of an estrogenized vaginal mucosa are more frequent in women with endometrial carcinoma than expected. Induction of endometrial carcinoma has occurred in rabbits treated with stilbestrol,[108] and chemical carcinogens introduced into the uteri of rabbits, cats, and mice produce endometrial carcinoma, an effect that is potentiated by estrogen and inhibited by progesterone and testosterone. Data obtained on the effects of steroids and carcinogens on the reproductive tracts of nonprimate species cannot be directly applied to women because of marked differences in physiology, anatomy, estrus, and gestational patterns, steroids, and life span. In humans, endometrial carcinomas tend to evolve in an environment of relative progesterone deficiency. Usually there is a gradual increase in cellular atypia associated with increasing complexity of the hyperplasia, as part of a gradual continuum between proliferative endometrium and invasive carcinoma.[40, 168, 191]

Ultrastructural studies also indicate a spectrum of change with progressive degrees of hyperplasia. The fine structure of endometrial hyperplasias reflects the progressive development of estrogen-related morphology in the gland cells.[16] There are increases in the complexity of the plasma and nuclear membranes, along with increases in surface microvilli, ciliated cells, autophagocytic activity, and pleomorphism of organelles, as well as alterations in the Golgi apparatus, lysosomal activity, and number and the appearance of lipid bodies (Fig. 13-10). A biologic progression from endometrial hyperplasia to carcinoma has not yet conclusively been demonstrated, however, varying degrees of hyperplasia are found in association with cancer in at least 40 percent of carcinoma cases, and many patients with endometrial carcinoma have had pre-existing endometrial hyperplasia.[45, 169, 191]

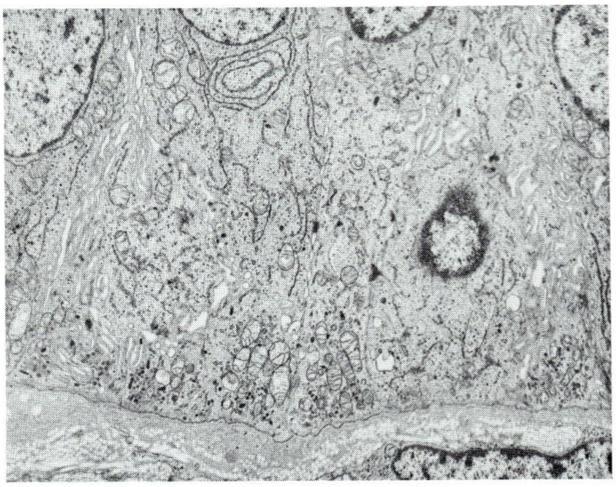

Fig. 13-10. Endometrial hyperplasia in a patient taking estrogen. Electron micrograph of the base of a gland showing palisaded nuclei, pleomorphic cellular organelles, and irregular rough endoplasmic reticulum. × 3150.

Progestogens, Antiestrogens, and Endometrial Neoplasia. Progestogen therapy in pharmacologic doses produces clinical regression in approximately one-third of patients with metastatic endometrial carcinoma.[1, 30, 49, 59, 69, 70, 72, 74, 78, 100, 136, 137, 156] and causes striking histologic changes in the carcinoma regardless of the clinical response.[1, 30, 78, 140, 156] The tumor response to progestogen therapy correlates best with the histologic grade of the tumor, the better differentiated carcinomas responding more frequently.[1, 30, 69, 74, 78, 100, 103, 156]

The histologic effect of progestins on endometrial hyperplasias and endometrial carcinomas closely parallels the response of the normal luteal phase endometrium. Mitotic activity is arrested, with inhibition of DNA and RNA synthesis, suppression of epithelial growth, conversion from nuclear hyperchromasia to normochromasia, and reversion of cells to the usual diploid state from their previously aneuploid one.[60] The stroma increases as the number, size, and crowding of epithelial cells decreases (Fig. 13-11).[1, 30, 70, 74, 78, 140] The glandular lining cells undergo secretory conversion, accumulate intracellular glycogen, and produce mucopolysacchacide-rich secretions (Fig. 13-12).[30, 48, 59, 140] This regressive remodeling process occurs via loss of apical cytoplasm, autophagocytosis, and apoptosis.[30, 31, 56, 140] Predecidual conversion of the stroma occurs invariably in gestin-

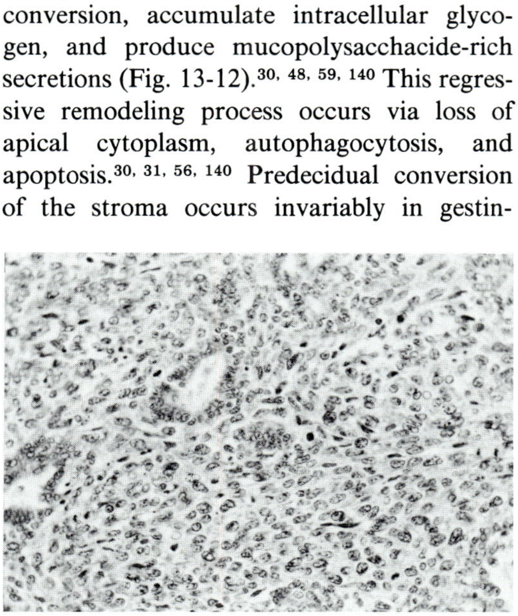

Fig. 13-11. Progestin effect on adenomatous hyperplasia of the endometrium. Note the increased stroma-to-gland ratio and the small atrophic glands. × 160.

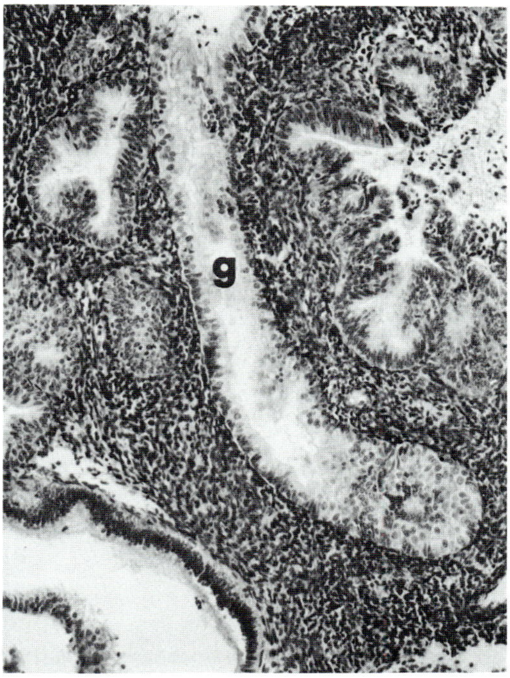

Fig. 13-12. Progestin effect on adenomatous hyperplasia of the endometrium. Note the secretory conversion of gland (g) surrounded by dense stroma and adenomatous glands. × 50.

treated endometrial hyperplasias, and is noted in 15 to 20 percent of patients with endometrial carcinoma (Fig. 13-13).[30, 59] Chronic therapy may result in complete glandular regression, stromal decidual transformation, and necrosis.

The late ultrastructural features of progestogen therapy also parallel those of the normal postovulatory secretory endometrium, and are characterized by glycogen deposition, increased granular endoplasmic reticulum, giant mitochondria, and "basket-like" nucleolar channel systems.[30, 48, 49, 140] The effect of progestogen therapy on responsive neoplastic tissue is a decrease in both estrogen receptors and progesterone receptors, with a more marked drop in progesterone receptor concentration. The disappearance of progesterone receptors is thought to be due to nuclear displacement and nonreplenishment.[103]

The concept of hormone receptor targets in carcinoma has led recent investigators to

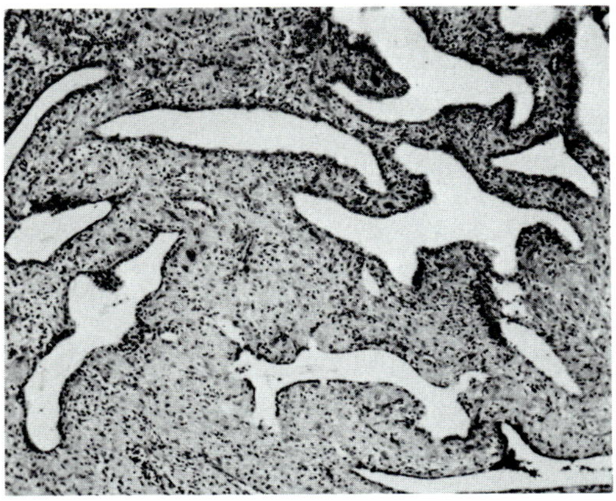

Fig. 13-13. Atypical hyperplasia of the endometrium treated with medroxyprogesterone acetate for 5 months. The irregular glandular outlines persist, but the epithelium is atrophic. The intervening stroma shows a marked decidual reaction. AFIP Neg. No. 2998.

add the nonsteroidal antiestrogens tamoxifen, nafoxidine, and clomiphene, to the chemotherapeutic regimen. The antiestrogens appear to function through the abnormal intranuclear processing of antiestrogen-estrogen receptor complexes, reducing the availability and replenishment of cytoplasmic estrogen receptors, thereby blocking binding and interaction with estrogen.[19, 20, 57] Tamoxifen inhibits the in vivo and in vitro uptake of tritiated estradiol by the endometrium and myometrium, and depresses estradiol receptor binding.[98] Tamoxifen is selectively taken up by the cells of the endometrium and corpus luteum, without quantitative variation during the menstrual cycle.[34] In rat uterine adenocarcinomas, tamoxifen and clomiphene were demonstrated, in vitro, to markedly reduce the colony-forming ability of tumor cells, an effect that was enhanced by the addition of progesterone.[150] Tamoxifen produces a progestational response in the endometrium, featuring decidual change and glandular inhibition. It has been reported to induce regression in some patients with metastatic endometrial carcinoma.[167] The various endometrial effects of antiestrogens are summarized in Table 13-2.

Table 13-2. Effects of Antiestrogens on the Endometrium

1. Block estrogen action	↓Receptor availability, limit receptor synthesis
2. Estrogenic effect	Induce transcription of proteins usually associated with estrogen stimulation Peroxidase synthesis
3. Progestogenic effect	Stimulate secretion of new protein
4. Antiuterotrophic effect	↓Mucosal hyperplasia

Myometrium

In various animal species, estrogen stimulates the myometrium to undergo hyperplasia and hypertrophy; this response is enhanced by progesterone.[90, 102, 145] The administration of estrogen results in increased RNA synthesis and myometrial growth because of increases in actin and collagen, and the synthesis of other proteins.[102] Ultrastructurally, under the influence of estrogen, the smooth muscle cells develop organelles to a degree not usually seen in smooth muscle cells in the uterus unless they have been estrogen-primed.[102] The increased size of fibroblasts may contribute to the increased uterine size. The response of the uterus to estrogen and progesterone varies in different species with the distensibility of the uterus and the dose of steroid that is given. Estradiol causes an increase in norepinephrine content and increases the innervation density of adrenergic nerves of the myometrium. Progesterone reduces and inhibits the effects of estrogen on the nerve endings.

Leiomyomas can be affected by oral contraceptives. Hemorrhagic degeneration occurs in some, along with focal increases in cellularity, edema, hyalinization, and myxoid degeneration (Fig. 13-14).[27, 28, 37, 134] Within the myometrium, arteries, veins and capillaries may show endothelial and intimal proliferation, as well as the deposition of an acid mucopolysaccharide. These findings are not specific for contraceptive steroids; they are also seen in patients who have recently been, or are, preg-

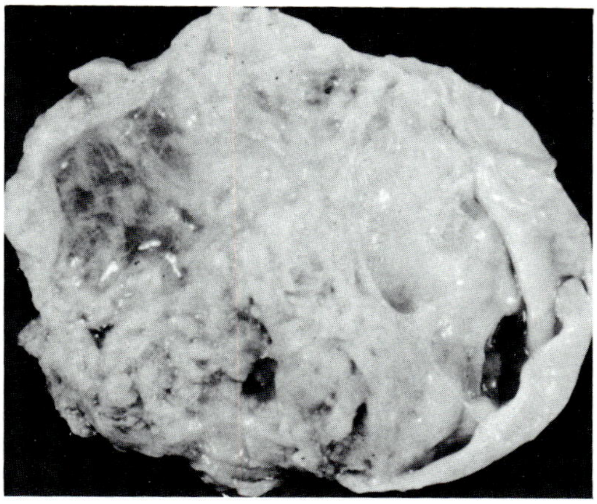

Fig. 13-14. Gross photograph of a leiomyoma showing cystic and myxoid degeneration.

nant. Hemorrhage within leiomyomas rarely occurs in the absence of exogenous steroids or pregnancy. Hemorrhagic degeneration is thought to be initiated by the development of central edema and hemorrhage followed by necrosis and scarring.[27, 37, 91] The mitotic activity in affected leiomyomas usually is low, and these lesions should not be confused with sarcomas.

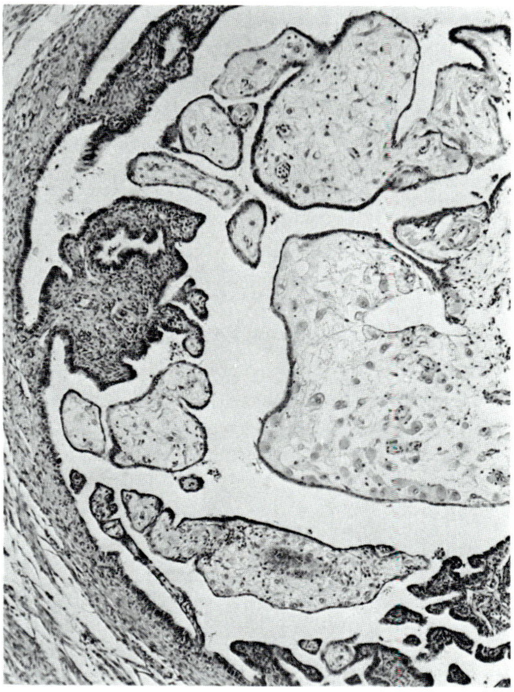

Fig. 13-15. Decidual transformation of the fallopian tube in a patient receiving progestin therapy. Normal-appearing tubular epithelium is seen at the left and lower right-hand portions of the photograph. × 60.

Fallopian Tube

Morphologic alterations of the fallopian tubes during the menstrual cycle are not consistently visible at the light-microscopic or ultrastructural level of examination.[111] Cyclic changes that have been reported to occur in the fallopian tube are inconsistent,[11] and there is disagreement over whether there are cyclic changes in the epithelium of the fallopian tube under the influence of oral contraceptives. Nevertheless, the reported effects of oral contraceptives can be summarized as follows: (1) Estrogens stimulate ciliated cells to produce cilia, while progestins inhibit this growth[2, 124]; (2) there is proliferation of the secretory and indifferent cells and an increase in the number of enlarged epithelial cells[38]; (3) combined preparations of oral contraceptives and progestins may cause focal increased height of the epithelium, enlargement of nuclei, and loss of cilia[33, 126]; (4) mild alterations of the epithelium occur in the infundibulum rather than in the ampulla[33]; and (5) tubal motility and ciliary activity decrease with combined agents, although they increase with estrogen alone.[7] A decidual reaction is observed in the serosal and mucosal layers of the fallopian tube in some patients undergoing exogenous progestin therapy (Fig. 13-15).

Ovary

The main effect of the oral contraceptive steroids on the ovary is the inhibition of ovulation. The combination oral contraceptives inhibit the secretion of hypothalamic releasing factors[163] and prevent ovulation by suppressing the synthesis of pituitary gonadotropins.[22] Follicle stimulating hormone (FSH) production is inhibited by estrogen, and progestin suppresses the midcycle surge of luteinizing hormone (LH). The low-dose or continuously administered progestins intermittently suppress ovulation. Histologic examination of the ovary in women receiving a combination oral contraceptive discloses the presence of inactive, small, uniformly sized follicles. A corpus luteum is usually not present. The number and appearance of the oocytes are unaffected. The cortical stroma is condensed and unstimulated,[146] but this is of no functional significance since the stroma becomes normal with restoration of normal pituitary function. After discontinuance of the oral contraceptive steroids, 98 percent of women resume ovulation and will have normal endometrial function within the first three cycles.[139]

Endometriosis

Endometriosis—the ectopic presence of endometrial lining and stroma in locations outside the uterine cavity—responds to the

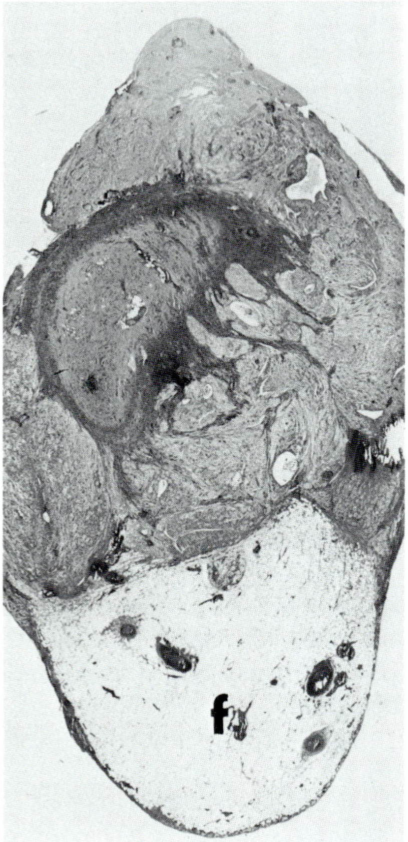

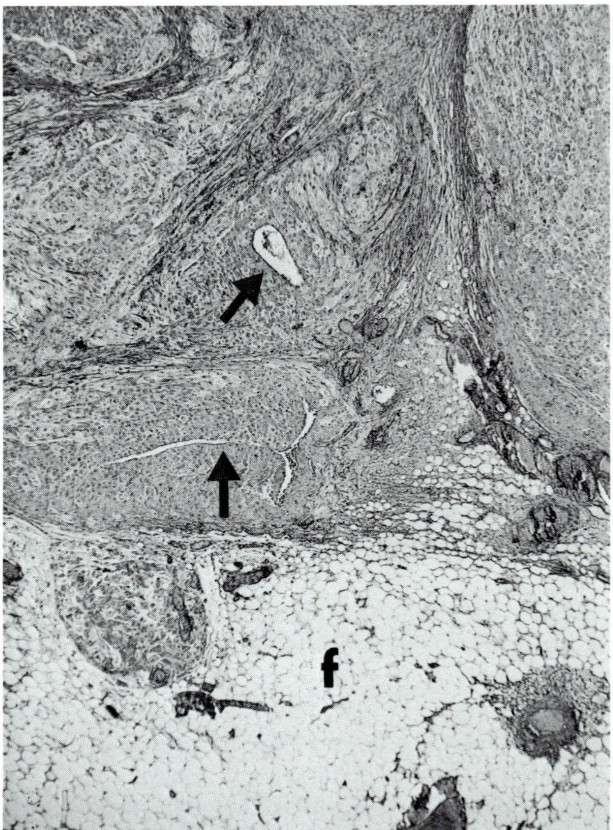

(A) **(B)**

Fig. 13-16. Endometriosis of the appendix with decidual response. (A) Cross-section of an appendix whose lumen is obliterated by endometriosis. (B) Higher magnification, wherein endometrial glands (arrows) are surrounded by a decidualized stroma; (f) represents the periappendiceal fat. (A): × 9; (B): × 25.

influence of steroid hormones in the same way in which the normal endometrium responds. The treatment of symptomatic endometriosis is directed toward manipulation of its hormonal responsiveness by eliminating or decreasing the proliferative influence of estrogens.[6] Progestational agents and pregnancy may produce a decidual response in endometriotic implants (Fig. 13-16). "Pseudopregnancy" regimens, with low-dose combination birth control pills, will induce glandular inhibition and pseudodecidual stromal changes in endometriosis, and gradual atrophy after the long-term use of such regimens.[4, 183]

Danazol, an impeded androgen with antigonadotropic, mild androgenic, and mild progestational properties is utilized in the "pseudomenopause" therapy of endometriosis.[4, 93] Within 4 to 8 weeks of chronic administration, it causes hypoestrogenicity, endometrial atrophy, amenorrhea and, in some women, menopausal symptoms.[3, 192] The ovaries, uterus, and fallopian tubes decrease in size and pelvic congestion diminishes. Ovarian biopsy during danazol therapy shows a small, inactive organ with a deeply corrugated cortex and no follicular or luteal activity.[23] The endometriotic implants undergo supression, with the development of small, inactive glands and a dense, inactive stroma. After prolonged therapy in mild and moderate cases, there may be complete resorption of the endometriosis or only a small residuum of iron pigment and adhesions in the location of previously active disease. In severe, chronic cases there may be residual endometriosis showing an atrophic histology.[23, 92, 182] Danazol administered to ovariectomized women or women with ovarian polycystic disease may produce atypical secretory changes in the endometrium (Fig. 13-17).

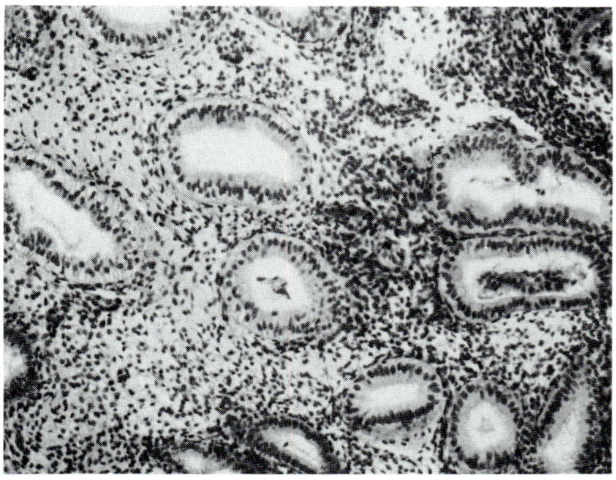

Fig. 13-17. Atypical secretory endometrium in a patient on danazol therapy. Note nonsynchronous secretory activity of the gland-lining cells on the right as compared to those in the center. × 100.

THE EFFECT OF PROSTAGLANDINS

Prostaglandins are present in semen and are also synthesized by the endometrium. Seminal fluid, when deposited in the vagina, is absorbed, causing an increase in uterine and fallopian tube motility. Prostaglandins stimulate the synthesis of RNA and of other proteins. They are thought to be involved in enzymatic and metabolic events that follow the action of estradiol on the endometrium and myometrium. Prostaglandin synthesis in the endometrium is stimulated in vitro by estradiol and inhibited by progesterone. Prostaglandins are believed to contribute to the effacement of the cervix during labor, but the mechanism of this is unknown.

INDUCTION OF OVULATION AND THE OVARIAN HYPERSTIMULATION SYNDROME

Human menopausal gonadotropin (HMG), human chorionic gonadotrophin (HCG), and clomiphene citrate are widely used in the treatment of infertility caused by secondary ovarian failure. Their use is occasionally complicated by the ovarian hyperstimulation syndrome. This syndrome, in its most fully developed state, is characterized by ovarian enlargement to over 10 cm in diameter, ascites, pleural effusions, clotting abnormalities, and serum electrocyte imbalance.[25, 62, 63, 117, 135] The syndrome is only rarely associated with clomiphine therapy,[62, 71, 160] but may occur with greater frequency during HCG and HMG administration. Morbidity and mortality associated with severe ovarian hyperstimulation, fortunately rare, may result from massive fluid shifts, electrolyte abnormalities and renal failure, arterial thrombosis, ovarian torsion, or ovarian rupture with hemorrhage.[25, 62, 63, 117, 135]

Pathologically, the ovaries are characterized by massive enlargement with multiple follicle cysts, stromal edema with hemorrhage and necrosis, and numerous, large cystic corpora lutea with hemorrhage (Fig. 13-18).[25, 62, 117, 147] The ovarian mass, volume, and surface area correlate with the amount of free peritoneal fluid.[25] Because of the increased number of corpora lutea and the progestins they produce, one may see an exaggerated secretory response in the endometrium (Fig. 13-19). The pathogenesis of the syndrome and the related conditions of Meigs and pseudo-Meigs syndrome is unknown, but may be related to increased capillary permeability secondary to estrogen excess.[25, 64, 147]

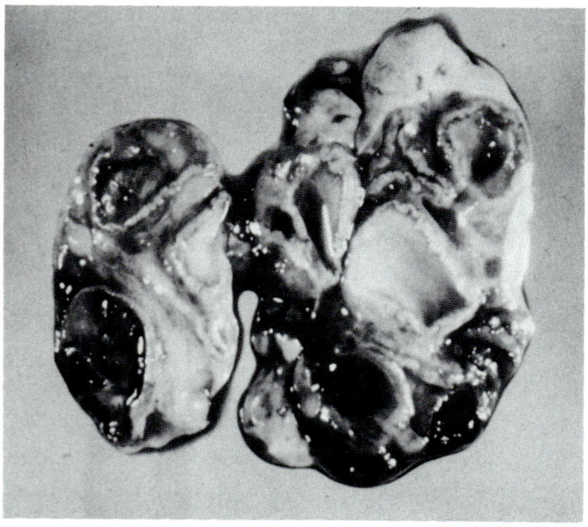

Fig. 13-18. Gross photograph of an ovary removed from a woman with ovarian hyperstimulation syndrome. Note the multiple hemorrhagic cystic corpora lutea and cystic follicles. (Courtesy of Dr. R. Vande Wiele, Columbia-Presbyterian Medical Center, New York.)

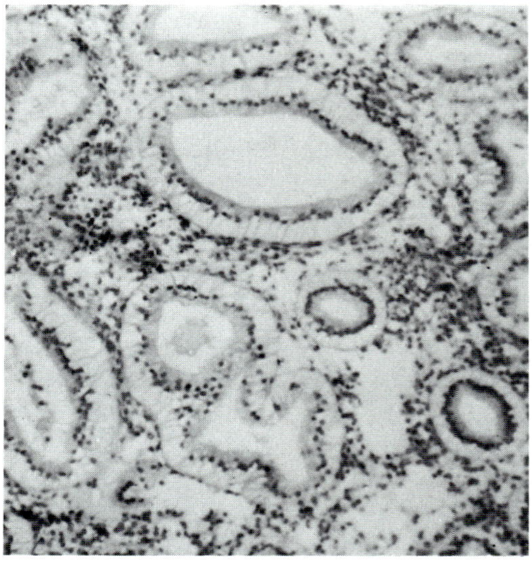

Fig. 13-19. Endometrial biopsy taken on day 17 of the cycle in a patient with ovarian hyperstimulation. Note the exaggerated subnuclear vacuolization in the glands. × 165.

THE EFFECT OF DIGITALIS

The long-term administration of digitalis produces estrogenic maturation of the squamous epithelium of the cervix and vagina in postmenopausal and oophorectomized women Fig. 13-20)[12, 55, 80]; it may also be associated with a proliferative endometrium in women and gynecomastia in men.[194] These side effects of digitalis are variable and appear to be re-

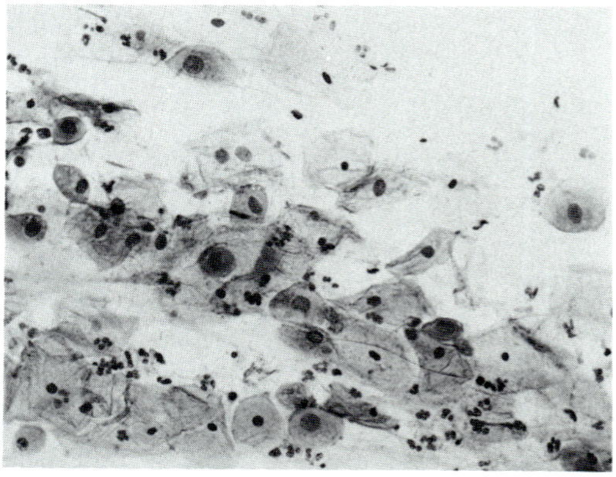

Fig. 13-20. Cytologic preparation showing abnormally estrogenized smear in a postmenopausal woman. × 200.

lated to the duration of therapy, with estrogenic effects occurring only after 2 years of chronic ingestion. In experimental animal models it was found that parenteral digitalis administration causes estrogenic cytologic changes in oophorectomized and adrenalectomized virgin female mice.[12,39,115,181]

The mechanism of the estrogenic effects of digitalis on the female genital squamous epithelium is uncertain. The molecular structure of digitalis is similar to that of some of the steroid hormones, raising the possibility of a direct "hormonal-like" action. An indirect mechanism may be modulated by the effect of digitalis on ACTH synthesis and release.[12]

CHEMOTHERAPEUTIC AGENTS

Effect in Cytologic and Epithelial Abnormalities

Alkylating agents and antifolates cause cytologic and epithelial abnormalities of the cervix and vagina.[29,32,44,80,81,86,116,143,185] The initial observations of the effect of chemotherapeutic agents on epithelial cells were made when urogenital atypia was found in association with cyclophosphamide therapy.[116] Subsequent surveillance has uncovered similar epithelial changes induced by other chemotherapeutic agents.

Epithelial dysplasia of the cervix and vagina, identical to that seen in women with megaloblastic anemia, has been reported in women treated with methotrexate for choriocarcinoma. The appearance of methotrexate-induced atypia correlates with dosage, and may be permanent and irreversible.[142] Methotrexate is a folate antagonist that binds to dihydrofolate reductase, blocking folate metabolism, and induces a state of folate deficiency which, if uncorrected, may lead to megaloblastosis. The cytologic abnormalities of folate deficiency are characterized by generalized enlargement of the intermediate squamous cells of the cervix and vagina, accompanied by nuclear enlargement. Other, less common features of megaloblastic cervical smears in folate deficiency include chromatin clumping, the presence of nucleoli, multinucleation, cytoplasmic vacuolization, and phagocytosis. The megaloblastic cellular alterations may be difficult to distinguish from early neoplastic changes; however, bizarre cell forms are absent in folate deficiency-induced cytologic atypia.[75,76,80,114,175,176] Cytologic changes in the cervical smear may be observed 8 to 10 weeks prior to the onset of clinically evident megaloblastic anemia.[76]

Numerous case reports describe diffuse cytomegalic changes of the squamous epithelium after the long-term administration of busulfan.[44,80,81,116,185] Cellular abnormalities secondary to busulfan therapy have been demonstrated at autopsy in the cells of many tissues, including sinusoidal endothelium, endometrium, columnar epithelium of the endocervix, and squamous epithelium of the cervix, vagina, and vulva.[29,32,44,80,81,116,185] The most pronounced cytologic changes occur in the epithelia of the lungs, urinary tract, and cervix.[81] A direct relationship between busulfan therapy and the appearance of cytologic atypia is supported by the demonstration of normal cervicovaginal smears prior to initial administration and during early usage of the drug.[44,80,81,116,152,185]

Cytomegalic epithelial alterations have been reported in an infant born to a leukemic mother who had received busulfan during pregnancy, an occurrence which negates the possibility that busulfan is only an additive factor in the development of dysplastic epithelium in an individual exposed to predisposing, antecedent environmental factors.[152]

Other alkylating agents, including thiotepa, chlorambucil and cyclophosphamide have been noted to induce epithelial abnormalities similar to those induced by busulfan.[80,81] The extent of the epithelial atypia correlates with the total dosage of the alkylating agent and the duration of therapy.[44,80,86,152,185] The abnormalities associated with busulfan are persistent after cessation of therapy, and appear to be irreversible.[80,81,185] Cytologic changes in smears from women under treatment with cyclophosphamide are frequent but may be less severe than those induced by busulfan, with reversion to normal after therapy is discontinued. When therapy with cyclophosphamide is recommenced, the cytologic changes will reappear, suggesting a direct causal relationship. Smears with characteristics identical to those of exfoliated neoplastic cells do not occur in association with cyclophosphamide therapy but may occur with busulfan-related lesions.[80, 81, 86] There has been no series documenting the progression of alkylating agent-induced dysplasia into carcinoma, although carcinoma-in-situ of the vulva and invasive cervical carcinoma have been reported in patients being treated with busulfan.[29, 80]

Abnormal exfoliative cytology induced by alkylating agents features cellular enlargement and an increased nuclear-to-cytoplasmic ratio. The cytoplasm is granular, with variable changes in staining intensity. Cytoplasmic vacuolization is common and occasionally marked. Hyperchromatism, nuclear pleomorphism, and wrinkling are prominent; nucleoli, chromocenters, and multinucleate forms may be seen. Bizarre cell forms may be present, but with the absence of mitoses. The same cytologic alterations are observed in the columnar cells of the endocervix.[32, 44, 80, 116, 152, 185] A generalized decrease in estrogen effect is seen in the smears.[185]

Histologic sections of cervices affected by alkylating agent therapy demonstrate a range of atypia, from isolated hypertrophic cells scattered within an atrophic epithelium to lesions indistinguishable from intraepithelial neoplasia.[29, 44, 80, 81, 116] The endocervical gland-lining epithelia may be multilayered, with decreased or absent mucus production.[29] More abundant cytoplasm, thinner, atrophic-appearing epithelium, and the absence of mitoses are the features that characterize alkylating agent-induced dysplasias.

The mechanism of action of alkylating agents in producing epithelial atypia has both direct and indirect effects. The indirect effects are hormonally mediated and related to the suppression of ovarian function[29, 44, 81, 198]; the direct effects are cytostatic and related to cell penetration, with the binding of alkylating agents to DNA strands, chromatid breakage, and inhibition of mitosis.[29, 42, 44, 86] Ultrastructural studies of the effect of cyclophosphamide on bladder epithelial cells of rats suggest an initial interaction with the plasma membrane and cytoplasmic matrix, and a subsequent interaction with intranuclear DNA, evidenced by nuclear granule formation.[79]

The important distinction with respect to alkylating agent-induced cellular abnormalities is that between a non-neoplastic cytotoxic or "cancer mimetic" process and a chemically induced premalignant or malignant transformation.[29, 80, 81, 82, 87, 116, 152, 198] Alkylating agents are recognized as having mutagenic, teratogenic, and carcinogenic properties in experimental systems.[29, 42, 86] In addition, they are identified as "radiomimetic" because their properties and effects bear similarities to those of radiation therapy. In terms of morphologic cytologic changes, it is perhaps best to consider this resemblance as being due to the limited reactive capabilities of cells to respond to injury.[42, 86] Case reports are accumulating which indicate an increased incidence of leukemia and other secondary malignancies in patients who have received alkylating-agent therapy.[66, 80, 89, 116, 138, 152]

Effect in Ovarian Toxicity

Chemotherapeutic agents may have a direct cytotoxic effect on ova and follicles. Alkylating agents, including mechlorethamine, phenylalanine mustard, busulfan, cyclophosphamide, thiotepa, and chorambucil cause menstrual abnormalities, and amenorrhea.[18, 26, 42, 50, 84, 88, 110, 144, 149, 152, 157, 173, 174, 186] Ovotoxicity caused by cyclophosphamide occurs because of the widespread use of this drug. In experimental animal systems, cyclophosphamide has been shown to cause severe chromosomal damage and to interfere with normal follicular and corpus luteum development.[109, 152, 186] In humans, the gonadotoxic effect of cyclophosphamide depends upon age, dosage, and duration of therapy.[53, 84, 88, 97, 129, 152] Long-term cyclophosphamide therapy has been reported to cause destruction of ova and follicles in prepubertal girls[42, 110, 186]; however, in larger series, ovarian function in girls treated with cyclophosphamide before and during puberty was found to be normal.[53, 97, 129] In contrast to radiotherapy, which causes permanent sterility and ovarian destruction, cyclophosphamide ootoxicity is cumulative, and varies with age and hormonal status.[53, 109, 186] In older women, cyclophosphamide causes amenorrhea in more than 80 percent within a few months of therapy.[84, 88, 129, 144, 152, 173, 186] Ovarian biopsy reveals an atrophic ovary, lacking ova and primary follicles.[129, 152, 186] The amenorrhea is reversible in some cases.[84, 88, 152]

Among the other alkylating agents, chlorambucil is also noted for the induction of ovarian failure via destruction of primordial follicles. Ovarian biopsy in chlorambucil-induced amenorrhea is reported to show thickening of the tunica albuginea, perioophoritis, stromal fibrohyalinization, and necrotic vasculitis and hemorrhage, suggesting diffuse ovarian toxicity.[113, 152] Busulfan therapy usually results in permanent amenorrhea, with only infrequent resumption of menstruation in patients treated with very low doses. In animal models, busulfan causes rapid destruction of follicles and oocytes.[50, 152] Mechlorethamine is reported to have a lesser ovotoxicity, which is manifested by menstrual irregularities and the arrest of graafian follicle formation, but no permanent damage to ovarian function.[13] The chronic administration of thiotepa in humans causes amenorrhea; in female mice the prolonged administration of this drug produces atrophy of the female reproductive tract, uterine hypoplasia, and ovarian tumors.[149] Mitomycin-C and methotrexate are also reported to cause ovarian ablation, which is mediated by defective oogenesis and chromosomal damage.[13,152] Alkylating agents are utilized in breast cancer therapy, where ovarian ablation has a beneficial effect in delaying the spread of recurrent carcinoma in premenopausal patients.[84, 144, 166, 186]

Aminoglutethimide, once in wide use as an anticonvulsant agent and presently used in the treatment of breast cancer, is associated with menstrual irregularities and ovarian dysfunction after its long-term administration.[58, 96] Ovarian biopsy of a patient with virilization occurring during anticonvulsant therapy with aminoglutethimide demonstrated the retarded involution of corpora lutea, with resultant corpus luteum cyst formation.[15] The ovarian effect of aminoglutethimide is mediated indirectly by its blockage of adrenal steroidogenesis.

THE EFFECT OF IMMUNOSUPPRESSIVE AGENTS

The use of immunosuppressive agents has become widespread in the treatment of transplant recipients and patients with various autoimmune diseases. With the increased use of immunosuppressive therapy, most commonly with azathioprine and corticosteroids, it has been recognized that patients undergoing long-term immunosuppression have an increased risk of developing malignancies[17, 87, 104, 128, 133]; most of the cancers reported have been lymphomas.

Numerous case reports have accumulated implicating a causal relationship between azathioprine administration and the development of squamous abnormalities in the vulva, vagina, and cervix similar to those seen during treatment with such chemotherapeutic agents as cyclophosphamide and busulfan.[9, 10, 43, 67, 94, 133, 148] Carcinoma of the cervix comprises 8 percent of de novo cancers in organ homograft recipients, among whom there is a 14-fold increase in the incidence of intraepithelial carcinoma of the cervix.[128, 133] The cytologic and histologic changes in the epithelium of women treated with azathioprine are virtually indistinguishable from spontaneously occur-

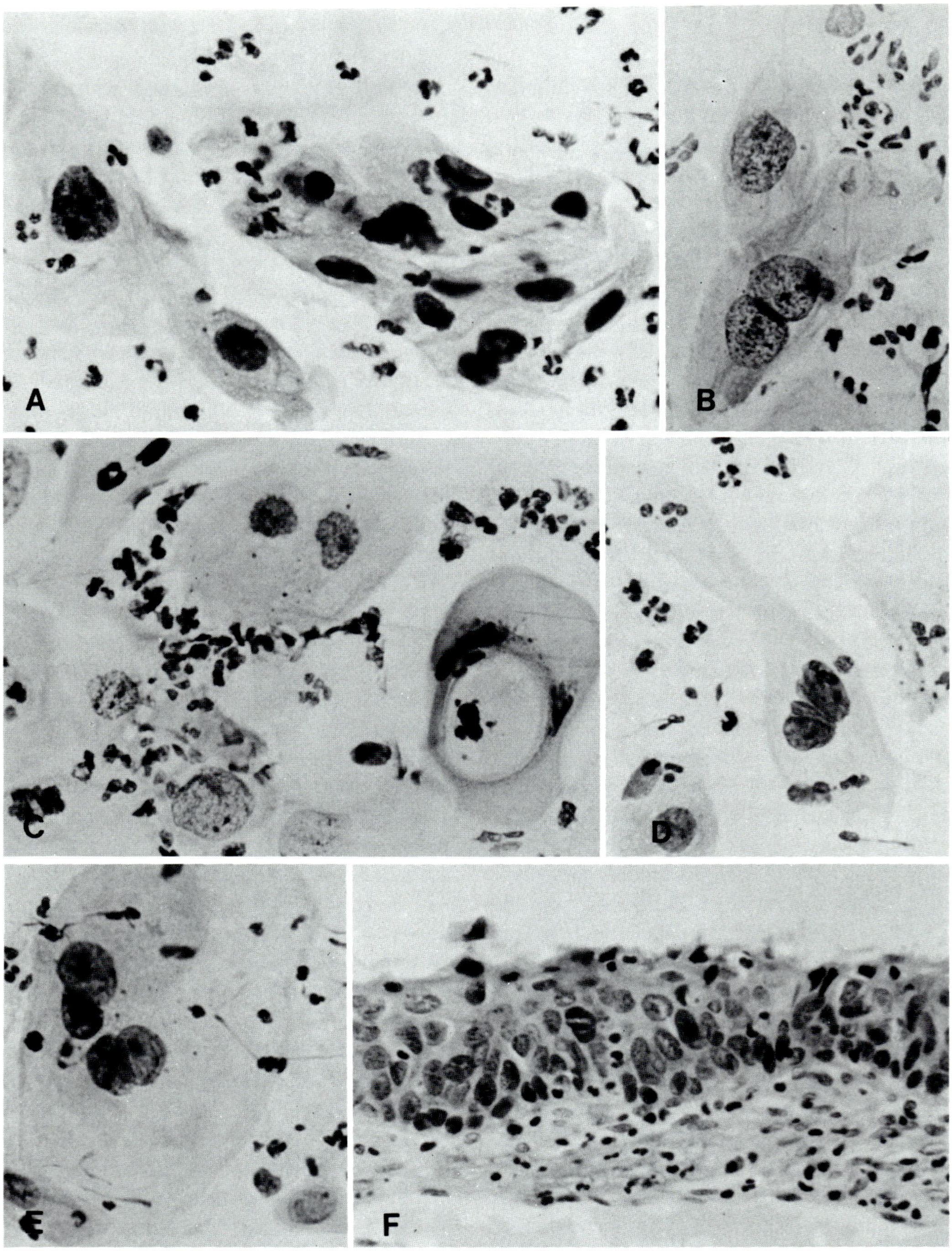

Fig. 13-21. Cervical smear and tissue from a young patient (age 25) with renal transplant (A, B, C, D, E) who was receiving immunosuppressive therapy. The abnormalities range from squamous cancer cells (A) to dyskaryotic cells of unusual configuration. Of note are cell gigantism (C, E), degenerative changes (C), and bizarre cell forms (D). Therapy was withheld because of the patient's general condition, but at the age of 28 the patient had to undergo hysterectomy for intractable bleeding. Histologic sections of the uterine cervix disclosed various levels of precancerous abnormalities, up to the level of carcinoma in situ (F). (A, B, C, D, E): × 560; (F): × 350. (Koss, L. G., Ed.: Diagnostic Cytology and Its Histopathologic Bases. 3rd Ed. Vol. 1, J. B. Lippincott Co., Philadelphia, 1979.)

ring cervical intraepithelial neoplasia and invasive carcinoma of the cervix. However, cellular gigantism and bizarre cell forms may be found more frequently in patients treated with azathioprine. (Fig. 13-21)[80] The intraepithelial neoplasms and squamous carcinomas developing in the genital tracts of women undergoing immunosuppressive therapy have similar prognoses and responses to therapy to those occurring in women not undergoing such therapy.[9, 10, 67, 80, 94, 133] The increased incidence of squamous neoplasia in association with immunosuppression should alert the clinician to careful follow-up of these patients with Pap smear, pelvic examination, and colposcopy.[24, 118, 133, 141]

In addition to squamous neoplasia, other types of gynecologic tumors have been reported in patients receiving immunosuppressive drugs; these have included ovarian carcinoma and endometrial carcinoma, and reticulum cell sarcoma of the vulva.[54, 170, 195, 196, 197] Because these reports are sporadic, no definite correlation can be made between the therapy and the development of the malignancy.

THE EFFECT OF TOPICAL ANTIBIOTIC THERAPY

Topical application of tetracycline compounds is associated with massive desquamation of the squamous epithelium of the vagina and cervix; cytologic preparations characteristically contain sheets of squamous cells with a yellowish discoloration of the cytoplasm.[80, 81] Desquamative reactions to other intravaginally applied antibiotics have not been reported.

Allergic dermatitides associated with local, oral, and parenteral antibiotic therapy may involve the vulva and, more rarely, the vagina.

In general, it should be noted that the use of antibiotic therapy in the eradication of infectious vaginitis improves the cytologic and hormonal interpretation of vaginal and cervical smears by eliminating debris associated with inflammation.

ANTICOAGULANT THERAPY AND CORPUS LUTEUM HEMORRHAGE

Ovarian hemorrhage is a relatively rare complication of anticoagulant therapy; however, it is a recognized clinical entity, especially in recent years. Numerous cases have been reported,[21, 45, 83, 85, 95, 101, 105, 130-132, 151, 159, 171, 187, 193] and they continue to accumulate as more premenopausal women receive anticoagulant therapy in the treatment of thrombophlebitis, pulmonary emboli, cardiac prostheses, and renal hemodialysis. Almost invariably a ruptured, hemorrhagic corpus luteum is documented pathologically as the source of bleeding, although bleeding follicular cysts and graafian follicles have also been reported (Fig. 13-22).[83, 131, 151, 171, 189] This hemorrhage is usually self-limited, but it may occasionally progress to hematoma formation (Fig. 13-23) and even to intraperitoneal hemorrhage. Even in the absence of anticoagulant therapy, ruptured, bleeding ovarian cysts have been recognized as uncommon causes of acute abdominal symptoms[45, 107, 162, 189]; with anticoagulant therapy, however, the hemorrhage may reach massive proportions.[85, 131, 151, 159, 171]

The diagnosis of a bleeding corpus luteum is rarely made preoperatively, but should be considered in all premenopausal women who are taking anticoagulants[21, 131, 151, 171, 187]; hemorrhage from a ruptured corpus luteum may occur in patients receiving heparin or coumadin. The incidence of corpus luteum hemorrhage does not correlate with the duration of anticoagulant therapy; such hemorrhage may occur in patients on either acute or chronic anticoagulant regimens. Among reported cases, the duration of anticoagulant therapy prior to ovarian hemorrhage has ranged from 36 hours to 10 years.[151] Suppression of ovulation or oophorectomy may be considered after

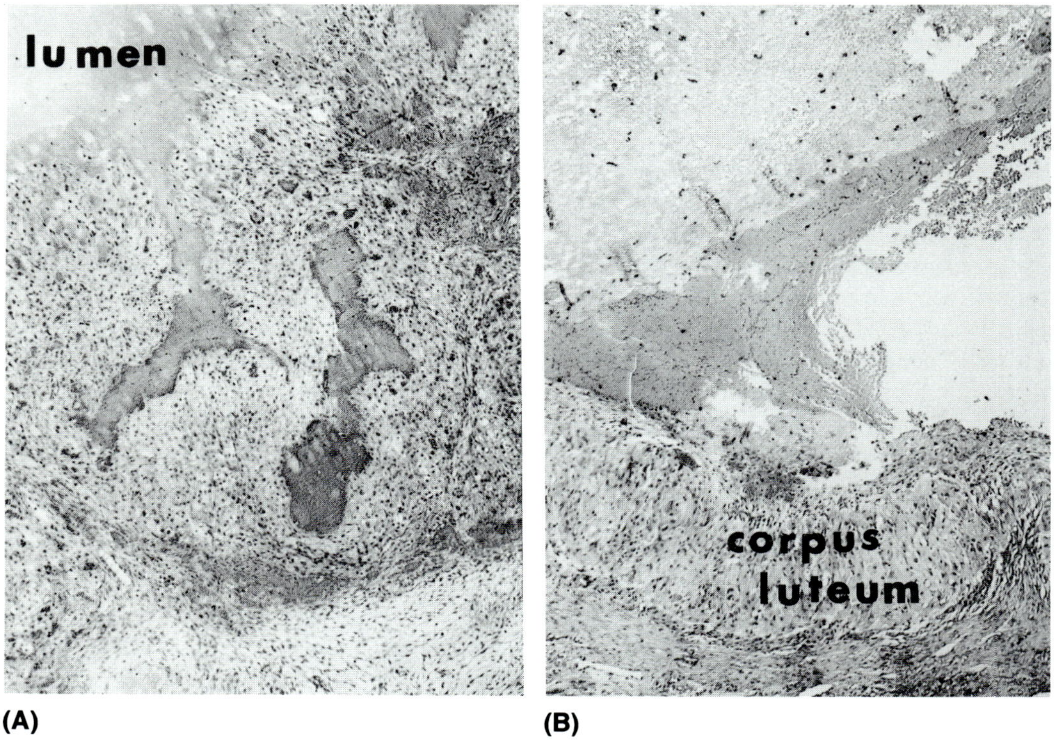

Fig. 13-22. Light micrographs of corpora lutea hemorrhages in various stages. (A) Large corpus luteum with numerous areas of extravasated hemorrhage. (B) Corpus luteum cyst with central hemorrhage. (A): × 55; (B): × 60.

recovery, in order to minimize the risk of recurrent corpus luteum bleeding.[151,171]

GOLD THERAPY AND VAGINITIS

Parenteral gold therapy for rheumatoid arthritis causes vaginitis characterized by acute inflammation.[47,188]

OVARIAN EFFECTS OF ALCOHOL AND HEROIN USE

Alcoholism in females has a deleterious effect on ovarian function, producing menstrual irregularities and alteration of secondary sex characteristics. This effect is most likely mediated by the toxicity of alcohol to the hypothalamic-pituitary-gonadal axis.[178-180] Alcohol is metabolized to acetaldehyde by ovarian alcohol dehydrogenase, with resultant NAD depletion and mitochondrial dysfunction.[177]

Heroin addiction is associated with a high incidence of menstrual irregularities, most

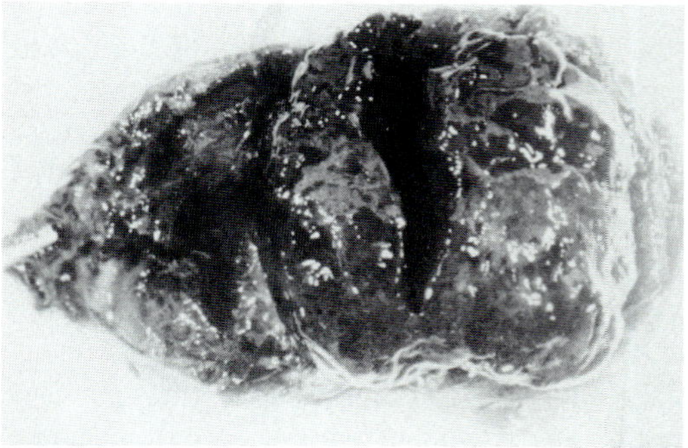

Fig. 13-23. Gross photograph of an ovarian hematoma removed from a patient with a cardiac valvular prostheses on chronic coumadin therapy. The hematoma measured 24 cm in diameter.

commonly amenorrhea and oligomenorrhea, which occur in as many as 60 to 90 percent of female heroin users.[36, 165, 184] The effect of heroin is thought to be due to interference at the hypothalamic level. Women who chronically use heroin have cytologic and serologic evidence of hormonal deficiency, characterized by low FSH and LH values and hypoestrogenism[36, 127, 165, 184]; ovarian biopsy demonstrates atrophic ovaries.[127] The menstrual irregularities are usually reversible after cessation of heroin use or after methadone therapy.

REFERENCES

1. Anderson, D.: Management of advanced endometrial adenocarcinoma with medroxyprogesterone acetate. Am. J. Obstet. Gynecol. 92:87, 1965.
2. Anderson, R. G. W., & Hein, C. E.: Estrogen dependent ciliogenesis in the chick oviduct. Cell. Tiss. Res. 171:459, 1976.
3. Andrews, M. C., & Wentz, A. C.: The effects of danazol on gonatotropins and steroid blood levels in normal and anovulatory women. Am. J. Obstet. Gynecol. 121:817, 1975.
4. Asch, R. H., & Greenblatt, R. B.: The use of an impeded androgen-danazol in the management of benign breast disorders. Am. J. Obstet. Gynecol. 127:130, 1977.
5. Beral, V.: Cardiovascular-disease mortality trends and oral contraceptive use in young women. Lancet 2:1047, 1976.
6. Betts, J. W., & Buttram, V. C.: A plan for managing endometriosis. Contemporary Ob/Gyn 15:121, 1980.
7. Boling, J. L.: Endocrinology of oviductal musculature. In: Hafez, E. S. E., & Blandau, R. J. Eds.: The Mammalian Oviduct: Comparative Biology and Methodology. p. 163. University of Chicago Press, Chicago, 1960.
8. Boutselis, J. G.: Histochemistry of the normal endometrium. In: Norris, H. J., Hertig, A. T., & Abell, M. R. Eds.: The Uterus. IAP Monograph. p. 175. The Williams and Wilkins Company, Baltimore, 1973.
9. Bowen-Simpkins, P., & Hull, M. G. R.: Intraepithelial carcinoma of the vagina following immunosuppression treated with topical 5-fluorouracil. Proc. R. Soc. Med. 67:589, 1974.
10. Bowen-Simkins, P., & Hull, M. G. R.: Intraepithelial vaginal neoplasia following immunosuppressive therapy treated with topical 5-fluorouracil. Obstet. Gynecol. 46:360, 1975.
11. Brenner, R. M.: The biology of oviductal cilia. In: Hafez, E. S. E., Blandau, R. J. Eds.: The Mammalian Oviduct: Comparative Biology and Methodology. p. 203. University of Chicago Press, Chicago, 1969.
12. Britssch, C. J., & Azar, H. A.: Estrogen effect in exfoliated vaginal cells following treatment with digitalis. A case report with experimental observations in mice. Am. J. Obstet. Gynecol. 85:989, 1963.
13. Calabresi, P., & Parks, Jr., R. E.: Alkylating agents, antimetabolites, hormones, and other antiproliferative agents. In: Goodman, L. S. and Gilman, A. Eds.: The Pharmacologic Basis of Therapeutics. 5th Ed. p. 1254. Macmillan, New York, 1975.
14. Candy, J., & Abell, M. R.: Progestogen-induced hyperplasia of the cervix. J.A.M.A. 203:323, 1968.
15. Cash, R., Petrini, M. A., & Brough, A. J.: Ovarian dysfunction associated with an anticonvulsant drug. J.A.M.A. 208:1149, 1969.
16. Cavazos, F., & Lucas, F. V.: Ultrastructure of the endometrium. In: Norris, H. J., Hertig, A. T., & Abell, M. R. Eds.: The Uterus. IAP Monograph Number 14. p. 136. Williams and Wilkins Co., Baltimore, 1973.
17. Cerilli, J., & Hattan, D.: Immunosuppression and oncogenesis. Am. J. Clin. Pathol. 62:218, 1974.
18. Chauvergne, M. J.: The gynecological and obstetrical risks of anti-cancer chemotherapy. Bord. Med. 4:1559, 1971.
19. Clark, J. H., Anderson, J. N., & Peck, E. J., Jr.: Estrogen receptor-antiestrogen complex: atypical binding by uterine nuclei and effects on uterine growth. Steroids 22:707, 1973.
20. Clark, J. H., Peck, E. J., & Anderson, J. N.: Oestrogen receptors and antagonism of steroid hormone action. Nature 251:446, 1974.
21. Dacus, R. M., III: Massive intraperitoneal hemorrhage from a corpus luteum hematoma in women taking anticoagulants. Obstet. Gynecol. 31:471, 1968.

22. Diczfalusy, E.: Mode of action of contraceptive drugs. Am. J. Obstet. Gynecol. 100:136, 1968.
23. Dmowski, W. P., & Cohen, M. R.: Treatment of endometriosis with an antigonadotropin, danazol. A laparoscopic and histologic evaluation. Obstet. Gynecol. 46:147, 1975.
24. Donohue, L. R.: Colposcopic and cytologic evaluation of women undergoing immunosuppressive therapy. J. Reprod. Med. 12:194, 1974.
25. Engel, T., Jewelewicz, R., Dyrenfurth, I. et al.: Ovarian hyperstimulation syndrome. Report of a case with notes on pathogenesis and treatment. Am. J. Obstet. Gynecol. 112:1052, 1972.
26. Fairley, K. F., Barrie, J. U., & Johnson, W.: Sterility and testicular atrophy related to cyclophosphamide therapy. Lancet 1:883, 1975.
27. Fechner, R. E.: Atypical leiomyomas and synthetic progestin therapy. Am. J. Clin. Pathol. 49:697, 1968.
28. Fechner, R. E.: The surgical pathology of the reproductive system and breast during oral contraceptive therapy. In: Sommers, S. C. Ed.: Genital and Mammary Pathology Decennial 1966-1975. p. 103. Appleton-Century Crofts, New York, 1975.
29. Feingold, M. L., & Koss, L. G.: Effects of long term administration of busulfan. Arch. Intern. Med. 124:66, 1969.
30. Ferenczy, A.: How progestogens affect endometrial hyperplasia and neoplasia. Contemporary Ob/Gyn 11:137, 1978.
31. Ferenczy, A., & Richart, R. M.: Female Reproductive System: Dynamics of Scan and Transmission Electron Microscopy. Wiley, New York, 1974.
32. Forni, A. M., Koss, L. G., & Geller, W.: Cytologic study of the effect of cyclophosphamide on the epithelium of the urinary bladder in man. Cancer 17:1348, 1964.
33. Fredricsson, B., & Bjorkman, N.: Morphologic alterations in the human oviduct epithelium induced by contraceptive steroids. Fertil. Steril. 24:19, 1973.
34. Fromson, J. M., & Sharp, D. S.: The selective uptake of tamoxifen by human uterine tissue. J. Obstet. Gynaecol. Br. Commonw. 81:321, 1974.
35. Frost, J. K.: Gynecologic and obstetric cytopathology. In: Novak, E. R., & Woodruff, J. D., Eds.: Novak's Gynecologic and Obstetric Pathology. 7th Ed. p. 634. W. B. Saunders, Philadelphia, 1974.
36. Gaulden, E. C., Littlefield, D. C., & Putoff, O. E., et al.: Menstrual abnormalities associated with heroin addiction. Am. J. Obstet. Gynecol. 90:155, 1964.
37. Goldzieher, J. W., Maqueo, M., Ricaud, L., Aguilar, J. A., & Canales, E.: Induction of degenerative changes in uterine myomas by high-dosage progestin therapy. Am. J. Obstet. Gynecol. 96:1078, 1966.
38. Gonzalez-Angulo, A., & Salazar, H.: Pathology of the reproductive system, breast, and liver in women during hormonal contraception. In: Josimovich, J. B. Ed.: Uterine Contraction. p. 210. John Wiley and Sons, Inc., New York, 1973.
39. Gordon, H. W., Rywlin, A. M., Sussman, H., et al.: The effect of digitalis therapy on the vaginal cytology in postmenopausal females. Am. J. Obstet. Gynecol. 94:524, 1966.
40. Gore, H.: Hyperplasia of the endometrium. In: Norris, H. J., Hertig, A. T., Abell, M. R., Eds.: International Academy of Pathology Monograph Number 14. The Uterus. p. 136. Williams and Wilkins, Baltimore, 1973.
41. Gray, L. A., Christopherson, W. M., & Hoover, R. N.: Estrogens and endometrial carcinoma. Obstet. Gynecol. 49:385, 1977.
42. Greenwald, E. S., Ed.: Cancer Chemotherapy. 2nd Ed. Medical Outline Series, New York, 1973.
43. Gupta, P. K., Pinn, V. M., & Taft, P. D.: Cervical dysplasia associated with azathioprine (Imuran) therapy. Acta. Cytol. 13:373, 1969.
44. Güreli, N., Denham, S. W., & Root, S. W.: Cytologic dysplasia related to busalfan (myleran) therapy. Report of a case. Obstet. Gynecol. 21:466, 1963.
45. Gurewich, V., & Thomas, D.: Massive intraperitoneal hemorrhage from a ruptured corpus luteum. N. Engl. J. Med. 263:909, 1960.
46. Gusberg, S. B., Chen, S. Y., & Cohen, C. J.: Endometrial cancer: factors influencing the choice of treatment. Gynecol. Oncol. 2:308, 1974.
47. Harvey, S. C.: Heavy metals. In: Goodman,

L. S. and Gilman, A., Eds.: The Pharmacological Basis of Therapeutics. 5th Ed. p. 931. Macmillan, New York, 1975.
48. Hayakawa, K.: Effects of dimethisterone on endometrial adenocarcinoma-electron microscopic study. Acta. Obstet. Gynaecol. Jap. 16:285, 1969.
49. Hayakawa, K., Okudaira, Y., & Nasu, K.: Effect of gestagen on uterine adenocarcinoma of the endometrium in the human, with special reference to electron microscope study. J. Jap. Obstet. Gynecol. Soc. 20:1528, 1968.
50. Hemsworth, B. N., & Jackson, H.: Effect of busulfan on the developing gonad of the male rat. J. Reprod. Fertil. 5:187, 1963.
51. Henzl, M. R., Smith, R. E., Boost, G., et al.: Lysosomal concept of menstrual bleeding in humans. J. Clin. Metab. 34:860, 1972.
52. Hilliard, G. D., & Norris, H. J.: The pathologic effects of oral contraceptives. In: Lingeman, C., Ed.: Recent Results in Cancer Research. Vol. 66. Carcinogenic Steroids. p. 49. Springer-Verlag, New York, 1979.
53. Himelstein-Braw, R., Peters, H., & Faber, M.: Influence of irradiation and chemotherapy on the ovaries of children with abdominal tumors. Br. J. Cancer, 36:269, 1977.
54. Hodgkinson, D. J., & Williams, T. J.: Endometrial carcinoma associated with azathioprine and cortisone therapy. A case report. Gynecol. Oncol. 5:308, 1977.
55. Hoffman, P., Höffele, R., & Buchholz, C.: Estrogen effects of glycoside therapy. Fortschr. Med. 93:1274, 1975.
56. Horowitz, R. I., & Feinstein, A. R.: Alternative analytic methods for case-control studies of estrogens and endometrial cancer. N. Engl. J. Med. 299:1089, 1978.
57. Horwitz, K. B., & McGuire, W. L.: Nuclear mechanisms of estrogen action. J. Biol. Chem. 253:8185, 1978.
58. Hughes, S. W. M., & Burley, D. M.: Aminoglutethimide: a "side effect" turned to therapeutic advantage. Postgrad. Med. J. 46:409, 1970.
59. Hustin, J.: Hormonal therapy of endometrial carcinoma: Effects of large doses given by parenteral or intracavitary routes. In: Brush, M. G., Taylor, R. W., Williams, D. C., Eds.: Symposium in Endometrial Cancer. p. 246. William Heinemann, London, 1973.
60. Hustin, J.: Morphology and DNA content of endometrial cancer nuclei under progestagen treatment. Acta. Cytol. 20:556, 1976.
61. Jensen, H. K., Hansen, P. A., & Blom, J.: Incidence of *Candida albicans* in women using oral contraceptives. Acta. Obstet. Gynecol. Scand. 49:293, 1970.
62. Jewelewicz, R.: Management of infertility resulting from anovulation. Am. J. Obstet. Gynecol. 122:909, 1975.
63. Jewelewicz, R., Dyrenfurth, I., Warren, M. P., et al.: Ovarian hyperstimulation syndrome—Relationship between preovulatory estrogen levels and ovarian hyperstimulation. In: Rosenberg, E., Ed.: Serono Foundation Workshop Conference on Gonadotropin Therapy in Female Infertility. p. 235. Excerpta Medical, Amsterdam, 1973.
64. Jewelewicz, R., & Vande Wiele, R.: Acute hydrothorax as the only symptom of ovarian hyperstimulation syndrome. Am. J. Obstet. Gynecol. 121:1121, 1975.
65. Jones, G. S., Sezer, A., & Wentz, A. C.: Serum progesterone values in the luteal phase defects. Obstet. Gynecol. 44:26, 1974.
66. Kaslow, R. A., Wisch, N., & Glass, J. L.: Acute leukemia following cytotoxic chemotherapy. J.A.M.A. 219:75, 1972.
67. Kay, S., Frable, W. J., & Hume, D. M.: Cervical dysplasia and cancer developing in women on immunosuppression therapy for renal homotransplantation. Cancer 26:1048, 1970.
68. Kelly, H. W., Moles, P. A., Buster, J. E., & Scragg, W. H.: Adenocarcinoma of the endometrium in women taking sequential oral contraceptives. Obstet. Gynecol. 47:200, 1976.
69. Kelley, R. M., & Baker, W. H.: The effect of 17-alpha-hydroxyprogesterone caproate on metastatic endometrial cancer. Natl. Cancer Inst. Monogr. 9:235, 1977.
70. Kistner, R. W.: Histologic effect of progestins on hyperplasia and carcinoma in situ of the endometrium. Cancer 12:1106, 1959.
71. Kistner, R. W.: Induction of ovulation with clomiphene citrate. In: Behrman, S. J., and Kistner, R W., Eds.: Progress in Infertility. p. 407. Little, Brown, New York, 1968.
72. Kistner, R. W.: Endometrial alterations associated with estrogen-progestin combinations. In: Norris, H. J., Hertig, A. T., & Abell, M. R., Eds.: The Uterus: IAP Monograph

14. p. 227. Williams and Wilkins, Baltimore, 1973.
73. Kistner, R. W., Duncan, C. J., & Mansell, H.: Suppression of ovulation by Tri-p-anisylchloroethylene (TACE). Obstet. Gynecol. 8:399, 1956.
74. Kistner, R. W., Griffiths, C. T., & Craig, J. M.: Use of progestational agents in the management of endometrial cancer. Cancer 18:1563, 1965.
75. Kitay, D. Z., & Wentz, W. B.: Cervical cytology in folic acid deficiency of pregnancy. Am. J. Obstet. Gynecol. 104:931, 1969.
76. Klaus, H.: Quantitative criteria of folate deficiency in cervico-vaginal cytograms, with report of a new parameter. Acta. Cytol. 50:50, 1971.
77. Knab, D. R.: Estrogen and endometrial carcinoma. Obstet. Gynecol. Surv. 32:267, 1977.
78. Kohorn, E. I.: Gestagens and endometrial carcinoma. Gynecol. Oncol. 4:398, 1976.
79. Koss, L. G.: A light and electron microscopic study of a single dose of cyclophosphamide on various organs in the rat. Lab. Invest. 16:44, 1967.
80. Koss, L. G., Ed.: Diagnostic Cytology and Its Histopathologic Bases. 3rd Ed. Vol. 1. J. B. Lippincott, Philadelphia, 1979.
81. Koss, L. G., Melamed, M. R., & Mayer, K.: The effect of busulfan on human epithelia. Am. J. Clin. Pathol. 44:385, 1965.
82. Koss, L. G., Stewart, F. W., Foote, F. W., et al.: Some histological aspects of behavior of epidermoid carcinoma in situ and related lesions of the cervix. Cancer 16:1160, 1963.
83. Kovalcik, P. J.: Massive hemoperitoneum from a ruptured ovarian graafian follicle while on oral anticoagulants. Milit. Med. 137:162, 1972.
84. Koyama, H., Wada, T., Nishizawa, Y., et al.: Cyclophosphamide induced ovarian failure and its therapeutic significance in patients with breast cancer. Cancer 39:1043, 1977.
85. Krause, J. R., & Amores, R.: Massive intraperitoneal hemorrhage from ruptured corpus luteum during anticoagulant therapy. South Med. J. 69:1220, 1976.
86. Kraus, H., Schuhmann, R., Ganol, M., et al.: Cytologic findings in vaginal smears from patients under treatment with cyclophosphamide. Acta. Cytol. 21:726, 1977.
87. Kripke, M. L., & Borsos, T.: Immunosuppression & carcinogenesis. A review. Israel J. Med. Sci. 10:888, 1974.
88. Kumar, R., Biggart, J. D., McEvoy, J., et al.: Cyclophosphamide and reproductive function. Lancet 1:1212, 1972.
89. Kyle, R. A., Pierre, R. V., & Bayrd, E. D.: Multiple myeloma and acute leukemia associated with alkylating agents. Arch. Intern. Med. 135:185, 1975.
90. Laguens, R., & Lagrutta, J.: Fine structure of human muscle in pregnancy. Am. J. Obstet. Gynecol. 89:1040, 1964.
91. Lamb, E. J., & Greene, R. R.: A microscopic study of the growth of leiomyomas of the uterus during pregnancy. Surg. Gynecol. Obstet. 108:575, 1959.
92. Lauerson, N. H., Wilson, K. H., & Birnbaum, S.: Danazol: An antigonadotropic agent in the treatment of pelvic endometriosis. Am. J. Obstet. Gynecol. 123:742, 1975.
93. Lauerson, N. H., & Wilson, K. H.: Evaluation of danazol as an oral contraceptive. Obstet. Gynecol. 50:91, 1977.
94. Leckie, G. B., & Cotton, R. E.: Simultaneous in situ carcinoma of the cervix, vulva and perineum after immunosuppressive therapy for renal transplantation. Br. J. Obstet. Gynaecol. 84:143, 1977.
95. Lee, R., & Kaznuer, F. J.: Ovarian hematoma complicating anticoagulant therapy. Mayo Clin. Proc. 52:19, 1977.
96. Legha, S. S., Davis, H. L., & Muggia, F. M.: Hormonal therapy of breast cancer: New approaches and concepts. Ann. Int. Med. 88:69, 1978.
97. Lentz, R., Bergstein, J., & Steffes, M. W., et al.: Postpubertal evaluation of gonadal function following cyclophosphamide therapy before and during puberty. J. Pediatr. 91:385, 1977.
98. Lunan, C. D., & Green, B.: 3H-oestradiol uptake in vivo by human uterine endometrium: effect of tamoxifen. Clin. Endocrinol. 3:465, 1974.
99. Lyon, F. A., & Frisch, M. J.: Endometrial abnormalities occurring in young women on long-term sequential oral contraception. Obstet. Gynecol. 47:639, 1976.
100. Malkasian, G. D., Decker, D. G., Mussey, E., et al.: Progesterone treatment of recurrent endometrial carcinoma. Am. J. Obstet. Gynecol. 110:15, 1971.

101. Manny, J., Merin, G., & Roziw, R. R.: Ovarian hemorrhage complicating anticoagulant therapy. Obstet. Gynecol. 41:512, 1973.
102. Marshall, J. M.: The physiology of the myometrium. In: Norris, H. J., Hertig, A. T., & Abell, M. R., Eds.: The Uterus: IAP Monograph Number 14. p. 89. Williams and Wilkins, Baltimore, 1973.
103. Mattin, P. M., Rolland, P. H., Gammere, M., et al.: Estradiol and progesterone receptors in normal and neoplastic endometrium: Correlations between receptors, histopathological examinations and clinical responses under progestin therapy. Int. J. Cancer 23:321, 1979.
104. Matas, A. J., Simmons, R. L., Kjellstrand, C. M., et al.: Increased incidence of malignancy during chronic renal failure. Lancet 1:883, 1975.
105. Matseoane, S., Batts, J. A., & Mandeville, E. O.: Ovarian hemorrhage complicating warfarin sodium anticoagulant therapy. Am. J. Obstet. Gynecol. 124:766, 1976.
106. McDonald, T. W., Annegers, J. F., O'Fallow, W. M., Dockerty, M. B., Malkasian, G. D., Jr., & Kurland, L. T.: Exogenous estrogen and endometrial carcinoma; case-control and incidence study. Am. J. Obstet. Gynecol. 127:572, 1977.
107. Meigs, J. V., & Hoyt, W. F.: Rupture of the graafian follicle, the corpus luteum and small follicle or lutein cysts simulating appendicitis. Am. J. Obstet. Gynecol. 25:532, 1933.
108. Meissner, W. A., Sommers, S. C., & Sherman, G.: Endometrial hyperplasia endometrial carcinoma, and endometriosis produced experimentally by estrogens. Cancer 10:500, 1957.
109. Miller, J. J., & Cale, L. J.: Changes in mouse ovaries after prolonged treatment with cyclophosphamide. Proc. Soc. Exp. Biol. Med. 133:190, 1970.
110. Miller, J. J., Williams, G. F., & Leissring, J. C.: Multiple late complications of therapy with cyclophosphamide including ovarian destruction. Am. J. Med. 50:530, 1971.
111. Moghissi, K. S.: Endometrium and endosalpinx of women treated with microdose progestogens. J. Reprod. Med. 14:217, 1975.
112. Moghissi, K. S., & Syner, F. N.: Contraceptive mechanism of microdose norethindrone. Obstet. Gynecol. 41:585, 1973.
113. Morgenfeld, M. C., Goldberg, V., Parisier, H., et al.: Ovarian lesions due to cytostatic agents during the treatment of Hodgkin's disease. Surg. Gynecol. Obstet. 134:826, 1972.
114. de Narvaez, F., & Blaustein, R.: Cytology of the female genital tract. In: Blaustein, A., Ed.: Pathology of the Female Genital Tract. p. 762. Springer-Verlag, New York, 1977.
115. Navab, A., Kross, L. G., & Jadue, J. S.: Estrogen-like activity of digitalis. J.A.M.A. 194:30, 1965.
116. Nelson, B. M., & Andrews, G. A.: Breast cancer & cytologic dysplasia in many organs after busulfan (Myleran). Am. J. Clin. Pathol. 42:37, 1964.
117. Neuwirth, R. S., Turksoy, R. N., & Vande Wiele, R.: Acute Meigs syndrome secondary to ovarian stimulation with human menopausal gonadotropins. Am. J. Obstet. Gynecol. 91:977, 1965.
118. Norfleet, R. G., & Sampson, C. E.: Carcinoma of the cervix after treatment with prednisone and azathioprine for chronic active hepatitis. Am. J. Gastroenterol. 70:383, 1978.
119. Noyes, R. W.: Normal phases of the endometrium. In: Norris, H. J., Hertig, A. T., & Abell, M. R., Eds.: The Uterus: IAP monograph Number 14. p. 110. Williams and Wilkins, Baltimore, 1973.
120. Noyes, R. W., Hertig, A. T., & Rock, J.: Dating the endometrial biopsy. Fertil. Steril. 1:3, 1950.
121. Ober, W. B.: Stilbestrol: a pathologist's view. In: Sommers, S. C., Ed.: Pathology Annual. p. 227. Appleton-Century Crofts, New York, 1976.
122. Ober, W. B.: Effects of oral and intrauterine administration of contraceptives on the uterus. Hum. Pathol. 8:513, 1977.
123. Ober, W. B., Decker, A., Clyman, M. J., & Roland, M.: Endometrial morphology after sequential medication with mestranol and chlormadinone. Obstet. Gynecol. 28:247, 1966.
124. Oberti, C., Dabancens, A., Garcia-Huidobro, M., Rodriquez-Bravo, R., & Zanartu, J.: Low-dosage oral progestogens to control fertility. II. Morphologic modifications in the gonad and oviduct. Obstet. Gynecol. 43:285, 1974.
125. Ory, H., Naib, Z., Conger, S. B., Hatcher, R. A., & Tyler, C. W., Jr.: Contraceptive choice and prevalence of cervical dysplasia and carcinoma in situ. Am. J. Obstet. Gynecol. 124:573, 1976.

126. Patek, E., Nilsson, L., Johannisson, E., Hellema, M., & Bout, J.: Scanning electron microscopic study of the human fallopian tube. Report III. The effect of midpregnancy and of various steroids. Fertil. Steril. 24:31, 1973.
127. Pelosi, M. A., Sama, J. C., Caterini, H., et al.: Galactorrhea-amenorrhea syndrome associated with heroin addiction. Am. J. Obstet. Gynecol. 118:967, 1974.
128. Penn, I., & Starzl, T. E.: A summary of the status of de novo cancer in transplant recipients. Transplant. Proc. 4:719, 1972.
129. Pennisi, A. J., Grushkin, C. M., & Lieberman, E.: Gonadal function in children with nephrosis treated with cyclophosphamide. Am. J. Dis. Child. 129:315, 1975.
130. Perlman, J. A., Barnes, A. B., & Demirjian, Z.: Corpus luteum hemorrhages complicating chronic anticoagulation. Obstet. Gynecol. 49: Suppl. 20, 1977.
131. Peters, W. A., Thiagarajah, M. B., & Thornton, W. N.: Ovarian hemorrhage in patients receiving anticoagulant therapy. J. Reprod. Med. 22:82, 1979.
132. Phillip, R. S.: Massive intraperitoneal hemorrhage from a ruptured ovarian cyst secondary to anticoagulant therapy for recurrent pulmonary emboli. Am. J. Obstet. Gynecol. 130:231, 1978.
133. Porreco, R., Penn, I., Droegemueller, W., et al.: Gynecologic malignancies in immunosuppressed organ homograft recipients. Obstet. Gynecol. 45:359, 1975.
134. Prakash, S., & Scully, R. E.: Sarcoma-like pseudogragnancy changes in uterine leiomyomas. Obstet. Gynecol. 24:106, 1964.
135. Rabau, E., Serr, D. M., Mashiah, S., et al.: Current concepts in the treatment of anovulation. Br. Med. J. 2:446, 1967.
136. Reifenstein, E. C.: Hydroxyprogesterone caproate therapy in advanced endometrial cancer. Cancer 27:485, 1971.
137. Reifenstein, E. C.: The treatment of advanced endometrial cancer with hydroxyprogesterone caproate. Gynecol. Oncol. 2:377, 1974.
138. Reimer, R. R., Hoover, R., Fraumeni, J., et al.: Acute leukemia after alkylating agent therapy of ovarian cancer. N. Engl. J. Med. 297:177, 1977.
139. Rice-Wray, E., Correu, S., Gorodovsky, J., Esquivel, J., & Goldzieher, J. W.: Return of ovulation after discontinuance of oral contraceptives. Fertil. Steril. 18:212, 1967.
140. Richart, R. M., & Ferenczy, A.: Endometrial response to hormonal environment. Gynecol. Oncol. 2:180, 1974.
141. Ringrose, C. A. D.: Carcinoma in situ of the cervix after amethopterin therapy. Am. J. Obstet. Gynecol. 119:1132, 1974.
142. Ritter, J., Bureau, J. P., & Bonhomme, J. S.: The effects of methotrexate on the cytology of the cervix and vagina. J. Gynecol. Obstet. Biol. Reprod. 4:507, 1975.
143. Roland, M., Clyman, M. J., Decker, A., & Ober, W. B.: Classification of endometrial response to synthetic progestogen-estrogen compounds. Fertil. Steril. 15:143, 1964.
144. Rose, D. P., & Davis, T. E.: Ovarian function in patients receiving adjuvant chemotherapy for breast cancer. Lancet 1:1174, 1977.
145. Ross, R., & Klebanoff, S. J.: Fine structural changes in uterine smooth muscle and fibroblasts in response to estrogen. J. Cell Biol. 32:155, 1967.
146. Ryan, G. M., Jr., Craig, J., & Reid, D. E.: Histology of the uterus and ovaries after long-term cyclic norethynodrel therapy. Am. J. Obstet. Gynecol. 90:715, 1964.
147. Schenker, J. G., & Polishuk, W. Z.: Ovarian hyperstimulation syndrome. Obstet. Gynecol. 46:23, 1975.
148. Schramm, G.: Development of severe cervical dysplasia under treatment with azathioprine (Imuran). Acta. Cytol. 14:507, 1970.
149. Sears, M. E., Eckles, N., & Kirschbaum, A.: Thiotepa-induced amenorrhea associated with prolonged regression of human breast cancer; similar ovarian alterations in mice. Proc. Am. Assoc. Cancer Res. 3:150, 1960.
150. Sekiya, S., & Takanrizawa, H.: Combined effect of nonsteroidal anti-oestrogens and sex steroids on the growth of rat uterine adenocarcinoma cells in tissue culture. Br. J. Obstet. Gynecol. 83:183, 1976.
151. Semchyshyn, S., & Zuspan, F. P.: Ovarian hemorrhage due to anticoagulants. Am. J. Obstet. Gynecol. 131:837, 1978.
152. Sieber, S. M., & Adamson, R. H.: Toxicity of antineoplastic agents in man: chromosomal aberrations, antifertility effects, congenital malformations & carcinogenic potential. Adv. Cancer. Res. 22:57, 1975.
153. Silverberg, S. G., & Makowski, E. L.: Endo-

metrial carcinoma in young women taking oral contraceptive agents. Obstet. Gynecol. 46:503, 1975.
154. Silverberg, S. G., Makowski, E. L., & Roche, W. D.: Endometrial carcinoma in women under 40 years of age. Cancer 39:592, 1977.
155. Smith, D. C., Prentice, R., Thompson, D. J., et al.: Association of exogenous estrogen and endometrial carcinoma. N. Engl. J. Med. 293:1164, 1975.
156. Smith, J. P., Rutledge, F., & Soffar, S. W.: Progestins in the treatment of patients with endometrial adenocarcinoma. Am. J. Obstet. Gynecol. 94:977, 1966.
157. Sobrinho, L. G., Levine, R. A., & DeConti, R. C.: Amenorrhea in patients with Hodgkins disease treated with antineoplastic agents. Am. J. Obstet. Gynecol. 109:135, 1971.
158. Sommers, S. C.: Carcinoma of the endometrium. In: Norris, H. J., Hertig, A. T., Abell, M. R. Eds.: The Uterus. IAP Monograph Number 14. p. 276. Williams and Wilkins, Baltimore, 1973.
159. Sopher, I. M., & Ming, S. C.: Fatal corpus luteum hemorrhage during anticoagulant therapy. Obstet. Gynecol. 37:695, 1971.
160. Southam, A. L., & Janovski, N. A.: Massive ovarian hyperstimulation with clomiphene citrate. J.A.M.A. 181:443, 1962.
161. Spellace, W. N.: Metabolic effects of oral contraceptives. Clin. Obstet. Gynecol. 17:53, 1974.
162. Speroff, L.: The bleeding corpus luteum. Analysis of 40 confirmed cases. Obstet. Gynecol. 28:416, 1966.
163. Speroff, L., Glass, R. H., & Kase, N. G.: Clinical Gynecologic Endocrinology and Infertility. Williams and Wilkins, Baltimore, 1973.
164. Stern, E., Forsythe, A. B., Youkeles, L., & Coffelt, C. F.: Steroid contraceptive use and cervical dysplasia: increased risk of progression. Science 196:1460, 1977.
165. Stoffer, S. S.: A gynecologic study of drug addicts. Am. J. Obstet. Gynecol. 101:779, 1968.
166. Stoll, B. A.: Ovarian function and adjuvant chemotherapy for breast cancer. Lancet 1:1159, 1978.
167. Swenerton, K. D., Shaw, D., White, G. W. et al.: Treatment of advanced endometrial carcinoma with tamoxifen. Letter to the Editor. N. Engl. J. Med. 301:105, 1979.
168. Tavassoli, F., & Kraus, F. T.: Endometrial lesions in uteri resected for atypical endometrial hyperplasia. Am. J. Clin. Pathol. 70:770, 1978.
169. Taylor, H. B., Irey, N. S., & Norris, H. J.: Atypical endocervical hyperplasia in women taking oral contraceptives. J.A.M.A. 202:637, 1967.
170. Thoua, Y., Dupont, E., Kinnaert, P. et al.: Endometrial carcinoma and amyloidosis after kidney transplantation. Transplantation 25:91, 1978.
171. Tresch, D. D., Halverson, G., Blick, M. et al.: Ovarian (corpus luteum) hemorrhage during anticoagulation therapy. Ann. Intern. Med. 88:642, 1978.
172. Tsukada, Y., Piver, M. G., & Barlow, J. J.: Microglandular hyperplasia of the endocervix following long-term estrogen treatment. Am. J. Obstet. Gynecol. 127:888, 1977.
173. Uldall, P. R., Feist, T. G., Morley, A. R. et al.: Cyclophosphamide therapy in adults with minimal change nephrotic syndrome. Lancet 1:1250, 1972.
174. Uldall, P. R., Kerr, D. N. S., & Tacchi, D.: Sterility and cyclophosphamide. Lancet 1:693, 1972.
175. Van Niekerk, W. A.: Cervical cells in megaloblastic anaemia of the puerperium. Lancet 1:1277, 1962.
176. Van Niekerk, W. A.: Cervical cytological abnormalities caused by folic acid deficiency. Acta. Cytol. 10:67, 1966.
177. Van Thiel, D. H., Gavaler, J. S., Lester, R. et al.: Alcohol-induced ovarian failure in the rat. J. Clin. Invest. 61:624, 1978.
178. Van Thiel, D. H., Gavaler, J., Vaitukaitis, J. et al.: Evidence for an isolated defect in pituitary secretion of LH in chronic alcoholic men. Gastroenterology 71:A40, 1976.
179. Van Thiel, D. H., Lester, R., & Sherins, R. J.: Hypogonadism in alcoholic liver disease: evidence for a double defect. Gastroenterology 67:1188, 1974.
180. Van Thiel, D. H., & Lester, R.: Alcoholism: its effect on hypothalamic-pituitary-gonadal function. Gastroenterology 71:318, 1976.
181. Vernikos-Danellis, J., & Marks, B. H.: Pituitary inhibitory effects of digitoxin and hydrocortisone. Proc. Soc. Exp. Biol. Med. 109:10, 1962.

182. Villee, C. A.: Biochemical aspects of the endometrium. Gynecol. Oncol. 2:198, 1974.
183. Wallach, E. E.: Finding the best therapy for endometriosis. A Symposium. Contemporary Ob/Gyn 15:70, 1980.
184. Wallach, R. C., Jerez, E., & Blinick, G.: Pregnancy and menstrual function in narcotic addicts treated with methadone. Am. J. Obstet. Gynecol. 105:1226, 1969.
185. Ward, H. N., Konikov, N., & Reinhard, E. H.: Cytologic dysplasia occurring after busulfan (Myleran) therapy. Ann. Intern. Med. 63:654, 1965.
186. Warne, G. L., Fairley, J. B., Hobbs, F. I. R. et al.: Cyclophosphamide-induced ovarian failure. N. Engl. J. Med., 289:1159, 1973.
187. Waxman, M. & Baird, G. J.: Corpus luteum hemorrhage. J.A.M.A. 239:2270, 1978.
188. Webster, J. C., & Guden, A. G.: Vaginitis complicating gold therapy for rheumatoid arthritis. Am. J. Obstet. Gynecol. 131:700, 1979.
189. Weil, A. M.: Ruptured graafian follicle and corpus luteum with intraabdominal hemorrhage. Am. J. Obstet. Gynecol. 38:288, 1939.
190. Weiss, N. S., & Sayvetz, T. A.: Incidence of endometrial cancer in relation to the use of oral contraceptives. N. Engl. J. Med. 302:551, 1980.
191. Welch, W. R., Scully, R. E.: Precancerous lesions of the endometrium. Hum. Pathol. 8:503, 1977.
192. Wentz, A. C., Jones, G. S., Sapp, K. C. et al.: Progestational activity of danazol in the human female subject. Am. J. Obstet. Gynecol. 126:378, 1976.
193. Weseley, A. C., Neustadter, M. I., & Levine, W.: Massive intraperitoneal hemorrhage of ovarian follicular origin during anticoagulant therapy. Am. J. Obstet. Gynecol. 73:683, 1957.
194. Winn, E. B.: Gynecomastia during digitalis therapy. N. Engl. J. Med. 248:316, 1953.
195. Wishart, J. M.: Reticulosarcoma of the vulva complicating azathioprine-treated dermatomyositis. Arch. Dermatol. 108:563, 1973.
196. Wishart, J. M.: Reticulosarcoma of the vulva complicating dermatomyositis treated by immunosuppression. Proc. R. Soc. Med. 66:330, 1973.
197. Yun-Hahk Kim, H., & Williams, T. J.: Endometrioid carcinoma of the uterus and ovaries associated with immunosuppressive therapy and anticoagulation. Mayo Clin. Proc. 47:39, 1972.
198. Zinca, V., & Strimbeanu, I.: Morphologic aspects in exfoliative cytology following anticancerous chemotherapy. Neoplasma 10:397, 1963.

Appendix to Chapter 13: Intrauterine Exposure to Diethylstilbestrol

Stanley J. Robboy, William R. Welch, and Jaime Prat

Intrauterine exposure to diethylstilbestrol (DES) has been linked to the development of clear-cell adenocarcinoma of the vagina and cervix in young women, and to non-neoplastic changes of the lower genital tract in both females and males. This section reviews the pathologic findings in DES-exposed subjects, new observations and recent advances in the study of the effects of DES, and the current status of attempts to develop animal models that mimic the DES-induced conditions of humans. The historical and current uses of DES and the management of exposed offspring are presented elsewhere.[5,31,37,40,51,55]

CLEAR-CELL ADENOCARCINOMA

More than 500 cases of clear-cell adenocarcinoma of the vagina or cervix in young women have been accessioned by the Clear Cell Carcinoma Registry at the University of Chicago through 1981.[25] The median age of the patients at the time of diagnosis was 19 years, and the age range from 7 to 29 years. After age 14, the age-incidence curve rises sharply to an irregular plateau which extends from the ages of 17 to 21 years, after which it declines rapidly. Approximately 61 percent of the patients have documented exposure in utero to DES or to the chemically related nonsteroidal estrogens, hexestrol and dienestrol; another 10 percent have been exposed to some form of medication for high-risk pregnancy, but in these cases the prenatal records have not been available. The majority of patients with negative histories for exposure to DES and its congeners have had cervical tumors,[27,28] a finding consistent with the observation that clear-cell adenocarcinoma of the cervix in young women was a well-recognized entity prior to the DES era, whereas clear-cell adenocarcinoma of the vagina was exceedingly rare.

It is estimated that the clear-cell adenocarcinoma of the cervix will develop in 0.014 to 0.14 percent of females exposed to DES and its congeners.[24] If the risk of development is calculated not for the exposed population, but rather for the entire United States female population, the highest risk is for daughters born from 1951 to 1953 since it was in these years that DES was most frequently prescribed.[25] The risk is much lower for daughters born before 1950, and declines progressively for women born in 1954 and thereafter. The risk is also highest when the intrauterine exposure was begun early in pregnancy, and declines to very small values if the exposure began during the 17th week of pregnancy or later.

The tumor may involve any portion of the vagina, cervix, or both.[28] Approximately 60 percent of lesions have been confined to the vagina (Fig. 13-24); the remainder have been limited to the cervix or have involved both the cervix and vagina. Most vaginal tumors arise on the anterior wall, usually in the upper third, a location corresponding to the most frequent site of adenosis. The lateral and posterior walls and, occasionally, the middle and lower third of the vagina may also be involved.

The tumors vary in size from a microscopic focus to more than 10 cm in greatest dimension. Most are polypoid and nodular but some are flat or ulcerated, with a granular or indu-

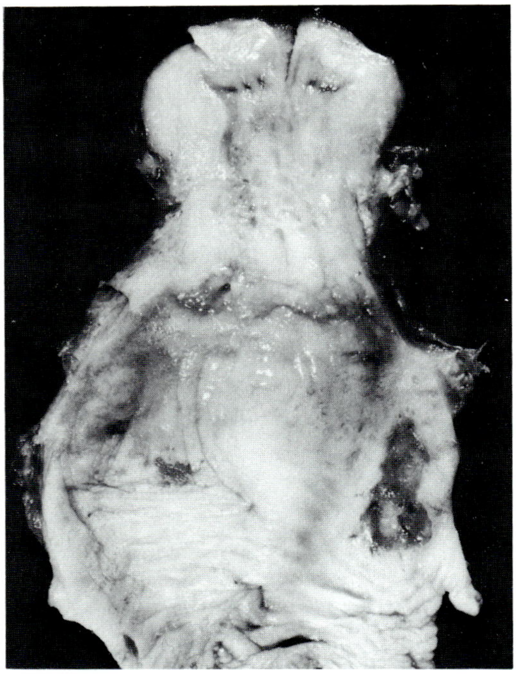

Fig. 13-24. Clear-cell adenocarcinoma bordered by dark zone of adenosis, which is circumferential about vagina. The vaginal adenosis and extensive ectropion of cervix appeared red in fresh state.

rated surface. A tumor that is tiny is usually palpable, but if confined to the lamina propria and covered by intact normal or metaplastic squamous epithelium, may be invisible to the naked eye or with the colposcope.[61] Although most of the cancers are superficial and invade only a few millimeters into the vaginal or cervical wall, some may penetrate more deeply or extend more centrifugally than can be ascertained by gross examination alone.[62]

By light- and electron microscopy, the clear-cell adenocarcinoma associated with DES exposure is identical to the clear-cell adenocarcinomas of the ovary and endometrium that occur sporadically in older women.[61] A characteristic pattern, for which the tumor is named, consists of solid sheets of clear cells, the clear appearance of the cytoplasm being due to the dissolution of glycogen as the tissue specimen is prepared for microscopic examination (Fig. 13-25). The second and most frequent pattern is characterized by tubules and cysts lined by "hobnail" cells (Fig. 13-26), flat cells, or by cells that resemble, to various degrees, the epithelium of the Mullerian tract, but lack features distinctive enough to warrant a special designation. The hobnail cell is characterized by a bulbous nucleus that protrudes into the lumen beyond the apparent cytoplasmic limits of the cell. Flat cells often appear deceptively innocuous; when only this type of epithelium is observed, for example, in a small biopsy, it may be very difficult to differentiate the tumor from adenosis, which is benign. Other patterns encountered include complex papillae and trabeculae. In any of the above patterns, the lumen may contain mucus. The cytoplasm, however, is mucin-free. By electron microscopy the neoplastic cells from each of the above patterns are of the same basic type; glycogen and microvilli

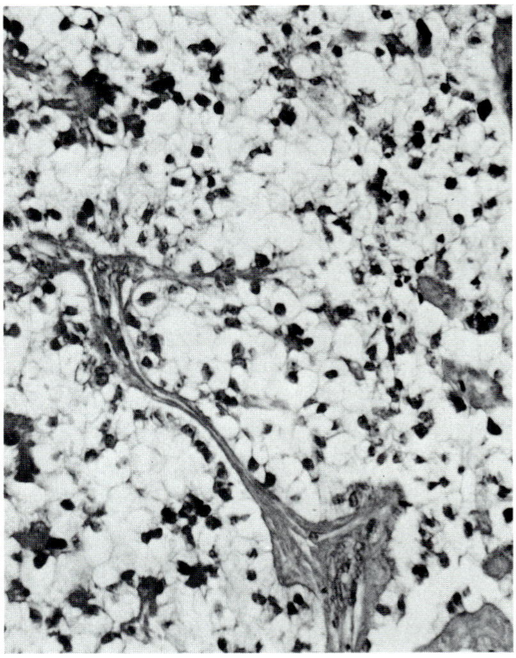

Fig. 13-25. Clear-cell adenocarcinoma. Clear-cell pattern of tumor resembles clear-cell carcinoma of ovary and endometrium. H&E, ×240. (Scully, R. E., Robboy, S. J., & Herbst, A. L.: Vaginal and cervical abnormalities, including clear cell adenocarcinoma related to prenatal exposure to stilbestrol. Ann. Clin. Lab. Sci. 4:222–233, 1974.)

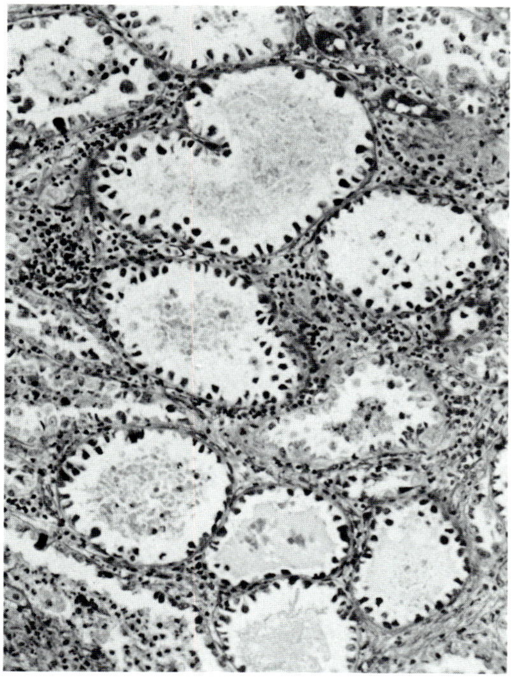

Fig. 13-26. Clear-cell adenocarcinoma. Tubules lined by hobnail cells. H&E, × 150. (Scully, R. E., Robboy, S. J., & Herbst, A. L.: Vaginal and cervical abnormalities, including clear cell adenocarcinoma related to prenatal exposure to stilbestrol. Ann. Clin. Lab. Sci. 4:222–233, 1974.)

are outstanding features.[14] Intracellular glycogen is abundant in the clear cells in the solid zones, and is present in varying but lesser amounts in the other cell types, including areas where it is not apparent at the light-microscopic level.

The cells of clear-cell adenocarcinoma can be detected cytologically, and a suspicious or positive smear may occasionally provide the first indication of an asymptomatic tumor.[58] With the use of circumferential vaginal and cervical scrapes and endocervical aspirations, a high percentage of tumors should probably be detected. The tumor cells often resemble large endocervical cells but vary greatly, and may appear even as undifferentiated carcinoma. False-negative results in one-fifth of cases are due to the difficulty in distinguishing tumor cells from endocervical cells, the heavy overlay of polymorphonuclear leukocytes, and the possibility that some of the neoplasms may not shed cells. Other cases of negative cell studies are those occasional ones in which the tumor is confined to the lamina propria, or has been extirpated in prior diagnostic biopsies.

The tumor spreads locally and also metastasizes via lymphatics and blood vessels.[48] Approximately one-sixth of tumors confined clinically to the vagina or cervix (stage I) metastasize to the pelvic lymph nodes.[28] The frequency of nodal involvement reaches approximately 50 percent when only stage II tumors are considered. Clear-cell adenocarcinoma extends outside the abdominal cavity more frequently than does squamous cell carcinoma of the vagina or cervix.[48] This distinction is illustrated by the fact that 36 percent of the first recurrences of clear-cell carcinomas are in the lung or supraclavicular lymph node, whereas these organs are involved in less than one-tenth of the recurrences of squamous cell carcinoma.

The 5-year actuarial survival rates for all patients with clear cell adenocarcinoma is 78 percent.[26] For patients with stage I tumor, it is 87 percent (vagina) and 91 percent (cervix). Factors associated with a worse prognosis are symptoms at the time of first detection of the tumor, and local excision, which cannot be guaranteed to remove the tumor.[26, 48] Large tumor size or deep invasion into the wall, or both, are often associated with a poor prognosis, but small or superficial tumors may also recur. Most of the patients with recurrences develop these within 3 years; after treatment, approximately one-fifth of these patients survive 3 years or more. Several patients have survived 2 or more years after treatment of a second recurrence.

NON-NEOPLASTIC CHANGES

Several DES-associated non-neoplastic changes of the vagina and cervix occur far more frequently than does clear-cell adenocarcinoma. These anomalies include epithelial changes of the vagina (VEC) and cervix, and structural abnormalities of these organs; the latter have been given such descriptive designations as ridges, hoods, collars, rims, cock's combs, and pseudopolyps (Fig. 13-27). Deformities of the uterine corpus, such as a T-shaped appearance of the cavity, constricting bands in the cavity, hypoplasia, and, rarely, synechiae have been observed with hysterosalpingographic studies,[21,32] but their physiologic significance has not yet been ascertained. Rare congenital anomalies of the cardiovascular system have also been reported,[55] but they have been associated with both steroidal and nonsteroidal estrogens and progestogens.

Various terms have been used in the medical literature to describe the changes in the vagina commonly observed in DES-exposed females.

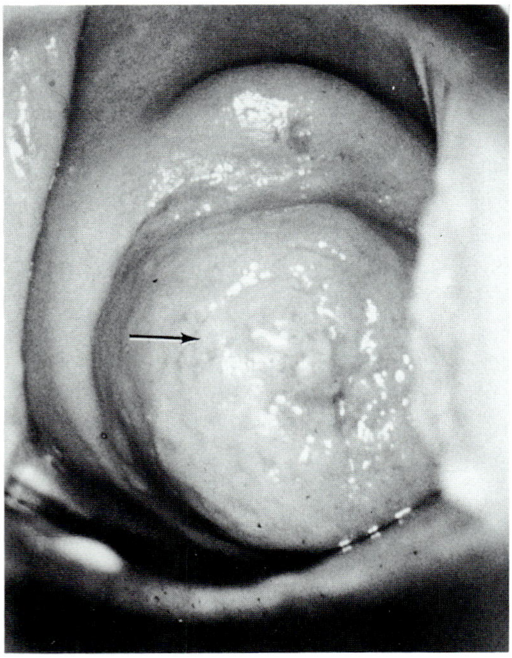

Fig. 13-27. Concentric ridge (arrow) in the cervix creates the appearance of a "pseudopolyp," in the center of which is the external os. A circular fold gives the appearance of a hood covering the cervix. (Robboy, S. J., Scully, R. E., & Herbst, A. L.: Pathology of vaginal and cervical abnormalities associated with prenatal exposure to diethylstilbestrol (DES). J. Reprod. Med. 15:13–18, 1975.)

The term "vaginal epithelial changes" (VEC) has been introduced recently[42,49] to encompass any mucosal change in the vagina observed macroscopically through examination with the colposcope or iodine staining, or microscopically in tissue sections. Colposcopic changes include columnar epithelium, gland, a "Nabothian" cyst, white epithelium, leukoplakia, mosaicism, and punctation. Microscopic changes include adenosis (the formation of columnar cells or the finding of their secretory products in the vagina) and squamous metaplasia (usually in the form of glycogen-poor squamous epithelium). The term "cervical epithelial change" denotes similar changes in the cervix.

Vaginal epithelial changes, especially adenosis, are a common finding in the DES-exposed female. In the pre-DES era, vaginal adenosis was a medical rarity detected only occasionally in women, usually in their 30s or 40s. Not surprisingly, it was found more frequently in autopsy studies in which the vagina was extensively sampled microscopically.[33,54] In about 4 percent of fetuses and infants who were unexposed, or exposed only to steroidal estrogens or progesterone,[29] colposcopic[45] and pathologic[29] examination at the time of autopsy revealed that the squamocolumnar junction lay in the vagina rather than in the cervix. VEC should be suspected clinically when the vaginal mucosa contains red granular spots or patches, does not stain with an iodine solution (Fig. 13-28), or is colposcopically abnormal. In 34 percent of all subjects, the changes involve the upper third of the vagina; the anterior wall is involved most frequently and the posterior wall least frequently.[49] The most distal part of VEC extends into the middle third of the vagina in 9 percent of subjects (26 percent of subjects with VEC), and into the lower third of the vagina in 2 percent of subjects (6 percent of subjects with VEC).

The glandular epithelium found in 62 percent of biopsy specimens with vaginal adenosis consists of mucinous columnar cells[49] which, by light- and electron microscopy,[15] resemble

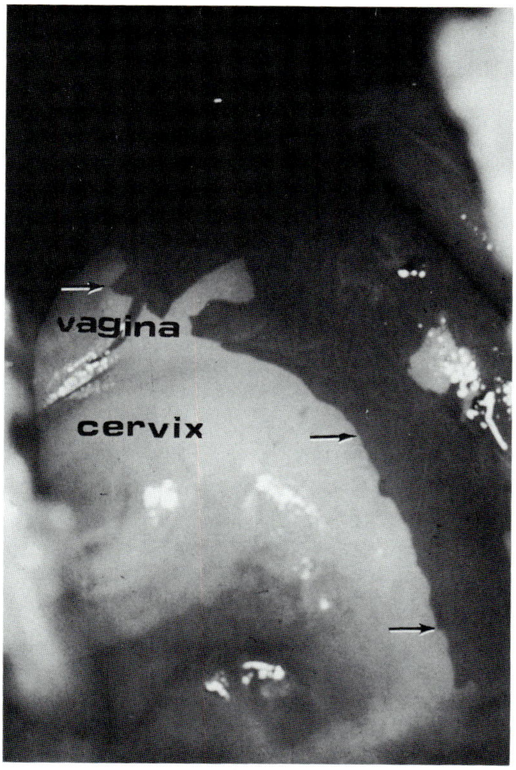

Fig. 13-28. Abnormal Schiller stain in which aglycogenated (nonstaining) areas in both the vagina and the cervix appear white in the photograph and represent the so-called transformation zone. The glycogenated vaginal epithelium stains black. Arrows demarcate the staining from the nonstaining areas. (Robboy, S. J., Scully, R. E., & Herbst, A. L.: Pathology of vaginal and cervical abnormalities associated with prenatal exposure to diethylstilbestrol (DES). J. Reprod. Med. 15:13–18, 1975.)

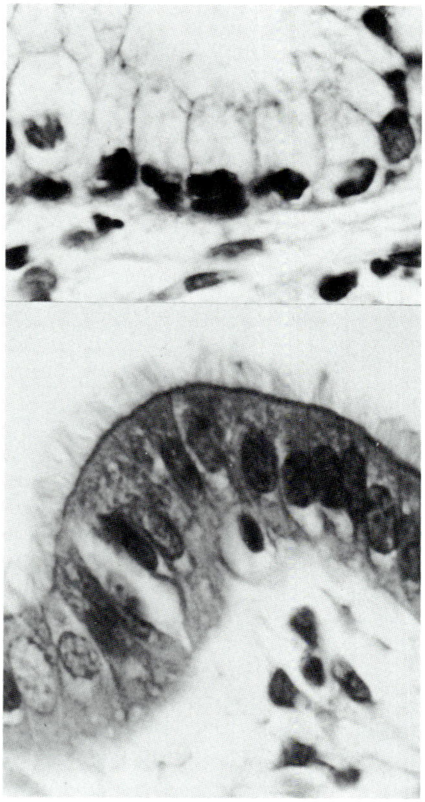

Fig. 13-29. Glandular epithelium of adenosis. Mucinous epithelium (top) resembles the normal endocervical mucosa. H&E, × 775. Ciliated epithelium (bottom) with dark cytoplasm resembles the normal lining of the tube or endometrium. H&E, × 890.

those of the normal endocervical mucosa (Fig. 13-29). Remnants of these cells, which appear as intracellular droplets of mucin in metaplastic squamous cells or as intercellular pools of mucin surrounded by metaplastic squamous cells (Figs. 13-30 and 13-31), account for 48 percent of biopsy specimens with adenosis[49] (vide infra). Dark or light cells, which are often ciliated and resemble the lining cells of the normal fallopian tube or endometrium, are found in 21 percent of specimens with adenosis (Fig. 13-29). Mucinous glands and mucinous pools or droplets are frequently encountered in the same biopsy specimen; mucinous and tuboendometrial-type glands are found together only occasionally.

In the majority of biopsy specimens with VEC, adenosis is replaced to various degrees by metaplastic squamous cells (Fig. 13-30), suggesting that the adenosis heals as a result of squamous metaplasia that begins as reserve-cell proliferation and progresses through the stages of immature and mature squamous metaplasia.[22, 49] During the course of replacement, the glandular epithelium becomes reduced, which accounts for the intercellular pools of mucin in which the cells lining the pool are flattened mucinous cells, which themselves are surrounded by metaplastic squa-

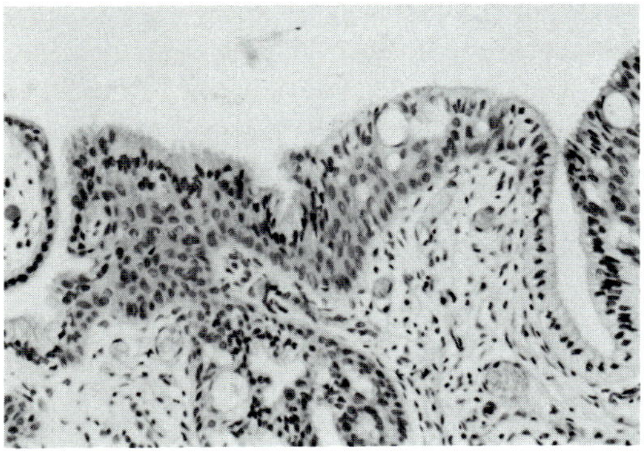

Fig. 13-30. Vaginal adenosis with mucinous columnar epithelium lying on the surface of metaplastic squamous epithelium (center and left). To the right, the mucinous epithelium appears to line the neck of a gland in the lamina propria. H&E, × 150. (Robboy, S. J., Scully, R. E., & Herbst, A. L.: Pathology of vaginal and cervical abnormalities associated with prenatal exposure to diethylstilbestrol (DES). J. Reprod. Med. 15:13–18, 1975.)

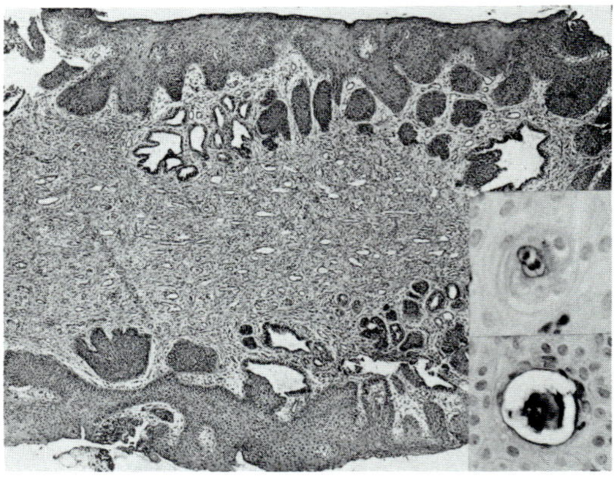

Fig. 13-31. Vaginal adenosis in the lamina propria of the vagina. Metaplastic squamous cells line the surface of the vagina and the squamous pegs continuous with it. H&E, × 25. Insets: Mucinous droplets (upper) and pools (lower) in metaplastic squamous epithelium. Mucicarmine stain, × 220 and × 150, respectively. (Robboy, S. J., Friedlander, L. M., Welch, W. R., et al: Cytology of 575 young females exposed prenatally to diethylstilbestrol (DES). Obstet. Gynecol. 48:511–517, 1976. Reprinted with permission from The American College of Obstetricians and Gynecologists.)

mous cells (Figs. 13-30 and 13-31). A final vestige consists of intracellular droplets of mucin in immature metaplastic squamous cells. When completely replaced by squamous epithelium, obliterated glands and their openings to the surface appear in the lamina propria as squamous pegs, which in serial sections are continuous with the metaplastic squamous epithelium covering the surface of the vagina.[49] Maturation of the metaplastic squamous epithelium, with the acquisition of glycogen, makes this epithelium indistinguishable from the normal squamous epithelium.

Clinically, the foregoing microscopic findings appear as abnormalities with the colposcope or with the iodine stain. The paucity or total lack of glycogen in the metaplastic squamous epithelium accounts for the abnormal iodine stain, while the increased vascularity, tortuous arrangement of the vessels that surround the pegs in the lamina propria, and the chronic inflammatory infiltrate are responsible for the atypical colposcopic patterns, such as mosaicism and punctation, seen so often in VEC. Hyperkeratosis accounts for the colposcopic finding of leukoplakia.[62]

Untreated VEC can disappear spontaneously with time. In part, the disappearance of changes is age related. For example, in the National Cooperative DES (DESAD) Project, the frequency of VEC declined dramatically for women age 26 years or older (Fig. 13-32).[42] In a second study, the relative percentages of columnar cells and immature metaplastic squamous cells in biopsies and smears shifted dramatically, from approximately 90 percent and 10 percent, respectively, in young women, to less than 20 percent and more than 80 percent, respectively, in subjects 30 years and older.[39] Preliminary reports from two centers in which the same subjects have been repeatedly examined over a period of several years have also indicated that the VEC may heal spontaneously and disappear.[2, 6a] Adenosis persisted in most women after 1 year of follow-up, but had undergone extensive squamous metaplasia in 75 percent of subjects who were followed for 3 years or longer.[2]

The frequencies of VEC observed in the exposed daughters of mothers who took DES

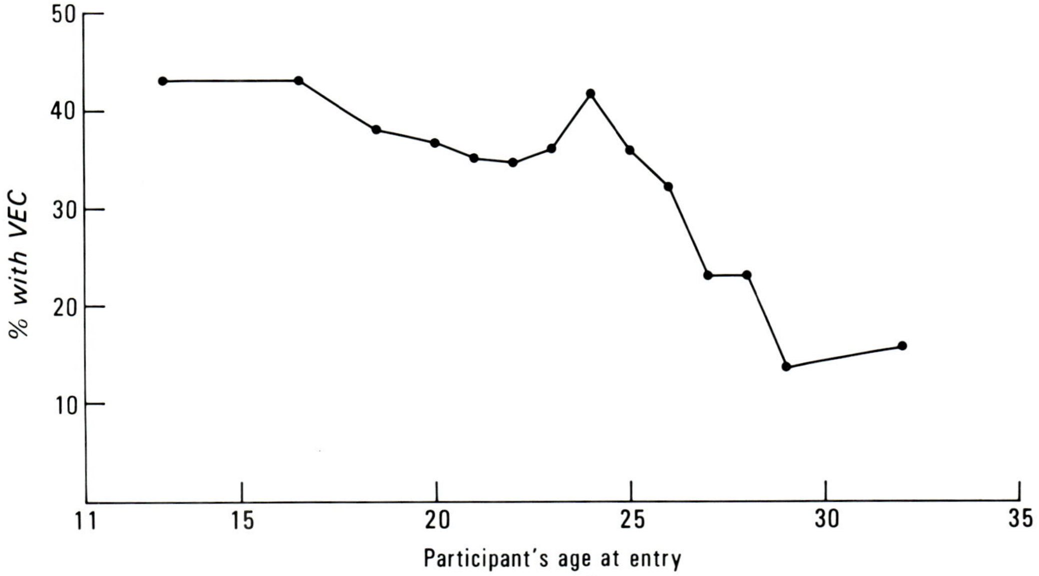

Fig. 13-32. Frequency of VEC as related to age of the participant at entry into the study. (O'Brien, P. C., Noller, K., Robboy, S. J., et al: Vaginal epithelial changes in young women enrolled in the national cooperative diethylstilbestrol adenosis (DESAD) project. Obstet. Gynecol. 53:300–308, 1979. Reprinted with permission from The American College of Obstetricians and Gynecologists.)

during pregnancy has varied markedly in the literature because of at least four important epidemiologic features: (1) selection bias of women examined; (2) the week during pregnancy in which the drug was first administered; (3) total drug dosage and duration of drug exposure; and (4) age of subject at the time of the examination.[34,42] For example, when women from various geographically distinct regions throughout the United States were identified through review of obstetric records, and were examined solely because of their history of DES exposure, the overall frequency of VEC was 34 percent. In contrast, the frequency was nearly twice as large for those women who referred themselves for examination (59 percent) or for women referred by their gynecologists (64 percent).[42] If the exposure occurred at a time during which the embryonic vagina was undergoing development, the frequency of VEC was as high as 48 percent (exposure at 8th week). If the initial exposure occurred after the time when vaginal development was complete (20th week or later), the frequency of VEC was less than 10 percent (Fig. 13-33). Figure 13-34 depicts the effect of total dosage on the frequency of VEC after adjustment for week of first exposure.

Cervical epithelial changes occur in nearly all DES-exposed females. Like VEC, with which they are probably closely related, the cervical changes include macroscopic changes found on the basis of colposcopy or with iodine stain, or microscopic squamous metaplasia or ectropion (the presence of glandular epithelium or its secretory products in the cervical portio). Although most of the features described for adenosis are applicable to ectropion, several observations suggest important differences exist between these processes; therefore, we prefer to consider them separately. First, tuboendometrial-type cells are found in only 3 percent of the cervical specimens with ectropion, in contrast to their much higher frequencies in specimens from the upper (20 percent), mid- (31 percent), and lower (100 percent) vagina.[49] Second, adenosis most often occurs in the form of glands in the lamina propria, whereas in ectropion, the

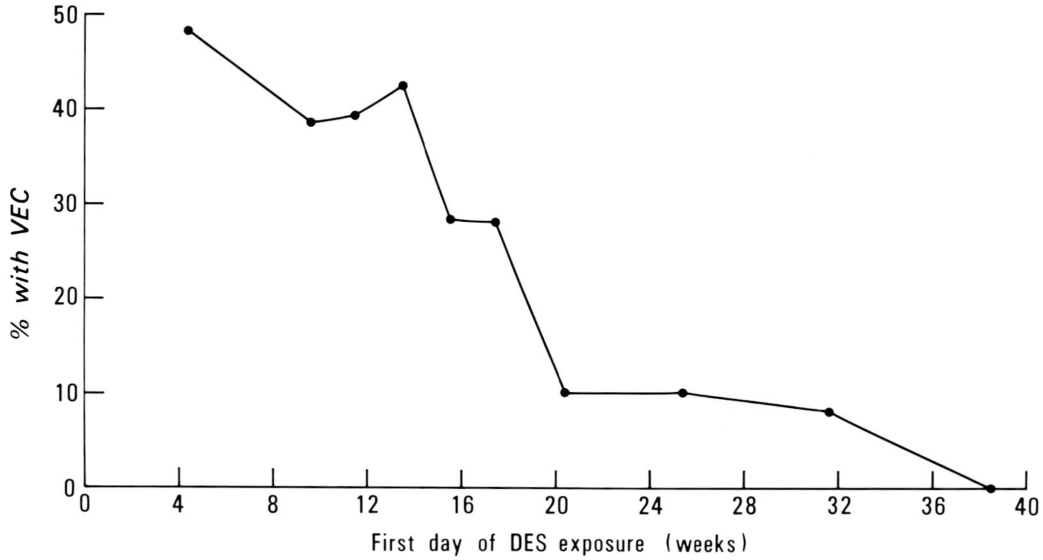

Fig. 13-33. Frequency of VEC as related to first day of DES exposure. (O'Brien, P. C., Noller, K., Robboy, S. J., et al: Vaginal epithelial changes in young women enrolled in the national cooperative diethylstilbestrol adenosis (DESAD) project. Obstet. Gynecol. 53:300–308, 1979. Reprinted with permission from The American College of Obstetricians and Gynecologists.)

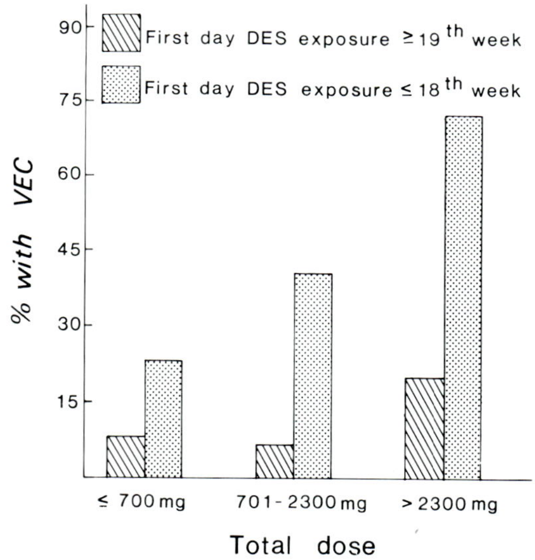

Fig. 13-34. Frequency of VEC according to the first day of DES exposure and total dose. Cross-hatching = first day DES exposure ≥ 19th week; dots = first day DES exposure ≤ 18th week. (O'Brien, P. C., Noller, K., Robboy, S. J., et al: Vaginal epithelial changes in young women enrolled in the national cooperative diethylstilbestrol adenosis (DESAD) project. Obstet. Gynecol. 53:300–308, 1979. Reprinted with permission from The American College of Obstetricians and Gynecologists.)

glandular epithelium commonly lines the surface of the cervix.[49] Until the pathogenesis, natural history, and responses to therapy of these changes are established, separation of adenosis and ectropion permits more accurate comparison of their features from one institution to another.

Cytologic studies, in addition to their usefulness in the detection of malignancy, are also helpful in detecting adenosis and in raising the suspicion that the individual might have been exposed in utero to DES. In smears obtained by scraping the middle and upper thirds of the entire circumference of the vagina, columnar cells with mucinous cytoplasm or metaplastic squamous cells have been found in more than 34 percent of cases; these cells are found in 54 percent of scrapes of the exocervix.[47] We have found that 3 percent of metaplastic cells from cases of in utero exposure to DES contain intracytoplasmic droplets of mucin (Fig. 13-35). Some investigators have encountered columnar cells with mucinous cytoplasm even more frequently (up to 78 percent in the vagina).[7,8,39] It is impor-

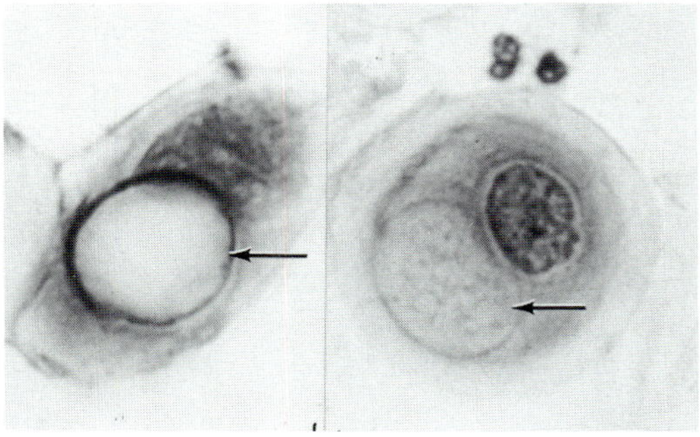

Fig. 13-35. Metaplastic squamous cells with a mucin droplet (arrow) in a vaginal scrape from a patient with vaginal adenosis. Papanicolaou stain; × 1,150. (Robboy, S. J., Scully, R. E., & Herbst, A. L.: Pathology of vaginal and cervical abnormalities associated with prenatal exposure to diethylstilbestrol (DES). J. Reprod. Med. 15:13–18, 1975.)

tant to recognize, however, that the foregoing cells are also found in the vagina in 11 percent of control subjects in whom the vagina is colposcopically unremarkable (unpublished data)—suggesting that the cervix either continually sheds cells or that the spatula used to obtain the vaginal smear has touched an ectropion of the cervix and thereby become contaminated. Furthermore, endometrial-type cells found in scrape smears of the vagina rarely originate from the tuboendometrial type of adenosis, but rather are shed from the uterine corpus (unpublished data).

COMPLICATIONS OF ADENOSIS AND ECTROPION

The glandular epithelium of adenosis and ectropion, and the metaplastic squamous epithelium that develops as a physiologic reaction to these glandular cell types, are susceptible to the same range of pathologic changes that have been encountered in the cervix of the non-DES-exposed female.

Atypical Adenosis

The glandular epithelium of adenosis is believed to provide the bed from which the clear-cell adenocarcinoma arises, possibly through the transitional state of atypical adenosis. Atypical adenosis, usually in the form of one or a few glands with cellular stratification, nuclear pleomorphism, and hyperchromasia and prominent nucleoli, has been identified near the periphery of several carcinomas (unpublished data). Atypical cells have also been identified in approximately 0.5 percent of cervical and vaginal smears as cells with nuclei that are larger and more irregular in outline than those seen either in normal endocervical cells or in the cells that line the glands of the adenosis.[3, 47, 49] The frequent finding of the tuboendometrial type of glandular cells and the rarity of the mucinous type of cells in adenosis immediately adjacent to the tumors, in addition to the occurrence in older women of clear-cell adenocarcinomas arising in the endometrium where mucinous cells are usually absent, have suggested that the tuboendometrial type of cell may be the anlage from which the clear-cell adenocarcinoma arises.

Dysplasia

Contrary to the prediction of some, squamous cell neoplasia has not developed with increasing frequency in the DES-exposed population.[11, 39, 49, 50, 52a, 52b] In the unexposed female, cervical ectropion heals by the formation of metaplastic epithelium, which eventually becomes mature and indistinguishable from normal squamous epithelium. Occasionally, immature metaplastic epithelium may not differentiate normally, but may instead evolve into dysplasia, carcinoma in situ (CIS), or squamous cell carcinoma. The frequency of extensive ectropion, adenosis, and colposcopic abnormalities, and the finding of squamous cell dysplasia in a small number of exposed subjects, led investigators several years ago to speculate that the incidence of in situ and invasive squamous cell carcinoma of the lower genital tract would rise greatly as the exposed population reached the peak ages at which these lesions are encountered in the cervices of unexposed women.[35, 56]

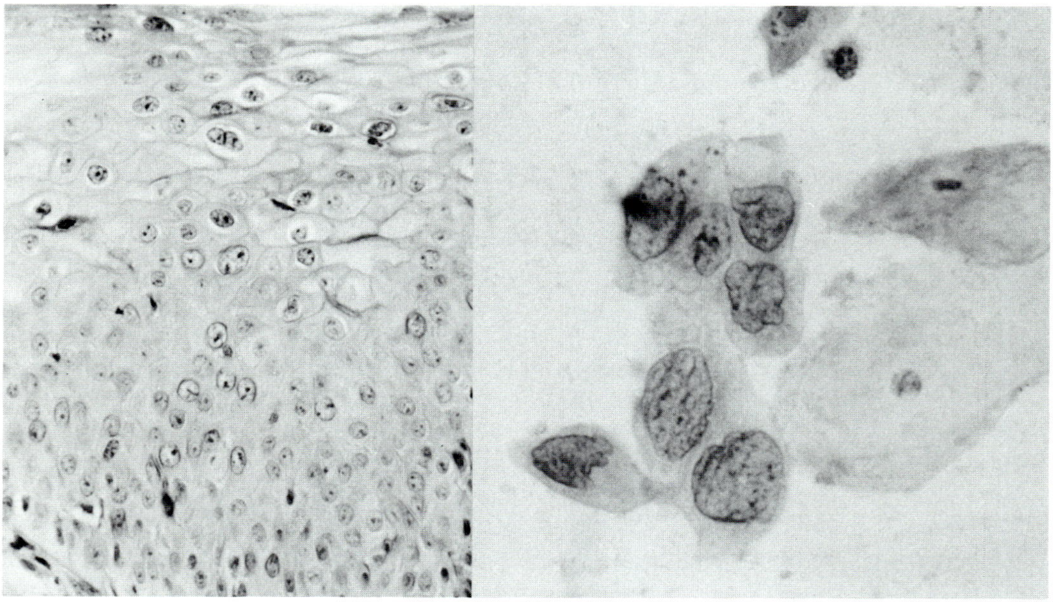

Fig. 13-36. Mild dysplasia. Left: biopsy. H&E, × 315. Right: Smear. Papanicolaou stain, × 640.

By 1978, 1,424 DES-exposed women had been examined and followed at the Massachusetts General Hospital, some since 1971. The prevalence of dysplasia was 2.1 percent and the incidence 0.85 per 100 person-years of follow-up.[50] The dysplasia was almost always mild (Fig. 13-36), and was slightly more frequent in the cervix than in the vagina. This study also indicated that the rates of dysplasia could be adversely affected if patients were included who had been specifically referred to the Massachusetts General Hospital because of dysplasia. In addition it was found that the more severe degrees of dysplasia and CIS were encountered only in subjects specifically referred because of these abnormalities. In the DESAD Project, in which data on dysplasia have been reported to date only for those participants with biopsy specimens, and not for the combined results of biopsy and cytology, the frequency of vaginal dysplasia was lowest when the patients were identified through a review of prenatal records (0.4 percent), was intermediate when women themselves requested examination (0.5 percent), and was highest (0.9 percent) when they were referred by other physicians because of a known exposure to DES.[42,49] Rates in the cervix were severalfold higher.

Another problem in the diagnosis of squamous cell neoplasia has been the misinterpretation of immature squamous metaplasia for dysplasia. Immature squamous metaplasia is characterized by increased cellularity, minimal differentiation of the cytoplasm, and the occasional presence of mitoses above the basal layer; however, the nuclei are not hyperchromatic, vary little in size and shape, and abnormal forms are not encountered. The DNA histogram of metaplastic squamous cells is one of euploidy or slight polypoidy.[18] On the basis of published photomicrographs in those series with the unusually high rates of precancerous changes, we would reclassify some of the cases illustrated as carcinoma in situ and dysplasia as falling in a range from immature squamous metaplasia to moderate dysplasia.[52]

Discordance between cytology and biopsy has been commonplace in the detection and follow-up of dysplasia, especially in the milder forms[50]; thus, the frequency of dysplasia is influenced by whether the patients are screened by cytology alone, biopsy alone, or both. Other factors that affect the rates of dysplasia include the sexual activity of the population studied and the misinterpretation of atypical columnar cells as dysplastic squamous cells.

Microglandular Hyperplasia

Microglandular hyperplasia is a benign, tumor-like condition, usually associated with the long-term ingestion of oral contraceptive agents and occasionally with pregnancy. When this lesion was first described in the cervix in 1967, it was emphasized that it could be easily confused with adenocarcinoma. Recently, there have been reported eight cases of microglandular hyperplasia arising in foci of adenosis in the vagina of young females, five of whom had been exposed prenatally to DES[53]; each of these lesions had been misinterpreted initially as clear-cell adenocarcinoma.

Grossly, the lesion in microglandular hypersplasia is soft, tan-yellow, and usually flat to granular. Occasionally, it may be cauliflower-like or multicentric (Fig. 13-37). On microscopic examination, myriads of tiny

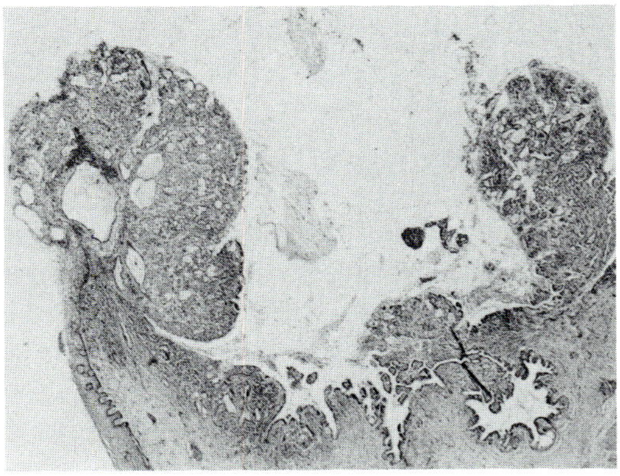

Fig. 13-37. Microglandular hyperplasia. Edges of polypoid mass in vagina where the empty space (center) is the biopsy site. At the base is a focus of adenosis. H&E, × 15. (Robboy, S. M., & Welch, W. R.: Microglandular hyperplasia in vaginal adenosis associated with oral contraceptives and prenatal diethylstilbestrol (DES) exposure. Obstet. Gynecol. 49:430–434, 1977. Reprinted with permission from The American College of Obstetricians and Gynecologists.)

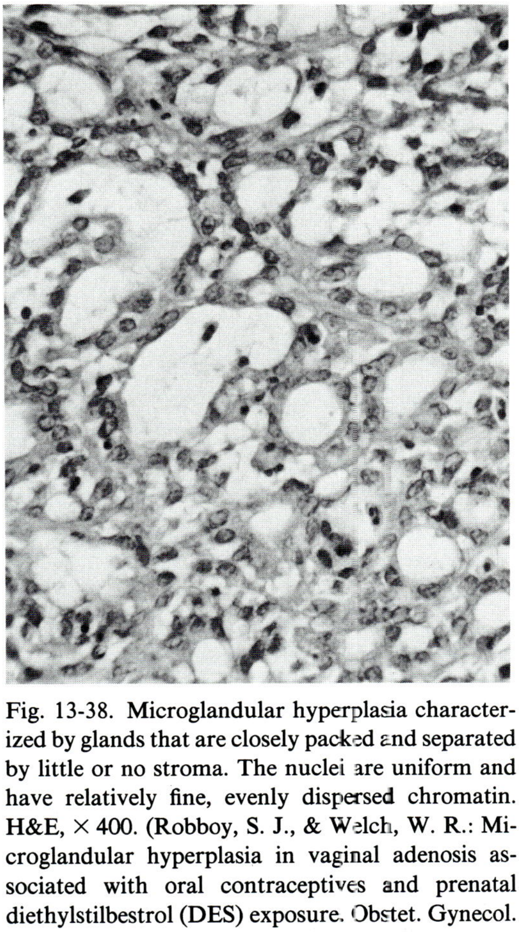

Fig. 13-38. Microglandular hyperplasia characterized by glands that are closely packed and separated by little or no stroma. The nuclei are uniform and have relatively fine, evenly dispersed chromatin. H&E, × 400. (Robboy, S. J., & Welch, W. R.: Microglandular hyperplasia in vaginal adenosis associated with oral contraceptives and prenatal diethylstilbestrol (DES) exposure. Obstet. Gynecol. 49:430–434, 1977. Reprinted with permission from The American College of Obstetricians and Gynecologists.)

glands that are devoid of intervening stroma are observed to be arranged in a reticular pattern (Fig. 13-38). The nuclei of the cells that line the glands are uniform in size and shape, and have finely dispersed chromatin. The glandular lumina contain mucin and an acute inflammatory cell infiltrate; intracellular mucin is variable. The presence of extensive nests of metaplastic squamous cells with filmy eosinophilic cytoplasm may make the lesion especially difficult to distinguish from the solid pattern of clear-cell carcinoma. A clue to the proper diagnosis is the presence of clefts lined by mucinous epithelium that course through the metaplastic squamous epithelium. The fact that the microglands have been observed in continuity with the clefts suggests that the former result from the budding and arborization of mucinous epithelium of the type that lines the normal endocervix and also constitutes one type of vaginal adenosis. Microglandular hyperplasia has not been observed to arise from the tuboendometrial type of adenosis. The lesion is generally reversed by discontinuance of oral contraceptive medication.

Functional Anomalies and Reproduction

Preliminary data about functional anomalies consequent upon DES exposure are, to date, conflicting. In a follow-up study of female offspring of mothers who participated in a double-blind, placebo controlled investigation during 1951-52, 18 percent of the DES-exposed-daughters had irregular menstrual cycles (usually characterized by oligomenorrhea) compared to 10 percent of unexposed females.[8] The menstrual flows were also shortened (less than 4 days) in DES-exposed women (60 percent versus 43 percent of controls).[7,8] In a second cohort-controlled investigation, no differences were found.[6] The frequency of menstrual irregularities was 12.4 percent in DES-exposed and 13 percent in unexposed daughters.

Unpublished data from the DESAD Project indicate that the frequency of conception is no different in DES-exposed and unexposed women. However, the ability of an exposed daughter to give birth to a full-term, live infant may be impaired. It is uncertain at this time whether the miscarriages, which occur late in pregnancy, are related to an incompetent cervix, grossly altered by structural changes such as ridges, pseudopolyps, and other aberrations, or whether some other, as yet undetermined factor, is responsible.[32]

Embryology

It is generally believed that the vagina has an ancestry in both Mullerian duct and urogenital sinus anlage; involvement of the Wolffian duct is controversial.[59] It has been postulated that in the normal female the Mullerian ducts extend caudally during early fetal life toward the level of the future hymen, where they fuse in their lower portions to form a muscular scaffold that meets the urogenital sinus; squamous cells, derived from the urogenital sinus, are thought to invade the fused tube from below, to completely replace the Mullerian epithelium up to the level of the external cervical os. Since the entire process begins sometime after the fourth or fifth week of intrauterine life and is not complete until sometime after the 20th week, it is possible that DES exposure inhibits the replacement of the Mullerian epithelium by squamous epithelium from the urogenital sinus, or that it stimulates the persistence of the Mullerian epithelium in the vagina. The fact that residual Mullerian epithelium on the portio vaginalis of the cervix differentiates almost exclusively into mucinous columnar epithelium, whereas tuboendometrial-type cells are found in progressively greater numbers in more caudal regions of the vagina, indicates that the factors that effect differentiation of the Mullerian epithelium must be complex.[49] Recent evidence in rodents suggests that the stroma in the wall of the vagina and the cervix plays an important role in the induction of the differentiation of surface epithelium.[13]

Anomalies in Males

To date, no definite association has been established between intrauterine DES exposure and neoplasia in males. Although preliminary findings from one study have suggested that there is an increased frequency (10.2 percent) of DES exposure in patients with testicular cancer in contrast to other, more common forms of cancers, such as lymphoma and leukemias (1.2 percent), the validity of the results is questionable because of methodologic faults in the design and execution of the investigation.[16] One study with animals reported the development of squamous cell carcinomas of the prostate and coagulating glands of the rat[4]; no cancers were of testicular origin.

Reports are also in conflict about the nonmalignant sequelae of DES exposure in male offspring of mothers who took this drug. In a follow-up study of mothers who were treated in 1951-52 with either DES or a placebo, epididymal cysts, anomalies of the penile urethra, microphallus, small testes, cryptorchidism, or "pathologic semen" were found in 32 percent of 308 exposed sons, in contrast to 8 percent of 307 controls.[7] The quality of the semen was "severely" pathologic in 18 percent of the exposed group, compared to 8 percent in the controls.[7, 19] In a second study, penile stenosis or hypospadias was found in 4.4 percent of DES-exposed male offspring but in no controls.[12] Yet in a third study just recently published,[1] no differences were observed in two groups of 24 exposed and 24 nonexposed male offspring with regard to their psychosexual history, medical history, genital examination, or semen analysis. For both groups the frequencies of severe oligospermia (9 percent versus 17 percent), abnormal sperm morphology (13 percent versus 17 percent), and abnormal motility (13 percent versus 17 percent) were not statistically different, resulting in nearly identical frequencies of severely pathologic semen (17 percent in exposed versus 20 percent in nonexposed male offspring, respectively). In addition, a rare patient has been born with hypospadias in whom the testes were apparently devoid of germ cells (reviewed in ref. 38). Experimentally, 60 percent of male mice exposed prenatally to DES are sterile and have testicular anomalies.[36] Undescended testes in rodents,[36, 41] nodular enlargment of the seminal vesicles and prostate, and the persistence of Mullerian structures[57] have also been observed, but the implications of these findings for human reproductive capacity will not be known until further follow-up data are available.

Anomalies in Mothers

The small amount of data collected on mothers treated with DES has not yet revealed a link between any pathologic condition and DES exposure. Breast cancer was found in one study only slightly more frequently in exposed (4.6 percent) than in unexposed (3.1 percent) mothers, but this difference is statistically insignificant.[9]

Animal Experimentation and Female Offspring

Several animal models have been developed that are believed to partly reproduce the consequence of prenatal exposure to DES. A condition that resembles adenosis of the vagina has been produced in mice treated prenatally or neonatally with a variety of different estrogens, including DES and synthetic estrogenic compounds.[17, 46] Unlike the human, in whom the glandular epithelium of adenosis may be composed of cells with intracellular mucin or dark cytoplasm, often with cilia, the glands in the mouse appear relatively immature, lacking distinctive cytoplasmic features. Jones and Bern have demonstrated that the adenosis in mice may proliferate markedly over long periods, and may resemble a neoplastic growth, with both squamous and glandular components.[30] Although well differentiated, the adenosis is transplantable and grows autonomously. This tumor, however, does not contain clear cells, and it is not certain whether it is analogous to that which occurs in humans. To date, the development of a clear cell adenocarcinoma has not been reported in animals.

Adenosis of the vagina has also been observed in monkeys exposed prenatally to DES[23]; the epithelium is composed of mucinous columnar cells, similar to that observed in humans. Preliminary data suggest that over time, the adenosis in the monkey undergoes replacement by metaplastic squamous cells, which is similar to the process in the human by which the adenosis resolves.

Gross structural changes analogous to those found in the cervix and vagina in humans have also been observed in DES-exposed animals. The cervix of the mouse is deformed and may become patulous (unpublished data of Dr.

Gerald Cunha), or may show a deficiency of the normally complex arrangement of mucosal folds.[46] Vaginal ridges and cervical hoods have been seen in monkeys.[23]

Results of animal studies must be viewed with caution, however, since many anomalies have been found that are not observed in humans. These have included a persistent urogenital sinus,[41, 60] precocious development of the breasts,[10] and a variety of neoplastic and non-neoplastic conditions in the ovary, endometrium, and vagina.[10]

As new models of DES-induced histologic change continue to be reported, one appears of particular interest, since it permits direct experimentation on human tissue in a controlled, in vivo environment. Athymic (nude) mice, which are immunologically deficient, have been shown to support the growth of explants of adenosis from humans.[43] Conceivably, this model can be used to investigate many aspects of the changes associated with DES exposure.

REFERENCES

1. Andonian, R. W., & Kessler, R.: Transplacental exposure to diethylstilbestrol in men. Urology 13:276-279, 1979.
2. Antonioli, D. A., Burke, L., & Friedman, E. A.: Natural history of diethylstilbestrol-associated genital tract lesions: cervical ectopy and cervicovaginal hood. Am. J. Obstet. Gynecol. 137:847-853, 1980.
3. Antonioli, D. A., Rosen, S., Burke, L., et al: Glandular dysplasia in diethylstilbestrol-associated vaginal adenosis. A case report and review of the literature. Am J Clin Pathol 71:715-721, 1979.
4. Arai, Y., Chen, C. Y., & Nishizuka, Y.: Cancer development in male reproductive tract in rats given diethylstilbestrol at neonatal age. Gann 69:861-862, 1978.
5. Barnes, A. B.: Ambulatory management of the DES-exposed patient. In: Ryan, G. M., Jr., Ed.: Ambulatory Care in Obstetrics and Gynecology, Grune and Stratton, New York (in press).
6. Barnes, A. B.: Menstrual history of young women exposed in utero to diethylstilbestrol. Fertil. Steril. 32:148-153, 1979.

6a. Barnes, A. B., Colton, T., Gundersen, J. H., et al.: Fertility and outcome of pregnancy in women exposed in utero to diethylstilbestrol: preliminary findings from the DESAD Project. N. Engl. J. Med. 302:609-613, 1980.

7. Bibbo, M.: Transplacental effects of diethylstilbestrol. In: Grundmann, E., & Kirsten, W. H. Current Topics in Pathology. pp. 191-211. Springer Verlag, New York, 1979.
8. Bibbo, M., Gill, W. B., Azizi, F., et al: Follow-up study of male and female offspring of DES-exposed mothers. Obstet. Gynecol. 49:1-8, 1977.
9. Bibbo, M., Haenszel, W. M., Wied, G. L., et al: A twenty-five-year follow-up study of women exposed to diethylstilbestrol during pregnancy. N. Engl. J. Med. 298:763-767, 1978.
10. Boylan, E. S.: Morphological and functional consequences of prenatal exposure to diethylstilbestrol in the rat. Biol. Reprod. 19:854-863, 1978.

10a. Brian, D. D., Tilley, B. C., Labarthe, D. R., et al.: Breast cancer in DES-exposed mothers. Absence of association. Mayo Clin. Proc. 55:89-93, 1980.

11. Burke, L., Antonioli, D., & Rosen, S.: Vaginal and cervical squamous cell dysplasia in women exposed to diethylstilbestrol in utero. Am. J. Obstet. Gynecol. 132:537-544, 1978.
12. Cosgrove, M., Benton, B., & Henderson, B.: Male genitourinary abnormalities and maternal diethylstilbestrol. J. Urol. 117:220-222, 1977.
13. Cunha, G. R., Shannon, J. M., Neubauer, B. L., et al.: Mesenchymal-epithelial interactions in sex differentiation. Hum. Genet. 58:68-77, 1981.
14. Dickersin, G. R., Welch, W. R., Erlandson, R., et al: Ultrastructure of 16 cases of clear cell adenocarcinoma of the vagina and cervix in young women. Cancer 45:1615-1624, 1980.
15. Fenoglio, C. M., Ferenczy, A., Richart, R. M., et al: Scanning and transmission electron microscopic studies of vaginal adenosis and the cervical transformation zone in progeny exposed in utero to diethylstilbestrol. Am. J. Obstet. Gynecol. 126:170-180, 1976.
16. Fink, D. J.: DES task force summary report. DHEW Publication No. 79-1688. National Institutes of Health, Bethesda, MD, 1978.
17. Forsberg, J. G.: Late effects in the vaginal and cervical epithelia after injections of diethylstilbestrol into neonatal mice. Am. J. Obstet. Gynecol. 121:101-104, 1975.

18. Fu, Y. S., Robboy, S. J., & Prat, J.: Nuclear DNA study of vaginal and cervical squamous cell abnormalities in DES exposed progeny. Obstet. Gynecol. 52:129-137, 1978.
19. Gill, W. B., Schumacher, G. F. B., & Bibbo, M.: Pathological semen and anatomical abnormalities of the genital tract in human male subjects exposed to diethylstilbestrol in utero. J. Urol. 117:477-480, 1977.
20. Goldstein, D. P.: Incompetent cervix in offspring exposed to diethylstilbestrol in utero. Obstet. Gynecol. 52(Suppl.):73s-75s, 1978.
21. Haney, A. F., Hammond, C. B., Soules, M. R., et al: Diethylstilbestrol-induced upper genital tract abnormalities. Fertil. Steril. 31:142-146, 1979.
22. Hart, W. R., Townsend, D. E., Aldrich, J. O., et al: Histopathologic spectrum of vaginal adenosis and related changes in stilbestrol-exposed females. Cancer 37:763-775, 1976.
23. Hendrickx, A. G., Benirschke, K., Thompson, R. S., et al: The effects of prenatal diethylstilbestrol (DES) exposure on the genitalia of pubertal Macaca Mulata I. Female offspring. J. Reprod. Med. 22:233-240, 1979.
24. Herbst, A. L., Cole, P., Colton, T., et al: Age-incidence and risk of diethylstilbestrol-related clear cell adenocarcinoma of the vagina and cervix. Am. J. Obstet. Gynecol. 128:43-48, 1977.
25. Herbst, A. L., Cole, P., Norusis, M. J., et al: Epidemiologic aspects and factors related to survival of 384 Registry cases of clear cell adenocarcinoma of the vagina and cervix. Am. J. Obstet. Gynecol. 135:876-886, 1980.
26. Herbst, A. I., Norusis, M. J., Rosenow, P. J., et al: An analysis of 346 cases of clear cell adenocarcinoma of the vagina and cervix with emphasis on recurrence and survival. Gynecol. Oncol. 7:111-122, 1979.
27. Herbst, A. L., Poskanzer, D. C., Robboy, S. J., et al: Prenatal exposure to stilbestrol. A prospective comparison of exposed female offspring with unexposed controls. N. Engl. J. Med. 292:334-339, 1975.
28. Herbst, A. L., Robboy, S. J., Scully, R. E., et al: Clear-cell adenocarcinoma of the vagina and cervix in girls: an analysis of 170 registry cases. Am. J. Obstet. Gynecol. 119:713-723, 1974.
29. Johnson, L. D., Driscoll, S. G., Hertig, A. T., et al: Vaginal adenosis in stillborns and neonates exposed to diethylstilbestrol and steroidal estrogens and progestins. Obstet. Gynecol. 53:671-679, 1979.
30. Jones, L. A., & Pacillas-Verjan, R.: Transplantability and sex steroid hormone responsiveness of cervicovaginal tumors derived from female BALB/cCrgl mice neonatally treated with ovarian steroids. Cancer Res. 39:2591-2594, 1979.
31. Jukes, T. H.: Diethylstilbestrol in beef production: What is the risk to consumers? Prev. Med. 5:438-453, 1976.
32. Kaufman, R. H., Adam, E., Binder, G. L., et al: Upper genital tract changes and pregnancy outcome in offspring exposed in utero to diethylstilbestrol. Am. J. Obstet. Gynecol. 137:299–308, 1980.
33. Kurman, R. J., & Scully, R. E.: The incidence and histogenesis of vaginal adenosis: an autopsy study. Hum. Pathol. 5:265-276, 1974.
34. Labarth, D. R., Adam, E., Noller, K. L., et al: Design and preliminary observations of national cooperative diethylstilbestrol adenosis (DESAD) project. Obstet. Gynecol. 51:453-458, 1978.
34a. Lawrence, W. D., Shingleton, H. M., Gore, H., et al.: Ultrastructural and morphometric study of diethylstilbestrol-associated lesions diagnosed as cervical intraepithelial neoplasia III. Cancer Res. 40:1558-1567, 1980.
35. Mattingly, R. F., & Stafl, A.: Cancer risk in diethylstilbestrol-exposed offspring. Am. J. Obstet. Gynecol. 126:543-548, 1976.
36. McLachlan, J. A., Newbold, R. R., & Bullock, B.: Reproductive tract lesions in male mice exposed prenatally to diethylstilbestrol. Science 190:991-992, 1975.
37. McMartin, K. E., Kennedy, K. A., Greenspan, P.: Diethylstilbestrol: a review of its toxicity and use as a growth promotant in food producing animals. J. Environ. Pathol. Toxicol. 1:279-313, 1978.
38. Mills, J. L., & Bongiovanni, A. M.: Effect of prenatal estrogen exposure on male genitalia. Pediatrics 62(Suppl.):1160-1165, 1978.
39. Ng, A. B. P., Reagan, J. W., Nadji, M., et al: Natural history of vaginal adenosis in women exposed to diethylstilbestrol in utero. J. Reprod. Med. 18:1-13, 1977.
40. Noller, K. L., & Fish, C. B.: Diethylstilbestrol usage: its interesting past, important present, and questionable future. Med. Clin. North Am. 58:793-810, 1974.
41. Nomura, T., & Kanzaki, T.: Induction of uro-

genital anomalies and some tumors in the progeny of mice receiving diethylstilbestrol during pregnancy. Cancer Res. 37:1099-1104, 1977.

42. O'Brien, P. C., Noller, K. L., Robboy, S. J., et al: Vaginal epithelial changes in young women enrolled in the national cooperative diethylstilbestrol-adenosis (DESAD) project. Obstet. Gynecol. 53:300-308, 1979.
43. Pienkowski, M. M., Mann, L. C., Rosloniec, E. F., et al: Accretion of biopsy specimens of vaginal adenosis from patients exposed in utero to diethylstilbestrol when transplanted to athymic nude mice. J. Natl. Canc. Inst. 62:521-523, 1979.
44. Pietras, R. J., Szego, C. M., Mangan, C. E., et al: Elevated serum cathepsin B1 and vaginal pathology after prenatal DES exposure. Obstet. Gynecol. 52:321-327, 1978.
45. Pixley, E.: Morphology of the fetal and prepubertal cervicovaginal epithelium, In: Jordon, J. A., & Singer, A., Eds.: The Cervix pp. 75-86. W. B. Saunders, Philadelphia, 1976.
46. Plapinger, L., Bern, H. A.: Adenosis-like lesions and other cervicovaginal abnormalities in mice treated perinatally with estrogen. J. Natl. Canc. Instit. 63:507-518, 1979.
47. Robboy, S. J., Friedlander, L. M., Welch, W. R., et al: Cytology of 575 young women with prenatal exposure to diethylstilbestrol. Obstet. Gynecol. 48:511-515, 1976.
48. Robboy, S. J., Herbst, A. L., & Scully, R. E.: Clear-cell adenocarcinoma of the genital tract in young females. Analysis of 37 tumors that persisted or recurred after primary therapy. Cancer 34:606-614, 1974.
49. Robboy, S. J., Kaufman, R. H., Prat, J., et al: Pathologic findings in young women enrolled in national cooperative diethylstilbestrol adenosis (DESAD) project. Obstet. Gynecol. 53:309-317, 1979.
50. Robboy, S. J., Keh, P. C., Nickerson, R. J., et al: Squamous cell dysplasia and carcinoma in-situ after prenatal exposure to diethylstilbestrol: examination and follow-up of 1,424 females. Obstet. Gynecol. 51:528-535, 1978.
51. Robboy, S. J., Noller, K. L., Kaufman, R. H., et al: Prenatal diethylstilbestrol (DES) exposure: recommendations of the diethylstilbestrol-adenosis (DESAD) project for the identification and management of exposed individuals. DHEW Publication No. 80-2049. U.S. Government, Washington, D.C., 1980.
52. Robboy, S. J., Prat, J., Welch, W. R., et al: Squamous cell neoplasia controversy in the DES-exposed female. Hum. Pathol. 8:483-485, 1977.

52a. Robboy, S. J., Szyfelbein, W. M., Goellner, J. R., et al.: Dysplasia and cytologic findings in 4,589 young women enrolled in diethylstilbestrol-adenosis (DESAD) project. Am. J. Obstet. Gynec. 140:579-586, 1981.

52b. Robboy, S. J., Truslow, G. Y., Anton, J., et al.: Role of hormones including diethylstilbestrol (DES) in the pathogenesis of cervical and vaginal intraepithelial neoplasia. Gynecol. Oncol. 12:S98-S110, 1981.

53. Robboy, S. J., & Welch, W. R.: Microglandular hyperplasia in vaginal adenosis associated with oral contraceptives and prenatal diethylstilbestrol exposure. Obstet. Gynecol. 49:430-434, 1977.
54. Sandberg, E. C.: The incidence and distribution of occult vaginal adenosis. Am. J. Obstet. Gynecol. 101:322-333, 1968.
55. Shapiro, S., & Slone, D.: The effects of exogenous female hormones on the fetus. Am. J. Epidemiol. (in press).
56. Stafl, A., & Mattingly, R. F.: Vaginal adenosis-a precancerous lesion? Am. J. Obstet. Gynecol. 120:666-677, 1974.
57. Suzuki, Y., & McLachlan, J. A.: Effects of sex hormones on mullerian duct derivatives in the genital tract of male mice exposed prenatally to diethylstilbestrol (DES). Biol. Reprod. 20(S1), A115, 1979 (Abstr).
58. Taft, P. D., Robboy, S. J., Herbst, A. L., et al: Cytology of clear-cell adenocarcinoma of the genital tract in young females. Report of 95 cases from the registry. Acta Cytol 18:279-290, 1974.
59. Ulfelder, H., Robboy, S. J.: The embryologic development of the human vagina. Am. J. Obstet. Gynecol. 126:769-776, 1976.
60. Vorherr, H., Messer, R. H., Vorherr, U. F., et al: Teratogenesis and carcinogenesis in rat offspring after transplacental and transmammary exposure to diethylstilbestrol. Biochem. Pharmacol. 28:1865-1877, 1977.
61. Welch, W. R., Prat, J., Robboy, S. J., et al: Pathology of prenatal diethylstilbestrol (DES) exposure. Pathol. Annu. 13:201-216, 1978.
62. Welch, W. R., Robboy, S. J., Townsend, D. E., et al: Comparison of histologic and colposcopic findings in DES-exposed females. Obstet. Gynecol. 52:457-460, 1978.

14

The Breast

Robert E. Fechner

INTRODUCTION

Many drugs, used for various therapeutic purposes, affect both the female and male breast. Some, such as estrogens, presumably exert part of their action directly on the breast parenchyma, whereas others, such as the neuroleptic agents, act through the hypothalamic-pituitary axis. Since many of these drugs are given for long periods, it is appropriate to consider that they may have an irreversible effect on the breast. Concern has been expressed regarding the carcinogenic potential for the vast number of women exposed for long periods to estrogens in postmenopausal replacement therapy, or to orally administered hormones for contraception. Additionally, questions have been raised as to whether or not estrogens modify the appearance of benign breast lesions. Similar questions arise when abnormal breast tissue is removed from men with prostatic cancer who have taken diethylstilbestrol (DES).

Besides the large number of drugs that affect the breast, it has become commonplace to introduce prosthetic materials into the female bosom. Some of the complications of this practice have culminated in histologic findings that may be confusing to the pathologist who is unfamiliar with the appearance and behavior of the synthetic substances.

THE MALE BREAST

The male breast responds to drugs by either undergoing enlargement (gynecomastia) or with galactorrhea. On several occasions, carcinoma of the male breast has been considered to be related to estrogen therapy, and there is one reported case of nipple papillomatosis in a man taking estrogens. Each of these lesions will be considered individually.

Gynecomastia

Gynecomastia may be produced by diethylstilbestrol,[77] androgens,[41] estradiol in combination with a progestin,[64] progestins alone,[6] conjugated estrogens,[6] digitalis,[53] phenothiazines,[58] spironolactone,[74] clomiphene,[11] methadone,[91] cimetidine,[16] and cytotoxic drug therapy.[80,81] In addition to gynecomastia caused by drugs administered directly, a young boy developed gynecomastia after exposure to dust generated in his home during the packaging of diethylstilbestrol pellets by his mother.[73] Finally, men undergoing chronic renal dialysis may develop enlarged breasts.[76]

Galactorrhea is rare in males, but has been reported in a few patients taking isoniazid, estrogens, or androgens, and occasionally occurs upon cessation of estrogen therapy.[50] Galactorrhea may or may not be accompanied by gynecomastia.[31] I am unaware of reports dealing with the histologic changes that accompany galactorrhea, although at least one reference provides illustrations of breast tissue from a man with gynecomastia secondary to androgen therapy who had a nipple discharge (not specifically galactorrhea); the tissue showed dilated ducts containing secretory material but no acinar development.[41]

The mechanisms of drug-induced gynecomastia are poorly understood. Even in the case of estrogen therapy, it is unclear as to how much of the effect is due to direct action on the breast and how much is mediated through the hypothalamic-pituitary axis, with a rise in serum prolactin promoting the breast growth.[34] Different drugs undoubtedly promote gynecomastia through different mechanisms. For example, gynecomastia secondary to digitalis might be due to the aglycone portion of the glycoside molecule, since it shares some structural similarity to steroidal hormones and may have estrogenic activity.[53] On the other hand, the phenothiazines act on the hypothalamus and initiate steps that ultimately increase serum prolactin.[58] Spironolactone and methadone lower serum testosterone levels, possibly by inhibiting the peripheral metabolism of testosterone.[12, 74] Gynecomastia in adolescent boys undergoing cytotoxic drug therapy is thought to be due to decreased androgen production by damaged Leydig cells.[80] Cimetidine has been reported by some to increase serum prolactin,[16] whereas others have not found an increase in this hormone.[57] In one study, gynecomastia developed in cimetidine users who had normal serum prolactin, androgen, and estrogen levels. The authors therefore hypothesized that the drug blockaded androgen receptors in the breast.[82]

Drug-related gynecomastia can be conveniently divided into three histologic categories: hyperplastic, fibrous, and an intermediate group with both hyperplastic and fibrous features. Parenthetically, these categories can be applied equally well to pubertal or senescent gynecomastia.[2] The hyperplastic group has stratification of the ductal epithelial cells, which often form small papillary protrusions into the lumen. The surrounding cuff of periductal stroma is cellular, but also has abundant hyaluronic acid, giving it a loose, myxomatous quality.[32] Conversely, the fibrous variant has a sparsely cellular, densely fibrotic stroma replacing the fat; the ducts are always dilated, and epithelial hyperplasia is less frequently seen than in the hyperplastic form. The intermediate type shows less epithelial hyperplasia and stromal cellularity than the hyperplastic form, and a tendency for broader zones of interductal fibrosis, approaching the fibrous type (Fig. 14-1); this probably represents a transition between the hyperplastic and fibrous categories. It is likely that these different histologic appearances are related to the duration of the gynecomastia, because the hyperplastic form tends to occur in patients whose gynecomastia has been present for less than 4 to 11 months, and the fibrous variant is usually found when the gynecomastia has been present more than a year.[2]

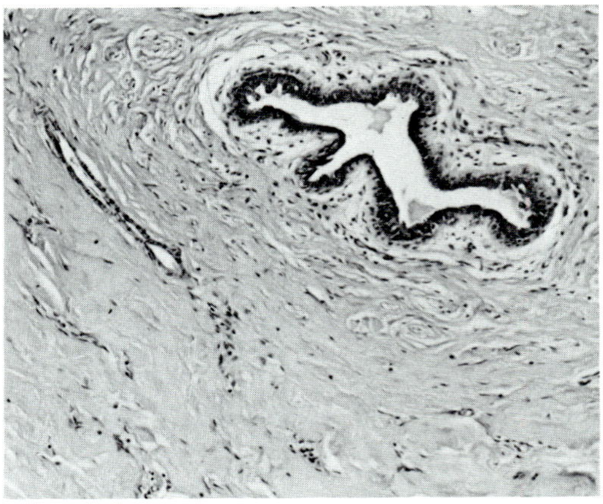

Fig. 14-1. Gynecomastia developed in a 58-year-old man taking digitalis. The breast tissue was removed 10 months after he first noted enlargement. The intermediate type of gynecomastia is present, with broad fibrous zones, epithelial hyperphasia, and slight periductal edema. H & E, × 90.

The histologic type of gynecomastia does not correlate with the inciting agent. The only change that may lead one to suspect a specific group of drugs as being causative is the formation of numerous lobules with secretory acini. Diethylstilbestrol can stimulate the formation of true acini that are histologically identical to those of a female lactating breast[77]; the secretions may be of sufficient quantity to be grossly visible on the cut surface of the tissue.[43] Neither the occurrence of gynecomastia nor the development of acini correlate well with the duration of therapy.[77]

Bannayan and Hajdu observed that gynecomastia secondary to estrogen therapy tended to be bilateral, whereas other drug-induced lesions were usually unilateral.[2] Moreover, in patients with bilateral involvement, the breasts tended to enlarge diffusely, whereas the mass in patients with unilateral disease formed a discrete lesion in most cases.

Pseudogynecomastia was described in a 50-year-old addict who had injected heroin into the subcutaneous tissue of the breast for 3 years.[9] Fat necrosis and a foreign body reaction was found in the tissue, but there was no evidence of increased or altered ductal tissue. Pseudogynecomastia may also occur as a result of leukemic infiltrates.[19]

Carcinoma

Since the late 1940s, many cases of supposed cancer of the breast have been described in men taking diethylstilbestrol for prostatic carcinoma. Most of the initially reported cases were thought to be primary breast tumors, but Campbell and Cummins felt that the cases were not sufficiently documented to warrant that conclusion.[7] Benson observed that when there was microscopic examination of both the prostate lesion and the breast tumor, there was histologic overlap in virtually every instance.[3] The confusion occurs because metastatic prostatic carcinoma may form a discrete mass in the breast,[79] and because microscopically the tumor often includes a poorly differentiated component similar to ordinary infiltrating ductal cancer of the breast. In addition, prostatic carcinoma metastatic to the breast can invade the stroma around and between the breast ducts, further simulating a primary cancer. One helpful way of identifying metastatic prostatic cancer is to demonstrate acid phosphatase in the malignant cells.[3] To be sure, both prostatic and breast cancer can develop in the same patient, but this is rare and probably occurs by chance alone. Treves and Holleb found only one case of prostatic cancer in 146 men with primary breast cancer.[92]

In patients with prostatic cancer, the primary breast cancer that can be accepted as such is one that has a histologic pattern that differs from that of the prostatic cancer, and resembles conventional primary infiltrating duct carcinoma of the breast. On the basis of adherence to these criteria, the best documented case of primary breast cancer in a patient with prostatic carcinoma is that of O'Grady and McDivitt, who described a primary infiltrating carcinoma of the breast in a 77-year-old man who had received unusually high doses of DES continuously for 6 years.[63] The carcinoma had an intraductal and intralobular component cytologically identical to the infiltrating lesion, and Paget's disease of the nipple was also present. Whether or not the DES contributed to the origin or growth of the carcinoma, this report is a model for adequate documentation of primary breast cancer occurring in a male patient treated with DES.

Regarding the relationship of estrogens and male breast cancer, Crichlow found that only 2 of 457 men with breast cancer gave a history of estrogen therapy, and that one of these had received estrogens for merely 5 months.[13] Liechty et al. noted no cases of breast cancer in more than 3,000 men treated with estrogens for prostatic carcinoma.[54] Under extraordinary circumstances, however, the role of estrogen in male breast cancer is unquestionable. Symmers described two transsexuals who developed breast cancer 5 years after they underwent sex change surgery followed by estrogen therapy that included the implantation of estrogen pellets into the breast. Both patients were 30 years old and had normal chromosomes.[87]

Even if exogenous estrogen is not a common factor in the pathogenesis of primary breast cancer, it may increase the frequency with which prostate cancer metastasizes to the breast, whereas in the absence of estrogen therapy, the male breast is rarely a site of metastatic disease.[10] Giarelli and Ferlito reported a case of pulmonary oat cell carcinoma that metastasized to both breasts in a man receiving DES for cancer of the prostate.[35]

They speculated that the estrogenic hormones make the breast more fertile for metastases from carcinoma of other types in addition to prostatic carcinoma; however, no systematic study has been done on this topic.

Florid Papillomatosis

Waldo et al. illustrate a case of florid papillomatosis of the nipple in an 83-year-old man who had taken DES for 10 years.[95] It is impossible to assess the role of estrogens on the basis of a single case such as this, but the extreme rarity of papillomatosis of the nipple in men makes the case intriguing.

THE FEMALE BREAST

A wide range of drugs affects the female breast. A few produce catastrophic damage, such as the necrosis caused by anticoagulant therapy, or the painful gigantic enlargement secondary to penicillamine treatment. A much more common effect is galactorrhea occurring during therapy with neuroleptic drugs or cimetidine.[16,45]

Steroidal hormones are by far the most widely used drugs with the theoretical potential to affect the breast. Estrogens have been available since the late 1930s for ovarian replacement therapy, but their widespread use did not begin until the early 1960s. By 1970, more than 2 million women in the United States were thought to be taking Premarin,[28] and this number has probably doubled in the last decade.[75] Oral contraceptive hormones were introduced in 1961; since then, an estimated 35 million women in the United States have used them.[30] Symptoms of fullness, pain, or slight enlargement of the breasts are common. Galactorrhea may occur during therapy with oral contraceptive hormones or become manifest for the first time when the hormones are withdrawn.

Because of the large number of women taking one or more of the above agents, it is inevitable that breast tissue should be obtained with considerable frequency from women taking drugs that may affect the breast. The potential effects on the female breast of each of several groups of drugs will be considered separately.

Oral Contraceptive Hormones

As one would expect, very little tissue is available from normal breasts of hormone users. Autopsies of five young women who had taken oral contraceptives disclosed that three had inactive breast tissue and two had lobular hyperplasia with varying degrees of secretion.[48] In one extraordinary case, lobular hyperplasia with secretion resulted in a palpable mass.[20] One study of tissue from nearly normal breasts has been reported by Erb and Kallenberger, who biopsied 12 women with "slight palpable alterations." They found lobular hyperplasia in 8.[22] With the use of nuclear labeling, Meyer found no difference between the proliferative activity of breast epithelium from women taking oral contraceptives and that of nonusers.[59]

Secretory changes indistinguishable from normal lactation have been found in women taking oral contraceptives who have never been pregnant.[23] Some of the cells in these cases have basally located nuclei and abundant foamy cytoplasm, while others have scant cytoplasm, with the nucleus protruding from the luminal side of the cell. The secretory changes are focal, and may involve only an occasional lobule, with adjacent lobules appearing normal. This selective susceptibility has been especially well discussed and illustrated by Kiaer and Andersen.[49]

Many series and individual case reports have dealt with possible changes in abnormal breast tissue from women taking oral steroids. The categories of fibroadenoma, fibrocystic disease, and carcinoma will be considered separately.

The earliest report of fibroadenomas showing changes attributed to hormone therapy described a florid hyperplasia that was characterized by complex bridges of epithelium.[36] However, an identical hyperplasia, was later reported in a teenager[38] and two young women who had never taken hormones.[94] Other observers have not seen florid hyperplasia in hormone users, and instead report only a simple hyperplasia, comparable to that found in fibroadenomas from nonusers of hormones.[71] In one study, the frequency of nonflorid epithelial hyperplasia in fibroadenomas was virtually the same in tumors from hormone users (9 percent) and nonusers (7 percent).[23] Prechtel and Seidel, however, found nonflorid hyperplasia twice as often in fibroadenomas from hormone users (25 percent) as in fibroadenomas from nonusers (12 percent).[72] Regardless of the degree of hyperplasia, all authors have noted the lack of cytologic atypia.[56]

The formation of acini with secretion was found in 4 of 54 fibroadenomas from women taking oral contraceptives (Fig. 14-2). All four of the patients were nulligravid. Two other patients had had fibroadenomas removed before they had ever taken hormones, and had then had fibroadenomas excised while using oral contraceptives. The stroma and epithelium were identical in the tumors removed before and after hormone therapy.[23]

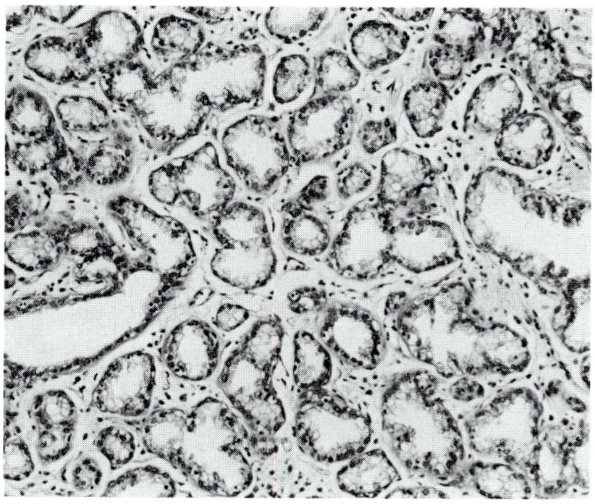

Fig. 14-2. An area of an otherwise typical fibroadenoma from a 24-year-old woman taking oral contraceptives contains numerous ductules with secretory activity. She had never been pregnant. H & E, × 135.

One study without controls concluded that there was an increased frequency of multiple fibroadenomas in users of oral contraceptives[96]; however, this is refuted by historical data showing that the frequency of multiple fibroadenomas long before the hormone era began was identical to that since the introduction of hormones.[62]

In addition to fibroadenomas, pure adenomas of the breast are also seen almost exclusively in young women. One such adenoma enlarged during the use of contraceptive hormones, but neither this lesion nor five others from women taking hormones showed unusual histologic features when compared with several lesions from nonusers.[44]

The wide spectrum of epithelial and stromal changes that are covered by the term "fibrocystic disease" makes this category more difficult to evaluate than fibroadenoma. Perhaps for this reason, no one has been able to ascribe changes to exogenous hormones.[38, 70, 97] In one study, specimens of fibrocystic disease from women taking hormones were compared with specimens from age-matched nonusers. A variety of changes were tabulated without knowledge of the status of hormone therapy, and no consistent stromal or epithelial differences were recognized.[24] Epithelial hyperplasia, a possible risk factor for subsequent cancer, was found in 32 percent of breast biopsies from hormone nonusers and in 24 percent of biopsies from users. Similar figures (30 percent and 34 percent, respectively) are reported by Gray and Robertson.[38] This range is in line with the percentages of hyperplasia in large series of fibrocystic disease reported prior to the use of oral contraception.

Epidemiologic data, on the other hand, have consistently shown that oral contraceptive use for 2 to 4 years or more is associated with a decreased frequency of fibrocystic disease. In light of the fact that fibrocystic disease is generally considered a risk factor for the subsequent development of carcinoma, especially when the disease is characterized by epithelial hyperplasia, it is surprising that there has been no reduction in the frequency of breast cancer in hormone users.[30] The apparent paradox between the decrease in the frequency of fibrocystic disease in contraceptive users and the absence of a corresponding decrease in breast cancer in this group may be explained by the meticulous study of LiVolsi et al.[55] They found that although the occurrence of hyperplasia in hormone users was similar to that in nonusers, there was a greater frequency of cytologic atypia in the hyperplastic foci in hormone users. It appears that benign breast disease may be mainly decreased in women who lack atypical hyperplasia, and who might have been at minimal risk for subsequent cancer in the first place. Conversely, women who develop or who have persistent fibrocystic disease despite hormone usage may be the women destined for cancer whether or not they are taking steroids. The hormones may offer no protective effect against carcinoma for this latter group of women.

Carcinomas of the breast in women taking oral contraceptive hormones have been the subject of several histologic studies. Spencer et al. found no difference in tumor size, histologic type, nuclear grade, presence or absence of lymphoid infiltrate, or nodal sinus histiocytosis in 44 women with cancer who were taking hormones compared with age- and parity-matched controls.[83] Penman, however, illustrated large numbers of colostrum-like foam cells in the intraductal component of a cancer from a woman taking oral contraceptives.[67] No foam cells were seen in the infiltrating part of the tumor nor in the metastases. This change is not limited to women taking hormones.[89] Gould et al. thought there was more secretory activity in the malignant cells of hormone users.[37] They also described widespread extension of cancer into lobules and throughout the ducts in hormone users; additionally, an increase in the mucosubstances in the stroma around neoplastic ducts was prominent (Fig. 14-3). This combination of changes was also noted by Norris and Taylor.[60] Such alterations are not specific for women taking oral contraceptives, however, since they may be seen in cancers from pregnant or lactating women. Moreover,

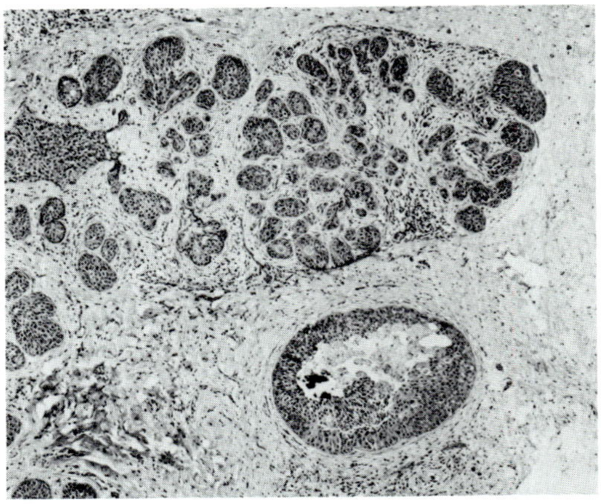

Fig. 14-3. A 34-year-old woman taking oral contraceptives had infiltrating ductal carcinoma. This field shows extensive intraductal and intralobular extension of carcinoma. Edema and mucinous change is seen in the stroma surrounding the lobules. H & E, × 40.

diffuse invasion of the lobules by cancer can occur in women of all ages, regardless of hormone usage, and is more frequent in premenopausal women.[26]

In addition to changes in the carcinoma itself, lobular sclerosis adjacent to carcinoma in a hormone user has been described.[52] In another study, however, 3 of 8 cancers in young women who had never taken oral contraceptives showed some degree of lobular sclerosis.[29] It is possible that young women with breast cancer who have a long history of steroid ingestion may attain a greater frequency of lobular sclerosis, but this hypothesis requires better data for confirmation. Parenthetically, one case of breast cancer, in a 28-year-old woman taking hormones for more than 7 years, failed to display sclerosis.[25]

Infiltrating ductal carcinoma, with or without an intraductal component, is the most frequently reported form of cancer in women taking hormones.

Carcinomas of the breast should be categorized accurately, because a shift in previously reported proportions of different types of carcinoma in hormone users would be evidence for a pathogenetic influence of hormones, even if no distinctive histologic feature can be identified in the individual case.

Despite the absence of consistent, hormone induced morphologic changes in breast cancers, the possibility exists that these cancers still may be affected by hormones. Both the estrogen and progestin components of oral contraceptives have been demonstrated, in isolated cases, to accelerate the growth of metastatic breast carcinoma.[30] On the other hand, a premenopausal woman has exhibited a temporary response to progestin therapy.[85] The use of commercially available oral contraceptive hormones in the therapy of breast cancer has been studied. Nine of 42 postmenopausal women responded, including some who had failed to respond to estrogens alone. The clinical improvement occurred in women treated at the contraceptive dose and in those who received higher doses.[84]

In summary, breast tissue of women taking contraceptive hormones does not undergo histologically distinctive changes. Nonetheless, oral contraceptives occasionally produce lobular hyperplasia with secretory activity either in the normal breast or within fibroadenomas. In addition, fibroadenomas may show a florid epithelial hyperplasia, although it is doubtful that this is qualitatively or quantitatively different from that seen in fibroadenomas from nonusers. Carcinomas from hormone users may also show diffuse invasion of the ducts and lobules, but this finding is similar to cancers in other young women, especially those who are pregnant or lactating. The failure to document specific alterations in women taking hormones should not deter pathologists from the continued close study of tissues from these patients; it is possible that late, unexpected effects of hormone usage will eventually appear, and histologic peculiarities may still play a role in the detection of such effects.

Estrogens

Breast tissue removed from women taking estrogens as ovarian replacement therapy has failed to show any consistent alterations. Swerdlow and Humphrey found large-duct epithelial hyperplasia in 50 percent of patients treated with replacement doses of estrogens, whereas their control group showed 55 percent with hyperplasia.[86] Lobular hyperplasia, however, was more frequent in the estrogen users. In another study, tissue sections from women with fibrocystic disease who were taking estrogens were compared with tissue sections from age-matched patients who denied hormone usage. A variety of epithelial patterns was tabulated without knowledge of the hormonal status. The patients taking estrogens had a slightly greater frequency of epithelial hyperplasia (39 percent) than did the controls (32 percent), but no qualitative differences were detected, and the slight variation in frequency was judged to be insignificant. Two fibroadenomas had no unusual features and specifically lacked epithelial hyperplasia.[27]

Obviously, the absence of specific histologic changes does not preclude an effect of estrogens on the breast; for example, changes are readily demonstrable by mammography and are reversible when hormone therapy ceases. The changes include formation of cysts as well as increases in the overall density of the breast.[66]

Estrogens given in high doses for the treatment of carcinoma almost always produce histologic changes in the contralateral, nonneoplastic breast. Huseby and Thomas found alterations in the nonneoplastic breast in all but 2 of 36 patients treated with either estradiol or diethylstilbestrol.[47] Epithelial and myoepithelial hyperplasia became evident within a month after starting therapy. Mitotic activity was increased and the ducts appeared to be elongated. Lobular hyperplasia, with the formation of true acini, was seen in nearly a third of the cases. The stroma had a loose appearance around large ducts as well as in the lobules. Both the stromal and epithelial alterations regressed after cessation of therapy.

The possibility of an increased frequency of carcinoma in estrogen users has only recently become the subject of adequate epidemiologic study. Hoover et al. found 49 cases of breast cancer in estrogen users, whereas 39 were expected.[46] Although this is not a statistically significant increase, the study at least showed that the use of estrogens did not have a protective effect. About 90 cases of fibrocystic disease and breast cancer in women who received DES while pregnant have been seen by Bibbo et al.[4]; they concluded that there was no increase in the frequency of breast cancer in these women. Nearly all of the cases had histologic confirmation of the diagnosis, but no details of the pathologic examinations are given. Thus far, there is no evidence that the daughters of mothers who took DES during pregnancy are at an increased risk for carcinoma of the breast.[40]

Mastectomy specimens from women with cancer who are taking estrogens have not shown distinctive microscopic features. The histologic types of cancers are roughly proportional to those found in large series of patients unselected for hormone therapy. In one small study, the frequency of lymph node metastases in estrogen users was similar to that in an unselected group. Interestingly, when tumor was present, it involved only a single, low axillary node. Another feature was the relatively large proportion of tumors with pushing margins and lymphocytic infiltrate.[28] The number of cases is small, and no significance can be assigned to these observations at the moment.

The effects of high doses of DES on carcinoma were described by Koller, who examined sequential biopsies from a single patient.[51] He found degenerating cells in which nuclear vacuolization was prominent. On the other hand, Taylor et al. saw no cytologic changes in two patients with breast cancer, 4 and 5 weeks after therapy with DES.[90] Emerson et al. described a decrease of cytoplasmic volume in tumor cells following DES treatment, plus nuclear karyolysis or pyknosis. The stroma appeared loosened and the collagen assumed a tangled appearance.[21]

Danazol

Danazol is an antigonadotropic compound used mainly to treat endometriosis; additionally, it produces dramatic relief in some women with severely symptomatic fibrocystic disease. Subjective improvement is often accompanied by objective decreases in the nodularity of the breasts.[1] The drug also diminishes the size of the breasts in males with gynecomastia and in females with virginal hypertrophy.[39]

I have personally reviewed breast tissue from 11 female patients who had generous incisional biopsies for fibrocystic disease, were subsequently treated with danazol, and were then rebiopsied. Clinically, the patients had decreased nodularity after taking the drug. The post-treatment biopsies were done under local anesthesia and yielded small amounts of tissue; nonetheless, they were sufficient to show the same microscopic spectrum of fibrocystic disease as seen in the larger pretreatment biopsies. The only difference noted was in two cases that showed lobular atrophy in the post-treatment tissue, whereas no atrophic lobules were present in the initial biopsy. This may only be a manifestation of a very small sample; additional tissue might have shown other alterations. No unusual histologic or cytologic abnormalities were present.

Danazol has caused regression of carcinoma in rats; the neoplastic cells undergo flattening and atrophy. The change is similar to that found in cancers treated with oophorectomy.[68]

Neuroleptic Drugs

Several antidepressant drugs and other tranquilizers increase serum prolactin levels and cause galactorrhea. Drugs specifically responsible for these effects include chlorpromazine (Thorazine), prochlorperazine (Compazine), thioridazine (Mellaril), trifluoperazine (Stelazine), imipramine (Tofranil), amitriptyline (Triavil), meprobamate, and haloperidol (Haldol).[45] I am unaware of histologic studies on tissue from women taking these drugs, although fully developed secretory acini would presumably be found. This assumption is based on the effect of neuroleptic drugs given to rats and rabbits. Changes are produced that are identical to those in the normal lactating breast when examined either by light or electron microscopy.[69]

It is possible that the secretory changes occasionally seen in one or two lobules of surgical or autopsy specimens are produced by neuroleptic or other drugs. Such focal involvement would not be expected to result in clinically apparent galactorrhea. If secretory changes are seen in the breasts of women who are not lactating, pregnant, or receiving hormones, a history of nonhormonal drug therapy should be sought.

Serum prolactin levels are elevated in some patients with carcinoma of the breast, and for this reason, there is concern that drugs which chronically increase prolactin might be carcinogenic. Indeed, some studies did conclude that reserpine was associated with an increased frequency of breast cancer, but more recent studies have not substantiated this.[78]

Anticoagulants

The female breast shares the same susceptibility to necrosis induced by coumadin or dicumarol as does fatty tissue in other parts of the body, such as the buttock or thigh; the subcutaneous fat of the breast may, in a manner analogous to these latter sites, be the area initially involved. Even if this is the case, the necrosis quickly extends into the substance of the breast so that the entire organ is affected. The process begins suddenly, 3 to 10 days after starting anticoagulant therapy, and progresses relentlessly even if the drug is stopped. Histologically there is a triad of acute necrotizing arteritis, venous thrombosis, and necrosis.[14, 61] The pathogenesis of the condition is unknown. Although there is extravasation of blood as a part of the tissue necrosis, it is obvious that the process is not merely a massive hemorrhage into the breast. The timing and the vasculitis suggest an allergic effect, but it is unclear why this would be localized. The possibility has been raised that the condition is a manifestation of disseminated intravascular coagulation, but this has not been confirmed.[18]

Miscellaneous Agents

Synchronous, bilateral breast cancers developed in two young women, aged 28 and 29, who had used clomiphene.[5] The details of clomiphene dosage in these two cases are not clearly stated, but it is implied that the women received the agent for only several cycles, over a relatively short period of time. Both patients had lymph node metastases, but no histologic particulars are given. Although a cause and effect relationship cannot be established from anecdotes, these cases serve as a reminder to be alert for similar findings in other women taking clomiphene or other drugs that affect the breast.

A few women have experienced the abrupt onset of bilateral enlargement of the breast during treatment with penicillamine.[65] The process continues steadily for a few weeks, with the breasts attaining huge proportions. There has been no tendency for the enlargement to regress after the cessation of penicillamine use, but the reported follow-up periods are short. In one patient bilateral mastectomy was necessary. Increased fibrosis and duct dilatation were described in the resected tissue, but no other details are provided.[17]

Isoniazid was considered to be a factor in the onset of gigantic breast hypertrophy in a patient who was pregnant.[93] It is difficult to know whether or not this was a case of coincidental gigantic hypertrophy of pregnancy or whether the isoniazid contributed to the process. The hypertrophy regressed several months after delivery and cessation of the drug.

Rarely, a patient receives cytotoxic chemotherapy for breast cancer followed by a mastectomy. If tumor is recognizable in the resected specimen it can be drastically altered when compared to that in the original biopsy. Gigantic cells, with increases in both the volume of the cytoplasm and nucleus, can be

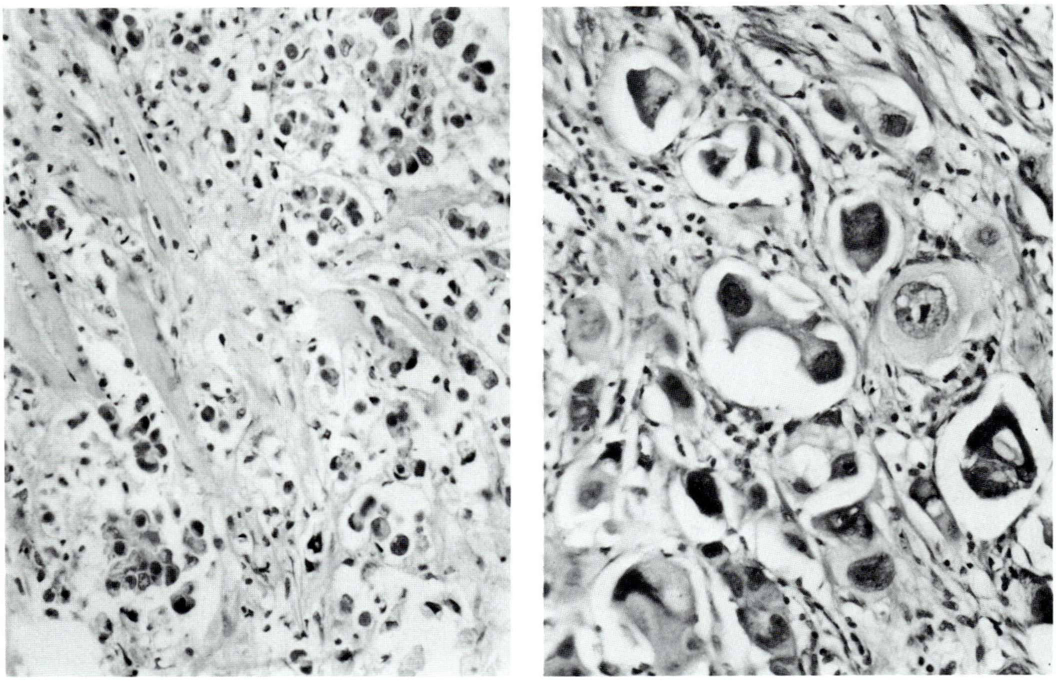

(A) **(B)**

Fig. 14-4. (A) Biopsy from an infiltrating ductal carcinoma prior to chemotherapy. (B) A simply mastectomy 7 weeks after Adriamycin therapy showed that the carcinoma had gigantic cells with correspondingly enlarged and bizarre nuclei. Both photographs are at same magnification. H & E, × 350.

encountered (Fig. 14-4). As in the case of irradiated tumor, the reproductive capacity—and therefore the neoplastic potential—cannot be determined despite the fact that the cells are intact. The pathologist can state only that tumor is present, and should not make a judgement regarding its capacity for replication.

Silicone

Although the injection of liquid silicone into the breast is no longer used in augmentation mammoplasties, many women carry this substance from procedures done as long as 15 years ago. The breast that contains silicone is susceptible to the development of new and different nodules as the material migrates and provokes additional inflammatory response. Silicone may also migrate through the subcutaneous tissue to areas as far away as the inguinal region.[15] Gross inspection of breast tissue containing silicone will disclose a thick, sticky, stringy material intermixed with the fat. If this has not been appreciated grossly, and the history of silicone injection is not given, the histologic sections may be difficult to interpret, because most or all of the silicone will be dissolved out. The silicone provokes a histiocytic and fibrous reaction. Mononuclear histiocytes predominate, although a few multinucleated forms may be present (Fig. 14-5). Individual histiocytes may contain silicone, or they may be stretched around large masses of silicone so that the stainable cytoplasm of individual cells is sparse. The fibrous reaction may be cellular, but eventually, bands of dense, acellular collagen are formed. All of these varying patterns of fibrohistiocytic reaction may be intermixed. This variable cellularity and the variation in the appearance of the individual histiocytes may be worrisome. The large ve-

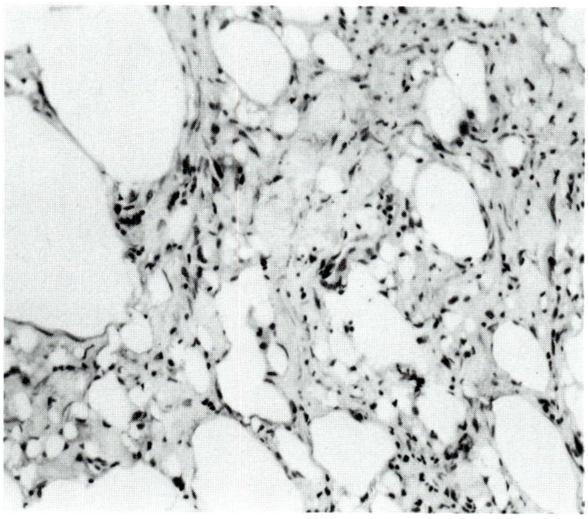

Fig. 14-5. Breast tissue 11 years after injection of silicone. The silicone is dissolved out, leaving clear spaces of varying size; the spaces are surrounded by an irregular fibrohistiocytic response. H & E, × 225.

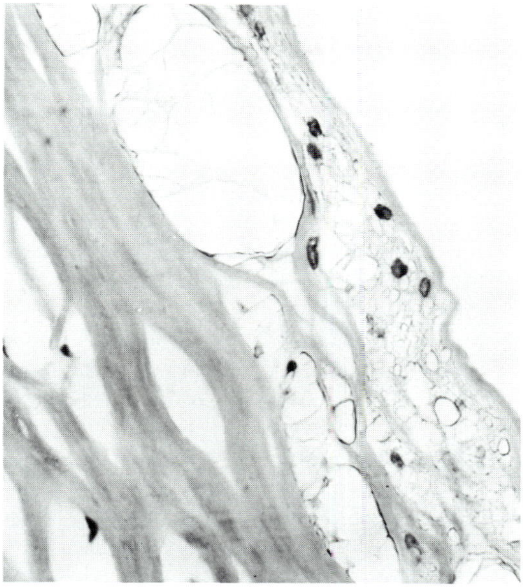

Fig. 14-6. Silicone is present as watery-appearing material or clear spaces in the fibrous capsule formed adjacent to silicone-gel prosthesis. H & E, × 335.

sicular nuclei of some histiocytes are similar to those of lipoblasts, and when the cytoplasm contains multiple vacuoles of silicone, the cells may closely resemble malignant lipoblasts. The distinction rests largely on the recognition of large, clear, coalescent areas of silicone with the vacuolated histiocytes located at the peripheries of these areas. Regional lymph nodes can also contain large histiocytes with a finely to coarsely vacuolated cytoplasm filled with transported silicone.[88]

In recent years, prostheses filled with silicone-gel have become widely used. Silicone leaks from these prostheses even when the envelope is grossly intact (Fig. 14-6). The histologic reaction to the silicone is similar to the reaction to liquid silicone injections. Histiocytes with vacuolated cytoplasm are found adjacent to the prosthesis in the region of the fibrous capsule that forms at the interface of the prosthesis and normal tissues. The prosthesis may rupture spontaneously, leading to the release of large quantities of the gel.[8] Even in the absence of rupture, the dense fibrous reaction frequently leads to deformity of the breast, requiring physical manipulation to break up the capsule. This may also lead to dispersion of silicone-gel beyond the immediate area of the prosthesis. Silicone may be found in the regional lymph nodes even in the absence of capsulotomy.[42]

A number of cases of carcinoma have been reported in patients with prosthetic implants. Thus far, there is no evidence of an increased incidence of cancer in these patients unless such other potential carcinogenic factors as irradiation are added.[33]

REFERENCES

1. Asch, R. H., & Greenblatt, R. B.: The use of an impeded androgen-danazol-in the management of benign breast disorders. Am. J. Obstet. Gynecol. 127:130, 1977.
2. Bannayan, G. A., & Hajdu, S. I.: Gynecomastia: Clinicopathologic study of 351 cases. Am. J. Clin. Pathol. 57:431, 1972.
3. Benson, W. R.: Carcinoma of the prostate with metastases to breast and testis. Critical review of the literature and report of a case. Cancer 10:1235, 1957.
4. Bibbo, M., Haenszel, W. M., Wied, G. L. et al.: A twenty-five-year follow-up study of women exposed to diethylstilbestrol during

pregnancy. N. Engl. J. Med. 298:763, 1978.
5. Bolton, P. M.: Bilateral breast cancer associated with clomiphene. Lancet 2:1176, 1977.
6. Byar, D. P.: VACURG studies on prostatic cancer and its treatment. In: Tannenbaum, M., Ed.: Urologic Pathology: The Prostate. Lea & Febiger, Philadelphia, 1977.
7. Campbell, J. H., & Cummins, S. D.: Metastases, simulating mammary cancer, in prostatic carcinoma under estrogenic therapy. Cancer 4:303, 1951.
8. Capozzi, A., DuBou, R., & Pennisi, V. R.: Distant migration of silicone gel from a ruptured breast implant. Case report. Plast. Reconstr. Surg. 62:302, 1978.
9. Carlson, R. H., Velez, R., & Rivlin, R. S.: Pseudogynecomastia secondary to injection of heroin into breast tissue. Arch. Intern. Med. 138:483, 1978.
10. Charache, H.: Metastatic tumors in the breast, with a report of ten cases. Surgery 33:385, 1953.
11. Check, J. H., Murdock, M. G., Caro, J. E. et al.: Case Report: Cystic gynecomastia in a male treated with clomiphene citrate. Fertil. Steril. 30:713, 1978.
12. Cicero, T. J., Bell, R. D., Wiest, W. G. et al.: Function of the male sex organs in heroin and methadone users. N. Engl. J. Med. 292:882, 1975.
13. Crichlow, R. W.: Carcinoma of the male breast. Surg. Gynecol. Obstet. 134:1011, 1972.
14. Davis, C. E., Jr., Wiley, W. B., & Faulconer, R. J.: Necrosis of the female breast complicating anticoagulant treatment. Ann. Surg. 175: 647, 1972.
15. Delage, C., Shane, J. J., & Johnson, F. B.: Mammary silicone granuloma. Migration of silicone fluid to abdominal wall and inguinal region. Arch. Dermatol. 108:104, 1973.
16. Della Fave, G. F., Tamburrano, G., de Magistris, L. et al.: Gynaecomastia with cimetidine. Lancet 1:1319, 1977.
17. Desai, S. N.: Sudden gigantism of breast: Drug induced? Br. J. Plast. Surg. 26:371, 1973.
18. DiCato, M. A., & Ellman, L.: Coumadin-induced necrosis of breast, disseminated intravascular coagulation, and hemolytic anemia. Ann. Intern. Med. 83:233, 1975.
19. DeVillez, R. L., Lufkin, E. G., & Bergin, J. J.: Symmetrical enlargement of breasts and testes due to leukemic infiltration. South. Med. J. 65:341, 1972.
20. Dito, W. R., & Batsakis, J. G.: Norethynodrel-treated endometriosis: A morphologic and histochemical study. Obstet. Gynecol. 18:1, 1961.
21. Emerson, W. J., Kennedy, B. J., Graham, J. N. et al.: Pathology of primary and recurrent carcinoma of the human breast after administration of steroid hormones. Cancer 6:641, 1953.
22. Erb, H., & Kallenberger, A.: The action of an oral high-dosed oestrogen-progestagen combination on the human breast. Acta Endocrinol. 70:143, 1972.
23. Fechner, R. E.: Fibroadenomas in patients receiving oral contraceptives: A clinical and pathologic study. Am. J. Clin. Pathol. 53:857, 1970.
24. Fechner, R. E.: Fibrocystic disease in women receiving oral contraceptive hormones. Cancer 25:1332, 1970.
25. Fechner, R. E.: Breast cancer during oral contraceptive therapy. Cancer 26:1204, 1970.
26. Fechner, R. E.: Ductal carcinoma involving the lobule of the breast. A source of confusion with lobular carcinoma in situ. Cancer 28:274, 1971.
27. Fechner, R. E.: Benign breast disease in women on estrogen therapy. A pathologic study. Cancer 29:273, 1972.
28. Fechner, R. E.: Cancer of the breast during estrogen replacement therapy. Cancer 29:566, 1972.
29. Fechner, R. E.: Oral contraceptive effects on the breast. J.A.M.A. 224:249, 1973.
30. Fechner, R. E.: Influence of oral contraceptives on breast diseases. Cancer 39:2764, 1977.
31. Finn, J. E., & Mount, L. A.: Galactorrhea in males with tumors in the region of the pituitary gland. J. Neurosurg. 35:723, 1971.
32. Fisher, E. R. & Creed, D. L.: Nature of the periductal stroma in gynecomastia. Lab. Invest. 5:267, 1956.
33. Frantz, P., & Herbst, C. A., Jr.: Augmentation mammoplasty, irradiation, and breast cancer. A case report. Cancer 36:1147, 1975.
34. Frantz, A. G.: Prolactin secretion in physiologic and pathologic human conditions measured by bioassay and radioimmunoassay. In: Josimovich, J. B., Reynolds, M., & Cobo, E., Eds.: Lactogenic Hormones, Fetal Nutrition, and Lactation. p. 379. John Wiley & Sons, New York, 1974.
35. Giarelli, L., & Ferlito, A.: Bilateral breast me-

tastases from oat-cell lung carcinoma in a man treated with diethylstilbestrol for prostatic adenocarcinoma. J. Am. Geriatr. Soc. 24:511, 1976.
36. Goldenberg, V. E., Wiegenstein, L., & Mottet, N. K.: Florid breast fibroadenomas in patients taking hormonal oral contraceptives. Am. J. Clin. Pathol. 49:52, 1968.
37. Gould, V. E., Wolff, M., & Mottet, N. K.: Morphologic features of mammary carcinomas in women taking hormonal contraceptives. Am. J. Clin. Pathol. 57:139, 1972.
38. Gray, L. A., & Robertson, R. W., Jr.: Estrogens, the pill, and the breast. In: Gallager, H. S., Ed.: Early Breast Cancer. Detection and Treatment. p. 27. John Wiley & Sons, New York, 1975.
39. Greenblatt, R. B., Dmowski, W. P., Mahesh, V. B. et al.: Clinical studies with an antigonadotropin—Danazol. Fertil. Steril. 22:102, 1971.
40. Greenwald, P., Nasca, P. C., Burnett, W. S., & Poland, A.: Prenatal stilbestrol experience of mothers of young cancer patients. Cancer 31:568. 1973.
41. Haagensen, C. D.: Diseases of the Breast. 2nd Ed. Philadelphia. W. B. Saunders, 1971.
42. Hausner, R. J., Schoen, F. J., & Pierson, K. K.: Foreign-body reaction to silicone gel in axillary lymph nodes after an augmentation mammoplasty. Plast. Reconstr. Surg. 62:381, 1978.
43. Hendrickson, D. A., & Anderson, W. R.: Diethylstilbestrol therapy gynecomastia. J.A.M.A. 213:468, 1970.
44. Hertel, B. F., Zaloudek, C., & Kempson, R. L.: Breast adenomas. Cancer 37:2891, 1976.
45. Hooper, J. H., Jr., Welch, V. C., & Shackelford, R. T.: Abnormal lactation associated with tranquilizing drug therapy. J.A.M.A. 178:506, 1968.
46. Hoover, R., Gray, L. A., Cole, P. et al.: Menopausal estrogens and breast cancer. N. Engl. J. Med. 295:401, 1976.
47. Huseby, R. A., & Thomas, L. B.: Histological and histochemical alterations in the normal breast tissues of patients with advanced breast cancer being treated with estrogenic hormones. Cancer 7:54, 1954.
48. Irey, N. S., Manion, W. C., & Taylor, H. B.: Vascular lesions in women taking oral contraceptives. Arch. Pathol. 89:1, 1970.
49. Kiaer, H. W., & Andersen, J. A.: Focal pregnancy-like changes in the breast. Acta Pathol. Microbiol. Scand. 85:931, 1977.
50. Kleinberg, D. L., Noel, G. L., & Frantz, A. G.: Galactorrhea: A study of 235 cases, including 48 with pituitary tumors. N. Engl. J. Med. 296:589, 1977.
51. Koller, P. C.: Cytology of serial biopsies from a case of carcinoma of the breast treated with stilboestrol. Br. Med. J. 2:298, 1944.
52. Kovi, J., & Viola, M. V.: Oral contraceptives and breast histology. J.A.M.A. 223:802, 1973.
53. LeWinn, E. B.: Gynecomastia during digitalis therapy. Report of eight additional cases with liver-function studies. N. Engl. J. Med. 248:316, 1953.
54. Liechty, R. D., Davis, J., & Gleysteen, J.: Cancer of the male breast. Forty cases. Cancer 20:1617, 1967.
55. LiVolsi, V. A., Stadel, B. V., Kelsey, J. L. et al.: Fibrocystic breast disease in oral-contraceptive users. A histopathological evaluation of epithelial atypia. N. Engl. J. Med. 299:381, 1978.
56. LiVolsi, V. A., Stadel, E. V., Kelsey, J. L. et al.: Fibroadenoma in oral contraceptive users. A histopathologic evaluation of epithelial atypia. Cancer 44:1778, 1979.
57. Majumbar, S. K., Thomson, A. D., & Shaw, G. K.: Cimetidine and serum prolactin. Br. Med. J. 1:409, 1978.
58. Margolis, I. B., & Gross, C. G.: Gynecomastia during phenothiazine therapy. J.A.M.A. 199:942, 1967.
59. Meyer, J. S.: Cell proliferation in normal human breast ducts, fibroadenomas, and other ductal hyperplasias measured by nuclear labeling with tritiated thymidine. Effects of menstrual phase, age, and oral contraceptive hormones. Hum. Pathol. 8:67, 1977.
60. Norris, H. J., & Taylor, H. B.: Carcinoma of the breast in women less than thirty years old. Cancer 26:953, 1970.
61. Nudelman, H. L., & Kempson, R. L.: Necrosis of the breast. A rare complication of anticoagulant therapy. Am. J. Surg. 111:728, 1966.
62. Oberman, H. A.: Hormonal contraceptives and fibroadenomas of breast. N. Engl. J. Med. 284:984, 1971.
63. O'Grady, W. P., & McDivitt, R. W.: Breast cancer in a man treated with diethylstilbestrol. Arch. Pathol. 88:162, 1969.
64. Orentreich, N., & Durr, N. P.: Proceedings:

Mammogenesis in trans-sexuals. J. Invest. Dermatol. 63:142, 1974.

65. Passas, C., & Weinstein, A.: Breast gigantism with penicillamine therapy. Arthritis Rheum. 21:167, 1978.
66. Peck, D. R., & Lowman, R. M.: Estrogen and the postmenopausal breast: Mammographic considerations. J.A.M.A. 240:1733, 1978.
67. Penman, H. G.: The effect of oral contraceptives on the histology of carcinoma of the breast. J. Pathol. 101:66, 1970.
68. Peters, T. G., Lewis, J. D., Wilkinson, E. J. et al.: Danazol therapy in hormone-sensitive mammary carcinoma. Cancer 40:2797, 1977.
69. Pier, W. J., Jr., Garancis, J. C., & Kuzma, J. F.: Fine structure of tranquilizer-induced changes in rat mammary gland. Am. J. Pathol. 60:119, 1970.
70. Prechtel, K.: Ovulationshemmer und Brustdrüsenveränderungen bei Frauen im geschlechtsreifen Alter. Munch. Med. Wochenschr. 111:2443, 1969.
71. Prechtel, K., & Seidel, H.: Brustdrüsenveränderungen nach Langzeitbehandlung mit sogennannten Ovulationschemmern. Verh. Dtsch. Ges. Pathol. 56:529, 1972.
72. Prechtel, K., & Seidel, H.: Der Einfluss oraler Steroidkontrazeptiva auf das Fibroadenom der Mamma. Dtsch. Med. Wochenschr. 98:698, 1973.
73. Proutz, M.: Gynecomastia with pigmentation in a four year old male following stilbestrol exposure. Pediatrics 9:55, 1952.
74. Rose, L. I., Underwood, R. H., Newmark, S. R. et al.: Pathophysiology of spironolactone-induced gynecomastia. Ann. Intern. Med. 87:398, 1977.
75. Ross, R., Mack, T., Gerkins, V. et al.: Breast cancer and menopausal estrogens. In: Silverberg, S. G. and Major, F. J., Eds.: Estrogens and Cancer. p. 55. John Wiley & Sons, New York, 1978.
76. Sawin, S. T., Longcope, C., Schmitt, G. W. et al.: Blood levels of gonadotropins and gonadal hormones in gynecomastia associated with chronic hemodialysis. J. Clin. Endocrinol. Metab. 36:988, 1973.
77. Schwartz, I. S., & Wilens, S. L.: The formation of acinar tissue in gynecomastia. Am. J. Pathol. 43:797, 1963.
78. Schyve, P. M., Smithline, F., & Meltzer, H. Y.: Neuroleptic-induced prolactin elevation and breast cancer. An emerging clincial issue. Arch. Gen. Psychiatry. 35:1291, 1978.
79. Seipel, W. D., & Malamet, M.: Carcinoma of the prostate with bilateral breast metastases. J. Am. Geriatr. Soc. 20:510, 1972.
80. Sherins, R. J., Olweny, C. L. M., & Ziegler, J. L.: Gynecomastia and gonadal dysfunction in adolescent boys treated with combination chemotherapy for Hodgkin's disease. N. Engl. J. Med. 299:12, 1978.
81. Smith, R. H., & Barrett, O., Jr.: Gynecomastia associated with vincristine therapy. Calif. Med. 107:347, 1967.
82. Spence, R. W., & Celester, L. R.: Gynecomastia associated with cimetidine. Gut 20:154, 1979.
83. Spencer, J. D., Miller, R. R., & Hayward, J. L.: Contraceptive steroids and breast cancer. Br. Med. J. 1:1024, 1978.
84. Stoll, B. A.: Effect of Lyndiol, an oral contraceptive, on breast cancer. Br. Med. J. 1:150, 1967.
85. Stoll, B. A.: Hormonal Management in Breast Cancer. p. 73. Philadelphia, J. B. Lippincott, 1969.
86. Swerdlow, M., & Humphrey, L. J.: The relationship of breast disease to gynecologic disease. Cancer 17:1165, 1964.
87. Symmers, W. St. C.: Carcinoma of breast in trans-sexual individuals after surgical and hormonal interference with the primary and secondary sex characteristics. Br. Med. J. 2:83, 1968.
88. Symmers, W. St. C.: Silicone mastitis in "topless" waitresses and some other varieties of foreign-body mastitis. Br. Med. J. 3:19, 1968.
89. Taylor, H. B.: Oral contraceptives and pathologic changes in the breast. Cancer 28:1388, 1971.
90. Taylor, S. G., III, Slaughter, D. P., Smejkal, W., et al.: The effect of sex hormones on advanced carcinoma of the breast. Cancer 1:604, 1948.
91. Thomas, B. L.: Methadone-associated gynecomastia. N. Engl. J. Med. 294:169, 1976.
92. Treves, N., & Holleb, A. J.: Cancer of the male breast. Cancer 8:1239, 1955.
93. Van Der Meulen, A. J.: An unusual case of massive hypertrophy of the breasts. S. Afr. Med. J. 48:1465, 1974.
94. Vessey, M. P., Doll, R., & Sutton, P. M.: Oral

contraceptives and breast neoplasia: A retrospective study. Br. Med. J. 3:719, 1972.
95. Waldo, E. D., Sidhu, G. S., & Hu, A. W.: Florid papillomatosis of male nipple after diethylstilbestrol therapy. Arch. Pathol. 99:364, 1975.
96. Wiegenstein, L., Tank, R., & Gould, V. E.: Multiple breast fibroadenomas in women on hormonal contraceptives. N. Engl. J. Med. 284:676, 1971.
97. Zanartu, J., Onetto, E., Medina, E., et al.: Mammary gland nodules in women under continuous exposure to progestagens. Contraception 7:203, 1973.

15

The Nervous System

Barbara F. Smith

Drugs and toxins may produce cellular damage for a number of different chemical reasons. If, however, a substance solely or predominantly damages a particular cell or tissue, this must be either because the physiology of the body concentrates that substance in the tissue that is damaged, or because there is some special aspect of the metabolism of the damaged cell that is peculiarly sensitive to the substance.

The central nervous system is to a large extent protected by the blood brain barrier, which cannot be penetrated by many substances that can do damage elsewhere in the body; if this were not so, it would be impossible to use a number of drugs, particularly the antineoplastic agents. However, there are some structures, such as the posterior root ganglia and autonomic ganglia, which are not so protected, and peripheral neuropathy, usually mild but occasionally severe, is a side effect of many drugs.

Brain damage can result from changes in blood vessels, without the toxic substance entering the brain; monoamine oxidase (MAO) inhibitors can produce paroxysmal hypertension, which may occasionally result in cerebral hemorrhage; hypotensive agents can be factors in the causation of cerebral occlusive disease. Any toxic infectious material present in the circulating blood must pass through the capillaries before it can enter the brain parenchyma; if these capillaries are damaged, they leak producing a condition of dysoric encephalopathy. A common cause of this sort of damage is anoxia. Heavy metals also tend to localize in the cerebral capillaries, where they may or may not produce damage. This can sometimes be shown in patients with severe siderosis, in whom stainable iron can be demonstrated in the capillary walls of the brain and choroid plexus, whereas hardly any is seen in the cerebral parenchyma. Furthermore, even though this iron appears to be innocuous, other metals which behave in the same way, such as lead, may damage the capillary endothelium; in such cases the capillaries may leak, producing cerebral edema, and possibly failing to retain other substances which are normally kept out of the brain.

Drugs specifically damaging the brain cells may affect neurons or glia. A particular feature of neurons is their high content of nucleic acid, both DNA and RNA, compared with other cells; they are therefore particularly susceptible to substances which interfere in any way with nucleic acid synthesis. These include antineoplastic agents, isonicotinic acid hydrazide, and phenytoin. Nerve cells also contain neurotubules which are structurally somewhat similar to spindles, and are damaged by spindle poisons such as the vinca alkaloids.

Oligodendroglia can be specifically affected for reasons which are not well understood. Demyelination due to oligodendrocyte damage occurs in cyanide poisoning and methotrexate toxicity. The demyelination in chronic cyanide poisoning may occur because the oligodendrocyte is a very active cell metabolically, and depends upon the "hexose monophosphate shunt" rather than the glycolytic pathway for its energy. The Schwann cell appears to be sensitive to a number of toxic and metabolic conditions, and segmental demyelination is common.

Astrocytes are relatively insensitive to toxins but are affected in liver failure, possibly by the high levels of circulating ammonia. The brain, like the liver, can synthesize glutamine from glutamate and ammonia, and this is one way of removing ammonia from the circulation. If this is not being done by the liver, the astrocytes may be overloaded and the brain deprived of its glutamate, which is necessary for the synthesis of γ-aminobutyric acid (GABA).

Asparaginase causes two types of cerebral dysfunction, one occurring early and the other a week or so after treatment commences. Since asparaginase does not cross the blood-brain barrier, the lesion must be due to metabolic changes outside the brain. In the early phases of the dysfunction, the EEG changes may be similar to those in hepatic coma,[91] and the blood ammonia can rise to 900 μg percent. The later neurotoxicity may be due to L-asparagine deficiency.[99]

Cerebral changes may occur secondarily from toxic damage to other such tissues as those of the heart, kidneys, and liver. The cerebral changes caused by some substances may contribute to death.

METALS

Metals, particularly heavy metals, in large quantities can be toxic to both the central and peripheral nervous system. Metals are general protoplasmic posions and block a number of enzyme systems. Organic metal compounds can be even more dangerous than pure metals themselves, and in much smaller quantities. Some metals and metal compounds damage the vascular endothelium or Schwann cells, others damage nerve cells directly. On the other hand, some metals, such as inorganic mercury, are so rarely encountered as toxins nowadays that we do not know much about the pathology they produce.

Lead

The most important features of inorganic lead encephalopathy are: (1) that it mainly affects blood vessels, with damage to the cerebral parenchyma being secondary; and, (2) that, with the exception of enormous doses, only young individuals are susceptible.

The damage done by lead to cerebral blood vessels has been demonstrated both in neonatal rats and in young children. In neonatal rats, lead produces capillary damage and proliferation, with edema and hemorrhage, the changes being most severe in the cerebellum.[2,109,140] It has also been shown, by Pentschew and Garro,[105] that the blood-brain barrier is permeable to Evans blue. At the ultrastructural level, there is damage by lead to the capillary basement membrane and intercellular junctions, with escape of horseradish peroxidase into the tissue.[139] Ahrens and Vistica,[2] using day-old rats, found that after the administration of radioactive led (^{210}Pb), this isotope was present in the endothelial cells of capillaries, and that there was edema of the adjacent astrocytic foot processes. When given to nursing rats, lead produced developmental changes in the brains of the offspring[74]; the neurons were small, and proliferation of neuropil was retarded. There was also a reduction in the number of synapses in each neuron. Press[110] suggests that the brain is susceptible to lead for only a limited period, which in the rat is the first 20 days of life, and in the child, the first 3 to 4 years. In the rat the cerebellum is most susceptible because it develops last (Fig. 15-1).

In children, the symptoms of acute lead poisoning are headache, convulsions, meningism, and coma. There is usually papilledema. Pathologically there is a firm, dry brain swelling with congestion. The capillaries show endothelial swelling, and later proliferation or even necrosis with hemorrhage.[3,15,108] Later there is some hyalinization of the vessel walls, with perivascular fibrosis; these changes are very similar to those or arterial degenerative disease occurring with age. Raimondi et al.[112] did ultrastructural studies on six brain biopsies of children with lead poisoning; they found homogenization of the capillary basement membrane and swollen rough endoplasmic reticulum in the pericytes. The changes in the neurons and glia were less striking. When the effects of lead intoxication have become chronic, there may be a sudden flare-up following a new exposure. The pathology then consists of vascular proliferation with adventitial fibrosis and sometimes calcification. There may be secondary areas of focal necrosis.[102]

Lead poisoning in young children is thus a dysoric encephalopathy, with primary changes in the capillary wall. Initially this results in leakage through the capillary wall, and in severe cases results in petechial hemorrhages. When these changes occur at a very young age, before cerebral development is complete, the result may be smaller neurons and a reduction in the number of neuronal processes and synapses. This might mean that cerebration would never reach a normal potential.

Inorganic lead is also an important cause of peripheral neuropathy. The segmental demyelination of peripheral nerves that lead produces was originally described in 1880 by Gombault.[53a] He gave lead carbonate to guinea pigs and showed the loss of myelin in a single internodal segment with a normal myelin sheath above and below. He did not report any axonal pathology. Fullerton[51] also used guinea pigs, which she fed with lead acetate. There was a reduction in motor nerve conduction velocity. Pathologically, some nerves showed segmental demyelination, some showed axonal degeneration, and some showed both effects. Lampert and Schochet[76] studied the changes in the nerves of lead-treated rats with the electron microscope. They found that there was proliferation and degeneration of Schwann cells and that the myelin segments of damaged Schwann cells disintegrated. The myelin lamellae split and separated into discrete membranous blebs, which were engulfed by the proliferated Schwann cells. New myelin lamellae were formed from the proliferated Schwann cells to wrap the denuded axon. This process was repeated a number of times, with the production of "onion bulb" formations of myelin lamellae.

Arsenic

Arsenic can produce both an encephalopathy and a peripheral neuropathy. Its effect appears to be similar whether it is taken as inorganic arsenic, or trivalent or pentavalent organic arsenic. The cerebral symptoms of arsenic intoxication are more often associated with parenteral treatment, while the peripheral neuropathy is associated with ingested arsenic.

The symptoms of acute arsenical encephalopathy are those of intracranial hypertension: headache, vomiting, confusion, epilepsy, and coma. The pathology consists of cerebral edema and ring hemorrhages. These occur mainly in the subcortical white matter, the internal capsule, and the pons.[115] In addition to frank hemorrhage, there is perivascular demyelination, small vessel thrombosis and, later, some perivascular cuffing.[46] In experimental work on rabbits, Grzycki and Kobusowna[54] showed that arsenic fed to rabbits was picked up by the capillary endothelium, with destruction of the endothelial cells. In a series of 40 patients described by Chauttani et al.,[35] peripheral neuropathy developed within 2 hours of arsenic administration, and in 10 days the patients were bedridden; they complained of paresthesia, pain, and weakness. Some tendon jerks were lost, but cranial nerve palsies were rare. Histologic study of the nerves showed some increase in cellularity, with fibrosis, a reduction in myelinated fibers, and swelling and fragmentation of axons.

Bismuth

Bismuth is usually given by mouth, as a relatively insoluble salt, and very little is absorbed. The maximum blood level is only 10 to 50 μg percent. There have been a few cases of bismuth intoxication reported, mainly from France where bismuth is used more extensively than elsewhere, of patients absorbing much more; blood levels of bismuth of 400 to 1,500 μg percent have been reported,[27]

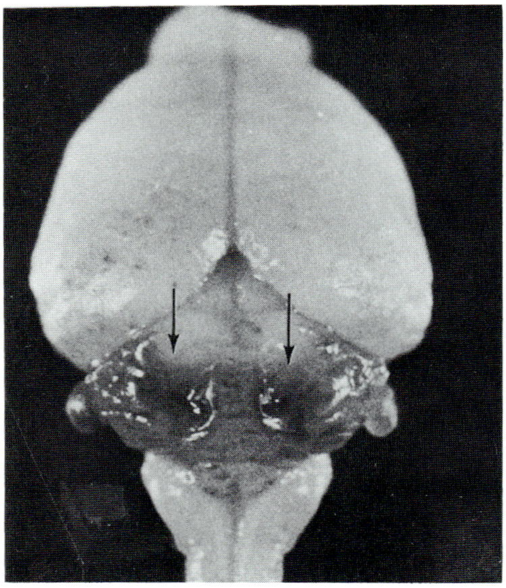

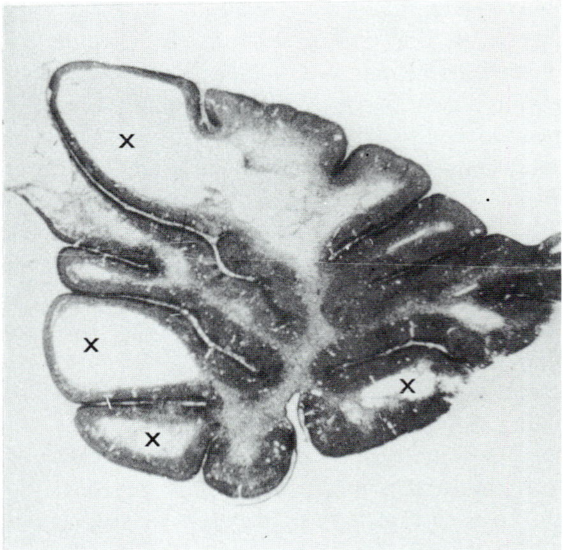

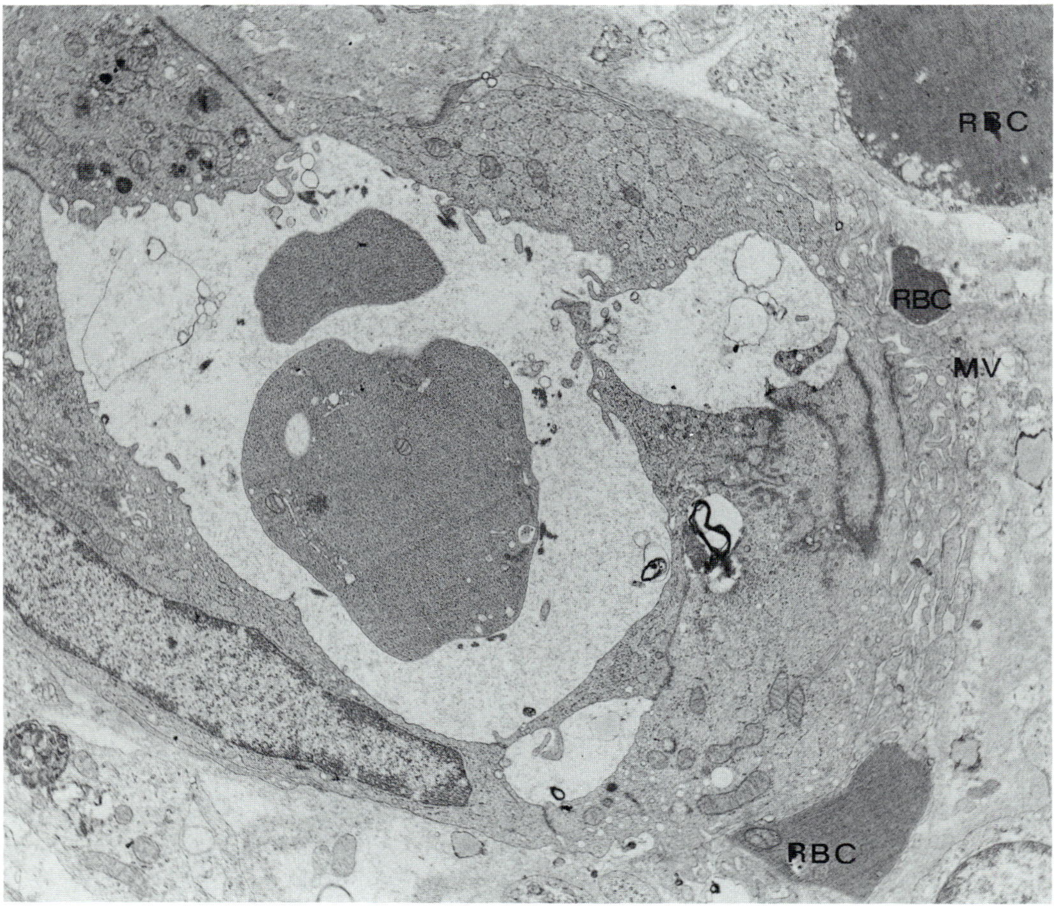
RBC
RBC
MV
RBC

which are reduced comparatively slowly by excretion of the metal. This is presumably due to some abnormality of absorption in the patient. These levels are associated with a syndrome of confusion, myoclonus, ataxia, dysarthria, and seizures, which remits spontaneously as the bismuth blood level falls.[88] The reversibility of the syndrome suggests that pathologic changes would be slight, and these appear to consist only of a slight reduction in numbers of Purkinje cells.[28]

Manganese

Manganese is an industrial poison that is carried to the central nervous system following its inhalation. Clinically there is a Parkinsonian syndrome with coarse tremor, and sometimes with dementia. The pathology of manganese intoxication in the human brain consists of loss of neurons and astrocyte proliferation. The most severe changes are in the globus pallidus and subthalamic nucleus, with some pathology in the rest of the basal ganglia; the cortex appears to be less affected.[30] Pentschew et al.[104] produced experimental manganese poisoning in monkeys that yielded lesions in the globus pallidus and subthalamic nucleus that were identical to those in the human brain; they considered that the primary damage is to glial cells, not neurons. The histology shows large immature astrocytes with very little chromatin.

Aluminium

Interest in the possible toxicity of aluminium has followed the introduction of chronic haemodialysis; very occasionally, patients undergoing this procedure develop an encephalopathy. Comparatively few histological studies have been done on the brains of such patients; Alfrey et al.[6] found no abnormality in those they studied. However, when the aluminium content of the brains was examined,[7] it was found that in the gray matter the level of aluminium in normal brains was 2.2 ppm, in dialysis patients without encephalopathy it was 6.5 ppm, and in encephalopathic brains 25 ppm. Somewhat similar figures were reported by McDermott et al.[85]

The brain pathology that has been suggested as a possible basis for dialysis encephalopathy is neurofibrillary change. This is the change produced in animals when aluminium salts are injected intracerebrally. De Boni et al.[43] injected aluminium salts subcutaneously into rabbits and increased the aluminium concentration of the gray matter from a normal level of 1.1 μg/gram to up to 47.9 μg/gram; there were silver and Congo red-positive deposits, and under the electron microscope 100Å-diameter filaments. Crapper et al.[41] assayed the aluminium content in normal brains and in Alzheimer's disease; the normal brains had 1.2 μg/gram and the Alzheimer brains 4.2μg/gram of aluminium.

There is suggestive evidence, but as yet no

Fig. 15-1. Lead encephalopathy in 10-day-old neonatal rats. (A) The cerebellum is the area of the brain most severely altered by lead intoxication. Hemorrhages are found throughout the central nervous system but are most prominent in the cerebellum. The cerebellar folia are distorted by the accumulation of large amounts of extravascular fluid (arrows). 3.8×. (Press, M. F.: Lead encephalopathy in neonatal Long-Evans rats: Morphologic studies. J. Neuropath. Exp. Neurol. 36:169–193, 1977.) (B) This sagittal section through the vermis shows the characteristic fluid-filled spaces (x) which form deep in the cerebellar folia. 15.7×. (Modified from Press, M. F.: Neuronal development in the cerebellum of lead poisoned neonatal rats. Acta Neuropath. 40:259–268, 1977.) (C) The small blood vessels of the developing cerebellum are often abnormal in lead encephalopathy. This electron micrograph shows three extravascular red blood cells (RBC) related to two distorted interendothelial junctions. This capillary is probably a growing blood vessel as is indicated by the richness of endothelial cytoplasmic organelles, lack of a capillary basement membrane and the presence of microvillus-like (MV) processes along the abluminal surface. 7,200×. (Modified from Press, M. F.: Lead encephalopathy in neonatal Long-Evans rats. Morphologic studies. J. Neuropath. Exp. Neurol. 36:169–193, 1977.)

proof, that dialysis encephalopathy may be related to high serum levels of aluminium.

Mercury

Clinically, inorganic mercury poisoning has occurred in persons involved in hat manufacture; the symptom seen is a "mercury tremor." The lesion appears to be in the basal ganglia and cerebellum, but there are no really adequate pathologic studies of the brain in cases of inorganic mercury poisoning; the intoxication may be accompanied by a peripheral neuropathy, also of unknown pathology.

Pink disease is a neuropathy caused by teething powders containing mercury sublimate; the lesion is a demyelination with retrograde cell change in the neurons of the anterior horns and posterior root ganglia.[103, 157]

Thallium

Thallium salts are used as depilators in the treatment of ringworm, and can be obtained over the counter as rodenticides; they are very toxic, and even at depilatory doses used for children (8 mg/kg), some mild symptoms are frequently observed.

The main toxic effect of thallium on the nervous system is a peripheral neuropathy and retrobulbar neuritis, but changes occur in the brain following larger doses. Bunch et al.[26] described cerebral congestion with chromatolysis of neurons, especially in the third nerve nucleus, the substantia nigra, and the globus pallidus. The patients had hyperpyrexia, possibly due to hypothalamic damage. Osetowska[102] had a case of thallium poisoning in which there was myelin pallor with perivascular loss of myelin and some changes in cortical neurons. Prick et al.[111] found small areas of cortical softening with pyramidal degeneration. Cavanagh et al.[34] described the changes in thallium-induced peripheral neuropathy, which consisted of chromatolysis of the anterior horn cells with distal breakdown of the axon and myelin sheath; Bredemann[14] showed changes in the cells of the posterior root ganglia.

ORGANIC METAL COMPOUNDS

Mercury

In 1954 Hunter and Russell[63] described the changes in the brain of a patient who had inhaled both methylmercury phosphate and nitrate. At about the same time, fishermen and their families around Minimata Bay in Japan began to develop the signs and symptoms of a condition which has become known as Minimata disease; mercury compounds contained in the effluent from a plastics factory had entered the food chain through contaminated bacteria, which methylated the inorganic mercury salts in the effluent.

The main symptoms of Minimata disease are ataxia, slurred speech, tremor, hypersalivation and hyperhidrosis, constricted visual fields, and deterioration of the intellect and personality. The damage to the brain is to the neurons themselves and has a rather specific distribution[127]; it is maximal in the cerebellum and occipital lobe, with less extensive damage in the pre- and postcentral cortex, the insula and adjacent temporal lobe, and the basal ganglia. In all of the affected areas the smaller neurons seem to be those that are involved. In the cerebellum the granule cells are extensively damaged, with sparing of the Golgi type II cells; in severe cases, the Purkinje cells are eventually also destroyed. The basket fibers are affected, with the production of torpedoes, and there is consecutive gliosis. The damage is greater at the depths of the sulci than superficially. In the cerebral cortex there is loss of nerve cells and disintegration of myelin. In the occipital lobe the periphery of the visual cortex is more affected than the central projection, resulting in field restriction. There may be extensive spongy change with gliosis.

Lead

Ethylated and methylated compounds of lead occur in petrol, and appear to be much more toxic than inorganic lead, producing an entirely different clinical and pathologic picture. Toxic damage has occurred in persons who have sniffed gasoline. The lead that issues from the exhaust of the internal combustion engine is inorganic.

The pathologic changes of organic lead intoxication in the brain have been described in humans[146] and in the rabbit.[95] Organic lead produces necrosis of nerve cells, particularly in the cerebellum, the basal ganglia, and the hypothalamus. This is in contrast to the effects of inorganic lead, described earlier. The amount of research that has been done on organic lead is much less than that done on the inorganic metal, and we do not know much about interconversion of the two. It is possible that bacteria can methylate inorganic lead, and also that the organic salt may split producing the inorganic metal.

ETHYL ALCOHOL

Ethyl alcohol has been used as a euphoriant, often to considerable excess, for hundreds of years. Gross overdosage can produce coma and death, but this is rare; the more usual acute fatalities are associated with the inhalation of vomit or exposure.

Alcoholism is associated with a number of general diseases that may affect brain pathology, such as hepatic cirrhosis with the sludging of blood in small vessels,[89] fat embolism from the liver,[81] and deficiency diseases. Neurons cannot metabolize ethanol and may suffer from hypoglycemia. These, as well as changes following cerebral arterial disease, may make the interpretation of brain pathology difficult in cases of alcohol intoxication.

Ethyl alcohol consists of "empty calories" so that, although it will maintain life for some time, the association of its consumption with an inadequate diet can produce deficiency syndromes, particularly of thiamine. The most important of these syndromes is Wernicke's encephalopathy. In this condition the pathology is maximal in the hypothalamus and mamillary body, consisting of small hemorrhages and vascular proliferation. There may be an associated gliosis, but neuronal damage is secondary and often not very severe.

The Marchiafava-Bignami syndrome also occurs in persons with alcoholism. It consists of partial demyelination of the corpus callosum, leaving some axons intact.[82] It may also affect parts of the centrum semiovale and other commissures, such as the anterior commissure. In severe cases the oligodendrocytes are reduced in number. The syndrome was originally thought to be due to the substance present in cheap Italian wine; it has since been seen in nonalcoholic individuals, and is rare in non-Latin peoples. The syndrome appears to involve a disease of oligodendrocytes, and it has been suggested that there is a racial or genetic weakness in these cells in some individuals.[19,66] Central pontine myelinolysis is a lesion that is histologically similar to that in Marchiafava-Bignami syndrome, but is not confined to alcoholics.

The pathology of direct neuronal damage by ethyl alcohol is more difficult to establish. There have been comparatively few published attempts to produce experimental damage to the brain with ethanol; Lhermitte et al.[78] fed absinthe to rabbits, but the relatively slight changes they produced could be reversed by thiamine.

Cortical atrophy from ethanol has been shown by air encephalography,[22,58] although numbers of patients were small, and normal variations in brain size are considerable. A number of pathologists have described cortical atrophy particularly in the frontal areas of the brain[5,40,143]; degenerative changes in the cerebellum, in both Purkinje cells and the granular layer, have also been seen.[8,93] These changes were examined in detail by Victor et al.,[148] who described damage, particularly in the anterior and superior parts of the vermis, but came to the conclusion that although such damage occurred in alcoholics, it was not necessarily due to alcohol, but could also be due to some associated deficiency disorder. Allsop and Turner[8] describe seven cases of alcoholic cerebellar atrophy which came to postmortem; in 6 of these there were pathologic changes of Wernicke's encephalopathy, suggesting that thiamine deficiency played a part in the etiology.

Peripheral neuropathy occurs in alcoholics and is probably due to thiamine deficiency. Walsh and McCleod[152] showed this neuropathy to be an axonal degeneration, with a reduction in the numbers of fibers of all diameters. This was confirmed by Tredici and Minazzi[142] with the electron microscope; they described Wallerian degeneration in myelinated and unmyelinated fibers. The peripheral neuropathy is thus probably due to the effect of thiamine deficiency on the neurons in the posterior root ganglia.

METHYL ALCOHOL

Because it is cheaper than ethyl alcohol, a considerable amount of methyl alcohol is drunk by down-and-out individuals. In large quantities it appears to have a rather specific effect on the neurons of the retina, producing blindness; it is converted in the body to formic acid and formaldehyde, which probably do the damage to the retina. The conversion is catalyzed by the same enzyme, alcohol dehydrogenase, that converts ethanol to acetic acid and acetaldehyde. There is, therefore, substrate competition, and the amount of retinal damage will depend on the amount of ethyl alcohol drunk simultaneously or subsequently. Ethyl alcohol can be used to treat methyl alcohol poisoning.

In fatal cases of methyl alcohol poisoning, the pathology of the brain itself is rather nonspecific, consisting of small hemorrhages, edema, and some neuronal degeneration.[13] There is chromatolysis and fallout of retinal neurons.

STEROIDS

Benign intracranial hypertension is a condition in which there is headache, papilledema, and occasionally other clinical manifestations of increased intracranial pressure. The condition sometimes occurs spontaneously, nearly always in women, who may be overweight. In one woman it occurred with every menstrual period, subsiding in between.[138] Another factor associated with benign intracranial hypertension is otitis media. In those cases that have been investigated, the ventricular system is normal.

Benign intracranial hypertension has been reported in a number of instances in relation to corticosteroid therapy. It is somewhat paradoxical that steroids are also used to treat the condition[97]; however, some cases have occurred when long-term steroid treatment has been reduced or modified.[56,150] Other authors have reported recovery after steroid treatment has been stopped.[135] Most steroid-associated cases have occurred in children. The condition has also been reported in cases of Addison's disease.[69,151] Investigations on six females with the spontaneous disease[100] and one steroid-associated case in an adult[67] have shown that although ACTH stimulation tests are normal, there is no response to metyrapone, suggesting that the lesion in benign intracranial hypertension is pituitary/hypothalamic rather than adrenal.

ORAL CONTRACEPTIVES

There have been a number of reports suggesting that oral contraceptives may produce cerebrovascular occlusion. In women of childbearing age with "strokes," more than expected were found to have been taking the "pill."

In particular, there have been reports of vertebrobasilar lesions—which are otherwise rather uncommon—among oral contraceptive users.[84,116] However, although some angiograms were done, many patients were diagnosed on clinical evidence alone. The presence or absence of hypertension is not always stated. Against this, Jennett and Cross[70] reported a series of 146 patients between the ages of 15 and 45, of whom 44.5 percent were female; 40 out of 42 nonpregnant women in the series were known not to be taking contraceptives, 20 were pregnant or puerperal. Angiography was done on 142 and autopsy on the remaining 4 fatal cases. Two-thirds showed major arterial occlusion. In addition to Jennett and Cross's study, Illis et al.[64] published a small series showing no significant increase in arterial occlusion in patients taking oral contraceptives. Markush and Seigel[83] have published the American figures of deaths from thromboembolism in women of childbearing age; they show no increase in the incidence of such deaths since oral contraceptives became available, and no alteration in the male/female ratio. This would suggest that if oral contraceptives are a precipitating factor of death from thromboembolism, there must be a reduction in mortality elsewhere. Most authors supplying figures for the incidence of cerebral occlusion in patients taking oral contraceptives do not supply the figures for the incidence in the same age group before contraceptives were available.

Oral contraceptives produce platelet aggregation, which would be an obvious factor in the production of thrombosis. Kjae et al.[72] has suggested that platelet destruction releases the level of 5-hydroxytryptamine, which produces vasospasm in the cerebral vessels, with resultant occlusion. Some patients who have had angiograms have had multiple lesions, as shown in one case described by Jacobs et al.[68] Although good postmortem studies are scarce, Altschuler et al.[9] described one fatal case in detail. They showed fibrinoid swelling of small arteries, with narrowing of the lumen. Unfortunately, the patient had been in a respirator for 5 days and this may have added to the vascular damage. Irey et al.[65] described vascular lesions associated with the use of female reproductive steroids, although they did not discuss cerebral vessels. They found intimal proliferation, with reduction in the size of the lumens of arteries. There was some increase in intercellular stroma, both myxomatous and fibrous. Irey et al. suggest that these changes, together with a labile clotting system, may result in thrombosis.

It would appear that oral contraceptives may be a factor in cerebral arterial occlusive disease, but we do not yet know whether this is purely a coagulation abnormality or whether there are also changes in the blood vessel walls.

Cortical venous thrombosis and thrombosis of venous sinuses occurs in patients taking oral contraceptives, as it does in pregnancy.[10,25,48,107] Benign intracranial hypertension, which is discussed in the section on steroids, may also be associated with oral contraceptives, remitting when the drug is stopped.[39]

ANTIBIOTICS AND ANTIBACTERIAL AGENTS

Penicillin given in very large quantities can produce seizures.[17,38,131] The dose given in the cases reported was in excess of 25 million units a day, and in the majority of cases renal failure was an additional complication. A cerebrospinal fluid penicillin concentration of more than 10 units/ml is considered the danger level; the mortality in humans has been very low, and no neuropathology is available. Topical applications of penicillin to the brain have been shown to produce seizures in animals,[53] particularly when given into the ventricle.

NITROFURANTOIN

Nitrofurantoin is used mainly as a urinary antiseptic. Attempts have been made to use it in trypanosomiasis, but the dose required appears to be too high to be tolerated. Polyneuropathy has been reported in patients given the drug, and the worst cases are those in which there is renal impairment.[47,136,141] Graebner and Heskowitz[55] have described cerebellar dysfunction during nitrofurantoin therapy. They suggest that the changes could be similar to those produced by phenytoin, and could be related to folate deficiency. Briand and Tygstrup[23] described the disintegration of myelin sheaths in the nerves and nerve roots in patients given nitrofurantoin. Behar et al.[12] gave nitrofurantoin to rats and produced axonal breakdown in the sciatic and brachial nerves.

ISONIAZID

Isoniazid can produce both peripheral neuropathy and encephalopathy. The former is much more common, and can be prevented by the simultaneous administration of pyridoxine. The peripheral nerves from patients with isoniazid neuropathy have been studied ultrastructurally by Ochoa,[96] who found a loss of both myelinated and unmyelinated fibers, with some regeneration. Experimental work with animals has shown Wallerian degeneration of axons[118] and retrograde cell change in the nerve cells of the spinal ganglia.[119]

The damage done by isoniazid to the central nervous system, if the dose is large, results in coma and seizures.[50,106] Normal doses have been reported to result in some degree of memory impairment.[101] These changes are less easily reversed by pyridoxine.[1] The only pathologic changes reported are swelling of the large neurons of the cortex, with peripheral displacement of the nucleus.[147] These are similar to the changes in pellagra. Toxic changes appear to occur only in patients who are "slow activators" of isoniazid.

ANTINEOPLASTIC AGENTS

Drugs given for their antimitotic activity may affect neurons either by their effect on nucleic acids, of which neurons contain a large amount, or by their effect on neurotubules.

Daunomycin

Daunomycin is an antineoplastic agent that binds specifically to DNA[29]; it inhibits DNA-dependent RNA polymerase and possibly intercalates between the base pairs of DNA.[45] The use of daunomycin in cancer chemotherapy has been limited by its cardiotoxicity, and some newer compounds, such as Adriamycin, are slightly less dangerous in this respect. The neurotoxicity of daunomycin, however, appears to be similar to that of Adriamycin. Daunomycin does not cross the blood-brain barrier, and the damage so far described has been in autonomic and posterior root ganglia. Loss of neurons has been seen in human cardiac ganglia.[129] Cho[36] did an ultrastructural study of the posterior root ganglia in rats given Adriamycin. There was some necrosis of neurons, and the less severely damaged cells showed an increase in neurofibrils. The peripheral nerves showed axonal degeneration, and there was some loss of fibers in the posterior columns.

Methotrexate

Methotrexate is a very useful antineoplastic agent, but it does not cross the blood-brain barrier. It has been used increasingly in leukemia and other malignancies by the intrathecal and occasionally by the intraventricular route. In leukemia, methotrexate is also used prophylactically, since it is thought that residual neoplasm, untreatable by other systemic drugs, may remain in the nervous system. Methotrexate was given intraventricularly to treat brain tumours by Wilson and Norrell,[156] Bresnan et al.[21] and Shapiro et al.[123] There was extensive coagulative necrosis of the white matter, but some of their patients had obstruction to the ventricular system, which might have resulted in a higher local concentration of the drug. Kay et al.[71] described encephalopathy following intrathecal methotrexate for leukemia. One brain was examined histologically; this showed infarcts, with fibrinoid necrosis of blood vessel walls. In 1975, Smith[130] described the brain pathology in 10 cases of leukemia given intrathecal methotrexate and craniospinal irradiation. Two patients showed large areas of white matter in which the oligodendrocytes had been destroyed. The myelin was pale but there was no breakdown and no fat granule cells were seen. A third patient showed areas of coagulative necrosis. Six others showed severe astrocytosis without much glial fiber formation (Fig. 15-2).

The main toxic effect of methotrexate appears to be on the oligodendrocyte; neuronal damage has not been described. The oligodendrocyte differs from the neuron in that it depends for its energy on the hexose monophosphate shunt, and is low in Krebs cycle enzymes.[87] However, this does not explain why the oligodendrocyte should be more sensitive to folate antagonists. It may be that the cell damage is due to synergism between methotrexate and radiotherapy. A chromosome fracture produced by the latter requires DNA-dependent RNA synthesis for repair[158]; methotrexate, by inhibiting nucleic acid synthesis, might prevent this repair, whereas neither agent alone would do significant damage. The time relationship between the administration of the two types of therapy could be critical; thus, only an occasional patient will receive fatal damage. Perhaps more worrying is the astrocytosis that appears to occur in most cases treated with methotrexate and radiotherapy, since this is likely to produce some impairment of cerebration in long-term survivors.

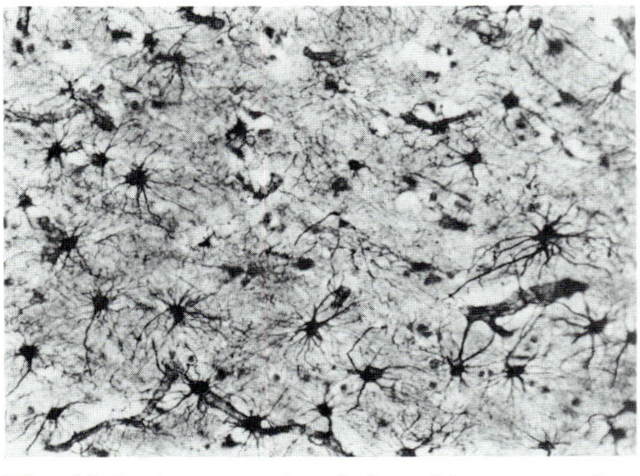

Fig. 15-2. Astrocytosis of the white matter in a patient with acute lymphatic leukemia given methotrexate intrathecally. Cajal × 115.

Vinca Alkaloids

The vinca alkaloids, vincristine and vinblastine, are spindle poisons like colchicine. They have a useful antimitotic effect, arresting the cell in metaphase.[32] Neurotubules, which are morphologically somewhat similar to the tubules of the mitotic spindle, appear to be the neuronal structures affected by the vinca alkaloids; however, these drugs do not normally cross the blood-brain barrier. On one occasion, vincristine was given intrathecally[117] and produced extensive neuronal damage, particularly to anterior horn cells. Shelanski and Wisniewski[124] showed, under the electron microscope, that in rabbits the first neuronal change produced by vincristine was a breakdown in the neurotubules, with a disruption of axoplasmic flow. Later, the tubules were replaced by neurofibrillary tangles similar to those seen in Alzheimer's disease. The changes were most marked in the posterior root ganglia.

Clinically, vincristine neurotoxicity presents with a predominantly autonomic or sensory neuropathy. The former may produce intestinal pseudo-obstruction.[16] Later there may be some muscle weakness which is reversed when the drug is stopped; the decrease in the amplitude of the sensory action potential persists after cessation of vincristine therapy.[33] Nerve biopsy shows mainly axonal degeneration.[86]

The vinca alkaloids damage the neurotubules of cells such as those of the posterior root ganglia and autonomic ganglia, which are outside the blood-brain barrier. With higher doses the anterior horn cells may also suffer, although less severely.

ANTICOAGULANTS

Patients on poorly controlled anticoagulant therapy can bleed anywhere, and although bleeding within the skull or spinal column is uncommon, the results may be unfortunate. The bleeding may be intracerebral,[11,154] and in such cases the mortality has been much higher in patients with hypertension. Subdural hematoma, either above or below the tentorium, is probably the most common complication, and in many instances has been precipitated by minor head injury.[31,134,155] Epidural spinal hematoma also occurs, and may result in paraplegia.[4,122,133] In 1963, Mosley et al. reviewed long-term anticoagulant therapy in 978 patients.[90] Among these, there were 15 major complications, of which 1 was a subdural hematoma. At that time, therefore, the incidence of neurologic complications from anticoagulants was about one per thousand patients treated; it is probably less now.

CARBON MONOXIDE

Carbon monoxide, whose affinity for hemoglobin is 200 times that of oxygen, combines with hemoglobin to form carboxyhemoglobin. Carbon monoxide thus replaces oxygen so that less is available for the tissues; in addition, it shifts the dissociation curve of oxyhemoglobin to the left, so that the oxygen that is available is released less easily. The blood flow in carbon monoxide poisoning is initially normal, and at this stage the condition is a true anoxic anoxia. However, anoxia also affects the capillary endothelium, causing edema because of increased permeability. If the damage is severe there may be thrombosis of small vessels. Carbon monoxide also has an affinity for cytochrome oxidase, and may produce some cellular damage.

The clinical effects of carbon monoxide poisoning, which consist of headache and exertional dyspnea, begin to occur when 20 percent of the hemoglobin has combined with carbon monoxide. Consciousness is lost at 60 to 70 percent carboxyhemoglobin and death ensues at higher concentrations.[24]

The pathology in acute cases of carbon monoxide poisoning is mainly related to vascular endothelial damage, consisting of edema and pinpoint hemorrhages in the white matter, the corpus callosum, and the basal ganglia. Thrombi can be seen in small vessels. The whole brain shows the pink color common to all viscera affected by carboxyhemoglobin.

If the patient survives, there may be a number of neurologic sequelae, including epilepsy, dementia and Parkinsonism; these sequelae are given in detail by Garland and Pearce.[52] The pathology in long-surviving cases particularly shows cortical atrophy and necrosis of the globus pallidus. The cortical damage may be laminar, from the direct effect of anoxia on neurons, and there is loss of nerve cells in the hippocampus and the Purkinje layer of the cerebellum. In addition to this damage to areas of selective vulnerability, there is necrosis due to focal vascular ischemia. All of these changes are accompanied by extensive gliosis. A characteristic finding in survivors of carbon monoxide poisoning is softening of the globus pallidus, which is usually bilateral. It affects the anteromedial parts of the nucleus and may be accompanied by other areas of necrosis in the striatum, thalamus, subthalamic nucleus, and substantia nigra. In most cases there is white matter loss leading to ventricular enlargement. Sometimes the white matter damage is more severe, with patchy, coalescing demyelination and fat-granule cells throughout the centrum semiovale.[120]

The effect of carbon monoxide on the infant brain, and particularly on that of the fetus, is much more severe than on the adult brain.

HYPOGLYCEMIA

Hypoglycemic brain damage usually follows injected insulin or occurs in insulinomas; however, occasional cases occur in pituitary and adrenal insufficiency. In many fatal cases the pure hypoglycemic cerebral pathology is modified by damage to cardiac and respiratory function, and sometimes by epileptic fits.

The appearances of the brain in fatal cases of hypoglycemia vary with the time of survival after the hypoglycemic episode; brain swelling is not a striking feature in the early stages. With increasing survival time, there is ventricular enlargement, cortical atrophy, and loss of structure in the hippocampus. Histologically, many neurons show ischemic change, progressing to fallout. However, although the areas of selective vulnerability are damaged, the extent of the injury in each area is somewhat different from that seen in other types of anoxia. The cortical necrosis is usually laminar, mainly affecting the third and fifth layers, but areas of full thickness necrosis or focal damage are seen, with microglial and astrocytic proliferation.[24, 77] The major damage is to the hippocampus, which may be completely necrotic. Lesions in the globus pallidus are unusual,[149] but the thalamus, and especially the lateral nucleus, may be involved. Purkinje cell loss is sometimes quite slight. Diffuse loss of myelin may accompany the cortical damage,[114] and there may be marked white matter gliosis.

Peripheral neuropathy in hypoglycemia is rare and mild. There are no pathologic studies, but the clinical picture has been reviewed by Wanchode[153] and Ziegler.[159]

PHENYTOIN

Diphenylhydantoin (DPH) seems to be a drug whose dosage must be very carefully controlled, preferably by serum levels; there have been instances of poisoning due to a change in the type of capsule used.[18] DPH can cause trouble when given together with other drugs, such as isoniazid, particularly in people who are "slow inactivators" of the latter.[20] In animals to which isoniazid was given together with DPH, the peak concentration of the latter was raised, and there was prolonged persistence of unmetabolized DPH.[75]

Clinically, DPH intoxication presents with nystagmus, ataxia, impaired intellectual performance, bizarre behavior, impaired speech, and an increased incidence of fits.[145] The main pathologic change is a loss of Purkinje cells, with gliosis, and a less significant loss of granule cells.[60, 73, 145] There may be difficulties in interpreting the specific effects of DPH intoxication, since the patients are likely to be epileptics, and repeated fits may produce a similar pathologic picture, although loss of Ammon's horn cells is not a feature of DPH intoxication.

Experimental studies of DPH intoxication in animals have produced conflicting results. Some have shown Purkinje cell damage and loss,[73, 144] while others have denied any change[42, 94] after DPH administration.

The neuronal loss produced by DPH is probably due to folate deficiency. In the normal individual, the folate level in the CSF is three times that in the serum; in phenytoin-treated epileptics, however, the CSF folate level is very low.[113] Therefore, if patients receiving DPH are given folate, it may improve cerebral retardation. The localization of most of the neuronal change produced by DPH to the cerebellum may be the result of the way in which the drug is localized in the brain. Kokenge et al.[73] found that when DPH was given to cats, more of the drug was found in the cerebellum than the cerebrum.

In addition to cerebellar change, DPH can produce peripheral neuropathy.[80, 121]

PSYCHOTROPIC DRUGS

Abnormal movements in patients taking phenothiazines were described by Hunter et al. in 1964;[61] these seem to occur only in patients taking large doses for long periods, and sometimes persist after the drug has been stopped. Yet despite the striking clinical picture, pathologic studies of the effects of phenothiazines have been few and not entirely satisfactory.

The clinical efficiency of drugs such as chlorpromazine is said to be related to their effect on dopamine receptors.[49, 132] One would therefore, perhaps, expect to find pathology in dopaminergic pathways. de Jaramillo and Guth[44] used dogs to show the intracerebral distribution of phenothiazines. They found concentrations of these drugs—in descending order—in the medulla, hypothalamus, basal ganglia, thalamus, hippocampus, pons, amygdala, and midbrain. Two varieties of cerebral pathology have been found in humans; Christensen et al.[37] found degeneration in neurons of the substantia nigra and gliosis in the brain stem; Greiner and Nicholson[57] found deposits of a pigment similar to lipofuscin in cortical neurons, the meninges, and cells of the choroid plexus. This pigment was also seen in the viscera. However, these sorts of changes are difficult to assess in patients of this group, and in the view of Hunter et al.[62] the changes they found were nonspecific.

Other psychotropic drugs are known to produce clinical neurologic side effects, but the pathology of these is unknown.

QUINOLINES

Quinolines and related cyclic compounds, when given by mouth, usually pass either through the alimentary canal without absorption or are conjugated to harmless and ineffective compounds. It is likely that most of them are neurotoxic when given parenterally, and most intravenous or intramuscular preparations have been withdrawn by the manufacturers.

A patient given many times the therapeutic dose of pamaquine developed nuclear cranial nerve palsies.[79] In animals, nitroxoline and mepacrine damage myenteric neurons when given intraperitoneally, without other ill-effects.[98, 128] A much more controversial quinoline is clioquinol (iodochlorhydroxyquin), which has been thought to produce subacute myelo-opticoneuropathy (SMON).

SMON was first recognized in Japan in the mid-1950s. It reached a peak in 1969 and has since declined. Only a handful of authenticated cases appear to have occurred outside Japan. SMON presents clinically with such abdominal symptoms as pain, diarrhea, and constipation, with dysesthesia, weakness, and visual loss. There is sometimes a greenish discoloration of the dorsum of the tongue, which is based on the ferric ion chelate of 5-chloro,7-iodo,8-hydroxyquinoline.

The pathology in SMON has been described by Nelson[92] and Shiraki;[126] it consists of demyelination of the posterior columns of the spinal cord, the medial fibers being more affected than the lateral, and with some involvement of the lateral and anterior columns and the spinocerebellar tracts. There is disintegration of neurons in the posterior root ganglia and the sympathetic ganglia. There is loss of ganglion cells of the inner layer of the retina, and demyelination of the optic nerve. It is not clear whether there is a primary demyelinating lesion or whether the loss of myelin in the optic nerve is secondary. Within the brain there are no lesions above the tentorium, but changes have been seen in the neurons of the olive, the Purkinje cells of the cerebellum, and the pyramidal cells of the reticular formation. These findings suggest that most of the damage in SMON occurs in structures outside the blood-brain barrier, and that the amounts of clioquinol that get through the barrier may be small.

Japanese workers[125] are convinced that SMON is the result of poisoning by clioquinol. The majority of patients with the condition have taken the drug, often in large doses; however, since the drug has been withdrawn from use, the condition is disappearing. Some workers, including Tateishi and Otsuki,[137] have been able to reproduce the disease in animals. There seems to be a species difference in susceptibility; dogs and cats develop spinal cord and optic nerve demyelination, while rats, mice, and rabbits develop only a peripheral neuropathy. Workers at Ciba-Geigy, who market one brand of clioquinol,[59] have failed to produce any neurotoxic effects in animals with similar doses to those used by Tateishi and Otsuki.

One difficulty in ascribing the cause of

SMON to clioquinol is that there appear to be about 15 percent of patients with the condition who have not taken the drug. Even allowing for poor historians and mistakes in diagnosis, this suggests that there may be unrelated cases. Another curious feature is that, although clioquinol can be bought without prescription in many Western countries, it is only in Japan that the disease has become important. One explanation for this may be that in the West clioquinol is usually taken for traveller's diarrhea, which means that it is likely to be taken for short periods only. In Japan, long-lasting diarrhea may be more common than in the West, where it tends to be related to infection, and is self-limiting. Certainly there is evidence that large numbers of people in Japan were taking the drug in high doses over long periods.

The amount of clioquinol that is absorbed may be affected by the bacterial content of the gut, which may also influence its conjugation and inactivation. There could also be a genetic difference in the enzyme activity of intestinal cells. Alternatively, the drug could be one factor in a multifactorial disease, potentiating a virus or other environmental factor. The clinical, experimental, and epidemiologic evidence suggests that clioquinol plays a predominant role in the causation of SMON.

REFERENCES

1. Adams, P. & White, C.: Isoniazid-induced encephalopathy. Lancet 1:680-682, 1965.
2. Ahrens, F. A., & Vistica, D. A.: Microvascular effects of lead in the neo-natal rat *1* Histochemical and light microscopic studies. Exp. Mol. Pathol. 26:129-138.
3. Akelaitis, A. J.: Lead encephalopathy in children and adults; Clinicopathological study. J. Nerv. Ment. Dis. 93:313-332, 1941.
4. Alderman, D. B.: Extradural spinal cord hematoma. Report of a case due to dicumarol and review of the literature. N. Engl. J. Med. 255:839-842, 1956.
5. Alexander, I.: Neuropathological findings in the brain and spinal cord of chronic alcoholics. Quart. J. Stud. Alc. 2:260-262, 1941.
6. Alfrey, A. C., Mishell, J. M., Burke, J., et al.: Syndrome of dyspraxia and multifocal seizures associated with chronic haemodialysis. Trans. Am. Soc. Artif. Intern. Organs 18:257-261, 1972.
7. Alfrey, A. C., LeGendre, G. R., & Kaehny, W. D.: The dialysis encephalopathy syndrome. N. Engl. J. Med. 294:184-188, 1976.
8. Allsop, J., & Turner, B.: Cerebellar degeneration associated with chronic alcoholism. J. Neurol. Sci. 3:238-258, 1966.
9. Altshuler, J. H., McLoughlin, R. A., & Neuberger, K. T.: Neurological catastrophe related to oral contraceptives. Arch. Neurol. 19:264-273, 1968.
10. Atkinson, E. A., Fairburn, B., & Heathfield, K. W.: Intracranial venous thrombosis as complication of oral contraception. Lancet 1:914-918, 1970.
11. Barron, K. D., & Ferguson, G.: Intracranial haemorrhage as a complication of anti-coagulant therapy. Neurology 9:447-455, 1959.
12. Behar, A., Rachmilewitz, E., Rahamimoff, R., & Deman, M.: Experimental nitrofurantoin neuropathy in rats. Arch. Neurol. 13:160-163, 1965.
13. Bennett, I. L., Cary, F. H., Mitchell, G. L., & Cooper, M. N.: Acute methyl alcohol poisoning. A review based on experiences in an outbreak of 323 cases. Medicine 32:431-463, 1953.
14. Bredemann, W.: Zur Histopathologie der Thalliumvergiftung im Bereich des Nervensystem. Arch. Psychiatr. Nervenkr. 192:393-404, 1954.
15. Blackman, S. S., Jr.: The lesions of lead encephalitis in children. Bull. Johns Hopkins Hosp. 61:1-61, 1937.
16. Bleehan, N. M., & Jeliffe, A. M.: Vinblastine sulphate in the treatment of malignant disease. Br. J. Cancer 19:268-273, 1965.
17. Bloomer, H., Barton, L., & Maddock, R.: Penicillin induced encephalopathy in uraemic patients. J.A.M.A. 200:121-123, 1967.
18. Bochner, F., Hooper, W. D., Tyrer, J. H., & Eadie, M. J.: Factors involved in an outbreak of phenytoin intoxication. J. Neurol. Sci. 16:481-487, 1972.
19. Bohrod, M. G.: Primary degeneration of the corpus callosum (Marchiafava's disease). Arch. Neurol. Psychiatr. 47:465-473, 1942.
20. Brennan, R. W., Dehejia, H., Kutt, H.,

Veresely, K., & McDowell, F.: Diphenyl hydantoin intoxication attendant to show inactivation of isoniazid. Neurology 20:687-693, 1970.

21. Bresnan, M. J., Giles, F. H., Lorenzo, A. V., Watters, G. V., & Barlow, C. F.: Luro-encephalopathy following combined irradiation and intraventricular Methotrexate therapy of brain tumours in children. Trans. Am. Neurol. Assoc. 97:204-206, 1972.
22. Brewer, C., & Perrett, L.: Brain damage due to alcohol consumption. An air-encephalographic psychometric and electro-encephalographic study. Br. J. Addict. 66:170-182, 1971.
23. Briand, P., & Tygstrup, I.: Polyneuritis efter behandlung med. nitrofurantoin (Furadantin) Agesk. Laege 121:664, 1959.
24. Brierley, J. B.: Cerebral hypoxia. In: Blackwood, W., & Corsellis, J. A. N., Eds.: Greenfield's Neuropathology. 3rd Ed.: Edward Arnold, London, 1976.
25. Buchanan, D. S., & Brazinsky, J. M.: Dural sinus and cerebral venous thrombosis. Incidence in young women receiving oral contraceptives. Arch. Neurol. 22:440-444, 1970.
26. Bunch, J. C., Ginsberg, H. M., & Nixon, C. E.: The 1932 Thallotoxicosis outbreak in California. J.A.M.A. 100:1315-1319, 1933.
27. Burge, A., et al.: Twenty cases of acute encephalopathy with myoclonus during treatments with orally administered bismuth salts. Ann. Med. Interne (Paris) 125:877-888, 1974.
28. Burns, R., Thomas, D. W., & Barron, V. J.: Reversible encephalopathy possibly associated with bismuth subgallate ingestion. Br. Med. J. 1:220-223, 1974.
29. Calendi, E., Di Marco, A., Reggiani, M., Scarpinato, B., & Valentini, L.: On physico-chemical interaction between daunomycin and nucleic acids. Biochim. Biophys. Acta 103:25-49, 1965.
30. Canavan, M., Cobb, S., & Drinker, C. K.: Chronic manganese poisoning. Arch. Neurol. 32:501-512, 1934.
31. Capistrant, T., Goldberg, R., Shibsaki, H., & Castle, D.: Posterior fossa subdural haematoma associated with anticoagulant therapy. J. Neurol. Neurosurg. Psychiatry 34:82-85, 1971.
32. Cardinali, G., Cardinali, G., & Blair, J.: The stathmokinetic effect of vincaleukoblastine on normal bone marrow and leukaemic cells. Cancer Res. 21:1542-1544, 1961.
33. Casey, E. B., Jellife, A. M., LeQuesne, P. M., & Millett, Y. L.: Vincristine neuropathy. Clinical and electrophysiological observations. Brain 96:69-86, 1973.
34. Cavanagh, J. B., Fuller, N. H., Johnson, H. M., & Rudge, P.: The effects of thallium salts with particular reference to the nervous system changes. Q. J. Med. 43:293-319, 1974.
35. Chuttani, P. N., Chawla, L. S., & Sharma, T. D.: Arsenical neuropathy. Neurology (Minneap) 17:269-274, 1967.
36. Cho, E. S.: Toxic effects of adriamycin on the ganglia of the peripheral nervous system. A neuropathological study. J. Neuropath. Exp. Neurol. 36:907-915, 1977.
37. Christensen, E., Moller, J. E., & Fayrbye, A.: Neuropathological investigation of 28 brains from patients with dyskinesia. Acta Psychiat. Scand. 46:14-23, 1970.
38. Conway, H., Beck, E., & Somerville, J.: Penicillin encephalopathy. Postgrad. Med. J. 44:891-897, 1968.
39. Cosnett, J. E.: Strokes and the pill. Br. Med. J. 2:450, 1969.
40. Courville, C. B.: Effects of Alcohol on the Nervous System of Man. San Lucas Press, Los Angeles, 1966.
41. Crapper, D. R.: Neuronal correlates of an encephalopathy associated with aluminium neurofibrillary degeneration. Brain Res. 97:253-264, 1975.
42. Dam, M.: Number of Purkinje cells after diphenylhydantoin intoxication in pigs. Arch. Neurol. 22:64-67, 1970.
43. DeBoni, V., Otvos, A., Scott, J. W., & Crapper, D. R.: Neurofibrillary degeneration induced by systemic aluminium. Acta Neuropathol. (Berlin) 35:285-294, 1976.
44. de Jaramillo, G. A. V., & Guth, P. S.: A study of the localisation of phenothiazines in dog brain. Biochem. Pharmacol. 12:525-532, 1963.
45. Di Marco, A.: Daunomycin pharmacological activity at the cellular level. Pathol. Biol. (Paris) 15:897-902, 1967.
46. Ecker, A. D., & Kernohan, J. W.: Arsenic as a possible cause of subacute encephalomyelitis. Arch. Neurol. 45:24-43, 1941.
47. Ellis, F. G.: Acute polyneuritis after nitrofurantoin therapy. Lancet 2:1136-1138, 1962.
48. Fairburn, B.: Intracranial venous thrombosis

complicating oral contraception. Treatment by anti-coagulant drugs. Br. Med. J. 2:647, 1973.

49. Feinberg, A. P., & Snyder, S. H.: Phenothiazine drugs structure activity relationships explained by a conformation that mimics dopamine. Proc. Natl. Acad. Sci. U.S.A. 72:1899-1903, 1975.
50. Friedman, S. A.: Death following massive ingestion of isoniazid. Am. Rev. Resp. Dis. 100:859-862, 1969.
51. Fullerton, P. M.: Chronic peripheral neuropathy produced by lead poisoning in guinea pigs. J. Neuropathol. Exp. Neurol. 25:214-231, 1966.
52. Garland, H., & Pearce, J.: Neurological complications of carbon monoxide poisoning. Q. J. Med. 36:445-455, 1967.
53. Gloor, P.: Epileptogenic agent of penicillin. Ann. N.Y. Acad. Sci. 166:350-360, 1969.

53a. Gombault, A.: Contribution à l'étude anatomique de la névrite parenchymateuse subaigüe ou chronique: Névrite segmentaire péri-axile. Arch. Neurol. 1:11-38, 1880.

54. Grzycki, S., & Kobusowna, B.: Histophysiological effects of arsenic and its derivatives on the central nervous system, and particularly on the third element of the central nervous system. J. Neuropathol. 10:325-337, 1951.
55. Graebner, R. W., & Heskowitz, A.: Cerebellar Toxic effects from nitrofurantoin. Arch. Neurol. 29:195-196, 1973.
56. Greer, M.: Benign intracranial hypertension II following corticosteroid therapy. Neurology (Minneap) 13:439-441, 1963.
57. Greiner, A. C., & Nicholson, G. A.: Pigment deposition in the viscera associated with prolonged chlorpromazine therapy. Can. Med. Assoc. J. 91:627-635, 1964.
58. Haug, J. O.: Pneumo-encephalographic evidence of brain damage in chronic alcoholics. Acta Psychiat. Scand. (Suppl.) 203:135-143, 1968.
59. Hess, R., Keberle, H., Koella, W., Schmidt, K., & Gelzer, J.: Clioquinol; absence of neurotoxicity in laboratory animals. Lancet 2:424-425, 1972.
60. Hofman, W. W.: Cerebellar lesions after parenteral dilantin administration. Neurology (Minneap) 8:210-214, 1958.
61. Hunter, R., Earl, C. J., & Thornicroft, S.: An apparently irreversible syndrome of abnormal movements following phenothiazine medication. Proc. R. Soc. Med. 57:758-762, 1964.
62. Hunter, R., Blackwood, W., Smith, M. C., & Cumings, J. N.: Neuropathological findings in three cases of persistent dyskinesia following phenothiazine medication. J. Neurol. Sci. 7:263-273, 1968.
63. Hunter, D., & Russell, D. S.: Focal cerebral and cerebellar atrophy in a human subject due to organic mercury compounds. J. Neurol. Psychiatr. 17:235-241, 1954.
64. Illis, L., Kocken, R. S., McDonald, W. I., & Mondkar, V. P.: Oral Contraceptives and cerebral arterial occlusion. Br. Med. J. 2:1164-1166, 1965.
65. Irey, N. B., & Norris, H. J.: Intimal vascular lesions associated with female reproductive steroids. Arch. Pathol. 96:227-234, 1973.
66. Ironside, R., Bosanquet, F. D., & McMenemey, W. H.: Central demyelination of the corpus callosum (Marchiafava-Bignami disease). Brain 84:212-230, 1961.
67. Ivey, K., & Den Besten, L.: Pseudotumour cerebri associated with corticosteroid therapy in an adult. J.A.M.A. 208:1698-1700, 1969.
68. Jacobs, G. B., Warren, H. F., Ladenheim, J. C., & Pillone, P. R.: Angiographically verified cerebrovascular disease in young women on oral contraceptives without previous neurological illness. Angiology 22:511-520, 1971.
69. Jefeerson, A.: Clinical correlation between encephalopathy and papilloedema in Addison's disease. J. Neurol. Neurosurg. Psychiatry 19:21-27, 1956.
70. Jennet, W. B., & Cross, J. N.: Influence of pregnancy and oral contraception on the incidence of strokes in women of child-bearing age. Lancet 1:1019-1023, 1967.
71. Kay, H. E. M., Knapton, P. J., O'Sullivan, J. P., et al.: Encephalopathy in acute leukaemia associated with methotrexate therapy. Arch. Dis. Child. 47:344-354, 1972.
72. Kjae, M., de Fine, Olivarius, B., & Waarst, A.: Cerebral ischaemic lesions and oral contraception. Dan. Med. Bull. 18:129-137, 1971.
73. Kokenge, R., Kuk, H., & McDowell, F.: Neurological sequelae following dilantin overdose in a patient and in experimental animals. Neurology 15:823-829, 1965.
74. Krigman, M. R.: Lead Encephalopathy in the

developing rat: effect on cortical ontogenesis. J. Neuropathol. Exp. Neurol. 33:671-686, 1974.
75. Kutt, H., Brennan, R., Dehejia, H., & Verebely, K.: Diphenylhydantoin intoxication. A complication of isoniazid therapy. Am. Rev. Resp. Dis. 101:377-384, 1970.
76. Lampert, P. W., & Schochet, S. S.: Demyelination and remyelination in lead neuropathy. Electron microscope studies. J. Neuropathol. Exp. Neurol. 27:527-545, 1968.
77. Lawrence, R. D., Meyer, A., & Nevin, S.: The pathological changes in the brain in fatal hypoglycaemia. Q. J. Med. 11:181-202, 1942.
78. Lhermitte, J., de Ajuriaguerra, J., & Garnier, J.: Les lesions du système nerveux dans l'intoxication alcoholique experimentale. C.R. des Scéances de la Soc. Biol. Paris 128:386-388, 1938.
79. Löken, A. C., & Haymaker, W.: Pamaquine poisoning in man with a clinicopathologic study of one case. Austr. J. Trop. Med. 29:341-352, 1949.
80. Lovelace, R. E., & Horwitz, S. J.: Peripheral neuropathy in long-term diphenylhydantoin therapy. Arch. Neurol. 18:69-77, 1968.
81. Lynch, M. J.: Brain lesions in chronic alcoholism. Arch. Pathol. 69:342-353, 1960.
82. Marchiafava, E., & Bignami, A.: Sopra un'alterazione del corpo calloso osservata in sogetti alcoolisti. Rivista di Patologia Neurosa e Mentale 8:544-549, 1903.
83. Markush, R. E., & Seigel, D. G.: Oral contraceptives and mortality trends from thromboembolism in the United States. Am. J. Publ. Health 59:418-434, 1969.
84. Masi, A. T., & Dugdale, M.: Cerebrovascular diseases associated with the use of oral contraceptives. A review of the English language literature. Ann. Intern. Med. 72:111-121, 1970.
85. McDermott, J. R., Smith, A., Ward, M. K., Parkinson, I. S., & Kerr, D. N. S.: Brain aluminium concentration in dialysis encephalopathy. Lancet 1:901-904, 1978.
86. McLeod, J. G., & Penny, R.: Vincristine neuroapthy: an electrophysiological and histological study. J. Neurol. Neurosurg. Psychiat. 32:297-304, 1969.
87. Meyer, I., & Meyer, P.: Enzyme histochemistry of the growing and adult oligodendrocyte. Acta Neurol. Scand. 40:89-90, 1964.
88. Monsen, G., Struelens, M., & Roland, M.: Bismuth encephalopathy. Acta. Neurol. Belg. 76:301-308, 1976.
89. Moskow, H. A., Pennington, R. C., & Knisely, M. H.: Alcohol, sludge and hypoxic areas of nervous system, liver and heart. Microvasc. Res. 1:174-185, 1968.
90. Mosley, D. H., Schatz, I. J., Breneman, G. M., & Keyes, J. W.: Longterm anticoagulant therapy. Complications and control in a review of 978 cases. J.A.M.A. 186:914-916, 1963.
91. Moure, J. M. B., Whitecar, J. P., & Bodey, G. P.: Electroencephalogram changes secondary to asparaginase in man. Arch. Neurol. 23:365-368, 1970.
92. Nelson, E.: Subacute myelo-optico-neuropathy. Ann. Intern. Med. 77:468-470, 1972.
93. Neuberger, K. T.: The changing neuropathologic picture of chronic alcoholism. Arch. Pathol. 63:1-6, 1957.
94. Nielsen, M. H.: The ultrastructure of Purkinje cells in diphenylhydantoin intoxicated rats. Exp. Brain. Res. 12:447-456, 1971.
95. Niklowitz, W. J.: Ultrastructural effects of acute tetraethyl lead poisoning on nerve cells of the rabbit brain. Environ. Res. 8:17-36, 1974.
96. Ochoa, J.: Isoniazid neuropathy in man: Quantitative E.M. study. Brain 93:831-850, 1970.
97. Odelowo, E. O. O., & Barber, J. B.: Another look at pseudotumour cerebri. J. Natl. Med. Assoc. 69:513-517, 1977.
98. O'Grady, F., & Smith, B.: Neuromyopathy in the mouse produced by the antimicrobial agent Nitroxoline. J. Pathol. Bacteriol. 92:43-48, 1966.
99. Ohnuma, T., Holland, J. F., & Freeman, A.: Biochemical and pharmacological studies with asparaginase in man. Cancer Res. 30:2297-2305, 1970.
100. Oldstone, M. B. A.: The endocrinological aspects of benign intracranial hypertension. Arch. Neurol. 15:362-366, 1966.
101. Olsen, P. Z., & Torning, K.: Isoniazid and loss of memory. Scand. J. Resp. Dis. 49:1-8, 1968.
102. Osetowska, E.: In: Mickler, J., Ed. Pathology of the Nervous System Vol. 2. Ch. 123. McGraw Hill, New York, 1971.
103. Paterson, D., & Greenfield, J. G.: Eryth-

roedema polyneuritis (the so-called pink disease). Q. J. Med. 17:6-18, 1923-4.
104. Pentschew, A., Elsner, F. F., & Kovatch, R. M.: Experimental manganese encephalopathy in monkeys. J. Neuropathol. Exp. Neurol. 22:488-499, 1963.
105. Pentschew, A., & Garro, F.: Lead encephalomyelopathy of the suckling rat and its implications on the porphyrinopathic nervous diseases. Acta Neuropathol. 6:266-278, 1966.
106. Phatak, A. T., & Shah, S. H.: Encephalopathy following accidental isoniazid poisoning. Clin. Pediatr. 10:356-358, 1971.
107. Poltera, A. A.: The pathology of intracranial venous thrombosis in oral contraception. J. Pathol. 106:209-219, 1972.
108. Popoff, N., Weinberg, S., & Feigin, S.: Pathologic observation in lead encephalopathy with special reference to vascular changes. Neurology 13:101-112, 1963.
109. Press, M. F.: Lead encephalopathy in neonatal Long-Evans rats: Morphologic studies. J. Neuropathol. Exp. Neurol. 36:169-193, 1977.
110. Press, M. F.: Animal model lead encephalopathy in neonatal Long-Evans rats poisoned via an esophageal catheter. Am. J. Pathol. 86:485-488, 1977.
111. Prick, J. J. G., Sillevis, W. G., & Muller, L.: Thallium Poisoning. Elsevier, Amsterdam, 1955.
112. Raimondi, A. J., Beckman, F., & Evans, J. P.: Fine structural changes in human lead encephalopathy. J. Neuropathol. Exp. Neurol. 27:154, 1968.
113. Reynolds, E. H.: Mental effects of anticonvulsants and folic acid metabolism. Brain 91:197-214, 1968.
114. Richardson, J. E., & Russell, D. S.: Cerebral disease due to functioning islet-cell tumours with pathological reports. Lancet 2:1054-1059, 1952.
115. Russell, D. S.: Changes in the central nervous system following arsphenamine medication. J. Pathol. Bacteriol. 45:357-366, 1937.
116. Salmon, M. L., Winkelman, J. Z., & Gay, A. J.: Neurophthalmic sequelae in uses of oral contraceptives. J.A.M.A. 206:85-91, 1968.
117. Schochet, S. S., Jr., Lampert, P. W., & Earle, K. M.: Neuronal changes induced by intrathecal vincristine sulphate. J. Neuropathol. Exp. Neurol. 27:645-656, 1968.
118. Schröder, J. M.: Ultrastructure of unmyelinated (Remak) nerve fibres in isoniazid neuropathy. Acta Neuropathol. (Berlin) 15:156-175, 1970a.
119. Schröder, J. M.: The pathogenesis of I.N.H. neuropathy II Phase & electron microscopic studies of spinal cord, spinal ganglia and muscle spindles. Acta Neuropathol. (Berlin) 16:324-341, 1970b.
120. Schwedenberg, T. H.: Leukoencephalopathy following carbon monoxide asphyxia. J. Neuropathol. 18:597-608, 1959.
121. Selhorst, J. B.: Diphenylhydantoin-induced cerebellar degeneration. Arch. Neurol. 27:453-455, 1972.
122. Senelick, R. C., Norwood, C. W., & Cohen, G. H.: Painless spinal epidural hematoma during anticoagulant therapy. Neurology 26:213-225, 1976.
123. Shapiro, W. R., Chernik, N. L., & Posner, J. B.: Necrotizing encephalopathy following intraventricular instillation of methotrexate. Arch. Neurol. 27:96-102, 1973.
124. Shelanski, M. L., & Wisniewski, H.: Neurofibrillary degeneration induced by vincristine therapy. Arch. Neurol. 20:199-206, 1969.
125. Shigematsu, I.: Subacute myelo-optic-neuropathy (SMON) and clioquinol. Jap. J. Med. Sci. Biol. (Suppl.) 28:35-52, 1975.
126. Shiraki, H.: The neuropathy of subacute myelo-optico-neuropathy. Jap. J. Med. Sci. Biol. (Suppl.) 28:101-164, 1975.
127. Shiraki, H., & Takeuchi, T.: In: Mickler, J., Ed.: Pathology of the Nervous System. Ch. 124 Vol. 2. McGraw Hill, New York, 1971.
128. Smith, B.: The Myenteric plexus in drug-induced neuropathy. J. Neurol. Neurosurg. Psychiatry 30:506-510, 1967.
129. Smith, B.: Damage to the intrinsic cardiac neurones by rubidomycin (daunorubicin). Br. Heart J. 31:607-609, 1969.
130. Smith, B.: Brain damage after intrathecal methotrexate. J. Neurol. Neurosurg. Psychiatry 38:810-815, 1975.
131. Smith, H., Lerner, P. I., & Weinstein, L.: Neurotoxicity and massive intravenous therapy with penicillin. Arch. Intern. Med. 120:47, 1967.
132. Snyder, S. H., Bannerjee, S. P., Yam Amua, H. I., & Greenberg, D.: Phenothiazines, amphetamines and enzymes synthesizing psychomimetic drugs and schizophrenia research. Science 184:1243-1253, 1974.

133. Spurny, O. M., Rubin, S., Wolf, J. W., & Wu, W. Q.: Spinal epidural haematoma during anticoagulant therapy. Report of two cases. Arch. Intern. Med. 114:103-107, 1964.
134. Sreerama, V.: Neurosurgical complication of anticoagulant therapy. Can. Med. Assoc., J. 108:305-307, 1973.
135. Sternberg, T. H., & Bierman, S. M.: Corticosteroids. Pseudotumour cerebri. Arch. Dermatol. 92:746, 1965.
136. Suchenwirth, R., & Dahl, P.: Nitrofurantoin polyneuritis. Fortschr. Neurol. Psychiatr. 36:100-115, 1968.
137. Tateishi, T., & Otsuki, S.: Experimental reproduction of SMON in animals by prolonged administration of clioquinol. Clinicopathological findings. Jap. J. Med. Sci. Biol. (Suppl.) 28:165-183, 1975.
138. Thomas, W. A.: Generalized oedema occurring only at the menstrual period. J.A.M.A. 101:1126, 1933.
139. Thomas, J. A., Dallenbach, F. D., & Thomas, I. M.: The distribution of radio-active lead ($^{21}O_{Pb}$) in the cerebellum of developing rats. J. Pathol. 109:45-50, 1973.
140. Thomas, J. A., & Thomas, I. M.: The pathogenesis of lead encephalopathy. Indian. J. Med. Res. 62:36-41, 1974.
141. Toole, J. F., & Parrish, M. L.: Nitrofurantoin polyneuropathy. Neurology 23:554-559, 1973.
142. Tredici, G., & Minazzi, M.: Alcoholic Neuropathy. An electron-microscopic study. J. Neurol. Sci. 25:333-346, 1975.
143. Tumarkin, B., Wilson, J., & Snyder, G.: Cerebral atrophy due to alcoholism in young adults. U.S. Armed Forces Med. J. 6:67-74, 1955.
144. Utterback, R. A., Ojeman, R., & Malek, J.: Parenchymatous cerebellar degeneration with dilantin intoxication. J. Neuropathol. Exp. Neurol. 17:516-517, 1958.
145. Vallarta, J. M., Bell, D. B., & Reichert, A.: Progressive encephalopathy due to chronic hydantoin intoxication. Am. J. Dis. Child. 128:27-34, 1974.
146. Valprey, R., Sumi, M., Sopass, M. K., & Goble, P. D.: Acute and chronic progressive encephalopathy due to gasoline sniffing. Neurology 28:507-510, 1978.
147. Victor, M., & Adams, R. D.: Symposium on role of some newer vitamins in human metabolism and nutrition. The neuropathy of experimental vitamin B6 deficiency in monkeys. Am. J. Clin. Nutr. 4:346-353, 1956.
148. Victor, M., Adams, R. D., & Mancall, E. L.: A restricted form of cerebellar cortical degeneration occurring in alcoholic patients. Arch. Neurol. 1:579-688, 1959.
149. Vital, C. I., Picard, J., Arne, L., Aubertin, J., Fenelon, J., & Monton, L.: Etude anatoclinique de 3 cas d'encephalopathie hypoglycemique (dont un apres sulfamidotherapie). Le Diabete 12 F:291-296, 1967.
150. Walker, A. E., & Adamkiewicz, J. J.: Pseudo tumour cerebri associated with prolonged cortico steroid therapy. J.A.M.A. 188:779-784, 1964.
151. Walsh, F. B.: Papilloedema associated with increased intracranial pressure in Addison's disease. Arch. Ophthalmol. 47:86, 1952.
152. Walsh, J. C., & McCleod, J. G.: Alcoholic neuropathy: an electrophysiological and histological study. J. Neurol. Sci. 10:457-469, 1970.
153. Wanchope, G. M.: Hypoglycaemia: critical review. Q. J. Med. 26:117-156, 1933.
154. Wells, C. E., & Urrea, D.: Cerebrovascular accidents in patients receiving anti-coagulant drugs. Arch. Neurol. 3:553-556, 1960.
155. Wiener, L. M., & Nathanson, M.: The relationship of subdural hematoma to anti-coagulant therapy. Arch. Neurol. 6:282-686, 1963.
156. Wilson, C. B., & Norrell, H. A.: Brain Tumour chemotherapy with intrathecal methotrexate. Cancer 23:1038-1045. 1969.
157. Wyllie, W. G., & Stern, R. O.: Pink disease. Its morbid anatomy with a note on treatment. Arch. Dis. Child. 6:137-155, 1931.
158. Zeman, W.: Pathogenesis of radio lesions in the mature central nervous system. In: Lüthy, F., & Biscoff, A., Eds.: Proceedings of 5th International congress of Neuropathology, Zurich. pp. 302-8. Excerpta Medica, Amsterdam, 1966.
159. Ziegler, D. K.: Minor neurologic signs and symptoms following insulin coma therapy. J. Nerv. Ment. Dis. 120:75-78, 1954.

16

The Eye

Ramesh C. Tripathi and Brenda J. Tripathi

INTRODUCTION

From the viewpoints of morphology and physiology, it is aptly noted that the eye (Fig. 16-1) is a sequestered microcosm of the tissues of the body; it represents examples of a variety of structures derived from the layers of surface ectoderm, neuroectoderm, and mesoderm. The skin and appendages with and without modifications are characterized by the lids, by the mucous membrane of the conjunctiva, and by the bony tissue of the orbit; a variety of generalized and specialized connective tissues compose the orbit, ocular adnexa, cornea, sclera, uveal tract, and vitreous body; pigment-containing cells are seen throughout the uveal tract and pigmented epithelium of the retina; striated muscles are represented in the lids and ocular recti, and smooth muscles in the ciliary body, iris, and certain parts of the lids; examples of secretory glands are typified by the lacrimal system and by the neuroepithelium of ciliary processes; nervous tissues of the retina and optic nerve are extensions of the central nervous system; and illustrations of fenestrated and nonfenestrated vessels, as well as somatic and autonomic nerves, are apparent throughout the eye.

In many instances, however, the eye represents the highest degree of specialization of function in the body, as is strikingly exemplified by the photoreceptor outer segments, by the transparent, avascular cornea, lens, and vitreous humor, by Descemet's membrane and lens capsule, which are the thickest basement membranes in the body, and by the light-absorping retinal pigment epithelium. The blood/tissue ratio in the choroid is the highest of all of the body tissues.

Because of the diversity of its structure, and the active biochemical processes that take place both independently of and in conjunction with the systemic metabolism, the eye is second only to the liver in showing the manifestations of drug toxicity. Since the eye is located externally in the body, and since most of its structures are extremely delicate, it is equally vulnerable to insults by chemical agents, toxins, poisons, nonmechanical agents, and foreign bodies. However, while the ocular tissues provide a unique opportunity for studying the toxicity of drugs, biopsies of these tissues are rarely possible, and the study of autopsy material from the eye is complicated by the rapid postmortem changes that occur in the specialized ocular tissues. On the other hand, the eye is readily accessible to biomicroscopic examination, thus providing a unique opportunity for documenting dynamic pathology. In this chapter, many of the gross morphologic changes described in the eye are representative of the biomicroscopic and ophthalmoscopic appearances of toxic lesions. The pathologic changes described are those seen in human eyes; reference to animal work is made where the experimental evidence has clearly enhanced our knowledge of the pathogenesis of the toxic lesions in humans.

In order to provide readers with a ready reference to the specialized structures of the eye and the fundamental pathologic reactions involved in toxic insults to this organ, a brief description, containing definitions of specialized terms, is appended at the beginning of each section. The literature included is necessarily selective since it is beyond the scope of this chapter to document in detail the pathologic reaction of the eye to every drug, chemical, toxin, poison, and nonmechanical agent. Interested readers are

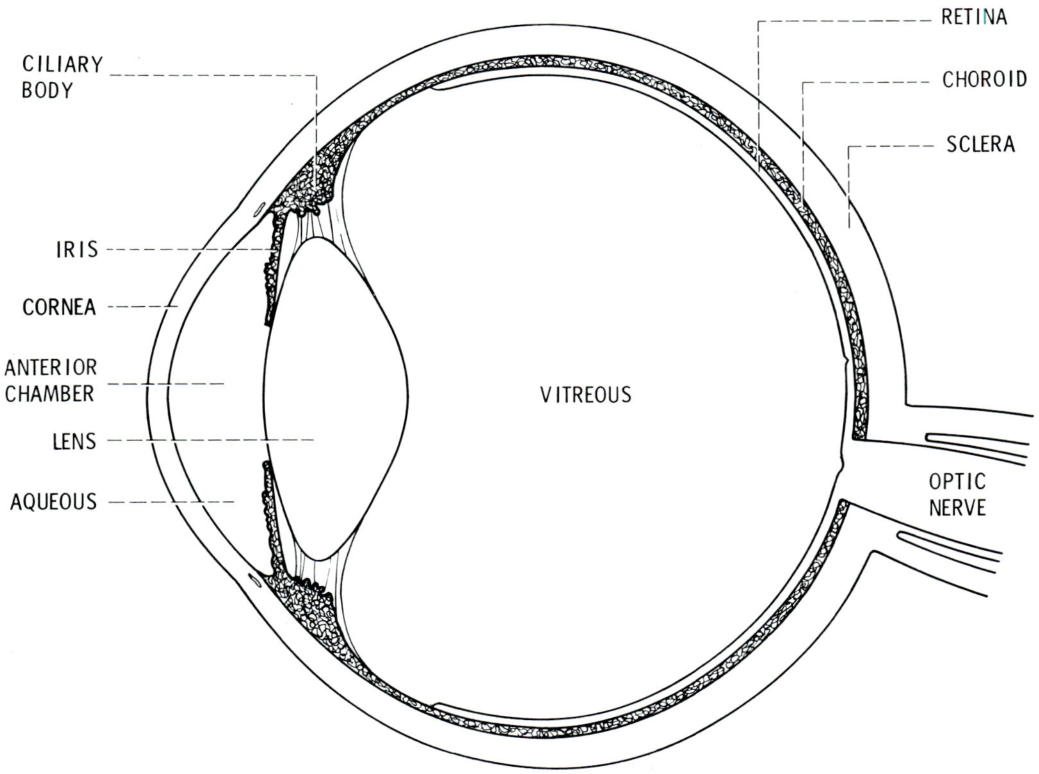

Fig. 16-1. Diagrammatic representation of human eye and its main structural components.

referred to several monographs on this subject.[114, 134, 137, 156, 333]

A glossary of ocular structures involved in the pathologic reactions of drugs, chemicals, toxins, poisons, and nonmechanical agents (Table 16-1) is presented at the end of this chapter.

CONJUNCTIVA

The conjunctiva is a thin, transparent mucous membrane that lines the posterior surface of the eyelids (palpebral conjunctiva), from which it is reflected upon itself as the fornices (loose, redundant portion), and lines the anterior surface of the eyeball (bulbar conjunctiva) (Fig. 16-2A). At the lid margin, the conjunctiva is continuous with the skin, and at the corneal margin, it is structurally continuous with the corneal epithelium. On the nasal side of the globe and at the edge of the caruncle, the conjunctiva forms a crescent (plica semilunaris), which represents the third eyelid or nictitating membrane of many animals. At the lacrimal puncta, the mucous membrane is continuous with that lining the lacrimal passages. The whole of the conjunctiva forms a cul-de-sac, with the large opening of the palpebral fissure. The bulbar conjunctiva is loosely connected to the underlying sclera and episclera, thus allowing free mobility to the eye.

The epithelial lining of the conjunctiva and the cornea form the external protective covering of the open eye, and are constantly kept moist by the secretory fluid of the tears, thus preventing keratinization. The conjunctiva, like all other mucous membranes in the body, consists of epithelium and substantia propria (Fig. 16-2B). The thickness of the epithelium (from two to five cell layers) varies from region to region, being thinnest in the bulbar region and thickest at the mucocutaneous junction of the lid. In the cuboidal basal cells, and occa-

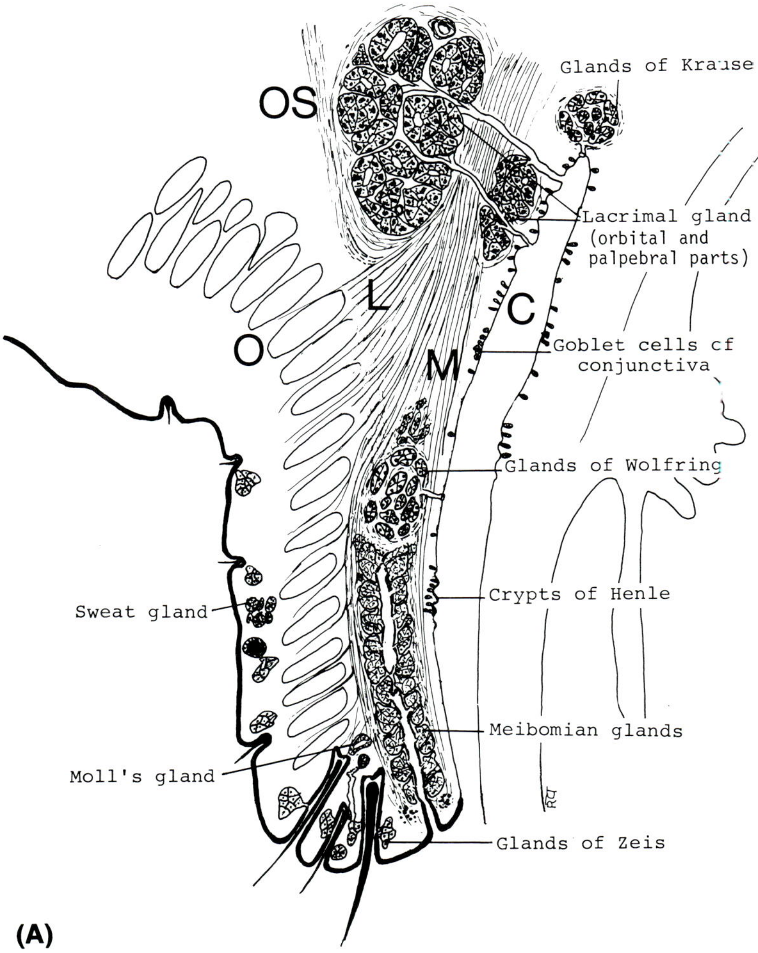

(A)

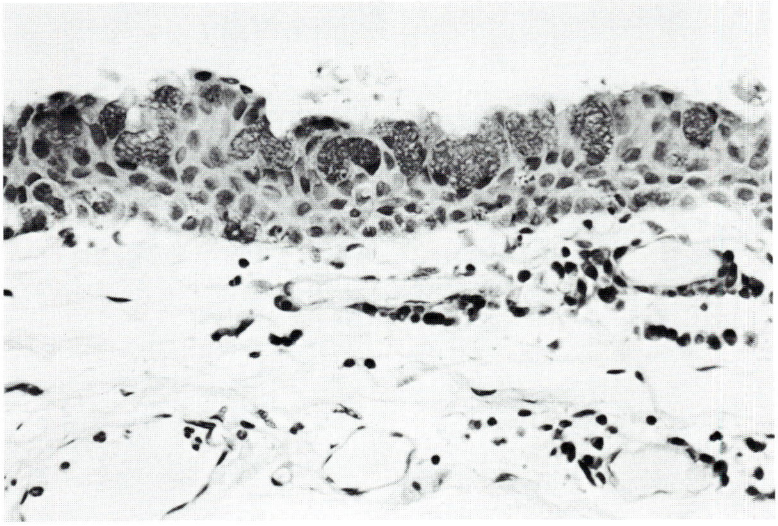

(B)

Fig. 16-2. (A) Diagrammatic representation of main components of human upper eyelid. L, levator muscle; M, smooth muscle of Muller; O, orbicularis oculi muscle; OS, orbital septum; S, skin; C, conjunctival cul-de-sac. (B) Light micrograph of conjunctiva consisting of substantia propria and epithelium, the latter containing several goblet cells. ×275.

sionally in the prickle cells, melanin granules are seen; the pigment is produced by melanocytes in the basal layer and is transferred to the epithelial cells. Mucous-secreting goblet cells are irregularly distributed in the conjunctiva, being abundant in the fornices and sparse in the bulbar conjunctiva; their secretion is responsible for wetting of the keratoconjunctival epithelium. The connective tissue of the conjunctival stroma, which contains blood vessels, nerves, and conjunctival glands, varies in its compactness, depending upon topography. The superficial layer is a fine, fibrous, reticular network having nodules of lymphoid tissue (after 3 months of age), a few mast cells, and histiocytes. The vascularized, deeper layers are constituted by irregularly arranged bundles of collagen and some elastic tissue, and randomly distributed fibroblasts, melanocytes, mast cells, lymphocytes, and plasma cells. The fibrous layer is continuous with the attached margin of the upper and lower tarsal plates and contains the smooth palpebral muscle of Müller.

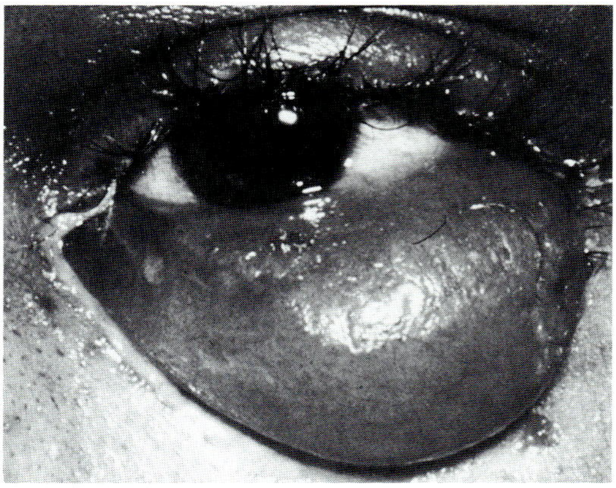

Fig. 16-3. Gross appearance of conjunctival edema with ecchymosis.

Pathologic Reactions

The metabolism of the conjunctiva is predominantly aerobic, and drugs, toxins, and chemicals interfering with glycolytic enzymes cause anoxic injury to the cells, hydropic degeneration, devitalization, and cellular necrosis. Suppression of secretory activity, and loss of goblet cells and of the accessory and main lacrimal glands, results in dryness, keratinization, or epidermalization. Many drug-induced mucocutaneous disorders will manifest themselves in the conjunctiva. Because of its exposed location, the conjunctiva is also subject to accidental toxic and chemical insults.

Hyperemia is a basic pathologic response of the conjunctiva to irritants and substances acting directly on blood vessels. The vascular engorgement and ecchymosis, with or without edema, may be mediated through the degranulation of the mast cells that are present locally (Fig. 16-3). Damage to the vascular integrity may cause frank or petechial hemorrhages. The chronic inflammatory response may manifest itself as papillary hypertrophy in which the hyperplastic epithelium is thrown into folds containing a core of vessels, surrounded by subepithelial edematous tissue and infiltrated with chronic inflammatory cells—predominantly lymphocytes and plasma cells (Fig. 16-4).

As a response to chronic irritation, the conjunctiva may undergo follicular formations or lymphoid hyperplasia with secondary vascularization (Fig. 16-5A, B). In allergic reactions, eosinophil infiltration may predominate. Drug-induced and toxic pemphigoid lesions

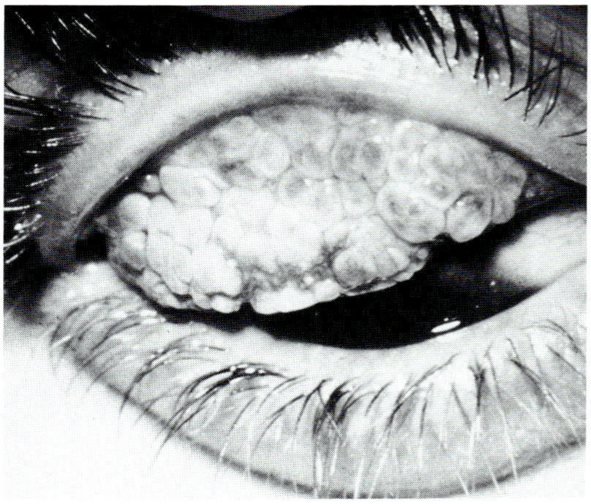

Fig. 16-4. Gross appearance of marked papillary hypertrophy of the conjunctiva.

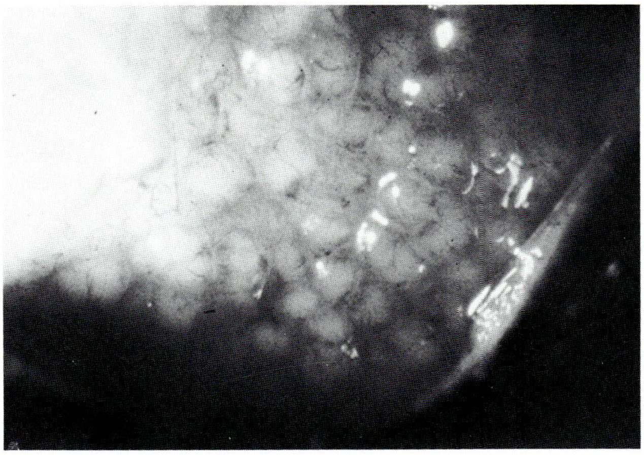

(A)

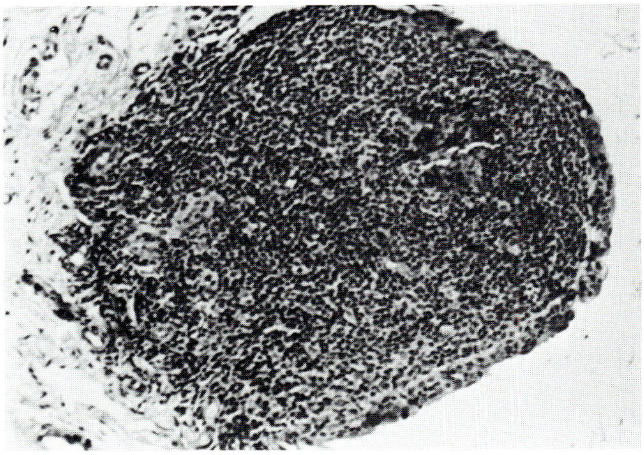

(B)

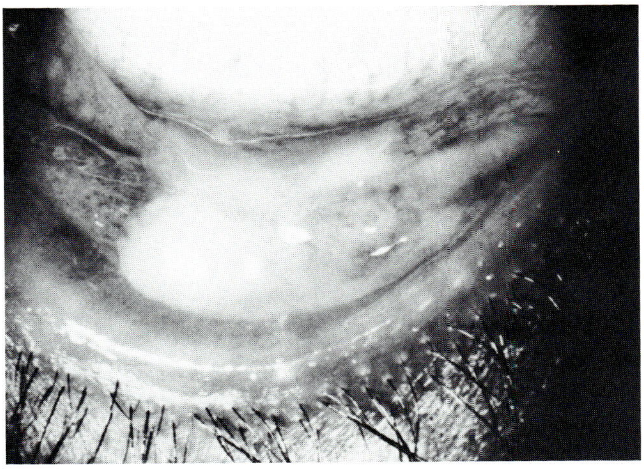

(C)

Fig. 16-5. (A) Gross appearance of conjunctival follicles. (B) Histologic section of a conjunctival follicle showing lymphoid hyperplasia. ×140. (C) Gross appearance of conjunctival pseudomembrane, which consists of loose fibrin, cellular debris, and exudate that can be easily stripped off from the underlying epithelium. Pseudomembranes may be seen in chemical burns (especially alkali) and Stevens-Johnson syndrome.

of the conjunctiva are characterized by subepithelial conjunctival bullae and epithelial replacement by fibrovascular tissue containing lymphocytes and plasma cells, followed by the contracture of fibrous tissue, shrinkage, scarring, and symblepharon and ankyloblepharon. Pseudomembrane and secondary scarring of the conjunctiva may occur with chemical burns and Stevens-Johnson type lesions (Fig. 16-5C). The latter are characterized by conjunctival bullae due to detachment of the epithelium from the subepithelial tissue, healing, and cicatrization, leading to symblepharon and entropion. In this process, goblet cells of the conjunctiva and the openings of the accessory lacrimal glands are frequently destroyed, leading to marked dryness of the conjunctiva with subsequent epidermalization. The conjunctiva may undergo extensive necrosis associated with a purulent inflammatory reaction or with a chronic, nongranulomatous reaction (Fig. 16-6A, B).

The conjunctiva is a frequent site for the deposition of drugs, toxins, and their derivatives and metabolites; in many instances these desposits appear as pigmented lesions. The deposits are usually subepithelial or are enclosed in epithelial cysts, but may be contained in

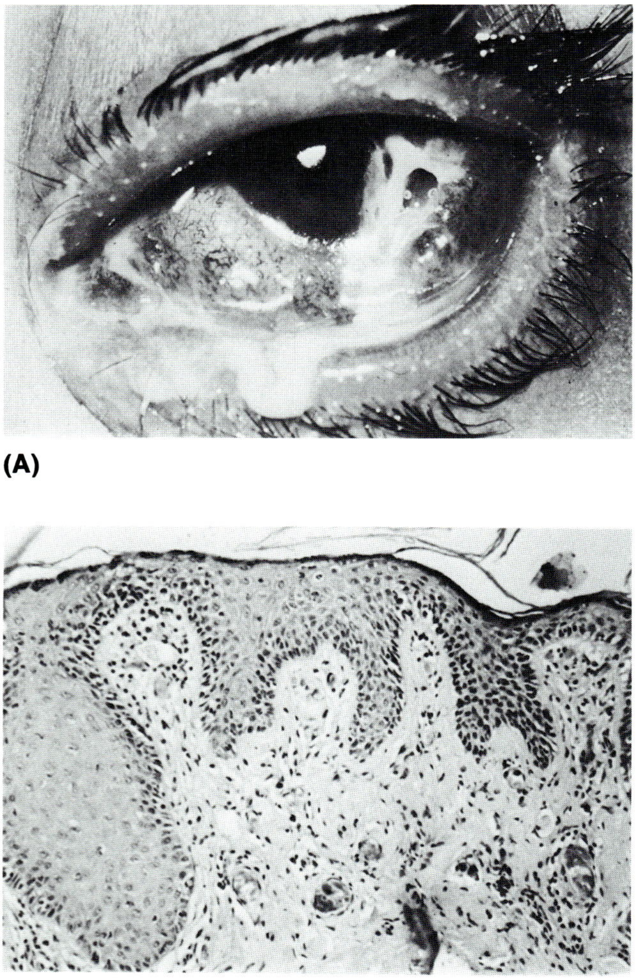

(A)

(B)

Fig. 16-6. (A) Gross appearance of Stevens-Johnson type lesion associated with purulent inflammatory reaction. (B) Light micrograph of conjunctiva in Stevens-Johnson syndrome showing epidermalization following marked drying due to loss of goblet cells and destruction of accessory lacrimal gland openings. Substantia propria shows cicatrization and chronic inflammatory reaction. ×135.

the intra- or extracellular spaces of the cells, especially in the basal region.

LIDS, ORBIT, AND ADNEXA

The eyelids consist of skin, muscles, and fibrous tissue, and are lined internally by the mucous membrane of the conjunctiva. The skin of the eyelid is the thinnest in the body, and has no subcutaneous fat, but does contain sebaceous and sweat glands. The muscles of the eyelids are the striated orbicularis oculi and levator palpebrae superioris, and the small, palpebral smooth muscle of Müller. Internally, a compact, fibrous tissue contains modified sebaceous glands (the Meibomian glands), which open at the lid margin. Associated with the eyelashes are the glands of Moll (sudiferous) and of Zeis (sebaceous). The main lacrimal gland (tubuloalveolar type) is located in the anterior lateral portion of the roof of the orbit and, together with the palpebral portions, opens in the superior temporal fornix (Fig. 16-2A).

The orbit of the eye is filled with a semispecialized, fibro-fatty tissue. The four recti and two oblique muscles which insert into the sclera are responsible for the movement of the globe. The extraocular muscles, which contain both fast and slow fibers corresponding to white and red muscle fibers, respectively, are the most highly organized of all striated muscles.

Pathologic Reactions

The lids are among the eye structures most frequently involved in drug toxicity and related injuries. Inflammation of the eyelid (blepharitis) is synonymous with dermatitis or eczema. Erythema multiforme is an acute, self-limiting dermatosis with the multiform lesions of macules, papules (the most common lesions in this condition), and bullae. In its most severe form, that starts suddenly with high fever and prostration, a predominantly bullous eruption of the skin and mucous membrane occurs and is referred to as Stevens-Johnson syndrome. Drug-related Lyell's syndrome (toxic epidermal necrolysis or scalded-skin syndrome) is an acute disease characterized in the eyelids by severe degeneration and necrosis of epidermal cells, resulting in detachment or exfoliation of large areas of entire epidermis (Fig. 16-7); the dermis is uninvolved or shows only mild lymphocytic infiltration. Contact dermatitis is one of the most common conditions affecting the eyelids; it can manifest in acute, subacute, or chronic form. Angioneurotic edema may result from hypersensitivity (Fig. 16-8).

The extraocular muscles are commonly af-

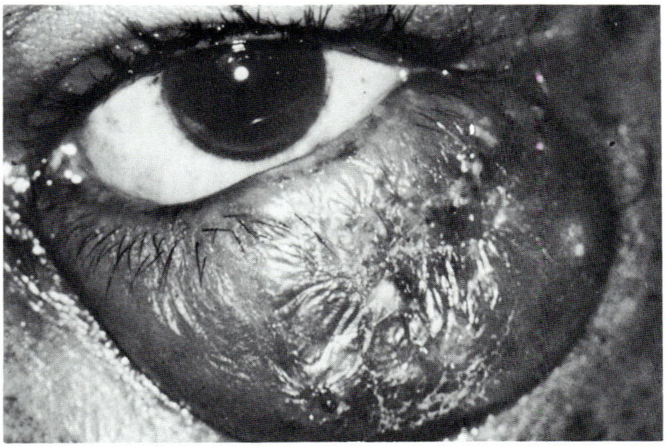

Fig. 16-7. Gross appearance of epidermonecrolysis associated with lid edema.

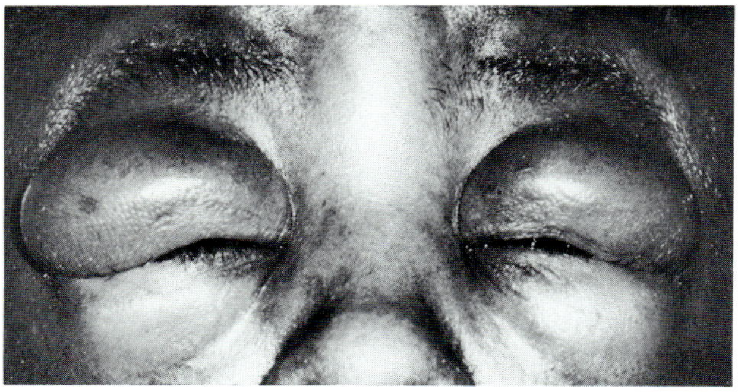

Fig. 16-8. Bilateral massive lid edema causing almost total closure of palpebral apertures. This reaction may be attributable in part to the loose aerolar tissue of the lid and high concentration of mast cells in this region.

fected by drugs; in most cases the responsible agents cause a weakness or imbalance in the action of these muscles. To a great extent, the effect is functional and reversible on withdrawal of the drug; rarely, permanent defects occur. For this reason, pathologic studies of the ocular muscles are sparse, and the mechanism by which drugs primarily affect these muscles remains obscure.

Drugs Affecting the Conjunctiva, Lids, Orbit, and Adnexa

Aminosalicylic acid (PAS). Together with isoniazid and pyridoxine, PAS produces chronic keratoconjunctivitis. The punctate devitalization of cells in the conjunctiva may be associated with filaments composed of degenerate epithelial cells and mucus. Subconjunctival hemorrhages may occur secondary to drug-induced anemia. There is also a questionable incidence of blepharitis, edema, Stevens-Johnson syndrome, and exfoliative dermatitis.[5, 114, 137, 177, 254]

Amphotericin B. Topical or subconjunctival injection of amphotericin B may produce an irritative inflammatory response, allergic reaction, ulceration, and follicular conjunctivitis. Occasionally, subconjunctival nodules have been reported.[5, 34, 114]

Arabinoside (Ara-A), Idoxuridine (IDU), Trifluorothymidine (TFT). Topical use of these antiviral agents may cause conjunctival hyperemia, edema, allergic reaction, follicular conjunctivitis, thickening of the eyelids, and narrowing or occlusion of the lacrimal punctum.[156, 200, 221]

Arsenicals. Used in therapeutic doses in some countries, arsenic is deposited as a toxic, insoluble compound in mucocutaneous tissue, including that of the eye. Conjunctival congestion may be the presenting pathology; exfoliative dermatitis may also occur.[146, 198]

Aspirin (Sodium Salicylate, Acetylsalicylic Acid). Ocular side effects of aspirin are rare. However, in susceptible patients, allergic reactions, nonspecific conjunctivitis, angioneurotic edema, urticaria, and subconjunctival and eyelid hemorrhages may occur.[140, 286]

Atropine, Scopolamine, Homatropine. Contact dermatitis is not an uncommon ocular side effect of atropine, scopolamine, and homatropine. Hypersensitivity reactions usually manifest as papillary hyperplasia together with eosinophilic reaction, and rarely with mucopurulent discharge, whereas toxic or irritative reactions give rise to the formation of follicles. Allergic dermatoconjunctivitis occurs less frequently with scopolamine and homatropine than with atropine.[156, 307]

Barbiturates. Functional ocular defects—and especially muscular weakness—are among the most frequently reported side effects of barbiturates; the microscopic pathology of barbiturate effects on the eyes has, however, only been rarely documented. In one reported case, the chronic use of barbiturates led to conjunctivitis followed by symblepharon. In cases of barbiturate-associated ocular toxicity, residues of barbiturate drugs may be detected in the conjunctiva, and may be responsible for the persistence of an ocular reaction for several months after the drug is discontinued. Eyelid reactions to barbiturates include allergic and irritative responses, angioneurotic edema, exfoliative dermatitis, Lyell's syndrome, and conjunctival hyperemia.[114, 137, 279, 343]

Benzalkonium. Topical application of benzalkonium to the eyelids causes hyperemia, edema, desquamation of superficial epithelial cells, and the formation of pseudomembrane.[134, 301]

Bismuth Compounds. Rarely, exfoliative dermatitis, a blue discoloration, and subconjunctival hemorrhage are seen as a consequence of the use of bismuth compounds on the eyelids.[78]

Bromides. Occasionally, the systemic administration of bromides produces blepharoconjunctivitis, Stevens-Johnson syndrome, erythema, and allergic reaction.[114, 137, 333]

Busulfan, Chlorambucil, Cyclophosphamide, Mechlorethamine, Melphalan, Triethylenemelamine, Uracil Mustard. Systemic administration of these drugs may cause allergic reactions, erythema, nonspecific conjunctivitis, hyperpigmentation of the eyelid and mucous membrane (busulfan, cyclophosphamide, and uracil mustard), exfoliative dermatitis, and Lyell's syndrome. There is a questionable incidence of madarosis.[114, 174]

Carbonic Anhydrase Inhibitors. Allergic reactions, urticaria, purpura, and Lyell's syndrome may become manifest in the eyelids and conjunctiva with the use of carbonic anhydrase inhibitors. Subconjunctival hemorrhages are associated with anemia induced by these drugs.[114, 156]

Chloral Hydrate. As with the barbiturates, the systemic administration of chloral hydrate may cause hyperemia, edema, and an allergic reaction of the conjunctiva (see p. 384).[114, 137, 343]

Chloroquine, Hydroxychloroquine. These drugs may produce an allergic reaction, erythema multiforme, Stevens-Johnson syndrome, and exfoliative dermatitis, as well as subconjunctival hemorrhages secondary to drug-induced anemia. The typical microscopic deposits of chloroquine and hydroxychloroquine (see p. 403) may be found in the conjunctiva (Fig. 16-9) and the recti muscles, which could account for their paralysis.[39, 264]

Chlorpromazine. Conjunctival and palpebral involvement by chlorpromazine may include allergic reaction, edema, purpura, and Stevens-Johnson syndrome. With large doses, finely pigmented, melanin-like deposits appear in the substantia propria, in the interpalpebral fissure area as well as in the lens (see p. 409). Conjunctival biopsy of patients treated with large doses of chlorpromazine has shown a markedly increased deposition of pigment granules in the basal layers of the epithelium, in the stroma, and around the vessels. In one report, the granules, varying in size (0.2 to 2 μm), were located in the endothelial cells of capillaries, in macrophages, and in fibroblasts, as well as extracellularly. Histochemically, there is an increase in tyrosinase concentration in the basal epithelial cells; an increase of melanosomes in melanocytes suggests enhanced melanocytic activity. In skin biopsies, the pigment shows all of the histochemical characteristics of melanin, but ultrastructurally, the typical internal striated matrix of true melanin granules is absent. Extraction studies suggest that these granules probably contain chlorpromazine or a related metabolite, and represent a melanin-chlorpromazine moiety. It is possible that melanin granules selectively bind chlorpromazine or its metabolites.[67, 219, 282, 349, 351]

Chlorpropamide. Systemic administration of chlorpropamide induces an exudative conjunctivitis and stomatitis, with scarring of the palpebral conjunctiva and pannus formation simulating trachomatous lesions.[86, 343]

Chrysarobin. Systemic absorption from topical application of chrysarobin to the skin may cause ocular irritation, conjunctival hyperemia, and a brown-violet discoloration. Inadvertent ocular exposure to this drug produces hyperemia, allergic reactions, nonspecific conjunctivitis, edema, and a brown-violet discoloration.[14, 137, 343]

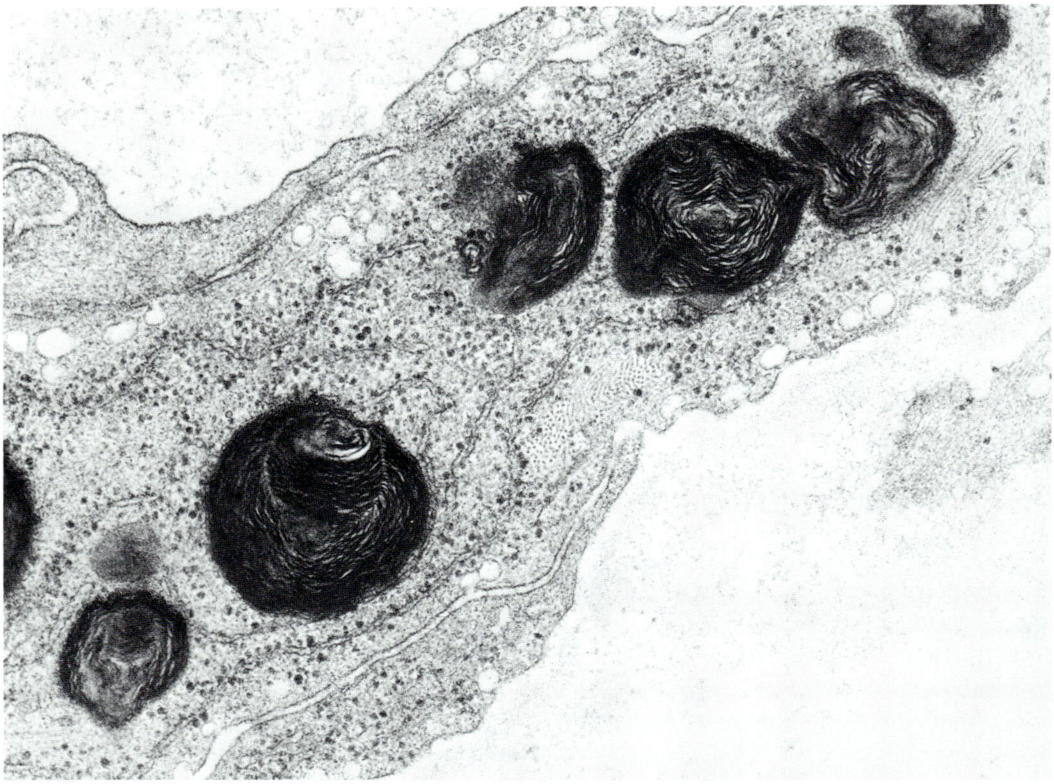

Fig. 16-9. Chloroquine toxicity. Laminated, dense inclusions in endothelial cell of a conjunctival blood capillary. Electron micrograph. ×48,000. (Courtesy Jacques Libert, M.D., University of Brussels.)

Copper salts. Topical application of copper salts to the eye may lead to conjunctivitis and lid edema, and may be accompanied by corneal ulceration.[314, 333]

Corticosteroids. Retrobulbar and depot injection of corticosteroids may cause a fibrotic reaction and degeneration of fatty tissue. Intralesional injection of fluorinated steroids, especially in susceptible black patients, can cause lid depigmentation because of corticosteroid inhibition of melanosome synthesis, impaired transfer of melanosomes to the keratinocyte, or melanocyte ischemia (Fig. 16-10). Topical application of corticosteroids to the eye may cause an allergic reaction, petechiae, and punctate keratitis, although the reaction may vary from one corticosteroid preparation to another. Systemic administration of corticosteroids may produce hyperemia, angioneurotic edema, Lyell's syndrome, and subconjunctival hemorrhage.[77, 87, 114]

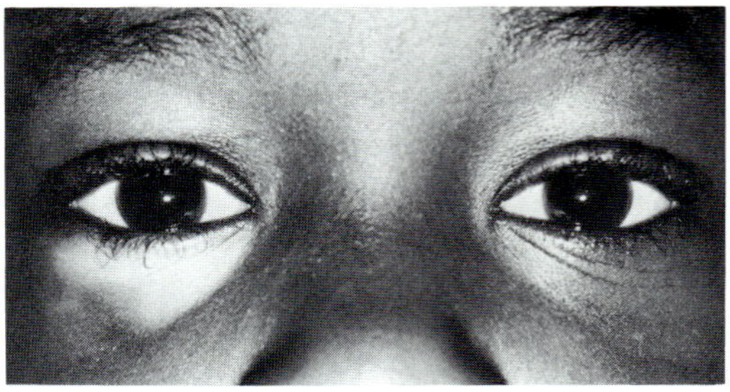

Fig. 16-10. Depigmentation of right lower lid in a black boy who had received intralesional injection of fluorinated steroid for chalazion.

Cytosine Arabinoside (Cytarabine). Topical application of this drug may induce an allergic reaction, nonspecific conjunctivitis, hyperpigmentation, and purpura. Subconjunctival hemorrhage is secondary to the associated drug-induced anemia. There is probably loss of eyelashes and eyebrows, and the drug has the potential for ocular teratogenic effects.[102, 114, 156, 180]

Diphenazine (1,4-bis-(Phenylisopropyl)-Piperazine). Systemic administration of diphenazine has caused photosensitized dermatitis of the eyelids, as well as a reversible depigmentation of the eyebrows and hair.[137]

Epinephrine (Adrenalin). Commonly used in the form of eyedrops in the treatment of glaucoma, epinephrine causes reactive or rebound hyperemia of the superficial conjunctival vessels. Many patients also develop an allergic or contact sensitivity characterized by itching, burning, epiphoria, and hyperemia of the conjunctiva and eyelids. More often this reaction is due to the preservative and the vehicle used in epinephrine preparations rather than to the drug itself. Rarely, subconjunctival hemorrhage may occur with epinephrine-containing eyedrops. Occasionally, follicular conjunctivitis and epithelial keratitis may be seen. These reactions are thought to arise from the low pH required to maintain the stability of the drug.

Chronic use of epinephrine results in a brown-black discoloration of the conjunctiva, cornea, and eyelid margins, resembling eye makeup; soft contact lenses may be similarly discolored. The newer drug, dipivalyl epinephrine, does not cause this discoloration. More commonly, sharply defined rounded black, melanin-like areas of adenochrome pigmentation develop, owing to oxidation products of epinephrine in the conjunctiva and cornea; histologically, these areas are enclosed in translucent epithelial cysts (Fig. 16-11A, B). The deposits disappear gradually after treatment with epinephrine is stopped.

That epinephrine allergy truly represents a sensitization phenemenon has been demonstrated by the presence of circulating antibodies to epinephrine and by animal experiments.

With prolonged topical use of epinephrine, the eyelid may manifest an allergic reaction and blepharoconjunctivitis, among other effects. A single case of loss of the eyelashes (madarosis) has been reported. Adenochrome deposits at the mucocutaneous junction and in the nasolacrimal passages have been observed in eyes treated with epinephrine, and rarely, nasolacrimal obstruction has also occurred.[14, 32, 61, 83, 156, 179, 294, 317]

Ethanol. Local use, exposure, or retrobulbar injection of ethanol causes hyperemia, edema, epithelial erosion, keratitis, corneal ulceration, necrosis, or opacities, as well as retrobulbar fibrosis and temporary ophthalmoplegia.[156, 227, 333]

Gentamicin. Subconjunctival injection of gentamicin in humans as well as in rats and rabbits induces a lysosomal storage process within the conjunctival fibroblasts. Electron microscopy shows the accumulated substance to consist of a granular material and pleomorphic lamellar structures corresponding to the presence of complex lipids (Fig. 16-12).[208]

Gold (Systemic: Gold Thiosulfate or Thiomalate; Topical: Gold Chloride). In crysiasis, red, violet, purple, or brown deposits of gold occur either within and deep to the epithelium and in wandering histiocytes, or as free particles fixed in the connective tissue. Alternatively, a phlyctenular bulbar conjunctivitis and a type of conjunctivitis with pseudomembrane formation in the superior palpebral region may develop. Allergic reactions, edema, conjunctival hyperemia, chronic inflammatory reactions, exfoliative dermatitis, Stevens-Johnson syndrome, and symblepharon may also occur as accompanying features.[114, 137, 270, 333, 343]

Griseofulvin. Systemic administration of griseofulvin may produce an allergic reaction, edema, angioneurotic edema, lupoid syndrome, and exfoliative dermatitis.[5, 114, 134]

Indomethacin (Indocin). Systemic administration of indomethacin may induce angioneurotic edema and subconjunctival hemorrhage secondary to drug-induced anemia, and may also produce madarosis.[93, 114]

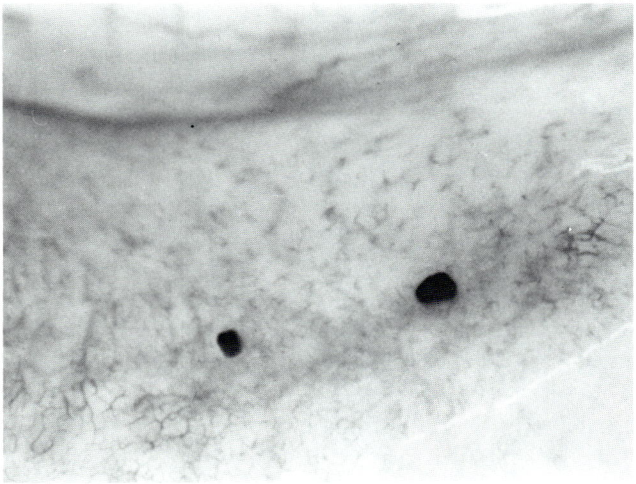

(A)

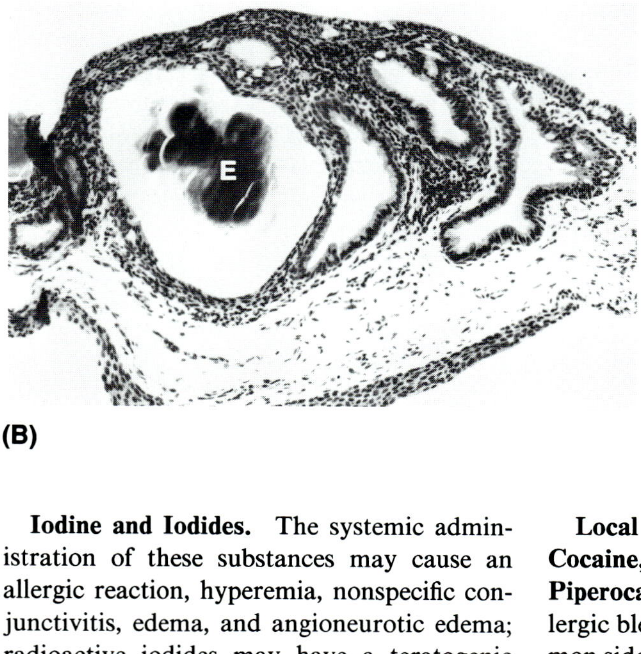

(B)

Fig. 16-11. (A) Gross appearance of palpebral conjunctival deposits of epinephrine (two black spots) following long-term topical use of drops. (B) Histologic section showing deposits of epinephrine derivative (E) in a conjunctival cyst. The deposits stain like melanin (i.e., bleaches and reduces silver salts). ×60. (Yanoff, M. & Fine, B. S.: Ocular Pathology. A Text and Atlas. Harper and Row, MD, 1975.)

Iodine and Iodides. The systemic administration of these substances may cause an allergic reaction, hyperemia, nonspecific conjunctivitis, edema, and angioneurotic edema; radioactive iodides may have a teratogenic effect.[114, 134, 156, 343]

Iron Compounds (Cholinate, Fumarate, Gluconate, Succinate, and Sulfate Salts of Ferrous, Iron Dextran, and Sorbitex, and Polysaccharated Iron Complex). Erythema, edema, and angioneurotic edema, as well as iron pigmentation of the conjunctiva, may occasionally be seen with the prolonged systemic administration of these agents.[71, 100]

Local Anesthetics (Benoxinate, Butacaine, Cocaine, Dibucaine, Dyclonine, Phenacain, Piperocaine, Proparacaine, Tetracaine). Allergic blepharoconjunctivitis is not an uncommon side effect of topical anesthetics, although the frequency of this condition may vary with the individual drug. Topical use of cocaine may additionally produce an exudative conjunctivitis and, rarely, ptosis.[156, 307, 343]

Mepacrine (Quinacrine). Systemic administration of mepacrine may produce variably colored (yellow, white, clear, brown, blue, or grey) punctate deposits in the conjunctiva. The deposits are due either to the drug itself

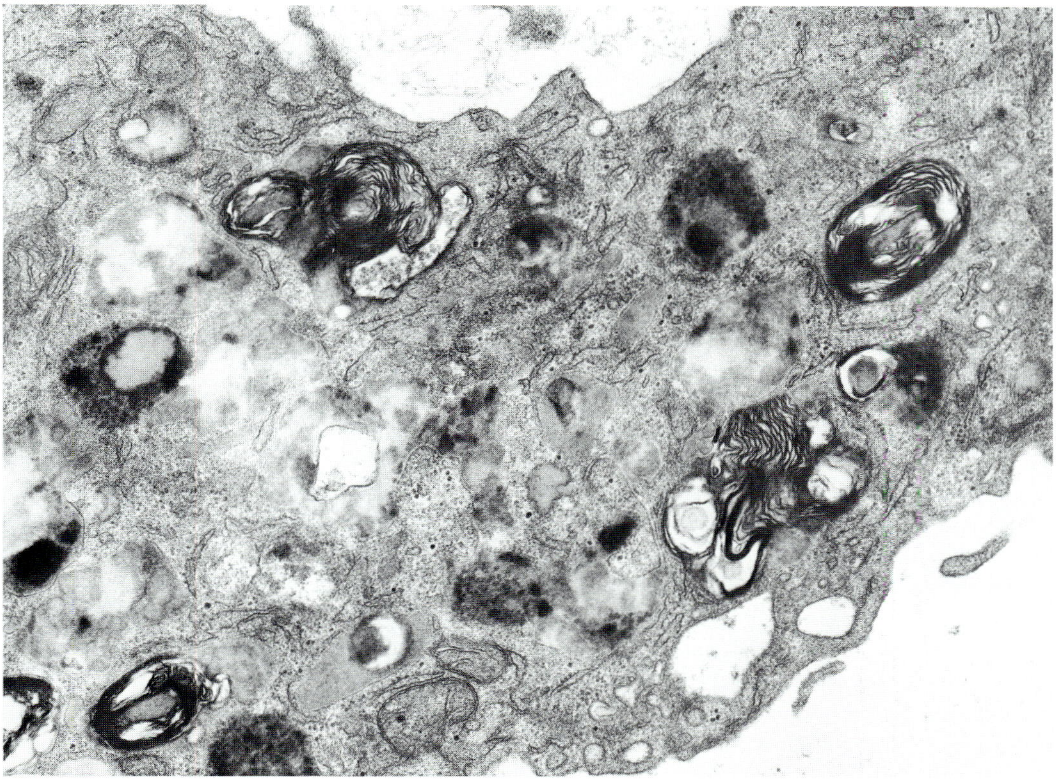

Fig. 16-12. Gentamicin toxicity. Granular and lamellar lipoidal structures in a conjunctival fibroblast following subconjunctival injection of gentamicin. Electron micrograph, ×33,000. (Courtesy Jacques Libert, M.D., University of Brussels.)

or to its metabolites within the basal conjunctival epithelial cells, as well as in the plica semilunaris and caruncle. Subconjunctival hemorrhages may occur secondary to mepacrine-induced anemia. The eyelid manifestations of mepacrine toxicity include exfoliative dermatitis, eczema, punctate deposits, and yellow discoloration.[137, 298]

Mercurial Compounds (Nitromersol Ointment, Ammoniated Mercury, Thimerosal). The chronic use of mercurial compounds causes conjunctival pigmentation with bluish-grey mercurial deposits, especially around blood vessels near the cornea. Blepharoconjunctivitis, erythema, and allergic reactions also occur. Delayed hypersensitivity to mercurial preservatives is not uncommon.[114, 306, 307, 343]

Miotics (Pilocarpine, Neostigmine, Physostigmine, Demercarium, Ecthothiophate, Isoflurophate). Topical application of these agents causes allergic reaction, follicular conjunctivitis, and conjunctival thickening. Physostigmine may also induce palpebral depigmentation. Punctal and lacrimal canalicular occlusion may occur with all of these drugs except pilocarpine.[114, 137, 156, 307]

Neomycin. Sensitivity to the topical application of neomycin is common, manifesting as a contact dermatitis and occasionally with angioneurotic edema of the eyelid. Withdrawal of the drug leads to slow clearing of the blepharitis, which may take several months, probably because the accumulated neomycin is released gradually from the stratum corneum.[104, 191]

Penicillin Derivatives (Semisynthetic or Natural). Systemic administration of penicillin derivatives may cause allergic reaction, nonspecific conjunctivitis, angioneurotic edema, Stevens-Johnson syndrome, exfoliative dermatitis, and Lyell's syndrome in the eye; subconjunctival hemorrhages may occur secondary to drug-induced anemia. Local subconjunctival injection of penicillin derivatives may produce irritation, hyperemia, allergic reaction, and angioneurotic edema. The incidence of allergic skin reactions to penicillin and ampicillin is high.[114, 137, 156, 307]

Phenacetin, Acetaminophen, Acetanilid. Rarely, allergic reactions, angioneurotic edema, urticaria, erythema multiforme, Stevens-Johnson syndrome, and subconjunctival hemorrhage secondary to drug-induced anemia occur with these drugs. This group of drugs can also produce sulfhemoglobinemia, which tends to give the conjunctival vessels a greenish tinge.[137, 337]

Phenazone (Antipyrine). This analgesic and antipyretic drug frequently causes a sensitivity reaction in the eye, manifesting as conjunctivitis together with edematous lid swelling, discoloration, and dermatitis. Toxic epidermal necrolysis caused by phenazone may be accompanied by ulcerative or pseudomembranous lesions of the conjunctiva or by Stevens-Johnson syndrome. In the eyelids, phenazone may produce discoloration, urticaria, an allergic reaction, and Lyell's syndrome.[114, 336, 343]

Phensuximide (Milontin). One case of phensuximide-induced oculotoxicity has been recorded, with induction of the typical ocular manifestations of Stevens-Johnson syndrome. Subconjunctival hemorrhage secondary to drug-induced anemia, and an allergic reaction, may be associated with palpebral involvement and periorbital edema.[173]

Phenylbutazone (Butazolidin). This drug may produce a Stevens-Johnson syndrome with typical conjunctival involvement. A greyish-yellow pseudomembrane may develop on the conjunctiva, together with an ischemic ring around the limbus and with severe dermatitis. Allergic reactions, hyperemia, edema, urticaria, and exfoliative dermatitis are frequent adverse ocular reactions to phenylbutazone. In some cases, Lyell's syndrome may manifest; subconjunctival hemorrhages secondary to drug-induced anemia may also occur. Ten to 15 percent of patients taking pyrazolon derivatives must discontinue their use of the drug because of a toxic reaction. Side effects of phenylbutazone are more common in patients older than 60 years.[53, 114, 134, 333]

Phenytoin (Diphenylhydantoin). Systemic administration of diphenylhydantoin may produce an allergic reaction, chronic conjunctivitis, ulceration, Stevens-Johnson syndrome, exfoliative dermatitis, and Lyell's syndrome in the eye. Subconjunctival hemorrhages, secondary to drug-induced anemia, are also seen. In the most toxic state, paralytic changes of the extraocular muscles may also occur. The drug may have a possible teratogenic effect.[326, 333, 343]

Practolol. Systemic administration of practolol may cause atrophy of the lacrimal glands, keratoconjunctivitis sicca, hyperemia, papillary eruptions, conjunctival scarring and cicatrix, and keratinization. The eyelids may show thickening, redness, "cafe au lait" pigmentation, and lupoid syndrome. Immunoperoxidase studies show fixation of a specific antibody, with an affinity for the intercellular spaces, in the conjunctival epithelium. Electron microscopy demonstrates electron-dense deposits in the intercellular spaces, which probably correspond to fixed immunoglobulins (Fig. 16-13). Practocol-associated epidermalization and necrolysis of the conjunctiva are probably related to destruction of the lacrimal glands.[121, 263, 314, 348]

Quinine. Systemic administration of this drug may cause an allergic reaction, angioneurotic edema, purpura, erythema multiforme, and Stevens-Johnson syndrome in the eye.[114]

Silver Compounds. Systemic absorption or topical application of these compounds (such as silver nitrate, colloidal silver, and mild silver proteinate) induce a nonspecific chemical conjunctivitis. Chronic use of silver-contain-

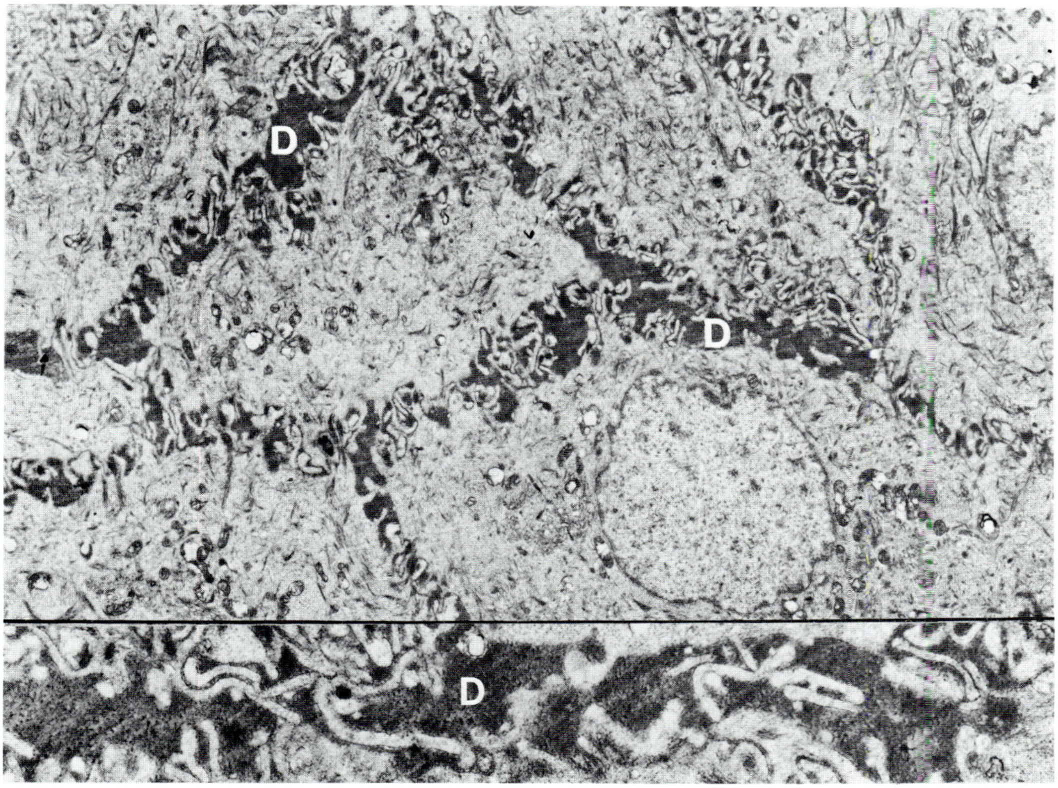

Fig. 16-13. Practolol toxicity. Intercellular deposits (D) of immunogobulins in conjunctival epithelium following systemic administration of practolol. Electron micrographs. ×4,750. Inset, ×12,050.

ing compounds may cause a slate-grey to black discoloration (argyrosis) of the mucous membranes, particularly in the fornices, as well as discoloration of the lids and nasolacrimal passages. One percent silver nitrate, as in crede prophylaxis for ophthalmia neonatorum, precipitates protein, including bacterial protein; the silver in this preparation reacts with sodium chloride of the tissue to form insoluble silver chloride. Stronger concentrations of silver nitrate cause epithelial coagulation and extensive scar formation.

Histologically, the metallic silver is deposited in closely packed dots of grey-black matter in the epithelial basement membrane, subepithelial reticulin fibers, and elastic tissue, as well as in the adventitia of the blood vessels (Fig. 16-14A, B, C).[149, 156, 223, 349]

Streptomycin. Systemic use of streptomycin may produce an allergic reaction, nonspecific conjunctivitis, angioneurotic edema, and a lupoid syndrome. Subconjunctival hemorrhages may occur as a result of drug-induced anemia. Topical application of streptomycin causes irritation, allergic reaction, and periorbital edema.[114, 307, 314]

Sulfonamide Drugs. Most commonly (in about 4 percent of patients), conjunctivitis, with or without follicles, appears between the 5th and 9th day of systemic administration of sulfonamides particularly with sulfathiazole. The manifestations of this condition include inflammation and chemosis of the conjunctiva accompanied by lid swelling, periorbital edema, photophobia, lacrimation, and discharge; in more severe cases, the changes resemble pemphigus and produce symblepharon, especially with the use of sulfadiazine and sulfamerazine. The conjunctival pathology may be combined with skin changes tak-

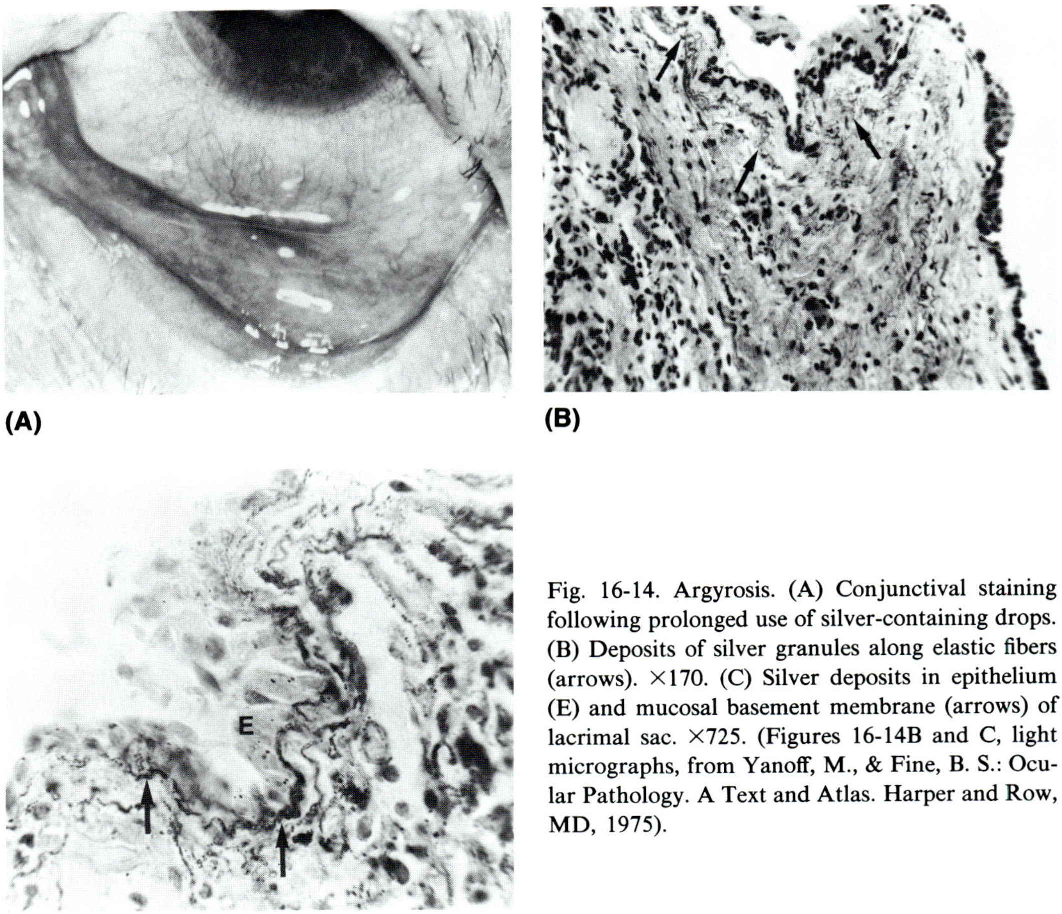

(A) (B) (C)

Fig. 16-14. Argyrosis. (A) Conjunctival staining following prolonged use of silver-containing drops. (B) Deposits of silver granules along elastic fibers (arrows). ×170. (C) Silver deposits in epithelium (E) and mucosal basement membrane (arrows) of lacrimal sac. ×725. (Figures 16-14B and C, light micrographs, from Yanoff, M., & Fine, B. S.: Ocular Pathology. A Text and Atlas. Harper and Row, MD, 1975).

ing the form of a Stevens-Johnson or Lyell syndrome. The foregoing reactions are usually reversible after discontinuing the causative drug. Subconjunctival hemorrhages may be associated with agranulocytosis and hemolytic anemia. Occasionally, keratitis may occur.

Topical application of sulfadiazine ointment for 1 year caused the formation of multiple, small white concretions within cysts of the palpebral conjunctiva. Sulfadiazine was identified in these concretions by spectroscopic studies.[44, 64, 237, 331]

Suxamethonium. In a 48-year-old woman with a 15-year history of progressive ocular myopathy, intravenous injection of 20 mg of succinylcholine resulted in succinate dehydrogenase-rich granules and bizarre mitochondria in the rectus muscle as demonstrated by light- and electron microscopy.[206]

Tetracycline. Systemic administration of tetracycline may produce erythema multiforme, angioneurotic edema, and Stevens-Johnson syndrome, whereas topical application of this drug may give rise to irritation and an allergic reaction in the eye.[114, 314]

Thiotepa. The topical use of thiotepa has been noted to produce depigmentation of the eyelids, particularly in darkly pigmented people; the process continues after the drug is discontinued. The pigment of the iris is apparently not affected. An allergic reaction, keratoconjunctivitis, loss of the eyelashes or eyebrows, and subconjunctival hemorrhages secondary to drug-induced anemia may also occur with thiotepa.[37, 137, 157]

Vincristine, Vinblastine. These chemotherapeutic agents may cause ptosis and ophthalmopelgia. Histologic examination of nerves and teased muscle fibers in cases of these conditions has indicated a primary axonal degeneration. Ocular signs of gout, which may include conjunctival hyperemia, uveitis, scleritis, and corneal deposits or ulceration, can also occur in association with vincristine or vinblastine therapy. In many cases, the changes are reversible when the drug is discontinued. There is questionable evidence of madarosis and teratogenic effects with the use of vincristine and vinblastine.[4, 46, 114]

Vitamin A. Hypervitaminosis A effects are more frequent in infants and children than in adults. Yellow discoloration of the eyelids may be associated with loss of the eyelashes or eyebrows, subconjunctival hemorrhage secondary to drug-induced anemia, and exophthalmos.[156, 233, 244, 320]

CORNEA AND SCLERA, INCLUDING THE DRAINAGE CHANNELS

The cornea and sclera together form the tough, fibrous protective coat for the internal structures of the eye. The cornea is a highly specialized, avascular structure almost unique in its transparency; complex physicochemical factors and a complex metabolism govern the degree of its hydration. Because of its exposed anatomic location, the cornea is frequently subjected to exogenous insults; endogenous affections start either in situ or spread from adjacent structures.

The corneal epithelium, the most sensitive structure in the body, is derived from surface ectoderm and is continuous with the conjunctival epithelium. It is regularly organized, consisting of five to six layers of stratified epithelial cells, covered anteriorly by a precorneal tear film that keeps the cells constantly moist and prevents keratinization (Fig. 16-15A, B). The anterior epithelial layers of the cornea are made up of flattened squamous cells, the intermediate layers are composed of transitional wing cells, and the columnar basal cells form the germinal layer. The adjacent interdigitating cell borders are joined by myriad desmosomes. The basal cells are attached by hemidesmosomes to a basal lamina (10 to 30 nm thick), which in turn is adherent to the modified zone of the anterior stroma—an acellular, collagenous feltwork known as Bowman's zone (Fig. 16-15C). The remainder of the corneal stroma, occupying some 85 percent of the total corneal thickness, consists of regularly arranged and equally-spaced collagen fibrils of nearly uniform diameter (Fig. 16-15D). The interfibrillar matrix is formed by glycosaminoglycans (keratan and chondroitin sulfates) thus sharing certain features in common with cartilage. The stroma contains scattered, modified fibroblasts or keratocytes, and is limited posteriorly by the predominantly collagenous, cuticular layer called Descemet's membrane, one of the thickest basement membranes in the body (Fig. 16-15E). The endothelial lining, the internal coat of the cornea, is formed by a unicellular layer of hexagonal cells that have a high metabolic activity. The secretory activity of the internal coat is responsible for the increasing thickness of Descemet's membrane. The factors determining corneal transparency include the structural organization, nature, and hydration of the collagen and ground substance, stromal avascularity, activity of the keratocytes, and the integrity and metabolism of the barrier layers of epithelium and endothelium.

The cornea is continuous posteriorly with the dense, fibrous coat of the sclera, which comprises some five-sixths of the eye (Fig. 16-16). The sclera is composed almost entirely of variable-diameter, interlacing bundles of collagen fibrils and scanty sclerocytes, a ground substance consisting of dermatan and chondroitin sulfates, and few blood vessels.

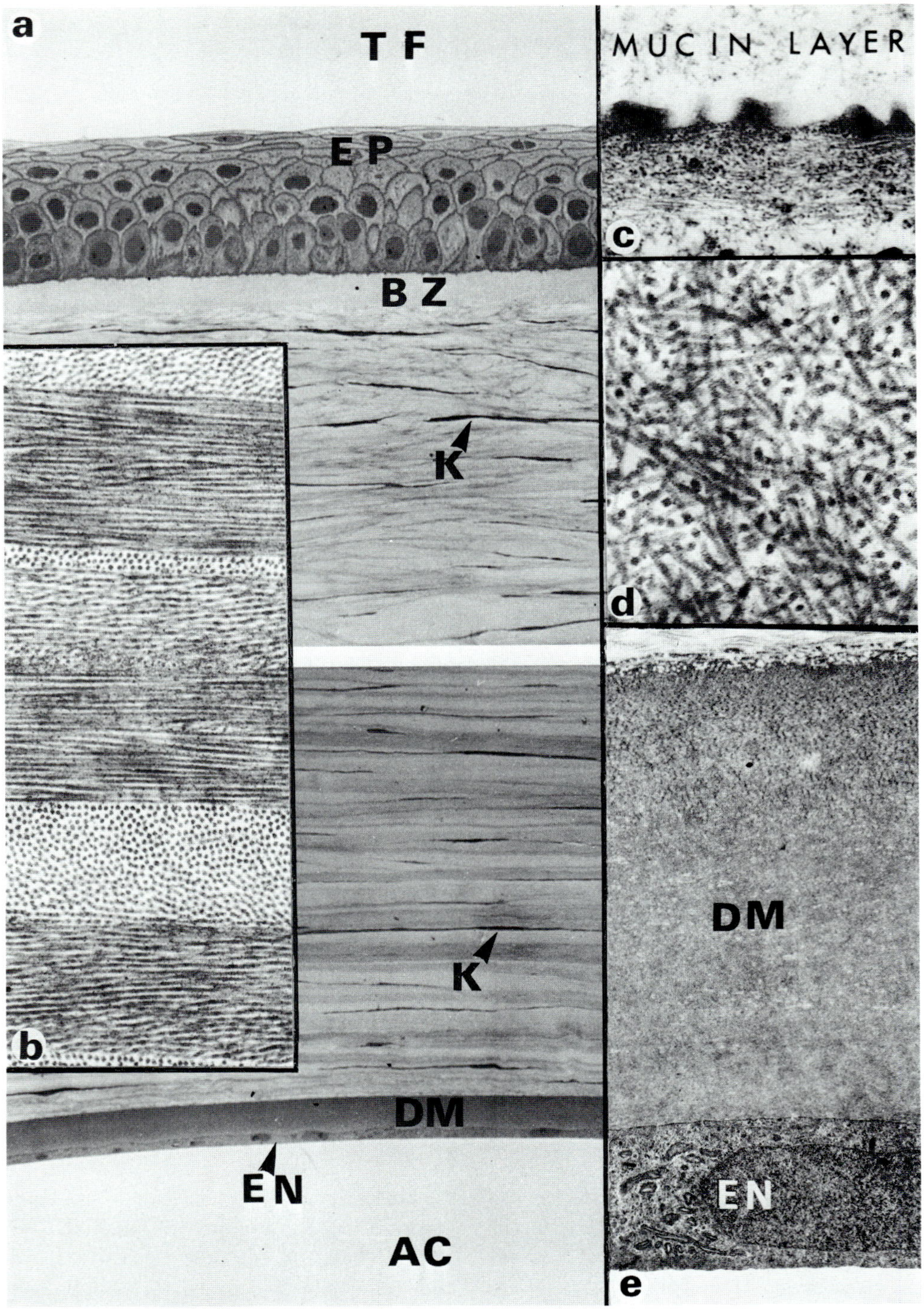

Fig. 16-15. (a) Light micrograph of cornea showing its layered architecture. EP, multilayered squamous epithelium; BZ, Bowman's zone of stroma; K, keratocytes in anterior and posterior stroma; DM, Descemet's membrane; EN, endothelium. The cornea is bathed anteriorly by tear fluid (TF) and posteriorly by aqueous humor of the anterior chamber (AC). ×400. (b) Corneal stroma showing regular and parallel arrangement of collagen fibrils in individual lamellae that cross each other at right angles. ×26,000. (c) A superficial cell of corneal epithelium showing microvillous surface projections covered by mucinous layer of the tear film. ×33,200. (d) Bowman's zone of stroma constituted by a feltwork arrangement of collagen fibrils. ×40,000. (e) Descemet's membrane (DM) is the thickened basement membrane of the endothelium (EN). ×7,250. Figures 16-15b through e are electron micrographs.

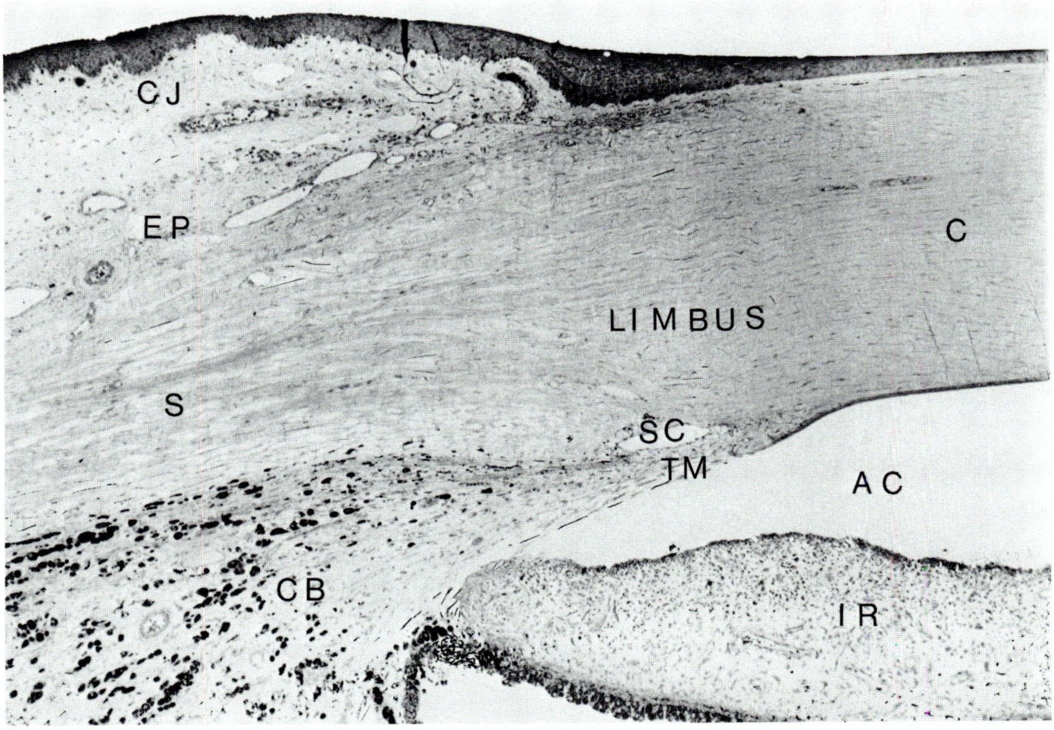

Fig. 16-16. Light micrograph of limbal region showing transition of regularly arranged collagen lamellae of cornea (C) into randomly arranged collagen lamellae of sclera (S). TM, trabecular meshwork; SC, Schlemm's canal; CB, ciliary body; IR, iris; AC, anterior chamber; EP, episclera; CJ, conjunctiva. ×50.

Anteriorly, the sclera is covered with the richly vascular episclera, Tenon's capsule (the fascia bulbi), and the conjunctiva. The transitional zone between the cornea and sclera, called the limbus, contains the aqueous drainage channels of the eye (Fig. 16-16). The internal limbus is occupied by superimposed, perforated sheets or beams known as the trabecular meshwork. The core of each beam is formed by fibrous tissue covered all around by flattened endothelial cells that are continuous internally with the corneal endothelium. The trabecular meshwork is separated from the compact corneosclera by a slit-like, endothelial-lined structure called Schlemm's canal. The extracellular spaces of the meshwork provide the pathway for the bulk flow of aqueous humor. The trabecular meshwork/Schlemm's canal system is subject to mechanical blockade and fibrocellular alterations in response to certain drugs, leading to glaucomatous disease of the eye.

Pathologic Reactions

The cornea is frequently involved in drug reactions and toxic insults. In such conditions, the pathologic alterations in the cornea and sclera vary, depending upon topical versus systemic administration and the nature of the causative drugs, toxins, poisons, and chemicals, and upon the nature of nonmechanical injuries. The corneal endothelium has a high aerobic metabolism, and is accordingly readily influenced by drugs, toxins, and other insults that affect the glycolytic pathway. The basic epithelial pathology includes intracellular edema (hydropic degeneration), extracellular edema (spongiosis), cystic and bullous

(Text continues on p. 399.)

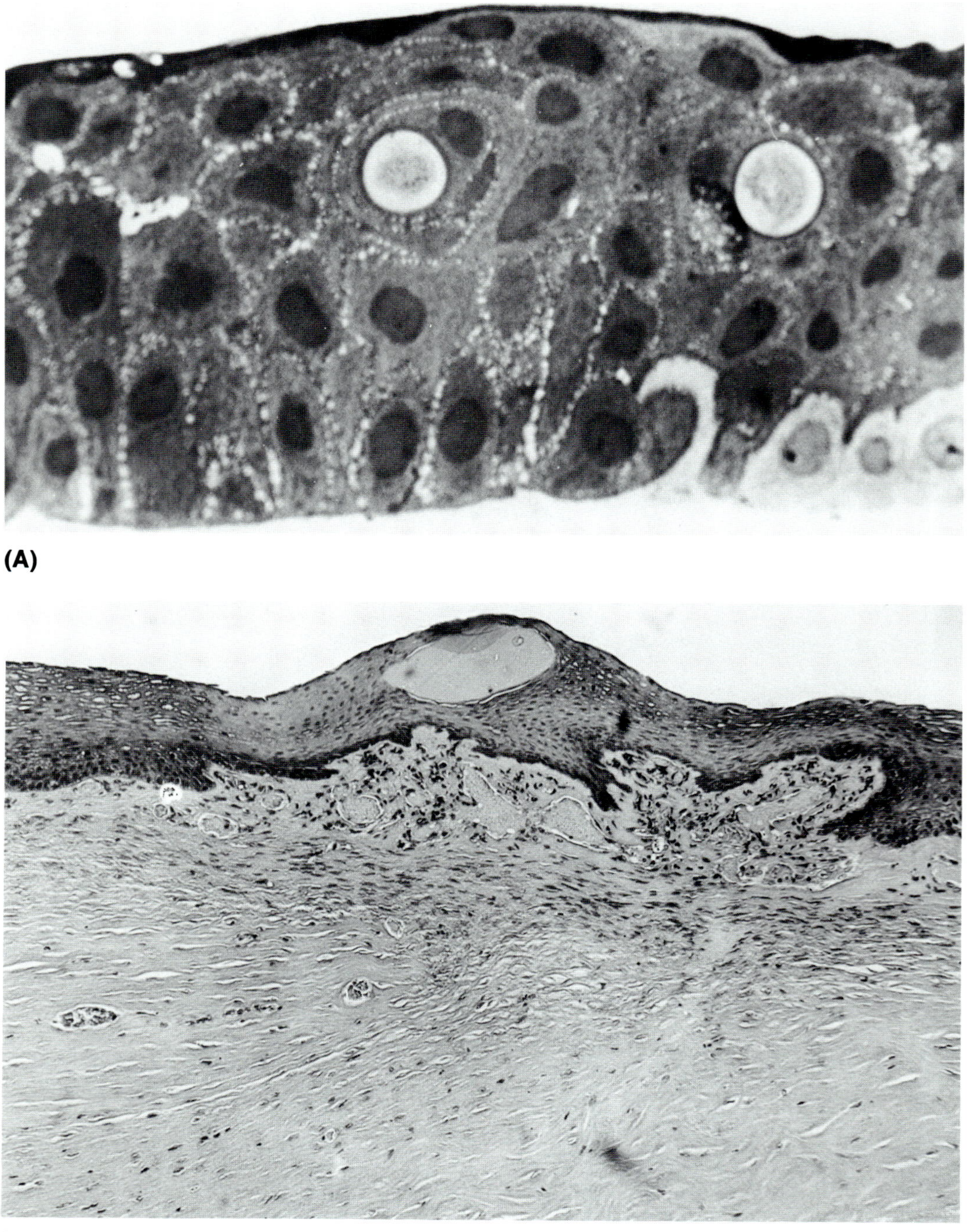

(A)

(B)

Fig. 16-17. (A) Edematous reaction of corneal epithelium manifesting as extracellular edema (spongiosis) and intracellular edema ("pale" cells) associated with cystic degeneration of cells. ×1,350. (B) Epidermalization of corneal epithelium characterized by rete peg formation, thickening, and keratinization. Bowman's zone is completely destroyed and the scarred anterior stroma is infiltrated with new blood vessels and chronic inflammatory cells. ×125.

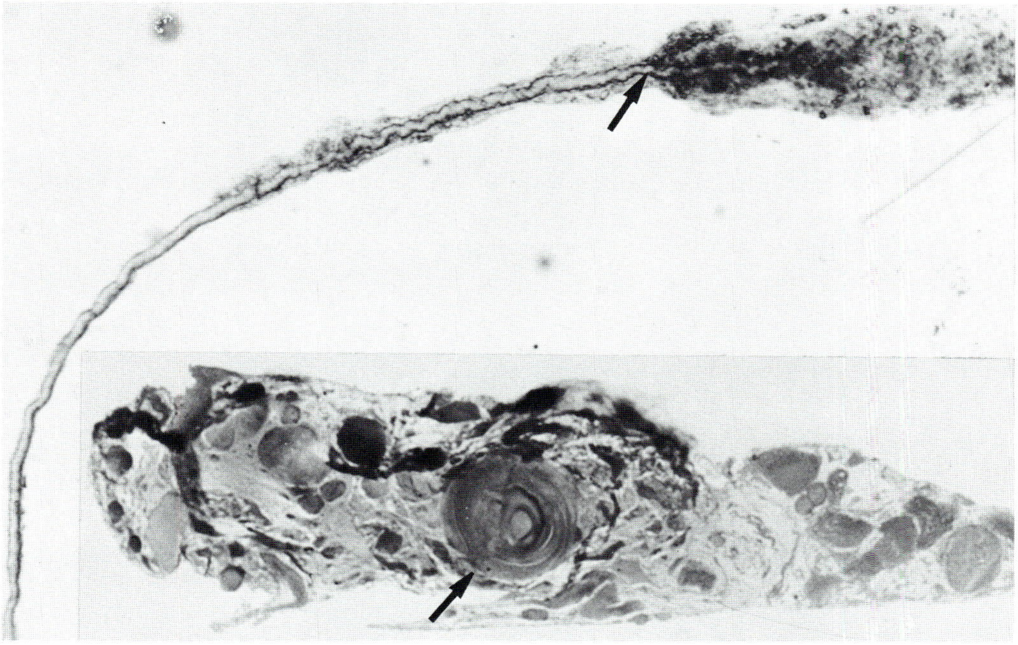

(C)

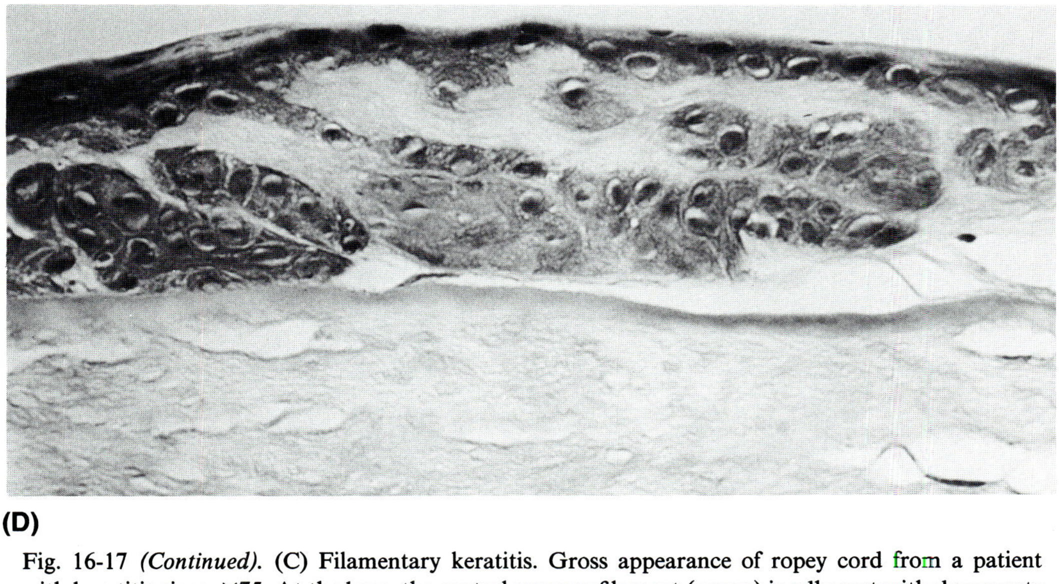

(D)

Fig. 16-17 *(Continued)*. (C) Filamentary keratitis. Gross appearance of ropey cord from a patient with keratitis sicca. ×75. At the base, the central mucous filament (arrow) is adherent with degenerate epithelial cells, glycoprotein, and lipoidal material, as seen in cross-section in the inset. ×760. (D) Extensive intraepithelial proliferation of basement membrane and fibrous tissue that may result from chronic degenerative changes of the corneal epithelium and hydrokeratopathy. ×450. Figures 16-17A through D are light micrographs.

(A)

(B)

(C)

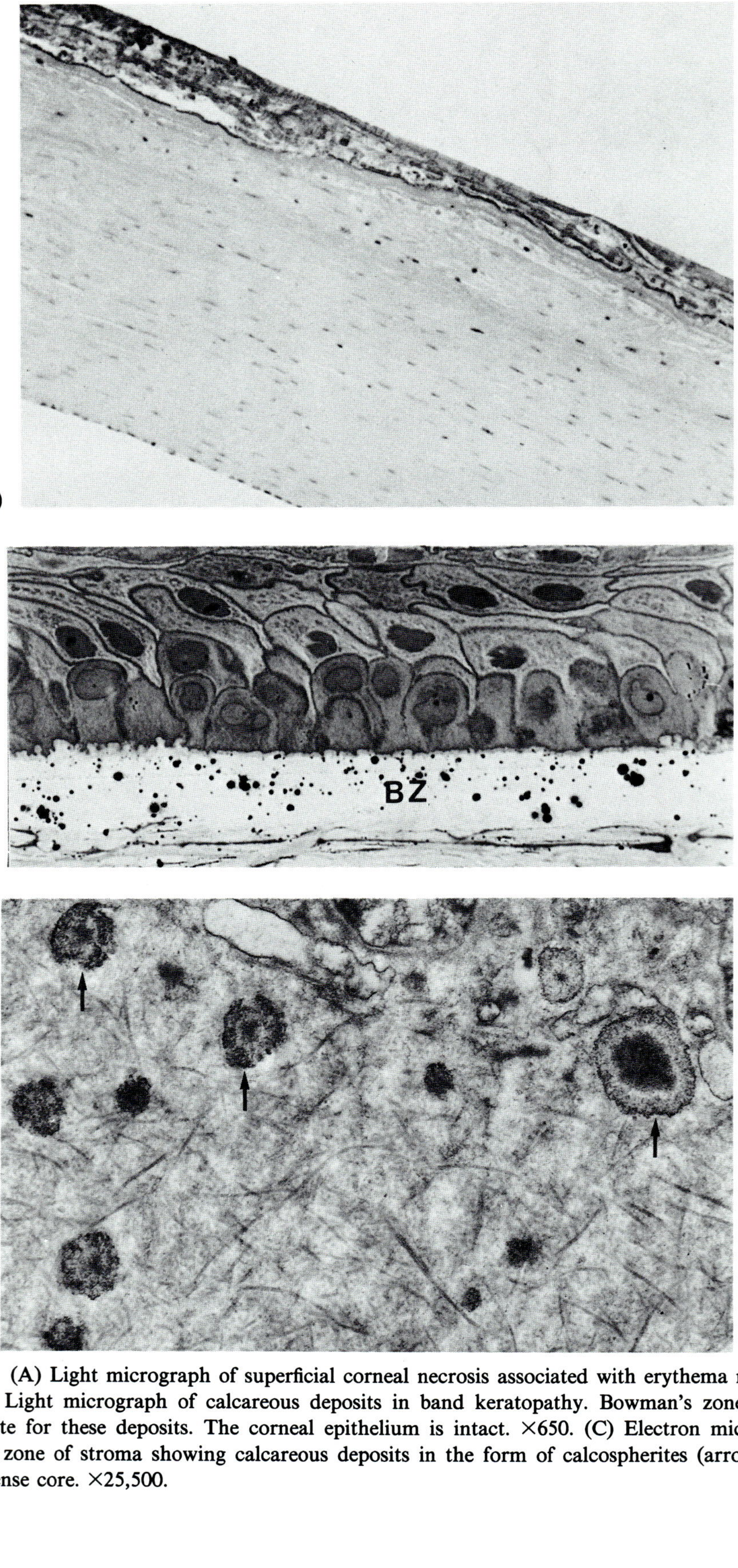

Fig. 16-18. (A) Light micrograph of superficial corneal necrosis associated with erythema multiforme. ×200. (B) Light micrograph of calcareous deposits in band keratopathy. Bowman's zone (BZ) is a frequent site for these deposits. The corneal epithelium is intact. ×650. (C) Electron micrograph of Bowman's zone of stroma showing calcareous deposits in the form of calcospherites (arrows) having electron-dense core. ×25,500.

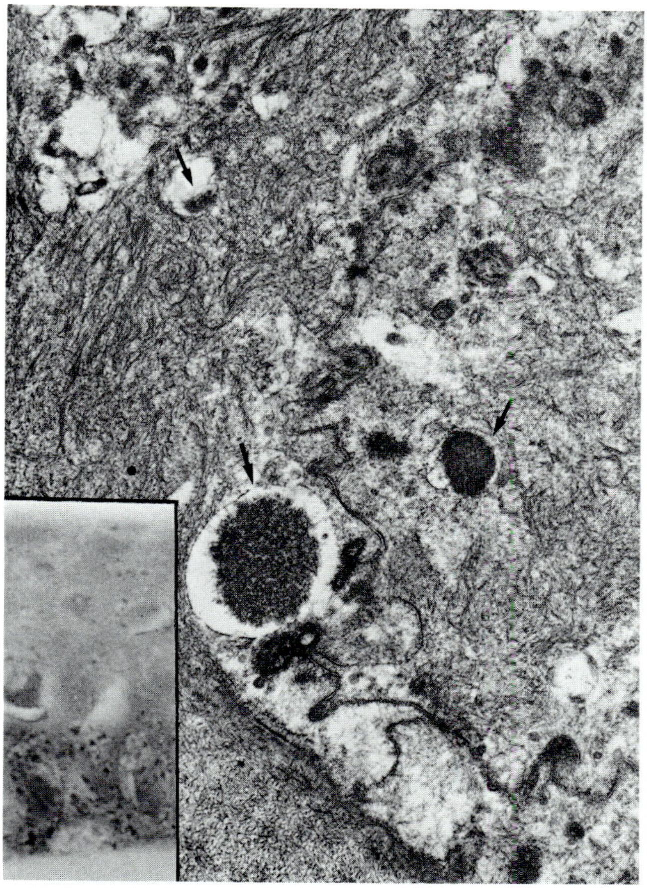

Fig. 16-18 *(Continued).* (D) Electron micrograph of granular electron-dense deposits of iron in membrane-bound structures (arrow) in the epithelium. ×15,000. Inset shows light microscopic appearance of corneal epithelium from a case of Fleischer ring. Prussian blue positive granules are seen predominantly in the basal cells. ×600.

changes, irregularity in cellular arrangement, dryness (keratitis sicca), keratinization (xerophthalmia), epidermalization and filament formation (filamentary keratitis, as in sicca and Sjogren's syndrome), cellular necrosis, focal or generalized loss (erosion) of epithelium, aberrant basement membrane/fibrous tissue formation, and pannus (subepithelial fibrous issue proliferation with or without vascularization) (Fig. 16-17A–D). Abnormal deposits and pigmentation may be seen within the cells or in the extracellular spaces, and the epithelium may participate in immunologic processes.

The basic stromal reactions include edematous changes, inflammation or interstitial keratitis (where inflammatory cells infiltrate the tissue), ulceration, necrosis, scarring (formation of haphazardly arranged collagen fibers of variable diameter), and vascularization, as well as degeneration, abnormal deposits, and pigmentation (such as the Fleischer ring, Hudson-Stahli line, or other regular, irregular, or generalized pigmentation) (Fig. 16-18A–D). The main changes in Descemet's membrane include physical alterations such as thickening, wrinkling, folds, or abnormal deposits, especially of heavy metals (Fig. 16-19A–C). Alterations in the integrity of the corneal endothelium and its metabolic activity readily influence the corneal hydration and transendothelial flux or penetration of toxic substances, whether these are secreted into the aqueous humor or penetrate the corneal thickness from outside.

Once the causative drug is discontinued,

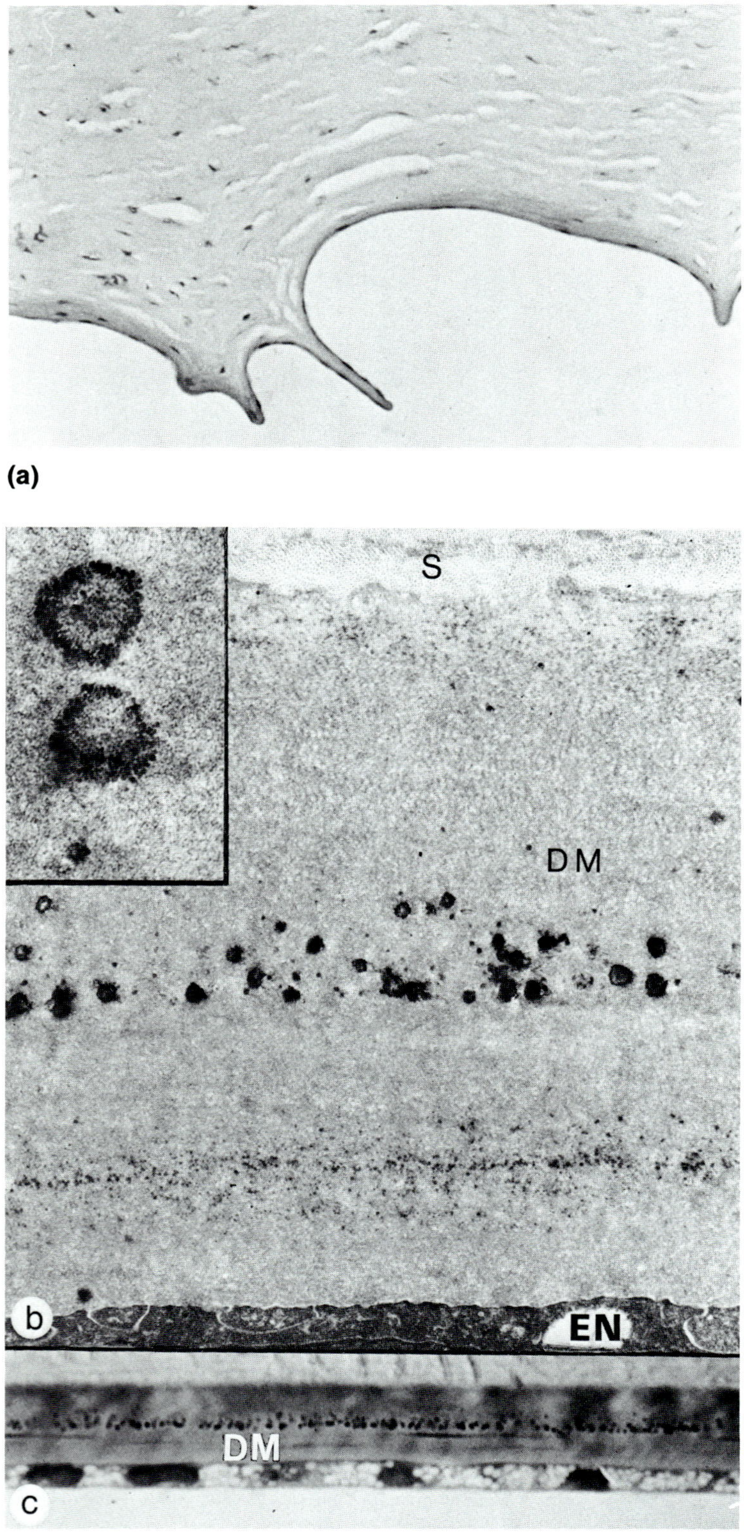

Fig. 16-19. (a) Light micrograph showing folds in Descemet's membrane and posterior stroma. ×200. (b) Pattern of copper deposits in Descemet's membrane (DM). Closer to the endothelium (EN), the deposits form fine granules. In the midregion of Descemet's membrane, larger deposits are seen with a central nidus (inset). S, posterior stroma. Electron micrographs. ×8,625. Inset ×56,925. (c) Light micrograph of peripheral Descemet's membrane (DM) showing histochemically demonstrable granular deposits of copper arranged in a linear fashion. In argyrosis, silver deposits show a similar pattern. ×900.

and provided there are no depots of the drug in the body, the epithelial deposits of the drug and its metabolites usually disappear within a few months to a year; the epithelial clearance is related to a continuous turnover of the actively metabolic epithelium. Stromal deposits, however, tend to remain for a long time, and are cleared mainly by diffusion and wandering macrophages.

The sclera is less commonly involved in drug reactions and toxic insults than the cornea. The manifestations of scleritis and episcleritis may be focal or extensive. Brawny scleritis (granulomatous inflammation) is more serious than anterior scleritis. Sclerokeratitis combines severe annular scleritis with a marked sclerosing keratitis; scleromalacia perforans may be the end result.

Drugs Affecting the Cornea and Sclera

Alcian Blue. In corneas with denuded epithelium, topical application of alcian blue may cause long-term staining of the basement membrane and the anterior stroma. The dye preferentially binds to the mucopolysaccharide component. Deposits of alcian blue in the basement membrane weaken the attachment of the regenerating epithelium since, in contrast to its behavior in normal regions, this epithelium can be easily dislodged even after several weeks of surface restoration. It is thought that the defect involves an alteration in the nature of the hemidesmosomes of the basal cells. In the stroma, the alcian blue particles are seen in the intercollagenous matrix and in the phagosomes of the corneal cells (Fig. 16-20).[50, 239, 314]

Alpha Chymotrypsin. This enzyme can digest the cement substance of the cellular attachment bodies. The direct effect of alpha-chymotrypsin injected into the anterior chamber of the eye is swelling and desquamation of the corneal endothelium, with resulting keratopathy; such injection also delays wound healing.

Approximately one-third of patients undergoing lens extraction with the use of alpha-

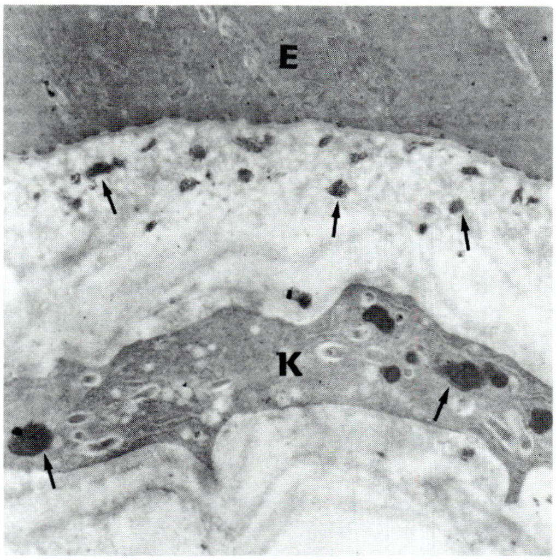

Fig. 16-20. Electron micrograph showing deposits of alcian blue granules (arrows) in the superficial stroma and keratocytes (K) following experimental application of alcian blue to a deepithelialized rabbit cornea. Many granular deposits of the dye persist for several months after restoration of the epithelium (E). ×7,000.

chymotrypsin show an increase in intraocular pressure 2 to 5 days postoperatively. Scanning electron microscopy has shown, in both monkeys and humans, that fragments of zonular fibers become trapped in the trabecular meshwork, causing a temporary blockade (1 to 3 weeks) to the egress of the aqueous humor (Fig. 16-21).[10, 70, 156, 190, 347]

Anesthetics, Local (Benoxinate, Butacaine, Cocaine, Dibucaine, Dyclonine, Phenacain, Piperacaine, Proparacaine, Tetracaine). Punctate keratitis, softening, erosion and sloughing of the epithelium, filaments, and ulceration are the oculotoxic effects of these agents. Repeated application of topical anesthetics to an already injured cornea produces erosion of the corneal epithelium and clouding and edema of the stroma, finally resulting in chronic keratitis and possibly in permanent opacification. Animal studies indicate that anesthetics depress the respiration and glycolysis of the epithelium, reduce its regenerative ability, increase its permeability, and render it sensitive. The primary toxic reaction appears

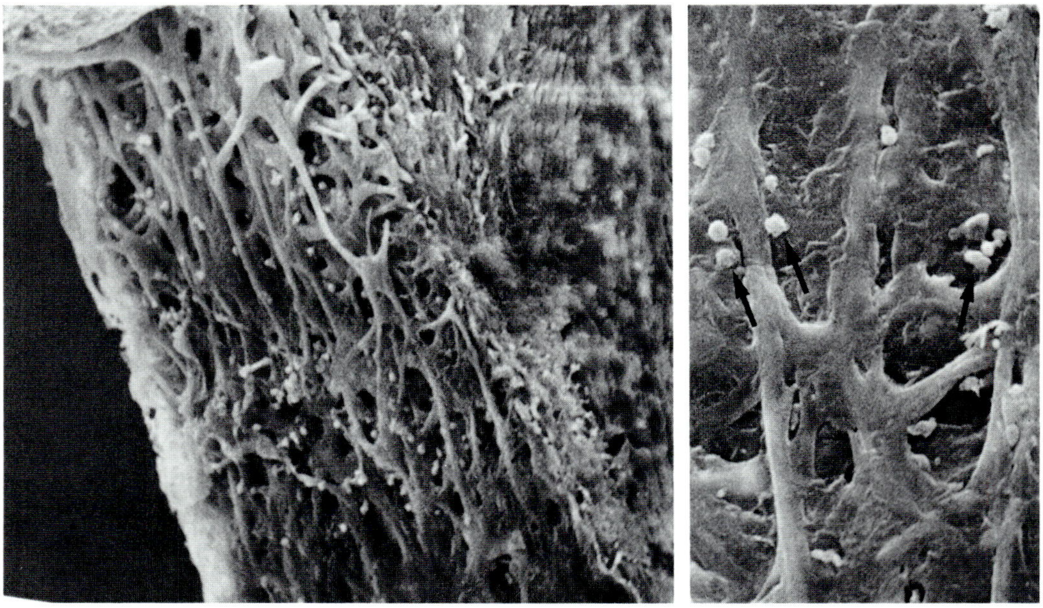

(A) **(B)**

Fig. 16-21. Scanning electron micrographs showing zonular fragments (arrows) deposited in the trabecular meshwork following experimental use of alpha-chymotrypsin in monkey. (A) ×1,000. (B) ×2,500. (Courtesy Douglas R. Anderson, M.D., Bascom Palmer Eye Institute.)

to be damage to the plasma membrane of the cell. The microvilli of the surface cells are affected, and the stability of the precorneal tear film may therefore be interrupted.[65, 103, 160, 290, 291, 314]

Anesthetics, General (Chloroform, Ether). Inadvertent exposure to these agents leads to hyperemia and edema of the conjunctiva. A splash of chloroform in the eye or prolonged exposure to ether during anesthesia causes keratitis, loss of corneal epithelium, ulceration, and corneal opacities.[100, 134, 137, 314]

Amidarone (Cordarone). Deposits of amidarone in the keratoconjunctiva occur after the systemic administration of this drug for periods of from 1 to 4 months; the deposits usually disappear within a few months following the withdrawal of the medication. The deposits consist of fine, yellowish-brown dots, sometimes condensed in a linear fashion, confined mainly to the palpebral fissure (Fig. 16-22A). Ultrastructural study suggests that the deposits are lysosomal inclusions, probably lipofuscins, in the epithelial cell cytoplasm, most likely occurring due to altered cellular metabolism (Fig. 16-22B). Corneal ulceration is rare.[47, 311]

Amodiaquine (Systemic). The metabolic products of amodiaquine are deposited in the corneal epithelium, which may be somewhat edematous. The deposits have also been observed in the sclera. In one patient, an acute toxicity reaction manifested with involvement of Bowman's zone and an associated discoloration of the skin and sclera not unlike icterus.[42, 137, 159]

Arabinoside (Ara-A), Idoxyuridine (IDU), Trifluorothymidine (TFT). Topical use of these agents causes punctate keratitis, corneal erosion, and delayed wound healing.[200, 201]

Arsenicals. Epithelial exfoliation and toxic degeneration of the corneal epithelium caused by arsenical agents may be followed by necrosis, ulceration, and perforation.[146, 187, 314, 333]

Aspirin (Sodium Salicylate, Acetylsalicylic Acid). Administered systemically, aspirin may occasionally cause keratitis. Inadvertent local exposure may cause keratitis with or

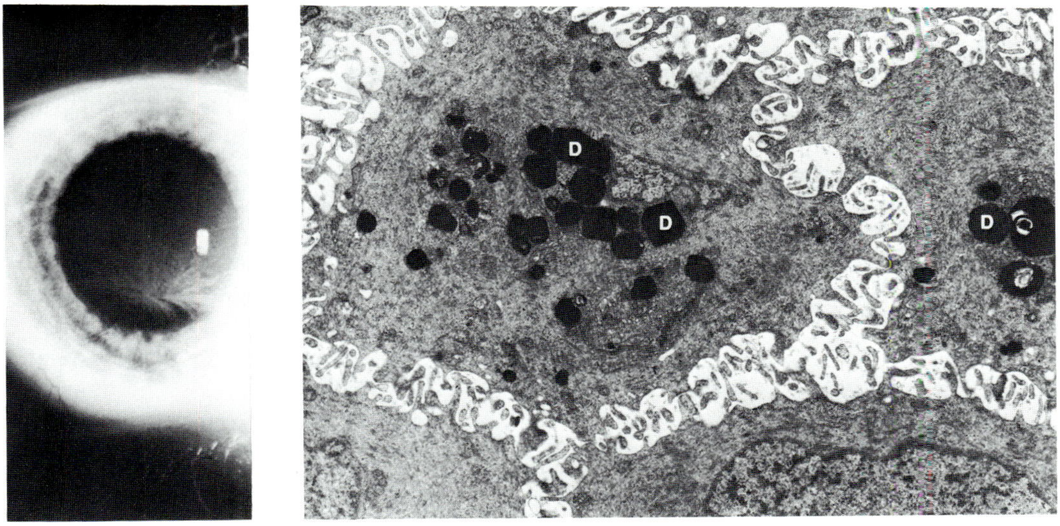

(A) **(B)**

Fig. 16-22. (A) Clinical photograph of cornea manifesting amidarone toxicity. (Courtesy Anthony J. Bron, M.D., F.R.C.S., University of Oxford.) (B) Electron micrograph of amidarone deposits in conjunctival epithelium. ×6,000. (Courtesy Jacques Libert, M.D., University of Brussels.)

without ulceration with systemic administration. The incidence of rebleed in traumatic hyphema is increased significantly.[84, 114, 314, 333]

Atropine. Local ophthalmic use, exposure, or subconjunctival injection of atropine may cause brawny scleritis.[114]

Benzalkonium. Topical use of benzalkonium in the eye may cause loss of epithelial microvilli and produce the fine grey dots of keratitis epithelialis. Damage to the cell plasma membrane by emulsification may occur with even an 0.01 percent solution of benzalkonium. Higher concentrations (such as 10 percent) cause corneal edema, vascularization, and scarring.[301]

Bismuth Compounds (Systemic). Corneal deposits of bismuth may occur as fine white crystals which clear when bismuth-containing medications are stopped.[108]

Chloroquine, Hydroxychloroquine (Systemic). Dose- and time-related corneal changes are fairly common with these drugs, and may appear in 3 weeks with high doses, and as late as 6 years with low doses. Deposits of chloroquine or its metabolites occur in the corneal epithelium, where they appear as numerous fine white or yellowish dots, often in the region corresponding to the palpebral fissure, arranged in a vortex-like pattern. The deposits are intracellular and are recognized by their strong autofluorescence. The corneal changes are reversible upon cessation of medication, and are not related to the retinal pathology.[39, 59, 159, 162, 242, 289, 314]

Chlorpromazine. Large oral doses (total 500 to 1,000 grams) of chlorpromazine produce the deposition of yellowish-white granules in the deepest layers of the stroma just anterior to Descemet's membrane, and fine deposits in the corneal endothelium. These deposits occur mainly in the region of the palpebral fissure, and when dense may give the cornea a brownish haze. Patients on larger doses of chlorpromazine may also have fine pigmented lines or streaks in the corneal epithelium. The distribution of these deposits has led to the suggestion that light may be a factor in their genesis, especially since chlorpromazine is a well-known photosensitizing agent.[95, 133, 219, 260, 340]

Chlorprothixene (Systemic). Corneal deposits, with or without keratitis, may occur with chlorprothixene. The deposits are similar to those seen in the lens (see p. 411).[114]

Chrysarobin. Systemic absorption of chrysarobin through the skin produces superficial grey opacities, together with a marked keratoconjunctivitis. Resolution generally occurs within 2 weeks. Inadvertent ocular contamination with chrysarobin produces punctate defects in the corneal epithelium.[5, 100, 343]

Corticosteroids. With the topical use of corticosteroids, thinning of the cornea and sclera, as well as punctate keratitis and delayed healing, may occur. Subconjunctival injection of corticosteroids into a diseased cornea and sclera may enhance thinning and even cause rupture of these structures.

Topical application of corticosteroids is far more effective in producing adverse changes in intraocular pressure than is its systemic administration. The corticosteroid-induced increase in intraocular pressure is markedly greater in glaucomatous eyes than in a normotensive eye; there is, however, a genetic predisposition to this corticosteroid response. The exact mechanism by which the increase in intraocular pressure is brought about is not clear; speculated mechanisms have ranged from swelling and excessive production of glycosaminoglycans to deposits of amorphous and fibrous material in the extracellular spaces of the trabecular meshwork and juxtacanalicular tissue. The changes reported are, however, indistinguishable from those seen in chronic simple glaucoma.[114, 156, 181, 245, 273, 313]

Cytosine Arabinoside (Cytarabine). Given topically at a concentration of 0.5 to 0.1 percent, cytosine arabinoside may cause development of glittering opacities in the deeper layers of the corneal epithelium, as well as keratitis and ulceration. The changes are reversible with discontinuation of the drug.[102, 156, 180]

Diiodohydroxyquine, Iodochlorohydroxyquine. Systemic administration of these agents may produce corneal opacities.[335]

Echothiophate. Corneal deposits may occur with the long-term topical use of echothiophate.[114]

Epinephrine (Adrenalin). With prolonged topical use of epinephrine, brown or black discoloration of the cornea develops. Oxidized epinephrine products may accumulate in roughened and edematous corneal areas, particularly gaining entry through ulcerated or bullous epithelium, and occurring with the use of discolored solutions of the drug. Circumscribed, black nodular, superficial corneal deposits or dense, brown-black discoloration of the entire cornea, resembling severe blood staining, may occur. Histologically, granular deposits may be found not only in the epithelium and subepithelial region of the cornea, but also in Bowman's zone and the deeper stroma (Fig. 16-23). In long-term topical therapy with epinephrine, degenerative corneal endothelial changes have been noted. Prolonged use of epinephrine causes discoloration of soft contact lenses; immersion of discolored contact lenses in 3 percent hydrogen peroxide for several hours will bleach the lenses back to their original state, but soaking in 2.5 percent sodium thiosulfate for 15 minutes and a thorough rinsing are required before reuse.[98, 107, 139, 214, 268, 317, 334]

Estrogen-Progestin Combination Products (Oral Contraceptives). Thickening of the corneal stroma, punctate keratitis, and epithelial edema may occur with these products, ac-

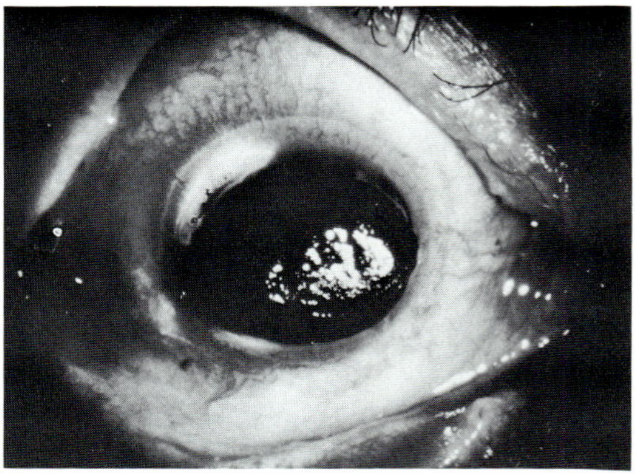

Fig. 16-23. Gross appearance of an advanced case of epinephrine keratopathy showing blackened central cornea. (Nicholson, D. H.: Ocular Pathology Update. pp. 253–259. © 1981 Masson Publishing USA, Inc., New York.)

counting for intolerance to contact lenses. Allergic reactions may manifest in the conjunctiva and eyelid.[114, 316]

Gold (Systemic: Gold Thiosulfate or Thiomalate; Topical: Gold Chloride). At moderate doses and after several months of therapy with gold compounds, gold deposition in the axial corneal epithelium appears as tiny punctate, glittering, golden-yellow, crystal-like opacities (Fig. 16-24). On cessation of treatment, the epithelial deposits disappear in a few months to a year. When gold compounds are given in high and cumulative doses, deposits of gold particles appear as fine, dust-like granules throughout the stroma, especially in the deeper layers including Descemet membrane; under such conditions the cornea may develop a red to purple color. Exposure to light favors the deposition. The lesions are asymptomatic.

In several patients treated with gold compounds, a more severe ulcerative keratitis has occurred, particularly in patients treated for pulmonary tuberculosis and rheumatoid arthritis. The keratitis first manifests as a superficial white opacity close to the limbal margin, that then spreads over the entire cornea and along the limbus. A pannus-like vascularization may develop if healing is delayed.[49, 155, 234, 270, 308, 314]

Indomethacin (Indocin). Systemic use of this drug may lead to an indomethacin-induced keratopathy, resembling chloroquine keratopathy, with a whorl-like pattern; alternatively, the corneal changes may appear only as fine, speckled opacities superficially and deep in the stroma. The opacities disappear upon discontinuing the medication.[58, 309]

Iodine and Iodides. Local application of these agents may cause keratitis bullosa,

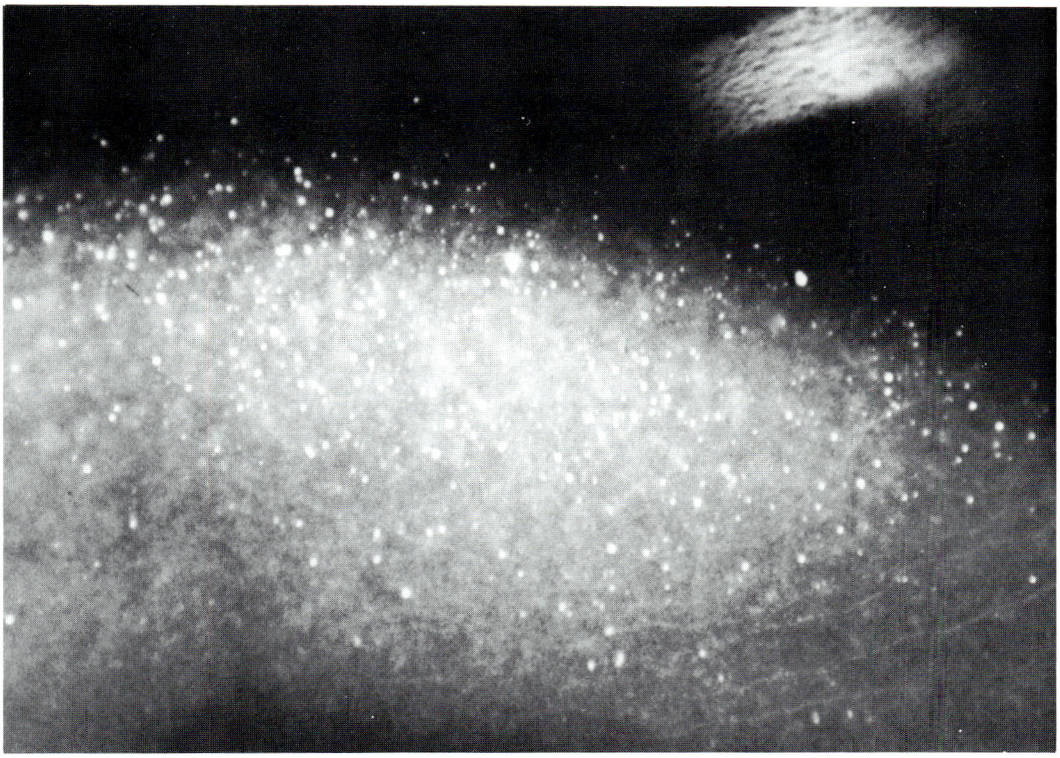

Fig. 16-24. Gold toxicity. With slit-lamp biomicroscopy, the epithelial deposits of gold appear as glittering specules. (Courtesy Anthony J. Bron, M.D., F.R.C.S., University of Oxford.)

brown discoloration, vascularization, stromal scarring, folds in Descemet's membrane, and delayed healing of corneal wounds.[129, 137, 314]

Iron Compounds (Cholinate, Fumarate, Gluconate, Succinate, and Sulfate Salts of Ferrous, Iron Dextran, and Sorbitex, and Polysaccharated Iron Complex). Prolonged systemic use of iron compounds may rarely cause a yellow-brown discoloration of the sclera.[114, 137]

Mepacrine (Quinacrine). Systemic administration of mepacrine produces deposits in and a yellow discoloration of the cornea, as well as epithelial edema. Direct contact of mepacrine powder, however, produces a severe striate keratopathy or wrinkling of the posterior corneal surface, presumably due to edema, in addition to the yellow-green staining of the cornea. The cornea returns to normal in both cases upon discontinuing the drug.[11, 69, 293, 333]

Mercurial Compounds (Nitromersol Ointment, Ammoniated Mercury, Thimerosal). Deposits of mercuric oxide, which may appear as a greyish ring, are seen in the peripheral Descemet's membrane in patients treated with mercurial compounds. Dense particles in the cytoplasm of the corneal epithelium and in the stromal cells of the superficial cornea have been reported in many patients who for several years used eyedrops containing phenylmercuric nitrate as a preservative. Experimental perfusion of the cornea with 0.005 to 0.001 percent thimerosal has resulted in increased corneal thickness and ultrastructural damage to the endothelial cells (vacuoles and swollen mitochondria).[122, 137, 325]

Penicillin Derivatives (Semisynthetic and Natural). Subconjunctival injection of cloxacillin may produce corneal opacities.[114]

Phenylbutazone (Butazolidin). With systemic use, phenylbutazone, in addition to producing a severe keratoconjunctivitis, may produce opacification and permeation of the cornea by new blood vessels, and symblepharon. The corneal changes regress after cessation of the drug.[7, 266, 314, 333, 343]

Phenytoin (Diphenylhydantoin). Administered systemically, this drug is believed to stimulate collagen production and may have a role in the formation of corneal keloids (Fig. 16-25).[315]

Practolol (Systemic). Practolol-induced, dense white or yellow stromal opacities, together with stromal thinning, may lead to corneal perforation. An intercellular antibody has been found in the serum of several patients, and intercellular deposits of specific antibody have been demonstrated by immunoperoxidase staining, suggesting a possible immunologic mechanism for practolol toxicity.[6, 121, 263, 314, 348]

Pyridine-3-Aldehyde-Thiosemicarbazone. Since this agent is used in combination with other antituberculous drugs, its ocular toxicity is not clear. Vacuoles in the corneal epithelium

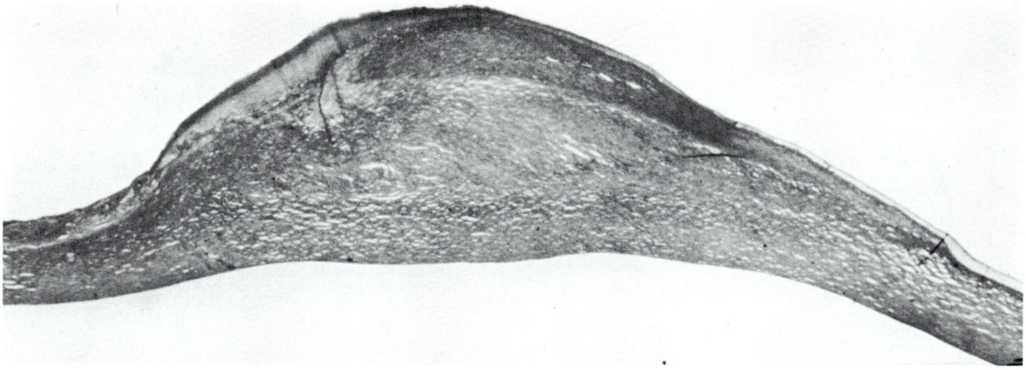

Fig. 16-25. Histologic appearance of corneal keloid in a patient receiving phenytoin therapy. The etiologic significance of the drug in this case is, however, not finally established. ×45.

(from a few to several hundred) have been reported, together with conjunctival hyperemia.[255]

Silver Compounds (Topical). Granular deposits of silver in Descemet's membrane produce a greenish-blue or grey hue at the limbus. A 6 to 12 percent silver nitrate solution may cause epithelial loss and extensive scar formation.[63, 138, 143, 149, 314]

Sodium Bisulfite. Used as an antioxidant in commercially available epinephrine solutions, sodium bisulfite may cause toxic damage to the corneal endothelium. Since pure epinephrine (1:1,000) did not cause endothelial damage even after 5 minutes of perfusion, sodium bisulfite has been suggested to be the main toxic agent in such preparations (see p. 387).[156]

Trichloroethylene (Inhalation Anesthetic). Systemic administration of trichloroethylene may cause corneal anesthesia and ulceration. Inadvertent ocular exposure to this substance produces punctate keratitis and corneal opacities.[137]

Vitamin D. In hypervitaminosis D, calcareous band keratopathy and diffuse, granular deposits may extend to other locations in the conjunctiva and even into the sclera (Fig. 16-18B,C).[123, 314, 337]

LENS

The crystalline lens is a biconvex, transparent structure (9 mm in diameter and 4 mm in central thickness) located behind the iris in a shallow depression of the anterior vitreous humor (Fig. 16-1). It is held in place by the zonular fibers extending between the lens capsule and the ciliary epithelium. The capsule, which completely encloses the lens, is a transparent, smooth, reflective, elastic, and indigestible, PAS-positive, thick collagenous basement membrane. Anteriorly beneath the lens capsule there is a single layer of cuboidal epithelial cells which continue posteriorly as far as the equator.

The lens increases in size throughout life because new cells are constantly added to it, owing to the mitotic activity of the epithelial cells in the equatorial region. The newly formed cells elongate, sending processes both anteriorly and posteriorly to form the so-called lens fibers which, at maturity, measure some 7 to 10 mm in length, 8 to 10 μm in width, and 2 to 5 μm in thickness. The nuclei of the cells migrate somewhat anterior to the equator to form the nuclear bow (Fig. 16-26), and eventually disappear. Owing to the superimposition of new cells, the older fibers become progressively displaced toward the center of the lens. Since the lens cells or fibers grow from all around the equator toward the anterior and posterior poles of the lens, they meet along radiating lines or sutures. Adjacent fibers interdigitate by complex ball-and-socket joints.

Several zones or nuclei may be distinguished in the adult lens. The embryonic nucleus is formed by the posterior primordial lens cells, which elongated rapidly to fill the lens vesicle and lose their cell nuclei; hence there is no epithelial cell layer beneath the posterior capsule similar to that present anteriorly. The fetal nucleus has two distinctive Y-shaped sutures (erect anteriorly and inverted posteriorly) to which the lens fibers join. The sutures formed after birth become more complex as the eye ages, having branches and further radial subdivisions. The adult nucleus is formed by the increasing density of the older lens fibers. A zone of external fibers show, on slit-lamp examination, a refractive index less than that of the nucleus; this zone is distinguished as the cortex. Histologically, the outlines of individual cells in the nucleus are indistinguishable.

Pathologic Reactions

Because new lens fibers are formed throughout life, it is possible to approximate the time in life at which the toxic effects of a specific agent may have become manifest. Thus, cataract may be classified as embryonic, fetal, or

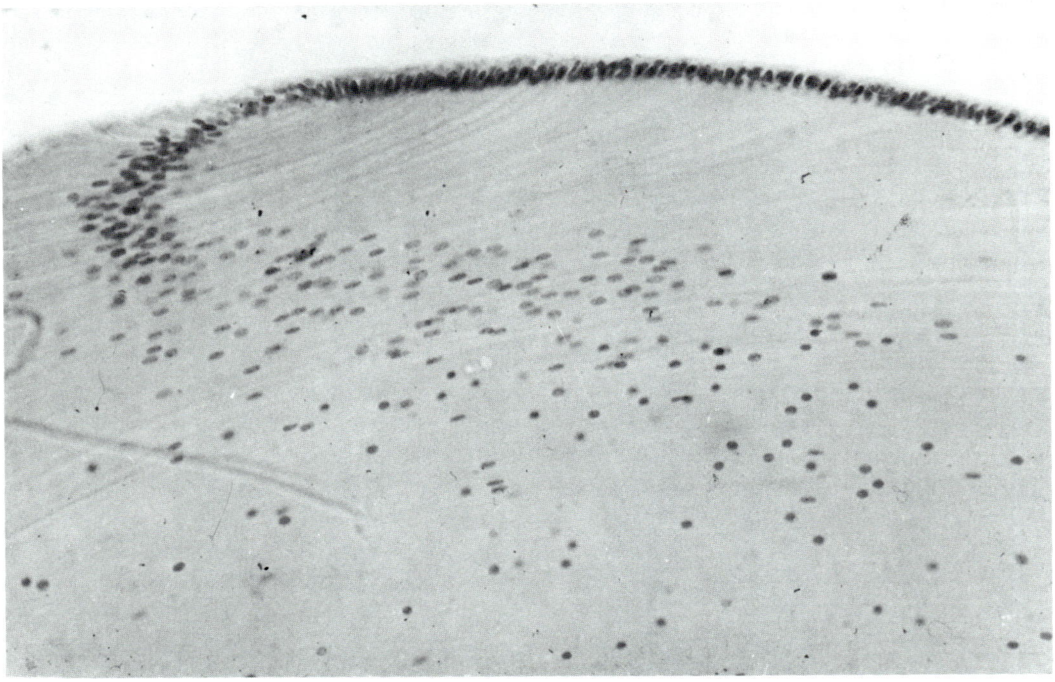

Fig. 16-26. Light micrograph of the equatorial region of the lens showing proliferative activity of the lens epithelium at the nuclear bow. ×200.

adult. Further designation of the cataract is often made according to its anatomic location. Many clinical types of cataracts are recognized (such as cuneiform, coronal, spoke-like, clefts), but their pathologic counterparts are nonspecific.

Histopathologically, most toxic changes seen in the lens cortex include clefts (diffuse watery or eosinophilic material derived from altered or denatured cell proteins), complex cellular tangles, and cell fragments (disrupted cortical cells); these lead to the formation of morganian globules (rounded fragments of cortical cells) (Fig. 16-27A–C). Excessive morganian globules together with denatured protein cause increasing hyperosmolarity of the cortex, resulting in the absorption of fluid; an intumescent, mature, liquefied, or morganian cataract may form. The entire lens may appear clinically as a milk-filled sac with a free-floating, small shrunken nucleus. The escape of liquefied lens material through the capsule results in a small lens with a wrinkled capsule, known as a hypermature cataract. In long-standing cataract, numerous crystals (calcium oxalate and cholesterol) and relatively insoluble amino acids may become deposited. Cataracta calcaria is an example of dystrophic calcification. It is to be noted that some changes (for example, vacuoles) in the lens cortex could be reversible once the toxic insult is withdrawn (Fig. 16-27D).

Densification and color changes (cataracta brunescence, cataracta nigra) increasing the refractive index of the nucleus and impeding light transmission, constitute what is known as a nuclear (hard) cataract. The histologic changes in this condition are subtle, consisting of absence of the usual artifactitious nuclear clefts and the formation of amorphous, homogenous, eosinophilic material. Electron microscopically, the lens fibers appear electron dense, extremely folded, and tightly packed, with obliteration of intercellular spaces.

Noxious insults may almost exclusively affect the lens epithelium. Anterior subcapsular cataract results from necrotic changes in the epithelium of the anterior pole. The adjacent epithelial cells migrate into the area, proliferate, and become metaplastic to form a subcapsular connective tissue plaque, which may be demarcated by the restoration of epithelial continuity beneath the plaque. With anterior subcapsular cataract, an anterior cortical cataract (duplication cataract) may form, depending upon the extent of the injury (Fig. 16-28A).

In posterior subcapsular cataract, the degeneration of the subcapsular posterior lens fibers is followed by proliferation and migration of epithelial cells from the equator. The abnormally positioned cells enlarge to contain abundant, pale-staining vesicular cytoplasm and small nuclei, and are known as bladder cells. Extension of similar changes to involve the deeper posterior cortex constitutes posterior cortical cataract (Fig. 16-28B,C).

Because of the proximity of the epithelium and its capsule to the aqueous humor and the high cellular metabolic activity, drugs and noxious substances as well as heavy metals may be physically deposited in the lens capsule or actively taken up by the lens epithelium.

To a great extent, the location of opacities in the lens may be determined by the route of drug administration. For example, equatorial changes are more common with systemically administered drugs that cross the blood-aqueous barrier, whereas centrally located anterior lens changes (corresponding to the pupillary area) are more common with topically administered drugs. Posterior subcapsular and cortical changes occur more often as a result of diffusion of noxious substances from the posterior chamber; by crossing the blood-aqueous barrier, and through disturbances of the vitreous humor, agents capable of penetrating the blood-retinal barrier may have a similar effect. The onset of deeper lens changes depends upon the permeability characteristics of the agent and the barrier function of the lens structures. The lens capsule offers little barrier to diffusion, other than to the diffusion of large proteins and macromolecules. Agents interfering with the glycolytic pathway could be expected to have little effect because of the predominantly anaerobic metabolism of the lens. Since the lens epithelium, located anteriorly and equatorially, is the site of active cation transport and of mitotic activity, it is often affected by noxious agents.

Drugs Affecting the Lens

Alpha Chymotrypsin. Posterior chamber injection of this proteolytic enzyme causes lysis of amino acid linkages of the zonular fibers of the lens, fragmenting them to about 100-nm units.[10, 156, 346]

Anticholinesterases (Topical Miotics: Demecarium, Echothiophate, Isoflurophate). The strongest concentrations of these miotic agents are suspected of producing cataracts. The anterior lens changes begin as subcapsular and epithelial vacuoles, which aggregate into irregular streaks or patches followed by the development of posterior subcapsular and nuclear opacities. The fundamental toxicologic or biochemical basis for these changes is not understood; an inhibition of cholinesterase activity in the lens epithelium and capsule has been suggested. Animal experiments show that minimal accumulation of echothiophate occurs in the lens.[1, 21, 96, 145, 152, 238, 304]

Busulfan (Myleran). Used systemically in the treatment of chronic myelogenous leukemia, busulfan is known to produce cataracts. Animal studies suggest that the cataractous changes may be related to interference of the drug with nucleic acid production during mitosis of the lens epithelium.[147, 210, 253, 265]

Carbromal, Bromisovalum. Cataract formation is suspected with the systemic administration of these brominated monoureides.[85]

Chlorpromazine. Systemic administration of chlorpromazine leads to the accumulation of fine, white to yellowish-brown granules covering more than a 2 mm area in the pupillary region of the lens beneath the anterior capsule. Later, the granules become arranged in a stel-

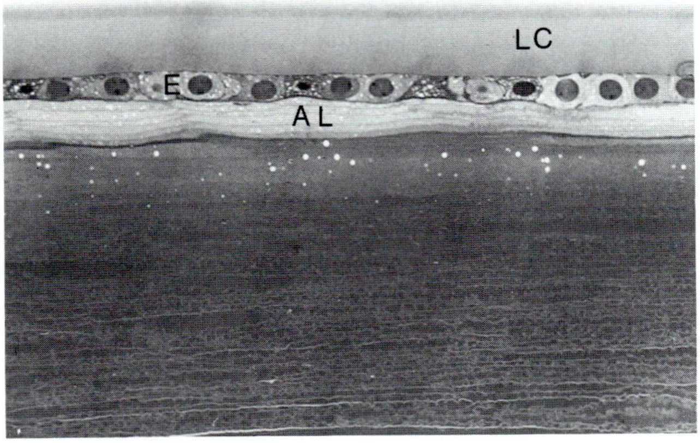

(A)

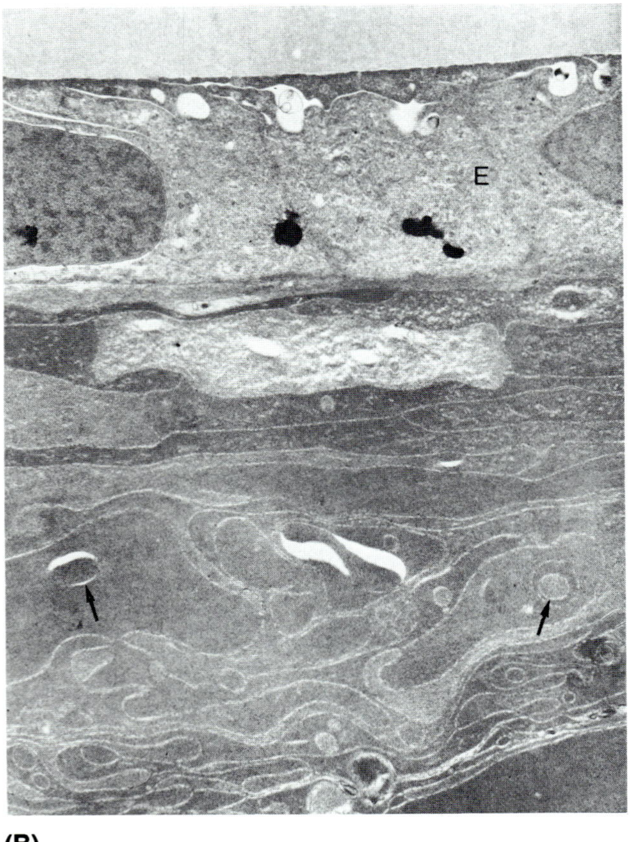

(B)

Fig. 16-27. (A) Light micrograph of a lens showing early histologic changes manifesting as hydropic degeneration in the anterior cortical lens fibers (AL) and in the lens epithelium (E). LC, lens capsule. ×400. (B) Electron micrograph showing cataractous changes in the epithelium (E) and lens fibers manifesting as globular configurations (arrows), clefts, and variations in cytoplasmic density. ×7,500.

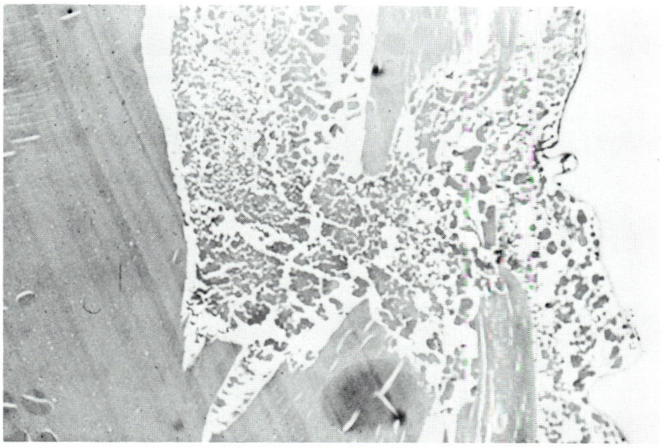

(C)

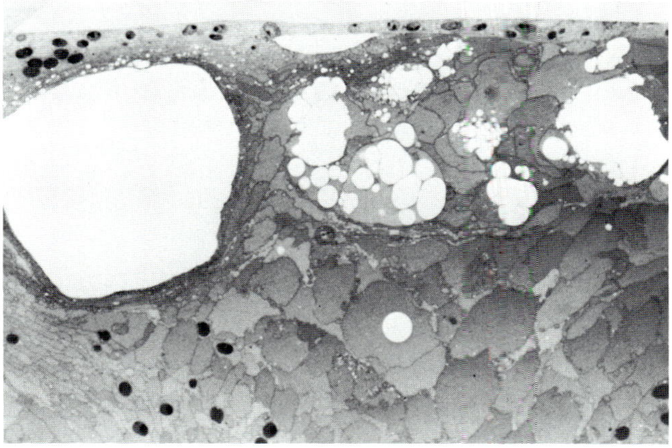

(D)

Fig. 16-27 *(Continued).* (C) Light micrograph of a mature cataract showing morganian globules. ×45. (D) Light micrograph showing optically empty vacuoles in the periequatorial region of the anterior lens cortex. These vacuolar changes may be reversible. ×250.

late pattern (following the lines of the lens sutures), and develop into true anterior polar capsular cataract. Chlorpromazine also produces cataracts in experimental animals. The mechanism of the deleterious effect of chlorpromazine on the cell is discussed on p. 385.[95, 137, 165, 340]

Chlorprothixene. Long-term systemic therapy with chlorprothixene may cause deposits of fine particulate pigmentary matter in the lens. Star-shaped lens opacities may also develop.[114]

Corticosteroids. Systemic administration of corticosteroids produces posterior subcapsular cataract, the incidence of which is related to dosage and duration, and which occurs more frequently in children than in adults. The opacity begins at the posterior pole as very refractile, multicolored dots. Although characteristic of corticosteroid oculotoxicity, the posterior subcapsular cataract that develops and gradually spreads towards the equator in a subcapsular location as a result of use of this drug cannot be differentiated from complicated cataracts, radiation cataracts, cataract associated with other ocular disease (retinitis pigmentosa), or from senile cataract. Animal experiments have tended to suggest that the mechanism of formation of the cataract may involve biochemical changes in the aqueous humor owing to corticosteroid therapy. The lens opacities may progress or remain stationary, but rarely regress upon withdrawal of the offending corticosteroid. The link be-

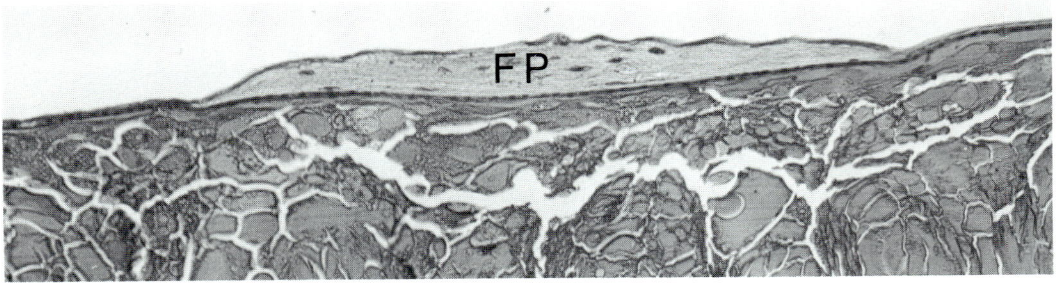

(A)

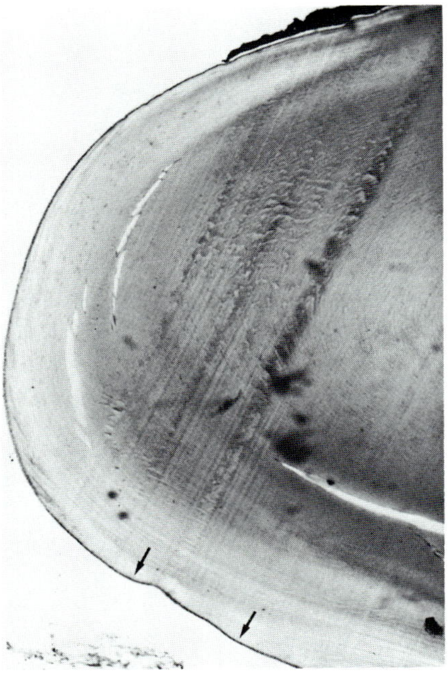

(B)

Fig. 16-28. (A) Anterior subcapsular cataract consisting of a subcapsular fibrous plaque (FP) separated from the lens cortex by secondary proliferation of epithelium and capsule. ×140. (B) Posterior proliferation of lens epithelium (arrow) in cataracta complicata. ×40. (C) Posterior subcapsular cataract with cortical "bladder" cell formation. ×165. Figures 16-28A through C are light micrographs.

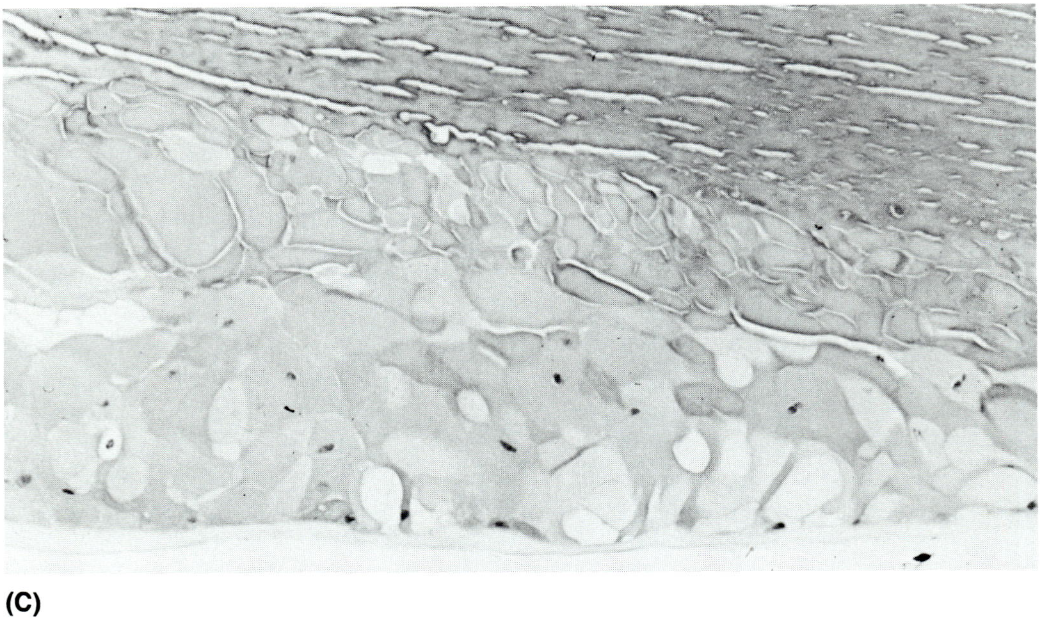

(C)

tween the development of congenital cataract and maternal steroid ingestion is not clearly understood.

Prolonged topical application of corticosteroids can also cause posterior subcapsular cataract; however, individual variations in ocular reaction to this drug are wide, and glaucoma is a much more frequent complication than cataract.[157, 196, 198, 240, 252, 295, 299, 342, 344]

Dimethylsulfoxide (DMSO). A very controversial agent, at one time banned from human use, DMSO is now released on a limited scale. Although no significant DMSO-associated lens changes have been confirmed in humans, DMSO given systemically is well known to produce cataracts in animals; these manifest as pronounced nuclear sclerosis and loss of normal lucency of the cortex.[135, 341]

2,4-Dinitrophenol (DNP). Formerly used in the treatment of obesity, DNP was withdrawn from the market because of its cataractogenic effect. In patients, the formation of DNP-induced bilateral cataracts usually began after several months of drug administration. The changes first appeared in the anterior cortex as fine grey cloudy opacities associated with scattered anterior capsule alterations. Posteriorly, golden granular opacities appeared, together with polychromatic specular reflections. The DNP-induced cataracts progressed rapidly, accompanied by lens swelling and by separation of embryonic suture lines by dark celfts; thus a mature cataract developed rapidly. Electron microscopy of experimentally induced cataract in rabbits has shown that vacuoles and opacitites develop as early as 3 hours after the systemic administration of DNP. The vacuoles originate in the mitochondria and endoplasmic reticulum of the lens epithelial cells, at the equator. The nuclear membranes are destroyed and the cell membranes separate. It is thought that a phenolic hydroxyl and at least one nitro group (in the para first position) are essential for cataract formation.[60, 163, 232, 269, 302, 336]

Mercurial Compounds. In one study, 31 patients using eyedrops containing the preservative phenylmercuric nitrate for between 3 and 15 years developed a brownish pigmentation of the anterior capsule of the lens in the pupillary region. Light- and electron microscopic studies on two lenses demonstrated deposits of dense particulate matter resembling melanin pigment on and in the anterior capsule of the lens in the area of the pupil. Special studies, including electron microprobe analysis and neutron activation analysis established the presence of mercury in a lens with mercurialentis (see also p. 406).[122]

Phenmetrazine. Two cases of phenmetrazine-induced oculotoxicity have been reported in which posterior subcapsular cataracts have developed rapidly and were extensive enough to require lens extraction.[202]

Piperazine Derivatives (1,4-bis-(Phenylisopropyl)-Piperazine or Diphenazine). After daily systemic use, diphenazine has produced cataracts in many patients. The changes include anterior cortical, radial, and glittering punctate opacities, as well as foaming posterior subcapsular opacities which may develop rapidly, eventually requiring surgery. Pathologically, the cataracts resemble senile cataracts, but contain granular cortical material which stains blue with hematoxylin. The mechanism of action of the drug is unknown.[226, 262]

Silver Compounds. In generalized argyrosis, greenish, iridescent discoloration under the anterior lens capsule has been reported.[30]

Triparanol. Systemic administration of triparanol produces cataracts in humans. Because of its undesirable ophthalmologic and dermatologic side effects, this drug was withdrawn from the market. Initially, the opacities occur in both anterior and posterior subcapsular locations. The posterior opacities resemble cataracta complicata in that they appear as amber or brownish granules. The anterior opacities appear as fine, white delicate branches. They may also be accompanied by cortical opacities extending from the equator. Vacuoles are more often seen posteriorly. The biochemical basis for the cataract formation remains to be determined. Histologic examination of experimentally produced cataracts in rats showed phospholipids and cholesterol-like substance in and between the lens fibers.[35, 188, 189, 330]

RETINA

The retina, derived from neuroectoderm, represents an invaginated portion of the brain. The outer unicellular layer is formed by the retinal pigment epithelium, whereas the inner or sensory retina is stratified. From outside inwards the layers are: receptor layer, external limiting membrane, outer nuclear layer, outer plexiform layer, inner nuclear layer, inner plexiform layer, ganglion cell layer, nerve fiber layer, and internal limiting membrane (which abuts onto the vitreous humor). Muller cells extend from the internal to the external limiting membranes, and together with astrocytes and accessory glia provide skeletal support for the retina. The outer segments of the rods and cones are intimately related to the retinal pigment epithelium and consist of a cell membrane enclosing a stack of membranous discs that are continuously renewed during the visual process. The external limiting membrane is formed by attachment bodies between the Muller cells and the outer segments of the receptor cells (Fig. 16-29A).

Acid mucopolysaccharide surrounds the photoreceptor outer segments. A cilium connects the outer and inner segments, the inner myoid region of which extends to the outer nuclear layer, accommodating the receptor cell nuclei. Synaptic connections between the visual cells and the bipolar cells, as well as with the horizontal cells, are made at the outer plexiform layer of the retina. The inner nuclear layer chiefly houses the nuclei of the bipolar cells, horizontal cells, amacrine cells, and Muller fibers. At the inner plexiform layer, the bipolar cells make synaptic contact with amacrine processes and the dendrites of the ganglion cells, the main cell bodies of which form the ganglion cell layer. The axons of the ganglion cells aggregate into nerve fiber bundles located in the nerve fiber layer. The axons acquire a myelin sheath as they pass through the cribriform plate of the optic nerve. The internal limiting membrane is composed of the plasma membrane of the Muller cells, their basement membrane, and the insertion of the condensed cortical fibers of the vitreous humor.

The structure and organization of the retina shows some variation, depending upon the topography. It is thickest at the margin of the optic disc (about 0.5 mm), and thinnest at the fovea (between 0.2 and 0.3 mm) and ora serrata (0.1 mm). The central retina, a specialized region approximately 6 mm in diameter (15 degrees of the visual field), has a central region, fovea, 1.5 mm in diameter (5 degrees of the visual field). Because of its yellow tinge, the central area is called the macular lutea. The cell layers present at the fovea are the pigment epithelium, the photoreceptors (exclusively cones, which are tall and slender in the human eye), the outer nuclear layer, and the outer plexiform layer (designated as the layer of Henle). The nerve fibers arising from the fovea are directed to the temporal region of the optic disc and constitute the papillomacular bundle. At the edge of the fovea, the retina regains full thickness (abundant ganglion cells are multilayered, Henle's layer is thick, and the cones become less slender and intermixed with rods) (Fig. 16-29B).

Except for the foveola (0.4 mm in diameter), the retina is permeated by blood vessels, to the level of the innermost part of the outer plexiform layer. Due to the structural and functional characteristics of these vessels, a competent blood-retinal barrier is normally maintained (Fig. 16-30A,B,C). The extra-retinal component of the blood-retinal barrier is constituted by the retinal pigment epithelium. The diameter of individual epithelial cells may vary from 14 to 60 μm, and their height from 10 to 14 μm, depending on the region of the retina (Fig. 16-31).

The cuboidal cells of the retinal pigment epithelium are narrow, tall, and uniform in the foveal region, and wide, low, and irregular toward the ora serrata. The interdigitating cell

(Text continues on p. 418.)

Fig. 16-29. (A) Histologic section passing through paracentral region of retina showing its normal constitution. 1, retinal pigment epithelium; 2, receptor layer; 3, external limiting membrane; 4, outer nuclear layer; 5, outer plexiform layer; 6, inner nuclear layer; 7, inner plexiform layer; 8, ganglion cell layer; 9, nerve fiber layer; 10, internal limiting membrane. Ch, choroid. ×160. (B) Histologic section passing through the fovea centralis of retina. At the foveola (F, 0.4 mm diameter), the layers present are retinal pigment epithelium, photoreceptors (cones), external limiting membrane, outer nuclear layer, outer plexiform layer (layer of Henle), and internal limiting membrane. The retinal thickening at the clivus (C) is due to addition of the ganglion cell layer and inner plexiform and nuclear layers. Ch, choroid. Compare with Fig. 16-29A. ×175.

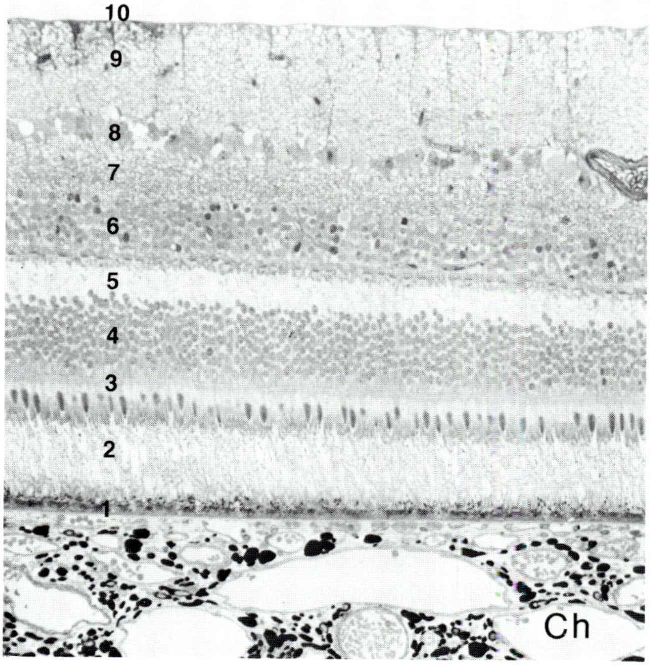

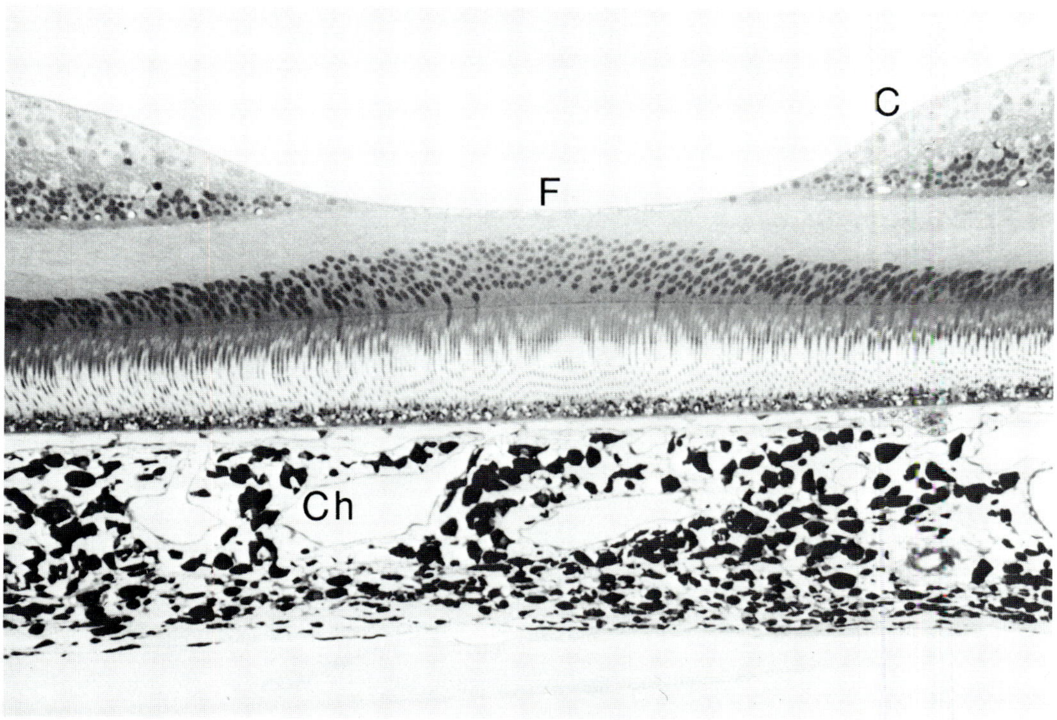

(B)

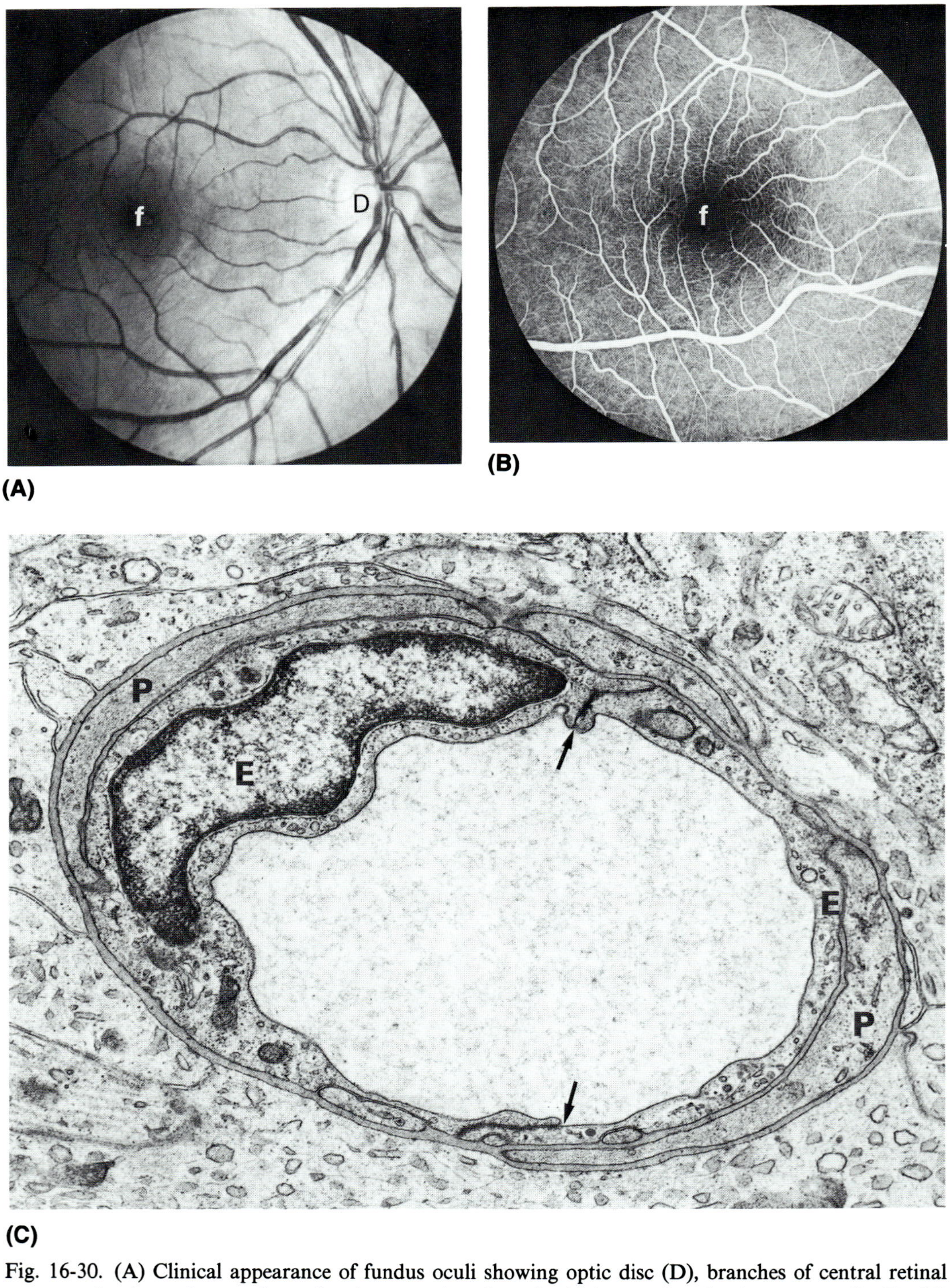

Fig. 16-30. (A) Clinical appearance of fundus oculi showing optic disc (D), branches of central retinal artery and vein, and posterior pole, the central region of which contains the fovea centralis (f). (B) Fluorescein angiogram of the macula showing the vascular pattern and capillary-free zone around the foveola (f). Nonextravasation of fluorescein dye into the retina is due to integrity of the intraretinal component of blood-retinal barrier. (C) Electron micrograph of retinal capillary showing its typical architecture. The blood-retinal barrier is maintained by the structural and functional integrity of the endothelial cells (E), the adjacent cell borders being joined by zonulae occludens (arrow). The pericytes (P), enclosed by basement membrane, form a discontinuous layer. The basal lamina of the capillary demarcates the vessel from the surrounding retinal tissue. ×17,800.

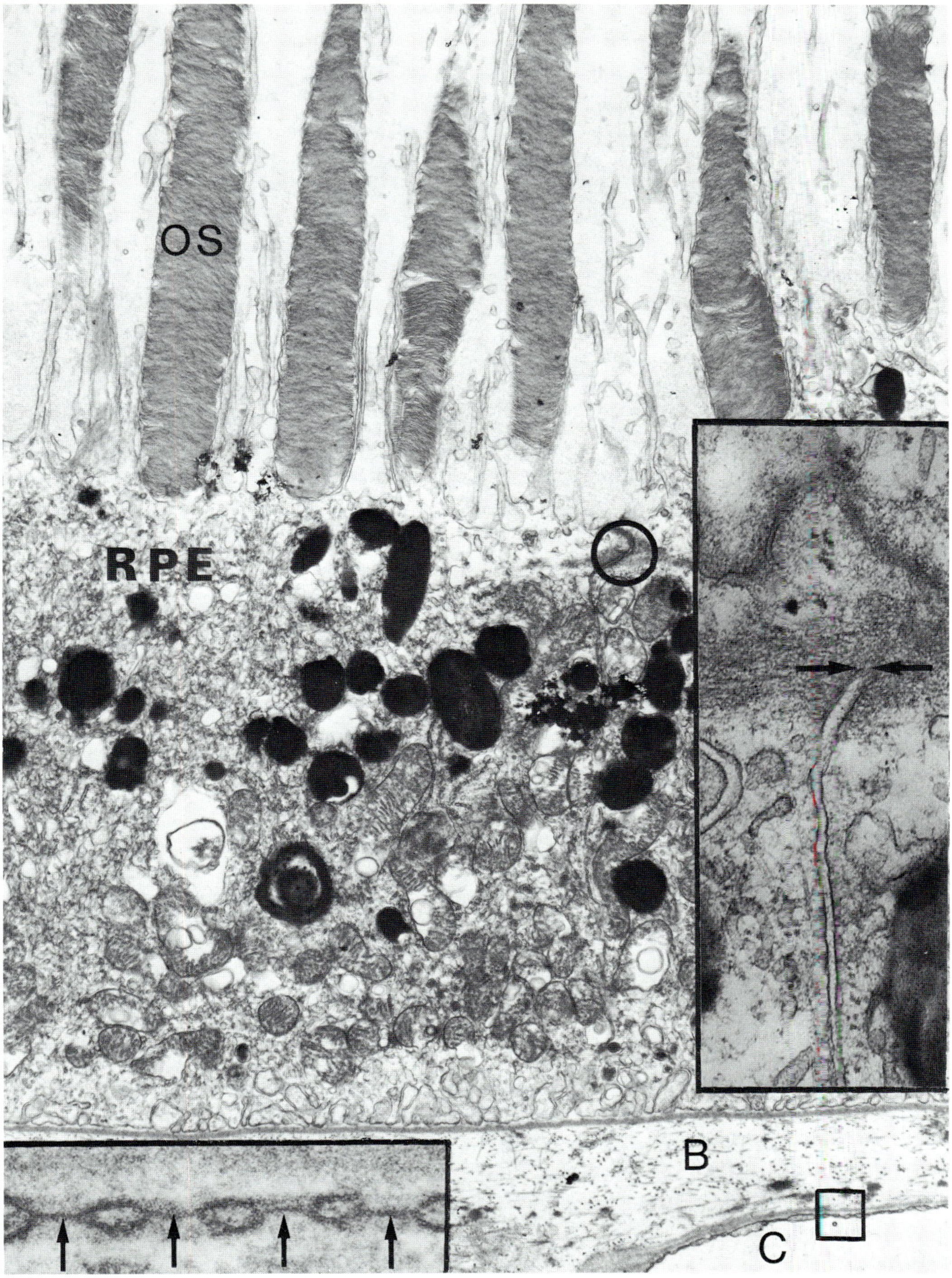

Fig. 16-31. Electron micrograph of retinal pigment epithelium (RPE) with outer segments of photoreceptor cells (OS) and Bruch's membrane (B). ×8,250. The outer blood-retinal barrier is constituted by structural and functional integrity of retinal pigment epithelial cells together with terminal bar and occluding zonule type junctional complexes (encircled and shown at higher magnification in inset right, ×48,500). In contrast to this, the endothelial lining of the choriocapillaris (C) located on the posterior aspect of Bruch's membrane has numerous diaphragmed fenestrations (arrows—inset left, ×126,000) that allow ready passage of macromolecules and particulate matter from plasma.

borders are irregular and are joined in the apical region by zonulae occludens. The cells, together with their apical junctions, form the external component of the blood-retinal barrier. The pigmented epithelium secretes a basement membrane which is an integral part of Bruch's membrane. The apical aspect of the cells in the retinal pigment epithelium is thrown into villous projections that enclasp the outer segments of the photoreceptors. Pigment granules (melanin), which absorb excess light, are concentrated mainly in the apical region of the cells. The retinal pigment epithelial cells are responsible for delivering nutrients from the choroidal vasculature to the photoreceptors, as well as for the collection and disposal of metabolic wastes. They are actively phagocytic, routinely engulf the shed outer segment discs, and recycle components of the visual pigment. Since the choriocapillaris is fenestrated, it allows easy passage of drugs and toxins circulating in the blood. The substances may accumulate in their original or metabolized form, alter the high metabolic activity of the pigment epithelial cells, or cause proliferative or degenerative changes.

The optic nerve is a collection of axons (1.1 to 1.4 million) extending from the retinal ganglion cells to the lateral geniculate body. The axons are arranged in bundles, with supporting astroglia and oligodendroglia, and pass through sieve-like openings in the sclera (lamina cribrosa). At this level the axons become myelinated. Like the brain, the optic nerve is covered by a pia mater, arachnoid mater, and dura mater. The central retinal artery and vein pass through the optic nerve and branch at the disc. The intact endothelial lining, joined by zonulae occludens, constitutes the internal component of the blood-retinal barrier (Fig. 16-30).

Pathologic Reactions

Noxious substances reach the retina and optic nerve mainly through the vascular supply. If the agents are able to cross the blood-retinal barrier without disrupting the blood vessels (intraretinal component) or the blood-pigment epithelial barrier (extraretinal component), the pathology primarily begins within the cells of the nervous tissue. There may be degenerative changes and intracellular deposits of the original substances or their metabolized products. In the event that the blood-retinal barriers are disrupted, the retinal pathology may be accelerated by hemorrhage, exudates, and edema.

In the early stage of an ischemic reaction, irrespective of its etiology, the retina shows coagulative necrosis of its inner layers. The neuronal cells become edematous, accounting for the grey retinal opacities seen clinically. In the late stages, the inner half of the retina presents a homogenized, relatively acellular appearance; the blood vessels show a thickened wall. Coagulative necrosis resulting from a microinfarct in the nerve fiber layer manifests as swollen interrupted axons, seen clinically as cotton-wool spots. Because the swollen end-bulbs of the axons superficially resemble a cell, they are termed cytoid bodies (Fig. 16-32A,B). The swelling is accelerated by an obstruction in the ortho- and retrograde axoplasmic flow. Complete coagulative necrosis of the posterior pole, as in central artery occlusion, causes little swelling of the foveola (since this central region of the fovea is free of retinal blood vessels); the appearance of a cherry-red spot is imparted by the red choroid shining through the foveola.

Obstruction to the central retinal vein, branch, or venule causes retinal hemorrhage and hemorrhagic infarct. Hemorrhagic necrosis may involve all retinal layers and be accompanied by papilledema. Hemorrhage in the nerve fiber layer spreads along the interaxonal space and presents clinically as a flame or splinter shape. Accumulation of blood in the inner nuclear and outer plexiform layers appear as dot-and-blot hemorrhage. Collection of blood beneath the internal limiting membrane gives rise to subhyaloid hemorrhage. In hemorrhagic necrosis, cytoid bodies are a common histologic finding. As the hemor-

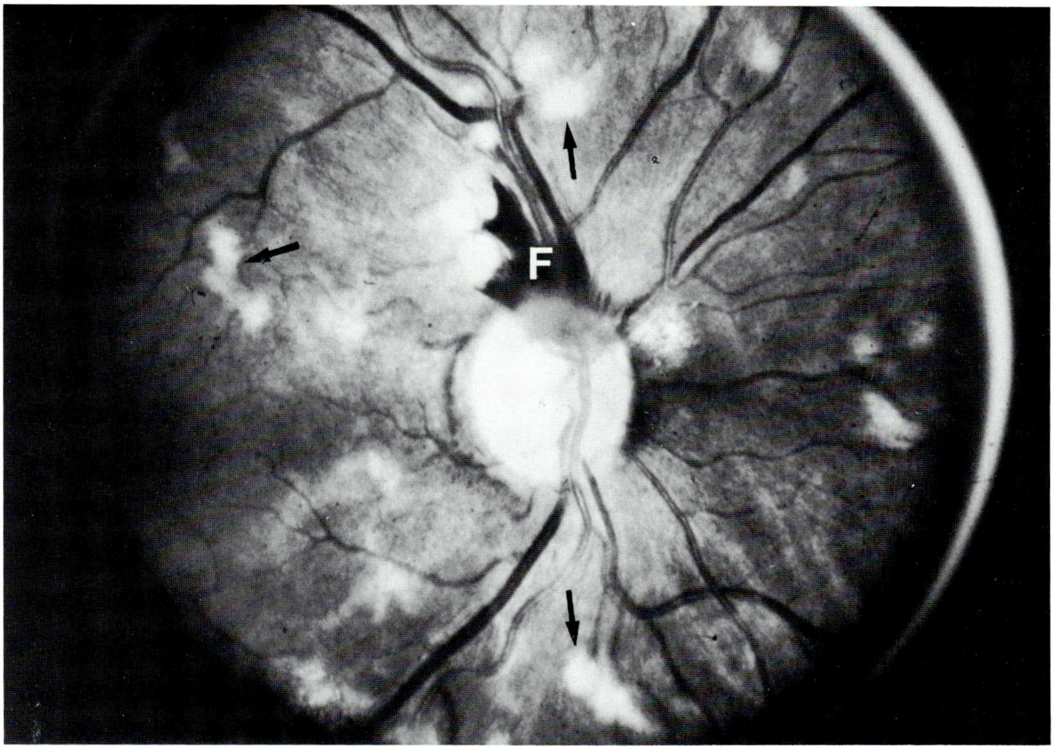

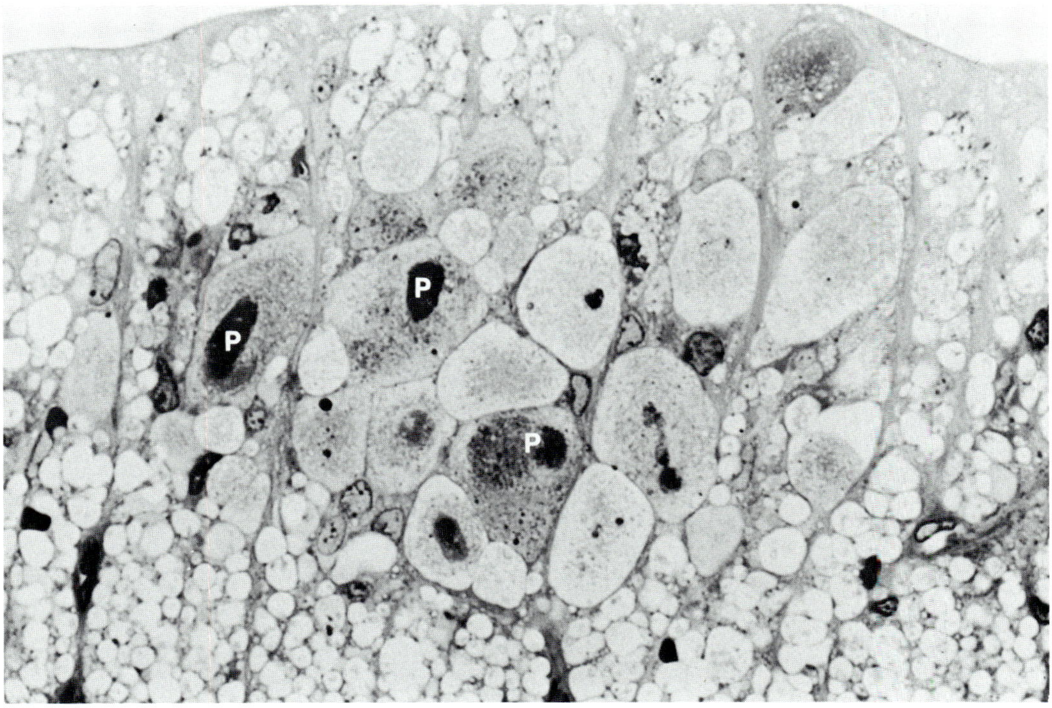

(B)

Fig. 16-32. (A) Gross appearance of "cotton-wool" spots (cytoid bodies, arrows) resulting from microvascular infarcts in the nerve fiber layer. A flame-shaped hemorrhage (F) is also seen at the superior edge of the optic disc. (B) Histologic section of cytoid bodies in the nerve fiber layer of retina. The axons are markedly swollen and some contain a central accumulation of degenerating cytoplasmic organelles forming pseudonuclei (p). ×650.

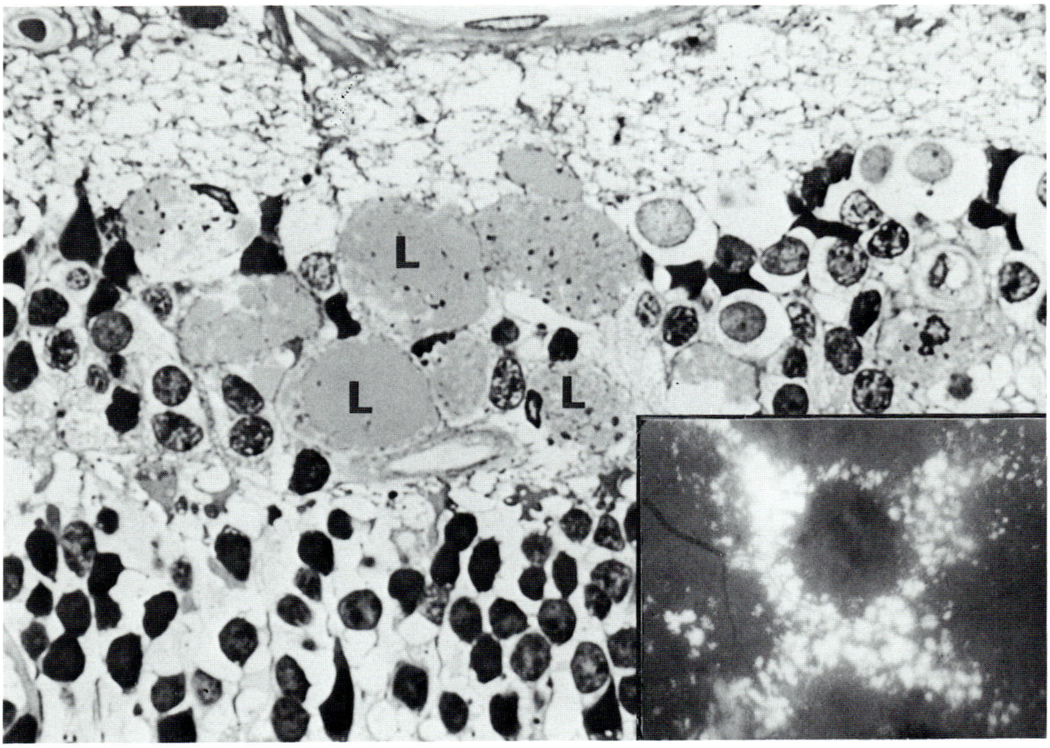

(A)

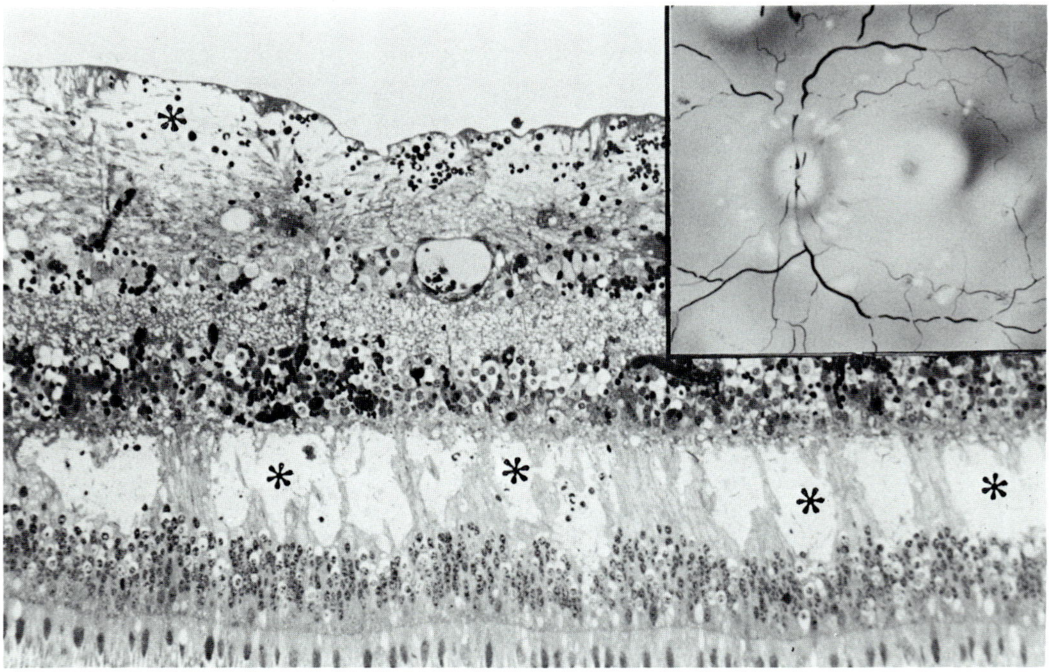

(B)

Fig. 16-33. (A) Lipoprotein deposits ("hard exudates", L) partly engulfed by macrophages in the deep layers (particularly outer plexiform) of the retina. ×715. Inset: gross appearance of hard exudates. (B) Histologic section of retina showing edematous disorganization and degeneration. The cystoid spaces (asterisks) are predominantly seen in the outer plexiform layer. Scattered hemorrhages are also present in the inner retinal layers. ×65. Inset: gross appearance of retinal edema.

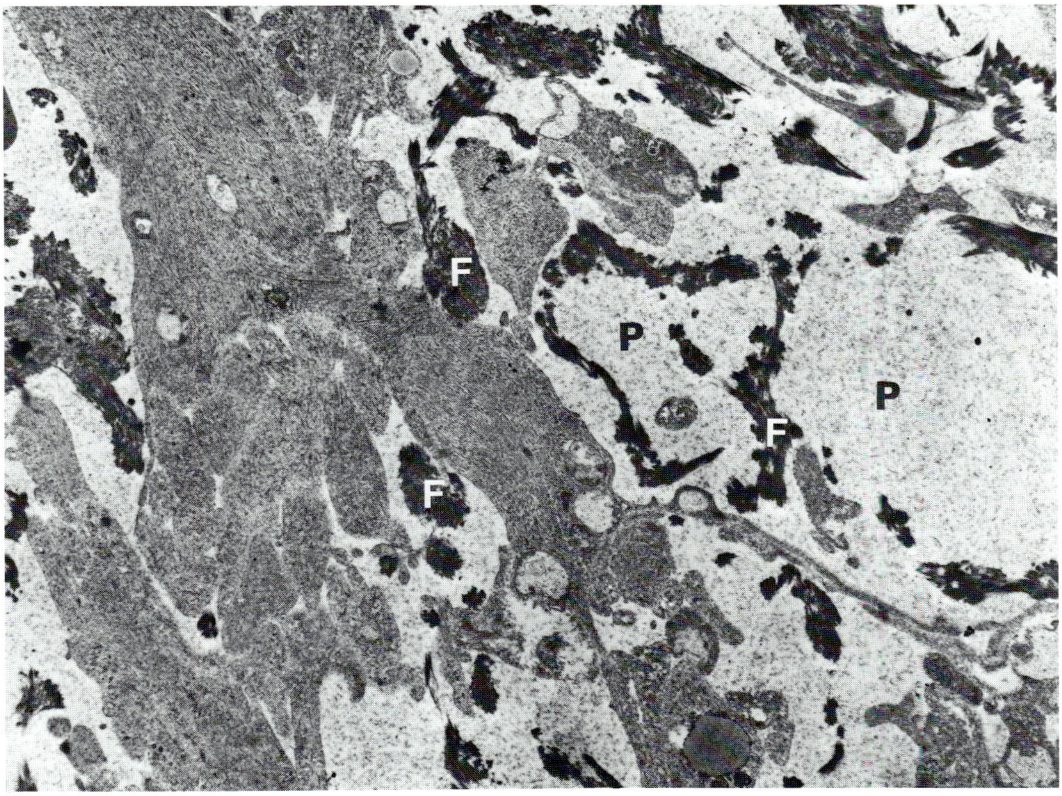

(C)

Fig. 16-33 *(Continued).* (C) Electron micrograph showing plasma proteins (P) and fibrin deposits (F) in the disorganized retina following branch vein occlusion. ×7,400.

rhage resolves, collections of lipoprotein residues and glial and neuronal breakdown products are seen clinically as hard, waxy exudates. Histologically, in the late stages of hemorrhagic resolution, architectural disruption—especially of the inner layers of the retina—gliosis, hemosiderosis with a macrophage reaction, and thick-walled vessels are seen. Hard or waxy exudates are usually located in the outer plexiform layer, and when occurring around the fovea produce a macular star; their removal by macrophages may take from a few months to more than a year (Fig. 16-33A).

Intracellular edema of the retina is a process of hydropic degeneration and is reversible in its early stages. Extracellular edema is more strictly a transudate and may develop in the presence of an intact endothelial lining of the vasculature. In superficial locations, it is seen histologically as a separation of nerve elements, and empty spaces filled with edema fluid. Deep edema is located in the outer retinal layers, giving rise to cysts which may rupture into the vitreous humor to cause a partial or full-thickness hole (Fig. 16-33B,C).

Intraretinal neovascularization is rare. New vessels (retinitis proliferans, rete mirabile) often grow into the vitreous humor or along the retinal surface, especially if the internal limiting membrane is breached; the vessels arise from the venous side in response to a hypoxic stimulus, and are accompanied by fibrous tissue proliferation. The new vessels are usually thin-walled, with the endothelial lining having diaphragmed fenestrations, and leak and bleed readily. Cicatrization of the fibrous tissue eventually causes retinal detachment.

The clinical terms optic neuritis, retrobulbar neuritis, papillitis, and neuroretinitis are not specific. Drug-induced changes may be secondary to vascular pathology, or may be due to primary involvement of nerve parenchyma.

Papilledema may be secondary to increased intracranial pressure, or may be due to local vascular, inflammatory, or obstructive phenomena. In the acute stage, an increased volume of nerve-head tissue results from edema and vascular congestion with or without hemorrhage (Fig. 16-34A,B). The surrounding sensory retina is displaced away from the edge of the disc, with resultant retinal and choroidal folds. In the chronic stage, degeneration of nerve fibers, gliosis, and optic atrophy result.

In optic neuritis, there may be breakdown or loss of the myelin sheath (Fig. 16-35), with

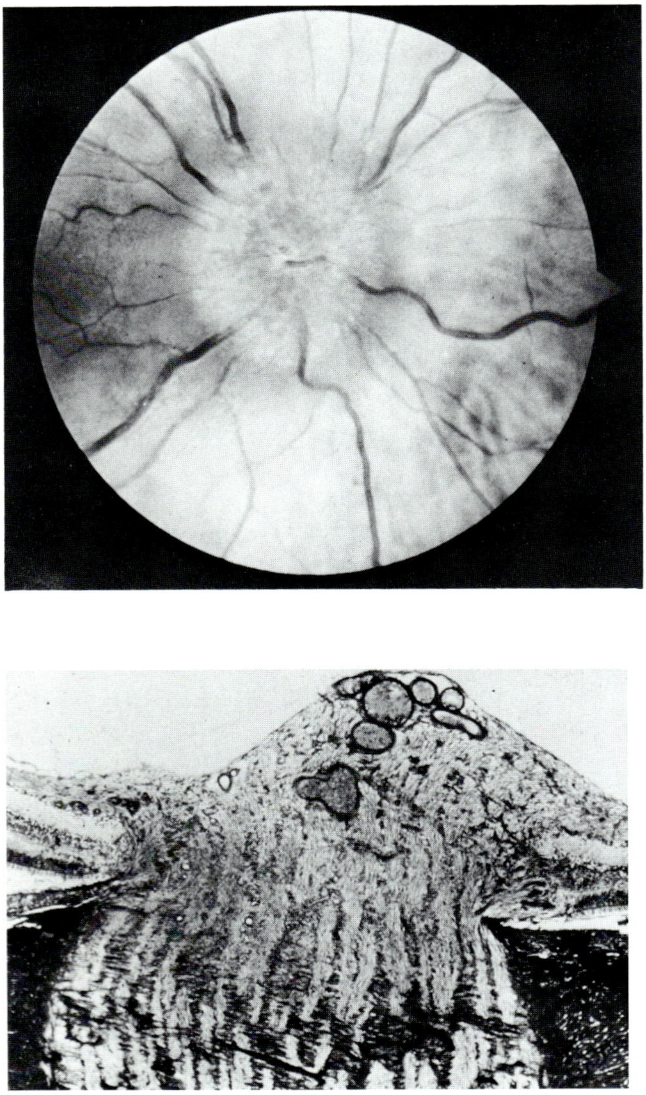

(B)

Fig. 16-34. (A) Gross appearance of optic disc edema (papilledema). Note the fluffy disc margin, occasional hemorrhages, and vascular tortuosity. (B) Histologic section of papilledema (choked disc) showing swollen, edematous disc tissue, dilated vessels, and displacement of retinal tissue at the disc edges. ×30.

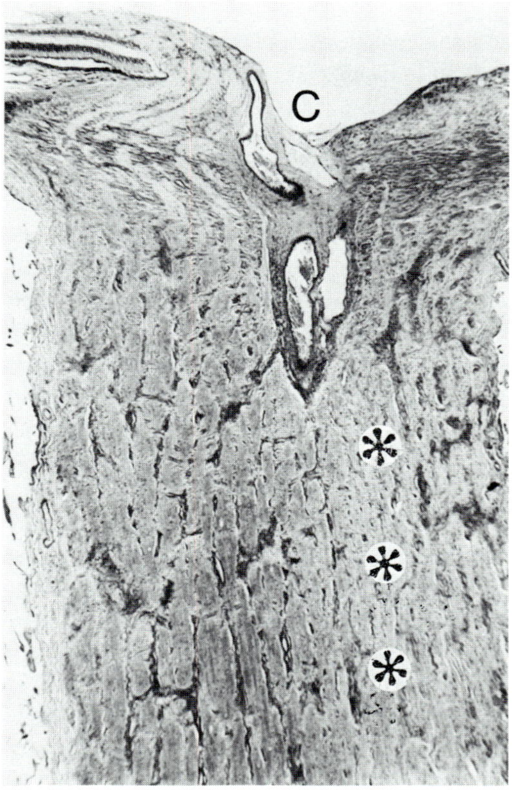

Fig. 16-35. Histologic section of optic nerve cut longitudinally. Demyelination of the nerve is particularly noticeable on the right side (asterisk). In contrast to papilledema (Fig. 16-34B), the disc shows partial cupping (C). ×27.

or without a macrophage reaction, and infiltration with lymphocytes and plasma cells as well as fluid exudation. In the healing stage, an astrocytic response and gliosis occur. Very little is known of acute reactions due to toxins, but destruction of the optic nerve parenchyma eventually results in optic atrophy, which may be of the ascending (primary pathology in the retina and optic nerve) or descending (primary pathology in the brain or optic nerve) type. At the optic disc, this destruction may manifest as a widening or deepening of the physiologic cup, with baring of the lamina cribrosa, and with or without glial proliferation. In optic atrophy there is loss or shrinkage of nerve parenchyma, widening of the pial septa, gliosis with proliferation of astrocytes, and widening of the subarachnoid space and redundant dura.

Drugs Affecting the Retina and Optic Nerve

Aminosalicylic Acid (PAS). Used in combination with other drugs against *Mycobacterium tuberculosis,* PAS may produce optic neuritis and atrophy. Retinal hemorrhages are probably secondary to PAS-induced anemia.[114]

Amphotericin B. Systemic administration of amphotericin B has, although rarely, been known to cause retinal exudates and hemorrhages secondary to the anemia induced by the drug.[114]

Anticholinesterases (Topical Miotics: Neostigmine, Physostigmine, Demercarium, Echothiophate, Isoflurophate). These drugs may exert traction on the peripheral retina and cause retinal detachment.[156, 193, 338]

Arsacetin. In a manner similar to that of the other derivatives of arsanilic acid, systemic administration of this drug causes optic neuritis and atrophy, together with degenerative changes in the retinal ganglion cells and nerve fibers. There is least damage to the papillomacular bundle, and no signs of inflammation.[283]

Arsphenamine. In contrast to Arsacetin, systemic administration of arsphenamine produces papilledema owing to raised intracranial pressure. In rare instances, neuroretinitis and retrobulbar neuritis (which may be questionably attributed to this agent) have been documented.[137]

Aspirin (Sodium Salicylate, Acetylsalicylic Acid). Occasionally, retinal hemorrhage, edema, papilledema, and optic neuritis and atrophy may occur with aspirin. Most changes are reversible upon early withdrawal of the drug.[100, 134, 314]

Barbiturates (Systemic). Retrobulbar/optic neuritis, papilledema, and optic atrophy may occur with barbiturate use. Retinal hemorrhages are probably secondary to drug induced anemia.[114, 137]

Carbon Dioxide. Cerebroretinal degeneration due to carbon dioxide poisoning has been reported. Carbon dioxide may have a specific toxicity for the retinal ganglion cells, thus accounting for the severe visual defects seen clinically.[100, 287]

Carbromal, Bromisovalum. Systemic administration of these brominated monoureides causes retrobulbar neuritis together with either pallor or hyperemia of the optic nerve head.[81, 283]

Cephaloridine. Systemic administration of cephaloridine has been suspected of inducing papilledema and retinal pigmentary changes.[25, 88]

Chloramphenicol. Systemic administration of chloramphenicol produces optic neuritis, particularly in children maintained on high doses for long periods. The pathology includes hyperemia of the papillae, peripapillary edema together with congestion, retinal pigmentary changes, and tortuosity of retinal veins. Hemorrhage on and around the optic disc is probably secondary to drug-induced anemia. In many instances, improvement occurs when chloramphenicol is discontinued, although in some cases optic atrophy persists. Histologically, the atrophy of the optic nerve fibers, particularly of the papillomacular bundle, continues as far back as the chiasm, with demyelinating changes and loss of retinal ganglion cells. While the toxic effects of chloramphenicol may be directly on the nerve cells, it is suggested that its effect may be mediated through interference with metabolism of B vitamins.

Inadvertent access of a 20 percent solution of chloramphenicol to orbital tissues (during lacrimal irrigation) has caused optic atrophy, probably through a central retinal artery occlusion.[76, 151, 192, 201, 209, 280, 345, 346]

Chloroquine, Hydroxychloroquine. Prolonged use of these drugs causes degenerative changes in the pigment epithelium and retina. Chloroquine retinopathy is classically recognized by the bull's eye pattern (Fig. 16-36A) that results from thinning and clumping of the retinal pigment epithelium, and may be partly due to inclusions in the ganglion cells. Histopathologically, there is depigmentation of the pigment epithelium, destruction of the receptor elements of the rods and cones, accumulation of pigment in the cells of the nuclear and plexiform layers of the retina, and subretinal clumping of pigment. By electron microscopy, damage to the ganglion cells as well as some of the inner nuclear cells is also seen. The characteristic findings in human eyes include membranous cytoplasmic bodies (myeloid bodies) and clusters of curvilinear tubules in the ganglion cells, in some inner nuclear layer cells, in connecting fibers, in the inner segments of photoreceptors, and frequently in the retinal pigment epithelium. Experimental evidence shows that the chloroquine is concentrated in the retinal pigment epithelium and choroid, and remains there long after the cessation of treatment; this may account for the progressive nature of the macular pathology. Whether or not this is due to binding of the drug to melanin pigment is uncertain. Animal experiments have revealed that chloroquine causes lysosomal overloading, producing myeloid bodies analogous to those seen in storage diseases (Fig. 16-36B,C). In isolated cases, optic neuritis, retinal exudates, and hemorrhages, as well as retinal detachment, may also occur.[38, 39, 40, 59, 141, 166, 264, 278, 339]

Clioquinol (Iodochlorohydroxyquin). This drug is suspected of causing optic atrophy in some patients. In Japan, the use of clioquinol and the occurrence of subacute myelo-opticoneuropathy has been noted. The histopathology in such cases showed degeneration of nerve fibers in the chiasm and optic tracts, and occasionally in the optic nerves and retina. Since attempts to produce this syndrome in experimental animals have failed, it has been suggested that the syndrome may have been caused by a virus.[235, 243, 322]

Corticosteroids. Inadvertent ocular exposure to or intraocular injection of corticosteroids may cause retinal hemorrhage, retinal degeneration, ascending optic atrophy, retinal detachment, and global atrophy. It is suggested that blindness probably occurs as a con-

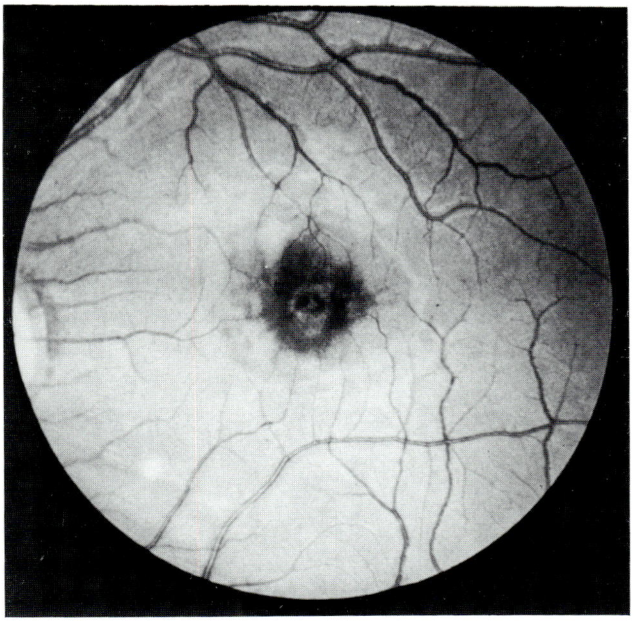

(A)

Fig. 16-36. Chloroquine toxicity. (A) Gross appearance of fundus with "bull's eye" fovea. (B) and (C) Electron micrographs of lamellar membranous bodies (MCBs) deposited in ganglion cell (G) of retina of experimental chloroquine retinopathy in monkey. (B) ×2,500. (C) ×36,800. (Fig. 16-36B and C from Rosenthal, A. R., Kolb, H., Bergsma, D., et al. Chloroquine retinopathy in the rhesus monkey. Invest. Ophthalmol. Vis. Sci. 17: 1158, 1978.)

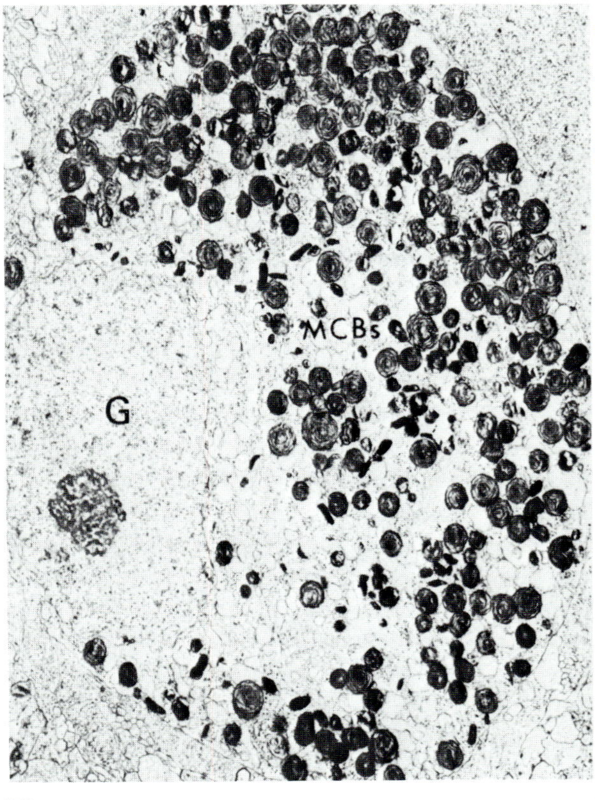

(B)

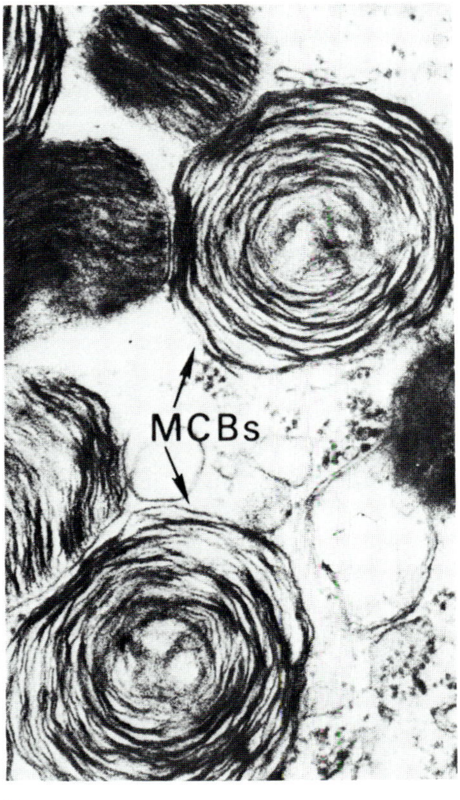

(C)

sequence of a direct toxic action of corticosteroids on the retina and optic nerve.[87,92]

Digitalis and Related Glycosides. With this group of drugs, reversible disturbances of vision are well recognized. The action may be directly on the retinal photoreceptor cells rathèr than on the optic nerve. Animal studies with radioactively labeled digoxin have shown greater concentration of this drug in the retina and ciliary body than in other parts of the eye, optic nerve, or brain.[212,271,272,337]

Diiodohydroxyquine. Systemic administration of diiodohydroxyquine causes optic neuritis, subacute myelo-optico-neuropathy, optic atrophy, and edema and degeneration of the macula.[33]

Epinephrine (Adrenalin). With epinephrine (used as a treatment for glaucoma), a cystoid maculopathy may develop in 20 to 30 percent of aphakic patients within a few weeks to many months. The edematous appearance of the macula may be accompanied occasionally by small grey or yellow cysts or flame-shaped hemorrhages close to the fovea or at the posterior pole. Since intravenous injection of epinephrine in rabbits transiently abolishes the C-wave of the electroretinogram, which originates from the retinal pigment epithelium, it has been hypothesized that epinephrine maculopathy is probably related to toxicity to the pigment epithelium. Based on fluorescein angiographic studies, however, it has been suggested that the cystoid collection of fluid in the macular area in epinephrine maculopathy is secondary to altered capillary permeability of the intraretinal vessels. While the mechanism of action of the drug in causing the maculopathy remains to be determined, the occurrence of pathology limited to aphakic eyes suggests that absence of the lens allows rapid posterior diffusion of epinephrine from the anterior chamber to the retina.[112,124,171,195,228]

Ergotamine Tartrate. Although far less toxic to the eye than its parent ergot, ergotamine tartrate was reported to have caused an occlusion of the central retinal artery in one patient, following an injection of ergotamine for headache.[86]

Estrogen and Progestin Combination Products (Oral Contraceptives). There is a higher incidence of thrombosis and occlusion of retinal vessels, perivasculitis, retinal edema, retrobulbar neuritis, papilledema secondary to pseudotumor cerebri, and optic atrophy in women taking oral contraceptives than in a comparable population not taking these drugs. We have observed a 22-year-old woman without apparent systemic abnormality who had been on oral contraceptives for 4 years and who developed central retinal vein occlusion followed by neovascular glaucoma. Upon histopathologic examination of the globe, no specific retinal pathology was attributable to the drug.[72,119,136,251,297,314]

Ethanol (Ethyl Alcohol). Chronic alcoholism is responsible for an amblyopia that is probably secondary to a vitamin B or other nutritional deficiency and may be partially or completely reversible. Although temporal pallor of the optic nerve head may be observed, there are, grossly, no other characteristic changes. Histologically, an interstitial inflammatory process may be seen in the optic nerve. There are degenerative changes in the papillomacular bundle of nerve fibers, and in late stages, the associated ganglion cells are similarly affected. However, it is not certain that a distinct entity of alcohol-induced amblyopia exists. At times, this amblyopia has been linked with tobacco amblyopia as a "tobacco-alcohol ambylopia" (see p. 437), but most likely the condition should be regarded as a nutritional retrobulbar neuropathy. The large number of ocular side effects reported with ethanol may be due to the fact that this agent is second only to water in the volume consumed by humans.

Retrobulbar injection of 25 to 100 percent alcohol (0.5 to 2 ml) to relieve ocular pain may permanently damage the optic nerve or its blood supply, impairing vision. Irrigation of the orbit with absolute alcohol during operative removal of a hydatid cyst resulted in optic atrophy and paralysis of the extraocular muscles, requiring corrective surgery.[23, 114, 137, 156, 227, 261, 333]

Ethambutal, Systemic. Many patients receiving ethambutal develop macular edema, retinal vasodilatation, retrobulbar neuritis with hyperemia of the optic nerve head, and occasional small surrounding hemorrhages; the pathology is dose-related. In a few cases, optic atrophy has followed the retrobulbar neuritis, with subsequent incomplete recovery of vision. Although no human ocular tissue has been examined from patients with ethambutal toxicity, experimental studies in monkeys have shown demyelinating lesions in the optic nerves, chiasm, and lower medulla, and in the pyramidal tracts.[29, 67, 203, 246, 281, 285, 350]

Ethylhydrocupreine Hydrochloride. Although blindness occurs with systemic use of this drug, often no obvious pathology is seen in the eye. In some cases, retinal edema and narrowing of the arteries occurs; rarely, pigmentary changes take place. Discontinuation of the medication often brings about reversal of these effects. In some cases, however, optic atrophy develops, leading to permanent blindness; in these cases, there is degeneration of the retinal ganglion cells and optic nerve fibers.[137, 284]

Griseofulvin. Systemic administration of griseofulvin may cause macular degeneration and edema, retinal hemorrhage secondary to drug-induced anemia, and papilledema due to pseudotumor cerebri.[94]

Hexamethonium. In rare cases, systemic administration of hexamethonium has caused visual loss. Optic atrophy subsequently developed in one case, with an appearance of hypertensive retinopathy characterized by hemorrhage and exudates, leading to permanent blindness. In other cases, a transient macular edema has been reported.[28, 52]

Hyaluronidase. Use of hyaluronidase with local retrobulbar anesthesia can cause an increased incidence of cystoid macular edema. Although the mechanism of action producing this effect is unknown, speculations on it include intraocular inflammation, vasodilatation, and alterations in the blood-retinal barrier for exogenous inflammatory agents.[18, 156, 230, 274]

Indomethacin (Indocin). Systemic administration of indomethacin may induce pigmentary changes, cystoid degeneration, macular edema and degeneration, and a central serous retinopathy with pallor of the disc. Hemorrhages may also occur secondary to the associated drug-induced anemia.[58, 158, 247]

Iodine and Iodides. Systemic administration of these substances may cause retinal or macular edema, vasoconstriction, retrobulbar neuritis, and optic atrophy, together with vitreous opacities.[129, 333]

Iron Compounds (Cholinate, Fumarate, Gluconate, Succinate, and Sulfate Salts of Ferrous, Iron Dextran and Sorbitex, and Polysaccharated Iron Complex). Sytemic administration of these compounds seldom causes retinal degeneration; they may possibly induce optic neuritis and optic atrophy.[114, 137]

Isoniazid (Systemic Administration Usually with Aminosalicyclic Acid and Streptomycin). Large doses of isoniazid, especially in combination therapy, result in optic neuritis and atrophy. Pathologic examination of the optic nerves shows softening and demyelination of the superior and medial portions of the optic tracts. Papilledema often precedes the optic atrophy, and there may be complete loss of vision.[97, 178, 182]

Mepacrine (Quinacrine). Retinal hemorrhages secondary to mepacrine-induced anemia may occur. High systemic dosage can produce optic neuritis.[90, 105]

Methoxyflurane, Systemic. Prolonged use of this substance causes oxalosis for unknown reasons. Calcium oxalate crystals deposit throughout the body, including the retinal pigment epithelium. Deposits of these crystals in the retina gives a clinical picture of "flecked retina syndrome."[56]

Methylene Blue. Systemic adminstration of methylene blue may produce blue-grey discoloration of the ocular tissues, especially the retina and vitreous humor, as well as papilledema and optic atrophy.[128, 333]

Nalidixic Acid. Systemic administration of nalidixic acid to children and infants produces edema of the optic nerve head, apparently due to the associated increase in intracranial pressure. The effect is reversible upon discontinuing the drug. Retinal hemorrhages may also occur secondary to drug-induced anemia.[45, 93]

Nicotinic Acid and Its Derivatives. An atypical cystoid macular edema has been attributed to systemic nicotinic acid therapy.[125]

Oxygen. The toxic manifestations of oxygen are most commonly seen in premature infants given oxygen in greater than a 30 percent concentration. The literature on this subject is vast. Clinical observations and experimental evidence have shown a severe constriction of the retinal blood vessels leading to total vaso-obliteration and destruction of the growing vessels, at which stage the changes are irreversible. Upon return of the patient to air, a vasoproliferative phase is characterized by haphazard growth of blood vessels from the remaining vessels at the disc, together with fibrous tissue proliferation, vitreous traction, and retinal detachment, which in its most severe form occurs as a morning-glory type of detachment. Thus, the association of the detached retina with the retrolental fibrous tissue gave rise to the name retrolental fibroplasia (Fig. 16-37A). In some cases, secondary glaucoma, complicated cataract, and atrophia bulbi ensue. The exact mechanism of oxygen toxicity on the developing retinal capillaries is not clearly understood. In vivo and in vitro studies have shown a selective involvement of lysosomes, with the formation of phagosomes, cellular retraction, elaboration of superoxide free radicals, and eventual degeneration of the endothelial cells (Fig. 16-37B,C).

Hyperbaric oxygen can affect any age group. In susceptible individuals, severe vasoconstriction or even direct retinal toxicity may occur from such therapy; permanent bilateral blindness due to 80 percent oxygen administered during general anesthesia has also been reported.[15, 16, 17, 194, 238, 250, 312]

Pheniprazine. Systemic administration of pheniprazine induces visual disturbances in about 1 percent of patients, and for this reason the drug is no longer used in many countries. The reduced visual acuity may be accompanied by a central scotoma, and partial optic atrophy may also develop. Histologically demonstrable lesions have been reported in one case, although animal studies suggest that the initial site for the toxic action of this drug is in the retina.[176]

Phenylbutazone (Butazolidin). Retinal hemorrhage secondary to phenylbutazone-induced anemia is the most frequent adverse reaction to this drug, next to those occurring in the eyelid and conjunctiva (see p. 390). Optic neuritis and optic atrophy may also occur in some cases.[114, 310]

Piperidylchlorophenothiazine. A phenothiazine derivative, similar to chloropromazine, this drug causes retinal degeneration in many patients. Abnormal retinal pigmentation develops first, giving the fundus a salt-and-pepper appearance. The progression of pigmentary changes gives rise to a picture similar to retinitis pigmentosa. The photoreceptors are also affected.[57, 131]

Quinine. Visual disturbances occur in a small proportion of patients taking average systemic doses of quinine. The toxic effect causes degeneration—especially of the macula, retinal ganglion cells, and nerve fibers—which may be accompanied or followed by optic atrophy and papilledema, as well as atrophy of the rods and cones. Retinal vasodilatation is followed by marked vasoconstriction, and macular edema and retinal exudates develop. Retinal hemorrhage is probably related to the drug-induced anemia or to idiosyncrasy.[27, 66, 68, 110, 120]

Streptomycin. Systemic administration of streptomycin may produce retrobulbar or optic neuritis, optic atrophy, and retinal vasospasm. Retinal hemorrhages can occur secondary to drug-induced anemia.[303]

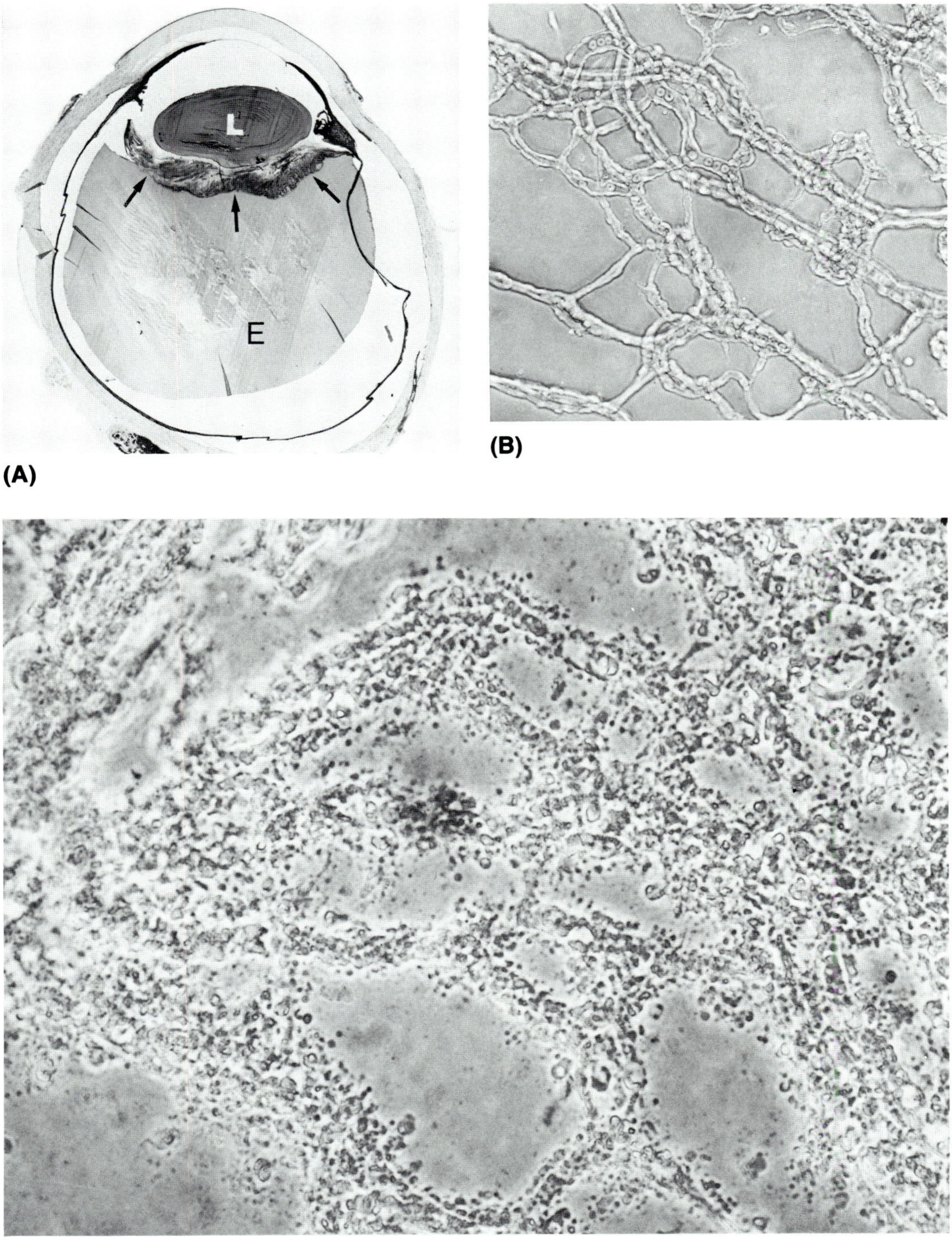

Fig. 16–37. Oxygen toxicity. (A) Section of human infant eye showing total retinal detachment. The gliosed retina (arrows) is adherent to the posterior aspect of the lens (L), hence the term retrolental fibroplasia. The anterior chamber is partially obliterated due to anterior displacement of iris diaphragm. E, subretinal exudate. ×4. (B) and (C) Exposure of immature retinal vasculature in vitro to 95 percent oxygen causes contraction followed by retraction and complete disintegration of the vessels resulting in cellular debris. (B) Initial vascular explant incubated at 37°C in tissue culture medium. ×150. (C) Vascular explant after 30 hours of oxygen exposure. Phase-contrast micrograph, ×310. The retinal vessels in vivo undergo a similar process when premature infants are exposed to hyperoxia.

Sulfonamide Drugs. Rarely, systemic administration of this group of drugs may cause retinal and preretinal hemorrhage. Occasionally, toxic amblyopia attributable to optic neuritis and papilledema is associated with administration of low doses of sulfonamides, but the pathology of this toxicity is not well documented. As part of the systemic manifestation of toxicity, the retinal vessels may appear a vivid, light lavender color.[55, 132, 305]

Thioridazine (Mellaril) is one of the few phenothiazine derivatives known to cause pigmentary retinopathy, and toxicity is probably related to high doses. It appears as a coarse black pigmentary stippling of the central retina and extends to the periphery, sparing the papillomacular bundle. With time, the dots of pigmentation coalesce to form contiguous areas of depigmentation. Retinal edema ensues, with accompanying impairment of vision. It is known that thioridazine has an affinity for melanin granules and accumulates in association with uveal pigment, but how this is related to the retinal pathology is not clear.[13, 80, 225, 258]

Trichloroethylene, Systemic. Retrobulbar or optic neuritis followed by optic atrophy can occur with this substance; it may also cause retinal edema, vasoconstriction, and peripapillary hemorrhage. Most adverse effects are due to toxic decomposition of the drug.[100]

Tryparasamide. Systemic administration of tryparasamide may cause optic neuritis and subsequent optic atrophy. Experimental studies in monkeys have produced lesions in the optic tracts.[170]

Vitamin D. Adverse reactions with hypervitaminosis D are more often seen in infants than in children or adults. Narrowing of the optic foramina may occur with calcium deposition, leading to papilledema and optic atrophy.[150]

UVEAL TRACT

The iris, ciliary body, and choroid constitute the uveal tract. The choroid lies behind the retina, separated from it by Bruch's membrane, and continues anteriorly as the ciliary body, together with the pigment epithelium. The nonpigmented epithelium is a continuation of the sensory retina, beginning at the ora serrata. The choroid is extremely rich in vessels arbitarily arranged in three layers, and has a connective tissue stroma of collagen fibrils, fibrocytic cells, and melanocytes. It also contains an elastic network and smooth muscle "stars." Beneath Bruch's membrane is the layer of the choriocapillaris, comprising the largest, flattened and fenestrated capillaries in the body, that is responsible for supplying of nutrients and oxygen to the retinal pigment epithelium and outer sensory retina, and exclusively to the vessel-free region of the fovea (Figs. 16-29A,B, and 16-31).

The bulk of the ciliary body is formed by smooth muscle fibers arranged meridionally, radially, and circumferentially. The bilayered ciliary epithelium is smooth posteriorly (pars plana) but becomes markedly convoluted anteriorly (pars plicata) to form the ciliary processes. The fenestrated capillaries of the choriocapillaris continue in the ciliary processes and are responsible for origin of aqueous humor, the final product being modified by the metabolic activity of the nonpigmented epithelium.

On the posterior aspect of the iris, the nonpigmented epithelium of the ciliary body continues as a pigmented layer, the central one-third of which glides on the anterior lens surface. The pigmented epithelium of the ciliary body continues as the myoepithelium that forms the dilator pupillae muscle of the iris. The smooth muscle sphincter pupillae is located in the iris stroma around the pupil. The remainder of the iris is formed by fibrovascular tissue. The collagen fibrils are arranged in a lattice pattern, thus providing a scaffold during pupillary dilatation and constriction. While the fibrocytic and melanocytic cells are randomly distributed in the stroma, they form an interlacing, discontinuous (because of crypts) network on the anterior iris stroma. In addition, within the stroma there are clump cells, mast cells, macrophages, and lymphocytes.

Pathologic Reactions

The main changes seen in the uveal tract are nonspecific inflammation (acute, subacute, or chronic), degenerative and atrophic changes, epithelial and vascular proliferation, alteration in muscular activity, and deposition of noxious substances as well as of their metabolic products. The sensitivity of the uveal tissue is mediated through its immunologic competency and by biogenic amines liberated by native and inflammatory cells. They may cause breakdown of the blood-tissue barrier, producing exudation or even frank hemorrhage. These changes in turn may affect the retina, vitreous humor, lens, cornea, and sclera. Substances brought through the circulation, secreted with the aqueous humor, or entering exogenously may accumulate in the intra- and extracellular spaces and can impart a characteristic hue to the iris. Certain agents may cause reactive changes in the epithelial lining of the iris and ciliary body to induce formation of epithelial cysts or disruptions of the pigmented epithelium, which appear as pigment floaters in the aqueous humor.

Drugs Affecting the Uveal Tract

Amphotericin B. Iridocyclitis may develop with the systemic administration of this drug.[114]

Chloroquine, Hydroxychloroquine. Typical deposits of chloroquine (see p. 424) may occur in the smooth muscle cells of the ciliary body as well as the choroid (Fig. 16-38).[264]

Cholinergic Agents (Topical Miotics: Pilocarpine, Neostigmine, Physostigmine, Demecarium, Echothiophate, Isoflurophate). Repeated topical application of these agents often causes the formation of cysts or nodules ("miotic cysts") in the pigment epithelium, most commonly in the iris and rarely in the ciliary processes. The iris blood vessels may also become dilated, and fine pigment granules may be released into the aqueous humor.

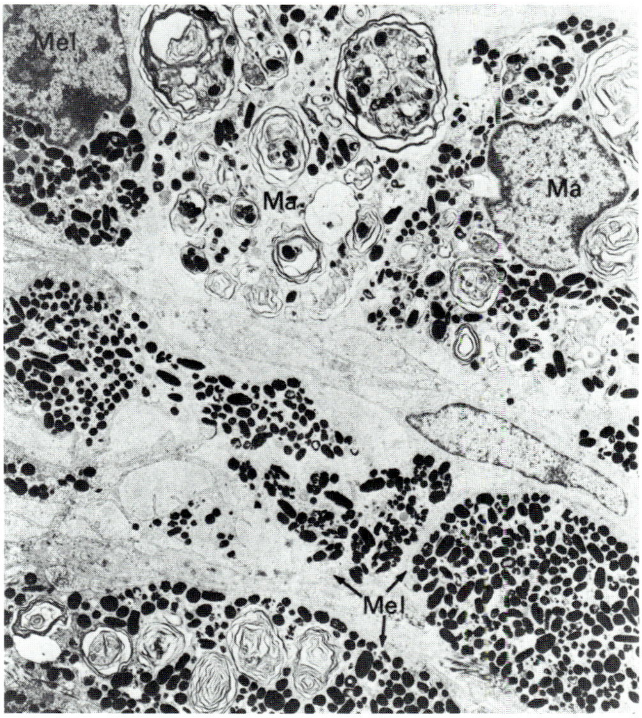

Fig. 16–38. Chloroquine toxicity. Electron micrograph showing membranous body inclusion in the melanocytes (Mel) and macrophages (Ma) of choroid. ×2,150. (Rosenthal, A. R., Kolb, H., Bergsma, D., et al.: Chloroquine retinopathy in the rhesus monkey. Invest. Ophthalmol. Vis. Sci. 17: 1158, 1978.)

Rarely, iritis manifests in association with ciliary spasm.[73,256]

Epinephrine (Adrenalin). Topical use of epinephrine in the eye may cause release of pigment from the posterior surface of the iris; on slit-lamp examination of the anterior chamber, the striking appearance of this is often mistaken for inflammatory cells seen in iritis.[137,156]

Nitrogen Mustard, Systemic. This antineoplastic agent may cause necrotizing uveitis associated with edema of the lid, conjunctiva, and cornea.[8]

Quinine. Atrophy of the iris has been reported with systemic use of this drug.[120,137,199]

CHEMICAL INJURIES, TOXINS, AND POISONS

Acetone. Acetone is a strong lipid solvent which extracts tissue lipid. While its vapors are not dangerous to the eye, a splash of liquid acetone into the human eye causes microscopic grey dots in the corneal and conjunctival epithelium. If washed out immediately, healing usually occurs in 1 or 2 days. Prolonged contact produces epithelial loss, temporary stromal haziness, and edema, which tend to disappear in 4 to 6 days. Since acetone is used as a solvent for the removal of cyanoacrylate inadvertently introduced into the eye tissues (see p. 434), it can gain entry into the eye through perforated wounds. Introduction of acetone into the anterior chamber causes immediate corneal opacity followed by severe iritis, glaucoma, and corneal necrosis.[137,156]

Acid Burns. The severity of the damage caused by acid varies with the quantity, concentration, and duration of contact. Acid exposure to the eye causes an instantaneous coagulative necrosis and precipitation of protein—mainly at the epithelial layer of the keratoconjunctiva—that helps to buffer the effect of the acid and limits its further penetration, so that damage is usually superficial. If the corneal epithelium is already defective and the amount of acid is excessive, the acid can penetrate into the eye and cause extensive damage, including coagulative necrosis of the corneal endothelium and lens epithelium. The damaged corneal epithelium eventually sloughs and is replaced by new epithelial cells. The acute phase lasts about 3 days. In the intermediate phase (3 to 7 days after injury), there is a period of active inflammation with uveitis. In severe burns, corneal ulceration and perforation occur. In the chronic phase, which occurs in severe burns, vascularization of the cornea, cicatrix formation, and symblepharon may result. In contrast to alkali burns, there is histologically no early loss of metachromatic staining or of hexosamine in acid burns of the eye. These changes do, however, occur later in scarred areas injured by acid.[99,100,118,248]

Alkali Burns. Alkali burns to the eye are more severe than other chemical injuries; they inflict damage rapidly, and there is a tendency for late complication even years after the injury. The concentration of alkali and duration of exposure are more important factors in determining the extent of damage than the character of the cations. In general, however, the higher the pH, greater is the damage to the eye. On the basis of measurements (comparing penetration rates of solutions of similar concentration and alkalinity through excised ox corneas with intact epithelium), alkalies have been graded from slowest to fastest in the following order: calcium hydroxide, tetraethylammonium hydroxide, barium hydroxide, strontium hydroxide, lithium hydroxide, potassium hydroxide, sodium hydroxide, and ammonium hydroxide.

In contrast to acid injury, which coagulates cellular protein, alkali tends to react with the lipid of the cellular structures, forming soluble compounds that rapidly penetrate the ocular tissues. Penetration of alkali into the cell causes dissociation of compounds and emulsification of lipid in the cell membrane, which disrupts the cell wall barrier. Cellular death occurs from dehydration as well as from the destruction of enzymes and proteins. After an alkali burn, the corneal epithelial cells, invading polymorphonuclear leukocytes, and possibly keratocytes release the enzyme collagenase, which digests the corneal stroma to produce corneal melting or keratomalacia. There is a strong tendency for corneal infiltration to develop from 1 to 3 weeks after injury.

The acute stage of alkali burn is characterized by immediate thrombosis of the conjunctival and episcleral blood vessels, ischemic necrosis, and edema of the conjunctiva and of the limbal region of the sclera, giving rise to a porcelain-white appearance. There is sloughing of the corneal epithelium, necrosis of stromal and endothelial cells, loss of corneal ground substance, and edema of the stroma and of the ciliary processes. Inflammatory cells infiltrate into the cornea and iris. Access of alkali inside the eye causes loss of nuclei in the lens epithelium, cortical degeneration, and a chronic nongranulomatous iridocyclitis, with frequent formation of peripheral anterior synechiae. The critical period for corneal ulceration is from 1 to 3 weeks after injury. Experimental studies suggest that the basal cells at the edge of the ulcer increase in number but have no basement membrane, and that their cytoplasmic processes project into the damaged stroma.

Late complications of severe alkali burns include persistent corneal edema, vascularization, scarring, pannus formation, staphyloma, cataract, secondary glaucoma, and symblepharon.[51, 137, 169, 217]

Arsenic Poisoning (Inorganic). Both local contact and systemic absorption of a variety of arsenical compounds induce pathology in the eye. Dusts such as arsenic trioxide and copper acetoarsenite (encountered in industry) produce hyperemia and chemosis of the conjunctiva, and corneal ulceration, together with the clinical symptoms of itching, burning, lacrimation, and photophobia. A similar reaction is seen with chronic systemic poisoning, in which there may also be formation of pigment spots in the corneal and conjunctival epithelium. The exact nature of the pigmentation has not been determined, but it is thought that the pathology occurs from the secretion of arsenic in the tears.[146, 224, 333, 343]

Benzene. Systemic benzene poisoning occasionally produces hemorrhages in the retina and conjunctiva. Rarely, edema of the retina and papilledema have been concomitant findings.[137]

Botulism. In addition to a paralysis of both intra- and extraocular muscles that accompanies other systemic findings, botulinus toxin may occasionally cause hyperemia of the optic papillae, retinal vessel engorgement and hemorrhage, and optic neuritis and atrophy. One histologically documented case had lymphocytic infiltration of the retrobulbar tissue and of the optic nerve. Other pathologic findings have included degenerative changes and hemorrhages in the ocular motor nuclei, optic nerve and tract, optic chiasm, retina, choroid, and in the ciliary body. These findings are thought to be secondary to the primary mechanism of poisoning, whereby the toxin acts at the terminal ends of the cholinergic autonomic nerve and at neuromuscular junctions.[26, 300]

Carbon Disulfide. Severe chronic poisoning from vapors of carbon disulfide may produce retrobulbar neuritis with temporal pallor of the optic nerve head corresponding to the papillomacular bundle. Rarely, optic atrophy has been recorded. There is some clinical evidence that this poison may also cause retinal hemorrhages as well as the formation of microaneurysms. The mechanism of action of carbon disulfide in inducing these changes is not known.[164, 328]

Cyanides. Acute cyanide poisoning affects the optic nerve and retina, although histopathologic examination has revealed only a marked central retinal edema.[3]

Dimethyl Sulfate. Vapors from this chemical cause eyelid edema and conjunctival hyperemia, irregularity of the corneal epithelium, and clouding of the superficial stroma. In severe cases, the poisoning causes grey necrosis of the epithelium, infiltration of the corneal stroma, and permanent opacification. The stromal edema is due to the selective injurious action of dimethyl sulfate on the corneal endothelium, whereby this substance causes denaturation and enzyme inhibition by methylation. Recovery of the endothelium relieves the stromal edema, although a mottled cloudiness may remain.[142]

Ethylene Glycol. Ingestion of ethylene glycol produces edema of the optic nerve head and marked dilatation of the retinal veins, probably secondary to the induced cerebral edema and increased cerebrospinal fluid pressure produced by this substance. Although every year some 40 to 60 deaths occur due to ingestion of antifreeze in the United States alone, there are apparently no pathologic descriptions of the eye changes in these cases.[116]

Euphorbia peplus, E. lactea,* and *E. tirucalli. Upon ocular contact, the sap or latex from these tropical, cactus-like plants causes conjunctival hyperemia, swelling of the lids, diffuse epithelial defects in the cornea, stromal edema, keratitis with fine keratic precipitates, and folds in Descemet's membrane. An associated iritis is responsible for a thick, serofibrinous exudate in the anterior chamber. Histopathologic examination shows infiltration of the stroma with inflammatory cells and damage to the corneal endothelium.[89, 154]

Formaldehyde, Glutaraldehyde, and Paraformaldehyde. The general action of these aldehydes is to fix or denature the tissues; the stronger the concentration, the more damaging is the effect. A splash of 26 percent formalin causes conjunctival hyperemia, severe inflammation, epithelial edema of the cornea, wrinkling of Descemet's membrane, and iritis. A 40 percent solution, in addition, produces lid swelling, loss of corneal epithelium, and ischemia of the conjunctiva. If not washed out of the eye immediately, degeneration and opacification of the cornea, damage to the irides, cataract, glaucoma, and eventually atrophia bulbi may ensue.[161, 183, 314]

Galactose. A natural hexose sugar, galactose in normal individuals produces no pathology. However, in patients with an inborn error of metabolism or galactose kinase (galactose-1-phosphate uridyltransferase) deficiency, ingestion of galactose in infants leads to the formation of cataracts.

The earliest change in the lens in metabolic galactose oculotoxicity occurs at about 3 weeks of age, and appears as an oily drop in the center of the lens or as a central refractile ring around the fetal nucleus. A zonular or nuclear cataract may follow, together with faint striae and dust-like opacities in the anterior cortex. These changes may be reversible if galactose is eliminated from the diet, particularly before 3 months of age. Histologic examination of the lens from a 5-month aborted fetus with a history of familial galactosemia showed extensive vacuolation and degeneration of the epithelial cells and lens fibers, indicating the onset of cataract even before birth.

Numerous experimental studies have been done to elucidate the pathogenesis of galactosemic cataracts. Animal experiments have shown that aldose reductase converts excess galactose into galactose alcohol (dulcitol), which is retained within the lens. This sugar alcohol is hyperosmotic and attracts water into and between the lens cells; the lens secondarily becomes abnormally permeable, so that potassium leaks out and sodium leaks in, attracting chloride ions. With hydrolysis, swelling, and alterations in the lens proteins, the lens fibers eventually disintegrate and show the general features of cortical cataract.[82, 185, 204, 323, 324, 327]

Glue (Cyanoacrylate). Besides various general uses, cyanoacrylate derivatives have been evaluated for sutureless surgery on the eye. Methyl forms are more toxic than butyl, hexyl, octyl, or decyl forms. Penetration of cyanoacrylate adhesives through the intact cornea and sclera is limited.

Irritative reactions (granulomatous or nongranulomatous) in the conjunctiva and cornea are common with cyanoacrylate contact, leading to a variable degree of vascularization, ulceration, edema, and inflammatory reaction. The introduction of 0.1 ml into the rabbit anterior chamber causes endothelial necrosis, moderate iritis, and permanent corneal opacity and vascularization. Choroidal penetration causes localized disorganization and retinal degeneration, together with vitreous inflammation and band formation.

The toxicity of cyanoacrylate adhesives is directly related to the amount present in the tissue. A forceful separation of tissue bonding may result in mechanical tissue disruption. Acetone, when used as a solvent for acrylate tissue adhesions, may cause its own tissue toxicity (see p. 432).[106, 156, 267, 314]

Hydrogen Sulfide. Low concentrations of this gas produce characteristic pathologic changes in the cornea and conjunctiva. Initially, biomicroscopy reveals scattered, fine grey dots of keratitis epithelialis, as well as conjunctival hyperemia and eyelid edema. As the severity of poisoning increases, the corneal epithelium becomes irregular, lusterless, and eroded, with death and loss of epithelial cells. The postulated mechanism of action of hydrogen sulfide is via an enzyme inhibition, possibly of cytochrome oxidase.[31, 113]

Hydroquinones. Acute exposure to hydroquinone vapors causes injury to the corneal epithelium, and even ulceration. In severe cases, the cornea may develop superficial opacities in the palpebral fissure area, as well as folds on the posterior corneal surface.

Chronic exposure to vapors of benzoquinone or to the dust of hydroquinone causes a brownish discoloration of the sclera and conjunctiva in the palpebral region, which over the course of years may be observed biomicroscopically as brown globules or granules in the deeper conjunctival layers. The conjunctiva becomes thickened and dry. Pigment has been seen to migrate from the limbus onto the cornea. After further exposure, in addition to the darker staining of the conjunctiva, diffuse brown staining of the cornea occurs, together with scarring beneath the corneal epithelium. These grey-white opacities are associated with a greenish-yellow staining of the anterior stroma and fine wrinkles in Descemet's membrane. In the late stages of chronic exposure, Hudson-Stähli pigment lines are seen in the epithelium.

Polymerized products of benzoquinone or hydroquinone are thought to deposit directly in the cells to produce the brown granules. Biopsies of the conjunctiva from such cases have revealed the presence of small granules in the superficial epithelium and larger conglomerates in the basal cells.[9, 236, 296]

Lead Poisoning, Systemic. Lead poisoning commonly involves several parts of the eye, which may include any of the following sites: the lens (rarely, cataracts are observed), intra- and extraocular muscles (swelling and degeneration of the fibers), the retina, optic nerve (bulbar and retrobulbar), visual cortex, and suprageniculate pathways. Pathologic examination, however, has contributed little information. Optic nerve damage manifesting as optic neuritis and optic atrophy may result either from increased intracranial pressure or from the direct toxic effect of lead. Some cases develop vasoconstriction of the retinal vessels with vasculitis, white ensheathing, and changes in the vascular walls associated with inflammatory and degenerative changes in the optic nerve.[22, 321]

Mercurial Poisoning. Chronic absorption of mercury, either as the metal or as an inorganic salt, leads to characteristic discoloration of the anterior lens surface, the condition being known as mercurialentis. The anterior surface takes on a pink or rose-brown hue due to fine deposits of black or dark brown pigmented particles beneath the lens epithelium. It has been shown chemically that these particles are mercurial in nature.

Discoloration of the cornea may lead to an opacity in the form of band keratopathy, but the mechanism of the toxicity is not understood. Droplets of metallic mercury have been observed within the epithelial cells of the cornea, but they are rapidly extruded without further pathologic reaction. (see also p. 406).[2, 19, 109, 122, 153, 275]

Methanol. Systemic methanol poisoning results in hyperemia of the optic nerve heads. Edema of the optic disc margins and of the adjacent retina develops rapidly (within 24 hours), and subhyaloid or flame-shaped hemorrhages may occur. Severe poisoning results in persistent retinal edema and eventually in optic atrophy. The latter may appear grossly as a white nerve head with distinct margins, and in some cases the atrophic disc is deeply cupped.

Pathologic examination of the eye in the early stages of methanol poisoning shows edema in the retinal nerve fiber layer, with proteinaceous subretinal fluid between the retina and choroid, as well as disruption in the pigment epithelium. In the late stages, the retinal ganglion cells and optic nerve fibers show degenerative changes. Similar changes have been found in experimental investigations using monkeys.

It would appear that the toxicity of methanol is due to its physiologic oxidation by the enzyme alcohol dehydrogenase to give formaldehyde. The reaction occurs within the retina, and the formaldehyde production inhibits retinal respiration, glycolysis, oxidative phosphorylation, and the formation of ATP.[24, 36, 222, 231, 257]

Methyl Bromide. Exposure to this gas produces hemorrhages in the retina which, on pathologic grounds, are insufficent to explain the visual disturbances. The basis for the toxicity appears to be a methylation (alkylation) reaction.[329]

Mustard Gas. Ocular exposure to this gas causes conjunctival hemorrhage, vascular thrombosis, edema of lids and corneal epithelium, and stromal opacification. In some cases, neovascularization of the cornea has occurred. The episcleral tissues adjacent to the cornea develop porcelain-white areas, with the formation of grossly enlarged, sausage-shaped vessels. In these regions, recurring ulceration may continue over several years. The toxicity of mustard gas is due to its prompt chemical reaction with tissues to form very stable bonds; the action denatures proteins and inactivates enzymes.[43, 168, 186]

Naphthalene. Although the oculotoxic effect of naphthalene in experimental animals is well established, injury to human eyes from systemic poisoning is uncertain. Naphthalene has, however, been suspected of causing cataract which manifests as brown discoloration of the lens with numerous, small white opacities around the nucleus and a narrow clear zone at the equator. In rabbits, lens changes can be produced rapidly. Swelling of the lens is followed by vacuoles first in the periphery and then toward the center. Biochemical studies have shown, among other changes, decreased glutathione and protein content, with increased ascorbate.[130, 207, 324]

Osmium Tetroxide (Osmic Acid). Osmic acid, employed in histology laboratories and in industry, produces damage to the eye by its vapors and by direct contact. Exposure to the vapors causes conjunctival hyperemia, epithelial edema, and death of the superficial cells of the keratoconjunctiva; recovery occurs in 24 to 48 hours. Experimental application of single drop of 1 percent osmic acid to the rabbit eye causes immediate brown staining of the epithelium. Epithelial regeneration may be complete, but in the stroma, moderate opacity persists together with superficial vascularization. Although osmic acid is an excellent fixative, its tissue penetration is slow and poor, affecting maximally to a depth of about 1 mm in moderately dense tissue. Osmic acid selectively binds to the double carbon bonds of unsaturated lipids and also denatures proteins.[54, 249, 314]

Phenol. Exposure of the eye to phenol causes conjunctival chemosis and lid edema, and renders the cornea white, accompanied by iritis. Chronic exposure causes carbolchronosis characterized by grey discoloration of the sclera with brown spots near the insertions of the rectus muscles. A melanin-like pigment forms from phenol and other phenolic substances.[292]

Snake Venom. Snake bites may cause a variety of changes, but most commonly retinal hemorrhage occurs. Instances of optic neuritis, optic atrophy, and extraocular muscle palsy have also been reported, depending upon the species of snake.[91, 144]

Tatoo. Corneal tatooing is generally done to disguise white corneal leukoma or nebulae, pupillary membrane, or mature cataract in a blind eye. Various coloring agents have been used. In situ precipitation of platinium chloride into black pigment by hydrazine hydrate is least toxic. Gold chloride reduced by epinephrine gives rise to a dark brown tatoo. Substances such as India ink may produce a chronic inflammatory reaction in the cornea and anterior chamber. Histologically, foreign body material is seen in the scarred corneal stroma.[314, 349]

Thallium. Systemic poisoning by this heavy metal and its salts produces retrobulbar optic neuritis, which is usually reversible, but in some cases permanent optic atrophy may develop. Severe poisoning causes selective loss of the retinal ganglion cells, with atrophy of the nerve fibers and of the optic nerve. The outer nuclear layer as well as the rod and cone photoreceptors appear normal, as does the anterior segment of the eye. Disturbance of the lens has been reported rarely; small, snowflake opacities seen in the deeper anterior and posterior cortex are usually regressive in nature. Ptosis may also occur. Since thallium poisoning in experimental animals induces an ocular pathology different from that seen in humans, the mechanism of thallium toxicity remains obscure.[137, 215]

Toad Poison. Contact of the eye with secretions from certain toads causes corneal clouding associated with a central nebula, corneal anesthesia, and conjunctival hyperemia. Biomicroscopically, the epithelium appears normal but Descemet's membrane shows folds and breaks, and the stroma is edematous. The central retina shows edematous changes, and whitish dots (of unknown etiology) appear on the posterior vitreous humor just in front of the retina.[79]

Tobacco. There is an extensive literature on tobacco smoking and vision, and on so-called tobacco amblyopia. It is, however, not clear whether retrobulbar neuritis and optic atrophy is caused by the tobacco per se or secondarily by nutritional deficiency, poor absorption, and low serum levels of vitamin B_{12}. The association of amblyopia with tobacco and alcohol has often been noted (see p. 426). Ophthalmoscopically, temporal pallor of the nerve heads is seen in some cases involving the papillomacular bundle. It is not known whether the primary disturbance is in the nerve fibers, in the retina, or in the associated blood vessels.[48, 100, 101, 137, 259]

Trinitrotoluene (TNT). Chronic exposure to this substance has caused cataract in several cases in the United States and in the U.S.S.R. The opacities initially begin axially and progress to spoke-like opacities in the cortex and the equator. Chemical investigations of one extracted lens has shown the presence of trinitrotoluene in the lens. In some instances, retrobulbar neuritis has also been reported.[137]

Zinc Disulfide and Barium Sulfate. These chemical particles are contained under enormous pressure in the core of golf balls, and

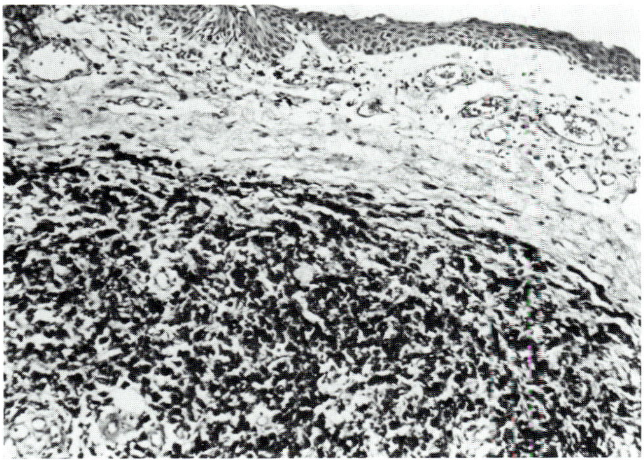

Fig. 16-39. Barium sulfate granuloma of conjunctiva following accidental injury with exploded golf ball. ×100.

if the latter are opened they can penetrate deeply into the tissues of the lids and conjunctiva without being felt. Histologically, a resulting amorphous mass, without much inflammatory reaction, shows birefringence under polarized light. The foreign material is white when viewed directly, but appears pigmented under transmitted light of the microscope. A macrophage reaction may, however, produce a foreign body granuloma (Fig. 16-39).[175, 241]

NONMECHANICAL INJURIES AND FOREIGN BODIES

Radiational Injuries

Ionizing Radiation (X-Rays and Gamma Rays). The eye may be involved as a result of inadequate protection during radiotherapy or by direct exposure in ocular therapy. Ionizing radiations usually have a latent period for biologic effect, and may cause a variety of lesions throughout the eye, depending upon the dose. Lens changes leading to cataract formation are the primary ocular effect. Other ocular and periocular manifestations may include chronic blepharitis, ectropion, entropion, madarosis, hyperemia, cicatrization, and symblepharon in the conjunctiva, atrophy of the lacrimal glands, keratoconjunctivitis sicca, orbital necrosis, punctate keratitis, epithelial loss, ulceration, necrosis, opacification, and vascularization of the cornea, anterior uveitis, atrophy, ciliary spasm, retinal burns, exudates, hemorrhages, macular degeneration and holes, vascular occlusion, neovascularization, and secondary glaucoma.[100, 126, 205, 220]

Laser Photocoagulators. Lasers essentially produce radiation energies that cause rapid thermal coagulation and tissue explosion, depending upon the dose. Pigmented tissues of the eye preferentially absorb energy, although at higher doses the transparent tissue of the cornea, lens, and retina may be affected. The corneal epithelial and endothelial damage is usually reversible. Lenticular damage may lead to a localized cataract. Retinal damage causes degenerative changes, especially in the receptor elements and in other inner layers, followed by glial proliferation. The affected pigment epithelium degenerates, while adjacent cells may show proliferative activity (Fig. 16-40A–C). Laser application to vessels causes spontaneous, temporary or permanent intravascular coagulation of blood and endothelial damage, with consequent ischemic and hemorrhagic necrosis (see p. 418). Inadequate coagulative changes may, however, cause vascular rupture and hemorrhage. With high energy emissions, the choroidal tissue as well as the outer retina may be directly affected.[205, 211, 216, 314]

Ultraviolet Waves (180 to 390 nm). The cornea and conjunctiva generally absorb ultraviolet waves which, depending on the wavelength (maximally sensitive to 288 nm) and dose, may cause punctate keratitis and conjunctivitis. Moderately damaged corneal epithelium may take 5 to 7 days to return to normal. Waves of sufficent power, such as ultraviolet laser waves, can reach the lens.[167, 205, 213]

Infrared Waves. Prolonged infrared exposure (as in glassblowers and steel workers) can cause true exfoliation of the lens capsule in which the anterior layers of the capsule split and may curl into the anterior chamber. It is suggested that the iris absorbs the infrared energy and transmits it to the lens capsule.[100, 205]

Microwaves. Although posterior cortical cataracts have been produced in experimental animals, the cumulative effect of microwaves on human lenses has yet to be documented.[12, 205]

Visible Light Waves. Sufficient intensity of visible light can cause chorioretinal lesions, and is exploited in the xenon arc photocoagulator. The projected beam radiance of several common ophthalmologic instruments carries potential hazards to patients from light exposure.[62, 117, 205, 319, 332]

Electrical Injury

Injury to the eye may occur with current arcing between an electrode and the body at voltages ranging from that of lightning, which

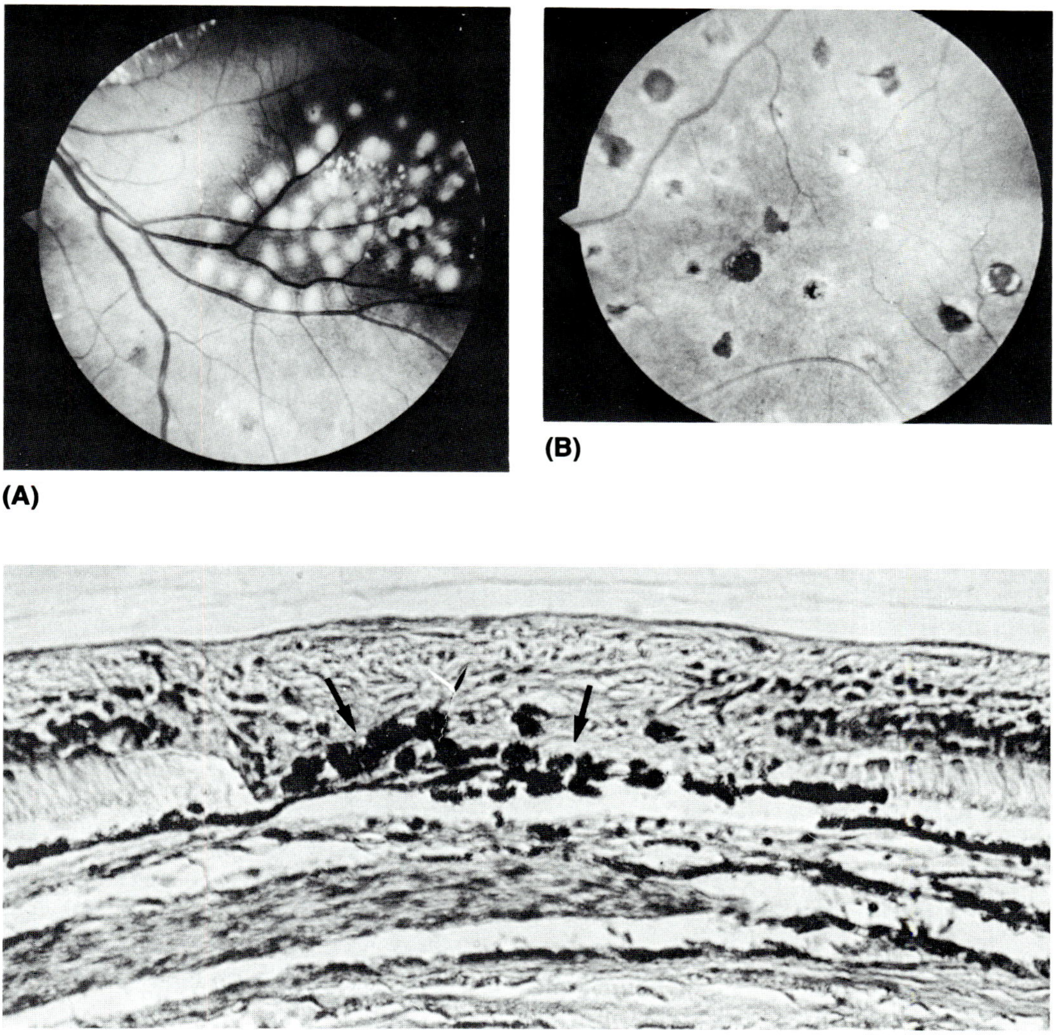

(A) **(B)** **(C)**

Fig. 16-40. Gross appearance of retina (A) immediately after laser application (white burn spots), and (B) a few days after laser application. Note the darkened appearance of burn spots due to pigment epithelium proliferation. The retinal reaction may, however, vary depending upon the duration and intensity of laser energy delivered. (C) Histologic section of retina showing retinal gliosis and proliferative changes in the retinal pigment epithelium (arrows) corresponding to the area of laser application. The retinal architecture is, however, preserved on either side of the laser burn. ×200.

may be 100 million volts, to as low as 380 volts. The most common ocular injury is opacification of the lens, which often appears after the flow of current through the head or near the eye. Cataract formation is usually unilateral, on the side proximal to the point of contact, although the contralateral eye may also be involved. Initially, multiple vacuoles are formed beneath the anterior capsule, to be subsequently replaced by anterior subcapsular streaks in an irregular pattern. Scale-like grey opacities may also appear in the anterior cortex. Vesicles and amorphous opacities may also occur in the posterior cortex or subcapsular area. These changes may ensue almost immediately or over several years, the average time of onset being 2 to 6 months. The lens changes are generally progressive.

Other periocular manifestations of electric shock include burns and necrosis of the eyelids, cicatrization, necrosis and perforation of the cornea, hyphema, paralysis of the extraocular muscles, anterior uveitis, atrophy and rupture of the choroid, and optic neuritis or optic atrophy. Retinal changes include attenuated arteries, dilated veins, cysts, edema, exudates, hemorrhage, holes, and pigmentary degeneration.[41, 111, 127, 148]

Foreign Bodies

Copper (Chalcosis). Retained copper foreign bodies in the eye cause gradual ionization, with deposition of copper throughout the limiting membranes of the eye, producing the characteristic picture of chalcosis. This is most noticeable in the iris (greenish color), but may also be observed in the lens, vitreous humor (yellowish-green and bluish color), and cornea (blue-green color). An iridescent reflection appears beneath the lens capsule with a sunflower appearance similar to that seen in Wilson's disease. Histologically, copper deposits are seen between the capsule and the epithelial layers.

In the cornea, deposits resembling a Kayser-Fleischer ring are seen in the periphery of Descemet's membrane (Fig. 16-19B, C), and in the deepest layers of the corneal stroma. In the retina, copper deposits may give a copper-colored sheen or appear as shiny granular deposits in the macula or along the vessels. In chalcosis, the predominant extracellular rather than intracellular deposition of copper may account for the tolerance of the eye to these foreign bodies for many years without serious toxicity to the retina or lens.[172, 276, 277]

Iron (Siderosis). Siderosis is produced by oxidation and absorption of iron or steel, with the distribution of ferrous compounds throughout the eye. The tissues surrounding the particle become rust-brown colored. The site of the foreign body determines the extent and intensity of the spread of the siderosis.

Histologically, deposits of iron are detected in the external limiting membrane and perivascular tissue of the retina. Narrowing of the vascular lumens, degeneration of the internal and external nuclear layers, and proliferation of the pigment epithelium have been reported; this may lead to complete degeneration of the retina, atrophy of the optic nerve, and gliosis. Vitreous reaction may cause bands, retinitis proliferans, and retinal detachment. It is possible that a histochemical binding occurs between iron and the acid muopolysaccharide in the retina and vitreous humor, accounting for the predominantly significant pathology in the posterior segment of the eye. In severe siderosis, obstruction of capillaries in the choriocapillaris layer occurs.

Deposits of iron in the lens cause brown discoloration and cataractous change. The iris may show rusty discoloration and an inflammatory reaction as well as iridoplasia. Rusty discoloration may also spread to the conjunctiva and lid. In the cornea, siderosis manifests as a Fleischer ring (Fig. 16-18D) and Hudson-Stähli line, and reactive changes may lead to interstitial keratitis, stromal edema, neovascularization, and opacification. The trabecular meshwork may be scarred and obliterated, or infiltrated with phagocytic cells containing siderin or hemosiderin. As opposed to copper,

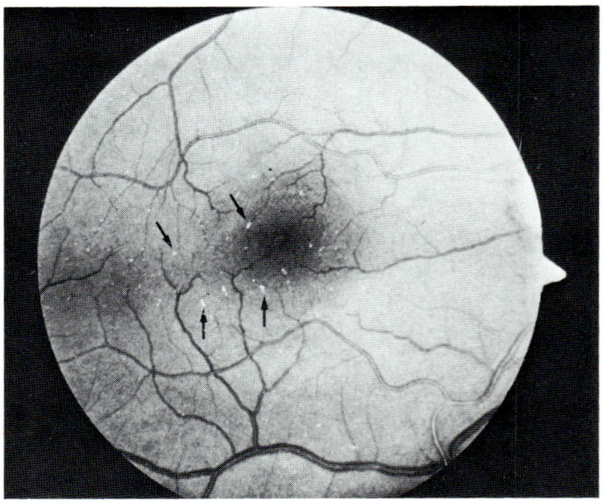

Fig. 16-41. Gross appearance of talc emboli (arrows) in the capillaries of the macular area.

iron deposits are largely intracellular and occur in phagocytic vacuoles.

Inadvertent ocular exposure to iron compounds causes an irritative reaction, yellow-brown discoloration or deposits in the eyelids, conjunctiva, cornea, and sclera, and may even cause ulceration of these structures if the eye is exposed to acidic ferrous salts.[71, 74, 75, 218, 352]

Talc and Cornstarch. Solutions of drugs (methylphenidate, cocaine, and heroin) injected by abusers are frequently contaminated with talc (hydrous magnesium silicate), cornstarch, and other materials that can travel to the retina, where they become lodged as microemboli. The particles are seen in the retina as tiny, glistening crystals, mainly in the paramacular vessels (Fig. 16-41). The retinopathy that develops may be characterized by punctate hemorrhages, irreversible macular ischemia, peripheral retinal neovascularization, and optic disc neovascularization. Escape of the particles into the retina and choroid may cause a granulomatous reaction.[20, 115, 197, 229, 314, 318]

ACKNOWLEDGMENT

This work was carried out in part with the grant provided by the National Institutes of Health (#EY-02046) and by the Block Fund of the University of Chicago. We thank F. T. Fraunfelder, M.D., C. Hanna, Ph.D., and F. W. Newell, M.D., for their encouragement and support.

Table 16-1. Glossary of Ocular Structures Involved in Pathologic Reactions of Drugs, Chemicals, Toxins, Poisons, and Nonmechanical Agents

Agent	Conjunctiva Lid Other Adnexa	Cornea Sclera	Lens	Retina Optic Nerve	Uveal Tract	References
Acetaminophen (paracetamol)	+	–	–	–	–	137, 337
Acetanilid	+	–	–	–	–	137, 337
Acetone	+	+	–	–	–	137, 156
Acids	+	+	+	–	+	99, 100, 118, 248
Alcian blue	–	+	–	–	–	50, 239, 314
Alkalis	+	+	+	–	–	51, 137, 169, 217
Alpha chymotrypsin	–	+	+	–	–	10, 70, 156, 190, 346, 347
Amidarone	–	+	–	–	–	47, 311
Aminosalicylic acid	+	+	–	+	–	5, 114, 137, 177, 254
Amodiaquine	+	+	–	–	–	42, 137, 159
Amphotericin B	+	–	–	+	+	5, 34, 114
Anesthetics, local	+	+	–	–	–	65, 103, 156, 160, 290, 291, 307, 314, 343
general	+	+	–	–	–	100, 134, 137, 314
Arabinoside	+	+	–	–	–	156, 200, 201, 221
Arsacetin	–	–	–	+	–	283
Arsenicals	+	+	–	–	–	146, 187, 198, 224, 314, 333, 343
Arsphenamine	–	–	–	+	–	137
Aspirin (sodium salicylate, acetylsalicylic acid)	+	+	–	+	–	84, 100, 114, 134, 140, 286, 314, 333
Atropine	+	+	–	–	–	114, 156, 307
Barbiturates	+	–	–	+	–	114, 137, 279, 343
Benzalkonium	+	+	–	–	–	134, 301
Benzene	+	–	–	+	–	137

Continued

Table 16-1 *(continued)*

Agent	Conjunctiva Lid Other Adnexa	Cornea Sclera	Lens	Retina Optic Nerve	Uveal Tract	References
Bismuth compounds	+	+	−	−	−	78, 108
Botulism	−	+	−	+	+	26, 300
Bromides	+	−	−	−	−	114, 137, 333
Busulfan	+	−	+	−	−	114, 147, 174, 210, 253, 265
Carbon dioxide	−	−	−	+	−	100, 287
Carbon disulfide	−	−	−	+	−	164, 328
Carbonic anhydrase inhibitors	+	−	−	−	−	114, 156
Carbromal, bromisovalum	−	−	+	+	−	81, 85, 283
Cephaloridine	−	−	−	+	−	25, 88
Chloral hydrate	+	−	−	−	−	114, 137, 343
Chloramphenicol	−	−	−	+	−	76, 151, 192, 201, 209, 280, 345, 346
Chloroquine, hydroxychloroquine	+	+	−	+	+	38, 39, 40, 59, 141, 159, 162, 166, 242, 264, 278, 289, 314, 339
Chlorpromazine	+	+	+	−	−	67, 95, 133, 137, 165, 219, 260, 282, 340, 349, 351
Chlorpropamide	+	−	−	−	−	86, 343
Chlorprothixene	−	+	+	−	−	114
Chrysarobin	+	+	−	−	−	5, 100, 114, 137, 343
Clioquinol	−	−	−	+	−	235, 243, 322
Copper (salts)	+	−	−	−	−	314, 333
Copper (metallic)	+	+	+	+	+	172, 276, 277
Corticosteroids	+	+	+	+	−	77, 87, 92, 114, 157, 181, 196, 198, 240, 245, 252, 273, 295, 299, 313, 342, 344
Cyanides	−	−	−	+	−	3
Cyanocrylate (glue)	+	+	−	+	+	106, 156, 267, 314
Cytosine arabinoside	+	+	−	−	−	102, 114, 156, 180
Digitalis	−	−	−	+	−	212, 271, 272, 337
Diiodohydroxyquine, iodochlorohydroxyquine	−	+	−	+	−	33, 335
Dimethyl sulfate	+	+	−	−	−	142
Dimethyl sulfoxide	−	−	+	−	−	135, 341
Dinitrophenol	−	−	+	−	−	60, 163, 232, 269, 302, 336
Diphenazine	+	−	+	−	−	137, 226, 262
Echothiophate, isoflurophate, demecarium	+	+	+	+	+	1, 21, 73, 96, 114, 137, 145, 152, 156, 193, 256, 288, 304, 307, 338
Electrical injury	+	+	+	+	+	41, 111, 127, 148
Epinephrine	+	+	−	+	+	14, 32, 61, 83, 98, 107, 112, 124, 137, 139, 156, 171, 195, 214, 228, 268, 294, 317, 334
Ergotamine tartrate	−	−	−	+	−	86
Estrogen/progestin combination products	+	+	−	+	−	72, 114, 119, 136, 251, 297, 314, 316
Ethanol	+	−	−	+	−	23, 114, 137, 156, 227, 261, 333

Continued

Table 16-1 ***(continued)***

Agent	Conjunctiva Lid Other Adnexa	Cornea Sclera	Lens	Retina Optic Nerve	Uveal Tract	References
Ethambutol	−	−	−	+	−	29, 67, 203, 246, 281, 285, 350
Ethylene glycol	−	−	−	+	−	116
Ethylcupreine hydrochloride	−	−	−	+	−	137, 284
Euphorbia sp. sap	+	+	−	−	−	89, 154
Formaldehyde, paraformaldehyde, glutaraldehyde	+	+	+	−	+	161, 183, 314
Galactose	−	−	+	−	−	82, 185, 204, 323, 324, 327
Gentamicin	+	−	−	−	−	208
Gold	+	+	−	−	−	49, 114, 137, 155, 234, 270, 308, 314,
Griseofulvin	+	−	−	+	−	5, 94, 114, 134
Hexamethonium	−	−	−	+	−	28, 52
Homatropine	+	+	−	−	−	156, 307
Hyaluronidase	−	−	−	+	−	18, 156, 230, 274
Hydroquinone	+	+	−	−	−	9, 236, 296
Hydrogen sulfide	+	+	−	−	−	31, 113
Idoxuridine (IDU)	+	+	−	−	−	156, 200, 201, 221
Indomethacin	+	+	−	+	−	58, 93, 114, 158, 247, 309
Iodine, iodides	+	+	−	+	−	114, 129, 134, 137, 156, 314, 333, 343
Iron (compounds)	+	+	+	+	−	71, 100, 114, 137
Iron (metallic)	+	+	+	+	−	71, 74, 75, 218, 352
Isoniazid	−	−	−	+	−	97, 178, 182
Lead poisoning	+	−	+	+	−	22, 321
Mepacrine (quinacrine)	+	+	−	+	−	11, 69, 90, 105, 137, 293, 298, 333
Mercurial compounds	+	+	+	−	−	2, 19, 109, 114, 122, 137, 153, 275, 306, 307, 325, 343
Methanol	−	−	−	+	−	24, 36, 222, 231, 257
Methoxyflurane	−	−	−	+	+	56
Methyl bromide	−	−	−	+	−	329
Methylene blue	−	−	−	+	−	128, 333
Mustard gas	+	+	−	−	−	43, 168, 186
Naldixic acid	−	−	−	+	−	45, 93
Naphthlene	−	−	+	−	−	130, 207, 324
Neomycin	+	−	−	−	−	104, 191
Nicotinic acid	−	−	−	+	−	125
Nitrogen mustard	+	−	−	−	+	8
Nitrogen mustard derivatives (chlorambucil, cyclophosphamide, mechlorethamine, melphalagen, uracil mustard)	+	−	−	−	−	114, 174
Osmium tetroxide	+	+	−	−	−	54, 249, 314
Oxygen	−	−	−	+	−	15, 16, 17, 194, 238, 250, 312
Penicillin and derivatives	+	+	−	−	−	114, 137, 156, 307
Phenacetin	+	−	−	−	−	137, 337

Continued

Table 16-1 *(continued)*

Agent	Conjunctiva Lid Other Adnexa	Cornea Sclera	Lens	Retina Optic Nerve	Uveal Tract	References
Phenazone (antipyrine)	+	−	−	−	−	114, 336, 343
Pheniprazine	−	−	−	+	−	176
Phenmetrazine	−	−	+	−	−	202
Phenol	+	+	−	−	+	292
Phensuximide (milontin)	+	−	−	−	−	173
Phenylbutazone (butazolidin)	+	+	−	+	−	7, 53, 114, 134, 266, 310, 314, 333, 343
Phenytoin	+	+	−	−	−	315, 326, 333, 343
Physostigmine, neostigmine	+	+	+	+	+	73, 114, 137, 156, 193, 256, 338
Pilocarpine	+	+	−	+	+	73, 114, 137, 156, 256, 307
Piperdylchlorophenothiazine	−	−	−	+	−	57, 131
Practolol	+	+	−	−	−	6, 121, 263, 314, 348
Pyridine-3-aldehyde-thio-semicarbazone	−	+	−	−	−	255
Quinine	+	−	−	+	+	27, 66, 68, 110, 114, 120, 137, 199
Radiation:						
x-and gamma-rays	+	+	+	+	+	100, 126, 205, 221
Lasers	+	+	+	+	+	205, 211, 216, 314
Ultraviolet	+	+	−	−	−	167, 205, 213
Infrared	−	−	+	−	−	100, 205
Microwaves	−	−	+	−	−	12, 205
Visible light	−	−	−	+	+	62, 117, 205, 319, 332
Scopolamine	+	+	−	−	−	156, 307
Silver compounds	+	+	+	−	−	30, 63, 138, 143, 149, 156, 223, 314, 349
Sodium bisulfite	−	+	−	−	−	156
Snake venom	−	−	−	+	−	91, 144
Streptomycin	+	−	−	+	−	114, 303, 307, 314
Sulfonamide	+	−	−	+	−	44, 55, 64, 132, 237, 305, 331
Suxamethonium	+	−	−	−	−	206
Talc, cornstarch	−	−	−	+	−	20, 115, 229, 314, 318
Tatoo	−	+	−	−	−	314, 349
Tetracycline	+	−	−	−	−	114, 314
Thallium	−	−	+	+	−	137, 215
Thiotepa	+	+	−	−	−	37, 137, 156
Thioridazine	−	−	−	+	−	13, 80, 225, 258
Toad poison	+	+	−	+	−	79
Tobacco	−	−	−	+	−	48, 100, 101, 137, 259
Trichloroethylene	−	+	−	+	−	100, 137
Triethylenemelamine	+	−	−	−	−	114, 174
Trifluorothymidine	+	+	−	−	−	156, 200, 201, 221
Trinitrotoluene	−	−	+	+	−	137
Triparanol	−	−	+	−	−	35, 188, 189, 330
Tryparasamide	−	−	−	+	−	170

Continued

Table 16-1 *(continued)*

Agent	Conjunctiva Lid Other Adnexa	Cornea Sclera	Lens	Retina Optic Nerve	Uveal Tract	References
Vinblastine, vincristine	+	+	−	−	?	4, 46, 114
Vitamin A	+	−	−	−	−	156, 233, 244, 320
Vitamin D	−	+	−	+	−	123, 150, 314, 337
Zinc sulfide and barium sulfate	+	−	−	−	−	175, 241

REFERENCES

1. Abraham, S. V., & Teller, J. J.: Influence of various miotics on cataract formation. Br. J. Ophthalmol. 53:833, 1969.
2. Abrams, J. D., & Majzoub, U.: Mercury content of the human lens. Br. J. Opthal. 54:59, 1970.
3. Alagna, G.: Intossicazione da acido cianidrico ed occhio. Ann. Ottal. 72:217, 1946.
4. Albert, D. M., Wong, V. G., & Henderson, E. S.: Ocular complications of vincristine therapy. Arch. Ophthalmol. 78:709, 1967.
5. American Medical Association Drug Evaluations, 3rd Ed. Publishing Sciences Group, Acton, Massachusetts, 1980.
6. Amos, H. E., Brigden, W. D., & McKerron, R. A.: Untoward effects associated with practolol: Demonstration of antibody binding to epithelial tissue. Br. Med. J. 1:598: 1975.
7. Anderes, W.: Uber einen Fall von "Toxic Epidermal Necrolysis" (Lyell) mit schweren Augenkonplikationen. Ophthalmologica 145: 291, 1963.
8. Anderson, B., & Anderson, B. Jr.: Necrotizing uveitis incident to perfusion of intracranial malignancies with nitrogen mustard or related compounds. Trans. Am. Ophthalmol. Soc. 58:95, 1960.
9. Anderson, B., & Oglesby, F.: Corneal changes from quinone-hydroquinone exposure. Arch. Ophthalmol. 59:495, 1958.
10. Anderson, D. R.: Scanning electron microscopy of zonulysis by alpha-chymotrypsin. Am. J. Ophthamol. 71:619, 1971.
11. Ansdell, V. E., & Common, T. D.: Corneal changes induced by mepacrine. J. Trop. Med. Hyg. 82:206, 1979.
12. Appleton, B., & McCrossan, G. C.: Microwave lens effects in humans. Arch. Ophthalmol. 88:259, 1972.
13. Apt, L.: Complications of phenothiazine tranquilizers–ocular side effects. Surv. Ophthalmol. 5:550, 1960.
14. Aronson, S. B., & Sassaetti, R.: Experimental ocular hypersensitivity to polyepinephrine and its analogs. Invest. Ophthalmol. Vis. Sci. 9:12, 1970.
15. Ashton, N.: Pathological basis of retrolental fibroplasia. Br. J. Ophthalmol. 38:385, 1954.
16. Ashton, N., Tripathi, B., & Knight, G.: Effect of oxygen on the developing retinal vessels of the rabbit. II. In vivo experiments. Exp. Eye Res. 14:221, 1972.
17. Ashton, N., Ward, B., & Serpell, G.: Role of oxygen in the genesis of retrolental fibroplasia. A preliminary report. Br. J. Ophthalmol. 37:513, 1953.
18. Atkinson, W. S.: Use of hyaluronidase with local anesthetics in ophthalmology. Arch. Ophthalmol. 42:628, 1949.
19. Atkinson, W. S., & von Sallman, L.: Mercury in the lens. Trans. Am. Ophthalmol. Soc. 44:65, 1946.
20. Atlee, W. E. Jr.: Talc and cornstarch emboli in eyes of drug abusers. J.A.M.A. 219:49, 1972.
21. Axelsson, U.: Glaucoma, miotic therapy, and cataract. Acta Ophthalmol. (Suppl.) 102:1-37, 1969.
22. Baghdassarin, S. A.: Optic neuropathy due to lead poisoning. Arch. Ophthalmol. 80:721, 1968.
23. Baghdassarin, S. A., & Zakharia, H.: Report of three cases of hydatid cyst of the orbit. Am. J. Ophthalmol. 71:1081, 1971.
24. Baumbach, G. L., Cancilla, P. A., Martinamat, G., et al.: Methyl alcohol poisoning. IV. Alterations of the morphological findings of the retina and optic nerve. Arch. Ophthalmol. 95:1859, 1977.
25. Ballingall, D. L. K., & Turpie, A. G. G.:

Cephaloridine toxicity. Lancet 2:835, 1967.
26. Bär, A.: Augenveränderungen bei Botulismus. Klin. Monatsbl. Augenheilkd. 72:675, 1924.
27. Bard, L. A., & Gills, A. P.: Quinine ambylopia. Arch. Ophthalmol. 72: 329, 1964.
28. Barnett, A. J.: Ocular effects of methonium compounds. Br. J. Ophthalmol. 36:593, 1952.
29. Barron, G. J., Tepper, L., & Lovine, G.: Ocular toxicity from ethambutal. Am. J. Ophthalmol. 77:256, 1974.
30. Bartlett, R. E.: Generalized argyrosis with lens involvement. Am. J. Ophthalmol. 38:402, 1954.
31. Beasley, R. W. R.: The eye and hydrogen sulfide. Br. J. Indust. Med. 20:32, 1963.
32. Becker, B., & Morton, W. R.: Topical epinephrine in glaucoma suspects. Am. J. Ophthalmol. 62:272, 1966.
33. Behrens, M. M.: Optic atrophy in children after diiodohydroxyquin therapy. J.A.M.A. 228:693, 1974.
34. Bell, R. W., & Ritchey, J. P.: Subconjunctival nodule after Amphotericin B injection. Medical therapy for *Aspergillus* corneal ulcer. Arch. Ophthalmol. 90:402, 1973.
35. Bellows, J. G.: Lens opacities produced by cataractogenic agents. Am. J. Ophthalmol. 55:537, 1963.
36. Benton, C. D., & Calhoun, F. P.: The ocular effects of methyl alcohol poisoning (Report of a catastrophe involving 320 persons). Am. J. Ophthalmol. 36:1677, 1953.
37. Berkow, J. W., Gills, J. P., & Wise, J. B.: Depigmentation of eyelids after topically administered thiotepa. Arch. Ophthalmol. 82:415, 1969.
38. Bernstein, H.N.: Chloroquine ocular toxicity. Surv. Ophthalmol. 12:415, 1967.
39. Bernstein, H. N.: Ocular Side Effects of Drugs. In: Dikstein, S. (ed.): Drugs and Ocular Tissues. Ch. 10, p. 560-643. Karger, Basel, 1977.
40. Bernstein, H. N., & Ginsberg, J.: The pathology of chloroquine retinopathy. Arch. Ophthalmol. 71:238, 1960.
41. Black, J.: Physical and chemical agents. Section I: General injuries in: Sorsby, A. (ed.): Modern Ophthalmology, 2nd Ed., Vol. 2. pp. 617-634. Lippincott, Philadelphia, 1972.
42. Bleil, D. C.: Unusual toxic manifestations of amodiaquin (Camoquin) Arch. Dermatol. 77:106, 1958.
43. Blodi, F. C.: Mustard gas keratopathy. Int. Ophthal. Clin. 11:1, 1971.
44. Boettner, E. A., Fralick, F. B., & Wolter, J. R.: Conjunctival concretions of sulfadiazine. Arch. Ophthalmol. 92:446, 1974.
45. Boreus, L. O., & Sundstrom, B.: Intracranial hypertension in a child during treatment with nalidixic acid. Br. Med. J. 2:744, 1967.
46. Bradley, W. G., Lassman, L. P., Pierce, G. W., & Walton, J. N.: The neuromyopathy of vincristine therapy in man. J. Neurol. Sci. 10:107, 1970.
47. Brini, A., Porte, A., & Flament, J.: Corneal lesions caused by cordarone (amidarone). Electron microscopy study. Bull. Soc. Ophthalmol. Fr. 72:83, 1972.
48. Bron, A. J.: Mechanisms of ocular toxicity. In: Garrad, J. W. (ed.): Aspects of Drug Toxicity. Ch. 13, p. 229–253. Taylor and Francis Ltd., London, 1979.
49. Bron, A. J., McLendon, B. F., & Camp, A. V.: Epithelial deposition of gold in the cornea in patients receiving systemic therapy. Amer. J. Ophthalmol. 88:354, 1979.
50. Bron, A. J., McLendon, B., Buckley, C., & Tripathi, R. C.: Retardation of corneal resurfacing. An experimental model using Alcian blue. Proc. VIth European Congress of Ophthalmology, Brighton, 1981. Royal Society of Medicine, London. p. 203–208.
51. Brown, S. I., Weller, C. A., & Akiyas, S.: Pathogenesis of ulcers of the alkali-burned cornea. Arch. Ophthalmol. 83:204, 1970.
52. Bruce, G. M.: Permanent bilateral blindness following use of hexamethonium chloride. Arch. Ophthalmol. 54:422, 1955.
53. Bruna, F.: Un caso mortale di sindrome di Stevens-Johnson da fenilbutazone. Boll. Ocul. 37:3, 1958.
54. Brunot, F. R.: The toxicity of osmium tetroxide. J. Indust. Hyg. 15:136, 1933.
55. Bucy, P. C.: Toxic optic neuritis resulting from sulfanilamide. J.A.M.A. 109:1007, 1937.
56. Bullock, J. D., Albert, D. M.: Flecked retina. Arch. Ophthalmol. 93:26, 1975.
57. Burian, H. M., & Fletcher, M. C.: Visual functions in patients with retinal pigmentary degeneration following the use of NP 207. Arch. Ophthalmol. 60:612, 1958.
58. Burns, C. A.: Indomethacin, reduced retinal sensitivity, and corneal deposits. Am. J. Ophthalmol. 66:825, 1968.

59. Burns, R. P.: Delayed onset of chloroquine retinopathy. N. Engl. J. Med. 275:693, 1966.
60. Buschke, W.: Acute reversible cataract in chickens due to various nitrocompounds. Am. J. Ophthalmol. 30:1356, 1947.
61. Byron, H. M.: Conjunctival reaction due to 1-epinephrine bitartrate. Arch. Ophthalmol. 63:567, 1960.
62. Calkins, J. L., & Hochheimer, B. F.: Retinal light exposure from ophthalmoscopes, slit lamps, and overhead surgical lamps. An analysis of potential hazards. Invest. Ophthalmol. Vis. Sci. 19:1009, 1980.
63. Calvery, H. O., Lightbody, H. D., & Rones, B.: Effects of some silver salts on the eye. Arch. Ophthalmol. 25:839, 1941.
64. Cameron, A.J., Baron, J. H., & Priestly, B. L.: Erythema multiforme drugs and ulcerative colitis. Br. J. Med. 2:1174, 1966.
65. Campinchi, R., Dhermy, P., Pouliquen, Y., & Hamard, H.: Keratite par usage prolonge de collyre anethesique. Bull. Soc. Opthalmol. Fr. 65:120, 1965.
66. Carapancea, M.: Etude physio-pathologique clinique et experimentale sur les troubles oculaires dans l'intoxication quinique. Arch. Ophthalmol. (Paris) 19:841, 1959.
67. Carr, R. E., & Henkind, P.: Ocular manifestations of ethambutal. Arch. Ophthalmol. 67:566, 1962.
68. Casini, F.: Il metabolismo respiratorio della retina nel'intossicazione sperimentale da chinino. Arch. Ottol. 46:263, 1939.
69. Chamberlain, W. P., & Boles, D. J.: Edema of the cornea precipitated by quinacrine. Arch. Ophthalmol. 35:120, 1946.
70. Chee, P., & Hamasaki, D. I.: The basis for chymotrypsin-induced glaucoma. Arch. Ophthalmol. 85:103, 1971.
71. Chisholm, J. F.: Iron pigmentation of palpebral conjunctiva. Amer. J. Ophthalmol. 33:1108, 1950.
72. Chizek, D. J., & Franceschetti, A. T.: Oral contraceptives: their side effects and ophthalmological manifestations. Surv. Ophthalmol. 14:90, 1969.
73. Christensen, L., Swan, K. C., & Huggins, H. D.: Histopathology of iris pigment changes induced by miotics. Arch. Ophthalmol. 55:666, 1956.
74. Cibis, P. A., Brown, E. B., & Hong, S. M.: Ocular effects of systemic siderosis. Amer. J. Ophthalmol. 44:158, 1957.
75. Cibis, P. A., Yamashita, T. & Rodriques, F.: Clinical aspects of ocular siderosis and hemosiderosis. Arch. Ophthalmol. 62:180, 1959.
76. Cocke, J. G., Brown, R. E., & Geppert, L. J.: Optic neuritis with prolonged use of chloramphenicol. J. Pediatr. 68:27, 1966.
77. Cohen, B., & Tripathi, R. C.: Eyelid depigmentation after intralesional injection of a fluorinated corticosteroid. Am. J. Ophthalmol. 88:269, 1979.
78. Cohen, E. L.: Conjunctival hemorrhage after bismuth injection. Lancet 1:627, 1945.
79. Collier, M.: Alterations oculaires par venin de crapand. Bull. Soc. Ophthalmol. Fr. 65:129, 1965.
80. Connell, M. M., Poley, B. J., McFarlene, J. R.: Chorioretinopathy associated with thioridazine therapy. Arch. Ophthalmol. 71:816, 1964.
81. Copas, D. E., Kay, W. W., & Longman, V. H.: Carbromal intoxication. Lancet 1:703, 1959.
82. Cordes, F. C.: Galactosemia cataract: a review. Am. J. Ophthalmol. 50:1151, 1960.
83. Corwin, M. E., & Spencer, W. H.: Conjunctival melanin depositions. Arch. Ophthalmol. 79:317, 1963.
84. Crawford, J. S., Lewandowski, R. L., & Chan, W.: The effect of aspirin rebleed in traumatic hyphema. Am. J. Ophthalmol. 80:543, 1975.
85. Crawford, R.: Toxic cataract. Br. Med. J. 2:1231, 1959.
86. Crews, S. J.: Toxic effects on the eye and visual apparatus resulting from systemic absorption of recently introduced chemical agents. Trans. Ophthalmol. Soc. U. K. 82:387, 1963.
87. Crews, S. J.: Adverse reactions to corticosteroid therapy in the eye. Proc. Roy. Soc. Med. 58:533, 1965.
88. Crosbie, R. B: Cephaloridine toxicity. Lancet 1:422, 1968.
89. Crowder, J. I., & Sexton, E. R.: Keratoconjunctivitis resulting from sap of candleabra cactus and the pencil tree. Arch. Ophthalmol. 72:476, 1964.
90. Dame, L. R.: The effect of Atabrine in human visual system. Am. J. Ophthalmol. 29:1432, 1946.
91. Davenport, R. C., & Budden, F. H.: Loss of

sight following snake bite. Br. J. Ophthalmol. 37:119, 1953.
92. David, D. S., & Berkowitz, J. S.: Ocular effects of topical and systemic corticosteroids. Lancet 2:149, 1969.
93. Davidson, S. I.: Reports of ocular adverse reactions. Trans. Opthalmol. Soc. U. K. 93:495, 1973.
94. Delman, M., & Leubuscher, K.: Transient macular edema due to griseofulvin. Am. J. Ophthalmol. 56:658, 1963.
95. DeLong, S. L.: Incidence and significance of chlorpromazine-induced eye changes. Dis. Nerv. Syst. (Suppl.) 29(3):19–22, 1968.
96. de Roetth, A.: Lens opacities in glaucoma patients on phospholine iodide therapy. Am. J. Ophthalmol. 62:619, 1966.
97. Dixon, G. J., Roberts, G. B. S., & Tyrrell, W. F.: The relationship of neuropathy to the treatment of tuberculosis with isoniazid. Scot. Med. J. 1:350, 1956.
98. Donaldson, D. D.: Epinephrine pigmentation of the cornea. Arch. Opthalmol. 78:74, 1967.
99. Duke-Elder, S.: Chemical Injuries: Textbook of Ophthalmology, Vol. 6. C. V. Mosby, St. Louis. 1954.
100. Duke-Elder, S.: System of Ophthalmology, Vol. 14, Pt. 2. C. V. Mosby, St. Louis, 1972.
101. Dunphy, E.: Alcohol and tobacco amblyopia. Historical review. Am. J. Ophthalmol. 68:569, 1969.
102. Elliott, G. A., & Schut, A. L.: Studies with cytarabine HCl in normal eyes of man, monkey and rabbit. Am. J. Opthalmol. 60:1074, 1965.
103. Epstein, D. L., & Paton, D.: Keratitis from misuse of corneal anesthetics. N. Engl. J. Med. 279:396, 1968.
104. Epstein, S.: Dermal contact dermatitis from neomycin. Ann. Allergy. 16:268, 1958.
105. Ferrara, A.: Optic neuritis from high doses of Atebrine. Rass. Ital. Ottalmol. 12:123, 1943.
106. Ferry, A. P., & Barnet, A. H.: Granulomatous keratitis resulting from use of cyanoacrylate adhesive for closure of perforated corneal ulcer. Am. J. Opthalmol. 72:538, 1971.
107. Ferry, A. P., & Zimmerman, L. E.: Black cornea: A complication of topical use of epinephrine. Am. J. Ophthalmol. 58:205, 1964.
108. Fisher, F. B.: Bismuthiase secondaire de la cornee. Ann. Ocul. (Paris) 183:615, 1950.
109. Fleischanderl, A.: Impregnation of the cornea with mercury. Klin. Monatsbl. Augenheilkd. 104:432, 1940.
110. Francois, J., De Rouck, A., & Cambie, E.: Retinal and optic evaluation in quinine poisoning. Ann. Ophthalmol. 4:177, 1972.
111. Fraunfelder, F. T., & Hanna, C.: Electric cataracts. Arch. Ophthalmol. 87:179:1972.
112. Francois, J., Jonsas, C., & De Rouck, A.: Studies of the effect of levorenine. Am. J. Ophthalmol. 68:119, 1969.
113. Frankisek, M. V.: Lesions of the eye due to hydrogen sulfide. Cs. Oftal. 6:5, 1950.
114. Fraunfelder, F. T.: Drug-Induced Ocular Side Effects and Drug Interactions. Lea and Febiger, Philadelphia. 1976.
115. Friberg, T. R., Gragoudas, E. S., & Regan, C. D. J.: Talc emboli and macular ischemia in intravenous drug abuse. Arch. Ophthalmol. 97:1089, 1979.
116. Friedman, E. A., Greenberg, J. B., Merrill, J. P., et al.: Consequences of ethylene glycol poisonings. Am. J. Med. 32:891, 1962.
117. Friedman, E., & Kuwabara, T.: The retinal pigment epithelium. IV. The damaging effects of radiant energy. Arch. Ophthalmol. 80:265, 1968.
118. Friedenwald, J. S., Hughes, W. F., & Herrmann, H.: Acid burns of the eye. Arch. Ophthalmol. 35:98, 1946.
119. Fulmek, R.: Occlusion of a branch of central retinal artery after prolonged use of ovulation inhibitors. Klin. Monatsbl. Augenheilkd. 164:371, 1974.
120. Gangitano, J. L., & Keltner, J. L.: Abnormalities of the pupil and visual-evoked potential in quinine amblyopia. Am. J. Ophthalmol. 89:425, 1980.
121. Garner, A., & Rahi, A. H. S.: Practolol and ocular toxicity. Br. J. Ophthalmol. 60:684, 1976.
122. Garron, L. K., Wood, I. S., Spencer, W. H., et al.: A clinical pathologic study of mercurialentis medicalentosus. Trans. Am. Ophthalmol. Soc. 74:295, 1977.
123. Gartner, S., & Rubner, K.: Calcified scleral nodule in hypervitaminosis D. Am. J. Ophthalmol. 39:658, 1955.
124. Gass, D., & Norton, E.: Cystoid macular edema and papilledema following cataract extraction. Arch. Ophthalmol. 76:646, 1966.

125. Gass, J. D.: Nicotinic acid maculopathy. Am. J. Ophthalmol. 76:500, 1973.
126. Geeraets, W. J.: Radiation effects on the eye. Indust. Med. 39:441, 1970.
127. Geeraets, W. J., & Nooney, T. W. Jr.: Retinal injury due to electric current. A clinical study. Ann. Ophthalmol. 5:265, 1973.
128. Gerber, A., & Lambert, R. K.: Blue appearance of fundus caused by prolonged ingestion of methylthionine chloride. Arch. Ophthalmol. 16:443, 1936.
129. Gerber, M.: Ocular reactions following iodide therapy. Am. J. Ophthalmol. 43:879, 1957.
130. Ghetti, G., & Mariani, L.: Eye changes due to naphthlene. Med. Lav. 47:533, 1956.
131. Goar, E. F., & Fletcher, M. C.: Toxic chorioretinopathy following the use of NP 207. Trans. Am. Ophthalmol. Soc. 54:129, 1956.
132. Goar, E. L.: Retinal hemorrhages following the ingestion of sulfathiazole. Am. J. Ophthalmol. 25:332, 1942.
133. Goldstein, J. H.: Effects of drugs on cornea, conjunctiva, and lids. Int. Ophthalmol. Clin. 11(2): 13, 1971.
134. Goodman, L. S., & Gilman, S.: The Pharmacological Basis of Therapeutics, 4th Ed. Macmillan, New York, 1970.
135. Gordon, D. M., Kleberger, K. E.: The effect of dimethylsulfoxide (DMSO) on animal and human eyes. Arch. Ophthalmol. 79:423, 1968.
136. Gorin, S. B.: Retinal edema secondary to oral contraceptives. Am. J. Ophthalmol. 64:447, 1967.
137. Grant, W. M.: Toxicology of The Eye, 2nd Ed., Charles C. Thomas, Springfield, Illinois, 1974.
138. Grayson, M., & Pieroni, D.: Severe silver nitrate injury to the eye. Am. J. Ophthalmol. 70:227, 1970.
139. Green, W. R., Kaufer, G. J., & Dubroff, S.: Black cornea: A complication of topical use of epinephrine. Ophthalmologica 154:88, 1967.
140. Greer, H. D., Ward, H. P., & Corbin, K. B.: Chronic salicylate intoxication in adults. J.A.M.A. 193:85, 1965.
141. Gregory, M. H., Rutty, D. A., & Wood, R. D.: Retinal changes and chloroquine. Br. Med. J. 2:428, 1968.
142. Grosz, S. de: Dimethyl sulphate poisoning in relation to ophthalmology. Am. J. Ophthalmol. 20:700, 1937.
143. Gutman, F. A., & Croswell, H. H.: Argyrosis of the cornea without clinical conjunctival involvement. Am. J. Ophthalmol. 65:183, 1968.
144. Guttman-Friedman, A.: Blindness after snakebite. Br. J. Ophthalmol. 40:57, 1956.
145. Haddad, H., & Leopold, I.: Rabbit lens uptake of tritium-labelled phospholine iodide. Am. J. Ophthalmol. 68:123, 1969.
146. Hallum, A.: Involvement of the cornea in arsenic poisoning. Arch. Ophthalmol. 12:93, 1934.
147. Hamming, N. A., Apple, D. J., & Goldberg, M. F.: Histopathology and ultrastructure of busulfan-induced cataract. Albrecht von Graefes Arch. Klin. Ophthalmol. 200:139, 1976.
148. Hanna, C., & Fraunfelder, F. T.: Electric cataracts. II. Ultrastructural lens changes. Arch. Ophthalmol. 87:184, 1972.
149. Hanna, C., Fraunfelder, F. T., & Sanchez, J.: Ultrastructural study of argyrosis of the cornea and conjunctiva. Arch. Ophthalmol. 92:18, 1974.
150. Harley, R. D., Di George A. M., Mabry, C. C., et al.: Idiopathic hypercalcemia of infancy: Optic atrophy and other ocular changes. Trans. Am. Acad. Ophthalmol. Otolaryngol. 69:977, 1965.
151. Harley, R. D., Huang, N. N., Macri, C. H., et al.: Optic neuritis and optic atrophy following chloramphenicol in cystic fibrosis patients. Trans. Am. Acad. Ophthalmol. Otolaryngol. 74:1011, 1970.
152. Harrison, R.: Bilateral lens opacities associated with use of diisopropyl fluorophosphate. Am. J. Ophthalmol. 50:153, 1960.
153. Harrison, W. J.: Primary zonular opacity of the cornea. Arch. Ophthalmol. 16:469, 1936.
154. Hartmann, K.: Augenschädigungen durch der Saft der Euphorbia peplus. Klin. Monatsbl. Augenheilkd. 104:324, 1940.
155. Hashimoto, A., Maeda, Y., Ho, H., et al.: Corneal chrysiasis. A clinical study in rheumatoid arthritis patients receiving gold therapy. Arthritis Rheum. 15:309, 1972.
156. Havener, W.: Ocular Pharmacology, 4th Ed. C. V. Mosby, St. Louis. 1978.
157. Havre, D. C.: Cataracts in children on long-term corticosteroid therapy. Arch. Ophthalmol. 73:818, 1965.
158. Henkes, H. E., Van Lith, G. H. M., & Canta,

L. R.: Indomethacin retinopathy. Am. J. Ophthalmol. 73:846, 1972.

159. Henkind, P., & Rothfield, N. F.: Ocular abnormalities in patients treated with synthetic antimalarial drugs. N. Engl. J. Med. 269:433, 1963.

160. Henrotte, J., & Weekers, J. F.: Clinical study of corneal lesions due to local and prolonged application of anesthetics. Arch. Ophthalmol. (Paris) 32:449, 1972.

161. Hisatomi, Y.: Ein selterner Fall von Augenverätzung durch Formalinlosung. Zentralbl. Gesamte Ophthalmol. 44:671, 1940.

162. Hobbs, H. E., Adeadie, S. P., & Sommerville, F.: Ocular lesions after treatment with chloroquine. Br. J. Ophthalmol. 45:284, 1961.

163. Horner, W. D.: Dinitrophenol and its relation to cataract. Arch. Ophthalmol. 27:1097, 1942.

164. Hotta, R., and Goto, S.: A fluorescein angiographic study on microangiopathia sulfocarbonica. Acta Soc. Ophthalmol. Jap. 74:1463, 1970.

165. Howard, R. O., MacDonald, C. J., Dunn, B., et al.: Experimental chlorpromazine cataracts. Invest. Ophthalmol. Vis. Sci. 8:413, 1969.

166. Hruban, Z., Slesers, A., & Hopkins, E.: Drug-induced and naturally occurring myeloid bodies. Lab. Invest. 27:62, 1972.

167. Hudnell, A. B., & Chick, E. W.: Corneal ultraviolet phototherapy. Arch. Ophthalmol. 68:304, 1962.

168. Hughes, W. F.: Mustard gas injuries to the eye. Arch. Ophthalmol. 27:582, 1942.

169. Hughes, W. F.: Alkali burns of the eye. Arch. Ophthalmol. 35:423, 1946.

170. Hurst, E. W.: The lesions produced in the central nervous system by certain organic arsenical compounds. J. Pathol. Bacteriol. 77:523, 1959.

171. Irvine, A. R.: Cystoid maculopathy. Surv. Ophthalmol. 21:1, 1976.

172. Jess, A.: Das histologische Bild der Kupfertrubung der Linse, eine Beitrag zue Frage der Linsenemährung. Klin. Monatsbl. Augenheilkd. 68:433, 1922.

173. Jensen, A.: A case of Stevens-Johnson syndrome following antiepileptic medication. Acta Ophthalmol. 45:576, 1967.

174. Johnson, D. R., & Burns, R. P.: Blepharoconjunctivitis associated with cancer chemotherapy. Trans. Pac. Coast Otolaryngol. Ophthalmol. Soc. 46:43, 1965.

175. Johnson, F. B., & Zimmermann, L. E.: Barium sulfate and zinc disulfide deposits resulting from golf-ball injury to the conjunctiva and eyelid. Am. J. Clin. Pathol. 44:533, 1965.

176. Jones, O. W. III: Toxic amblyopia caused by pheniprazine. Arch. Ophthalmol. 66:29, 1961.

177. Kalinowski, S. J., Lloyd, T. W., & Moyes, P. N.: Complications in the chemotherapy of tuberculosis. A review with analysis of the experience of 3148 patients. Am. Rev. Resp. Dis. 83:359, 1961.

178. Kass, I., Mendel, W., Cohen, H., et al.: Isoniazid as a cause of optic neuritis and atrophy. J.A.M.A. 164:1740, 1957.

179. Kass, M. A., Stamper, R. L., & Becker, B.: Madarosis in chronic epinephrine therapy. Arch. Ophthalmol. 88:429, 1972.

180. Kaufman, H. E., Capella, J. A., Maloney, E. D., et al.: Corneal toxicity of cytosine arabinoside. Arch. Ophthalmol. 72:535, 1964.

181. Kayes, J., & Becker, B.: The human trabecular meshwork in corticosteroid-induced glaucoma. Trans. Am. Ophthalmol. Soc. 67:339, 1969.

182. Keeping, J. A., & Searle, C. W. A.: Optic neuritis following isoniazid therapy. Lancet 2:278, 1955.

183. Kelecom, J.: Les bru lures oculaires par le formol. Arch. Ophthalmol. (Paris) 22:259, 1962.

184. Kini, M. M., & Cooper, J. R.: Biochemistry of methanol poisoning. Biochem. Pharmacol. 8:207, 1961.

185. Kinoshita, J. H., Dvornik, D., Kraml, M., et al.: The effect of an aldose reductase inhibitor on the galactose-exposed rabbit lens. Biochem. Biophys. Acta 158:472, 1968.

186. Kinsey, V. E., & Grant, W. M.: Determination of the rate of disappearance of mustard gas and mustard intermediate in the corneal tissue. J. Clin. Invest. 25:776, 1946.

187. Kirby, D. B.: Keratitis exfoliativa complicating dermatitis exfoliativa (arsphenamine). Arch. Ophthalmol. 2:661, 1929.

188. Kirby, T. J., Jr.: Cataracts as possible complications of treatment with triparanol. Arch. Ophthalmol. 67:543, 1962.

189. Kirby, T. J., Jr.: Cataracts produced by triparanol (MER/29). Trans. Am. Ophthalmol. Soc. 65:493, 1967.

190. Kirsch, R. E.: Glaucoma following cataract

extraction associated with alpha-chymotrypsin. Arch. Ophthalmol. 75:774, 1966.

191. Kirton, V., & Munro-Ashman, D.: Contact dermatitis from neomycin and framycetin. Lancet 1:138, 1965.

192. Kittel, V., & Cornelius, C.: Sehnervenschädigung durch Chloramphenicol. Klin. Monatsbl. Augenheilkd. 155:83, 1969.

193. Klendshoj, N. C., & Olmsted, E. P.: Observations of a dangerous side effect of phospholine iodide in glaucoma therapy. Am. J. Ophthalmol. 56:247, 1963.

194. Kobayashi, T., & Murakami, S.: Blindness of an adult caused by oxygen. J.A.M.A. 279:741, 1972.

195. Kolker, A. E., Becker, B.: Epinephrine maculopathy. Arch. Ophthalmol. 79:552, 1968.

196. Krause, A. M.: Congenital cataract and maternal steroid ingestion. J. Pediatr. Ophthalmol. 12:107, 1975.

197. Kresca, L. J., Goldberg, M. F., & Jampol, L. M.: Talc emboli and retinal neovascularization in a drug abuser. Am. J. Ophthalmol. 87:334, 1979.

198. Kristensen, P.: Posterior subcapsular cataract (P.S.C.) and systemic steroid therapy. Acta Ophthalmol. 46:1025, 1968.

199. Knox, D. L., & Palmer, C. A. L.: Iris atrophy after quinine amblyopia. Arch. Ophthalmol. 76:359, 1966.

200. Laibson, P.: Current therapy of herpes simplex virus infection of the cornea. Int. Ophthalmol. Clin. 13:39, 1973.

201. Lamda, P. A., Sood, N., & Moorthy, S. S.: Retinopathy due to chloramphenicol. Scot. Med. J. 13:166, 1968.

202. Le Grand, J., & Chevannes, H.: Les opacifications du cristallins dans les traitments contre l'obesite. Bull. Soc. Ophthal. Fr. 65:943, 1965.

203. Leibold, J. E.: Ocular toxicity of ethambutal and its relation to dose. Ann. N.Y. Acad. Sci. 135:904, 1966.

204. Lerman, S.: Pathogenetic factors in experimental galactose cataract. Arch. Ophthalmol. 65:331, 1961.

205. Lerman, S.: Radiant Energy and the Eye. Macmillan Publishing Co., New York, 1980.

206. Lessell, S., Kuwabara, T., & Feldman, R. G.: Myopathy and succinylcholine sensitivity. Am. J. Ophthalmol. 68:789, 1969.

207. Lezenhuis, A.: Ein Fall von Naphthalinkatarakt am Menschen, Klin. Monatsbl. Augenheilkd. 40:129, 1902.

208. Libert, J., Ketelbant-Balasse, P. E., Van Hoof, F., et al.: Cellular toxicity of gentamicin. Am. J. Ophthalmol. 87:405, 1979.

209. Lietman, P. S., De Santagnes, P. A., & Wong, V.: Optic neuritis in cystic fibrosis of the pancreas—Role of chloramphenicol therapy. J.A.M.A. 189:924, 1964.

210. Light, A. E.: Additional observations of the effects of Busulfan on cataract formation, duration of anesthesia, and reproduction in rats. Toxicol. Appl. Pharmacol. 10:459, 1967.

211. Little, H. L., Zweng, H. C., & Peabody, R. R.: Argon laser slit-lamp retinal photocoagulation. Trans. Am. Acad. Ophthalmol. Otolaryngol. 74:85, 1970.

212. Lufkin, M. W., Harrison, C. E., Henderson, J. W., et al.: Ocular distribution of digoxin-^{3}H in the cat. Am. J. Ophthalmol. 64:1134, 1967.

213. MacKeen, D., Fine, S., & Fine, B. S.: Production of cataract in rabbits with ultraviolet laser—a preliminary report. Ophthalmol. Res. 5:317, 1973.

214. Madge, G. E., Geeraets, W. J., & Guerry, D. III: Black cornea secondary to topical epinephrine. Am. J. Ophthalmol. 71:402, 1971.

215. Manschot, W. A.: Ophthalmic pathology findings in a case of thallium poisoning. Ophthalmol. Addit. Ad. 158:348, 1969.

216. Marshall, J., & Bird, A.: A comparative histopathological study of argon and krypton laser irridiations of the human retina. Br. J. Ophthalmol. 63:657, 1979.

217. Matsuda, H., & Smelser, G. K.: Epithelium and stroma in alkali-burned corneas. Arch. Ophthalmol. 89:396, 1973. Endothelial cells in alkali-burned corneas. Arch. Ophthalmol. 89:402, 1973.

218. Matsuo, N., & Hasegawa, E.: Histochemical and electron microscopical studies on the retinal siderosis. Acta Soc. Ophthalmol. Jap. 68:1702, 1964.

219. McClanhan, W. S., Harris, J. E., Knobloch, W. H., et al.: Ocular manifestation of chronic phenithiazine derivative administration. Arch. Ophthalmol. 75:319, 1966.

220. McFaul, P. A., & Bedford, M. A.: Ocular complications after therapeutic irridations. Br. J. Ophthalmol. 54:237, 1970.

221. McGill, J., Fraunfelder, F. T., & Jones, B.:

Current and proposed management of ocular herpes simplex. Surv. Ophthalmol. 20:358, 1976.
222. McGregor, I. S.: A study of the histopathological changes in the retina and late changes in the visual field in acute methyl alcohol poisoning. Br. J. Ophthalmol. 27:523, 1943.
223. McKee, S. H.: Severe argyrosis of the conjunctiva. Can. Med. Assoc. J. 39:474, 1938.
224. Meesmann, A.: Ein Fall von Arsenmelanose. Klin. Monatsbl. Augenheilkd. 64:548, 1920.
225. Meredith, T. A., & Aaberg, T. M.: Progressive chorioretinopathy after receiving thioridazine. Arch. Ophthalmol. 96:1172, 1978.
226. Mezey, P.: The significance of piperazine derivatives in the morphogenesis of cataracts. Klin. Monatsbl. Augenheilkd. 151:885, 1967.
227. Michels, R. G., & Maumenee, A. E.: Retrobulbar alcohol injection in seeing eyes. Trans. Am. Acad. Ophthalmol. Otolaryngol. 77:164, 1973.
228. Michaels, R. G., & Maumenee, A. E.: Cystoid macular edema associated with topically applied epinephrine in aphakic eyes. Am. J. Ophthalmol. 80:379, 1975.
229. Michelson, J. B., Whitcher, J. P., Wilson, S., et al.: Possible foreign body granuloma of the retina associated with intravenous cocaine addiction. Am. J. Ophthalmol. 87:278, 1979.
230. Moore, D. C.: Use of hyaluronidase in local and nerve block analgesia other than spinal block, 1520 cases. Anesthesiology 12:611, 1951.
231. Muller, H.: Histologische Untersuchung eines Auges bei akuter tödlicher Methylakoholvergiftung. Klin. Monatsbl. Augenheilkd. 116:135, 1950.
232. Muller, H. K., Kleifeld, O., Fuchs, R., et al.: The effect of age, poisoning with naphthlene, dinitrophenol, and alloxan upon the incorporation of phosphorus-32 in the electrophoretically separable phosphate fractions. Albrecht von Graefes Arch Klin. Ophthalmol. 156:460, 1955.
233. Munter, M. D., Perry, H. O., & Ludwig, J.: Chronic vitamin A intoxication in adults. Hepatic, dermatologic, and neurologic complications. Am. J. Med. 50:129, 1971.
234. Mylius, K.: Uber eine toxische Hornhautentzundung. Dtsch. Ophthalmol. Gesamte 56:265, 1950.
235. Nakae, K., Yamamoto, S., & Igata, A.: Subacute myelo-opticoneuropathy (SMON) in Japan. Lancet 2:510, 1971.
236. Naumann, G.: Corneal damage in hydroquinone workers. Arch. Ophthalmol. 76:189, 1966.
237. Newell, F. W., & Greentham, J. S.: Pemphigus conjunctivae. Am. J. Ophthalmol. 29: 1426, 1946.
238. Nichols, C. W., & Lambertsen, C.: Effect of high oxygen pressure on the eye. N. Engl. J. Med. 281:25, 1969.
239. Norn, M. S.: Vital staining of cornea and conjunctiva. Acta Ophthalmol. (Suppl.) 113:1-64, 1972.
240. Oglesby, R. B., Black, R. L., von Sallman, L., et al.: Cataracts in rheumatoid arthritis patients treated with chloramphenicol. Arch. Ophthalmol. 66:97, 1961.
241. O'Grady, R., & Shoch, D.: Golf-ball granuloma of the eyelids and conjunctiva. Am. J. Ophthalmol. 76:148, 1973.
242. Okuda, K.: Electron microscopy of chloroquine-induced corneitis. Jap. J. Clin. Med. 26:1655, 1968.
243. Okuda, K., & Ueno, H.: Histopathology of the optic nerve and eyeball in S.M.O.N. Acta Soc. Ophthalmol. Jap. 74:1145, 1970.
244. Oliver, T. K., & Havener, W. H.: Eye manifestation of chronic vitamin A intoxication. Arch. Ophthalmol. 60:19, 1958.
245. Opelt, W. W., White, E. D., & Halpert, E. S.: The effect of corticosteroids on aqueous humor formation rate and outflow facility. Invest. Ophthalmol. Vis. Sci. 8:535, 1969.
246. Pahlitzsch, H., & Tiburtius, H.: Augenuntersuchungen bei Behandlung mit dem neuen Tuberkulostakum Ethambuto-dihydrochloride Lederle (Myambutol). Klin. Monatsbl. Augenheilkd. 154:228, 1969.
247. Palimeris, G., Koliopoulis, J., & Velissaropoulos, P.: Ocular side effects of indomethacin. Ophthalmologica 164:339, 1972.
248. Paton, D., and Goldberg, M. F.: Management of Ocular Injuries, 2nd Ed. W. B. Saunders, Philadelphia, 1976.
249. Patty, E. A.: Industrial Hygiene and Toxicology. Intersciences, New York, 1949.
250. Patz, A., Eastham, A., Higgenbotham, D. H., & Kleh, T.: Oxygen studies in retrolental fibroplasia. Production of microscopic changes in retrolental fibroplasia in experimental animals. Am. J. Ophthalmol. 36:1511, 1953.

251. Perry, H. D., & Mallen, F. J.: Cilioretinal artery occlusion associated with oral contraceptives. Am. J. Ophthalmol. 84:56, 1977.
252. Pfahl, S. B., Makley, T. A., Rothermich, N., et al.: The relationship of steroid therapy and cataracts in patients with rheumatoid arthritis. Am. J. Ophthalmol. 52:831, 1961.
253. Podos, S. M., & Canellos, G. P.: Lens changes in chronic granulocytic leukemia. Possible relationship to chemotherapy. Am. J. Ophthalmol. 68:500, 1969.
254. Pohjola, S., & Horsmanheimo, A.: Keratitis sicca after erythema exudatum multiforme caused by PAS (A case report). Acta Ophthalmol. 44:415, 1966.
255. Popp, C.: Keratitis superficialis punctata intraepithelialis nach enteraler Arzneimittelverabreichung. Klin. Monatsbl. Augenheilkd. 126:754, 1955.
256. Posner, A.: Toxic action of miotics on the uveal pigment epithelium. Eye, Ear, Nose, Throat Monthly 41:547, 1962.
257. Potts, A. M.: Retinotoxic and choriodotoxic substances. Invest. Ophthalmol. Vis. Sci. 1:290, 1962.
258. Potts, A. M.: Drug-induced macular disease. Trans. Am. Acad. Ophthalmol. Otolaryngol. Soc. 70:1054, 1966.
259. Potts, A. M.: Tobacco amblyopia. Surv. Ophthalmol. 17:313, 1973.
260. Pouliquen, Y., Graf, B., Bisson, J., et al.: Etude ultrastructurale d'une surcharge corneenee au cours d'un traitement par la chlorpormazine. Arch. Ophthalmol. (Paris) 30:769, 1970.
261. Quatermass, M.: Amblyopia due to ethyl alcohol. Br. J. Ophthalmol. 42:628, 1958.
262. Radnot, M., & Varga, M.: Structure histologique de la cataracta causee par la piperazine. Ann. Oculist (Paris) 202:325, 1969.
263. Rahi, A. H. S., Chapman, C. M., Garner, A., et al.: Pathology of practolol-induced ocular toxicity. Br. J. Ophthalmol. 60:312, 1976.
264. Ramsey, M. S., & Fine, B. S.: Chloroquine toxicity in the human eye. Am. J. Ophthalmol. 73:229, 1972.
265. Ravindranathan, M. P., Paul, V. J., & Kuriakose, E. T.: Cataract after busulfan treatment. Br. Med. J. 1:218, 1972.
266. Raymond, L. F.: Neovascularization of the cornea due to butazolidin toxicity. Am. J. Ophthalmol. 43:287, 1957.
267. Refojo, M. F., Dohlman, C. H., & Koliopoulos, J.: Adhesives in ophthalmology, a review. Surv. Ophthalmol. 15:217, 1971.
268. Reinecke, R. D., & Kuwabara, T.: Corneal deposits secondary to topical epinephrine. Arch. Ophthalmol. 70:170, 1963.
269. Rigdon, R. H., Feldman, G. L., Ferguson, T. M., et al.: Cataracts produced by dinitrophenol. Arch. Ophthalmol. 61:249, 1959.
270. Roberts, W. H., & Wolter, J. R.: Ocular chrysiasis. Arch. Ophthalmol. 56:48, 1956.
271. Robertson, D. M., Hollenhorst, R. W., & Callahan, J. A.: Ocular manifestations of digitalis toxicity. Arch. Ophthalmol. 76:640, 1966.
272. Robertson, D. M., Hollenhorst, R. W., & Callanhan, J. A.: Receptor function in digitalis therapy. Arch. Ophthalmol. 76:852, 1966.
273. Rohen, J. W., Linner, E., & Witmer, R.: Electron microscopic studies on the trabecular meshwork in two cases of corticosteroid glaucoma. Exp. Eye Res. 17:19, 1973.
274. Roper, D. L., & Nisbet, R. M.: Effect of hyaluronidase on the incidence of cystoid macular edema. Ann. Ophthalmol. 10:1673, 1978.
275. Rosen, E.: Mercurialentis. Am. J. Ophthalmol. 33:1287, 1950.
276. Rosenthal, A. R., Appleton, B., & Hopkins, J. L.: Intraocular copper foreign bodies. Am. J. Ophthalmol. 78:671, 1974.
277. Rosenthal, A. R., & Appleton, B.: Histochemical localization of intraocular copper foreign bodies. Am. J. Ophthalmol. 79:613, 1975.
278. Rosenthal, A. R., Kolb, H., Bergsma, D., et al.: Chloroquine retinopathy in the rhesus monkey. Invest. Ophthalmol. Vis. Sci. 17:1158, 1978.
279. Roth, J. H.: Luminal poisoning with conjunctival residue. Am. J. Ophthalmol. 9:533, 1926.
280. Rothkoff, L., Biedner, B., Shoham, K., et al.: Optic atrophy after irrigation of the lacrimal ducts with chloramphenicol. Ann. Ophthalmol. 11:105, 1979.
281. Roussos, T., & Tsolkas, A.: The toxicity of myambutol on the human eye. Ann. Ophthalmol. 2:578, 1970.
282. Satanove, A.: Pigmentation due to phenothiazines in high and prolonged doses. J.A.M.A. 191:263, 1965.
283. Sattler, C. H.: Bromural-und Adalinvergiftung des Auges. Klin. Monatsbl. Augenheilkd. 70:149, 1929.
284. Sattler, C. H.: Augenveränderungen bei In-

toxikationen. In: Kurzes Handbuch der Ophthalmologie, Vol. 7. pp. 229-290. Springer, Berlin, 1932.
285. Schmidt, I. G.: Central nervous system effect of ethambutal in monkeys. Ann. N.Y. Acad. Sci. 135:759, 1966.
286. Sedan, J.: Papillite aigue hemorragique au cours d'une intoxication suraigue par l'aspirine. Bull. Soc. Ophthalmol. Fr. 58:333, 1958.
287. Seville, D., & Freedman, A.: Cerebroretinal degeneration due to carbon dioxide poisoning. Br. J. Ophthalmol. 51:475, 1967.
288. Shaffer, R. N., & Hetherington, J., Jr.: Anticholinesterase drugs and cataracts. Am. J. Ophthalmol. 62:613, 1966.
289. Shearer, R. B., & Dubois, E. L.: Ocular changes induced by long-term hydroxychloroquine (Plaquenil) therapy. Am. J. Ophthalmol. 64:245, 1967.
290. Skalska-Rakowska, J.: The effect of cocaine and tetracaine (pantocaine) on histochemically demonstrable phosphatases in the rat corneal epithelium. Folia Histochem. Cytochem. (Krakow) 6:269, 1968.
291. Smelser, G. K., & Ozanics, V.: Effect of local anesthetics on cell division and migration following thermal burns of the cornea. Arch. Ophthalmol. 34:271, 1965.
292. Smith, J. W.: Ochronisis of sclera and cornea complicating alkaptinuira. J.A.M.A. 120: 1282, 1942.
293. Somerville-Large, L. B.: Mepacrin and the eye. Br. J. Ophthalmol. 31:191, 1947.
294. Spaeth, G. L.: Nasolacrimal duct obstruction caused by topical epinephrine. Arch. Ophthalmol. 77:355, 1967.
295. Spencer, R. W., & Andelman, S. Y.: Steroid cataracts. Arch. Ophthalmol. 74:38, 1965.
296. Sterner, J. H., Oglesby, F. L., & Anderson, B.: Quinone vapors and their harmful effects. J. Indust. Hyg. 29:60, 1947.
297. Stowe, G. C., Zakov, Z. N., & Albert, D. M.: Central retinal vascular ocular occlusion associated with oral contraceptives. Am. J. Ophthalmol. 86:798, 1978.
298. Sugar, H. S., & Waddell, W. W.: Ochronosis-like pigmentation associated with use of atabrine (quinacrine). Illinois Med. J. 89:234, 1946.
299. Sundmark, E.: The cataract-inducing effect of systemic corticosteroid therapy. Acta Ophthalmol. 44:291, 1966.
300. Swab, C. M., & Gerald, H. F.: The ophthalmic lesions of botulism; additional notes and research. Br. J. Ophthalmol. 17:129, 1933.
301. Swan, K. C.: Reactivity of the ocular tissues to wetting agents. Am. J. Ophthalmol. 27:1118, 1944.
302. Swett, W. F.: Eye complications following the use of reducing agents. Am. J. Ophthalmol. 19:796, 1936.
303. Sykowski, P.: Streptomycin causing retrobulbar optic neuritis. Am. J. Ophthalmol. 34:1446, 1951.
304. Tarkkanen, A., & Karjalainen, K.: Cataract formation during miotic treatment for open-angle glaucoma. Acta Ophthalmol. 44:932, 1966.
305. Taub, R. G., & Hollenhorst, R. W.: Sulfonamides as a cause of toxic amblyopia. Am. J. Ophthalmol. 40:486, 1955.
306. Taub, S. J.: Delayed hypersensitivity to Mertholate preservative. Eye, Ear, Nose, Throat Monthly 49:235, 1970.
307. Theodore, F. H.: Drug sensitivities and irritation of the conjunctivia. J.A.M.A. 151:25, 1953.
308. Thiel, H. J., & Langness, U.: Augensymptome bei parenteraler Goldtherapie der chronischen Polyarthritis. Med. Klin. 65:1366, 1970.
309. Tillman, W., & Keital, L.: Indomethacine induced corneal deposits. Klin. Monatsbl. Augenheilkd. 170:756, 1977.
310. Tostevin, A. L.: Retinal hemorrhages associated with the administration of butazolidin. Med. J. Aust. 7:69, 1961.
311. Toussaint, D., & Pohl, S.: Aspect histologique et ultrastructure des depots corneens dus au chlorhydrate d'amiodarone. Bull. Soc. Belge Ophthalmol. 153:676, 1969.
312. Tripathi, B., Ashton, N., & Knight, G.: Effect of oxygen on the developing retinal vessels of the rabbit. IV. Effect of hyperoxia on rabbit retinal vessels in tissue culture. Exp. Eye Res. 19:449, 1974.
313. Tripathi, R. C.: Functional Anatomy of the Human Anterior Chamber Angle. In: Jakobiec, F., and Duane, T. (eds.): Biomedical Foundations of Ophthalmology. Harper and Row, Gaithersburg, Maryland (In press.)
314. Tripathi, R. C.: Personal observations.
315. Tripathi, R. C., Cibis, G. W., & Tripathi, B. J.: Corneal keloid in Lowe's syndrome. Arch. Ophthalmol. (In press).

316. Tripathi, R. C., & Tripathi, B. J.: Applied Physiology and Anatomy: Tears, Cornea, Conjunctiva and Ocular Adnexa. In: Ruben, M. (ed.): Contact Lens Practice. Ch. 3. p. 24-55. Bailliere Tindall, London, 1975.
317. Tripathi, R. C., Tripathi, B. J., & Ruben, M.: The pathology of soft contact lens spoilage. Ophthalmology 87:365, 1980.
318. Tse, D. T., & Ober, R. R.: Talc retinopathy. Am. J. Opthalmol. 90:624, 1980.
319. Tso, M. O. M., Fine, B. S., & Zimmerman, L. E.: Photoic maculopathy in rhesus monkey. A light and electron microscopic study. Invest. Ophthalmol. Vis. Sci. 12:17, 1973.
320. Turtz, C. A., & Turtz, A. I.: Vitamin A intoxication. Am. J. Ophthalmol. 50:165, 1960.
321. Uhtoff, W., & Metzer, E.: Die Sehgifte und die pharmakologische Beeinflussung des Sehens. Handb. Norm. Pathol. Physiol. 12:812, 1931.
322. Van Balen, A. T. M.: Toxic damage to the optic nerve caused by iodochlorhydroxyquinoline (Enterovioform). Ophthalmologica 163:8, 1971.
323. van Heyningen, R.: Metabolism of xylose by the lens. 2. Rat lens in vivo and in vitro. Biochem. J. 73:197, 1959.
324. van Heyningen, R.: The Lens: Metabolism and Cataract. In: Davson, H. (ed.) The Eye. 2nd Ed. Vol. 1, Ch. 6. p. 381. Academic Press, London, 1969.
325. Van Horn, D. L., Edlehauser, H. F., Prodanovich, G., et al.: Effect of the ophthalmic preservative thimerosal on rabbit and human corneal endothelium. Invest. Ophthalmol. Vis. Sci. 16:273, 1977.
326. Van Huyssteen, M. P.: Conjunctival ulceration as a complication in the treatment of epilepsy. S. Afr. Med. J. 27:626, 1953.
327. Vannas, A., Hogan, M. J., Golbus, M. S., et al.: Lens changes in a galactosemic fetus. Am. J. Ophthalmol. 80:726, 1975.
328. Vigiliani, E. C.: Clinical observations on carbon disulfide intoxication in Italy. Indust. Med. Surg. 19:240, 1950.
329. von Oettingen, W. F.: The Toxicity and Potential Dangers of Methyl Bromide. N.I.H. Bull. No. 185, Washington, D.C., 1946.
330. von Sallman, L., Grimes, P., & Collins, E.: Triparanol-induced cataract in rats. Arch. Ophthalmol. 70:522, 1963.
331. Wagener, H. P.: Toxic effects of sulfonamides on the eyes. Am. J. Med. Sci. 206:261, 1943.
332. Wallow, I. H. L., & Tso, M. O. M.: Repair after xenon arc photocoagulation. 3. An electron microscopic study of the evolution of retinal lesions in rhesus monkeys. Am. J. Ophthalmol. 75:957, 1973.
333. Walsh, F. B., & Hoyt, W. F.: Clinical Neurophthalmology, 3rd Ed., Vol. 3. Williams and Wilkins, Baltimore, 1969.
334. Waltman, S. R., Yarian, D., Hart, W., Jr., et al.: Corneal endothelial changes with long-term epinephrine therapy. Arch. Ophthalmol. 95:1357, 1977.
335. Warshawsky, R. S., Hill, C. W., Doughman, D. J., & Harris, J. E.: Acrodermatitis enteropathica. Corneal involvement with histochemical and electron micrographic studies. Arch. Ophthalmol. 93:194, 1975.
336. Watanabe, T.: Electron microscopic studies of the lens and the ciliary body of rabbits with experimental dinitrophenol cataract. Acta Soc. Ophthalmol. Jap. 73:393, 1969.
337. Wegner, H. P., Smith, H. L., & Nickesen, R. W.: Retrobulbar neuritis and complete heart block caused by digitalis poisoning. Arch. Ophthalmol. 36:478, 1946.
338. Westsmith, R. A., & Abernathy, R. E.: Detachment of retina with use of diisopropyl fluorophosphate (Flurópryl) in treatment of glaucoma. Arch. Ophthalmol. 52:779, 1954.
339. Wetterholm, D. H., & Winter, F. C.: Histopathology of chloroquine retinal toxicity. Arch. Ophthalmol. 71:82, 1964.
340. Wetterholm, D. H., Snow, H., & Winter, F.: A clinical study of pigmentary changes in cornea and lens in chronic chlorpromazine therapy. Arch. Ophthalmol. 74:55, 1965.
341. Weyer, E. M. (ed.): Biological actions of dimethylsulfoxide. Ann. N.Y. Acad. Sci. 141, 1967.
342. Wiesinger, H., & Irby, R.: Posterior subcapsular cataract (PSC) in patients with rheumatoid arthritis treated with corticosteroids. Invest. Ophthalmol. Vis. Sci. 2:294, 1963.
343. Willetts, G. J.: Ocular side effects of drugs. Br. J. Ophthalmol. 53:252, 1969.
344. Wirno, M., Schirru, A., Pecori-Giraldi, J., et al.: Aqueous humor alkylosis and marked reduction in ocular ascrobic acid content following long-term topical cortisone (9A-fluoro-16a-methyl-prednisolone). Ann. Ophthalmol. 6:983, 1974.

345. Woolington, S. S., Adler, S. J., & Bower, R. G.: 5 years experience with chloramphenicol. Antibiotics Ann. p. 365, 1956-7.
346. Wong, V., & Collins, E.: Optic atrophy in cystic fibrosis. Am. J. Ophthalmol. 59:763, 1965.
347. Worthen, D. M.: Scanning electron microscopy after alphachymotrypsin perfusion in man. Am. J. Ophthalmol. 73:637, 1972.
348. Wright, P.: Untoward effects associated with practolol administration. Oculomucocutaneous syndrome. Br. Med. J. 1:595, 1975.
349. Yanoff, M., & Fine, B. S.: Ocular Pathology. A Text and Atlas. Harper and Row, Gaithesburg, Maryland, 1975.
350. Yonekura, Y., Mori, T., & Kondo, N.: Optic nerve complications of ethambutal. Folia Ophthalmol. Jap. 20:545, 1969.
351. Zelickson, A.: Skin changes and chlorpromazine. Some hazards of long-term therapy. J.A.M.A. 198:341, 1966.
352. Zuckerman, B. D., & Lieberman, T. W.: Corneal rust ring. Arch. Ophthalmol. 63:254, 1960.

17

The Liver

Kamal G. Ishak

INTRODUCTION

Many drugs and toxins are known to cause liver injury, as attested to by a constant flood of published reports. In most instances such reports represent continued studies of drugs known to be hepatotoxic or of those recently introduced into clinical practice; however, some of these reports are about established drugs suddenly recognized as causes of hepatic injury, as was the case with papaverine, aspirin, and disulfiram. The effects of chemical agents on the liver may complicate therapy (by qualified practitioners of medicine, in folk medicine, and in self medication) or may result from drug addiction, suicide or homicide attempts, or exposure to toxins.

Although many surveys of adverse drug reactions and drug-related deaths have been conducted, the conclusions from most of these have been severely criticized, particularly in view of the lack of controls and the fact that the majority have focused on hospitalized patients in acute medical wards.[278] For example, while a recent study of 26,462 medical patients showed a death rate of 0.9 per 1,000[454]—a rate that appears alarmingly high—most of the patients who died were seriously ill prior to the event that caused death. With reference to the liver, drug reactions have been incriminated in about 2 percent of all cases of jaundice in hospitalized patients.[42,303] Evidence of the importance of drugs in the etiology of some drug reactions affecting the liver is provided by a study in which it was found that about one quarter of the cases of fulminant hepatic failure in the United States may be related to drug injury.[603]

The general methodology for evaluating drug injury is discussed elsewhere in this monograph (see Chapter 1). With regard to the liver,[116,247] the pathologist, in studying hepatic biopsy or autopsy material, should always consider a possible drug reaction when making a differential diagnosis. If a drug injury is suspected the case should be discussed with the patient's clinician in the light of all available clinical and biochemical data. The following considerations in evaluating drug- or toxin-related hepatic injury are based on the author's experience:

1. An adequate drug or toxin history must be available in any suspected case. When the injury is suspected of coming from a therapeutic drug this history must include the dosage, route of administration, and duration of therapy of that drug and other, concomitantly administered drugs. When a toxin is being considered the dose, duration, and route of exposure (ingestion, inhalation, absorption from the skin or mucous membranes), if known, are all extremely important in the evaluation of a given case.
2. The interval of time from the beginning of drug therapy or exposure to a toxin to the development of symptoms or signs heralding the onset of the injury must be estimated. In some instances, it is possible to pinpoint the onset by the occurrence of a symptom complex, such as a "flu-like" syndrome, various gastrointestinal complaints, or fever followed by a rash while the patient is taking a drug. On the other hand, such symptoms and signs may be difficult to unravel from those of the underlying disease, in which case reliance must be placed on the subsequent appearance of jaundice or abnormal findings from tests

of hepatic function. The latent period should fall within the previously accepted range of time for injury from a particular drug, as, for example, from 2 to 4 weeks for injury associated with chloropromazine or diphenylhydantoin to anywhere from 5 weeks to 1 year for a drug such as isoniazid.

3. Other major causes of liver disease should be ruled out by careful assessment of the clinical, morphologic and biochemical findings. The pathologist plays a key role in this regard since: (1) some patients may withhold critical information, such as a history of alcoholism, from their clinician; (2) the histologic changes may be clearly related to a disease, such as alpha-1 antitrypsin deficiency, for which tests are not routinely made; (3) the pattern of injury, particularly when correlated with the biochemical data, may strongly favor a non-drug etiology; for example, the findings of acute cholangitis and bile plugs in the interlobular ducts can suggest extrahepatic rather than intrahepatic biliary obstruction.

4. The possibility of a drug or toxic insult superimposed on another, pre-existing liver disease, should always be considered. An example is the occurrence of centrilobular necrosis from acetaminophen overdose in a patient with alcoholic steatonecrosis.

5. Although most drugs or toxins generally lead to one type of injury, the simultaneous occurrence of two or more types of injury should be borne in mind. The anabolic steroids, for example, can lead to peliosis hepatis and intrahepatic cholestasis, and some affected livers may also show hemosiderosis from multiple blood transfusions used in the treatment of an underlying anemia. Another example of simultaneous multiple injury occurs with phenylbutazone, which may induce hepatic granulomas that, in some patients, may be associated with a hepatocellular/cholestatic injury.

6. If the clinicopathologic correlation establishes with reasonable certainty that a drug is a possible or probable cause of a hepatic injury, then use of the offending drug must be immediately discontinued. More often than not, this is followed by prompt clinical and biochemical improvement, providing further presumptive evidence of a drug etiology. Ultimate proof of a cause-and-effect relationship requires re-challenge with the suspected drug; the pros and cons of re-challenge must be considered by the clinician and the patient. It is highly probable that other, less risky and more sensitive methods of diagnosis will be increasingly utilized in the future; examples of the latter are lymphocyte transformation studies or a macrophage inhibition factor test, as used in the diagnosis of hepatic injury related to propylthiouracil[376] or cloxacillin,[152] respectively.

Zimmerman[666] classifies hepatotoxic agents into two main categories, intrinsic and idiosyncratic (Table 17-1). The intrinsic ("true" or "predictable") hepatotoxins are further subdivided into direct and indirect types, the damage being related to a direct physicochemical effect in the former and to interference with a specific metabolic pathway or process in the latter. Idiosyncratic reactions also appear to fall into two categories, hypersensitivity-related and toxic metabolite-dependent (Table 17-1). Differences between the two types of idiosyncratic reactions are summarized in Table 17-2.

The clinical and biochemical aspects of drug-induced injury are beyond the scope of this presentation. Zimmerman's[666] classification of the various types of injury into hepatocellular, hepatocanalicular, and canalicular types has gained wide acceptance (Table 17-3). Hepatocanalicular and canalicular injury leads to a clinical picture resembling that of extrahepatic obstruction, while the hepatocellular type of injury closely mimics viral hepatitis. Mixed subtypes (mixed-hepatocellular and mixed-hepatocanalicular) of injury are also recognized.[666]

The morphologic lesions caused by drugs and toxins may resemble those of any known

Table 17-1. Classification of Hepatotoxic Agents and Major Characteristics of Each Group

Category	Incidence	Experimental Reproducibility	Dose-Dependent	Mechanism	Histologic Lesion	Example
Intrinsic toxicity Direct	High	Yes	Yes	Direct physico-chemical effect	Necrosis and/or steatosis	CC14; phosphorus
Indirect Cytotoxic	High	Yes	Yes	Interference with hepatocellular metabolic pathways	Steatosis or necrosis	Tetracycline; ethyl alcohol
Cholestatic	High	Yes	Yes	Interference with bile excretory pathway		Anabolic and contraceptive steroids
Host idiosyncrasy Hypersensitivity	Low	No	No	Drug allergy	Necrosis or cholestasis	Chlorpromazine; phenytoin;
Metabolic	Low	No	No	Production of toxic metabolites (?)	Necrosis or cholestasis	Isoniazid; halothane (?)

Modified from Zimmerman, H. J.: Hepatotoxicity. Appleton-Century-Crofts. New York, 1978.

type of liver disease, from benign cholestasis to malignant tumors. Most toxins and drugs produce similar lesions in exposed or susceptible individuals, but some may have more than one type of pathologic effect. For example, tetracycline and halothane generally lead to microvesicular steatosis or acute hepatocellular degeneration and necrosis, respectively; on the other hand, the oral contraceptives may be associated with a variety of lesions, such as acute cholestasis, sinusoidal dilation, hepatic vein thrombosis, or the development of benign and possibly malignant tumors.

The primary pathologic effects of drugs and toxins are discussed according to the various systems of the liver, with the exception of the section on adaptive changes and hyperplasia and neoplasia, which covers all systems. For additional sources on drug-induced hepatic injury the reader is referred to several review articles and monographs published in the last decade.[184, 293, 341, 436, 467, 476, 499, 529, 664, 666, 668] Valuable information on specific drug reactions is also included in Meyler's *Side Effects of Drugs*[137-139] and the American Medical Association *Drug Evaluations.*[10]

Table 17-2. Putative Types of Idiosyncratic Reactions to Drugs as Causes of Hepatic Injury

Type of Idiosyncrasy	Latent Period	Clinical Features of Hypersensitivity	Response to Challenge Dose
Hypersensitivity	1-5 weeks	Rash, fever, eosinophilia	Prompt: after 1 or 2 doses
Metabolic Aberration	Variable: 1 week to 12 or more months	No	Delayed: many days or weeks

Modified from Zimmerman, H. J., and Ishak, K. G.: Hepatic injury due to drugs and toxins. In: MacSween, R. N. M., Anthony, P. P. J., & Scheuer, P. J., eds.: Pathology of the Liver. Churchill Livingstone, Edinburgh, 1979.

Table 17-3. Types of Drug-Induced Jaundice

Features	Hepatocellular	Hepatocanalicular	Canalicular
Clinical			
Anorexia, nausea	+	+	−
Abdominal pain	+	+	−
Pruritis	−	+	+
Hepatic failure	+	−	−
Biochemical			
GOT, GPT	300-8,000 KU[a]	300 KU[a]	300 KU[a]
Alkaline phosphatase	Threefold increase	Threefold increase	Threefold increase
Cholesterol	< 300 mg %	> 300 mg %	< 300 mg %
Histologic	Necrosis + inflammation	Cholestasis + minor hepatocellular injury + portal inflammation	Cholestasis
Prognosis			
Mortality	10-50%	1%	Negligible
Possible Sequelae	Cirrhosis, macronodular or mixed	Chronic cholestatic syndrome resembling primary biliary cirrhosis	Negligible
Examples	Isoniazid, methyldopa, halothane, nitrofurantoin	Chlorpromazine, erythromycin estolate	C-17 anabolic and contraceptive steroids

[a]K.U. = Karmen Units (normal = 40).
Modified from Zimmerman, H. J.: Hepatotoxicity. Appleton-Century-Crofts, New York, 1978.

ADAPTIVE CHANGES

Ground-glass Transformation of Liver Cells

The ground-glass transformation of liver cells may result from long-term therapy with a number of drugs, such as chlorpromazine, barbiturates, azathioprine, steroids, resorcin, some analgesics, disulfiram, cyanamide, and diphenylhydantoin.[267, 297, 394, 616, 649] An example associated with long-term therapy with chlorpromazine is shown in Fig. 17-1. The change is attributable to marked diffuse hypertrophy of the smooth endoplasmic reticulum,[267, 297] and may be a cause of asymptomatic hepatomegaly.[436] Quantitative studies in patients on long-term anticonvulsant therapy have shown an eightfold increase in the amount of endoplasmic reticulum.[266] Experimentally, there is an associated increase in drug-metabolizing enzymes, such as P-450.[554] Drug-induced ground-glass transformation can be distinguished from a similar type of change associated with hepatitis B by its lack of staining with the Shikata stains,[532] such as the aldehyde fuchsin or orcein stains, by the absence of tissue immunoreactivity to antibodies directed against hepatitis B surface or core antigens and, ultrastructurally, by the absence of hepatitis B surface antigen particles within the proliferated smooth endoplasmic reticulum. In the author's experience the drug-induced change is usually zonal or panlobular, in contrast to the spotty distribution of the ground-glass cells in the carriers of hepatitis B. With most of the causative drugs the central zones tend to be more severely affected, but some drugs, such as disulfiram and cyanamide, may predominantly affect the peripheral zones,[616, 617] in which case the change resembles that of Lafora's disease (myoclonus epilepsy).

The prognostic significance of the ground-glass transformation remains conjectural. It is not usually accompanied by acute or chronic injury caused by the drug that produces it. There are no known chronic sequelae, but the borderland between adaptation and overt injury remains on uncharted terrain.[162, 267]

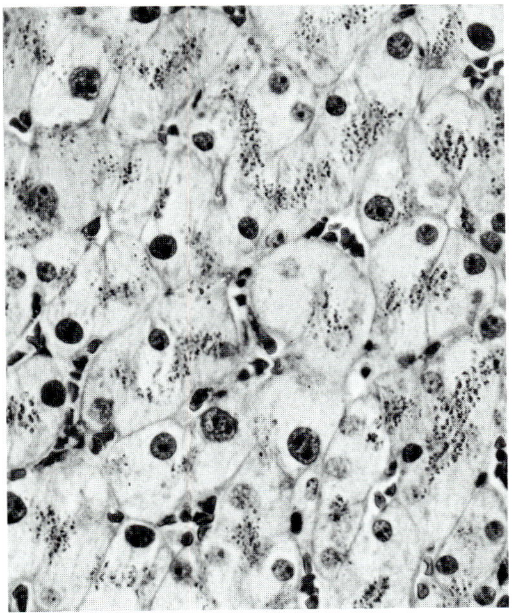

Fig. 17-1. Diffuse ground-glass transformation of liver cells associated with long-term therapy with chlorpromazine. Cells also contain an excessive amount of lipofuscin. H&E, × 350.

Before leaving this section it should be noted that the organochlorine pesticides (DDT, chlordane, heptachlor, dieldrin, and others) are potent stimulators of microsomal enzymes.[564] A recent study of workers industrially exposed to chlordecone (Kepone) has shown hepatomegaly without functional impairment[210]; the light-microscopic and ultrastructural changes in this condition are considered to be adaptive and reversible, the most notable change being the marked proliferation of smooth endoplasmic reticulum.[210]

Subcellular Adaptive Changes

Subcellular adaptive changes may involve hepatocytes or the bile secretory apparatus. Swelling or pleomorphism of mitochondria, with the formation of paracrystalline inclusions, have been reported in women using oral contraceptive agents.[198, 325, 355, 435] Similar hepatocellular changes have been noted during pregnancy and in women with trophoblastic growths,[197, 433] and also in the cells of hepatocellular adenomas and carcinomas in women on oral contraceptives.[18, 221] An increase in the number of peroxisomes in liver cells has been observed in pregnancy[433] and in patients treated with 6-mercaptopurine.[265] Various nonspecific changes have been noted in patients on chenodeoxycholic acid therapy.[219]

Subcellular alterations of the bile-secretory apparatus have been recognized in patients taking 17-α-alkyl-substituted anabolic steroids,[515] oral contraceptives,[325] azathioprine,[267] penicillin,[193] and nitrofurantoin.[194]

HEPATOCELLULAR REACTIONS

ACUTE HEPATOCELLULAR DEGENERATION AND NECROSIS

Predominantly Hepatocellular

Panlobular Degeneration. This type of injury is defined as acute hepatocellular degeneration resembling typical or "classical" viral hepatitis, and involves all zones of the lobule (Fig. 17-2). Zonal necrosis with "dropping-out" of cells is not evident. Cholestasis is absent to minimal. The degeneration may be of the ballooning or acidophilic type, or both (Figs. 17-2 and 17-3). Focal necrosis and sinusoidal acidophilic (free hyaline) bodies are scattered throughout the lobule. Kupffer cells are hypertrophied and often contain lipofuscin (or a mixture of that pigment and hemosiderin during the subsiding phase of the condition.) The inflammatory response in the lobule and portal areas is variable and may be minimal or totally lacking. A significant number of eosinophils may be present, usually in patients who also have peripheral eosinophilia. The presence of fatty metamorphosis in some cases points to a drug injury rather than viral hepatitis.[476] Examples of drugs leading to a hepatitis-like injury include isoniazid, paraminosalicyclic acid (PAS), the sulfonamides, many of the monoamine oxidase (MAO) inhibitors, methyldopa (Figs. 17-2 and 17-3),

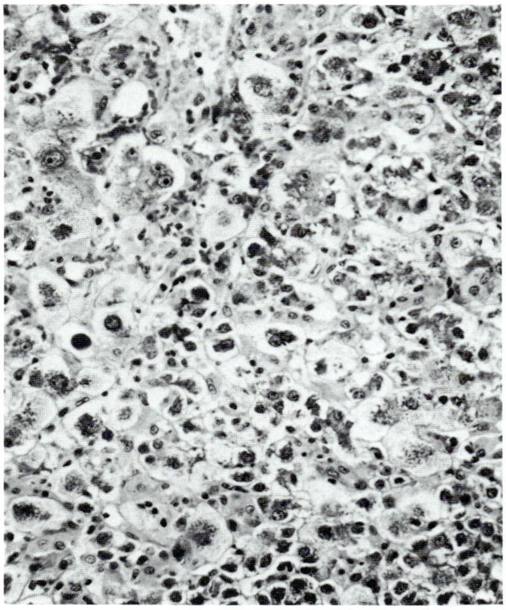

Fig. 17-2. Panlobular hepatitis-like injury associated with methyldopa therapy. There is a lobular disarray, ballooning degeneration, and a darkly-stained acidophilic body (right, center). H&E, × 200.

phenylbutazone, indomethacin, and diphenylhydantoin.

Submassive Degeneration and Necrosis. This is usually zonal in distribution, the central zones being more often affected.

Centrilobular with or without Midzonal Necrosis. The underlying change that eventually leads to the necrosis is predominantly ballooning degeneration, although scattered acidophilic bodies may be seen. A peculiar "hydropic" ballooning is characteristic of ethylene and diethylene glycol toxicity (Fig. 17-4). Injuries secondary to some toxins, such as ammatoxins or tannic acid, may lead to a coagulative type of degeneration. Cholestasis is variable but usually minimal. The biopsy or necropsy specimen will show dropping-out of most hepatocytes from central zones, with variable encroachment on the midlobular zones (Figs. 17-5 and 17-6). The zones of necrosis may be linked together (bridging necrosis) (Fig. 17-7). Variable numbers of inflammatory cells are seen infiltrating the collapsed stroma, and Kupffer cells are hypertrophied

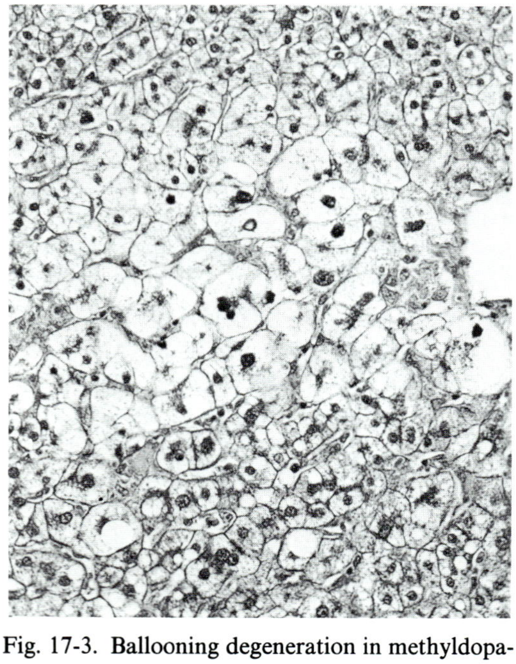

Fig. 17-3. Ballooning degeneration in methyldopa-associated injury. H&E, × 350.

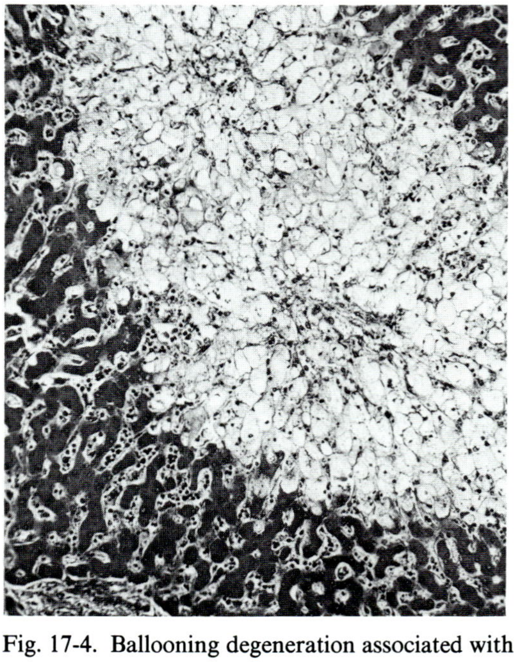

Fig. 17-4. Ballooning degeneration associated with diethylene glycol intoxication. PAS, × 85.

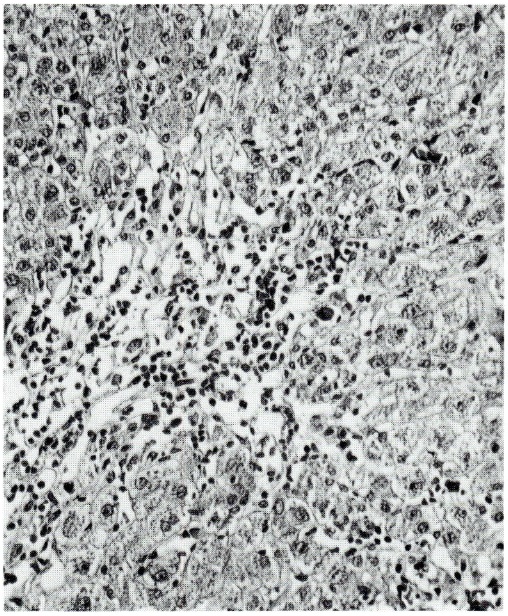

Fig. 17-5. Centrilobular necrosis associated with acetaminophen overdose. H&E × 200.

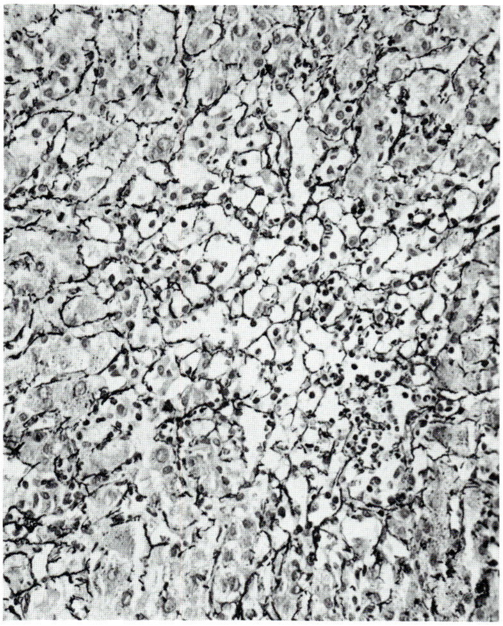

Fig. 17-6. Same case illustrated in Figure 17-5. Centrilobular "dropping-out" of cells with residual intact but empty reticulum framework. (Manuel's reticulum, × 200).

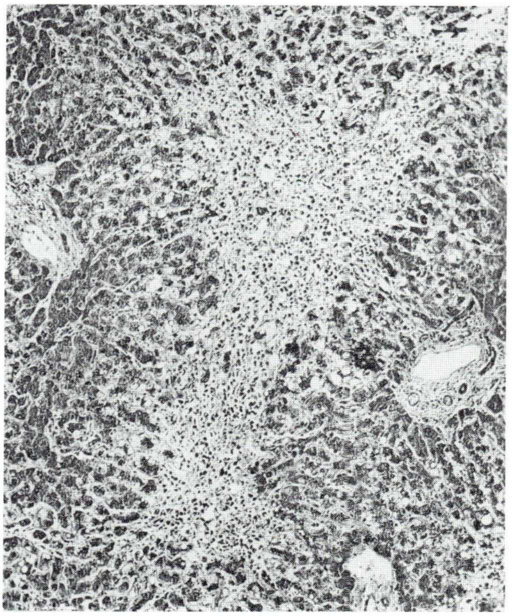

Fig. 17-7. Submassive necrosis associated with isoniazid chemoprophylaxis. Note central to central "bridging." (Masson's trichrome, × 55).

and packed with lipofuscin. When the injury is of the hypersensitivity type the eosinophilic leukocyte may predominate, both intralobularly and in portal areas. A variable degree of periportal cholangiolar proliferation may be evident. Cases related to halogenated hydrocarbon injury often show fat accumulation in the spared parenchyma (Fig. 17-8). Drugs and toxins that may lead to submassive necrosis include halothane, methoxyflurane, propylthiouracil, acetaminophen (paracetamol), allopurinol, dantrolene, copper sulfate, and trichlorethylene, to mention but a few.

Peripheral Zonal Necrosis. Ferrous sulfate toxicity can lead to coagulative degeneration in peripheral zones of the liver, with striking nuclear pyknosis and karyorrhexis and little or no inflammation (Fig. 17-9). Paraminosalicylic acid, phenylbutazone, and halothane may rarely cause peripheral lobular degeneration and necrosis (Fig. 17-10). Phosphorus intoxication results in marked (medium and large vacuolar) fat accumulation throughout

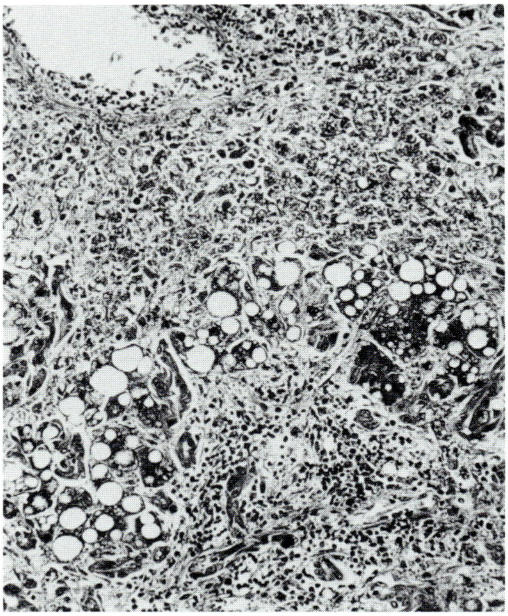

Fig. 17-8. Submassive necrosis secondary to carbon tetrachloride toxicity. Spared liver cells (lower half of field) show fat vacuolization. H&E, × 125.

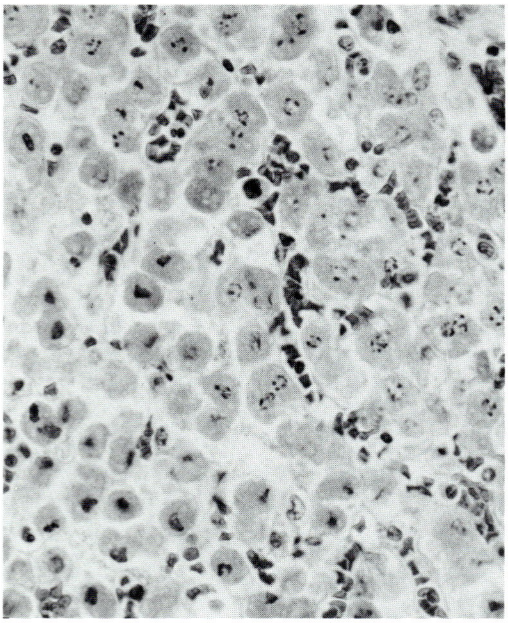

Fig. 17-9. Periportal coagulative degeneration with nuclear karyorrhexis or pyknosis of liver of child who died from accidental ferrous sulfate toxicity. H&E, × 385.

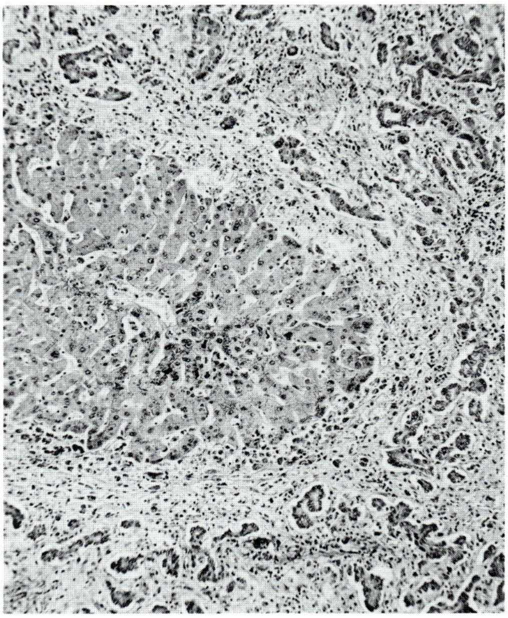

Fig. 17-10. Peripheral necrosis in hepatocellular injury following halothane anesthesia. H&E × 65.

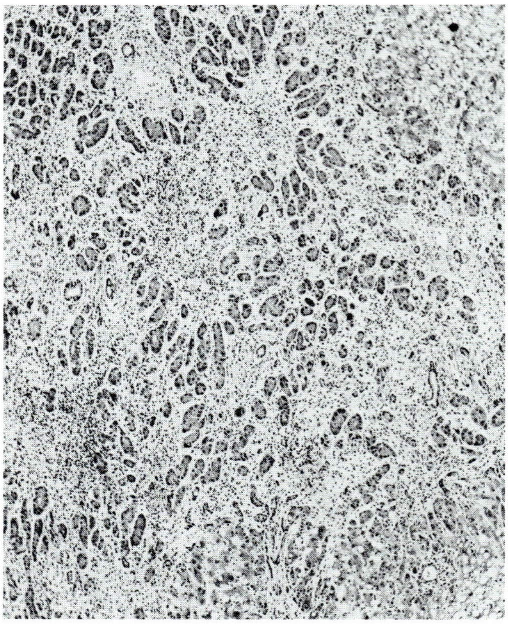

Fig. 17-11. Massive necrosis associated with isoniazid chemoprophylaxis. Peripheral lobular zones are outlined by proliferating pseudoductules. H&E, × 40.

the lobule, in addition to peripheral necrosis.

Massive Necrosis. This type of injury morphologically resembles that seen in fatal viral hepatitis. There is loss of liver cells throughout the lobule, condensation of the reticulum framework with infiltration by inflammatory cells, pseudoductular proliferation, and a variable degree of portal inflammation (Fig. 17-11). Central veins may show an endophlebitis, and Kupffer cells and portal macrophages are hypertrophied and full of lipofuscin, hemosiderin or both. All drugs that cause submassive necrosis may also lead to massive necrosis. Among the relatively more frequent causes of massive necrosis are halothane and isoniazid.

Combined Hepatocellular and Cholestatic Injury

In addition to hepatocellular degeneration, necrosis, or both, the injury in combined hepatocellular and cholestatic injury is accompanied by a significant degree of intrahepatic cholestasis (Fig. 17-12); the condition corresponds to the mixed-hepatocellular type of hepatotoxicity of the classification of Zimmerman.[666] Biochemically there are marked serum transaminase elevations, as well as significantly raised serum bilirubin and alkaline phosphatase levels. The hepatocellular degeneration (ballooning/acidophilic bodies) may be panlobular, or the injury may be more severe in central zones. Cholestasis of moderate or marked intensity is more prominent in central zones but may also have a panlobular distribution. The inflammatory response, whether intralobular or portal, is quite variable. Examples of drugs that could lead to this type of injury are isoniazid, PAS, phenylbutazone, the sulfonamides, methyldopa, carbamazepine, and diphenylhydantoin (Fig. 17-12). The cholestatic form of viral hepatitis must be distinguished from this type of drug injury by clinicopathologic correlation.

Listed below are examples of drugs that have been associated with acute hepatocellular injury. For convenience, and also for comparison with the drugs that lead to cholestatic type of injury (p. 475), they are grouped into broad categories related to therapeutic use.

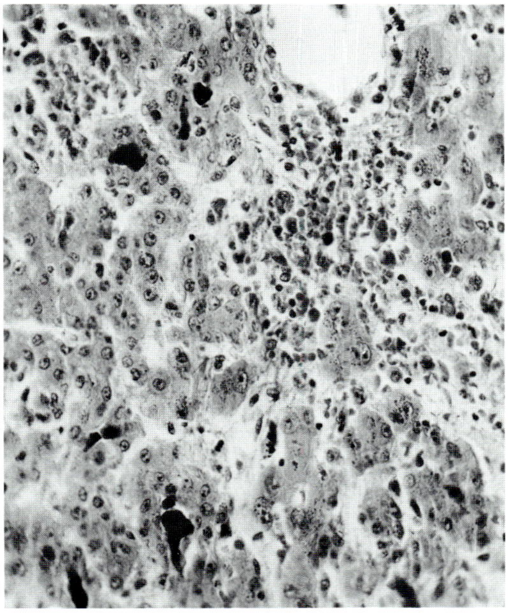

Fig. 17-12. Combined hepatocellular and cholestatic injury resulting from diphenylhydantoin therapy. There is necrosis near the central vein (top) and several pseudoglands contain large (black) canalicular bile plugs. H&E, × 200.

Anesthetic Drugs: Halothane[83, 102, 177, 298, 392, 442, 573, 646]; methoxyflurane[274]; fluroxene[477]; enflurane.[296]

Tranquilizer Drugs: chlordiazepoxide[448]; prochlorperazine.[362]

Antidepressant Drugs: Iproniazid[276, 493]; isocarboxazid[31]; phenelzine[100, 129, 234, 235, 270]; pheniprazine[29, 34, 164, 234, 494]; iproclozide[439]; tranylcypromine[19]; imipramine and desipramine[457]; amitryptyline.[656]

Anticonvulsant Drugs: Mephenytoin[79, 461]; phenacemide[104, 329]; trimethadione[666]; paramethadione[666]; carbamazepine[465, 669]; diphenylhydantoin (phenytoin).[215, 327, 394, 445]

Hypnotic and Sedative Drugs: Phenobarbital.[363, 636]

Analgesic Drugs and Drugs used in Musculoskeletal Disease: Acetaminophen (paracetamol)[43, 95, 159, 262, 328]; ibufenac[218, 588]; ibuprofen[179, 510, 547]; indomethacin[163, 280]; phenylbutazone[13, 84, 153, 167, 359, 396, 399]; salicylates[413, 444, 505, 523, 607]; phenazopyridine[191]; sulindac[11, 653]; naproxen.[326]

Drugs used in the Treatment of Gout: Probenecid[478]; allopurinol.[78, 657]

Muscle Relaxants: Dantrolene.[411, 520, 609, 643]

Drugs used in Cardiovascular Disease: Methyldopa[241, 246, 350, 486, 591, 597, 606]; hydralazine[21]; quinidine[181, 301]; procainamide[290]; aprindine[64]; nicotinic acid[88]; papaverine[289, 428, 490]; phenindione.[663]

Diuretics: Ethacrynic acid[114]; acetazolamide.[314]

Antimicrobial Drugs: Chloramphenicol[188, 663]; erythromycin[659]; isoniazid[44, 349, 381]; ethionamide[99, 437]; pyrazinamide[663]; paraminosalicylic acid[141]; rifampicin[519]; sulfonamides[136]; salicylazosulfapyridine[209, 549]; sulfones[141]; nitrofurantoin.[194]

Antihelminthic Drugs: Hycanthone.[160]

Antithyroid Drugs: Propylthiouracil.[376, 423, 634]

Laxative Preparations: Oxyphenisatin[121, 128, 192, 430, 480, 481, 654]; diacetoxydiphenolasatin[663]; triacetyldiphenolisatin[663]; 4,4′-(2-chinolyl-methylen)-diphenol hydrochloride[663]; dioctyl calcium sulfosuccinate.[598]

Cholecystographic Dyes: Meglumin—Ioglycamide.[648]

Antineoplastic and Immunosuppressive Agents: Methotrexate: (1) In the treatment of leukemia[228, 366, 503, 578]; (2) in the treatment of psoriasis.[106, 371, 407, 408, 452, 488, 518, 596, 632, 633] Cytosine arabinoside[371]; cytosine arabinoside, 6-thioguanine and other drugs[627]; L-asparaginase[371]; mithramycin[12, 283]; actinomycin D after irradiation[216, 367]; Adriamycin and 6-mercaptopurine.[380]

Miscellaneous Drugs: Disulfiram[150, 279, 390, 466]; lergotrile mesylate[587]; phenprocoumon[124, 540]; vasopressor amines.[74]

Hepatocellular injury associated with metallic compounds, various organic toxins and the natural hepatotoxins is listed in Tables 17-4 to 17-6. The majority of these substances act as direct hepatotoxins, although a few, such as gold salts, may lead to hepatic injury on the basis of a hypersensitivity reaction.

Mononucleosis-like Hepatitis

The reactions of mononucleosis-like hepatitis are characterized by fever, rash, lymphadenopathy, and lymphocytosis with atypical lymphocytes, but the serologic tests for infectious mononucleosis are negative. Histologically the liver shows sinusoidal and portal/periportal infiltration with lymphocytes as well as eosinophils, varying anisocytosis and anisonucleosis, sinusoidal acidophilic bodies, focal necrosis, and mitotic figures in both liver and Kupffer cells (Figs. 17-13 and 17-14). The Kupffer cells are hypertrophied and hyperplastic, with the formation of "retothelial"

Table 17-4. Hepatocellular Injury Associated with Metallic Compounds

Toxin	Type of Injury	References
Arsenic	Centrilobular necrosis; cholestasis; fatty metamorphosis	293, 498
Beryllium	Centrilobular necrosis	141, 613
Chromium	Fatty metamorphosis; focal necrosis	426
Copper	Centrilobular necrosis; focal necrosis; cholestasis	92
Gold	Cholestasis; ballooning; focal necrosis	440
Iron	Peripheral necrosis	345, 541
Lead	Resolving or persistent hepatitis	27
Phosphorous	Focal, peripheral or massive necrosis; fatty metamorphosis	73, 127, 168, 316, 508

Table 17-5. Miscellaneous Direct Hepatotoxins

Toxin	Type of Injury	References
Carbon tetrachloride	Centrilobular necrosis, steatosis	264, 281, 384, 558
Trichlorethylene	Centrilobular necrosis	16, 273
Tetrachlorethane	Submassive or massive necrosis	666
Chlorinated naphthalenes	Submassive or massive necrosis	202, 563
Trinitrotoluene	Submassive or massive necrosis; macronodular cirrhosis	666
Diethylene glycol	Centrilobular hydropic degeneration	56
Paraquat	Centrilobular necrosis	75, 302

Table 17-6. Hepatocellular Injury Associated with the Natural Hepatotoxins

Toxin	Type of Injury	References
Tannic acid	Centrilobular necrosis, steatosis	170, 340, 361
Aflatoxin	Centrilobular fibrosis; thickening of central veins; bile duct proliferation; cholestasis; giant cells	313, 581
	Microvesicular steatosis	57, 86, 233, 504
Ammatoxins (from toxic mushrooms)	Centrilobular or massive necrosis	217, 292, 337, 637
Pennyroyal oil	Centrilobular necrosis	572
Apiol	Hepatitis-like	339
Marihuana	Hepatitis-like	429

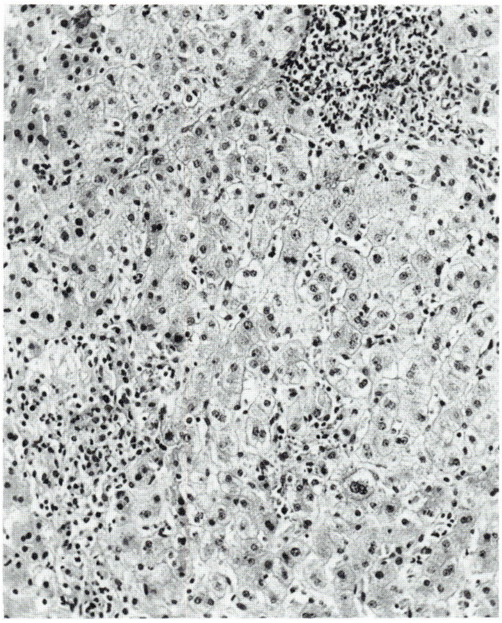

Fig. 17-13. Mononucleosis-like hepatitis associated with diphenylhydantoin. Portal areas (top, right and bottom, left) are moderately inflamed, and sinusoids contain an increased number of mononuclear cells. H&E, × 100.

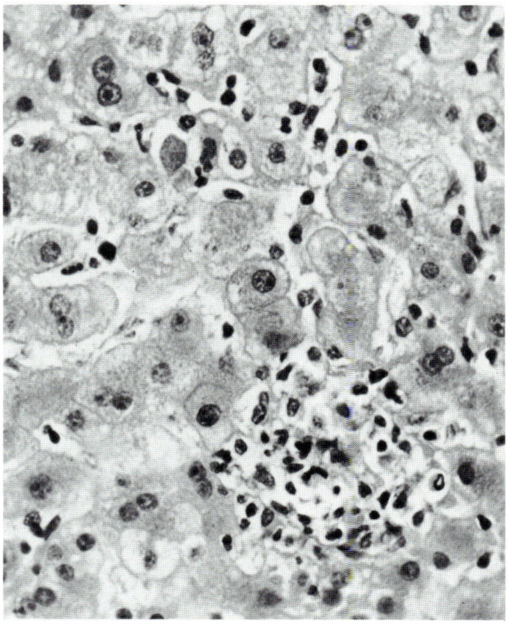

Fig. 17-14. Same case illustrated in Figure 17-13. There is a sinusoidal acidophilic body (top) and a focus of necrosis at the bottom of the field. H&E, × 320.

nodules; true epithelioid granulomas are rarely seen. Cholestasis is absent or minimal, as is ballooning, and there is no zonal necrosis. Drugs that could lead to this type of injury, which closely resembles infectious or cytomegalovirus mononucleosis, include paraminosalicylic acid[332] and diphenylhydantoin.[394]

CHRONIC HEPATOCELLULAR DEGENERATION AND NECROSIS

Chronic Persistent Hepatitis

Most reported cases of chronic necroinflammatory disease of the liver have been chronic active hepatitis or cirrhosis. Occasional examples of chronic persistent hepatitis have been attributed to oxyphenisatin[128] and diphenylhydantoin.[394] The histologic changes in chronic persistent hepatitis include scattered sinusoidal acidophilic bodies, focal necrosis, a generally mild degree of hepatocellular unrest, focal hypertrophy of Kupffer cells, mild to moderate portal inflammation with predominance of plasma cells and lymphocytes, preservation of the limiting plates, and little or no periportal fibrosis.

Chronic Active Hepatitis

The injury in chronic active hepatitis is morphologically indistinguishable from auto allergic ("lupoid") chronic active hepatitis or from chronic active viral hepatitis (hepatitis B or non-A, non-B). Most of the cases also have clinical, biochemical, and serologic similarities to chronic active hepatitis of other etiologies. Many of the patients will improve or recover completely when the causative drug is withdrawn. Changes seen on histologic examination in all cases include moderate to marked portal inflammation, with a predominance of plasma cells and lymphocytes (sometimes with lymphoid follicle formation), erosion of limiting plates (piecemeal peripheral necrosis), and varying degrees of periportal fibrosis. In the majority of cases the intralobular injury is spotty (focal necrosis, acidophilic bodies), but there may be more severe injury with centrilobular (with or without bridging) or multilobular necrosis. Drugs that have been etiologically linked to chronic active hepatitis are listed in Table 17-7. One example related to nitrofurantoin therapy is illustrated in Figures 17-15 to 17-17.

Table 17-7. Drug-induced Chronic Active Hepatitis

Drug	References
Oxyphenisatin	106, 121, 128, 187, 192, 479, 480, 481
Acetylsalicylic acid	317, 523
Acetaminophen	20, 54, 182
Alpha-methyldopa	192, 522
Isoniazid	44, 349, 381
Sulfonamides	599
Nitrofurantoin	45, 220, 258, 528
Propylthiouracil	161, 635
Dantrolene	609
Halothane	590
Chlorpromazine	501

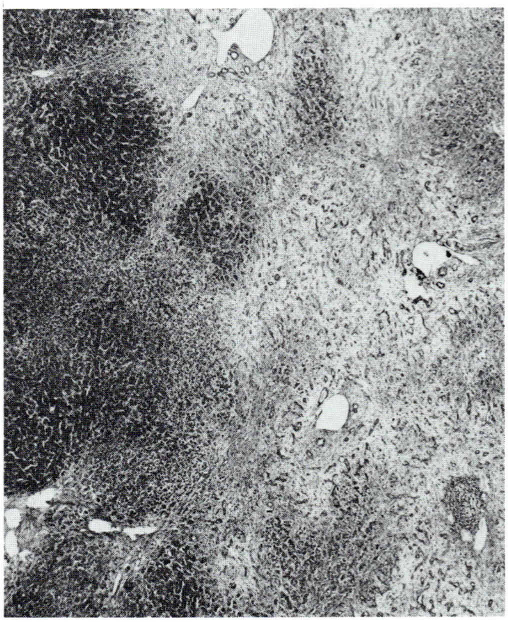

Fig. 17-15. Chronic active hepatitis associated with nitrofurantoin therapy. Section from liver biopsy specimen showing multilobular postnecrotic collapse and fibrosis. Masson's trichrome, × 20.

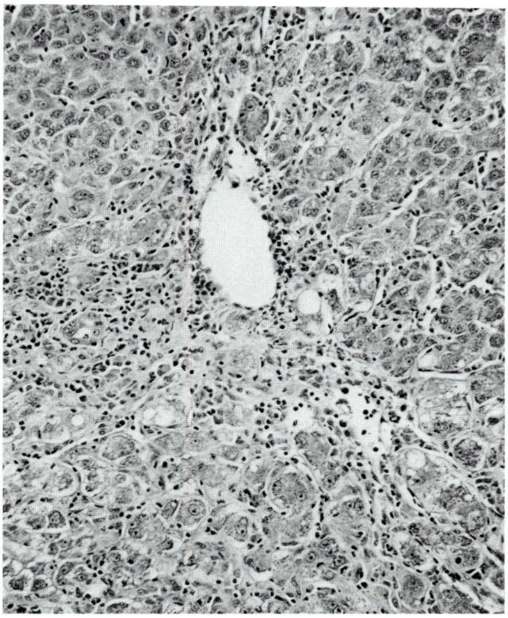

Fig. 17-16. Same case illustrated in Figure 17-15. Centrilobular postnecrotic fibrosis and inflammation. H&E, × 125.

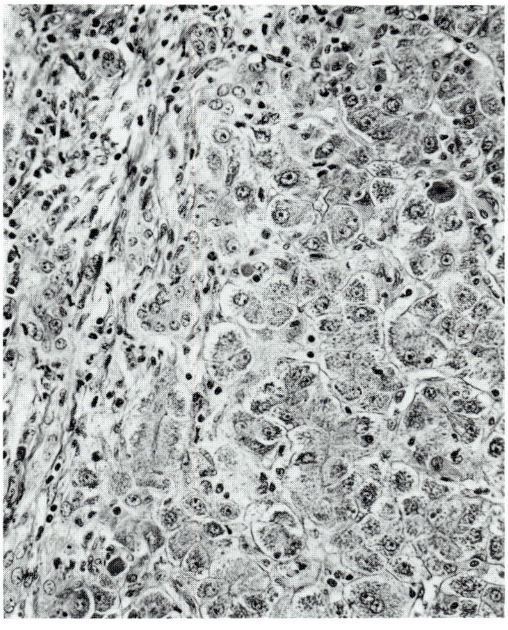

Fig. 17-17. Same case illustrated in Figure 17-16. Junction between lobule and portal area (left) is eroded. There are several sinusoidal acidophilic bodies, and liver cells show cytoplasmic dissociation. H&E, × 125.

Hepatic Fibrosis and Cirrhosis

Most hepatic drug reactions of minimal to moderate severity are followed by recovery and no significant fibrosis. Drug-induced chronic active hepatitis is associated with periportal (stellate) fibrosis, with central-to-portal and portal-to-portal linkage. There may also be multilobular fibrosis (Fig. 17-15). Irregular periportal and subcapsular fibrosis is seen in persons chronically exposed to vinyl chloride[33, 40, 47, 447, 516, 542, 592] or arsenical compounds, and in relation to thorotrast deposits[584] (Figs. 17-18 and 17-19). Exposure to vinyl chloride can also lead to intralobular pericellular fibrosis, as does hypervitaminosis A. The relationship of hepatic fibrogenesis to the perisinusoidal cell system is discussed in a later section. Periportal hepatic fibrosis has been reported in leukemic patients on methotrexate therapy.[228, 366, 578]

Any drug-induced or toxic injury that can cause submassive hepatocellular injury may, if the patient lives, lead to fibrosis, nodular regeneration, and eventually to cirrhosis. On

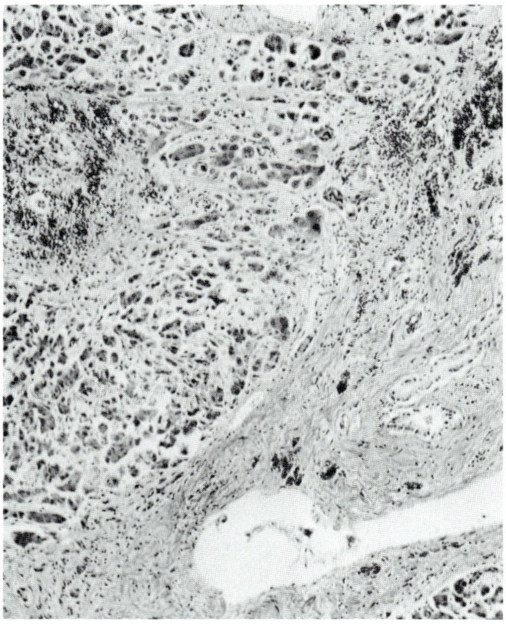

Fig. 17-18. Extensive fibrosis associated with thorotrast accumulation in the liver. H&E, × 45.

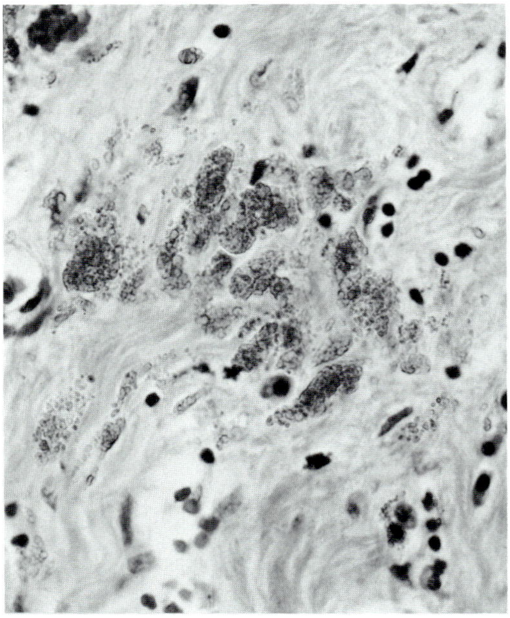

Fig. 17-19. Close-up of thorotrast granules in dense fibrous tissue from same liver illustrated in Figure 17-18. H&E, × 500.

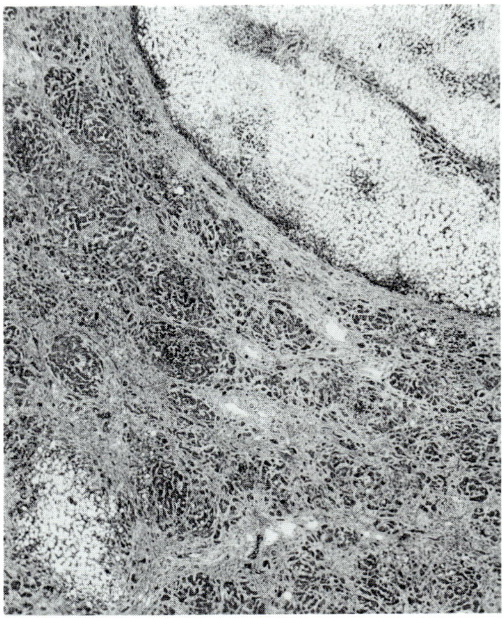

Fig. 17-20. Cirrhosis associated with long-term methotrexate therapy for psoriasis. The cirrhosis is predominantly micronodular, but shows occasional "adenomatoid" macronodules. H&E, × 20.

the other hand, cirrhosis may evolve more insidiously from drug-induced chronic active hepatitis. Few well-documented cases of drug-induced or toxic cirrhosis, particularly those in which serial biopsy and subsequent autopsy material have shown progression from the acute injury to cirrhosis, have been reported. Examples of drug-induced cirrhosis are listed in Table 17-8, and one case associated with methotrexate therapy is illustrated in Figures 17-20 and 17-21. Biliary cirrhosis following

Table 17-8. Drug-induced Cirrhosis

Drug	References
Oxyphenisatin	121, 128, 480, 645
Nicotinic acid	306
Perhexilene maleate	420, 438
Methyldopa	241, 246, 486, 591
Isoniazid	44, 349, 381
Nitrofurantoin	258, 528
Dantrolene	609
Methotrexate	407, 452, 488, 518
Total parenteral nutrition	96

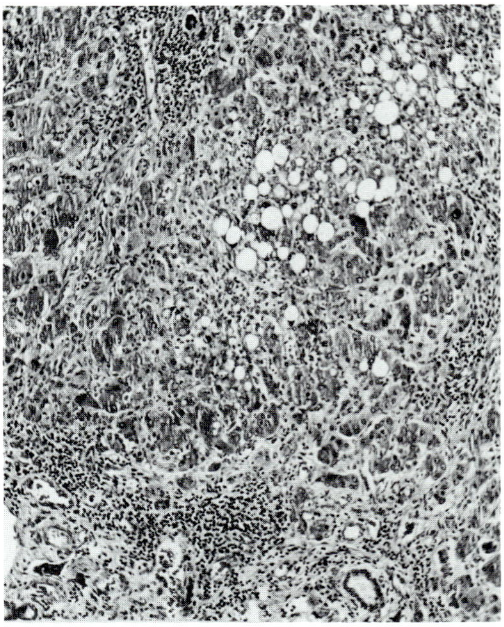

Fig. 17-21. Same case illustrated in Figure 17-20, showing fat vacuolization of liver cells and moderate septal inflammation. H&E, × 80.

drug-induced chronic intrahepatic cholestasis is discussed in the section on cholestasis.

LIPID AND PHOSPHOLIPID ACCUMULATION

Steatosis

Fatty metamorphosis that is iatrogenic or toxic may be conveniently divided into two types, depending on the size of the lipid droplets in the cytoplasm of liver cells.

Microvesicular Steatosis. This condition has been associated with the tetracycline group of drugs,[98, 577] valproic acid therapy,[183, 625] methyl salicylate toxicity,[148, 374] aflatoxin in children with Reye syndrome,[57, 86, 233, 504] and hypoglycin A (from ingestion of a ripe fruit called akee) toxicity in children with Jamaican vomiting sickness.[579] A fatal case of a Reye-like syndrome associated with use of an insect repellent (*N,N*-diethyltoluamide) in a presumed heterozygote for ornithine carbamoyl transferase deficiency was reported by Heick et al.[224]

With reference to tetracycline-induced steatosis, most of the reported cases have occurred after intravenous administration of the drug in doses of 1.5 grams or more per day. Underlying factors that predispose to the injury are pregnancy and poor renal function. Clinical findings include nausea, vomiting, and abdominal pain possibly related to acute pancreatitis; (see p. 614) jaundice is rarely intense. An associated coagulopathy may develop. Syncope, lethargy, and stupor are usually followed by death within 10 days of the onset. The hepatic injury has been reproduced in experimental animals.[577] It is postulated that tetracycline impairment of hepatic secretion of triglyceride is related to inhibition of synthesis of the apoprotein of very-low-density lipoprotein (VLDL).[577]

In microvesicular steatosis the triglyceride accumulates in the form of many small droplets in the cytoplasm of liver cells throughout the lobule. In routinely processed material the cells have a foamy cytoplasm and centrally located nuclei that are often hyperchromatic (Figs. 17-22 and 17-23). There may or may not be a mild degree of cholestasis, but degeneration or necrosis are very rare.

Macrovesicular Steatosis. This condition is characterized by the accumulation of medium and large fat droplets in liver cells, often with the peripheral displacement of nuclei. It is seen in patients receiving corticosteroids.[8, 555] Mild to moderate fatty metamorphosis, for example, is a frequent finding seen in the follow-up hepatic biopsy material of patients with chronic active hepatitis treated with corticosteroids. Fat embolism is a rare complication of steroid-induced fatty metamorphosis of the liver.[230, 271] Other drugs leading to macrovesicular steatosis include alcohol, L-asparaginase,[39, 318, 458, 640] mithramycin, colchicine (together with numerous mitoses arrested in metaphase),[140] and methotrexate (among other changes). Hepatic steatosis is an early change in the liver injury accompanying total parenteral nutrition in infants.[96] Numerous direct hepatotoxins can

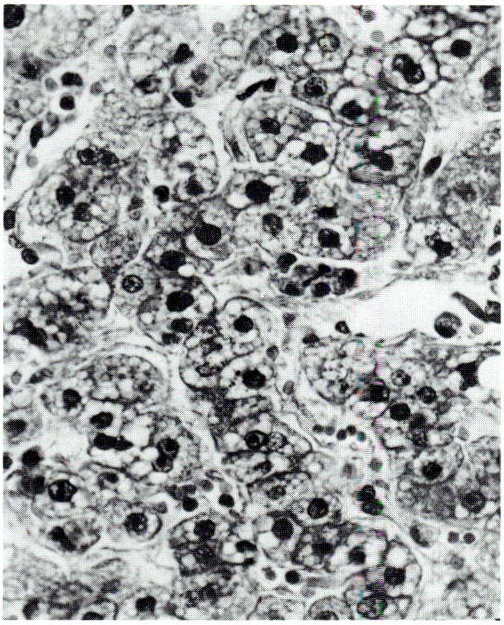

Fig. 17-22. Microvesicular steatosis associated with intravenously administered tetracycline. H&E, × 200.

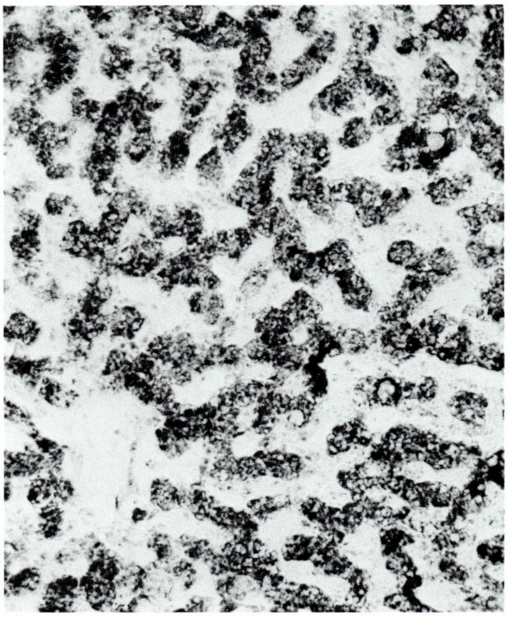

Fig. 17-23. Frozen section stained with oil red-O from same liver illustrated in Figure 17-22, showing positively stained small fat globules. H&E, × 85.

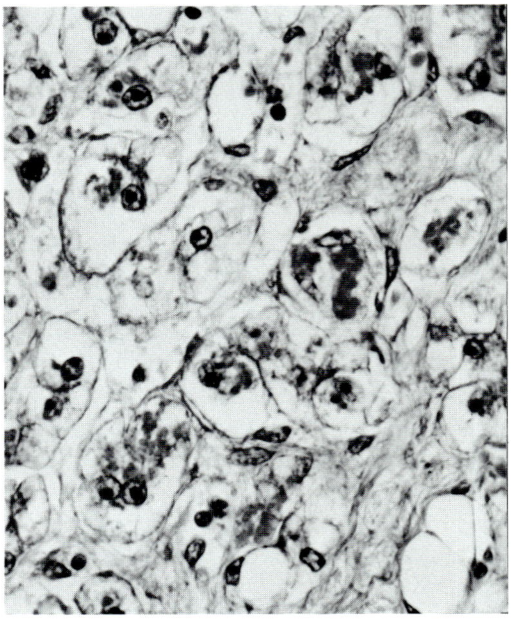

Fig. 17-24. Mallory bodies and large vacuolar fatty metamorphosis after jejunoileal bypass surgery. H&E, × 425.

induce fatty metamorphosis of the liver with or without associated necrosis. These toxins include carbon tetrachloride, tri- and tetrachlorethylene, chloroform, tannic acid, chromates, α-amanitin, and phosphorus. Several extensive reviews on toxic hepatic injury are recommended for further reading.[498, 665] Before leaving this section it should be noted that an important iatrogenic cause of fatty metamorphosis of the liver other than drugs is jejunoileal bypass surgery.[286, 441, 443, 509]

Steatonecrosis, Mallory-body Type

A hepatocellular injury resembling that of alcoholic hepatitis (with fatty metamorphosis, Mallory bodies, and associated neutrophilic focal necrosis, fibrosis, and even cirrhosis) has been reported as a complication of therapy with perhexilene maleate, a drug used in the treatment of angina pectoris.[420, 432, 438, 456] The term "nonalcoholic steatohepatitis" has also been used to refer to this type of injury.[342] Histochemical studies of some perhexilene maleate-related cases of this condition have shown increased amounts of triglyceride, phospholipids, free fatty acids, and gangliosides.[456] Ultrastructural studies by Pessayre et al.[438] have revealed, in the cytoplasm of hepatocytes, numerous myelin figures similar to those noted in the phospholipidoses caused by other drugs (vide infra).[438] Nonmedicinal iatrogenic steatohepatitis with Mallory bodies is a recognized complication of jejunoileal bypass surgery[441, 443] (Fig. 17-24) and massive small-bowel resection.[200, 456]

Phospholipidosis

The changes in drug-induced phospholipidosis resemble those in some inborn errors of lipid metabolism, such as Niemann-Pick or Tay-Sachs disease. The injury is thought to result from a direct interaction between phospholipids and the drug, leading to the formation of a complex that prevents the enzymatic degradation of the lipid molecules. Drugs that can induce a generalized phospholipidosis are all amphiphilic (that is, they have a high hydrophobic and a hydrophilic moiety in close proximity within the same molecule). Light-microscopy of biopsy specimens in the condition reveals the enlargement of hepatocytes and reticuloendothelial cells of the liver, lymphatic tissue, and bone marrow, all of the cells having a foamy appearance. Positive staining for phospholipids can be demonstrated by histochemical methods. Ultrastructurally, the drug-induced phospholipidoses are characterized by membrane-bound residual bodies with a lamellated structure (myelin figures, multilamellar bodies). Only two drugs, the coronary vasodilator 4, 4′,-diethylaminoethoxyhexestrol (Coralgil) and perhexilene maleate have been implicated in this change in humans.[120, 409, 415, 438, 456, 530, 531] I have seen this type of change in several patients receiving multiple drugs, making it difficult to incriminate a specific drug (Fig. 17-25). Among drugs that have induced a phospholipidosis in experimental animals are chlorphentermine, amitriptyline, l-chloroamitriptyline, iprindole, noxiptiline, and chlorpromazine.[134, 343] Myelin figures isolated from experimental animals with such drug-induced phospholipidoses have high acid phosphatase activity, contain large quantities of phospholipid, cholesterol, and cholesteryl ester, and are the sole site of bis-monoglycerophosphate and the enzyme that catalyzes its synthesis from phosphatidylglycerol.[358]

PIGMENT ACCUMULATION

Pigment accumulation in the liver and other organs has been reported after the prolonged or excessive use of the phenothiazines, in particular chlorpromazine,[125, 206] of analgesics containing phenacetin (Fig. 17-26),[3, 377] and of Cascara sagrada preparations.[143] The change is not accompanied by functional abnormalities or symptoms and signs referable to the liver. The pigment in the cytoplasm of liver cells has all the physical and tinctorial

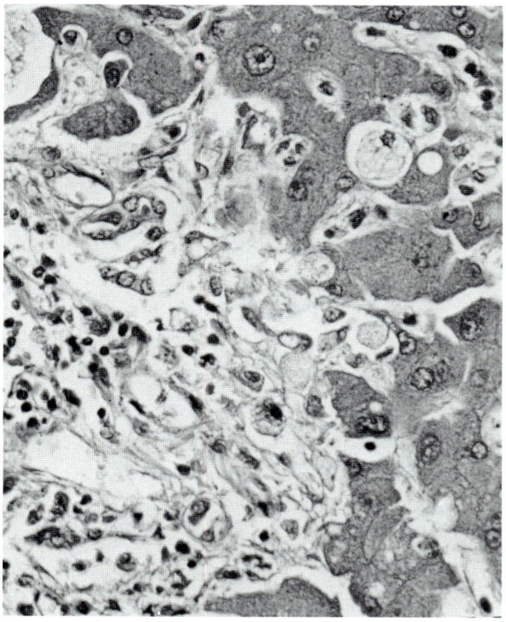

Fig. 17-25. Drug-induced phospholipidosis. Kupffer cells (right half of field) are hypertrophied and have a foamy cytoplasm. H&E, × 300.

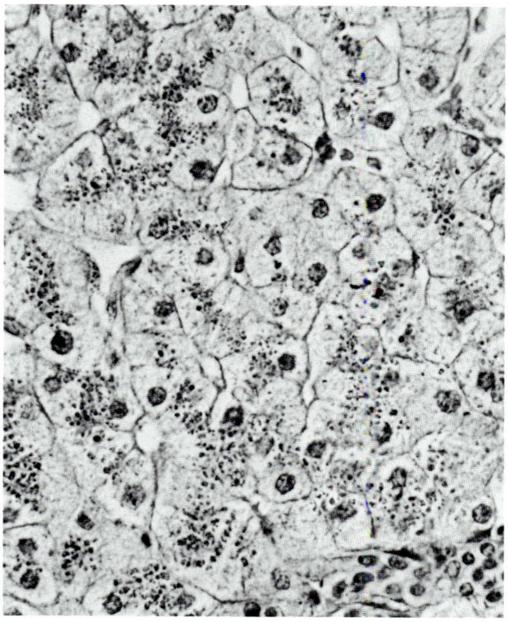

Fig. 17-26. Marked accumulation of coarsely granular lipofuscin in the cytoplasm of liver cells of patient who had chronically ingested *Cascara sagrada* for constipation. H&E, × 350.

characteristics of lipofuscin, including autofluorescence. Its chief significance is in the differential diagnosis of other conditions associated with excessive hepatic lipofuscin accumulation, such as the Dubin-Johnson syndrome.

In addition to transfusional hemosiderosis,[414] note should be taken of the accumulation of hemosiderin in liver cells in alcoholic liver disease,[667] or after excessive ingestion of dietary iron (as typically seen in the Bantu race)[55] or of iron-containing medications.[225] Hepatic hemosiderosis has been reported recently in patients on long-term hemodialysis who had received parenteral iron.[7,309]

Bile pigment accumulation in the cytoplasm of liver cells is considered in the section on cholestasis. Copper may accumulate in periportal hepatocytes in chronic cholestasis related to some drugs, such as chlorpromazine.

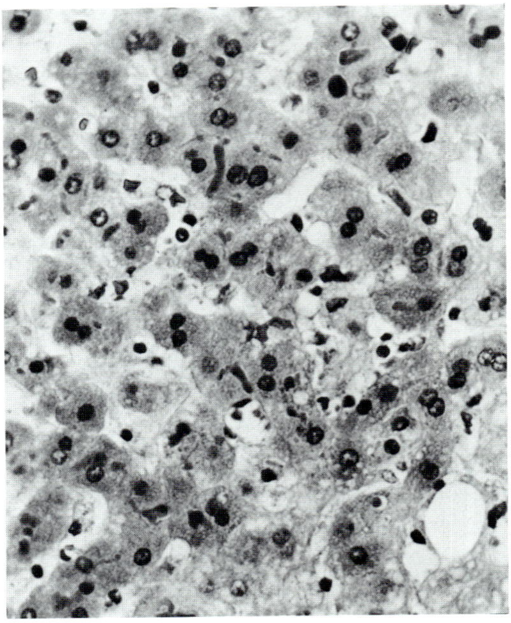

Fig. 17-27. Intrahepatic cholestasis associated with use of an oral contraceptive preparation containing norethindrone and mestranol. H&E, × 385.

CHOLESTATIC REACTIONS

ACUTE INTRAHEPATIC CHOLESTASIS

Bland or Pure Cholestasis

Bland or pure cholestasis is cytoplasmic, canalicular, and reticuloendothelial (Kupffer cells), and is initially centrilobular (Fig. 17-27); in severe cases bile plugs may be found in periportal cholangioles. Liver cells may show mild to moderate anisocytosis, but there is no degeneration, necrosis, or inflammation (intralobular or portal). This type of injury is most frequently associated with the anabolic or contraceptive steroids, but may also be seen with some drugs in the following section when hepatocellular injury is minimal.

Cholestasis with Mild Hepatocellular Injury

The hepatocytic injury in cholestasis with mild hepatocellular injury is unicellular (acidophilic degeneration or bodies or both, and ballooning) and of mild degree. In drug reactions assumed to occur on the basis of hypersensitivity, there may be a variable number of eosinophils in sinusoids, in foci of necrosis, and intermingled with other inflammatory cells in portal areas of the liver. Examples of drugs leading to this type of injury are some tranquilizers (chlorpromazine, prochlorperazine, chlordiazepoxide, thioridazine), antibiotics (oleandomycin, erythromycin estolate), sulfonylurea derivatives (tolbutamide, chlorpropamide) and total parenteral nutrition (particularly in infants).

Cholestasis with Mild Hepatocellular and/or Cholangiocellular Injury

In addition to cholestasis and unicellular hepatocytic injury some drugs may cause degeneration, inflammation, or both, of interlobular bile ducts. The injury associated with paraquat is manifested by acidophilic degeneration of the lining cells, with shrinkage and

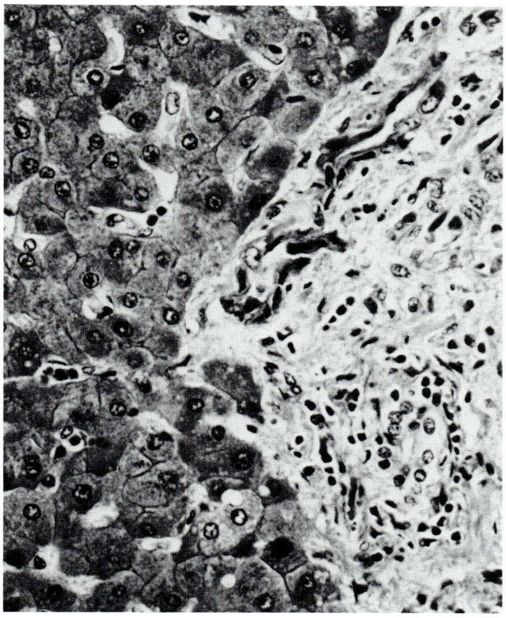

Fig. 17-28. Liver from fatal case of paraquat toxicity. Bile duct near limiting plate shows marked degeneration, with shrinkage of lining cells and nuclear pyknosis. H&E, × 320.

nuclear pyknosis, occasional vacuolization, accumulation of amorphous debris in the lumen, and variable inflammation, usually with infiltration of the wall by neutrophils, eosinophils, or both (Fig. 17-28). Drugs and toxins that may lead to an acute cholangitis include erythromycin estolate, allopurinol, chlorpropamide, and 4, 4′-diamino diphenylmethane (methylenediamine)—the cause of Epping jaundice.[421]

The drugs or toxins that can lead to the various types of cholestatic reactions are listed below:

Anabolic/Androgenic Steroidal Compounds[122, 172, 185, 199, 277, 514, 638, 642, 654]

Oral Contraceptives: numerous varieties.[51, 105, 109, 132, 312, 320, 324, 402, 416, 546, 561]

Tranquilizing Drugs: Chlorpromazine[254, 256, 662]; fluphenazine[624]; mepazine[382]; perphenazine[15, 100]; prochlorperazine[254]; promazine[281, 621]; thioridazine[48, 473, 582]; trifluoperazine[305, 353]; haloperidol[666]; chlordiazepoxide[1, 81, 335]; diazepam.[171, 553]

Antidepressant Drugs: Amitriptyline[38]; imipramine[238, 535]; iprindole.[5]

Analgesics and Drugs used in Musculoskeletal Disease: Naproxen[23, 618]; propoxyphene hydrochloride.[108, 295]

Drugs used in Cardiovascular Disease: Methyldopa[232]; ajmaline[30, 422]; disopyramide.[370, 482]

Diuretic Drugs: Furosemide[111]; chlorothiazide[135]; hydrochlorothiazide.[245]

Antimicrobial Drugs: Erythromycin[204, 571, 620, 659]; penicillins[28, 152, 193, 425]; oleandomycin[186, 595]; co-trimoxazole[412, 557]; sulfones[379]; nitrofurantoin.[194]

Antiparasitic Drugs: Thiobendazole.[261]

Antiviral Drugs: Idoxuridine.[118, 538]

Antifungal Drugs: Griseofulvin.[87]

Oral Hypoglycemic Drugs: Acetohexamide[195]; tolbutamide[17]; chlorpropamide.[472, 497]

Antithyroid Drugs: Methimazole[166, 354, 533, 585]; carbimazole.[344]

Immunosuppressive and Antineoplastic Agents: 6-mercaptopurine[149, 311, 534]; azathioprine[69, 117, 174, 371, 548, 550, 660]; Adriamycin and 6-mercaptopurine.[487]

Miscellaneous Drugs: Warfarin[471]; D-penicillamine[388]; nicotinic acid[424]; total parenteral nutrition.[26, 35, 351, 431, 455, 485, 545, 600]

Metallic Compounds: Arsenic: (a) carbarsone[403, 463]; (b) neoarsphenamine.[214] Copper[92]; gold.[440]

Miscellaneous Toxins: Methylenedianiline[307, 365]; paraquat.[395]

CHRONIC INTRAHEPATIC CHOLESTASIS

Most cases of drug-induced cholestasis are followed by rapid clinical and biochemical recovery upon withdrawal of the causative medication and supportive treatment for the condition. Occasional patients, however, continue to have abnormal tests of hepatic function for many months, as for example after chlorpromazine[254] or total parenteral nutrition.[455] Some patients (Table 17-9) will sooner or later develop clinical and biochemi-

Table 17-9. Drug-Induced and Toxic Chronic Intrahepatic Cholestasis

Drug or Toxin	References
Chlorpromazine	254, 397, 468, 623
Prochlorperazine	254
Imipramine	238
Tolbutamide	205
Thiobendazole	379
Methyl testosterone	189
Ajmaline	30
Organic arsenicals	222, 562

cal features indistinguishable from those of primary biliary cirrhosis, except that antibodies directed against mitochondria are not detectable in the serum. The histologic features of drug induced cholestasis include cholestasis (which may be central but is more typically periportal), pseudoxanthomatous transformation of hepatocytes and Kupffer cells, accumulation of copper in periportal liver cells, peripheral unicellular hepatocytic degeneration (piecemeal necrosis), mild to moderate patchy chronic portal inflammation, and a progressive reduction in the number of interlobular bile ducts (Figs. 17-29 and 17-30). The bile duct lesions of primary biliary cirrhosis (chronic nonsuppurative destructive cholangitis) are not seen.[254] The pathogenesis of the destruction of bile ducts is unclear, but I have observed occasional ducts showing a pseudoxanthomatous transformation of lining cells, suggesting that the accumulation of bile salts and perhaps cholesterol may be the culprit. A true cirrhosis has been reported in occasional cases of chronic intrahepatic cholestasis associated with chlorpromazine.[397, 623]

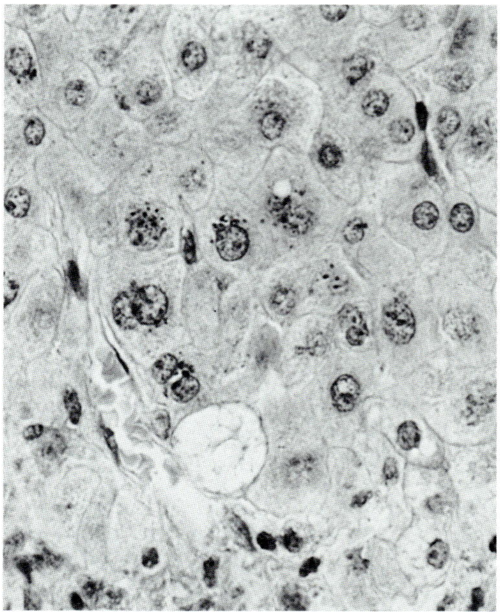

Fig. 17-30. Copper storage (black granules) in periportal liver cells in same case illustrated in Figure 17-29. Rhodanine, × 525.

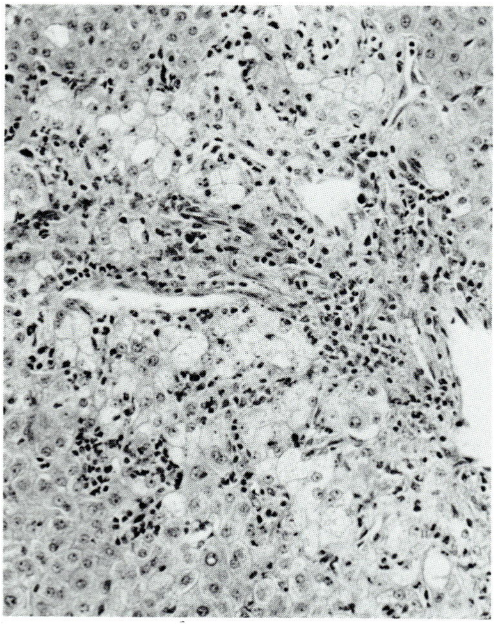

Fig. 17-29. Chronic cholestasis associated with chlorpromazine therapy. The expanded portal area is moderately infiltrated with mononuclear cells, lacks a bile duct, and is surrounded by numerous pseudoxanthomatous hepatocytes. H&E, × 180.

VASCULAR REACTIONS

SINUSOIDS

Sinusoidal Dilatation

Sinusoidal dilatation was first described in liver biopsy material from four women using oral contraceptives for periods varying from

11 to 36 months[650]; other cases have since been reported.[552] Patients with this condition have hepatomegaly but no symptoms, and few or no biochemical abnormalities. Histologically there is striking dilatation of sinusoids, predominantly in peripheral zones of the liver (zone 1), disruption of the reticulum framework, and varying atrophy of liver plates (Figs. 17-31 and 17-32). Ultrastructural studies have shown dilatation of endoplasmic reticula, with the accumulation of granular, electron-dense material, disruption of mitochondrial membranes, and deposition of collagen fibers in the spaces of Disse and interhepatocytic spaces.[552] The dilatation has not been complicated by peliosis hepatis or rupture. The long-term sequelae of oral-contraceptive-induced sinusoidal dilatation are not known, and the hepatomegaly may recede following discontinuation of oral contraceptive use.[650]

Sinusoidal dilatation has also been noted in some patients treated for 6 to 12 months with chenodeoxycholic acid for dissolution of gall stones.[330]

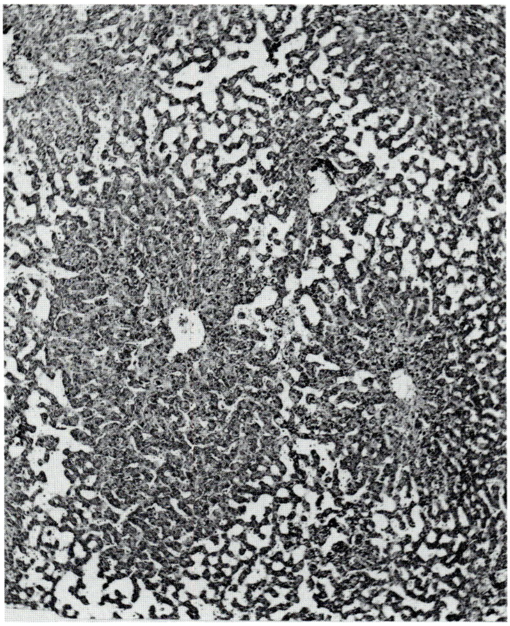

Fig. 17-31. Striking periportal sinusoidal dilatation associated with use of oral contraceptive. Masson's trichrome × 40.

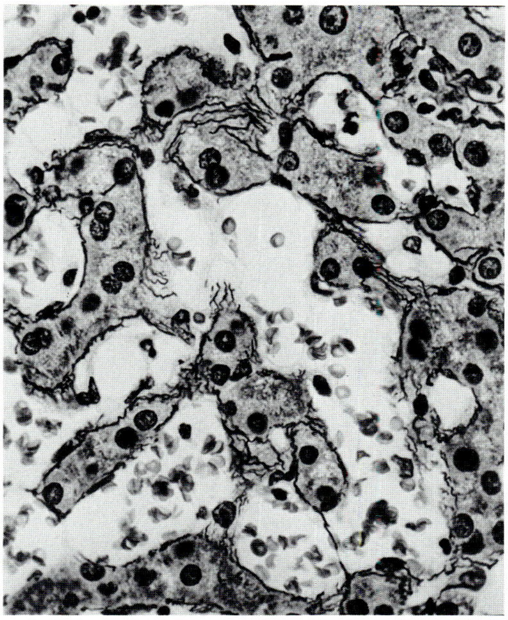

Fig. 17-32. Same case illustrated in Figure 17-31, showing disruption of reticulum framework. Manuel's reticulum, × 320.

Other Sinusoidal Changes

Drug-induced hepatic injury associated with peripheral eosinophilia, such as that related to chlorpromazine, may be accompanied by an increased number of eosinophilic leukocytes in sinusoids.[254] Many lymphocytes are seen in the lumen of sinusoids in drug-induced mononucleosis, as in the mononucleosis secondary to diphenylhydantoin.[394] Sinusoidal hematopoiesis may be a secondary effect of drug-induced damage to the bone marrow. Immunosuppressed patients, particularly those treated with corticosteroids, may develop disseminated strongyloidiasis, in which case strongyloides larvae may be found in hepatic sinusoids.[357, 375]

Peliosis Hepatis

Two recent reviews have dealt at length with peliosis hepatis—a complication of androgenic-anabolic steroid therapy[398, 60]; other cases have since been reported.[527, 583] The steroids implicated in this change have included oxymetholone, fluoxymesterone, norethandrolone, methandrostenolone, and testosterone. There is no relationship between the development of peliosis and the dose or duration of therapy with the androgenic-anabolic steroid.[398] Regression of the lesions has been documented following the discontinuation of therapy.[60] Peliosis hepatis has also been reported in renal transplant recipients treated with azathioprine,[119] and in two patients on diethylstilbesterol therapy.[462]

On gross examination, peliosis hepatis is marked by multiple, fluctuant-to-soft, blue-black projections studding the surface of the liver. The cut section shows varying-sized cavities filled with liquid or clotted blood. Microscopically, the cavities have a ragged lining of liver cells and no endothelium (Fig. 17-33). There may be organization of the contents of the cavities, with invasion by capillaries and fibroblasts from the periphery. The cavities may communicate with adjacent sinusoids. The liver between the peliotic cavities often shows varying degrees of sinusoidal dilatation of patchy distribution, and central and sublobular veins may also be dilated (Fig. 17-33). Intrahepatic cholestasis, also assumed to be due to the steroid therapy, and reticuloendothelial and even hepatocellular hemosiderosis (usually related to multiple transfusions or an underlying anemia) may be seen in some cases.[252] Occasional cases may show hyperplasia of liver cells[421, 639] or hepatocellular carcinoma.[36, 527] Extrahepatic peliotic lesions, as in the spleen, for example, have been observed rarely.[583]

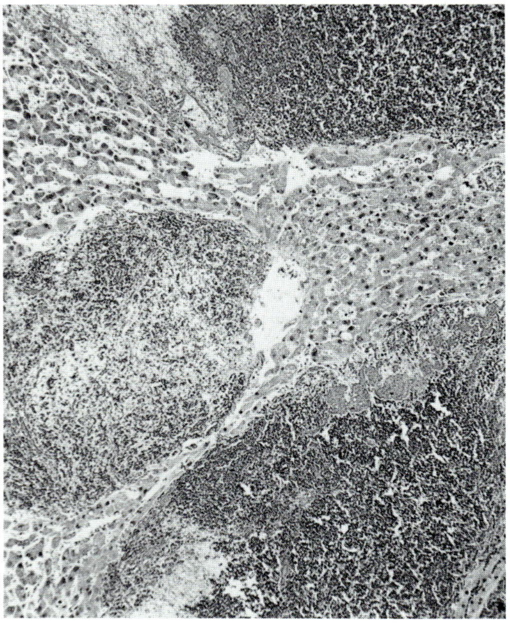

Fig. 17-33. Peliosis hepatitis in patient with aplastic anemia treated with oxymetholone. H&E, × 50.

Ultrastructural studies of human biopsy material[398, 495] and of endothelial cells exposed to oxymetholone in vitro[308] suggest that damage to the endothelial lining of sinusoids is the underlying pathogenetic mechanism of peliosis hepatis.

HEPATIC VEINS

Phlebosclerosis (Perivenular Sclerosis)

Alcohol appears to be the chief cause of this lesion.[145, 146, 615] The lesion may be of predictive value in identifying patients who may develop more severe liver disease with continued drinking.[615]

Veno-occlusive Disease

The majority of cases of veno-occlusive disease (Table 17-10) are the result of drinking tea brewed from the leaves of plants containing pyrrolizidine alkaloids, but recent outbreaks in Afghanistan and India[383, 580] were caused by the contamination of wheat or cereals by the seeds of *Heliotropium* or *Crotalaria* plants, respectively. The geographic pathology of veno-occlusive disease is discussed by Bras.[66]

With some exceptions, veno-occlusive disease differs from the Budd-Chiari syndrome in the lack of involvement of the larger hepatic veins.[524] The acute disease is usually followed

Table 17-10. Veno-occlusive Disease

Drug or Toxin	Underlying Condition	References
Pyrrolizidine alkaloids (*Senecio, Crotalaria* or *Heliotropium* plant species)	None	66, 67, 68, 72, 383, 524, 559, 569, 580
Oral contraceptives	None	9
Azathioprine	Renal transplantation	356
Urethane	Multiple myeloma	70, 368
6-Thioguanine/cytosine arabinoside	Leukemia	207
Busulfan	Bone marrow transplantation	37
Dimethylbusulfan/radiotherapy	Bone marrow transplantation	537

by rapid recovery, but some patients may succumb to liver failure. A subacute form may gradually merge with chronic veno-occlusive disease, with the development of cirrhosis.[66, 67] Histologically the central and sublobular veins in the acute disease show eccentric or concentric narrowing, to complete obliteration of the lumen by the accumulation of a loose (sometimes weblike) connective tissue in the intima (Fig. 17-34). This tissue is progressively collagenized and may contain newly formed, tiny vascular channels (recanalization) in the absence of previous thrombosis. There is widespread damage to the vascular endothelium in central zones, and extravasation of erythrocytes between liver cells and into the spaces of Disse.[67] The liver cells may undergo coagulative degeneration and necrosis. Subacute and chronic cases are associated with sinusoidal dilatation, atrophy of liver cell plates, and progressive fibrosis with central-to-central fibrous linkage and, ultimately, the development of a micronodular congestive cirrhosis.

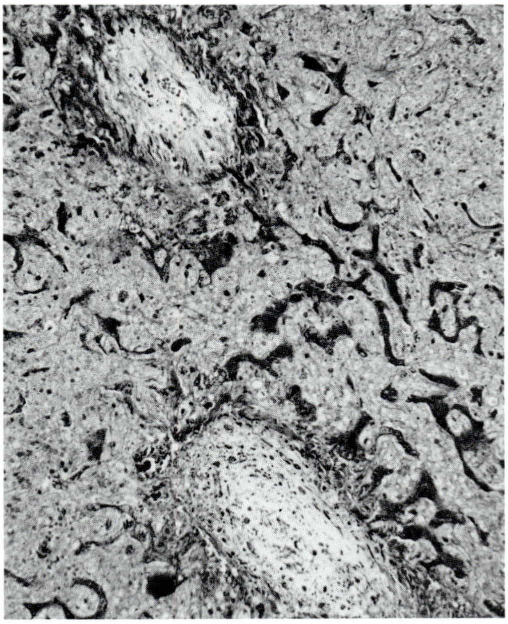

Fig. 17-34. Veno-occlusive disease due to ingestion of tea brewed from *Senecio formosus.* Two central veins show obliteration of the lumen by intimal fibrosis, with extravasation of red cells. All necrotic liver cells have dropped-out. Masson's trichrome, × 125.

Radiation injury to the liver leads to veno-occlusive disease with histopathologic changes indistinguishable from those caused by toxins or drugs.[322, 469, 631]

Hepatic Vein Thrombosis

Four patients with the Budd-Chiari syndrome attributed to the use of oral contraceptives have been reported since the review of 14 published cases and case report by Wu et al.[655] The duration of oral contraceptive use in patients developing the condition has varied from 2 weeks to 8 years, the mean latent period being 20.6 months.[655] Most of the cases have ended fatally, although survival after ceasing of use of oral contraceptives has been recorded.[242, 544] One patient whose liver ruptured recovered after lobectomy.[173]

Grossly there is enlargement of the liver and spleen, and thrombotic occlusion of hepatic veins, often at their junction with the inferior vena cava (with or without extension into that vessel). The liver has a "nutmeg" pattern, and in a cut section, red or white thrombi may be visible in interlobular veins. Microscopically, recent or old and recanalized thrombi are often seen in the same liver, suggesting that the thrombotic process had occurred at different times before the disease became clinically apparent (Figs. 17-35 and 17-36). Several of the cases on file at our institution have shown lesions resembling those of veno-occlusive disease in small central veins, in addition to the thrombotic changes. Besides the venous changes the liver shows severe sinusoidal dilatation and congestion, coagulative degeneration (in cases with recent thrombosis), and varying degrees of perivenular (and perisinusoidal) fibrosis (in subacute or chronic cases). Hemorrhagic infarcts were reported in one case[556] and calcification in two other cases.[202, 655] Regenerative nodules may be present.[242]

Other than the contraceptive steroids, only one agent—dacarbazine (dimethyltriazeno-imidazole-carboxamide)—has been implicated in the Budd-Chiari syndrome.[14, 500]

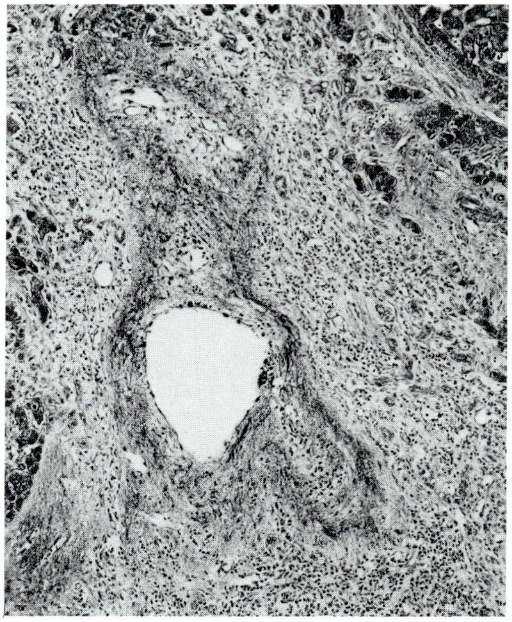

Fig. 17-36. Sublobular vein showing an old recanalized thrombus from same case illustrated in Figure 17-35. H&E, × 80.

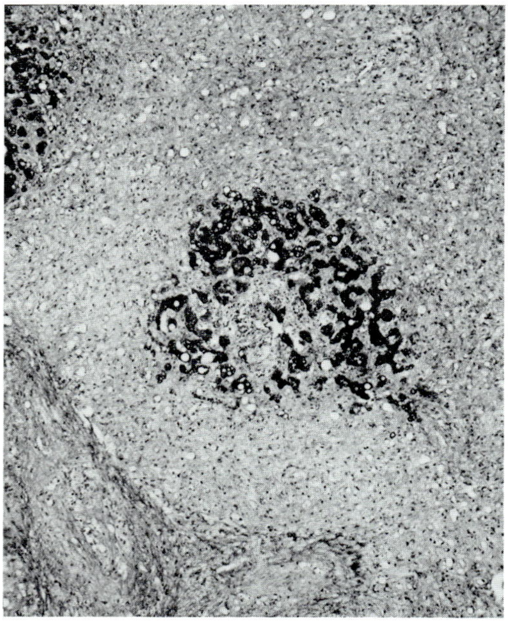

Fig. 17-35. Budd-Chiari syndrome in patient on oral contraceptive for about 2 years. The only surviving liver cells (darkly stained) are in the immediate vicinity of a portal area. PAS, × 60.

PORTAL VEIN

Thrombosis and Pyelephlebitis

Several patients with Budd-Chiari syndrome associated with oral contraceptives have also had thrombosis of the portal vein or other intra-abdominal vessels. Intimal hyperplastic lesions similar to those described in women taking oral contraceptives[248, 249] were noted in one patient with the Budd-Chiari syndrome.[252]

Numerous instances of portal vein thrombosis, pyelephlebitis, or both, have been reported as a complication of umbilical vein catheterization in newborn infants.[65, 147, 323, 417, 512, 526, 577, 641] The catheterization has been employed for exchange transfusion, the administration of fluids or drugs, and for drawing blood samples for biochemical tests. Important factors in the development of portal

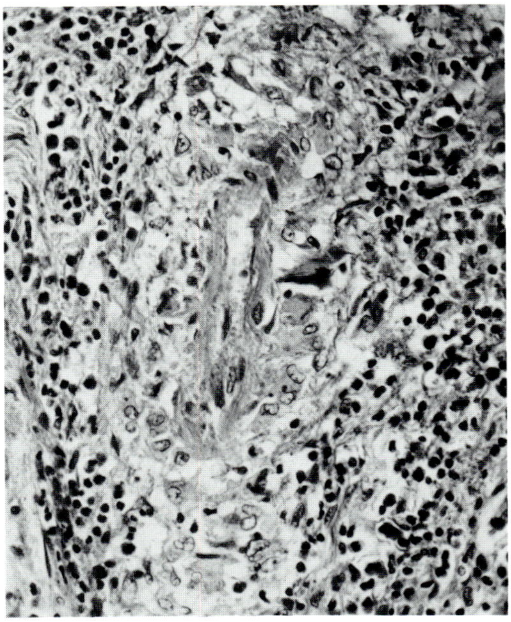

Fig. 17-37. Necrotizing granulomatous angiitis associated with diphenylhydantoin hypersensitivity reaction. H&E, × 240.

vein thrombosis or pyelephlebitis include the use of solutions that are hypertonic or have a different pH from that of blood; infection; duration of catheterization; and trauma from the improper placement of catheters. Of a series of 75 infants subjected to exchange transfusion, 53 percent had bacterially contaminated umbilical cords before insertion of the catheter, and 62 percent of the catheters were colonized upon removal.[4] Systemic antibiotic therapy has not been effective in sterilizing the cord or catheter or in combating bacteremia.[4,310]

The portal vein thrombosis developing in catheterized infants may be accompanied by extensive hepatic necrosis[323,641] or infarction.[147,577,641] Septic emboli to the liver and lung,[512] or hepatic abscesses[65] may complicate acute pyelephlebitis of the portal vein. Dystrophic calcification, presumed to be secondary to antecedent hepatic damage, has been reported in a few cases.[2] Infants who survive may subsequently develop portal hypertension.[417,526] Umbilical vein catheterization in adults may also be complicated by thrombosis, mainly in patients with cirrhosis.[287,288]

Hepatoportal Sclerosis

Hepatoportal sclerosis, a feature of noncirrhotic portal hypertension, is a recognized complication of chronic exposure to arsenic.[103,115,243,389,401,619,661] In reported cases the ingested arsenic was in the form of Fowler's solution (2 percent solution of arsenic trioxide), contaminated drinking water, or bhasams (folk medicines used in India). A variety of histologic changes have been described, including thickening of portal vein branches (intimal thickening, muscular hypertrophy), an increase in the number of vessels in portal areas, and periportal and intralobular (perisinusoidal) fibrosis. Nodular transformation and thrombosis of intrahepatic portal vein branches, with recanalization, have been observed in a series of cases, not specifically attributed to arsenic,[400] from India.

HEPATIC ARTERY

Angiitis

Drug-induced vasculitis usually affects multiple organs and tissues. In one series the liver was involved in the majority of cases; the responsible drugs included chlorpropamide, diphenylhydantoin, phenylbutazone, allopurinol, penicillin, and chlorothiazide.[393] All layers of arteries and veins were involved, the inflammatory response being predominantly mononuclear. In contrast to this type of vasculitis, which is not accompanied by necrosis of the vessel wall or thrombosis, a necrotizing angiitis (also referred to as polyarteritis nodosa) has been attributed to several drugs, including sulfathiazole,[331,386] penicillin,[628] diphenylhydantoin,[211,614] (Fig. 17-37) and allopurinol.[61,263] Most of these cases of necrotizing angiitis were systemic reactions involving multiple organs, including the liver, and were accompanied by a skin rash (often exfoliative), peripheral eosinophilia, and other manifestations of a hypersensitivity response.

A necrotizing angiitis indistinguishable from periarteritis nodosa, with the involvement of coronary, hepatic, renal, and other arteries, has been reported in intravenous drug abusers.[94] Methamphetamine alone or in combination with heroin or d-lysergic acid diethylamide, was the drug commonly used. A case of intrahepatic mycotic aneurysms (resulting from methylphenidate abuse) was reported by Maxwell et al.[360] in a series of 18 patients with vascular complications from drug abuse.

Thrombosis

Infarction of the liver, in one case associated with thrombosis of the celiac artery, has been reported as a rare complication of umbilical artery catheterization in children.[641]

Miscellaneous Arterial Lesions

A systemic arterial disease has been described in children in Northern Chile who were chronically exposed to high levels of arsenic in drinking water.[492] Arteries in portal areas of the liver showed fibrous intimal thickening, and one of the livers was also cirrhotic.

Intimal and other vascular lesions resembling those occurring in other organs and tissues of women taking oral contraceptives[248,249] have been observed in vessels, principally arteries, at the periphery of hepatocellular adenomas.[253] It is speculated that these lesions may be significant in the pathogenesis of the hemorrhages and infarcts frequently found in these contraceptive steroid-related tumors.[253]

PERISINUSOIDAL CELL REACTIONS

Although the perisinusoidal cells (perisinusoidal lipocytes, fat storing cells, Ito cells) are generally regarded as "sinusoidal" and discussed with endothelial cells and Kupffer cells, their pivotal role in vitamin A metabolism, hepatic fibrogenesis, and possibly other functions merits their separate consideration. The cells are located in the space of Disse, and contain fat globules; differences between them and sinusoidal lining cells have been reviewed recently.[257,651] Each perisinusoidal cell generally contains less than 10 fat droplets having a diameter varying from 0.8 μm to 2.9μm.[257] The cells may show transitions to fibroblasts, and are considered to participate in intralobular fibrogenesis,[285,364] although all of the current evidence for this is indirect, and other cells in the liver (including hepatocytes) may also be involved in fibrogenesis.[489] The perisinusoidal cells store vitamin A,[122] which can be detected by its autofluorescence upon ultraviolet microscopy. It has been postulated that the fat stored in these cells may serve as an energy source for hepatocytes.[257]

An increase in the number of perisinusoidal cells has been reported in patients treated with anabolic steroids or corticosteroids,[71] in one case of chlorpromazine jaundice,[71] and in patients receiving chenodeoxycholic acid therapy for the dissolution of gallstones.[24] An increase in both the number and size of the perisinusoidal cells has been observed in alcoholic hepatitis (both during and after recovery),[71] during methotrexate therapy for psoriasis,[237] in human[260,502] and experimental[142,604] hypervitaminosis A, and in experimental animals after long-term exposure to vinyl chloride.[513] Hepatomegaly, abnormal tests of hepatic function, and portal hypertension were reported in two patients with hypervitaminosis A,[502] one of whom subsequently developed cirrhosis.[260] Histologic findings in humans with hypervitaminosis A include an increase in the size and number of perisinusoidal lipocytes, an increase in fibrous tissue in the spaces of Disse, with disruption and atrophy of liver plates, sinusoidal dilatation that is more prominent in central zones, sclerosis of central veins, patchy periportal fibrosis, and chronic portal inflammation (Figs. 17-38 to 17-41). The liver of the

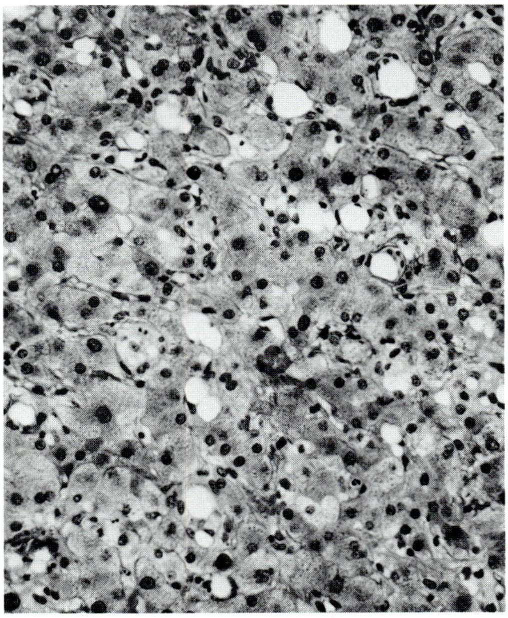

Fig. 17-38. Marked hypertrophy of perisinusoidal lipocytes (vacuolated cells) in hypervitaminosis A. H&E, × 200.

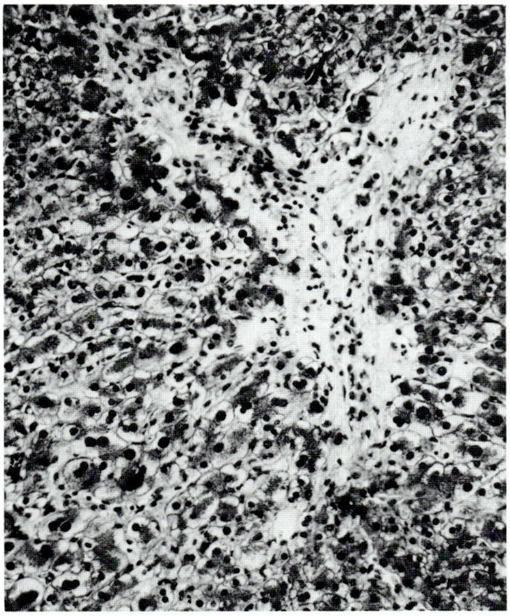

Fig. 17-40. Centrilobular fibrosis in patient with hypervitaminosis A. Masson's trichrome, × 125.

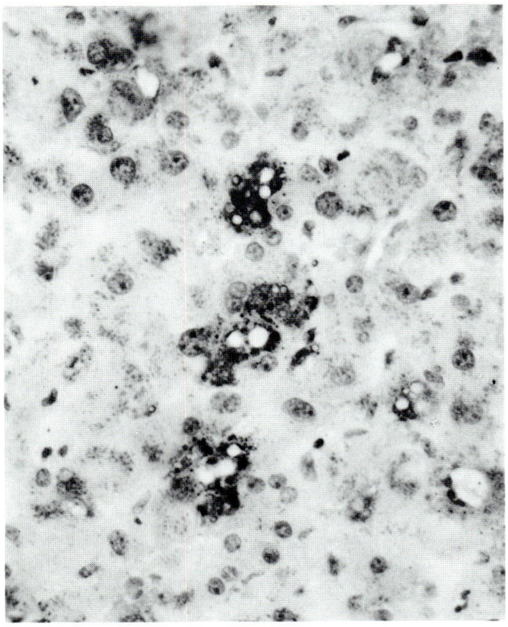

Fig. 17-39. Several darkly stained lipocytes are markedly hypertrophied in case of hypervitaminosis A. The granular pigment is lipofuscin. Frozen section stained with oil red-O, × 320.

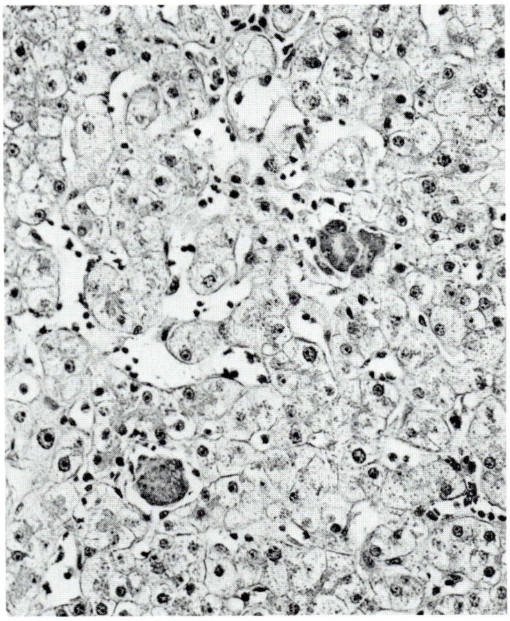

Fig. 17-41. Hypertrophied Kupffer cells contain polyvinylpyrrolidone. H&E, × 200.

cirrhosis patient reported by Jacques et al.[260] showed architectural distortion by the severe fibrosis.

RETICULOENDOTHELIAL REACTIONS

NONGRANULOMATOUS REACTIONS

A number of drugs and foreign materials that gain access to the circulation may be phagocytosed by the reticuloendothelial (RE) system of the liver where they may be retained for months or even years. Some of these substances are associated with no known effects, others may interfere with the phagocytic or immunologic functions of this system, while still others (after a long latent period) may be tumorigenic. Examples of exogenous substances that can accumulate in RE cells of the liver include polyvinyl pyrrolidone (at one time used as a plasma expander and later as a binder or retarding agent in some drugs) (Figs. 17-41 and 17-42), talc and other particulate contaminants in drugs used by intravenous drug abusers, silicone rubber (released into the circulation from damaged or cracked prosthetic devices), and thorotrast (at one time used as a contrast material in radiographic procedures) (Figs. 17-18 and 17-19). Aids in the identification of these materials in tissue sections include the physical appearance of the hypertrophied Kupffer cells and portal macrophages, electron microscopy, special microscopy (for example, phase-contrast or polarizing microscopy), special stains, autoradiography, or energy dispersive x-ray analysis (Table 17-11).

Reticuloendothelial hemosiderosis may be a component of drug-induced hepatocellular injury when such an injury is accompanied by a hemolytic reaction, may result from drug-induced (primaquine, phenylhydrazine) hemolysis in patients with G-6-PD deficiency, or may result from transfusion reactions.[414, 284]

Intravenous fat pigment may accumulate

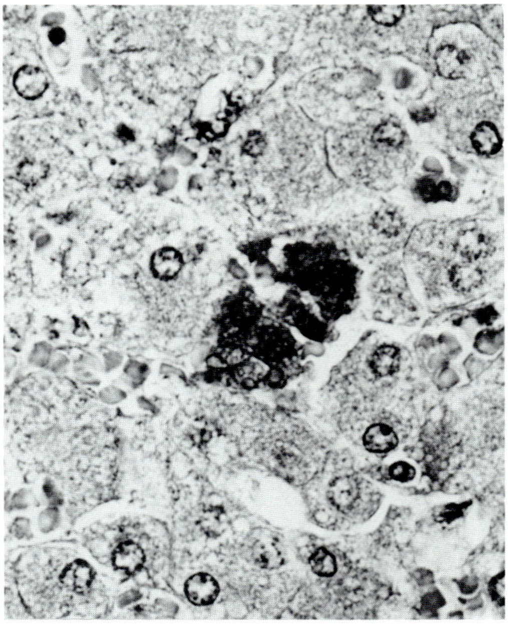

Fig. 17-42. Kupffer cells with polyvinylpyrrolidone show strongly positive staining (black) with Congo red stain. × 640.

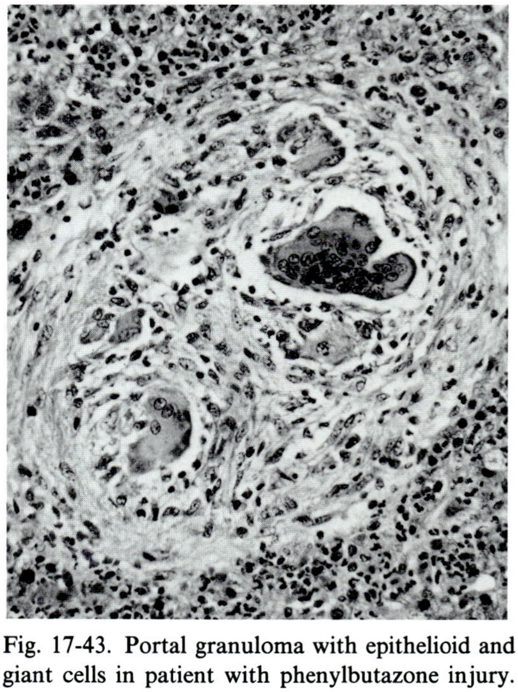

Fig. 17-43. Portal granuloma with epithelioid and giant cells in patient with phenylbutazone injury. H&E, × 200.

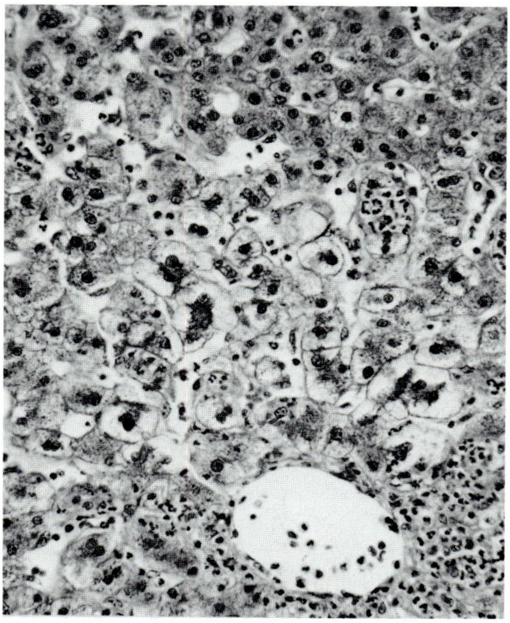

Fig. 17-44. Centrilobular ballooning degeneration in same liver illustrated in Figure 17-43. H&E, × 125.

in Kupffer cells and portal macrophages after infusions of lipid emulsions.[259, 427, 449, 450, 589] The pigment resembles lipofuscin in its physical and staining characteristics, but is said to be birefringent under polarized light.[449] Although the pigment remains in the liver for many months, its long-term sequelae are unknown. Interference with macrophage function has, however, been demonstrated in vitro.[612] More recently, Fischer et al.[304] showed impaired bacterial clearance and enhanced bacterial virulence in mice, as well as the inhibition of human neutrophil chemotaxis in vitro.

Silica, silicates, and anthracotic pigment may accumulate in reticuloendothelial cells of the liver, usually as a result of occupational exposure.[321, 568] In the author's experience, most of the cases of occupational silicosis with liver involvement also demonstrate accumulation of anthracotic pigment. The foreign material may incite the formation of granulomas, which ultimately undergo fibrosis.

Table 17-11. Hepatic Reactions with Reticuloendothelial Storage

Material	Light-microscopy (HE Stain)	Special Stains	Special Procedures	References
Talc	Colorless, needle-shaped or irregular, refractile	—	Polarizing microscopy: birefringent; EDXA*	77, 208, 212, 250
Polyvinyl pyrrolidine	Blue-grey, amorphous	PAS +; Congo red +; Sirius red +	Electron microscopy	80, 178, 475
Silicone rubber	Colorless to light tan, amorphous	—	Polarizing microscopy: birefringent; phase-contrast; EDXA*	213
Thorotrast	Pink-brown, coarsely granular, refractile	—	Autoradiography; EDXA*	58, 299, 586
Hemosiderin	Yellow brown, refractile	Prussian blue+	Atomic absorption; neutron activation analysis	414, 284
Copper	Yellow brown	Rhodanine +; rubeanic acid+	Atomic absorption; neutron activation analysis	449, 450
IV lipid pigment	Light tan, finely granular	PAS +; sudanophilic; autofluorescent	Electron microscopy; polarizing microscopy: birefringent	165, 259, 304, 427, 449, 450, 569, 589, 612
Silica, silicates	Colorless, needle shaped or amorphous	—	Polarizing microscopy: birefringent; EDXA*	93, 321, 347, 419
Anthracotic pigment	Black, finely granular	—	Microincineration	321

* EDXA = Energy-dispersive x-ray analysis.

Table 17-12. Toxic and Drug-Induced Granulomatous Reactions

Type of Injury	Location	Presumed Mechanism	Examples
Pure granuloma	Portal, lobular	Hypersensitivity response	Quinidine, phenylbutazone, gold, beryllium
		Foreign-body reaction	Talc, thorotrast, barium sulfate
Granuloma + hepatocellular injury	Portal, lobular	Hypersensitivity response	Phenylbutazone, hydralazine
Granuloma + hepatocellular + cholestatic injury	Portal, lobular	Hypersensitivity response	Phenylbutazone, diphenylhydantoin, chlordiazepoxide
Granulomatous vasculitis	Portal, perivascular	Hypersensitivity response	Diphenylhydantoin, allopurinol

GRANULOMATOUS REACTIONS

Granulomas may be the sole response to a drug-induced or toxic insult, or they may be a component of other types of injury (Table 17-12). In the majority of cases they are noncaseating or "sarcoid-like," and are scattered in a portal/periportal—and to a lesser extent intralobular—location (Figs. 17–43 and 17–44). An increased number of eosinophils within the granulomas, if present, helps to distinguish drug-induced granulomas from those due to other causes, except those associated with parasites. The presence of larvae, eggs, or parasitic pigment in the latter cases is helpful in making a differential diagnosis. Granulomas related to drugs or toxins are usually transient, and their long-term sequelae are not recorded in the literature. The medicinal and other causes of hepatic granulomas are listed in Tables 17-13 and 17-14.

Table 17-13. Hepatic Granulomas Associated with Therapeutic Agents

Drug	References
Sulfonamides	156, 175, 386, 464
Penicillin	628
Sulfonylurea derivatives	49, 50, 483
Phenylbutazone	255
Oxyphenbutazone	255
Allopurinol	61, 154, 369, 539, 574
Hydralazine	272
Quinidine	62, 85, 181, 226, 301
Halothane	133
Alpha methyldopa	378
Pronestyl	155
Nitrofurantoin	565
Mineral oil	53
BCG vaccination or immunotherapy	52, 176, 201, 244, 525, 551

HYPERPLASIA AND NEOPLASIA

The various benign and malignant tumors of the liver associated with drug therapy or exposure to toxins are listed in Table 17-15.

BENIGN HYPERPLASIA AND NEOPLASIA

Diffuse Hyperplasia

This condition has been noted with the anabolic/androgenic steroids.[421,575] It is postulated that this change could account for the prolapse of hepatocytes into hepatic veins during long-term methyltestosterone therapy.[421]

Nodular "Regenerative" Hyperplasia (Nodular Transformation)

This condition has been reported on patients on anabolic/androgenic steroids[507,576] or oral contraceptives.[63,566] Some cases have

Table 17-14. Hepatic Granulomas Caused by Nonmedicinal Agents

Agent	References
Beryllium	372, 560
Copper	449, 450
Barium	*
Silicone rubber	213
Thorotrast	*
Silica, silicates, anthracotic pigment	93, 165, 321, 347, 419, 451, 568

* Cases on file at the Armed Forces Institute of Pathology, Washington, D.C. 20306.

occurred in patients receiving a number of other drugs, as for example corticosteroids, immunosuppressive, antineoplastic, or antiepileptic drugs, and alcohol,[566] but a cause-and-effect relationship remains to be determined.

Focal Nodular Hyperplasia

An etiologic relationship between this tumor, which can occur in both sexes and at any age, and oral contraceptives is not established, but it is possible that oral contraceptive steroids can exert a trophic effect on pre-existing tumors.[252] Most of the published cases of focal nodular hyperplasia in women taking contraceptive steroids have been included in a number of recent reviews.[294, 300, 626] There are a few instances of this tumor in women who had taken conjugated estrogens.[90, 6]

Hepatocellular Adenoma

An etiologic relationship of hepatocellular adenoma to oral contraceptives is strongly supported by recent epidemiologic studies.[144, 491] Increasing duration of use of oral contraceptives is associated with an increased risk of development of hepatocellular adenoma to about 500-fold in women taking the steroids for 85 or more months.[491] Use of preparations with high hormonal potency and age over 30 years may further increase a woman's risk of developing the tumor.[491]

The annual incidence of hepatocellular adenoma is estimated to be 3 to 4 per 100,000

Table 17-15. Exposure to Drugs and Toxins and Hepatic Neoplasms

	Type of Tumor[a]						
Toxin or Drug	HCA	FNH	NRH	HCC	CCC	AGS	Other
Contraceptive steroids	+++	++	+	++	+	+	Hepatoblastoma, carcinosarcoma
Anabolic steroids	+	−	+	++	+	+	−
Estrogens	−	+	−	−	−	−	−
Corticosteroids	−	−	+	−	−	−	−
Diethylstilbesterol	−	−	−	−	−	+	−
Phenelzine	−	−	−	−	−	+	−
Methotrexate	−	−	−	+	−	−	−
Isoniazid	−	−	−	−	+	−	−
Alcohol	−	−	+	+++	−	−	−
Arsenic	−	−	−	+	−	+++	−
Copper	−	−	+	−	−	+	−
Vinyl chloride	−	−	+	+	−	+++	−
Thorotrast	−	−	+	+++	+++	+++	−
Aflatoxin	−	−	−	?	−	−	−
Polychlorinated biphenyls	−	−	−	+	−	−	−

+++ = well-established association; ++ = cases reported but relationship not definitely established; + = isolated case reports or lesion described with angiosarcoma; − = no cases reported.

[a] HCA = hepatocellular adenoma; FNH = focal nodular hyperplasia; NRH = nodular regenerative hyperplasia; HCC = hepatocellular carcinoma; CCC = cholangiocellular carcinoma; AGS = angiosarcoma.

per year in long-term users of oral contraceptives.[491] The clinicopathologic aspects of the tumor are described in a previous report.[252] It is worth nothing that oral contraceptives are not the sole hormone-associated cause of hepatocellular adenoma: some cases have been attributed to endogenous hyperestrogenemia[391, 629] while others have occurred in persons on anabolic/androgenic steroids.[41, 59, 227, 252, 421]

MALIGNANT NEOPLASIA

Hepatocellular Carcinoma

Hepatocellular carcinoma (HCC) has been reported following previous thorotrast administration,[22, 113, 157, 275, 348, 352, 543] with a mean induction period of 19.4 ± 4.0 years.[22] Experimental induction of HCC by ionizing radiation is well recognized,[410, 511, 608] but human cases (other than those related to internally emitted radiation from thorotrast) are rare.[91, 385]

A considerable number of hepatocellular carcinomas have occurred in women who had previously used oral contraceptives.[89, 252, 404, 611] In the reported cases I have reviewed, the average duration of use of oral contraceptives prior to the diagnosis of HCC was 45 months.[252] Of the 19 cases in the series studied by Christopherson and Mays,[89] 12 had died of their disease at the time of writing. There is general agreement that a cause- and effect-relationship of oral contraceptives with HCC remains to be established.

Cases of HCC following anabolic steroid therapy have been reviewed by several authors.[252, 269, 421] Most of the patients had had underlying anemias, especially Fanconi's anemia. While these tumors have been classified as histologically malignant, few have metastasized, and some have regressed following cessation of therapy.

At present, there is no convincing evidence incriminating pesticides (DDT, aldrin, dieldrin, heptachlor) in human hepatocarcinogenesis, although 16 of pesticides have been identified as carcinogens in animals, usually mice.[652] The same holds true for the naturally occurring carcinogens such as the mycotoxins (with the probable exception of aflatoxin,[460, 652]); pyrrolizidine alkaloids; cycasin; safrole; tannic acid[333]; the synthetic carcinogens such as the nitrosamines and nitrosamides; and the chlorinated hydrocarbons[152, 333, 460] (with the possible exception of the polychlorinated biphenyls).[610] Two cases of HCC were encountered during the long-term follow-up of the Yusho mass poisoning that resulted from contamination of cooking oil by polychlorinated biphenyls in Japan in 1968.[610] Some 1,665 persons were affected, and 51 deaths had occurred up to the end of 1977. Eleven of the deaths (35.4 percent) were due to neoplasms, a rate substantially higher than the 21.2 percent mortality rate from neoplasms in the same perfecture. There is one possible case of a hepatocellular carcinoma occurring some 7 years after toxic exposure to carbon tetrachloride.[601]

Considerable epidemiologic evidence implicating both hepatitis B and aflatoxins in the induction of HCC has accumulated in the last few years.[453] Recently, Lutwick[346] has postulated a new role for aflatoxin in the production of HCC. He suggested that in humans, aflatoxin suppresses cell-mediated immunity rather than acting as a primary carcinogen. This effect on the immune system would allow the hepatitis B virus to maintain itself more easily in the liver, with more chronic infection and cirrhosis, leading, in the long run, to a high incidence of HCC.

Exposure to vinyl chloride has generally been associated with angiosarcoma. There are, however, at least three instances of HCC (one occurring concomitantly with an angiosarcoma) recorded in the literature following chronic exposure to vinyl chloride.[123, 190, 447]

Chronic exposure to arsenical compounds (therapeutic or occupational) has been associated with several cases of hepatocellular carcinoma.[103, 126, 268, 658]

A recent survey of workers employed in petroleum refining and petrochemical plants has shown an increased proportionate mortality ratio for cancers of the liver and biliary passages.[593] In another study the proportional cancer mortality ratios for cancers of the esophagus and liver were moderately elevated in workers in the metal polishing and plating industries.[46]

The role of alcohol in hepatocarcinogenesis has recently been reviewed.[521, 605] The consensus is that chronic alcohol abuse is an important risk factor for HCC, but that the mechanism(s) of action remain unclear. Attempts to produce cancer in animals by prolonged feeding of pure alcohol have failed. Various alternative or associated mechanisms have therefore been proposed, such as the occurrence of other carcinogens (such as as fusel oil, nitrosamines) in alcoholic beverages, the effect of alcohol on detoxification and biotransformation by the endoplasmic reticulum, and the secondary effects of immunosuppression and nutritional deficiencies.[521, 605]

The occurrence of malignant tumors in long-term survivors of organ transplants is well established.[236, 433] Several hepatocellular carcinomas and a cholangiocarcinoma have been reported, although the most frequently occurring neoplasms are extrahepatic lymphomas. In the series of renal transplant recipients reported by Hoover and Fraumeni,[236] the risk of developing lymphomas was 35 times higher than normal, as compared to other cancers, which occurred from two-and-a-half to four times more frequently. No specific immunosuppressive measure, either singly or in combination with other factors, has been incriminated thus far in the development of malignant tumors in recipients of organ transplants. In the follow-up study of Kinlen et al.,[291] comparing renal transplant recipients and patients without transplants treated with immunosuppressive drugs (azathioprine, cyclophosphamide or chlorambucil), there was no clear-cut evidence that the drugs were the cause of the increased cancer risk in either group.

Cholangiocellular Carcinoma

Many cases of intrahepatic cholangiocellular carcinoma (CCC) and some carcinomas of the extrahepatic bile ducts following thorotrast administration are recorded in the literature.[22, 107, 113, 157, 196, 275, 387, 630, 647] In two of the cases the CCC had developed simultaneously with an angiosarcoma.[630, 647] External irradiation of rats has led to CCC.[410] An excess risk for intrahepatic CCC and adenocarcinoma of the biliary passages has been determined in workers in the nonelectrical machinery and primary metal industries.[239] Cases of intrahepatic CCC have been rarely reported in patients receiving contraceptive or anabolic steroids.[151, 157, 337, 567] Adenocarcinoma of the extrahepatic bile ducts have developed in two patients, 2 and 18 years, respectively, after therapy with isoniazid.[338] It should be noted, however, that a recent epidemiologic study has shown no difference in mortality from all cancer and from cancer in individual sites (except for esophageal cancer in males) between 41,226 tuberculous patients treated with isoniazid and controls.[240]

Combined Cholangiocellular and Hepatocellular Carcinoma

There are several published examples of this tumor in women who had been on oral contraceptives.[157, 418]

Carcinosarcoma

Tumors with sarcomatous and epithelial elements have been reported in two users of oral contraceptives.[315, 373]

Angiosarcoma

Angiosarcoma has been reported in patients who had received thorotrast, a contrast medium containing radioactive thorium dioxide, and the use of which was discontinued in the early 1950s. The latent period for induction of angiosarcomas is about 20 years[112]; most of the reported cases are included in a previous review.[251] The largest series have been reported from Portugal,[112,113] but relatively large series have been collected in other countries, including Japan,[387] Denmark,[157] the United Kingdom,[25] and the United States.[158,584]

There is a well-established association between long-term exposure to vinyl chloride and angiosarcoma of the liver.[223,261,592] In cases investigated in the United States, the average length of time between initial vinyl chloride work and the diagnosis of angiosarcoma has been 20.3 years.[223]

Other than cases related to previous exposure to thorotrast and vinyl chloride, there are multiple cases of angiosarcoma that have been related to arsenic.[268,319,470,474,496,658] Isolated cases have been attributed to exposure to copper[450] and a number of drugs such as diethylstilbesterol,[231] and to anabolic steroids,[22] oral contraceptives,[252] and phenelzine.[110]

The clinicopathologic aspects of 55 cases of angiosarcoma on file at this institution have been reviewed previously.[251] More recently, a comprehensive clinical review of 99 cases called from the literature, together with 4 new cases, was published by Locker et al.[336]

MISCELLANEOUS REACTIONS

Rupture of the Liver

Other than rupture secondary to drug-induced peliosis hepatis or neoplasms, there are several reports of spontaneous rupture of the liver in patients receiving various drugs. Fredrick et al.[668] reported rupture of the right lobe of the liver of a 28-year-old woman who had been on an oral contraceptive preparation for 1 year before, and for 3 months after, full-term pregnancy. Pathologic study of the surgically excised lobe showed necrosis and hemorrhage and hepatic vein thrombosis. In this context it is worth nothing that spontaneous rupture of the liver is a recognized but rare complication of pregnancy.[229,406]

Rupture of the liver of unclear pathogenesis has occurred in some patients on oral anticoagulants[131,484] or on streptokinase therapy for deep vein thrombosis.[405]

Abscess of the Liver

Liver abscesses are a serious complication of temporary hepatic dearterialization combined with the intra-arterial infusion of oncolytic drugs in the treatment of primary or secondary malignancies[32]; it is thought that they develop from secondary infection of the necrotic tumor masses. Several cases of liver abscess following umbilical vein catheterization have been reported in neonates[97,602,644]; it seems likely that these were secondary to portal pyelephlebitis, as was the case in the examples reported by Brans et al.[65]

REFERENCES

1. Abbruzzese, A., & Swanson, J.: Jaundice after therapy with chlordiazepoxide hydrochloride. N. Engl. J. Med. 273:321, 1965.
2. Ablow, R. C., & Effman, E. L.: Hepatic calcifications associated with umbilical vein catheterization in the newborn infant. Am. J. Roentgenol. 114:380, 1972.
3. Abrahams, C., Wheatley, A., Rubenstein, A. H., et al.: Hepatocellular lipofuscin after excessive ingestion of analgesics. Lancet 2:621, 1964.
4. Agnostakis, D., Kamba, A., Petrochilou, V., et al.: Risk of infection associated with umbilical vein catheterization. J. Pediatr. 86:759, 1975.
5. Ajdukiewicz, A. B., Grainger, J., Scheuer, P. J., et al.: Jaundice due to iprindole. Gut 12:705, 1971.
6. Aldinger, K., Ben-Menachem, Y., & Whalen, G.: Focal nodular hyperplasia of the liver associated with high-dosage estrogens. Arch. Intern. Med. 137:357, 1977.
7. Ali, M., Fayemi, A. O., Riolusi, R., et al.:

Hemosiderosis in hemodialysis patients: An autopsy study of 50 cases. J.A.M.A. 244:343, 1980.
8. Alpers, D. H., & Isselbacher, K. J.: Fatty liver: Biochemical and clinical aspects. In: Schiff, L., ed.: Diseases of the Liver, 4th Ed. p. 815. Lippincott, Philadelphia, 1975.
9. Alpert, L. I.: Veno-occlusive disease of the liver associated with oral contraceptives: Case report and review of literature. Hum. Pathol. 7:709, 1976.
10. AMA Drug Evaluations, 4th Ed. American Medical Association, Chicago, 1980.
11. Anderson, R. J.: Severe reaction associated with sulindac administration. N. Engl. J. Med. 300:735, 1979.
12. Ansfield, F. J.: Clinical studies with mithramycin. Oncology 23:283, 1969.
13. Antreasian, B., Roth, M. I., & Tavel, M. E.: Toxic hepatitis following the use of phenylbutazone (Butazoliden): Report of a fatal case. J. Indiana Med. Assoc. 51:761, 1958.
14. Asbury, R. F., Rosenthal, S. N., Descalzi, M. E., et al.: Hepatic veno-occlusive disease due to DTIC. Cancer 45:2670, 1980.
15. Ayd, F. J., Jr.: Perphenazine: A reappraisal after eight years. Dis. Nerv. Syst. 25:311, 1964.
16. Baerg, R. D., & Kimberg, D. V.: Centrilobular hepatic necrosis and acute renal failure in "solvent sniffers." Ann. Intern. Med. 73:713, 1970.
17. Baird, R. W., & Hull, J. G.: Cholestatic jaundice from tolbutamide. Ann. Intern. Med. 53:194, 1960.
18. Balazs, M.: Electron microscopic study of benign hepatoma and icterus in patients on oral contraceptives. Virchows Arch. [Pathol. Anat.] 381:97, 1978.
19. Bandt, C. J., & Hoffbauer, F. W.: Liver injury associated with tranylcypromine therapy. J.A.M.A. 188:752, 1964.
20. Barker, J. D., de Carle, D. J., & Anuras, S.: Chronic excessive acetaminophen use and liver damage. Ann. Intern. Med. 87:299, 1977.
21. Bartoli, E., Massarelli, G., Solinas, A., et al.: Acute hepatitis with bridging necrosis due to hydralazine intake. Arch. Intern. Med. 139:698, 1979.
22. Baserga, R., Yookoo, H., & Hennigar, G. C.: Thorotrast-induced cancer in man. Cancer 13:1021, 1960.
23. Bass, B. H.: Jaundice associated with naproxen. Lancet 1:998, 1974.
24. Bateson, M. C., Hopwood, D., & Bouchier, I. A. D.: Effect of gallstone-dissolution therapy on human liver structure. Am. J. Digest Dis. 22:293, 1977.
25. Baxter, P. J., Langlands, A. O., Anthony, P. O., et al.: Angiosarcoma of the liver: A marker tumour for the late effects of thorotrast in Great Britain. Br. J. Cancer 41:446, 1980.
26. Beale, E. F., Nelson, R. M., Bucciarelli, R. L., et al.: Intrahepatic cholestasis associated with parenteral nutrition in premature infants. Pediatrics 64:342, 1979.
27. Beattie, A. D., Mullin, P. J., Baxter, R. H., et al.: Acute lead poisoning: An unusual cause of hepatitis. Scot. Med. J. 24:318, 1979.
28. Beeley, L., Gourevitch, A., & Kendall, M. J.: Jaundice after oral penicillin. Lancet 2:1297, 1976.
29. Beer, D. T., & Schaffner, F.: Fatal jaundice after administration of betaphenylisopropylhydrazine: Report of a case. J.A.M.A. 171:887, 1959.
30. Beermann, B., Ericsson, J. L. E., Hellstrom, K., et al.: Transient cholestasis during treatment with ajmaline, and chronic xanthomatous cholestasis after administration of ajmaline, methyltestosterone and ethinylestradiol. Acta Med. Scand. 190:241, 1971.
31. Benack, R. T., & Lynch, V.: Jaundice associated with iso-carboxazid therapy. N. Engl. J. Med. 264:294, 1961.
32. Bengmark, S., & Fredlund, P. E.: Temporary dearterialization combined with intra-arterial infusion of oncolytic drugs in the treatment of liver tumors. Progr. Clin. Cancer 7:207, 1978.
33. Berk, P. D., Martin, J. F., Young, R. S., et al.: Vinylchloride-associated liver disease. Ann. Intern. Med. 84:717, 1976.
34. Berkowitz, D., Rotman, M., Greenstein, R. H., et al.: Occurrence of jaundice during perphenazine and betaphenylisopropyl-hydrazine. Am. J. Digest Dis. 6:160, 1961.
35. Bernstein, J., Chang, C. H., Brough, A. J., et al.: Conjugated hyperbilirubinemia in infancy associated with parenteral alimentation. J. Pediatr. 90:361, 1977.
36. Bernstein, M. S., Hunter, R. L., Yachnin, S., et al.: Hepatoma and peliosis hepatis develop-

ing in a patient with Fanconi's anemia. N. Engl. J. Med. 284:1135, 1971.
37. Beschorner, W. E., Pino, J. L., Boitnott, J. K., et al.: Liver pathology following bone marrow transplantation. Lab. Invest. 40:5A, 1979.
38. Biagi, R. W., & Bapat, B. N.: Intrahepatic obstructive jaundice from amitriptyline. Br. J. Psychiatry 113:1113, 1967.
39. Biggs, J. C., Chesterman, C. N., & Holliday, J.: L-asparaginase-clinical experience in leukemia, lymphoma and carcinoma. Aust. N.Z. J. Med. 1:1, 1971.
40. Binns, C. H. B.: Vinyl chloride: A review. J. Soc. Occup. Med. 29:134, 1979.
41. Bird, D., Vowles, K., & Anthony, P. P.: Spontaneous rupture of a liver cell adenoma after long term methyltestosterone. Br. J. Surg. 66:212, 1979.
42. Bjorneboe, M., Iversen, O., & Olsen, S.: Infective hepatitis and toxic jaundice in a municipal hospital during a five-year period. Acta Med. Scand. 182:491, 1967.
43. Black, M.: Acetaminophen hepatoxicity. Gastroenterology 78:382, 1980.
44. Black, M., Mitchell, J. R., Zimmerman, H. J., et al.: Isoniazid-associated hepatitis in 114 patients. Gastroenterology 69:289, 1975.
45. Black, M., Rabin, L., & Schatz, N.: Nitrofurantoin-induced chronic active hepatitis. Ann. Intern. Med. 92:62, 1980.
46. Blair, A.: Mortality among workers in the metal polishing and plating industry, 1951-1969. J. Occup. Med. 22:158, 1980.
47. Blendis, L., Smith, P. M., Lavine, B. W., et al.: Portal hypertension in vinyl chloride monomer workers. Gastroenterology 75:206, 1978.
48. Block, S. L.: Jaundice following thioridazine administration. Am. J. Psychiatry 119:77, 1962.
49. Bloodworth, J. M. B., Jr.: Morphologic changes associated with sulfonylurea therapy. Metabolism 12:287, 1963.
50. Bloodworth, J. M. B., Jr., & Hamwi, G. J.: Histopathologic lesions associated with sulfonylurea administration. Diabetes 10:90, 1961.
51. Boake, W. C., Schade, S. G., Morrissey, J. F., et al.: Intrahepatic cholestatic jaundice of pregnancy followed by Enovid-induced cholestatic jaundice. Ann. Intern. Med. 63:302, 1965.
52. Bodurtha, A., Kim, Y. H., Laucius, J. F., et al.: Hepatic granulomas and other hepatic lesions associated with BCG immunotherapy for cancer. Am. J. Clin. Pathol. 61:747, 1974.
53. Boitnott, J. K., & Margolis, S.: Saturated hydrocarbons in human tissues. III. Oil droplets in the liver and spleen. Johns Hopkins Med. J. 127:65, 1970.
54. Bonkowsky, H. L., Mudge, G. H., & McMurty, R. J.: Chronic hepatic inflammation and fibrosis due to low doses of paracetemol. Lancet 1:1016, 1978.
55. Bothwell, T. H., & Charlton, R. W.: Dietary iron overload. In: Kief, H., ed.: Iron Metabolism and Its Disorders. p. 221. American Elsevier, New York, 1975.
56. Boure, M. D., & McKenzie, D.: Diethylene glycol poisoning in children. S. Afr. Med. J. 46:931, 1972.
57. Bourgeois, C., Olson, L., Comer, D., et al.: Encephalopathy and fatty degeneration of the viscera: A clinicopathologic analysis of 40 cases. Am. J. Clin. Pathol. 56:558, 1971.
58. Bowen, J. H., Woodward, B. H., Mossler, J. A., et al: Energy dispersive x-ray detection of thorium dioxide. Arch. Pathol. Lab. Med. 104:459, 1980.
59. Boyd, P. R., & Mark, G. J.: Multiple hepatic adenomas and a hepatocellular carcinoma in a man on oral methyl testosterone for eleven years. Cancer 40:1765, 1977.
60. Boyer, J. L.: Androgenic-anabolic steroid associated peliosis hepatis in man: A review of 38 reported cases. In: Olive, G., ed.: Advances in Pharmacology and Therapeutics, Vol. 8. p. 175. Pergamon Press, Oxford, 1979.
61. Boyer, T. D., Sun, N., & Reynolds, T. B.: Allopurinol-hypersensitivity vasculitis and liver damage. West. J. Med. 126: 143, 1977.
62. Bramlet, D. E., Posalaky, Z., & Olson, R.: Granulomatous hepatitis as a manifestation of quinidine hypersensitivity. Arch. Intern. Med. 140:395, 1980.
63. Brander, W. L., Vosnides, G., Ogg, C. S., et al: Multiple hepatocellular tumours in a patient treated with oral contraceptives. Virchows Arch. [Pathol. Anat.] 370:69, 1976.
64. Brandes, J. W., Schintz-Moormann, P., Lehmann, F. G., et al: Gelbsucht nach Aprindin. Eine hepatitisahnliche Arzneimittel—schadigung. Dtsch. Med. Wochenschr. 101:111, 1976.

65. Brans, Y. W., Ceballos, R., Cassady, G., et al: Umbilical catheters and hepatic abscesses. Pediatrics 53:264, 1974.
66. Bras, G.: Aspects of hepatic vascular diseases. In: Gall, E. A. and Mostofi, F. K., eds.: The Liver. p. 406. Williams & Wilkins, Baltimore, 1973.
67. Bras, G., & Brandt, K. H.: Vascular disorders. In: MacSween, R. N. M., Anthony, P. P., & Scheuer, P. J., eds.: Pathology of the Liver. p. 315. Churchill Livingstone, Edinburgh, 1979.
68. Bras, G., Jeliffe, D. B., & Stuart, K. L.: Veno-occlusive disease of liver with non-portal type of cirrhosis, occurring in Jamaica. Arch. Pathol. 57:285, 1954.
69. Briggs, W. A., Lazarus, M., Birtch, A. G., et al: Hepatitis affecting hemodialysis and transplant patients. Arch. Intern. Med. 132: 21, 1973.
70. Brodsky, I., Johnson, H., Killman, S. A., et al: Fibrosis of central and hepatic veins and perisinusoidal spaces of the liver following prolonged administration of urethane. Am. J. Med. 30:976, 1961.
71. Bronfenmajer, S., Schaffner, F., & Popper, H.: Fat-storing cells (lipocytes) in human liver. Arch. Pathol. 82:447, 1966.
72. Brooks, S. E. H., Miller, C. G., McKenzie, K., et al: Acute veno-occlusive disease of the liver: Fine structure in Jamaican children. Arch. Pathol. 89:507, 1970.
73. Brown, C. A., & Halpert, B.: Poisoning with yellow phosphorous. South. Med. J. 50:740, 1957.
74. Brunson, J. G., Eckman, P. L., & Campbell, J. B.: Increasing prevalence of unexplained liver necrosis. N. Engl. J. Med. 257:52, 1957.
75. Bullivant, C. M.: Accidental poisoning by paraquat: Report of two cases. Br. Med. J. 1:1272, 1966.
76. Burkhardt, A., & Kloppel, G.: Unusual obliterative disease of the hepatic veins in an infant. Virchows Arch. [Pathol. Anat.] 375:225, 1977.
77. Buschmann, R. J., & Mir, J.: Electron microscopic identity of talc in the liver of a narcotic addict. Hum. Pathol. 10:736, 1979.
78. Butler, R. C., Shah, S. M., Grunow, W. A., et al: Massive hepatic necrosis in a patient receiving allopurinol. J.A.M.A. 237:473, 1977.
79. Butscher, W. C., & Gallager, H. S.: Fatal hepatic necrosis occurring during therapy with phethenylate sodium. J.A.M.A. 148, 535, 1952.
80. Cabanne, F., Michiels, R., Dusserre, P., et al: La maladie polyvinylique. Ann. Anat. Pathol. 14:419, 1969.
81. Cacioppo, J., & Merlis, S.: Chlordiazepoxide hydrochloride (Librium) and jaundice: Report of a case. Am. J. Psychiatry 117:1040, 1961.
82. Carmichael, G. P., Targoff, C., Pintar, K., et al: Hepatic silicosis. Am. J. Clin. Pathol. 73:720, 1980.
83. Carney, F. M. T., & Van Dyke, R. A.: Halothane hepatitis: A critical review. Anesth. Analg. (Cleve.) 51:135, 1972.
84. Catterall, R. D.: Fatal reaction to phenylbutazone in a patient with Reiter's disease. Brit. J. Vener. Dis. 44:151, 1968.
85. Chajek, T., Lehrer, B., Geltner, D., et al: Quinidine-induced granulomatous hepatitis. Ann. Intern. Med. 81:744, 1974.
86. Chaves-Carballo, E., Ellefson, R. D., & Gomez, M. R.: An alfatoxin in the liver of a patient with Reye-Johnson syndrome. Mayo Clin. Proc. 51:48, 1976.
87. Chiprut, R. O., Viteri, A., Jamroz, C., et al: Intrahepatic cholestasis after griseofulvin administration. Gastroenterology 70:1141, 1976.
88. Christensen, N. A., Anchor, R. W. P., Berge, K. G., et al: Nicotinic acid treatment of hypercholesterolemia. J.A.M.A. 177:546, 1961.
89. Christopherson, W. M., & Mays, E. T.: Relation of steroids to liver oncogenesis. In: Lapis, W., & Johannessen, J., eds.: Liver Carcinogenesis. p. 207. Hemisphere Publishing Corp., Washington, D.C., 1979.
90. Christopherson, W. M., Mays, E. T., & Barrows, G.: A clinicopathologic study of steroid-related tumors. Am. J. Surg. Pathol. 1:31, 1977.
91. Chudecki, B.: Primary cancer of the liver following treatment of polycythemia vera with radioactive phosphorus. Br. J. Radiol. 45:770, 1972.
92. Chuttanni, M. K., Gupta, P. S., Gulati, S., et al: Acute copper sulfate poisoning. Am. J. Med. 39:849, 1965.
93. Cisno, F., Azzaline, M., & Camagna, M. T.: Considerazioni su 16 casi di silicosi del fegato e della milza. Med. Lav. 62:378, 1971.

94. Citron, B. P., Halpern, M., McCarson, M., et al: Necrotizing angiitis associated with drug abuse. N. Engl. J. Med. 283:1003, 1970.
95. Clarke, R., Borirakchanyavat, V., Davidson, A. R., et al: Hepatic damage and death from overdose of paracetamol. Lancet 1:66, 1973.
96. Cohen, C., & Olsen, M. M.: Liver histopathology with pediatric total parenteral nutrition. Lab Invest. 42:98(A), 1980.
97. Cohen, J. J., & Presner, S.: Liver abscess following exchange transfusion for erythroblastosis fetalis. Q. Rev. Pediatr. 16:148, 1961.
98. Combes, B., Whalley, P. J., & Adams, R. H.: Tetracycline and the liver. Progr. Liver Dis. 4:589, 1972.
99. Conn, H. O., Binder, H. J., & Orr, H. O.: Ethionamide-induced hepatitis: A review with a report of an additional case. Am. Rev. Resp. Dis. 90:542, 1964.
100. Cook, G. C., & Sherlock, S.: Jaundice and its relation to therapeutic agents. Lancet 1:175, 1965.
101. Cooksley, W. G. E., Cowen, A. E., & Powell, L. W.: The incidence of oxyphenisatin ingestion in chronic active hepatitis: A prospective controlled study of 29 patients. Aust. N.Z.J. 3:124, 1973.
102. Cousins, M. J.: Halothane hepatitis: What's new? Drugs 19:1, 1980.
103. Cowlishaw, J. L., Pollard, E. J., Cowen, A. E., et al: Liver disease associated with chronic arsenic ingestion. Austral. N.Z.J. Med. 9: 310, 1979.
104. Craddock, W. L.: Use of phenacemide in epilepsy, with analysis of fatal reactions and case report. J.A.M.A. 159:1437, 1958.
105. Cullberg, G., Lundstrom, R., & Stenram, U.: Jaundice during treatment with an oral contraceptive, Lyndiol. Br. Med. J. 1:695, 1965.
106. Dahl, M. G. C., Gregory, M. M., & Schuer, P. J.: Liver damage due to methotrexate in patients with psoriasis. Br. Med. J. 1:625, 1971.
107. Dahlgren, S.: Thorotrast tumours. Acta Pathol. Microbiol. Scand. 53:147, 1961.
108. Daikos, G. K., & Kosmidis, J. C.: Propoxyphene jaundice. J.A.M.A. 232:835, 1975.
109. Dalén, E., & Westerholm, B.: Occurrence of hepatic impairment in women jaundiced by oral contraceptives and in their mothers and sisters. Acta Med. Scand. 195:459, 1974.
110. Daneshmend, T. K., Scott, G. L., & Bradfield, J. W. B.: Angiosarcoma of liver associated with phenelzine. Br. Med. J. 6:1679, 1979.
111. Dargie, H. J., & Dollery, C. T.: Adverse reactions to diuretic drugs. In: Dukes, M. N. G., ed.: Meyler's Side Effects of Drugs, Vol. 8. p. 483. American Elsevier, New York, 1975.
112. da Silva Horta, J., Abbott, J. D., da Motta, L. C., et al: Malignancy and other late effects following administration of thorotrast. Lancet 2:201, 1965.
113. da Silva Horta, J., da Silva Horta, M. F., da Motta, L. C., et al: Malignancies in Portuguese thorotrast patients. Hlth. Phys. 35:137, 1978.
114. Datey, K. K., Deshmukh, S. N., Dalvi, C. P., et al: Hepatocellular damage with ethacrynic acid. Br. Med. J. 2:152, 1967.
115. Datta, D. V., Mitra, S. K., Chhuttani, P. N., et al: Chronic arsenic intoxication as a possible aetiological factor in idiopathic portal hypertension (noncirrhotic portal fibrosis) in India. Gut 20:378, 1979.
116. Davidson, C. S., Leevy, C. M., & Chamberlayne, E. C.: Guidelines for Detection of Hepatotoxicity due to Drugs and Chemicals. U.S. Government Printing Office, Washington, D.C., 1978.
117. Davis, M., Eddleston, A. L. W. F., & Williams, R.: Hypersensitivity and jaundice due to azathioprine. Postgrad. Med. J. 56:274, 1980.
118. Dayan, A. D., & Lewis, P. D.: Idoxuridine and jaundice. Lancet 2:1073, 1969.
119. Degott, C., Rueff, B., Kreis, H., et al: Peliosis hepatis in recipients of renal transplants. Gut 19:748, 1978.
120. de la Iglesia, F. A., Feuer, G., Takada, A., et al: Morphologic studies on secondary phospholipidosis in human liver. Lab. Invest. 30:539, 1974.
121. Delchier, J. C., Métreau, J. M., Lévy, V. G., et al: L'oxyphenisatine, laxatif responsable d'hepatities chroniques et de cirrhoses—toujours commercialise en France. Presse Med. 8:2955, 1979.
122. deLorimier, A. E., Gordan, G. S., Lowe, R. C., et al: Methyltestosterone related steroids, and liver function. Arch. Intern. Med. 116:289, 1965.
123. Delorme, F.: Association d'un angiosarcome du foice et d'un hepatome chez un ouvrier

du chlorure de vinyle. Ann. Anat. Pathol. 23:105, 1978.

124. den Boer, W., & Loechiger, E. A.: Phenprocoumon-induced jaundice. Lancet 1:912, 1976.

125. Dencker, S. J., Enoksson, P., & Persson, S.: Pigment deposits in various organs during phenothiazine treatment. Acta Psychiatr. Scand. 43:21, 1967.

126. Denk, R., Holzmann, H., Lange, H. J., et al: Leber Arsenspatchaden bei obduzorten Moselwinzern. Die Med. Welt. 11:557, 1979.

127. Diaz-Rivera, R. S., Collazo, P. J., Pons, E. R., et al: Acute phosphorous poisoning in man: A study of 56 cases. Medicine 29:269, 1950.

128. Dietrichson, O., Juhl, F., Nielsen, J. O., et al: The incidence of oxyphenisatin-induced liver damage in chronic non-alcoholic liver disease: A controlled investigation. Scand. J. Gastroenterol. 9:473, 1974.

129. Dipple, P. E., & Williams, D. M.: Hepatitis caused by the newer amine-oxidase-inhibiting drugs. Lancet 2:1459, 1961.

130. Dirschmid, K., & Kiesler, J.: Die Morphologie der leber bei der Anthrakosilikose. Leber, Magen, Darm 10:115, 1980.

131. Dizadji, H., Hammer, R., Strazyz, B., et al: Spontaneous rupture of the liver: A complication of oral anticoagulant therapy. Arch. Surg. 114:734, 1979.

132. Dooner, H. P., Hoyl, C., Aliaga, C., et al: Jaundice and oral contraceptives. Acta Hepatosplenol. 18:84, 1971.

133. Dordal, E., Glagov, S., Orlando, R. A., et al: Fatal halothane hepatitis with transient granulomas. N. Engl. J. Med. 283:357, 1970.

134. Drenckhahn, D., Kleine, L., & Lullmann-Rauch, R.: Lysosomal alterations in cultured macrophages exposed to anorexigenic and psychotropic drugs. Lab. Invest. 35:116, 1976.

135. Drerup, A. L., Alexander, W. A., Lumb, G. D., et al: Jaundice occurring in a patient treated with chlorothiazide. N. Engl. J. Med. 259:534, 1958.

136. Duhovne, C. A., Chan, C. H., & Zimmerman, H. J.: Sulfonamide hepatic injury. N. Engl. J. Med. 277:785, 1967.

137. Dukes, M. N. G.: Meyler's Side Effects of Drugs, Vol. 8. Excerpta Medica, Amsterdam, Oxford, 1975.

138. Dukes, M. N. G.: Meyler's Side Effects of Drugs: Annual 1. Excerpta Medica, Amsterdam, Oxford, 1977.

139. Dukes, M. N. G.: Meyler's Side Effects of Drugs: Annual 2. Excerpta Medica, Amsterdam, Oxford, 1978.

140. Dustin, M. P.: Intoxication mortelle par la colchicine: Etude histologique et hématologique. Bull. Acad. R. Med. Belg. 6:505, 1941.

141. Dutra, F. R.: The pneumonitis and granulomatosis peculiar to beryllium workers. Am. J. Pathol. 24:1137, 1948.

142. Earnest, D., Chvapil, M., Kanun, C., et al: Treatment with vitamin A and BCG increases hepatic collagen. Gastroenterology 77:10(A), 1979.

143. Edmondson, H. A.: Seminar on Diseases of the Liver. American Society for Clinical Pathology, Chicago, 1968.

144. Edmondson, H. A., Henderson, B. E., & Benton, B.: Liver-cell adenomas associated with use of oral contraceptives. N Engl. J. Med. 294:470, 1976.

145. Edmondson, H. A., Peters, R. L., Frankel, H. H., et al: The early stage of liver injury in the alcoholic. Medicine 46:119, 1967.

146. Edmondson, H. A., Peters, R. L., Reynolds, T. B., et al: Sclerosing hyaline necrosis in the chronic alcoholic: A recognizable clinical syndrome. Ann. Intern. Med. 59:646, 1963.

147. Egan, E. A., & Eitzman, D. V.: Umbilical vessel catheterization. Am. J. Dis. Child. 121:213, 1971.

148. Eimas, A.: Methyl salicylate poisoning in an infant. J. Pediatr. 13:550, 1938.

149. Einhorn, M., & Davidsohn, I.: Hepatotoxicity of mercaptopurine. J.A.M.A. 188:802, 1964.

150. Eisen, H. J., & Ginsberg, A. L.: Disulfiram hepatotoxicity. Ann. Intern. Med. 83:673, 1975.

151. Ellis, E. F., Gordon, P. R., & Gottlieb, L. S.: Oral contraceptives and cholangiocarcinoma. Lancet 1:207, 1978.

152. Enat, R., Pollack, S., Ben-Arieh, Y., et al: Cholestatic jaundice caused by cloxacillin: Macrophage inhibition factor test in preventing rechallenge with hepatotoxic durgs. Br. Med. J. 1:982, 1980.

153. Engleman, E. P., Krupp, M. A., Rinehart, J. F., et al: Hepatitis following the ingestion of phenylbutazone. J.A.M.A. 156:98, 1954.

154. Espiritu, C. R., Alalu, J., Glueckauf, L. G.,

et al: Allopurinol-induced granulomatous hepatitis. Am. J. Digest. Dis. 21:804, 1976.
155. Espiritu, C. R., Alalu, J. V., & Lubin, J.: Pronestyl induced granulomatous hepatitis. Gastroenterology 73:1219A, 1977.
156. Espiritu, C. R., Kim, T. S., & Levine, R. A.: Granulomatous hepatitis associated with sulfadimethoxine hypersensitivity. J.A.M.A. 202:161, 1976.
157. Faber, M.: Malignancies in Danish thorotrast patients. Hlth. Phys. 35:153, 1978.
158. Falk, H., Telles, N. C., Ishak, K. G., et al: Epidemology of thorotrast-induced hepatic angiosarcoma in the United States. Environ. Res. 18:65, 1979.
159. Falk, H., Thomas, L. B., Popper, H., et al: Hepatic angiosarcoma associated with androgenic-anabolic steroids. Lancet 2:1120, 1979.
160. Farid, Z., Smith, J. H., Bassily, S., et al: Hepatotoxicity after treatment of schistosomiasis with hycanthone. Br. Med. J. 1:88, 1972.
161. Fedotin, M. S., & Lefer, L. G.: Liver disease caused by propylthiouracil. Arch. Intern. Med. 135:319, 1975.
162. Feinman, L., Rubin, E., & Lieber, C. S.: Adaptation of the liver to drugs. In: Orlandi, F., & Jezequel, A. M., eds.: Liver and Drugs. p. 41. Academic Press, London, 1972.
163. Fenech, F. F., Bannister, W. H., & Gretch, J. L.: Hepatitis with biliverdinemia in association with indomethacin therapy. Br. Med. J. 3:155, 1967.
164. Fenton, P. H., & Howitt, G.: Fatal jaundice after administration of pheniprazine. Br. Med. J. 2:1616, 1961.
165. Fischer, G. W., Hunter, K. W., Wilson, S. R., et al: Diminished bacterial defences with intralipid. Lancet 2:819, 1980.
166. Fischer, M. G., Nayer, H. R., & Miller, A.: Methimazole-induced jaundice. J.A.M.A. 223:1028, 1973.
167. Fisher, J. H.: Fatal phenylbutazone hepatitis. Can. Med. Assoc. J. 83:1211, 1960.
168. Fletcher, G. F., & Galambos, J. T.: Phosphorous poisoning in humans. Arch. Intern. Med. 112:846, 1963.
169. Flinn, F. B., & Jarvik, N. E.: Liver lesions caused by chlorinated naphthalene. Am. J. Hyg. 27:19, 1938.
170. Forbes, J. C., & Evans, E. I.: Tannic acid and liver necrosis. Surg. Gynecol. Obstet. 76:612, 1943.
171. Fors, B., & Nilsson, F.: Hepatitis probably induced by diazepam medication. Laekartidningen 65:4528, 1968.
172. Foss, G. L., & Simpson, S. L.: Oral methyltestosterone and jaundice. Br. Med. J. 1:259, 1959.
173. Fredrick, W. C., Howard, R. G., & Spatola, S.: Spontaneous rupture of the liver in patient using contraceptive pills. Arch. Surg. 108:93, 1974.
174. Freise, J., May, B., & Schmidt, E.: Cholestatischer Ikterus nach Azathioprin. Dtsch. Med. Wochenschr. 101:1223, 1976.
175. French, A. J.: Hypersensitivity in the pathogenesis of the histopathologic changes associated with sulfonamide chemotherapy. Am. J. Pathol. 22:679, 1946.
176. Freundlich, E., & Suprun, H.: Tuberculoid granulomata in the liver after BCG vaccination. Israel. J. Med. Sci. 5:108, 1969.
177. Gall, E. A.: Report of the pathology panel: National Halothane Study. Anesthesiology 29:233, 1968.
178. Gall, E. A., Altemeier, W. A., Schiff, L., et al: Liver lesions following intravenous administration of polyvinyl pyrrolidone (PVP). Am. J. Clin. Pathol. 23:1187, 1953.
179. Gasparetto, P.: Un caso di ittero apatocellulare in corso di trattamento con ibuprofen. Minerva Pediatr. 26:531, 1974.
180. Gedigk, P., Muller, R., & Bechtelsheimer, H.: Morphology of liver damage among polyvinyl chloride production workers: A report of 51 cases. Ann. N. Y. Acad. Sci. 246:278, 1975.
181. Geltner, D., Chajek, T., Rubinger, D., et al: Quinidine hypersensitivity and liver involvement: A survey of 32 patients. Gastroenterology 70:650, 1976.
182. Gerber, M. A., Kaufmann, H., Klion, F., et al: Acetaminophen associated hepatic injury: Report of two cases showing unusual portal tract reactions. Hum. Pathol. 11:37, 1980.
183. Gerber, N., Dickinson, R. C., Harland, R. K., et al: Reye-like syndrome associated with valproic acid therapy. J. Pediatr. 95:142, 1970.
184. Gerok, W., & Sickinger, K.: Drugs and the Liver. Schattauer-Verlag. Stuttgart, 1975.
185. Gilbert, E. F., DaSilva, A., & Queen, D. M.: Intrahepatic cholestasis with fatal termination following norethandrolone therapy. J.A.M.A. 185:538, 1963.

186. Gilbert, F. J.: Cholestatic hepatitis caused by esters of erythromycin and oleandomycin. J.A.M.A. 182:1048, 1962.
187. Gjone, E., Blomhoff, J. P., Ritland, S., et al: Laxative-induced chronic liver disease. Scand. J. Gastroenterol. 7:395, 1972.
188. Gjone, E., & Orning, O. M.: Jaundice due to chloramphemicol. Acta Hepatosplenol. 13:288, 1966.
189. Glober, G. A., & Wilkerson, J. A.: Biliary cirrhosis following the administration of methyltestosterone. J.A.M.A. 204:170, 1968.
190. Gokel, S. M., Liebezeit, E. & Eder, M.: Hemangiosarcoma and hepatocellular carcinoma of the liver following vinyl chloride exposure. Virch. Arch. [Pathol. Anat.] 372:195, 1976.
191. Goldfinger, S. E., & Marx, S. E.: Hypersensitivity hepatitis due to phenazopyridine hydrochloride. N. Engl. J. Med. 286:1090, 1972.
192. Goldstein, G. B., Lam, K. C., & Mistilis, S. P.: Drug-induced active chronic hepatitis. Am. J. Digest. Dis. 18:177, 1973.
193. Goldstein, L. I., & Ishak, K. G.: Hepatic injury associated with penicillin therapy. Arch. Pathol. 98:114, 1974.
194. Goldstein, L. I., Ishak, K. G., & Burns, W.: Hepatic injury associated with nitrofurantoin therapy. Am. J. Digest. Dis. 19:987, 1974.
195. Goldstein, M. J., & Rothenberg, A. J.: Jaundice in a patient receiving acetohexamide. N. Engl. J. Med. 275:97, 1966.
196. Gondos, B.: Late clinical and roentgen observations following thorotrast administration. Clin. Radiol. 24:195, 1973.
197. González-Angulo, A, Aznar-Ramos, R., Marquez-Monter, H., et al.: The ultrastructure of liver cells in women under steroid therapy. I. Normal pregnancy and trophoblastic growths. Acta Endocrinol. 65:193, 1970.
198. González-Angulo, A., & Salazar, H.: Pathology of the reproductive system, breast, and liver in women during hormonal contraception. In: Josimovich, J. B., ed.: Uterine Contraction. p. 343. John Wiley, New York, 1973.
199. Gordon, B. S., Wolf, J. Krause, T., et al: Peliosis hepatis and cholestasis following administration of norethandrolone. Am. J. Clin. Pathol. 33:156, 1960.
200. Graig, R. M., Neumann, T., Jeejeebhoy, K. N., et al: Severe hepatocellular reaction resembling alcoholic hepatitis with cirrhosis after massive small bowel resection and prolonged total parenteral nutrition. Gastroenterology 79:131, 1980.
201. Grant, R. M., Mackie, R., Cochran, A. J., et al: Results of administering BCG to patients with melanoma. Lancet 2:1096, 1974.
202. Grayson, M. J., & Reilly, M. C. T.: Budd-Chiari syndrome after oral contraceptives. Br. Med. J.: 1:512, 1968.
203. Greenburg, L., Mayers, M. R., & Smith, A. R.: The enzymatic effects resulting from exposure to certain chlorinated hydrocarbons. J. Indust. Hyg. Toxicol. 21:29, 1939.
204. Greenlaw, C. W., Henrietta, G. C., & Stolley, S. N.: Hepatotoxicity possibly associated with erytromycin ethylsuccinate. Drug. Intell. Clin. Pharmacol. 13:236, 1979.
205. Gregory, D. H., Zaki, G. F., Sarcosi, G. A., et al: Chronic cholestasis following prolonged tolbutamide administration. Arch. Pathol. 84:194, 1967.
206. Griener, A. C., & Nicolson, G. A.: Pigment deposition in viscera associated with prolonged chlorpromazine therapy. Can. Med. Assoc. J. 91:627, 1964.
207. Griner, P. F., Elbadawi, A., & Packman, C. H.: Veno-occlusive disease of the liver after chemotherapy of acute leukemia. Ann. Intern. Med. 85:578, 1976.
208. Groth, D. H., Mackay, G. R., Crable, J. V., et al: Intravenous injection of talc in a narcotics addict. Arch. Pathol. 94:171, 1972.
209. Gulley, R. M., Mirza, A., & Kelly, C. E.: Hepatotoxicity of salicylazosulfapyridine: A case report and review of the literature. Am. J. Gastroenterol. 72:561, 1979.
210. Guzelian, P. S., Vranian, G., Boylen, J. J., et al: Liver structure and function in patients poisoned with chlordecone (Kepone). Gastroenterology 78:206, 1980.
211. Haas, P.: Uber einen perakut verlau fenden Fall von Periarteritis nodosa nach Diphenylhydantoin. Wien. Klin. Wochenschr. 79:56, 1967.
212. Hahn, H. H., Schweid, A. I., & Beaty, H. N.: Complications of injecting methylphenidate tablets. Arch. Intern. Med. 123:656, 1969.
213. Hameed, K., Ashfaq, S., & Waugh, D. O. W.: Ball fracture and extrusion in Starr-Edwards aortic valve prosthesis with dissemination of ball material. Arch. Pathol. 86:520, 1968.

214. Hanger, F. M., & Gutman, A. B.: Postarsphenamine jaundice apparently due to obstruction of intrahepatic biliary tract. J.A.M.A. 115:263, 1940.
215. Harinasuta, U., & Zimmerman, H. J.: Diphenylhydantoin sodium hepatitis. J.A.M.A. 203:1015, 1968.
216. Harris, F., Cullity, G., & Lister, J.: Hepatitis following acitnomycin D and irradiation. Proc. R. Soc. Med. 67:756, 1974.
217. Harrison, D. C., Coggins, C. H., Welland, F. H., et al: Mushroom poisoning in five patients. Am. J. Med. 38:787, 1965.
218. Hart, F. D., & Boardman, P. L.: Ibufenac (4-isobutyl phenylacetic acid). Ann. Rheum. Dis. 26:61, 1965.
219. Hartmann, W., Paulini, K., & Goebell, H.: Light and electron microscopy of human liver before and during chenodeoxycholic acid therapy. Hepatol. Gastroenterol. 27:91, 1980.
220. Hatoff, D. E., Cohen, M., Schweigert, B. F., et al: Nitrofurantoin: Another cause of drug-induced chronic active hepatitis? A report of a patient with HLA-B8 antigen. Am. J. Med. 67:117, 1979.
221. Hatzibuyas, Von J., Ueberberg, H., Stoldt, R., et al: Elektron-microskopische Befunde eines malignen Hepatoms nach oraler Kontrazeption. Zeitschr. Gastroenterol. 16:616, 1978.
222. Haubrich, W. S., & Sancetta, S. M.: Spontaneous recovery from hepatobiliary disease with xanthomatosis. Gastroenterology 26:658, 1954.
223. Heath, C. W., Falk, H., & Creech, J. L.: Characteristics of cases of angiosarcoma of the liver among vinyl chloride workers in the United States. Ann. N.Y. Acad. Sci. 246:231, 1975.
224. Heick, H. M. C., Shipman, R. T., Norman, M. G., et al: Reye-like syndrome associated with use of insect repellent in a presumed heterozygote for ornithine carbamoyl transferase deficiency. J. Pediatr. 97:471, 1980.
225. Hennigar, G. R., Greene, W. B., Walker, E. M., et al: Hemochromatosis caused by excessive vitamin iron intake. Am. J. Pathol. 96:611, 1979.
226. Herman, J. E., & Bassan, H. M.: Liver injury due to quinidine. J.A.M.A. 234:310, 1975.
227. Hernandez-Nieto, L., Bruguera, M., Bombi, J. A., et al: Benign liver-cell adenoma associated with long-term administration of an androgenic-anabolic steroid (methandienone). Cancer 40:1761, 1977.
228. Hersh, E. M., Wong, V. G., Henderson, E. S., et al: Hepatotoxic effects of methotrexate. Cancer 19:600, 1966.
229. Hibbard, L. T.: Spontaneous rupture of the liver in pregnancy: A report of eight cases. Am. J. Obstet. Gynecol. 126:334, 1976.
230. Hill, R. B., Jr.: Fatal fat embolism from steroid-induced fatty liver. N. Engl. J. Med. 265:318, 1961.
231. Hoch-Ligeti, C.: Angiosarcoma of the liver associated with diethylstilbesterol. J.A.M.A. 240:1510, 1978.
232. Hoffbrand, B. I., Fry, W., & Bunton, G. L.: Cholestatic jaundice due to methyldopa. Br. Med. J. 2:559, 1974.
233. Hogan, G. R., Ryan, N. J., & Hayes, A. W.: Aflatoxin B, and Reye's syndrome. Lancet 1:561, 1978.
234. Holdsworth, C. D., Atkinson, M., & Goldie, W.: Hepatitis caused by the newer amine-oxidase-inhibiting drugs. Lancet 2:621, 1961.
235. Holdsworth, C. D., Atkinson, M., Dosset, J. A., et al: Hepatitis caused by the newer amine-oxidase-inhibiting drugs. Lancet 2: 1459, 1961.
236. Hoover, R., & Fraumeni, J. F.: Risk of cancer in renal-transplant recipients. Lancet 2:55, 1973.
237. Hopwood, D., & Nyfors, A.: Effect of methotrexate therapy in psoriatics on the Ito cells in liver biopsies, assessed by point-counting. J. Clin. Pathol. 29:698, 1976.
238. Horst, D. A., Grace, N. D., & LeCompte, P. M.: Prolonged cholestasis and progressive hepatic fibrosis following imipramine therapy. Gastroenterology 79:550, 1980.
239. Houten, L., & Sonnesso, G.: Occupational exposure and cancer of the liver. Arch. Environ. Hlth. 35:51, 1980.
240. Howe, G. R., Lindsay, J., Coppock, E., et al: Isoniazid exposure in relation to cancer incidence and mortality in a cohort of tuberculosis patients. Int. J. Epidemiol. 8:305, 1980.
241. Hoyumpa, A. M., & Connell, A. M.: Methyldopa hepatitis: Report of three cases. Am. J. Digest. Dis. 18:213, 1973.
242. Hoyumpa, A. M., Schiff, L., & Helfman, E. L.: Budd-Chiari syndrome in women tak-

ing oral contraceptives. Am. J. Med. 50:137, 1971.

243. Huet, P. M., Guillaume, E., Cote, J., et al: Noncirrhotic perisinusoidal portal hypertension associated with chronic arsenical intoxication. Gastroenterology 68:1270, 1975.
244. Hunt, J. S., Silverstein, J. J. Sparks, F. C., et al: Granulomatous hepatitis: A complication of BCG immunotherapy. Lancet 2:820, 1973.
245. Husebye, K. O.: Jaundice with persisting pericholangiolitic inflammaiton in a patient treated with chlorothiazide. Am. J. Digest. Dis. 9:439, 1964.
246. Hyer, S., & Knell, A. J.: Cirrhosis and haemolysis complicating methyldopa treatment. Br. Med. J. 1:879, 1977.
247. Irey, N. S.: Tissue reaction to drugs. Am. J. Pathol. 82:617, 1976.
248. Irey, N. S., Manion, W. C., & Taylor, H. B.: Vascular lesions in women taking oral contraceptives. Arch Pathol. 89:1, 1970.
249. Irey, N. S., & Norris, H. J.: Intimal vascular lesions associated with female reproductive steroids. Arch. Pathol. 96:227, 1973.
250. Ishak, B. W., & Ishak, K. G.: Foreign-body reaction in the liver of a drug-addict. J. Forensic Sci. 14:515, 1969.
251. Ishak, K. G.: Mesenchymal tumors of the liver. In: Okuda, K., & Peters, R. L., eds: Hepatocellular Carcinoma. p. 247. John Wiley, New York, 1976.
252. Ishak, K. G.: Morphologic hepatic lesions associated with oral contraceptives (O.C.) and anabolic steroids (A. S.). In: Olive, G., ed.: Advances in Pharmacology and Therapeutics, Vol. 8. p. 185. Pergamon Press, Oxford, 1979.
253. Ishak, K. G.: Hepatic neoplasms associated with contraceptive and anabolic steroids. In: Lingeman, C. H., ed.: Carcinogenic Hormones. p. 73. Springer-Verlag, Berlin, 1979.
254. Ishak, K. G., & Irey, N. S.: Hepatic injury associated with the phenothiazines. Arch. Pathol. 93:283, 1972.
255. Ishak, K. G., Kirchner, J. P., & Dhar, J. H.: Granulomas and cholestatic-hepatocellular injury associated with phenylbutazone: Report of two cases. Am. J. Digest. Dis. 22:611, 1977.
256. Isselbacher, J., & Lesser, P. B.: Phenothiazine jaundice. In: Gerok, W., & Sickinger, K., ed.: Drugs and the Liver. p. 359. Schattauer Verlag, Stuttgart, 1975.
257. Ito, T.: Recent advances in the study on the fine structure of the hepatic sinusoidal wall: A review. Gunma Rep. Med. Sci. 6:119, 1973.
258. Iwarson, S., Lindberg, J., & Lundsdin, P.: Nitrofurantoin-induced chronic liver disease: Clinical course and outcome of five cases. Scand. J. Gastroenterol. 14:497, 1979.
259. Jacobson, S., Ericsson, J. L. E., & Obel, A. L.: Histopathological and ultrastructural changes in the human liver during complete intravenous nutrition for seven months. Acta Clin. Scand. 137:335, 1971.
260. Jacques, E. A., Buschmann, R. J., & Layden, T. J.: The histological progression of vitamin A-induced hepatic injury. Gastroenterology 76:599, 1979.
261. Jalota, R., & Freston, J. W.: Severe intrahepatic cholestasis due to thiobendazole. Am. J. Trop. Med. 23:676, 1974.
262. James, O., Lesna, M., Roberts, S. H., et al: Liver damage after paracetamol overdose: Comparison of liver function tests, fasting serum bile acids and liver histology. Lancet 2:579, 1975.
263. Jarzobski, J., Ferry, J., Wombolt, D., et al: Vasculitis with allopurinol therapy. Am. Heart. J. 79:116, 1970.
264. Jennings, R. B.: Fatal fulminant acute carbon tetrachloride poisoning. Arch. Pathol. 59:269, 1955.
265. Jezequel, A. M.: Ultrastructural changes induced by drugs in the liver. In: Taylor, W., ed.: The Hepatobiliary System. p. 179. Plenum Press, London, 1976.
266. Jezequel, A. M., Koch, M. M., Galeazzi, R., et al: Liver response to drugs in man. A correlated morphometric and functional study. In: Leevy, C. M., ed.: Diseases of the Liver and Biliary Tract. p. 153. S. Karger, Basel, 1976.
267. Jezequel, A. M., & Orlandi, F.: Fine morphology of the human liver as a tool in clinical pharmacology. In: Orlandi, F., & Jezequel, A. M., eds.: Liver and Drugs. p. 145. Academic Press, London, 1972.
268. Jhaveri, S. S.: A case of cirrhosis and primary carcinoma of the liver in chronic arsenical intoxication. Br. J. Indust Med. 16:248, 1959.
269. Johnson, F. L.: Androgenic-anabolic steroids and hepatocellular carcinoma. In: Okuda, K.,

& Peters, R. L., eds.: Hepatocellular Carcinoma. p. 95. John Wiley, New York, 1976.
270. Jones, E. A., Clain, D., Clink, H. M., et al: Hepatic coma due to acute necrosis treated by exchange transfusion. Lancet 2:169, 1967.
271. Jones, J. P., Engelman, E. P., & Najarian, J. S.: Systemic fat embolism after renal homotransplantation and treatment with corticosteroids. N. Engl. J. Med. 273:1453, 1965.
272. Jori, G. P., & Peschle, C.: Hydralazine disease associated with transient granulomas in the liver. Gastroenterology 64:1163, 1973.
273. Joron, G. E., Cameron, D. G., Halpenny, G. W., et al: Massive necrosis of the liver due to trichlorethylene. Canad. Med. Assoc. J. 73:890, 1955.
274. Joshi, P. H., & Conn, H. O.: The syndrome of methoxyflurane—associated hepatitis. Ann. Intern. Med. 80:395, 1974.
275. Kahn, H. L.: Two cases of carcinoma after thorotrast administration. Ann. N.Y. Acad. Sci. 145:700, 1967.
276. Kahn, M., & Perez, V.: Jaundice associated with the administration of iproniazid: Report of nine cases. Am. J. Med. 25:898, 1958.
277. Kaplan, A. A.: Jaundice due to methyltestosterone therapy. Gastroenterology 31:384, 1956.
278. Karch, F. E. & Lasagna, L.: Adverse drug reactions: A critical review. J.A.M.A. 234:1236, 1976.
279. Keeffe, E. B., & Smith, F. W.: Disulfiram hypersensitivity hepatitis. J.A.M.A. 230:435, 1974.
280. Kelsey, W. M., & Scharyi, M.: Fatal hepatitis probably due to indomethacin. J.A.M.A. 199:586, 1967.
281. Kemp, J. A.: Jaundice occurring during administration of promazine. Gastroenterology 32:937, 1957.
282. Kennaugh, R. C.: CCl_4 overdosage: A case report. S. Afr. Med. J. 49:635, 1975.
283. Kennedy, B. J.: Metabolic and toxic effects of mithramycin tumor therapy. Am. J. Med. 49:494, 1970.
284. Kent, G., & Bahu, R. M.: Iron overload. In: MacSween, R. N. M., Anthony, P. P., & Scheuer, P. J., eds.: Pathology of the Liver. p. 148. Churchill Livingstone, Edinburgh, 1979.
285. Kent, G., Gray, S., Inouye, T., et al.: Vitamin A—containing hepatocytes and formation of type III collagen in liver injury. Proc. Natl. Acad. Sci. U.S.A. 73:3719, 1976.
286. Kern, W. H., Payne, J. H., & DeWind, L.: Hepatic changes after small-intestinal bypass for morbid obesity. Am. J. Clin. Pathol. 61:763, 1974.
287. Kessler, R. E., Tice, D. A., & Zimmon, D. S.: Value, complications, and limitations of umbilical vein catheterization. Surg. Gynecol. Obstet. 136:529, 1973.
288. Kessler, R. E., & Zimmon, D. S.: Umbilical vein catheterization in man. Surg. Gynecol. Obstet. 124:594, 1967.
289. Kiaer, H. W., Olson, S., & Ronnov-Jessen, V.: Hepatotoxicity of papaverine. Arch. Pathol. 98:292, 1974.
290. King, J. A., & Blount, R. E., Jr.: An unexpected reaction to procainamide. J.A.M.A. 186:603, 1963.
291. Kinlen, L. J., Sheil, A. G. R., & Doll, R.: Collaborative United Kingdom—Australian study of cancer on patients treated with immunosuppressive drugs. Br. Med. J. 2:1461, 1979.
292. Kisilevsky, R.: Hepatic nuclear and nucleolar changes in amanita poisoning. Arch. Pathol. 97:253, 1974.
293. Klatskin, G.: Toxic and drug-induced hepatitis. In: Schiff, L., ed.: Diseases of the Liver. p. 604. Lippincott, Philadelphia, 1975.
294. Klatskin, G.: Hepatic tumors: Possible relationship to use of oral contraceptives. Gastroenterology 73:386, 1977.
295. Klein, N. C., & Magida, M. G.: Propoxyphene (Darvon) hepatotoxicity. Am. J. Digest Dis. 16:467, 1971.
296. Kline, M. M.: Euflurane-associated hepatitis. Gastroenterology 79:126, 1980.
297. Klinge, O., & Bannasch, P.: Zur Vermehrung des glatten endoplasmatischen Retikulum in Hepatocyten Menschlicher Leberpunktate. Verhand. Dtsch. Gesellsch. Pathol 52:568, 1968.
298. Klion, F. M., Schaffner, F., & Popper, H.: Hepatitis after exposure to halothane. Ann. Intern. Med. 71:467, 1969.
299. Kluge, T., & Hovig, T.: Ultrastructural localization of thorotrast in the reticuloendothelial system. Am. J. Pathol. 54:355, 1969.
300. Knowles, D. M., & Wolff, M.: Focal nodular hyperplasia of the liver: A clinicopathologic

study and review of the literature. Hum. Pathol. 7:533, 1976.
301. Koch, M. J., Seeff, L. B., Grumley, C. E., et al.: Quinidine hepatotoxicity: A report of a case and review of the literature. Gastroenterology 70:1136, 1976.
302. Kodagoda, N., Jayewardene, R. P., & Attygalle, D.: Poisoning with paraquat. Forensic Sci. 2:107, 1973.
303. Koff, R. S., Gardner, R., Harinasuta, U., et al.: Profile of hyperbilirubinemia in three hospital populations. Clin. Res. 18:680, 1970.
304. Koga, Y., Svanson, V. L., & Hays, D. M.: Hepatic "intravenous fat pigment" in infants and children receiving lipid emulsion. J. Pediatr. Surg. 10:641, 1978.
305. Kohn, N., & Myerson, R. M.: Cholestatic hepatitis associated with trifluoperazine. N. Engl. J. Med. 264:549, 1961.
306. Kohn, R. M., & Montes, M.: Hepatic fibrosis following long acting nicotinic acid therapy: A case report. Am. J. Med. Sci. 258:94, 1969.
307. Kopelman, H., Scheuer, P. J., & Williams, R.: The liver lesion in Epping jaundice. Q. J. Med. 35:553, 1966.
308. Kosek, J. C., & Smith, D. L.: Cytotoxicity of oxymetholone to endothelial cells *in vitro*. Arch. Pathol. Lab. Med. 104:405, 1980.
309. Kothari, T., Swamy, A. P., Lee, J. C. K., et al.: Hepatic hemosiderosis in maintenance hemodialysis (MHD) patients. Digest. Dis. Sci. 25:363, 1980.
310. Krauss, A. N., Albert, R. F., & Kannan, M. M.: Contamination of umbilical catheters in the newborn infant. J. Pediatr. 77:965, 1970.
311. Krawitt, E. L., Stein, J. H., Kirkendall, M., et al.: Mercaptopurine hepatoxicity in a patient with chronic active hepatitis. Arch. Intern. Med. 120:729, 1967.
312. Kreek, M. J., Weser, E., Sleisenger, M. H., et al.: Idiopathic cholestasis of pregnancy: The response to challenge with the synthetic estrogen, ethinyl estradiol. N. Engl. J. Med. 277:1391, 1967.
313. Krishanmachari, K. A. V. R., Bhat, R. V., Nagarajan, V., et al.: Hepatitis due to aflatoxicosis: An outbreak in Western India. Lancet 1:1061, 1975.
314. Kristinnsson, A.: Fatal reaction of acetazolamide. Br. J. Ophthalmol. 51:348, 1967.
315. Ladaga, L., Kay, S., Melcher, M., et al.: Combined epithelial and sarcomatous elements in a liver cancer associated with oral contraceptive use. Am. J. Surg. Pathol. 3:185, 1979.
316. LaDue, J. S., Schenken, J. R., & Kuker, L. H.: Phosphorous poisoning: A report of 16 cases with repeated liver biopsies in a recovered case. Am. J. Med. Sci. 208:223, 1944.
317. Lai, M., Sung, J., Lin, W., et al.: Biochemical and morphological study of the liver injury induced by drugs and chemicals. J. Formosan Med. Assoc. 78:525, 1979.
318. Land, V. J., Sutow, W. W., Fernbach, D. J., et al.: Toxicity of L-asparaginase in children with advanced leukemia. Cancer 30:339, 1972.
319. Lander, J. J., Stanley, R., Sumner, H. W., et al.: Angiosarcoma of the liver associated with Fowler's solution (potassium arsenite). Gastroenterology 68:1582, 1975.
320. Langlands, A. O., & Martin, W. M. C.: Jaundice associated with norethisterone-acetate treatment of breast cancer. Lancet 1:584, 1975.
321. Langlois, S. de P., Sterrett, G. F., & Henderson, D. W.: Hepatosplenic silicosis. Aust. Radiol. 21:142, 1977.
322. Lansing, A. M., Davis, W. M., & Brizel, H. E.: Radiation hepatitis. Arch. Surg. 96:878, 1968.
323. Larroche, J. C.: Umbilical catheterization: Its complications. Biol. Neonate 16:101, 1970.
324. Larsson-Cohn, U., & Stenram, U.: Jaundice during treatment with oral contraceptive agents: Report of two cases. J.A.M.A. 193:422, 1965.
325. Larsson-Cohn, U., & Stenram, U.: Liver ultrastructure and function in icteric and non-icteric women using oral contraceptive agents. Acta Med. Scand. 181:257, 1967.
326. Law, L. P., & Knight, H.: Jaundice associated with naproxen. N. Engl. J. Med. 295:1201, 1974.
327. Lee, T. J., Carney, C. N., Lapis, J. L., et al.: Diphenylhydantoin-induced hepatic necrosis: A case study. Gastroenterology 70:422, 1976.
328. Lesna, M., Watson, A. J., Douglas, A. P., et al.: Evaluation of paracetamol-induced damage in liver biopsies: Acute changes and follow-up findings. Virchows Arch. [Pathol. Anat.] 370:333, 1976.
329. Levy, R. W., Simons, D. J., & Aronson, S.: Fatal hepatorenal syndrome associated with

phenurone therapy. N. Engl. J. Med. 242:933, 1950.

330. Levy, V. G., Bouma, M. E., Lageron, A., et al.: Hepatic sinusoidal dilatation after chenodeoxycholic-acid therapy. Lancet 1:206, 1978.
331. Lichtenstein, L., & Fox, L. J.: Necrotizing arterial lesions resembling those of periarteritis nodosa and focal visceral necroses following administration of sulfathiazole. Am. J. Pathol. 22:665, 1945.
332. Lichtenstein, M. R., & Cannemeyer, W.: Severe paraminosalicylic acid hypersensitivity simulating mononucleosis or hepatitis. J.A.M.A. 152:606, 1953.
333. Linsell, C. A.: Environmental chemical carcinogens and liver cancer. In: Lapis, K., & Johannessen, J. F., eds.: Liver Carcinogenesis. p. 173. Hemisphere Publishing, Washington, 1979.
334. Littlewood, E. R., Barrison, I. G., Murray-Lyon, I. M., et al.: Cholangiocarcinoma and oral contraceptives. Lancet 1:310, 1980.
335. Lo, K. J., Eastelvod, T. R., & Eidelman, S.: Cholestatic jaundice associated with chlordizepoxide hydrochloride therapy: Report of a case and review of the literature. Am. J. Digest Dis. 12:845, 1967.
336. Locker, G. Y., Doroshow, J. H., Zwelling, L. A., et al.: The clinical features of angiosarcoma: A report of four cases and a review of the English literature. Medicine 58:48, 1979.
337. Lough, J., & Kinnear, D. G.: Mushroom poisoning in Canada: Report of a fatal case. Canad. Med. Assoc. J. 102:858, 1970.
338. Lowenfels, A. B., & Norman, J.: Isoniazid and bile duct cancer. J.A.M.A. 240:434, 1978.
339. Lowenstein, L., & Ballew, D. H.: Fatal acute hemolytic anemia, thrombocytopenic purpura, nephrosis and hepatitis resulting from ingestion of a compound containing apiol. Canad. Med. Assoc. J. 78:195, 1958.
340. Lucke, H. H., Hodge, K. E., & Patt, N. L.: Fatal liver damage after barium enemas containing tannic acid. Canad. Med. Assoc. J. 89:1111, 1963.
341. Ludwig, J.: Drug effects on the liver: A tabular compilation of drugs and drug-related hepatic diseases. Digest Dis. Sci. 24:785, 1979.
342. Ludwig, J., Viggiano, T. R., McGill, D. B., et al.: Nonalcoholic steatohepatitis: Mayo clinic experience with a hitherto unnamed disease. Mayo Clin. Proc. 55:434, 1980.
343. Lullmann, H., Lullmann-Rauch, R., & Wassermann, O.: Drug induced phospholipidoses. Crit. Rev. Toxicol. 4:185, 1975.
344. Lunzer, M., Huang, S., Ginsburg, J., et al.: Jaundice due to carbimazole. Gut 16:913, 1975.
345. Luongo, M. A., & Bjornson, S. S.: The liver in ferrous sulfate poisoning: A report of three fatal cases in children and an experimental study. N. Engl. J. Med. 251:995, 1954.
346. Lutwick, L. C.: Relation between aflatoxin, hepatitis-B virus, and hepatocellular carcinoma. Lancet 1:755, 1979.
347. Lynch, K. M.: Silicosis of systemic distribution. Am. J. Pathol. 18:313, 1942.
348. MacKay, J. S., & Ross, R. C.: Hepatoma induced by thorium dioxide (thorotrast). Canad. Med. Assoc. J. 94:1298, 1966.
349. Maddrey, W. C., & Boitnott, J. K.: Isoniazid hepatitis. Ann. Intern. Med. 79:1, 1973.
350. Maddrey, W. C., & Boitnott, J. K.: Severe hepatitis from methyldopa. Gastroenterology 68:351, 1975.
351. Manginello, F. P., & Javitt, N. B.: Parenteral nutrition and neonatal cholestasis. J. Pediatr. 94:296, 1979.
352. Mann, N. S., Chandbry, A., Thaler, S., et al.: Hepatoma induced by thorium dioxide. South. Med. J. 69:510, 1976.
353. Margulies, A. I., & Berris, B.: Jaundice associated with the administration of trifluoperazine. Can. Med. Assoc. J. 98:1063, 1968.
354. Martinez-Lopez, J. I., Greenberg, S. E., & Kling, R. R.: Drug-induced hepatic injury during methimazole therapy. Gastroenterology 43:84, 1962.
355. Martinez-Manautou, J., Aznar-Ramos, R., Bautista-O'Farrill, J., et al.: The ultrastructure of liver cells in women under steroid therapy. II. Contraceptive therapy. Acta Endocrinol. 65:207, 1970.
356. Marubbio, A. T., & Danielson, B.: Hepatic veno-occlusive disease in a renal transplant patient receiving azathioprine. Gastroenterology 69:739, 1975.
357. Masur, H., & Jones, T. C.: Protozoal and helminthic infections. In: Grieco, M. H., ed.: Infections in the Abnormal Host. p. 406. Yorke Medical Books, New York, 1980.

358. Matsuzawa, Y., & Hostetler, K. Y.: Studies on drug-induced lipidosis: Subcellular localization of phospholipid and cholesterol on the liver of rats treated with chloroquine on 4, 4′-bis (diethylaminoethoxy) B-diethyldephenylethane). J. Lipid. Res. 21:202, 1980.
359. Mauer, E. F.: The toxic effects of phenylbutazone (Butazolidin): Review of the literature and report of the twenty-third death following its use. N. Engl. J. Med. 253:404, 1955.
360. Maxwell, T. M., Olcott, C., & Blaisdell, F. W.: Vascular complications of drug abuse. Arch. Surg. 105:875, 1972.
361. McAlister, W. H., Anderson, M. S., Bloomberg, G. R., et al.: Lethal effects of tannic acid in the barium enema: Report of three fatalities and experimental studies. Radiology 80:765, 1963.
362. McFarland, R. B.: Fatal drug reaction associated with prochloperazine (Compazine). Am. J. Clin. Pathol. 40:284, 1963.
363. McGeachy, T. E., & Bloomer, W. E.: The phenobarbital sensitivity syndrome. Am. J. Med. 14:600, 1953.
364. McGee, J. O., & Patrick, R. S.: The role of perisinusoidal cells in hepatic fibrogenesis: An electron microscopic study of acute carbon tetrachloride injury. Lab. Invest. 26:429, 1972.
365. McGill, D. B., & Mott, J. D.: An industrial outbreak of toxic hepatitis due to methylenediamine. N. Engl. J. Med. 291:278, 1974.
366. McIntosh, S., Davidson, D. L., O'Brien, R. T., et al.: Methotrexate hepatotoxicity in children with leukemia. J. Pediatr. 90:1019, 1977.
367. McVeagh, P., & Ekert, H.: Hepatotoxicity of chemotherapy following nephrectomy and radiation therapy for right-sided Wilm's tumor. J. Pediatr. 87:627, 1975.
368. Meacham, G. C., Tillotson, F. W., & Heinle, R. W.: Liver damage after prolonged urethane therapy. Am. J. Clin. Pathol. 22:22, 1952.
369. Medline, A., Cohen, L. B., Tobe, B. A., et al.: Liver granulomas and allopurinol. Br. Med. J. 5:1320, 1978.
370. Meinertz, T., Langer, K. H., Kasper, W., et al.: Disopyramide-induced intrahepatic cholestasis. Lancet 2:828, 1980.
371. Ménard, D. B., Gisselbrecht, C., Marty, M., et al.: Antineoplastic agents and the liver. Gastroenterology 78:142, 1980.
372. Metzner, F., & Lieben, J.: Respiratory disease associated with beryllium refining and alloy fabrication. J. Occup. Med. 3:341, 1961.
373. Meyer, P., LiVolsi, V. A., & Cornog, J. L.: Hepatoblastoma associated with an oral contraceptive. Lancet 2:1387, 1974.
374. Meyerhoff, I. S.: Methyl salicylate poisoning in infancy. J.A.M.A. 94:1751, 1930.
375. Meyers, W. M., Connor, D. H., & Neafie, R. C.: Strongyloidiasis. In: Binford, C. H., & Connor, D. H., eds.: Pathology of Tropical and Extraordinary Diseases, Vol. 2. Armed Forces Institute of Pathology, Washington, D.C., 1976.
376. Mihas, A. A., Holley, P., Koff, R. S., et al.: Fulminant hepatitis and lymphocyte sensitization due to propylthiouracil. Gastroenterology 70:770, 1976.
377. Mihatsch, M. J., Torhorst, J., Steinmann, E., et al.: The morphologic diagnosis of analgesic (phenacetin) abuse. Pathol. Res. Pract. 164:68, 1979.
378. Miller, A. G., & Reid, W. M.: Methyldopa-induced granulomatous hepatitis. J.A.M.A. 235:2001, 1976.
379. Milliken, L. E., & Harrell, E. R.: Drug reactions to the sulfones. Arch. Dermatol. 102:220, 1970.
380. Minow, R. A., Stern, M. H., Casey, J. H., et al.: Clinicopathologic correlations of liver damage in patients treated with 6-mercaptopurine and adriamycin. Cancer 38:1524, 1976.
381. Mitchell, J. R., Zimmerman, H. J., Ishak, K. G., et al.: Isoniazid liver injury: Clinical spectrum, pathology and probable pathogenesis. Ann. Intern. Med. 84:181, 1976.
382. Mitchell, P. H., Sykes, P., & King, A.: Effect of "Pactal" on symptoms in chronic psychotic female in-patients. Br. Med. J. 1:204, 1957.
383. Mohabbat, O., Srivastava, R. N., Younos, M. S., et al.: An outbreak of hepatic veno-occlusive disease in north-western Afghanistan. Lancet 2:269, 1976.
384. Moon, H. D.: The pathology of fatal carbon tetrachloride poisoning with special reference to the histogenesis of the hepatic and renal lesion. Am. J. Pathol. 26:1041, 1950.
385. Moore, T. A., Ferrante, W. A., & Crawson, T. D.: Hepatoma occurring two decades after

hepatic irradiation. Gastroenterology 71:128, 1976.
386. More, R. H., McMillan, G. C., & Duff, G. L.: The pathology of sulfonamide allergy in man. Am. J. Pathol. 22:703, 1946.
387. Mori, T., Sakai, T., Nozue, Y., et al.: Malignancies and other injuries following thorotrast administration: Follow-up study of 147 cases in Japan. Strahlentherapie 134:229, 1967.
388. Morotomi, I., Hirose, S., & Irisa, T.: A case of intrahepatic cholestasis due to D-penicillamine. Acta Hepatol. Jap. 20:616, 1979.
389. Morris, J. S., Schmid, M., Newman, S., et al.: Arsenic and noncirrhotic portal hypertension. Gastroenterology 64:86, 1974.
390. Morris, S. J., Kanner, R., Chiprut, R. O., et al.: Disulfiram hepatitis. Gastroenterology 75:100, 1978.
391. Mosonyi, L.: Multiple benign hepatomas and virilization by ovarian tumor. Lancet 2:1263, 1973.
392. Moult, P. J. A., & Sherlock, S.: Halothane-related hepatitis: A clinical study of twenty-six cases. Q. J. Med. 43:99, 1975.
393. Mullick, F. G., McAllister, H. A., Wagner, B. M., et al.: Drug related vasculitis. Hum. Pathol. 10:313, 1979.
394. Mullick, F. G., & Ishak, K. G.: Hepatic injury associated with diphenylhydantoin therapy: A clinicopathologic study of 20 cases. Am. J. Clin. Pathol. 74:442, 1980.
395. Mullick, F. G., & Ishak, K. G.: Hepatic injury associated with paraquat toxicity in humans. Liver 1:209, 1981.
396. Muscat-Baron, J. M.: Toxic hepatitis following phenylbutazone therapy. Br. J. Clin. Pract. 20:437, 1966.
397. Myers, J. D., Olson, R. E., & Moran, T. J.: Xanthomatous biliary cirrhosis following chlorpromazine with observations indicating overproduction of cholesterol, hyperprothrombinemia and the development of portal hypertension. Trans. Assoc. Am. Physicians 70:243, 1957.
398. Nadell, J., & Kosek, J.: Peliosis hepatis: Twelve cases associated with oral androgen therapy. Arch. Pathol. Lab. Med. 101:405, 1977.
399. Nassim, J. R.: Multiple visceral lesions due to phenylbutazone toxicity. Br. Med. J. 2:1028, 1954.
400. Nayak, N. C., & Ramalingaswami, V.: Obliterative portal venopathy of the liver associated with so-called idiopathic portal hypertension or tropical splenomegaly. Arch. Pathol. 87:359, 1969.
401. Neale, G., & Azzopardi, J. G.: Chronic arsenical poisoning and noncirrhotic portal hypertension: A case for diagnosis. Br. Med. J. 2:725, 1971.
402. Neilan, L.: Estrogen therapy intrahepatic cholestasis: Characteristics of high-risk patients. J. Am. Women's Assoc. 31:97, 1976.
403. Nelson, R. S.: Hepatitis due to carbarsone. J.A.M.A. 160:764, 1956.
404. Neuberger, J., Portmann, B., Nunnerly, H. B., et al.: Oral contraceptive associated liver tumours: Occurrence of malignancy and difficulties in diagnosis: Lancet 1:273, 1980.
405. Norgren, L.: Spontan rupture av lever och mjälte vid streptokinasbehandling av djup ventrombos. Läkartidningen 75:777, 1978.
406. Notelovitz, M., & Crichton, D.: Spontaneous rupture of the liver in pregnancy. S. Afr. Med. J. 1:476, 1965.
407. Nyfors, A., & Poulsen, H.: Liver biopsies from psoriasis related to methotrexate therapy. Acta Pathol. Microbiol. Scand. 84:253 and 262, 1976.
408. Nyfors, A., & Poulsen, H.: Morphogenesis of fibrosis and cirrhosis in methotrexate-treated patients with psoriasis. Am. J. Surg. Pathol. 1:235, 1977.
409. Oda, T., Shikata, T., Naito, C., et al.: Phospholipid fatty liver: A report of three cases with a new type of fatty liver. Jap. J. Exp. Med. 40:127, 1970.
410. Oehlert, W.: Radiation induced liver cell carcinoma in the rat. In: Remmer, H., Bannasch, P., & Popper, H., eds.: Primary Liver Tumors. p. 217. MTP Press, Lancaster, 1978.
411. Ogburn, R. M., Myers, R. L., & Burdick, G. E.: Hepatitis associated with dantrolene sodium. Ann. Intern. Med. 84:53, 1976.
412. Ogilvie, A. L., & Toghill, P. J.: Cholestatic jaundice due to cotrimoxazole. Postgrad. Med. J. 56:202, 1980.
413. O'Gorman, T., & Koff, R. S.: Salicylate hepatitis. Gastroenterology 72:726, 1977.
414. Oliver, R. A. M.: Siderosis following transfusion of blood. J. Pathol. Bacteriol. 77:171, 1959.
415. Onozawa, Y., Adachi, Y., Furusawa, S., et al.: Clinicopathological studies on the so-

called foam cell syndrome associated with a long-term use of a coronary dilating agent (in Japanese). J. Jap. Med. 59:1228, 1970.
416. Orellana-Alcade, J. M., & Dominguez, J. P.: Jaundice and oral contraceptive drugs. Lancet 2:1278, 1966.
417. Oski, F. A., Allen, D. M., & Diamond, L. K.: Portal hypertension—A complication of umbilical vein catheterization. Pediatrics 31:297, 1963.
418. O'Sullivan, J. P., & Roswick, R. P.: Oral contraceptives and malignant hepatic tumours. Lancet 1:1124, 1976.
419. Pacheco, G. O., & Nuno, A. S.: Silicosis hepatica: Analysis de 21 cases. Rev. Exp. Enf. Ap. Digest. 46:107, 1975.
420. Paliard, P., Vitrey, D., Fournier, G., et al.: Perhexilene maleate-induced hepatitis. Digestion 17:419, 1978.
421. Paradinas, F. J., Bull, D., Westaby, D., et al.: Hyperplasia and prolapse of hepatocytes into hepatic veins during long-term methyltestosterone therapy: Possible relationships of these changes to the development of peliosis hepatis and liver tumors. Histopathology 1:225, 1977.
422. Pariente, E. A., Pessayre, D., Bentata-Pessayre, M., et al.: Hepatite a l'Ajmaline: Description de 4 observations et revue de la litterature. Gastroenterol. Clin. Biol. 4:240, 1980.
423. Parker, L. N.: Hepatitis and propylthiouracil. Ann. Intern. Med. 82:228, 1975.
424. Parsons, W. B.: Studies of nicotinic acid use in hypercholesteremia. Arch. Intern. Med. 107:85, 1961.
425. Pas, A. T., & Quinn, E. L.: Cholestatic hepatitis following the administration of sodium oxacillin. J.A.M.A. 191:138, 1965.
426. Pascale, L. R., Waldstein, S. S., Engerling, G., et al.: Chromium intoxication with special reference to hepatitic injury. J.A.M.A. 149:1385, 1952.
427. Passwell, J. H., David, R., Katznelson, D., et al.: Pigment disposition in the reticuloendothelial system after fat emulsion infusion. Arch. Dis. Child. 51:366, 1976.
428. Pathy, M. S., & Reynolds, A. J.: Papaverine and hepatotoxicity. Postgrad. Med. J. 56:488, 1980.
429. Payne, R. J., & Brand, W. N.: The toxicity of intravenously used marihuana. J.A.M.A. 233:351, 1975.
430. Pearson, A. J. G., Grainger, J. M., Scheuer, P. J., et al.: Jaundice due to oxyphenisatin. Lancet 1:994, 1971.
431. Peden, V. H., Witzleben, C. L., & Skelton, M. A.: Total parenteral nutrition. J. Pediatr. 78:180, 1971.
432. Pelletier, M., Lambert, R., Paliard, P., et al.: Hépatite toxique subaiguë après traitement par maléate de perhexilène. Nouv. Presse Med. 5:1070, 1976.
433. Penn, I., & Starzl, J. E.: Malignant tumors arising *de novo* in immunosuppressed organ transplant recipients. Transplantation 14:407, 1972.
434. Perez, V., Gorodisch, S., Casavilla, F., et al.: Ultrastructure of human liver at the end of normal pregnancy. Am. J. Obstet. Gynecol. 110:428, 1971.
435. Perez, V., Gorodisch, S., de Martire, J., et al.: Oral contraceptives: Long-term use produces fine structural changes in liver mitochondria. Science 165:805, 1969.
436. Perez, V., Schaffner, F., & Popper, H.: Hepatic drug reactions. Progr. Liver Dis. 4:597, 1972.
437. Pernod, J.: Hepatic tolerance of ethionamide. Am. Rev. Resp. Dis. 92:39, 1965.
438. Pessayre, D., Bichara, M., Feldmann, G., et al.: Perhexilene maleate-induced cirrhosis. Gastroenterology 78:170, 1979.
439. Pessayre, D., de Saint-Louvent, P., Degott, D., et al.: Iproclozide fulminant hepatitis. Gastroenterology 75:492, 1978.
440. Pessayre, D., Feldmann, G., Degott, C., et al.: Gold salt-induced cholestasis. Digestion 19:56, 1979.
441. Peters, R. L.: Hepatic morphologic changes after jejuno-ileal bypass. Progr. Liver. Dis. 5:581, 1979.
442. Peters, R. L., Edmondson, H. A., Reynolds, T. B., et al.: Hepatic necrosis associated with halothane anesthesia. Am. J. Med. 47:748, 1969.
443. Peters, R. L., Gay, T., & Reynolds, T. B.: Post-jejunal bypass hepatic disease: Its similarity to alcoholic hepatic disease. Am. J. Clin. Pathol. 63:318, 1975.
444. Petty, B. G., Zahka, K. G., & Bernstein, M. T.: Aspirin hepatitis associated with encephalopathy. J. Pediatr. 93:881, 1978.

445. Pezzimenti, J. F., & Hahn, A. L.: Anicteric hepatitis induced by diphenylhydantoin. Arch. Intern. Med. 125:118, 1970.
446. Peura, D. A., Stromeyer, F. W., & Johnson, L. F.: Liver injury with alcoholic hyaline after intestinal resection. Gastroenterology 79:128, 1980.
447. Pialat, J., Pasquier, B., Pahn, M., et al.: Pathologie hepatique du chlorure de vinyle monomère (CVM). Arch. Anat. Cytol. Pathol. 27:361, 1979.
448. Pickering, D.: Hepatic necrosis after chlordiazepoxide therapy. N. Engl. J. Med. 274:1449, 1966.
449. Pimentel, J. C., & Menezes, A. P.: Liver granulomas containing copper in vineyard Sprayer's lung. Am. Rev. Resp. Dis. 111:189, 1975.
450. Pimentel, J. C., & Menezes, A. P.: Liver disease in vineyard sprayer's. Gastroenterology 72:275, 1977.
451. Pimentel, J. C., & Menzes, A. P.: Pulmonary and hepatic granulomatous disorders due to the inhalation of cement and mica dusts. Thorax 33:219, 1978.
452. Podurgiel, B. J., McGill, D. G., Ludwig, J., et al.: Liver injury associated with methotrexate therapy for psoriasis. Mayo Clinic Proc. 48:787, 1973.
453. Popper, H., Gerber, M. A., Schaffner, F., et al.: Environmental hepatic injury in man. Progr. Liver Dis. 6:605, 1979.
454. Porter, J., & Hick, H.: Drug-related deaths among medical inpatients. J.A.M.A. 237:879, 1977.
455. Postuma, R., & Trevenen, C. L.: Liver disease in infants receiving total parenteral nutrition. Pediatrics 63:110, 1979.
456. Poupon, R., Rosensztajn, L., de Saint-Maur, P. P., et al.: Perhexilene maleate-associated hepatic injury prevalence and characteristics. Digestion 20:145, 1980.
457. Powell, W. J., Koch-Weser, J., & Williams, R. A.: Lethal hepatic necrosis after therapy with imipramine and desipramine. J.A.M.A. 206:642, 1968.
458. Pratt, C. B., & Johnson, W. W.: Duration and severity of fatty metamorphosis following L-asparaginase therapy. Cancer 28:361, 1971.
459. Prescott, L. F., Roscoe, P., Wright, N., et al.: Plasma paracetamol half-life and hepatic necrosis in patients with paracetamol overdosage. Lancet 1:519, 1971.
460. Preussman, R.: Hepatocarcinogens as potential risk for human liver cancer. In: Remmer, H., Bolt, H. M., Bannasch, P., & Popper, H., eds.: Primary Liver Tumors. p. 11. MTP Press, Lancaster, 1978.
461. Pryles, C. V., Burnett, J. M., & Livingston, S.: Acute hepatic necrosis with death occurring during phethenylate sodium therapy: Report of two cases. J.A.M.A. 148:536, 1952.
462. Puppala, A. R., & Ro, J. A.: Possible association between peliosis hepatis and diethylstilbesterol. Postgrad. Med. 65:277, 1979.
463. Radke, R. A., & Baroody, W. G.: Carbarsone toxicity: A review of the literature and report of 45 cases. Ann. Intern. Med. 47:418, 1957.
464. Raforth, R. J.: Systemic granulomatous reaction of salicylazopyridine (Azulfidine) in a patient with Crohn's disease. Am. J. Digest Dis. 19:465, 1974.
465. Ramsay, I. D.: Carbamazepine-induced jaundice. Br. Med. J. 2:155, 1967.
466. Ranek, L., & Andreason, P. B.: Disulfiram hepatoxicity. Br. Med. J. 2:94, 1977.
467. Read, A. E.: The liver and drugs. In: Wright, R., Alberti, K. G. M. M., Karran, S., & Milward-Sadler, G. H., eds.: Liver and Biliary Disease. p. 822. Saunders, London, 1979.
468. Read, A. E., Harrison, C. U., & Sherlock, S.: Chronic chlorpromazine jaundice. Am. J. Med. 31:249, 1961.
469. Reed, G. B., & Cox, A. J.: The human liver after radiation injury: A form of veno-occlusive disease. Am. J. Pathol. 48:597, 1966.
470. Regelson, W., Kim, U., & Ospina, J.: Hemangioendothelial sarcoma of the liver from chronic arsenic intoxication by Fowler's solution. Cancer 21:514, 1968.
471. Rehnqvist, N.: Intrahepatic jaundice due to warfarin therapy. Acta. Med. Scand. 204:335, 1978.
472. Reichel, J., Goldberg, S. B., Ellenberg, M., et al.: Intrahepatic cholestasis following administration of chlorpropamide: Report of a case with electron microscopic observations. Am. J. Med. 28:654, 1960.
473. Reinhart, M. J., Benson, R. M., Kwass, S. K., et al.: Suggestive evidence of hepatoxicity concomitant with thioridazine hydrochloride use. J.A.M.A. 197:767, 1966.
474. Rennke, H., Prat, G. A., Etcheverry, R. B., et al.: Hemangioendothelioma maligno del hi-

gado of arsenicismo chronica. Rev. Med. Chil. 99:664, 1971.

475. Reske-Nielsen, E., Bojsen-Moller, M., Vetner, M., et al.: Polyvinyl pyrrolidone-storage disease. Acta Pathol. Microbiol. Scand. 84:397, 1976.

476. Review by International Group: Guidelines for diagnosis of therapeutic drug-induced liver injury in liver biopsies. Lancet 1:854, 1974.

477. Reynolds, E. S., Brown, B. R., & Vandam, L. D.: Massive hepatic necrosis after fluroxene anesthesia—a case of drug interaction? N. Engl. J. Med. 286:530, 1972.

478. Reynolds, E. S., Schlent, R. C., Gonick, H. C., et al.: Fatal massive necrosis of the liver as a manifestation of hypersensitivity to probenecid. N. Engl. J. Med. 256:592, 1957.

479. Reynolds, J. D. H., & Wilber, R. D.: Chronic active hepatitis associated with oxyphenisatin. Am. J. Gastroenterol. 57:566, 1972.

480. Reynolds, T. B.: Laxative liver disease. In: Gerok, W., & Sickinger, K., eds.: Drugs and the Liver. p. 319. Schattauer Verlag, Stuttgart, 1975.

481. Reynolds, T. B., Peters, R. L., & Yamada, S.: Chronic active and lupoid hepatitis caused by a laxative, oxyphenasitin. N. Engl. J. Med. 285:813, 1971.

482. Riccioni, N., Bozzi, L., Susini, N., et al.: Disopyramide-induced intrahepatic cholestasis. Lancet 2:1362, 1977.

483. Rigberg, L. A., Robinson, M. J., & Espiritu, C. R.: Chlorpropamide-induced granulomas: A probable hypersensitivity reaction in liver and bone marrow. J.A.M.A. 235:409, 1976.

484. Roberts, M. H., & Jonston, F. R.: Hepatic rupture from anticoagulant therapy. Arch. Surg. 110:1152, 1975.

485. Rodgers, B. M., Hollenbeck, J. I., Donnelly, W. H., et al.: Intrahepatic cholestasis with parenteral alimentation. Am. J. Surg. 131:149, 1976.

486. Rodman, J. S., Deutsch, D. J., & Gutman, S. I.: Methyldopa hepatitis: A report of six cases and review of the literature. Am. J. Med. 60:941, 1976.

487. Rodriguez, V., Bodey, G. P., McCredie, K. B., et al: Combination 6-mercaptopurine-adriamycin in refractory adult acute leukemia. Clin. Pharmacol. Ther. 18:462, 1975.

488. Roenigk, H. H., Jr., Bergfeld, W. F., Jacques, R. S., et al: Hepatotoxicity of methotrexate in the treatment of psoriasis. Arch. Dermatol. 103:250, 1971.

489. Rojkind, N., & Dunn, M. A.: Hepatic fibrosis. Gastroenterology 76:849, 1979.

490. Ronnov-Jessen, V., & Tgernlund, A.: Hepatotoxicity due to treatment with papaverine: Report of four cases. N. Engl. J. Med. 281:1333, 1969.

491. Rooks, J. B., Ory, H. W., Ishak, K. G., et al: Epidemiology of hepatocellular adenoma: The role of oral contraceptive use. J.A.M.A. 242:644, 1979.

492. Rosenberg, H. G.: Systemic arterial disease and chronic arsenicism in infants. Arch. Pathol. 97:360, 1974.

493. Rosenblum, L. E., Korn, R. J., & Zimmerman, H. J.: Hepatocellular jaundice as a complication of iproniazid therapy. Arch. Intern. Med. 105:583, 1960.

494. Ross, A. L.: Liver atrophy following pheniprazine. Br. Med. J. 2:606, 1962.

495. Ross, R. C., Kovacs, K., & Horvath, E.: Ultrastructure of peliosis hepatis in a percutaneous biopsy. Pathol. Europ. 7:273, 1972.

496. Roth, F.: The sequelae of chronic arsenic poisoning in Moselle vintners. Ger. Med. Mon. 2:211, 1957.

497. Rothfeld, E. L., Goldman, J., & Goldberg, H. H.: Severe chlorpropamide toxicity. J.A.M.A. 172:54, 1960.

498. Rouiller, C.: Experimental toxic injury of the liver. In: Rouiller, C. ed.: The Liver, Vol. 2. p. 335. Academic Press. New York, 1974.

499. Rubin, E.: Iatrogenic hepatic injury. Hum. Pathol. 11:312, 1980.

500. Runne, U., Doepfmer, K., Antz, H., et al: Budd-Chiari-syndrom unter Dacarbazin. Dtsch. Med. Wochenschr. 105:230, 1980.

501. Russell, R. I., Allan, J. G., & Patrick, R.: Active chronic hepatitis after chlorpromazine ingestion. Br. Med. J. 1:655, 1973.

502. Russell, R. M., Boyer, J. L., Bagheri, S. A., et al: Hepatic injury from chronic hypervitaminosis A resulting in portal hypertension and ascites. N. Engl. J. Med. 291:435, 1974.

503. Ruymann, F. B., Mosijczuk, A. A., & Sayers, R. J.: Hepatoma in a child with methotrexate-induced hepatic fibrosis. J.A.M.A. 238:2631, 1977.

504. Ryan, N. J., Hogan, G. R., Hayes, A. W., et al: Aflatoxin B_1: Its role in the etiology of Reye's syndrome. Pediatrics 64:71, 1979.

505. Sabarbaro, J. A., & Bennett, R. M.: Aspirin hepatotoxicity and disseminated intravascular coagulation. Ann. Intern. Med. 86:183, 1977.
506. Safouh, M., & Shehata, A.: Hepatic vein occlusion disease in Egyptian children. Arch. Pathol. 79:505, 1965.
507. Sale, G. E., & Lerner, K. G.: Multiple tumors after androgen therapy. Arch. Pathol. Lab. Med. 101:600, 1977.
508. Salfelder, K., Doehnert, H. R., Doehnert, G., et al: Fatal phosphorous poisoning: A study of forty-five autopsy cases. Beitr. Pathol. 147:321, 1972.
509. Salmon, P. A., & Reedyk, L.: Fatty metamorphosis in jejunoileal bypass. Surg. Gynecol. Obstet. 141:75, 1975.
510. Sasaki, S.: Clinical trials of ibuprofen in Japan. Rheumatol. Phys. Med. (Suppl.) 10:32, 1970.
511. Sasaki, S., Kasuga, T., Sato, F., et al: Induction of hepatocellular tumor by x-ray irradiation at perinatal stage of mice. Gann 69:451, 1978.
512. Scott, J. M.: Iatrogenic lesions in babies following umbilical vein catheterization. Arch. Dis. Child. 40:426, 1965.
513. Schaffner, F.: Effects of long-term vinyl chloride exposure on mouse liver structure. In: Remmer, H., Bolt, H. M., Bannasch, P. J., & Popper, H. eds.: Primary Liver Tumors. p. 189. MTP Press, Lancaster, 1978.
514. Schaffner, F., Popper, H., & Chesrow, E.: Cholestasis produced by administration of norethandrolone. Am. J. Med. 26:249, 1959.
515. Schaffner, F., Popper, H., & Perez, V.: Changes in bile canaliculi produced by norethandrolone: Electron microscopic study of human and rat liver. J. Lab. Clin. Med. 56:623, 1960.
516. Schattenberg, P. J., Totovic, V., Gredigk, P., et al: Die Ultrastruktur der Leberschadigung bei der chromischen Vinylchlorid-Intoxikation. Virchows Arch. [Pathol. Anat.] 373:233, 1977.
517. Schenker, S., Breen, K. J., & Heimberg, M.: Pathogenesis of tetracycline-induced fatty liver. In: Gerok, W., & Sickinger, K., eds.: Drugs and the Liver. p. 269. Schattauer Verlag, Stuttgart, 1975.
518. Scheuer, P. J.: Hepatotoxicity of methotrexate and azathioprine. In: Gerok, W., & Sickinger, K., eds.: Drugs and the liver. p. 281. Schattauer Verlag, Stuttgart, 1975.
519. Scheuer, P. J., Summerfield, J. A., Lal, S., et al: Rifampicin hepatitis: A clinical and histological study. Lancet 1:421, 1974.
520. Schneider, R. J., & Mitchell, D.: Dantrolene hepatitis. J.A.M.A. 235:1590, 1976.
521. Schottenfeld, D.: Alcohol as a co-factor in the etiology of cancer. Cancer 43:1962, 1979.
522. Schweitzer, J. L., & Peters, R. L.: Acute submassive hepatic necrosis due to methyldopa: A case demonstrating possible initiation of chronic liver disease. Gastroenterology 66: 1203, 1974.
523. Seaman, W. E., Ishak, K. G., & Plotz, P. H.: Aspirin-induced hepatotoxicity in patients with systemic lupus erythematosus. Ann. Intern. Med. 80:1, 1974.
524. Selzer, G., & Parker, R. G. F.: Senecio poisoning exhibiting as Chiari's syndrome. Am. J. Pathol. 27:885, 1951.
525. Serrou, B., Michel, H., Dubois, J. B., et al: Granulomatous hepatitis caused by BCG vaccination of a malignant melanoma. Biomedicine 23:236, 1975.
526. Shaldon, S., & Sherlock, S.: Obstruction to the extrahepatic portal system in childhood. Lancet 1:63, 1962.
527. Shapiro, P., Ikela, R. M., Ruebner, M. H., et al: Multiple hepatic tumors and peliosis hepatis in Fanconi's anemia treated with androgens. Am. J. Dis. Child. 131:1105, 1977.
528. Sharp, J. R., Ishak, K. G., & Zimmerman, H. J.: Chronic active hepatitis and severe hepatic necrosis associated with nitrofurantoin. Ann. Intern. Med. 92:14, 1980.
529. Sherlock, S.: Progress report: Hepatic reactions to drugs. Gut 20:634, 1979.
530. Shikata, T., Kanetaka, T., Endo, Y., et al: Drug-induced generalized phospholipidosis. Acta Pathol. Jap. 22:577, 1972.
531. Shikata, T., Oda, T., Naito, C., et al: Phospholipid fatty liver: A proposal of a new concept and its electron microscopical study. Acta Pathol. Jap. 20:467, 1970.
532. Shikata, T., Uzawa, T., Yoshiwara, N., et al: Staining methods of Australia antigen in paraffin section—Detection of cytoplasmic inclusion bodies. Jap. J. Exp. Med. 44:25, 1974.
533. Shipp, J. C.: Jaundice during methimazole ("Tapazole") administration. Ann. Intern. Med. 42:701, 1955.

534. Shorey, J., Schenker, S., Suki, W. N., et al: Hepatotoxicity of mercaptopurine. Arch. Intern. Med. 122:54, 1968.
535. Short, M. H., Burns, J. M., & Harris, M. E.: Cholestatic jaundice during imipramine therapy. J.A.M.A. 206:1791, 1968.
537. Shulman, H. M., McDonald, G. B., Matthews, D., et al: An analysis of hepatic veno-occlusive disease and centrilobular hepatic degeneration following bone marrow transplantation. Gastroenterology 79:1178, 1980.
538. Silk, B. R., & Roome, A. P. C. H.: Herpes simplex encephalitis treated with intravenous idoxuridine. Lancet 2:411, 1970.
539. Simmons, F., Feldman, B., & Gerety, D.: Granulomatous hepatitis in a patient receiving allopurinol. Gastroenterology 62:101, 1972.
540. Slagboom, G., & Lochiger, E. A.: Coumarin-associated hepatitis: Report of two cases. Arch. Intern. Med. 140:1023, 1980.
541. Smith, J. P.: The pathology of ferrous sulphate poisoning. J. Pathol. 64:467, 1952.
542. Smith, P. M., Grossley, I. R., & Williams, D. M. J.: Portal hypertension in vinyl-chloride production workers. Lancet 2:602, 1976.
543. Smoron, G. L., & Battifora, H. A.: Thorotrast-induced hepatoma. Cancer 30:1252, 1972.
544. Somayaji, B. N., Feles, G. H., Paton, A., et al: Budd-Chiari syndrome after oral contraceptives. Br. Med. J. 1:53, 1968.
545. Sondheimer, J. M., Bryan, H., Andrews, W., et al: Cholestatic tendencies in premature infants on and off parenteral nutrition. Pediatrics 62:984, 1978.
546. Somayaji, B. N., Price, J. H., & Flewett, T. H.: Norethisterone jaundice in two sisters. Br. Med. J. 1:281, 1968.
547. Sonnenblick, M., & Abraham, A. S.: Ibuprofen hypersensitivity in systemic lupus erythematosus. Br. M. J. 1:619, 1978.
548. Sopko, J., & Anuras, S.: Liver disease in renal transplant recipients. Am. J. Med. 64:139, 1978.
549. Sotolongo, R. P., Neefe, L. I., Rudzki, C., et al: Hypersensitivity reaction to sulfasalazine with severe hepatotoxicity. Gastroenterology 75:95, 1978.
550. Sparberg, M., Simon, N., & del Greco, F.: Intrahepatic cholestasis due to azathioprine. Gastroenterology 57:439, 1969.
551. Sparks, F. C., Silverstein, M. J., Hunt, J. S., et al: Complications of BCG immunotherapy in patients with cancer. N Engl. J. Med. 289:827, 1973.
552. Spellberg, M. A., Mirro, J., & Chowdhury, L.: Sinusoidal dilatation related to oral contraceptives. Am. J. Gastroenterol. 72:248, 1979.
553. Stacher, G.: Intrahepatische Cholestase nach einer hochdosierten Kombinationstherapie mit Diazepam and Barbituren bei Tetanus-Patienten. Wien. Klin. Wochenschr. 22:401, 1973.
554. Staubli, W., Hess, R., & Weibel, E. R.: Correlated morphometric and biochemical studies on the liver cell. II. Effects of phenobarbital on rat hepatocytes. J. Cell. Biol. 42:92, 1969.
555. Steinberg, H., Webb, W. M., & Rafsky, H. A.: Hepatomegaly with fatty infiltration secondary to cortisone therapy: Case report. Gastroenterology 21:304, 1952.
556. Sterup, K., & Mosbech, J.: Budd- Chiari syndrome after taking oral contraceptives. Br. Med. J. 2:660, 1967.
557. Stevenson, D. K., Christie, D. L., & Haas, J. E.: Hepatic injury in a child caused by trimethoprin-sulfamethoxazole. Pediatrics 61: 864, 1978.
558. Stewart, R. D., Boethner, E. A., Southsorth, R. R., et al: Acute carbon tetrachloride intoxication. J.A.M.A. 183:994, 1963.
559. Stillman, A. E., Huxtable, R., Consroe, P., et al: Hepatic veno-occlusive disease due to pyrrolizidine (Senecio) poisoning in Arizona. Gastroenterology 73:349, 1977.
560. Stoeckle, J. D., Hardy, H. L., & Weber, A. L.: Chronic beryllium disease: Long-term follow-up of sixty cases and selective review of the literature. Am. J. Med. 46:545, 1969.
561. Stoll, B. A., Andrews, J. T., & Motteram, R.: Liver damage from oral contraceptives. Br. Med. J. 1:960, 1966.
562. Stolzer, B. L., Miller, C., White, W. A., Jr., et al: Post-arsenical obstructive jaundice complicated by xanthomatosis and diabetes mellitus. Am. J. Med. 9:124, 1950.
563. Strauss, N.: Hepato-toxic effects following occupational exposure to Halowax (chlorinated hydrocarbons). Rev. Gastroenterol. 11:381, 1944.
564. Street, J. C.: Organochlorine insecticides and the stimulation of liver microsome enzymes. Ann. N.Y. Acad. Sci. 160:274, 1969.
565. Strohscheer, J., & Wegener, H. H.: Nitrofu-

rantoin-induzierte granulomatose Hepatitis. Munch. Med. Wochenschr. 119:1535, 1977.
566. Stromeyer, F. W., & Ishak, K. G.: Nodular transformation (nodular "regenerative" hyperplasia) of the liver: A clinicopathologic study of 30 cases. Hum. Pathol. 12:60, 1981.
567. Stromeyer, F. W., Smith, D. H., & Ishak, K. G.: Anabolic steroid therapy and intrahepatic cholangiocarcinoma. Cancer 43:440, 1979.
568. Strunk, R. C., Payne, C. M., Nagle, R. B., et al: Alteration of the structure and function of guinea pig peritoneal macrophages by a soybean oil emulsion. Am. J. Pathol. 96:753, 1979.
569. Stuart, K. L., & Bras, G.: Veno-occlusive disease of the liver. Q. J. Med. 26:291, 1957.
570. Sugar, J., Toth, K., Csuka, O., et al: Role of pesticides in hepatocarcinogenesis. In: Lapis, K., & Johannessen, J. V., eds.: Liver Carcinogenesis. p. 18. Hemisphere Publishing, Washington, D.C., 1979.
571. Sullivan, D., Csulka, M. E., & Blanchard, B.: Erythromycin ethylsuccinate hepatotoxicity. J.A.M.A. 243:1074, 1980.
572. Sullivan, J. B., Rumack, B. H., Thomas, H., et al: Pennyroyal oil poisoning and hepatotoxicity. J.A.M.A. 242:2873, 1979.
573. Summary of the National Halothane Study. J.A.M.A. 297:775, 1966.
574. Swank, L. A., Cheyfee, G., & Nemchausky, B. A.: Allopurinol-induced granulomatous hepatitis with cholangitis and a sarcoid-like reaction. Arch. Intern. Med. 138:997, 1978.
575. Sweeney, E. C., & Evans, J.: Liver lesions and androgenic steroid therapy. Lancet 2: 1042, 1975.
576. Sweeney, E. C., & Evans, D. J.: Hepatic lesions in patients treated with synthetic anabolic steroids. J. Clin. Pathol. 29:626, 1976.
577. Symansky, M. R., & Fox, H. A.: Umbilical vein catheterization: Indications, management, and evaluation of the technique. J. Pediatr. 80:820, 1972.
578. Taft, L. I.: Methotrexate-induced hepatitis in childhood leukemia. Israel. J. Med. Sci. 1:600, 1966.
579. Tanaka, K., Kean, E. A., & Johnson, B.: Jamaican vomiting sickness: Biochemical investigation of two cases. N. Engl. J. Med. 295:462, 1976.
580. Tandon, B. N., Tandon, R. K., Tandon, H. D., et al: An epidemic of veno-occlusive disease of liver in central India. Lancet 2:271, 1976.
581. Tandon, H. D., Tandon, B. N., & Ramalingaswami, V.: Epidemic of toxic hepatitis in India of possible mycotoxic origin. Arch. Pathol. Lab. Med. 102:372, 1978.
582. Tanikawa, K., & Tanaka, M.: Electron microscopic observations of thioridazine-induced hepatitis. Kurume Med. J. 13:15, 1966.
583. Taxy, J. B.: Peliosis: A morphologic curiosity becomes an iatrogenic problem. Hum. Pathol. 9:331, 1978.
584. Telles, N. C., Thomas, L. B., Popper, H., et al: Evolution of thorotrast-induced hepatic angiosarcomas. Environ. Res. 18:74, 1979.
585. Tennenbaum, J. I., & Dreskin, O. H.: Toxic hepatitis during treatment with methimazole (Tapazole): Report of a case with apparent recovery. Ohio State Med. J. 58:306, 1962.
586. Tessmer, C. F., Chang, J. P.: Thorotrast localization by light and electron microscopy. Ann. N.Y. Acad. Sci. 145:545, 1967.
587. Teychenne, P. F., Jones, E. A., Ishak, K. G., et al: Hepatocellular injury with distinctive mitochondrial changes induced by lergotrile mesylate: A dopaminergic ergot derivative. Gastroenterology 76:575, 1979.
588. Thompson, M., Stephenson, P., & Perry, J. S.: Ibufenac in the treatment of arthritis. Ann. Rheumat. Dis. 23:397, 1974.
589. Thompson, S. W.: The Pathology of Parenteral Nutrition with Lipids. Charles C Thomas, Springfield, Illinois, 1974.
590. Thomas, E. B.: Chronic aggressive hepatitis caused by halothane. Ann. Intern. Med. 81:487, 1974.
591. Thomas, E., Bhuta, S., & Rosenthal, W. S.: Methyldopa-induced liver injury. Arch. Pathol. Lab. Med. 100:132, 1976.
592. Thomas, L. B., Popper, H., Berk, P. D., et al: Vinyl-chloride-induced liver disease: From idiopathic portal hypertension (Banti's syndrome) to angiosarcoma. N. Engl. J. Med. 292:17, 1975.
593. Thomas, T. L., De Coufle, P., & Moure-Eraso, R.: Mortality among workers employed in petrochemical refining and petrochemical plants. J. Occup. Med. 22:97, 1980.
594. Thulin, K. E., & Nermark, J.: Seven cases of jaundice in women taking an oral contraceptive, Anovlar. Br. Med. J. 1:584, 1966.

595. Ticktin, H. E., & Zimmerman, H. J.: Hepatic dysfunction and jaundice in patients receiving triacetyloleandomycin. N. Engl. J. Med. 267:964, 1962.
596. Tobias, H., Auerbach, R.: Hepatotoxicity of long-term methotrexate therapy for psoriasis. Arch. Intern. Med. 132:391, 1973.
597. Toghill, P. J., Smith, P. G., Benton, P., et al: Methyldopa liver damage. Br. Med. J. 2:545, 1974.
598. Tolman, K. G., Hammer, S., & Sannella, J. J.: Possible hepatotoxicity of Doxidan. Ann. Intern. Med. 84:290, 1976.
599. Tonder, M., Nordoy, A., & Elgio, K.: Sulfonamide-induced chronic liver disease. Scand. J. Gastroenterol. 9:23, 1974.
600. Touloukian, R. J., & Seashore, J. H.: Hepatic secretory obstruction with total parenteral nutrition in the infant. J. Pediatr. Surg. 10:353, 1975.
601. Tracey, J. P., & Sherlock, P.: Hepatoma following carbon tetrachloride poisoning. N.Y. State J. Med. 68:2202, 1968.
602. Traga, J. R., Javate, B. A., & Venkatessan, S.: Liver abscess and sepsis due to *Klebsiella pneumoniae* in a newborn. Clin. Pediatr. 13:1081, 1974.
603. Trey, C., Lipworth, L., Chalmers, T., et al: Fulminant hepatic failure: Presumable contribution of halothane. N. Engl. J. Med. 279:798, 1968.
604. Tuchweber, B., Garg, B. D., & Salas, M.: Microsomal enzyme inducers and hypervitaminosis A in rats. Arch. Pathol. Lab. Med. 100:100, 1976.
605. Tuyns, A. J.: Epidemiology of alcohol and cancer. Cancer Res. 39:2840, 1979.
606. Tysell, J. E., & Knauer, M.: Hepatitis induced by methyldopa. Report of a case and review of the literature. Am. J. Digest. Dis. 16:849, 1971.
607. Ulshen, M. H., Grand, R. J., Crain, J. D., et al: Hepatotoxicity with encephalopathy associated with aspirin therapy in rheumatoid arthritis. J. Pediatr. 93:1034, 1978.
608. Upton, A. C., Kimball, A. W., Furth, J., et al: Some delayed affects of atom-bomb irradiations in mice. Cancer Res. 20:1, 1960.
609. Utili, R., Boitnott, J. K., & Zimmerman, H. J.: Dantrolene-associated hepatic injury: Incidence and character. Gastroenterology 72:610, 1977.
610. Urabe, H., Koda, H., & Asahi, M.: Present state of Yusho poisoning. Ann. N. Y. Acad. Sci. 302:273, 1979.
611. Vana, J., & Murphy, G. P.: Primary malignant liver tumors. N.Y. State J. Med. 79:321, 1979.
612. Van Haelst, U. J. G. M., & Sengers, R. C. A.: Effects of parenteral nutrition with lipids on the human liver: An electron-microscopic study. Virchows Arch. [Pathol. Anat.] 22:323, 1976.
613. Van Ordstrand, H. S.: Current concepts of beryllium poisoning. Ann. Intern. Med. 35: 1203, 1951.
614. Van Wyk, J. J., & Hoffman, C. R.: Periarteritis nodosa: Case of fatal exfoliate dermatitis resulting from "Dilantin sodium" sensitivity. Arch. Intern. Med. 81:605, 1948.
615. Van Waes, L., & Lieber, C. S.: Early perivenular sclerosis in alcoholic fatty liver: An index of progressive liver injury. Gastroenterology 73:646, 1977.
616. Vasquez, J. J., & Cervera, S.: Cyanamide-induced liver injury in alcoholics. Lancet 1:361, 1980.
617. Vasquez, J. J., & Pardo-Mindan, J.: Liver cell injury (bodies similar to Lafora's) in alcoholics treated with disulfiram (Antabuse). Histopathology 3:377, 1979.
618. Victorino, R. M. M., Silveira, J. C. B., Baptista, A., et al: Jaundice associated with naproxen. Postgrad. Med. J. 56:368, 1980.
619. Villeneuve, J. P., Huet, P. M., Joly, J. G., et al: Idiopathic portal hypertension. Am. J. Med. 61:459, 1976.
620. Viteri, A. L., Greene, J. F., Jr., & Dyck, W. P.: Erythromycin ethylsuccinate-induced cholestasis. Gastroenterology 76:1007, 1979.
621. Waitzkin, L.: Hepatic dysfunction during promazine therapy. N. Engl. J. Med. 257:276, 1957.
622. Wake, K.: "Sternzellen" in the liver: Perisinusoidal cells with special reference to storage of vitamin A. Am. J. Anat. 132:429, 1971.
623. Walker, C. O., & Combes, B.: Biliary cirrhosis induced by chlorpromazine. Gastroenterology 51:631, 1966.
624. Walters, G. M., Terrence, C., & Steckel, R.: Jaundice following administration of fluophenazine dihydrochloride. Am. J. Psychiatry 120:81, 1963.
625. Ware, S., & Millward-Sadler, G. H.: Acute

liver disease associated with sodium valproate. Lancet 2:1110, 1980.
626. Warren, B. L., & Bellward, G. D.: Benign liver tumors and oral contraceptive therapy. Drug. Intell. Clin. Pharmacol. 13:680 and 741, 1979.
627. Wasser, J. S., & Coleman, M.: Leukemia chemotherapy and centrilobular hepatic necrosis. Ann. Intern. Med. 86:508, 1977.
628. Waugh, D.: Myocarditis, arteritis and focal hepatic, splenic and renal granulomas due to penicillin sensitivity. Am. J. Pathol. 28:437, 1952.
629. Webster, M. W., Van Thiel, D. H., Bron, K. M., et al: Hepatic adenoma associated with portasystemic shunting. Digestion 19:328, 1979.
630. Wegener, K., & Leipolz-Angermuller, S.: Double tumors of the liver following intravenous thorotrast injection. Virchows Arch. [Pathol. Anat.] 382:63, 1979.
631. Weinbren, K.: Diseases of the liver. In: Harrison, C. U., ed.: Recent Advances in Pathology, 8th Ed. p. 185. Churchill, London, 1966.
632. Weinstein, G. D.: Methotrexate. Ann. Intern. Med. 86:199, 1977.
633. Weinstein, G. D., Cox, J. W., Suringa, D. W. R., et al: Evaluation of possible chronic hepatotoxicity from methotrexate for psoriasis. Arch. Dermatol. 102:613, 1970.
634. Weiss, M., Hassin, D., & Bank, H.: Propylthiouracil-induced hepatic damage. Arch. Intern. Med. 140:1184, 1980.
635. Weiss, M., Hassin, D., & Bank, H.: Propylthiouracil-induced hepatic damage. Arch. Intern. Med. 140:1184, 1980.
636. Welton, D. G.: Exfoliative dermatitis and hepatitis due to phenobarbital. J.A.M.A. 143:232, 1950.
637. Wepler, W., & Opitz, K.: Histologic changes in the liver biopsy in *Amanita phalloides* intoxication. Hum. Pathol. 3:249, 1972.
638. Werner, S. P., Hanger, F. M., & Kritzler, R. A.: Jaundice during methyltestosterone therapy. Am. J. Med. 8:325, 1950.
639. Westaby, D., Ogle, S. J., Paradina, J. B., et al: Liver damage from long-term methyltestosterone. Lancet 2:261, 1977.
640. Whitecar, J. P., Bodey, G. P., Harris, J. E., et al: L-asparaginase. N. Engl. J. Med. 282:732, 1970.
641. Wigger, H. J., Bransilver, B. R., & Blanc, W. A.: Thromboses due to catherization in infants and children. J. Pediatr. 76:1, 1970.
642. Wilder, E. M.: Death due to liver failure following the use of methandrostenolone. Can. Med. Assoc. J. 87:768, 1962.
643. Wilkinson, S. B., Portmann, B., & Williams, R.: Hepatitis from dantrolene sodium. Gut 20:33, 1979.
644. Williams, J. W., Rittenberry, A., Dillard, R., et al: Liver abscess in newborn: Complications of umbilical vein catherization. Am. J. Dis. Child. 125:111, 1973.
645. Willing, R. L., & Hecker, R.: Oxyphenisatin and liver damage. Med. J. Aust. 1:1179, 1971.
646. Wills, E. J., & Waltron, B.: A morphologic study of unexplained hepatitis following halothane anesthesia. Am. J. Pathol. 91:11, 1978.
647. Winberg, C. D. & Ranchod, M.: Thorotrast induced hepatic cholangiocarcinoma and angiosarcoma. Hum. Pathol. 10:108, 1979.
648. Winckler, K.: Lebernekrosen nach Infusionscholangiographie. Dtsch. Med. Wochenschr. 103:420, 1978.
649. Winckler, K., Junge, U., & Creutzfeldt, W.: Ground-glass hepatocytes in unrelated liver biopsies: Ultrastructure and relationship to hepatitis B surface antigen. Scand. J. Gastroenterol. 11:167, 1976.
650. Winkler, K., & Poulsen, H.: Liver disease with periportal sinusoidal dilatation: A possible complication to contraceptive steroid. Scand. J. Gastroenterol. 10:699, 1975.
651. Wisse, E., & Knook, D. L.: The investigation of sinusoidal cells: A new approach to the study of liver function. Progr. Liver Dis. 6:153, 1979.
652. Wogan, G. N.: Aflatoxins and their relationship to hepatocellular carcinoma. In: Okuda, K., & Peters, R. L., eds.: Hepatocellular Carcinoma. p. 25. John Wiley, New York, 1976.
653. Wolfe, P. B.: Sulindac and jaundice. Ann. Intern. Med. 91:656, 1979.
654. Wood, J. C.: Jaundice due to methyltestosterone therapy. J.A.M.A. 150:1484, 1952.
655. Wu, S., Spurny, O. M., & Klotz, H. P.: Budd-Chiari syndrome after taking oral contraceptives: A case report and review of 14 reported cases. Am. J. Digest Dis. 22:623, 1977.
656. Yon, J., & Anuras, S.: Hepatitis caused by amitryptyline therapy. J.A.M.A. 232:833, 1975.
657. Young, J. L., Boswell, R. B., & Nies, A. S.:

Severe allopurinol hypersensitivity. Arch. Intern. Med. 134:553, 1974.

658. Zachariae, H., Sogaard, H., & Nyfors, A.: Liver biopsy in psoriatics previously treated with potassium arsenite. Acta Dermatovener 54:235, 1974.
659. Zafrani, E. S., Ishak, K. G., & Rudzki, C.: Cholestatic and hepatocellular injury associated with erythromycin esters: Report of nine cases. Am. J. Digest. Dis. 24:385, 1979.
660. Zarday, Z., Veith, F. J., Gliedman, M. L., et al: Irreversible liver damage after azathioprine. J.A.M.A. 222:690, 1972.
661. Zeegan, R., Stansfeld, A. G., Dawson, A. M., et al: Prolonged survival after portal decompression of patients with non-cirrhotic intrahepatic portal hypertension. Gut 11:610, 1970.
662. Zelman, S.: Liver cell necrosis in chlorpromazine jaundice (allergic cholangiolitis). Am. J. Med. 27:708, 1959.
663. Zimmerman, H. J.: Clinical and laboratory manifestations of hepatotoxicity. Ann. N.Y. Acad. Sci. 104:954, 1963.
664. Zimmerman, H. J.: Hepatic injury caused by therapeutic agents. In: Becker, F. F., ed.: The Liver. Part A. p. 225. Marcel Dekker, New York, 1974.
665. Zimmerman, H. J.: Experimental hepatotoxicity. In: Eichler, O., ed.: Handbook of Experimental Pharmacology, Vol. 16. Springer-Verlag, Berlin, 1976.
666. Zimmerman, H. J.: Hepatotoxicity. Appleton-Century-Crofts, New York, 1978.
667. Zimmerman, H. J., Chomet, B., Kulesh, M. H., et al: Hepatic hemosiderin deposits: Incidence in 558 biopsies from patients with and without intrinsic hepatic disease. Arch. Intern. Med. 107:494, 1961.
668. Zimmerman, H. J., & Ishak, K. G.: Drug-induced and toxic liver injury. In: MacSween, R. N. M., Anthony, P. P., & Scheuer, P., eds.: Pathology of the Liver. p. 335. Churchill-Livingstone, Edinburgh, 1979.
669. Zucker, P., Daum, F., & Cohen, M. J.: Fatal carbamazepine hepatitis. J. Pediatr. 91:667, 1977.

18

The Gastrointestinal Tract

Robert H. Riddell

The actions of drugs and toxins on the gastrointestinal tract (GIT) can be considered within two broad categories: agents that may affect any part of the tract, and agents that tend to act predominantly on one part of the tract. While diseases will be considered within this framework, the framework has disadvantages in that the same disease may affect adjacent organs. Thus, caustic injury tends to affect the mouth and esophagus, but may, although less frequently, affect the stomach and, rarely, the small bowel. In the sections dealing with substances acting predominantly on one part of the tract, the discussion will include adjacent parts of the tract that may also be involved, where this is appropriate. Some drugs produce such a different morphologic picture in an adjacent part of the bowel that it seems best to consider them separately. In the section dealing with disease that may be generalized, only those substances that can involve the entire tract will be considered.

DISEASE AFFECTING ANY PART OF THE TRACT

Hemorrhage
Ischemia
Radiation injury and its sequelae
Antineoplastic and immunosuppressive agents and their sequelae
Radiologic contrast media
Obstruction
Sequelae of instrumentation
Extrinsic damage to the bowel

HEMORRHAGE

Although hemorrhage affecting the GIT may take several forms, the most frequent is an intramural hematoma. Much less frequently, retroperitoneal hemorrhage may occur and extend into the mesentery to reach the bowel wall directly, or may form a mass over which the bowel becomes stretched. In the general population, most hematomas follow abdominal trauma. While they tend to occur in patients taking anticoagulants or thrombolytic agents, many seem to occur spontaneously. Hemorrhage occurring with the use of antineoplastic agents is usually the result of low platelet counts. Although thrombolytic agents clearly have the potential for causing gastrointestinal hemorrhage, few such cases have been documented[266]; the vast majority of drug-associated cases of hemorrhage occur as a complication of standard anticoagulant therapy.

Intramural Hematoma

This is the most common GIT complication in patients taking anticoagulants, with several hundred cases appearing in the world's literature. It has been estimated that up to 40 percent of patients on anticoagulants bleed as a result of their medication, but the vast majority of these hemorrhages are relatively harmless, and serious complications are far less frequent. The Boston Collaborative Drug Surveillance Program found that in medical inpatients, the rate for major gastrointestinal complications was 1.2 percent for patients treated with heparin and 0.2 percent for those treated with warfarin.[303] Clinically such hematomas cause pain, frequently evidence of ileus, and, especially if the hematoma becomes circumferential, symptoms of obstruction. The most common site is in the small bowel, and in one series 9 percent of documented cases were duodenal, 59 percent were jejunal, 25 percent were ileal, and 7 percent were in the large bowel.[270] The average age of patients in the series just noted was 62, and males were affected more than three times as frequently as females. There appeared to be no relationship between the period of medication and bleeding. Similar figures have also been obtained in a more recent series in which coumarin anticoagulants were by far the most common anticoagulants being taken, mainly in males following myocardial infarction.[587] Since this latter study, it has become apparent that the stomach may also be the seat of intramural hematomas.[166]

Intramural hematomas are invariably well localized to a relatively short segment of bowel, and primarily involve the submucosa and external muscle coats. This often leaves doubt in the mind of the surgeon as to whether the bowel wall has actually been infarcted, but despite the fragmentation of muscle fibers, the mucosa is invariably intact, and pink when freshly observed, and even the occasional reports documenting apparent infarction show what appears to be normal mucosa. Since the mucosa is far more susceptible to hypoxia than the underlying muscle, true infarction is probably rare. Patients on anticoagulants presenting with abdominal pain or with obstructive symptoms, especially if the prothrombin time is prolonged, should therefore be managed conservatively, and should not be subjected to laparotomy unless other clinical indications are present. Occasionally, a more severe complication may occur, such as severe blood loss into the bowel lumen.[63]

Retroperitoneal Hematomas

These are considerably less common than intramural hematomas, but in one study almost a third of retroperitoneal hematomas occurring over a 10-year period in a University Hospital were related to anticoagulants.[446] Although hemorrhage from a small retroperitoneal vessel is an obvious cause of retroperitoneal hematoma, it has been shown that the fascial compartments of the thigh, while interconnected, can communicate with the retroperitoneal space either beneath Poupart's ligament or through the great sacrosciatic notch.[434] Injection of heparin into the thigh may therefore occasionally be associated with local hemorrhage that can extend into the retroperitoneal space. Although signs of shock are usually accompanied clinically by flank pain and masses or local hematomas, other, rare complications, such as intussusception, have been noted and may require more active clinical management.[385]

ISCHEMIA

Iatrogenic ischemia of the GIT can result from a variety of different insults that have in common the reduction of intestinal blood flow either partially or totally. Practically, these fall into two major categories: those secondary to arterial obstruction or constriction, and those caused by a reduction in blood volume, blood pressure, or both, with a subsequent reduction in perfusion pressure. It is important to realize that most ischemic bowel disease is multifactorial, and that one of the causative factors is invariably some form of intrinsic vascular disease. When further factors are added, an ischemic episode may result. Angiography and autopsy studies have shown the amazing ability of the body to compensate for severe vascular disease by forming numerous anastomotic channels bypassing the major obstruction, but this is sometimes so precari-

Table 18.1. Iatrogenic Methods of Causing or Potentiating Ischemia

Following angiography
Trauma to vessel wall
Arterial embolization for uncontrolled hemorrhage
Arterial or venous thrombosis
Drug-induced vasculitis (see Chapter 10)
Estrogens and oral contraceptives (OC)
Arterial spasm:
Vasopressin (Pitressin)
Ergot-containing preparations
Methysergide maleate
Stevens-Johnson syndrome
Hypotensive and hypovolemic agents
Diuretics, reserpine, hydralazine, methyldopa, digoxin
Ganglion blockers, alpha-adrenergic blockers and catecholamines
Antiarrhythmic drugs, some antidepressants

ous that a relatively minor additional insult may be the last straw. In elderly patients, even bowel transection may sufficiently reduce collateral blood supply to lead to ischemia. A variety of iatrogenic insults may have the same effect; these are listed in Table 18-1.

Following Angiography

Trauma to Vessel Wall

Contrast media may be injected into the wall of a vessel, or dislodge atheromatous plaques or thrombi, usually either in the aorta or superior mesenteric artery. This may cause thrombosis of the vessel, with subsequent small-bowel infarction and death. Other patients may develop an ileus and recover without operative intervention; presumably, this group does not experience thrombosis. Most of these side-effects have occurred with iodopyracet or acetrizoate.[554] Newer contrast media, such as sodium iothalamate (angio-Conray), are said to be safer. It should be borne in mind that these complications are rare, and occur in under 0.1 percent of angiograms.[352] (Intraluminal masses resulting from the use of intraluminal contrast media that may cause ischemia are discussed on p. 537.)

Arterial Embolization for Uncontrolled Hemorrhage

With the increasing use of embolization under radiologic control to manage intestinal bleeding, it is not surprising to find this technique occasionally complicated by infarction of the appropriate segment of bowel. In one patient, such infarction occurred in the duodenum following embolization of the gastroduodenal artery and its superior pancreaticoduodenal branch.[556] Since the duodenal arteries are said to be end arteries, this complication is perhaps not too surprising. In a second patient, extensive gastric necrosis followed embolization of the left gastric artery.[79]

Arterial or Venous Thrombosis

Drug-Induced Vasculitis

This is discussed in detail in Chapter 10.

Estrogens and Oral Contraceptives (OC)

The propensity of estrogens and OC to cause both arterial and venous thrombosis at a variety of anatomic sites is well documented. Most cases affecting the GIT occur almost exclusively in the small and large bowel. In a review of OC-induced small bowel ischemia, Hoyle[288] reconfirmed the increased predisposition of patients of blood group A (or more strictly, non-O[304]), cigarette smokers, and hypertensive patients to develop this complication. Of the 21 patients reviewed, thrombosis affected the superior mesenteric vein in 12 patients, the superior mesenteric artery in 7, the celiac axis in 1, and was not precisely located in the final patient. Ten of the patients died, 6 as a direct result of the infarction, the remainder from a secondary complication such as pulmonary embolus or bleeding following anticoagulation. The latter may be particularly hazardous in patients taking OC, in view of the potentiation of anticoagulants by OC.[622] Several of the patients surviving had short bowel syndrome.

There seems to be a general relationship between the amount of estrogen ingested and thrombotic sequelae, especially when the former exceeds 0.5 mg daily; but there has been little relationship to the duration of estrogen ingestion, although almost half of the thrombotic catastrophes in the study by de Teresa et al. occurred during the first year.[622]

Ischemic colitis has also been recently reviewed.[32] In this study of 26 patients, all 10 less than 50 years old were female, and 6 were taking OC, most for 2 years or more. However, the prognosis for ischemic colitis appeared to be much better than for small-intestinal disease, and the majority of patients recovered with conservative treatment. Most of the disease occurred in the left colon, but bleeding was sometimes severe.

Bonfils[74] recently reported 6 patients with acute, spontaneously remitting ulcerative colitis; 4 of these were young women taking OC. All of the patients recovered completely within a short period. No pathology was illustrated, but the possibility that the colitis might have been ischemic in etiology must be considered; however, it differed from that in other reports in involving almost the entire large bowel, so that the precise etiology, and whether this represents a new disease, awaits further confirmation.

Arterial Spasm

Vasopressin

This substance causes marked constriction of the vessel into which it is perfused, and of the branches of that vessel, hence its success in stopping or markedly reducing hemorrhage. One disadvantage is that such vasoconstriction may occasionally proceed to ischemic necrosis. If perfused through a peripheral vein, vasopressin may cause necrosis of part of the limb if it escapes into the tissues.[251] In the GIT, vasopressin is frequently administered directly into the appropriate artery under radiologic control, and sometimes produces similar complications. In one patient, a combination of partial gastrectomy, vasopressin, subsequent ligation of a branch of the left gastric artery, and further vasopressin was successful in producing an area of infarction in the lesser curve of the residual stomach.[16] In another study, Conn et al.[119] described a patient with severe atheroma that caused a cardiovascular accident, and who developed a bleeding stress ulcer postoperatively. Following vasopressin administration, the patient developed an extensive area of ileal and jejunal necrosis. Renert et al.[510] have reported a patient who developed thrombosis of numerous, small mesenteric veins following perfusion of vasopressin into the superior mesenteric artery; this resulted in an area of jejunal infarction.

Ergot

There are uncommon case reports of patients developing evidence of arterial spasm or frank intestinal ischemia following the excessive use of ergot. One patient developed pain in her feet as a result of excessive use of Cafergot (an ergotamine-caffeine combination), which she then tried to relieve with more ergot. Aortography showed marked spasm of the superior mesenteric artery and its branches, but this seems not to have caused overt GIT disease.[249] A second patient taking ergotamine tartrate for migraine developed typical ischemic colitis that ultimately proceeded to stricture formation.[594]

Methysergide

A patient was reported who took increasing doses of methysergide maleate for migraine. Originally she had taken ergot, but changed because this was no longer effective. Although only 38 years old at presentation, she had had postprandial pain for several years, and this had gradually increased in intensity. Arteriography done because of symptoms and an abdominal bruit showed a long tapering stenosis of the superior mesenteric artery, with complete occlusion just distal to the origin of the ileocolic artery. The patient recovered with glucagon treatment and cessation of the methysergide.[380] A similar case was described by Katz and Vogel.[315]

Stevens-Johnson Syndrome

Rarely, a Stevens-Johnson reaction to drugs progresses to intestinal involvement that may present as an abdominal emergency due to a marked hemorrhage that is primarily submucosal, but which also dissects through all muscle layers and may involve the mucosa. The skin lesions in Stevens-Johnson syndrome, and the drugs that may presumably cause both skin and GIT involvement, are discussed in Chapter 6. Nevertheless, the distinctive mucosal bullae that this condition produces in the GIT may be caused by drugs, with one such instance being due to co-trimoxazole.[630]

Hypotensive and Hypovolemic Agents

These are well known clinically, and some of the basic drug groups responsible for gastrointestinal ischemia are shown in Table 18-1. A more exhaustive list is hardly required, but an excellent review of intestinal blood flow and the substances that modify it is given by Granger et al.[244] Digoxin-induced ischemia is discussed in greater detail on p. 569.

PATHOLOGY

The pathology of ischemic bowel disease is familiar to most physicians, and is well documented in textbooks of pathology. If ischemia is sudden and complete, it results in full-thickness necrosis of the bowel wall. Less severe forms of ischemia may give rise to a spectrum of intestinal injury. In the early phase, this injury may take the form of a pseudomembranous enteritis or colitis. The mucosa is by far the most susceptible part of the bowel wall to ischemic insult, and the luminal surface is the most susceptible part of the mucosa, probably because it is also the most hypoxic. Consequently, the luminal surface is the first part of the mucosa to be injured. Surface ulceration is followed by an exudate of necrotic epithelial cells, polymorphs, and mucus, producing the characteristic pseudomembrane. This may ultimately involve the full thickness of the mucosa. If the bases of the crypts are spared, the mucosa will regenerate from these and will return to normal. However, if these bases are destroyed, and re-epithelialization occurs from viable epithelium at the margins of the areas of ulceration, the subsequent mucosa may vary from one that is indistinguishable from normal to a typically regenerated mucosa with crypt atrophy, glandular distortion, Paneth cell metaplasia (in the large bowel), and reduplication of the muscularis mucosae similar to that seen in quiescent ulcerative colitis. Submucosal edema may be marked, and gives rise to the characteristic "thumb-printing" seen radiologically. There may be marked congestion and hemorrhage, especially if the occlusion is on the venous side. There may also be varying degrees of myocytolysis, resulting in destruction of the muscle layers. If there is sufficient blood flow remaining to prevent infarction, this stage may ultimately resolve to produce a stricture.

Occasionally, ischemia may be severe enough to prevent the mucosa from regenerating adequately, but be insufficient to cause necrosis and perforation of the bowel wall. Under these circumstances there is only patchy and poor regeneration of the mucosa. Biopsy or examination of resected bowel shows some regenerated crypts, usually with an excess of chronic inflammatory cells; some crypts that are actively regenerating and which may have polymorphs passing through the epithelium; and moderate hemorrhage in the lamina propria. There is no evidence of the original pseudomembranous phase of the disease, and there may be considerable difficulty in distinguishing the condition from either Crohn's disease or ulcerative colitis. Occasionally, the presence of only small islands of residual mucosa, with areas of deep intervening ulceration, may even mimic an early fulminant stage of these two diseases.

Perhaps the most useful morphologic indication of an ischemic etiology under the foregoing circumstances is vascular proliferation involving capillary channels immediately beneath the luminal epithelium. This proliferation presumably occurs as a response to chronic ischemia, as a mechanism for increasing the blood flow to the most severely affected part of the mucosa. In some patients this proliferative lesion may partially or completely resolve, with the production of a layer of collagen immediately beneath the luminal epithelium, mimicking "collagenous colitis" in the large bowel.[61,463] Good clinical information may be required to arrive at a correct diagnosis. Capillary proliferation is an interesting complication of ischemia, because a similar picture was occasionally seen in antibiotic-induced pseudomembranous colitis that persisted before specific therapy was developed; some patients seen several weeks or months after the initial episode had a similarly frustrating and nonspecific biopsy. Although the antibiotic-induced disease may rarely be either focal or be an enterocolitis, usually it stops precisely at the ileocecal valve. This is in marked contrast to ischemic disease which, although characteristically affecting the "watershed" area in the vicinity of the splenic flexure, can affect any part of the bowel but tends not to affect the entire colon. If the ileocolic vessels are involved, ischemic disease will invariably cross the ileocecal valve. Angiographic studies may be helpful, particularly in young patients, but in the elderly, in whom extensive vascular disease may be present without bowel disease, these studies may be of limited value.

RADIATION INJURY

The GIT is said to have a tolerance of between 4,500 and 6,500 rads, but there is marked individual susceptibility. The effects of radiotherapy also depend on several other variables, particularly the duration of the therapy and the type of particles used. In some patients it is possible to protect exposed parts of the tract with a variety of maneuvers aimed at keeping as much bowel as possible out of the field of irradiation, but in other patients this is relatively futile because previous surgery has caused numerous adhesions, so that adjacent loops of bowel are adherent to each other. Previous surgery therefore increases the risk of potential damage by irradiation by a factor of two-and-a-half to three, because the same segment of bowel tends to get irradiated on each occasion. About 40 to 50 percent of patients receiving radiotherapy to the GIT get acute injury, but only about 5 to 10 percent develop chronic disease. Interestingly, in the opossum, radiation damage to the esophagus was reduced in animals receiving indomethacin and enhanced in those receiving 16,16-dimethylprostaglandin E_2.[466] Indomethacin also appears to have some protective effect in the healing of experimental esophagitis,[47] and may therefore be beneficial in treating some other types of esophagitis. However, other parts of the gastrointestinal tract may respond differently (see specific sections below).

Perhaps the most important point about radiation damage is that it produces no pathognomonic histologic features, although it is accompanied by many characteristic features. Thus, "typical" irradiation fibroblasts may be seen wherever a reparative process occurs, particularly if the site is secondarily infected. Such fibroblasts may therefore be found in the stroma of ulcerated infected tumors, particularly in the head and neck region, and also in the base of decubitus ulcers.

There are two excellent reviews of irradiation damage particularly involving the GIT.[59, 467] Clinically and pathologically, it is useful to divide the GIT changes caused by irradiation into "early" and "late." Irradiation damage is most frequently seen in the upper rectum of patients with stage II carcinoma of the uterine cervix, this being the subgroup that is treated aggressively with both external and intracavitary radiation, often to a combined dose in the vicinity of 8000 rads. This subgroup also has the best long-term prognosis because their relatively limited cervical carcinoma inevitably means that there are more survivors to develop the late complications resulting from radiation.

Acute Injury

This occurs within about 2 weeks of completing a course of radiotherapy, and consists of an acute enteritis or colitis due to damage to the mucosa. There are surprisingly few morphologic studies of this phase of irradiation damage in humans. The changes are best described in the large bowel, where crypts have bizarre nuclei, mucin depletion, show evidence of regeneration, and characteristically have eosinophils in the lamina propria and eosinophilic crypt abscesses.[657] These changes tend to subside within 1 to 2 months. Mitoses are usually conspicuous by their absence, but it is difficult to be certain what part this plays in the disturbance of crypt architecture that may be present.[663] An excess of what appear to be pyknotic nuclei may be found, particularly near the crypt base; these take the form of small supranuclear inclusions that have been called karyolytic[223, 289] or apoptotic bodies.[550] Although normally present, they are markedly increased in number following irradiation.[223, 289]

In the small bowel, Tarpila[612] performed biopsies before, immediately after, and several months after irradiation for carcinomas that did not originate in the GIT. In patients receiving more than 3,000 rads to the abdomen, there was either partial or total loss of villi, and an excess of chronic inflammatory cells in the lamina propria.

A further, poorly documented complication of radiotherapy in the acute phase of irradiation injury is perforation following the irradiation of tumors. The latter fall into two broad categories: (1) radiosensitive tumors, such as primary malignant lymphomas, treated with conventional radiotherapy (however, perforation may also follow chemotherapy [v.i]); and (2) conventional tumors treated relatively unconventionally. At the University of Chicago we have seen several patients with advanced tumors of the esophagus or gastroesophageal junction who were treated with neutron therapy and who, shortly after the termination of the course, presented with perforation at the site of the tumor. Histologically the effect of neutrons on the tumors was dramatic, often with little or no residual viable tumor. However, the mortality from perforation was exceedingly high.

Late Changes

These tend to occur many years following the course of radiation, although there is marked variation, ranging from a few months to more than 20 years. In the GIT, stromal changes persist longer than epithelial changes, although the mucosal damage is usually the most obvious. This is reflected by the red and inflamed macroscopic appearance of the mucosa (and often the serosa as well) in patients undergoing resection. However, the mucosal redness is rarely due to inflammation unless it occurs at or adjacent to a radionecrotic ulcer. Elsewhere it is due to mucin depletion and numerous telangiectatic vessels in the mucosa and submucosa. It should be noted that wherever it occurs, mucin loss imparts a red hue to the mucosa, and that the normal color of the mucosa is due in part to the presence of mucus-producing cells.

Histologically, mucosal atrophy is invariably present; this is seen as a reduction in the amount of epithelium per unit area of mucosa. It takes the form of a reduced number of crypts (or pits in the stomach), while those remaining are distorted and frequently show budding directed toward increasing the numbers of crypts. Paneth cell metaplasia is invariably present in the large bowel. Mucin depletion is obvious and is reflected by a reduction in the usual numbers of goblet cells, although this tends to be variable even within the same specimen. Nuclei are often larger than normal, and atypical features such as nuclear stratification, may be present; it is uncertain whether this is really a premalignant change. Additionally, both Paneth and argentaffin cells may have an excess number of granules, and these may be present on the wrong side of the nucleus. Thus, typical Paneth cells may exhibit large subnuclear granules in addition to those in the normal supranuclear distribution, while argentaffin cells may have typical fine granules in a supra- or peri-nuclear position. Telangiectatic capillary channels (discussed below) are present. The lamina propria may contain an excess of chronic inflammatory cells, but this also is very variable.

The stromal changes of late irradiation damage consist of edema and a fibrinous exudate which organizes by fibrosis, and are probably the result of initial endothelial damage. Histologically the edema is easily missed (a control should be used if there is doubt), while the exudate is irregular and has focal condensations resembling amyloid. Subsequent fibrosis is therefore also irregular, and focally replaces parts of such structures as the submucosa. Fibroblasts characteristically enlarge, their nuclei and nucleoli become enlarged and prominent, and their cytoplasm tends to be basophilic due to an increase in the rough endoplasmic reticulum, and may acquire a "swallow-tail" appearance. The most spectacular changes are usually seen in arterioles, particularly those in the submucosa. The arterioles frequently show intimal proliferation, sometimes with "foamy" endothelial cells—particularly relatively early in this phase of the disease—while the media may become hyalinized. Thrombosis, often becoming organized, may be found within the lumen, particularly in the region of an ulcer. At the capillary level of the mucosa, there are numerous telangiectatic blood vessels that are sometimes asymmetric (Fig. 18-1). These vessels may be found immediately beneath the luminal epithelium, and sometimes appear to open directly into the lumen. This is the usual cause of the bleeding found in long-standing radiation damage.

Late Complications

These usually involve the intrapelvic bowel. Complications other than hemorrhage from the telangiectatic vessels described above consist of radionecrotic ulcers (complicated, although rarely, by colitis cystica profunda),

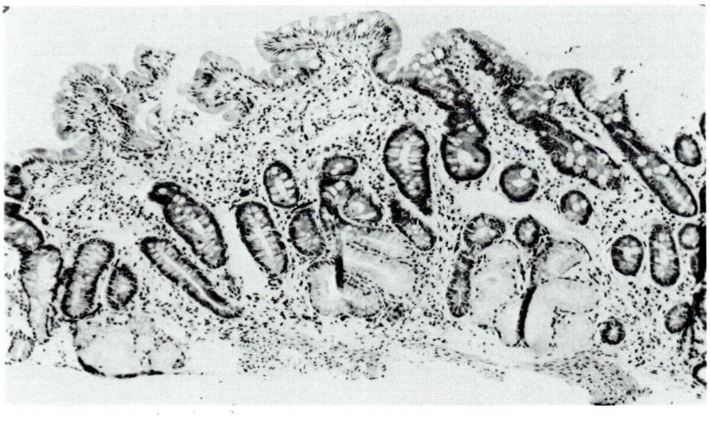

Fig. 18-1. Irradiation changes in the small intestine. There is loss of villi and regenerative changes in the crypts (they are irregular and also show pyloric metaplasia). The lamina propria contains numerous telangiectatic capillaries (H&E, × 80).

stenosis, obstruction, fistula formation, and carcinoma. Deitel and Vasic[149] reported 38 patients with late complications of radiotherapy: small-bowel injury was found in 27 patients in adherent loops of small bowel in the pelvis. All 15 patients with rectosigmoid stenosis had received intracavitary irradiation for carcinoma of the uterine cervix (13) or endometrium (2). Two patients had rectovaginal fistulas, and both required rectal excision. Three further patients required anterior resection, 8 required excision of loops of small bowel, while in a further 8 only lysis of adhesions was required. Four patients (19 percent) died in the perioperative period.

Two rare late complications of radiation injury are localized colitis cystica profunda and carcinoma. In the rectum, the former is usually a complication of the solitary ulcer syndrome of the rectum.[535] An appearance similar to that in colitis cystica profunda can be found as a sequel to irradiation therapy, but the mechanism in the latter is unknown.[30] The appearance of the rectal tissue most likely results from simple re-epithelialization of hemorrhagic pools in the submucosa following leakage from the abnormal blood vessels. Should these pools extend up to the overlying mucosa and an overlying ulcer be present, the regenerating epithelium could reline both the ulcerated area and the margins of the hemorrhagic cavity, producing the appearance of colitis cystica profunda. It is unclear from published papers whether the lamina propria has the characteristic fibromuscular proliferation seen in the solitary ulcer syndrome. If such proliferation is present, it would suggest that prolapse might be the cause of the injury in colitis cystica profunda complicating radiation therapy.

In view of the atypical nuclei that can be seen in colitis cystica profunda irrespective of its etiology, it is imperative that it be distinguished from a well-differentiated, mucin-producing adenocarcinoma. The presence of radiation-induced atypia in the epithelium could increase the difficulty in making this distinction.

Carcinoma, malignant lymphoma, and sarcoma are all rare complications of radiation therapy. Carcinoma affecting the GIT tends to be found mainly in the large bowel, and particularly following irradiation for female genital cancers; indeed, irradiation-induced large bowel carcinoma in males is exceedingly rare,[468] one patient developing a colon carcinoma following irradiation for testicular seminoma.[376] In their review, Martins et al.[402] found that 32 percent of rectal cancers developed between 3 and 10 years after irradiation, 40 percent between 11 and 20 years, 24 percent between 21 and 30 years, and 4 percent more than 30 years following irradiation, but the average was 15.2 years.

At the University of Chicago in the 1950s, many patients with peptic ulcers unresponsive to medical treatment were treated with gastric irradiation—treatment which temporarily reduced acid secretion and often promoted healing of the ulcers.[366] However, these effects were usually temporary, and in most patients the acid output returned to normal. Because some of these patients had subsequent surgery and others had gastric ulcers and gastritis, all of which predispose to the subsequent development of gastric carcinoma, attempts to analyze the data have been unsuccessful in reaching a conclusion about the role of irradiation, per se, in the development of such cancers (M. L. Griem, personal communication).

Malignant lymphomas are also increasing in frequency as a late complication of combined chemotherapy and radiotherapy, or the latter alone. These will be discussed further in the following sections.

ANTINEOPLASTIC AND IMMUNOSUPPRESSIVE AGENTS AND THEIR SEQUELAE

This will be discussed in three main parts: the direct effects of antineoplastic agents on the gut, the immediate sequelae of infection and bowel perforation, and the late sequel of neoplasia. Steroids will be included, insofar as they also predispose to infection, but their ulcerogenic effect on the gastric mucosa will be considered in the section on these drugs.

Direct Effects on the Mucosa

The variety of gastrointestinal side effects occurring in patients receiving antineoplastic agents is well known clinically, and many patients treated with these agents or combinations of them develop oral ulceration, diarrhea, nausea, vomiting, hemorrhage, ileus, or other symptoms as a result. Further, when mucosal ulcerations occur in these patients they are sometimes infected, and it is difficult to be certain whether the ulcers were initially caused by the drug and then became infected, or whether the organism was the initiating factor in an immunosuppressed individual. It is surprising that the genesis of these ulcers is so poorly documented in humans. Furthermore, although the pathology of antineoplastic drug-induced changes in the gut is fairly well documented in animal studies,[558] most of these were done using lethal doses of drugs, so that their significance in humans is questionable. Nevertheless, the few human studies done to date suggest similar conclusions, so that a fairly characteristic pattern of changes emerges. However, these vary considerably from patient to patient in their severity, and there appears to be a relatively poor correlation between the severity or extent of the pathology and clinical symptoms.

Perhaps not surprisingly, there are similarities between the acute effects of irradiation on the bowel mucosa and those of some antineoplastic agents. Further, there may in some intances be marked potentiation when both radiotherapy and chemotherapy are given together or sequentially. This seems to be especially true in the esophagus, where there appears to be marked potentiation, especially between actinomycin D or antineoplastic agents of the anthracycline group, particularly adriamycin, and radiotherapy.[462] Ulceration is seen at surprisingly low doses of irradiation (less than 2,000 rads), and not only recurs if the same combination is repeated, but also with further courses of chemotherapy in a patient who has been irradiated—a phenomenon known as "recall."[65,246] Further, this seems to be part of a more generalized phenomenon that affects tissues in the irradiation port, since the overlying skin may be similarly affected. However, this phenomenon does not seem to be limited to the skin or esophagus; it has also been described in the lung, small intestine, and heart.[22,62,418] In many of these patients the esophageal disease is so severe that the patient cannot swallow, and other forms of feeding may temporarily be required. As far as can be ascertained, infection plays no part in the genesis of this condition.

The effects of chemotherapy alone vary tremendously from patient to patient. Some patients with seemingly severe bowel disease tolerate these effects well and have surprisingly few symptoms. Others, with diarrhea, have had relatively normal biopsies from the left colon[437,662]; however the terminal ileum may be the most severely affected part of the intestinal tract,[661] which may offer at least a partial explanation of why some patients have diarrhea without obvious distal colitis. Of interest therapeutically is that patients whose large bowel tumors have responded to chemotherapy have invariably exhibited evidence of mucosal changes, although some primary tumors have appeared to be unaffected on the rare occasions when they were biopsied.[437] When mucosal effects of these drugs occur (Fig. 18-2), they can be considered as a continuum that starts with cessation of mitoses, causes progressive damage to the mucosa, and finally resolves.

In any part of the bowel the initial effect of an antineoplastic drug is to prevent mitotic activity, usually for several days, and often continuing for 2 days after the cessation of therapy. This is dramatic, and in one study, was apparent in the small intestine within a few hours of the administration of methotrexate, the nadir being reached on average about 21 hours after a single bolus of this drug was administered, returning to normal in 9 ± 5 days.[634] On electron microscopy, however, the same author demonstrated marked changes in the mitochondria, which were swollen and fragmented, while the Golgi showed severe cisternal dilatation. The same focality was also present at the electron microscopic level when normal cells were found immediately adjacent to damaged cells.[635] However, the underlying architecture of the mucosa, such as the villi in the small intestine, is often well preserved. At this stage, an excess of what appear to be pyknotic nuclei may be found, particularly near the crypt base; these take the form of small, supranuclear inclusions, and have been called karyolytic[223, 289] or apoptotic bodies.[550] They are normal but markedly increased in number following irradiation[223, 289] or chemotherapy,[550, 635] and appear to be phagolysosomes or large, membrane-bound vacuoles.[223, 289, 550]

There is marked, probably dose-related variation in the amount of epithelial damage, with some patients developing no change in either the villous architecture of the small intestine or breaches in the epithelial cells.[634] Mild changes in villous architecture may have to be treated with caution in patients with malignancies: in one study that attempted to define the cause of weight loss and malabsorption in these patients, it was found that about a third had some degree of villous loss, and that small-intestinal biopsies were normal in only a third.[151] However, since some patients had received either chemotherapy or radiotherapy, the question remains open. The association between villous loss and starvation is also well known. In another study, involving only 5-fluorouracil (5-FU), there was also relatively little epithelial loss, and only mild broadening and flattening of the villi.[662]

Nevertheless, where combination chemotherapy has been used, the changes are more marked, with focal reduction or loss of villi[572] which may proceed to complete superficial necrosis of the mucosa.[383] A similar spectrum of changes is also found in the large bowel in patients receiving 5-FU[437, 572] or its analogue Tagafor[496] (Fig. 18-3). In Milles study,[437] biopsies from colostomy mucosa were more severely affected than those from rectal mucosa, possibly because the trauma that usually occurs around colostomy sites, requiring increased reparative changes, predisposed the mucosa to severe injury when antimitotic agents were given.

The first description of epithelial changes occurring with antineoplastic therapy in humans seems to have been that of Weston and Guin in 1955, describing the appearances of bizarre mucosal changes in the intestine and lung that at the time were considered to be possibly precancerous.[661] Although called metaplasia, the changes described conform so closely to typical chemotherapy changes that there is little doubt that that was the cause. All of the patients studied were children with acute leukemia who had been treated with the early versions of combination chemotherapy.

The characteristic feature of antineoplastic drug-induced damage to the bowel seems to be the focal variation of the damage, even from crypt to crypt, some crypts being severely damaged while adjacent crypts remain relatively unaffected. Mucin depletion is typical, and is accompanied by attenuated cuboidal cells in the upper part of the crypt. In the affected crypts, the brunt of the damage is borne in the superficial portion, where the nuclei are large, pleomorphic, and often have a prominent nucleolus. After a few days the lamina propria becomes more vascular, and there is an increase in the content of lymphocytes and eosinophils. Where the changes are severe, virtually all of the crypts are affected, showing depletion of mucus and atypical nuclear features, but even at this stage there is variation in the disease from crypt to crypt. The cytoplasm may appear foamy, while the surface epithelial cells and the brush border may be lost. It is at this stage that frank erosion or ulceration may occur.

The foregoing phase of degeneration and progressive injury is followed by a regenerative phase that is heralded by a burst of mitotic activity. At this stage many of the crypts are

(Text continues on p. 529.)

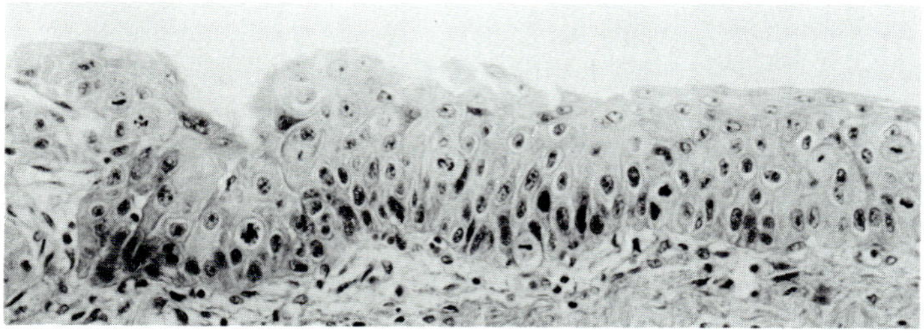

(A)

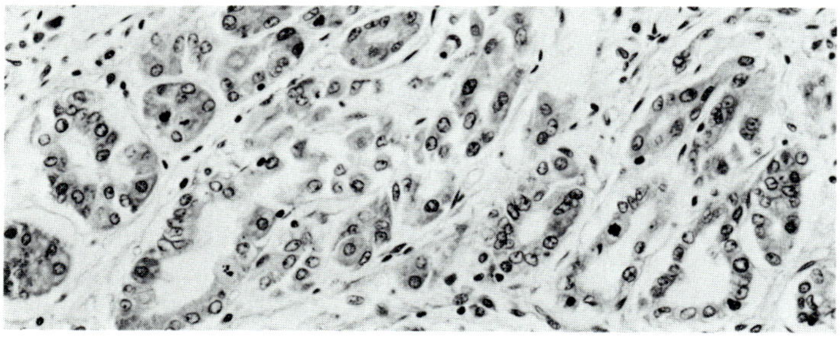

(B)

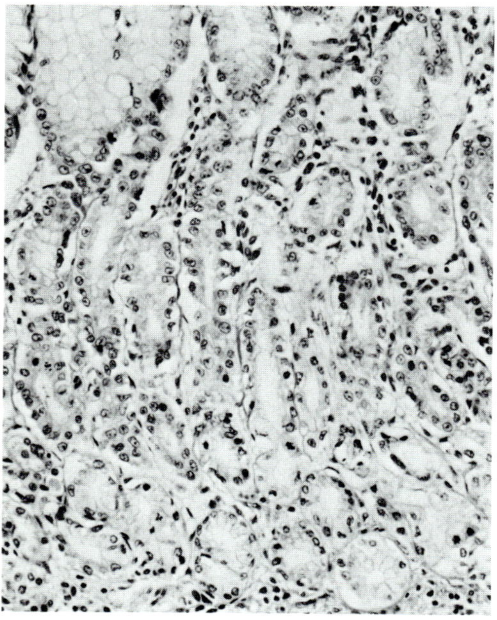

(C)

Fig. 18-2. Recovery from chemotherapy along the length of the intestinal tract. Despite affecting the entire length of the gastrointestinal tract, there was no abnormality in the pancreas. (A) Esophageal mucosa showing hyperplasia of the basal layer, mild atypia, and numerous mitoses, some of which are abnormal and close to the surface. (H&E, × 200). (B) Basal portion of gastric body mucosa. The specialized mucosa is partially lost, with only occasional recognizable parietal cells, but numerous mitoses. Normally, no mitoses are seen in this region. (H&E, × 200). (C) Gastric antrum. There is no apparent loss of glands, but many mitoses can be seen, mainly in the lower part of the mucosa. (H&E, × 160).

Fig. 18-2 (*Continued*). (D) Small intestine, showing only rudimentary villi with actively regenerating epithelium over their surface and a slight increase in acute and chronic inflammatory cells in the lamina propria. (H&E, × 125). (E) Large intestine, showing crypts at different stages of regeneration (H&E, × 80). (F) Higher power of (E), showing lack of maturation of crypts with little attempt at goblet cell formation, but with numerous mitotic figures. Cytomegalovirus infection is also present in the crypt just right of center. (H&E, × 160).

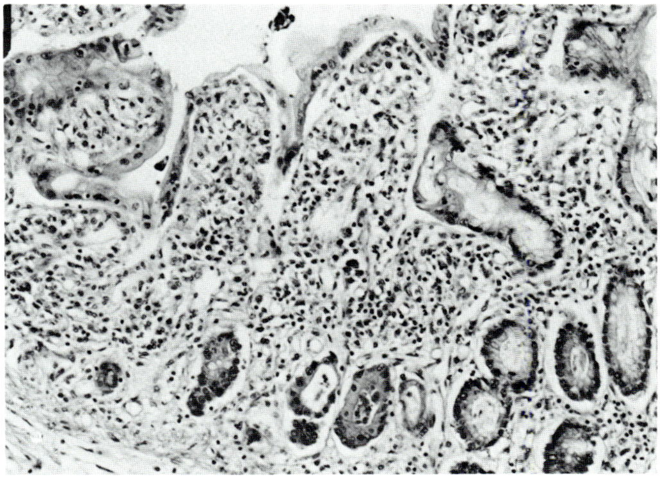

(D)

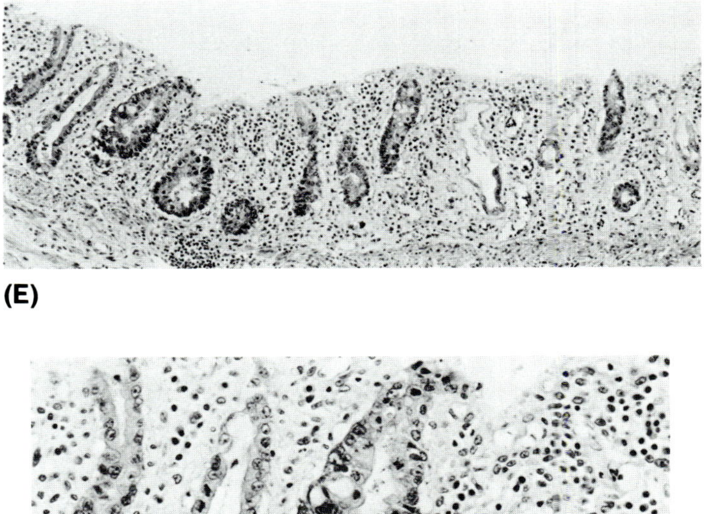

(E)

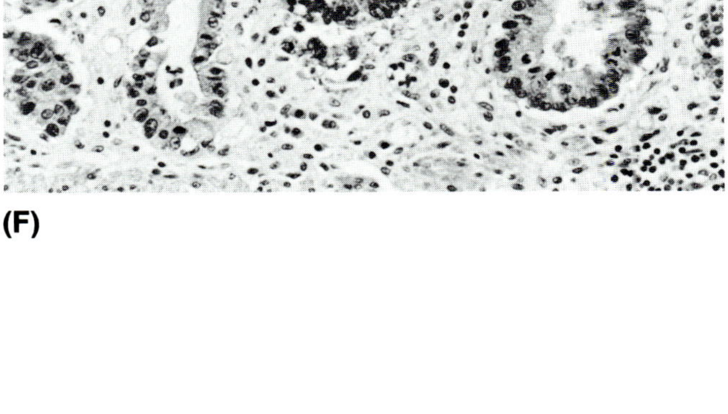

(F)

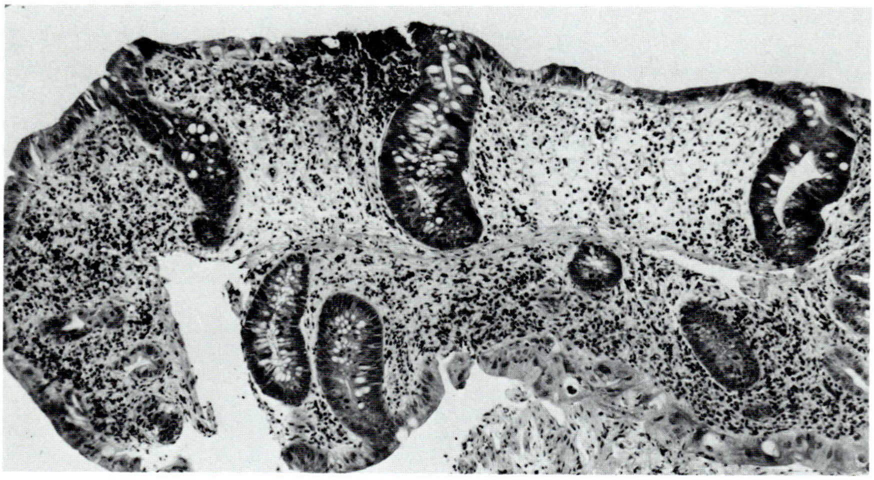

(A)

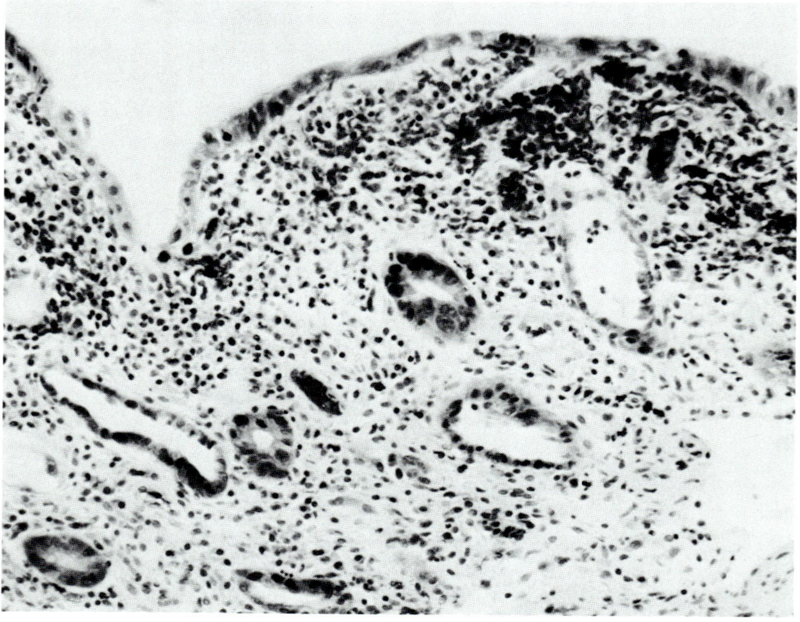

(B)

Fig. 18-3. Colonoscopic biopsy in a patient following colitis as a result of Tegafor, a long-acting 5-fluorouracil compound. (A) Note the obvious atrophy with marked reduction in the number of crypts present. Regeneration is present in the surface epithelium (lower right) and in the crypts on the extreme left (H&E, × 80). (B) Higher magnification of a further biopsy, showing marked variation in the degree of regeneration from crypt to crypt (H&E, × 175).

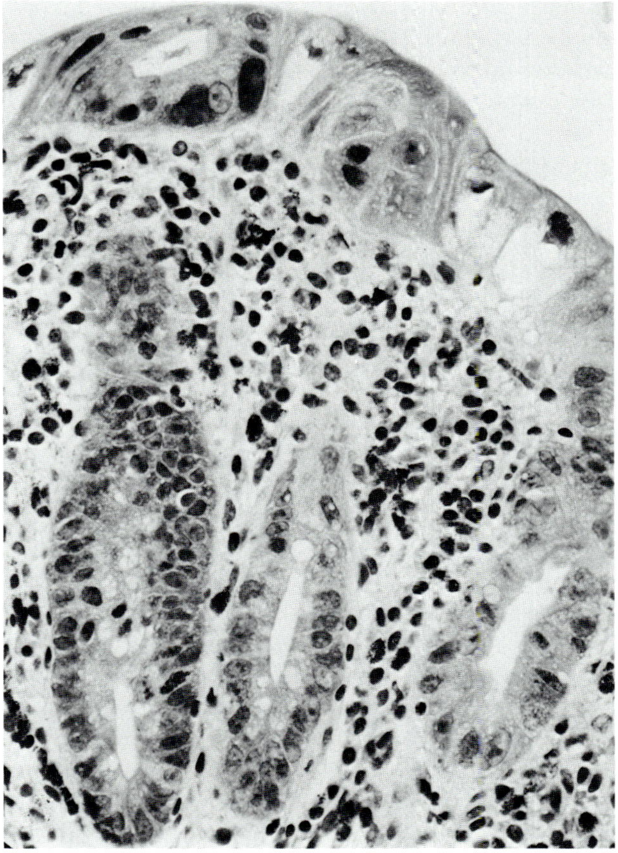

(C)

Fig. 18-3 (*Continued*). (C) High-power view of a third biopsy, showing crypts with no differentiation into goblet cells, but with enlarged nuclei. The crypt on the right still has the attenuated nuclei associated with active regeneration, while quite severe atypia is present in the surface nuclei. (H&E, × 350).

atrophic, cystically dilated, and lined by attenuated epithelium. There is marked variation in both nuclear size and staining, and little evidence of mucus production, although some crypts appear distended with mucus and sometimes with cellular debris. Mitoses are present at all levels of the crypt and even on the surface. The reparative changes maintain the focal characteristics seen in the earlier phases, the changes progressing more rapidly in some crypts than their neighboring crypts. Throughout the process, the cells at the bases of the crypts are the least affected, and may remain intact throughout the full episode. It is from these that the entire regenerative process occurs.

Changes in the bowel epithelium usually resolve within about 14 days, but the inflammatory and telangiectatic changes may persist for 3 to 4 weeks. In the esophagus, telangiectasia of the capillaries in the papillae may be pronounced.[572] Wherever telangiectatic changes occur, they are prone to rupture and cause intramucosal or submucosal hemorrhages. Occasionally, larger hematomas may form, especially in patients with marked depression of the platelet count.

As hinted at earlier, some drugs have a greater tendency to affect the GIT than others. Thus, cyclophosphamide appears to cause relatively little damage other than atypia in the esophageal mucosa.[571] On the basis of animal work, vincristine might be expected to cause an excess of mitotic figures in the early stages of GIT injury because of its effect on the mitotic spindle[279]; myenteric plexus damage following the use of this drug will be considered in the section below, on obstruction. Nitrogen mustard administered in doses from 60 to 90 mg with high-pressure limb tourniquets to prevent marrow damage in patients with Hodgkin's disease produced surprisingly little intestinal damage according to gastric and small-intestinal biopsies examined 48 to 72 hours after administration of the drug.[121] However, the most severe disease has been apparent with 5-FU and its analogues, and particularly with combination chemotherapy involving the use of cytosine arabinoside.[572] The latter study was of autopsy material from patients treated with this drug in combinations with cyclophosphamide, daunorubicin, and vincristine. While the study therefore incriminates cytosine arabinoside, it seems likely that combinations may be particularly likely to cause injury.

Finally, it would be remiss to finish without a word about colchicine, the antimitotic effects of which have been used experimentally for years. It is almost anachronistic that a drug with the known effects of colchicine, and which is also known to produce gastrointestinal side effects in humans, has very little pathologic documentation. In animals it is known to produce malabsorption, with some histologic changes.[456] In humans it produces variable changes, predominantly partial loss of villi with an excess of inflammatory cells in the lamina propria. There appeared to be little correlation of these changes with any malabsorption produced.[265, 503]

Long-term Effects

Malabsorption. Some children with acute leukemia, receiving maintenance chemotherapy, and particularly methotrexate, appear to develop a malabsorption syndrome that resolves when the offending drug is withdrawn.[131] One patient who underwent a jejunal biopsy was reported to have shown some loss of villi.[28] However, the change was not illustrated, and it is thus uncertain whether it was of the hypoplastic or hyperplastic type.

Megaloblastic Changes. The development of megaloblastic nuclei, as may be seen in the small and large intestine in patients with vitamin B_{12} or folate deficiency,[199, 267] might be expected fairly commonly in view of the number of patients now on chemotherapeutic protocols for extended periods, either as maintenance or adjuvant treatment. However, we have been surprised at how infrequently such changes are found, particularly at autopsy, in well-preserved bowel in patients known to have been receiving such therapy virtually up to the time of death.

Ulceration

Ulceration of all parts of the GIT may be observed in patients undergoing treatment with antimitotic agents and is very frequent at autopsy. Indeed, it is often a surprise to clinicians to see the extent of ulceration that may be present in immunosuppressed patients dying with sepsis and in whom an enterologic source of the latter was suspected but never documented. No part of the tract is spared. In his autopsy study of patients treated with combination chemotherapy that included cytosine arabinoside, Slavin[572] found esophageal ulcers in 55 percent of patients, gastric ulcers in 20 percent, small intestinal ulcers in 33 percent, and large intestinal ulcers in about 70 percent. Ulcers were multiple in a third of the patients. Throughout the tract, *Candida* was frequently associated with these ulcers, particularly in the stomach. In the large bowel it was often associated with Gram-negative bacilli or enterococci. In the esophagus and small intestine, *Candida* was present in half of the ulcers, the remaining organisms being Gram-negative organisms or, in the esophagus, herpes. Both pneumatosis cystoides intestinalis involving all parts of the tract and liver abscesses were among the more unusual complications of the sepsis.

Increasing numbers of patients treated with antimitotic agents both for tumors and for immunosuppression following transplantation have developed large-bowel complications. A variety of lesions may result, but the most common seem to be perforation of a diverticulum, particularly in the sigmoid colon and presumably as a result of diverticulitis that has not resolved and often has not been clinically recognized because of immunosuppression, and ulceration that has a distinct tendency to affect the right side of the colon, particularly the cecum (typhlitis). Ulceration may take the form of single or multiple ulcers that may perforate or cause severe blood loss and carry a high mortality. Quite why this area should be selectively affected is unknown. It is, however, intriguing that this is the same area in which angiodysplasia occurs in elderly patients, particularly those with low-output states or other forms of severe cardiovascular disease. It is also the same region in which neonatal enterocolitis tends to occur in the very young. The luminal PO_2 is also at its lowest in this region. It is therefore tempting to speculate that all of these conditions may be related, the common factor being mucosal ischemia or anoxia, which in patients with angiodysplasia is chronic but in the other groups is relatively acute. However, other factors, currently unknown, must also come into play. Some of the focal ulcers have been called "nonspecific" ulcers,[214, 395, 397] particularly in non-immunosuppressed individuals. Many immunosuppressed patients will show evidence of cytomegalovirus (CMV) infection around the base of the ulcer,[603] and particularly in endothelial cells, if this is carefully sought.

Some of the evidence that immunosuppression may be involved in the genesis of gastrointestinal ulcers is as follows:

Steroids

Although steroid-induced gastric disease is best considered in the section on gastric disease, it is appropriate to consider steroid-related ulceration of the intestines in this section. Since the association between intestinal ulceration and steroids was first postulated by Beck et al in 1950[48] there have been many documented occurrences of predominantly large-bowel, but also small-bowel, ulceration in patients treated with steroids.[234, 400, 427] Steroid-induced large-bowel disease usually takes the form of either a perforated diverticulum,[188, 477] usually in the sigmoid colon. Sometimes "nonspecific" ulcers occur in the right colon, particularly in the cecum and proximal ascending colon.[592, 650] The association between steroids and bowel perforation has been well investigated by ReMine and McIlrath,[509] who found that among 780 patients with gastrointestinal perforation, 79 cases were related to steroids. Dividing patients into those that received perioperative "cover," those regularly receiving less than 20 mg of prednisone per day, and those receiving more than 20 mg of prednisone per day revealed large differences in the last group. This last group was characterized by having a much longer delay from the onset of symptoms to treatment (8 versus 2 days), a lower white count, and a much higher mortality (85 versus 13 percent). The clinical symptoms of perforation were much less apparent in this group, and this factor was primarily responsible for the delay in operation. A further point of interest was that the duration of steroid therapy averaged almost 18 months in the low-dose group but only 4 months in the high-dose group. The sites of perforation were interesting in that only 3 of 79 were in the stomach. In the low-dose group, 7 perforations were in the small intestine (4 duodenal, 3 ileal) and 7 were in the large bowel (2 ascending, 1 transverse, 1 descending, 3 sigmoid colon). In the high-dose group 17 (36 percent) perforations were small-intestinal (8 duodenal, 2 jejunal, 7 ileal), and 29 (60 percent) were in the large bowel (4 ascending, 2 transverse, 2 descending, 20 sigmoid colon). In all groups it appeared that the first 3 weeks of treatment was the period when perforation was most likely to occur.

Antineoplastic Agents

When this group of agents is considered, a slightly different spectrum of disease becomes apparent, which has been best described in patients undergoing chemotherapy for malignancies that usually have involved the hematopoietic system. These disorders were well described by Amromin and Solomon[20] who invoked four pathogenetic mechanisms for bowel disease in their 69 patients. Some were in shock/ischemia (7); others had therapeutic necrosis of tumor or tumor infiltration (21), mucosal hemorrhage and necrosis (7), trauma (21—mainly peptic esophagitis and stercoral ulcers in the rectosigmoid), or combinations of these conditions (21). In all of the patients, mucosal erosions or frank ulceration created a potential port for infection, and many of the patients were also septic. Sixty patients had received some form of chemotherapy within the 2 weeks prior to death, steroids alone being used in 27 and steroids as part of combination chemotherapy in a further 28. The third group (those with mucosal hemorrhage and necrosis) has been called "agranulocytic necrosis,"[154] neutropenic enterocolitis,[444] necrotizing enteropathy,[20] agranulocytic lesion,[164, 502] and typhlitis,[645] and has been included in the ileocecal syndrome.[561]

Sherman et al.[561] pointed out that among 20 children with acute leukemia, many of the gastrointestinal complications of this disease tended to be localized to the right iliac fossa. Five of their patients had acute appendicitis and 5 had typhlitis. However, leukemic infiltration was found in only 2 patients. Although not stated, it is possible that the high mortality in this series occurred partly because patients were taking steroids that may have masked the symptoms of what was otherwise typical appendicitis. Typhlitis, however, is not a typical childhood disease, and either the leukemia or its treatment predisposed to the development of this unusual complication. It is apparent that this and other forms of focal intestinal ulceration can occur when patients are in remission as well as in relapse,[330, 381, 641] and that although the prognosis is poor, early surgical intervention when the ulceration is first suspected may be lifesaving.[327] Although the pathogenesis of these ulcers is multifactorial, the fact that some occur in patients in remission but on maintenance chemotherapy raises the question of an association with chemotherapy, on which many patients were maintained.

A somewhat similar group of disorders may be seen in patients with chronic renal disease, particularly those who have had transplants, while the same group of lesions is also being seen following liver transplantation.[340]

Immunosuppression Following Transplantation

A variety of gastrointestinal complications may follow renal transplantation, and may affect all parts of the GIT.[56, 255, 441, 484, 539, 603] A range of underlying lesions may occur, some of which have an ischemic basis, but ulceration with subsequent infection, hemorrhage, or perforation is the most common lesion.

In the paper by Sutherland et al.,[603] typhlitis was the cause of intestinal bleeding in 12 of 65 patients with gastrointestinal bleeding among 964 patients undergoing renal transplantation. The study showed that patients with this complication were likely to have had aggressive treatment for episodes of rejection immediately prior to the hemorrhage and in the face of CMV infection. Cytomegalovirus was found in 9 of the 12 ulcers. The mortality of this complication was high, only 2 patients surviving. It is difficult to speculate on whether the CMV in the etiology of typhlitis is causal or a secondary invader and, if the latter, whether it is innocent or potentiates underlying disease. Also of interest was that 5 of the 12 patients with typhlitic ulcers were diabetic; however, this was roughly the same proportion of diabetics that was present in the entire group, so that this statistic is of uncertain significance.

It is becoming increasingly apparent that typhlitis is not limited to renal transplant patients; it is also described following liver transplantation. In the Denver series, 8 of 157 patients developed large bowel complications following liver transplantation. In 3 of these, cecal ulceration occurred.[340]

In summary, when the three subgroups discussed above are considered together, a variety of intestinal complications may be seen with antineoplastic and immunosuppressive drugs, including steroids, but the causal relationship may not be immediately apparent. Thus, if a point source of bleeding is seen angiographically in the ascending colon, a clinical diagnosis of angiodysplasia may be made. It is only following resection that bleeding is found to be due to an ulcer or bleeding diverticulum that may be drug related. Similarly, stercoral ulceration (usually discovered at autopsy) may not immediately be causally related to preceding chemotherapy. Some patients in whom vincristine has been included as part of their treatment protocol may develop obstructive symptoms that may be secondary to damage to the myenteric plexus, with subsequent stercoral ulceration. Also it is worth remembering that since a transplanted kidney is usually placed in the left iliac fossa, it abuts directly onto the adjacent large bowel. This often causes constipation in the immediate postoperative period, but stercoral ulceration, with subsequent perforation may occasionally occur in this portion of bowel.[10] Significantly, "spontaneous" perforation of the colon caused by a barolith,[64] has also been reported in a patient on hemodialysis, thereby also increasing the spectrum of gastrointestinal diseases that may be seen in patients with chronic renal failure.

INFECTION

As was apparent in the previous section, it is difficult to easily separate ulceration and infection, because so many ulcers in immunosuppressed individuals become infected. Nevertheless, it is convenient to do so in order to deal with some of the more unusual infections that tend to affect this group of patients. The relationship between immunosuppression and herpes and *Candida* infection of the esophagus, and also between immunosuppression and large bowel ulcers and typhlitis in which CMV may be found, has already been mentioned above. However, as with other anatomic locations, a variety of organisms may be found. Not only do immunosuppressive drugs provide fertile soil for opportunistic infections not usually seen in humans, they may also lead to the reactivation of a variety of infections which, prior to therapy, were quiescent or producing relatively few symptoms.

Strongyloides

Symptoms from this nematode vary from none to severe diarrhea. However, there have been about 50 reports in the literature of intestinal involvement by *Strongyloides stercoralis* causing death, all of which have occurred in immunosuppressed patients. In about 20 percent of these, the infection was thought to have contributed to the patient's death. The infection causes diarrhea that may be bloody. Powell et al. also describe massive large-bowel hemorrhage, and provide adequate references to previous reports.[498]

Amebiasis

Amebiasis is among the many parasitic infections that may be reactivated by corticosteroids.[598] It has been suggested that patients from areas in which amebiasis is endemic, and who may require steroid therapy, should routinely be screened so that this complication can be avoided.

Cryptosporidiosis

Human infection by coccidial organisms was once thought to be confined to infection by *Isospora belli* or *hominis* occurring primarily in the tropics, and to be self-limiting. However, it has become apparent that a closely related organism, *Cryptosporidium,* can cause a profuse, watery diarrhea that may be fatal

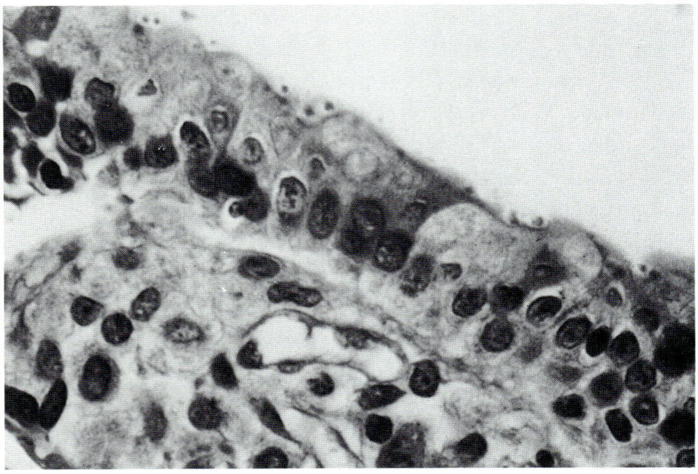

Fig. 18-4. Small-intestinal epithelium in a renal transplant patient with *Cryptosporidium* on the luminal surface (H&E, × 640). (Courtesy of Dr. J. Yardley, Baltimore, MD.)

in immunocompromised patients.[423, 464, 658] The diagnosis is readily made on a jejunal biopsy, provided that one takes the usual care to screen the enterocytes at high-power. This should routinely be done to detect *Giardia lamblia* infection, but the organisms of cryptosporidosis are also readily seen as small organisms adhering to enterocytes (Fig. 18-4).

Histoplasma Capsulatum

This is a further example of an organism that may occasionally be seen in the general population, but which acquires opportunistic properties in immunocompromised individuals[459] (including the very young and the very old). It can affect any part of the intestinal tract, although it has a distinct preference for the ileocecal region[156]; the infection may have a variety of gross appearances, including diffuse polyposis[57] or giant gastric[195] or duodenal[29] folds—appearances that occur when the organism has become disseminated.

Candida

As mentioned above, *Candida* infection may occur anywhere in the intestinal tract, although it is most common in the upper part of the tract and particularly in the esophagus.[339] It classically produces white plaques or pseudomembranes, and invasive, budding organisms can usually be detected on biopsy or brushing. In the stomach, infection may be associated with multiple erosions or ulcerations, penetrating ulcers, or tumor masses.[176] It is difficult to know whether the infection is a primary or secondary phenomenon; however, gastric ulcers infected with *Candida* appear to heal at a slower rate than noninfected ulcers.[316] *Candida* infection may also be a complication in patients receiving broad-spectrum antibiotics of any type, although in practice ampicillin seems particularly likely to be associated with the disease. However, this antibiotic is so widely used that it is difficult to know how great this risk is. *Candida* infection has also been seen following the inhalation of steroids in an asthmatic patient.[268]

Phycomycosis

Other fungal infections than candidiasis may affect the intestinal tract in immunosuppressed individuals. Phycomycetes are nonseptate fungi that include *Rhizopus, Mucor,* and a variety of other fungi that rarely affect humans. The major site of infection is the stomach, occasionally with a second infected site that is most frequently colonic. The subject is reviewed by Lyon et al.[386]

Cytomegalovirus (CMV)

Mention of the possible pathogenetic role of CMV in the genesis of cecal ulceration has already been made with regard to immunosuppressed patients. One of the problems in defining its exact role is that CMV infection may be relatively common in this group of patients without giving rise to any overt disease. Nevertheless, its presence is associated with a higher rate of renal graft failure.[410] Franzin et al.[204] performed gastroduodenoscopy randomly on 12 patients following renal transplantation, and found biopsy evidence of CMV infection in 7. In 4 of these 7, multiple inclusions were found, whereas in the other 3, only rare inclusions were seen. All of these patients had been endoscoped prior to transplantation; biopsies did not show the infection, and titers against CMV were not elevated at that time. When infection is present, typical inclusions may be found in the epithelial cells in any part of the tract. However, when ulceration is present, the inclusions may also often be found in mesenchymal and endothelial cells.[269] In one immunosuppressed patient, CMV infection following renal transplantation was not only associated with an area of ulceration, but also diffusely involved the entire myenteric and submucosal plexus of the resected colon and appendix.[499]

In an attempt to determine whether CMV was a primary or secondary factor, Goodman et al.[238] compared 3 patients with CMV associated with perforation with 10 others who also had colonic perforation. Of the total of 13 patients, 11 had an identifiable cause of perforation; CMV was present in 1 of these. Conversely, both patients in whom no cause of perforation could be found had CMV infection. In other cases of CMV infection, the authors confirmed the presence of inclusions in the vicinity of ulceration or perforation but, unlike Henson,[269] were unable to find inclusions in unaffected mucosa. They concluded that these findings were consistent with the theory that mucosal injury from any cause may be followed by CMV infection, which may then lead to further injury and perforation, while in their 2 cases in which no other cause was found, the CMV may well have been the primary factor. There is therefore an analogy to be drawn with gastric *Candida* infection, which seems to prolong and perhaps increase the damage in areas of ulceration.[316]

Herpesvirus

Although herpes infection may affect the esophagus of apparently normal patients, and may even cause bleeding,[194] it more commonly affects immunosuppressed individuals, and even those treated with steroid inhalation.[268] The usual site of involvement is the esophagus, although much less commonly the stomach alone may be affected[581]; the diagnosis may be made by biopsy or brushing of the pseudomembranes or ulcers involved,[372] at which time typical intranuclear inclusions may be found in cells that appear to be falling away from the usually tightly cohesive squamous epithelium. However, it has been repeatedly stressed that antemortem diagnosis of herpes infection, particularly esophageal, is still relatively uncommon,[93] although awareness appears to have improved considerably of late.

Neoplastic Sequelae

The development of a second neoplasm in patients who have undergone treatment for a prior neoplasm is well documented. Such neoplasms fall into two general categories: spontaneous tumors, in which case patients have a tendency, possibly inherited, to develop more than one tumor (thus, patients with ovarian carcinoma appear to be at increased risk of developing second primary cancers of the uterine corpus, colon, bladder, breast, and hematopoietic system[507]); and tumors that appear to be increased in incidence in those patients who have been treated with radiotherapy,[590] chemotherapy, or both. Tumors affecting the hematopoietic system are discussed in Chapter 5.

Since second neoplasms can occur anywhere, it is not surprising that they occasionally appear in the intestinal tract. If only those occurring initially in the intestinal tract are considered, most are malignant lymphomas of large-cell type.[312] The entire subject of drug-induced cancer is reviewed by Hoover and Fraumeni.[284]

RADIOLOGIC CONTRAST MEDIA

A variety of complications have been described following the use of contrast media in the intestinal tract. These will be discussed under the major categories of perforation, granuloma formation, ischemic necrosis, acute appendicitis, and bezoar or mass formation with subsequent obstruction, mucosal injury, or both.[403]

Perforation

This is an uncommon complication of the use of contrast media, with an incidence that varies from about 1 in 3000 to 1 in 40,000 barium enemas.[236] Such perforations tend to occur under three different conditions: (1) mechanical damage, which may be caused by the introduction of enema tips, balloons, catheters, and so forth, and which may occur with normal mucosa; (2) perforation following damage caused by previous mucosal biopsy[18, 406] (rarely does perforation occur in the normal intestinal tract); and (3) perforation among patients who have pre-existing disease such as peptic ulceration, active colitis, irradiation damage, diverticulitis, and ischemia in which the mucosa is already damaged and the pressure causes perforation. Perforation of the esophagus may cause barium pleuritis and mediastinitis.[66] Perforation of duodenal ulcers[232] or the large bowel is serious, and carries a mortality of about 40 to 70 percent if not treated rapidly; the mortality increases if faecal material is also spilled.[549] Interestingly, Zheutlin reported 53 cases in which the mortality was 47 percent in the surgically treated group and 42 percent in patients treated conservatively[677]; however, about a third developed late complications of repeated small-bowel obstruction due to adhesions. In an interesting review, Rosenoer[526] mentions 3 neonates with obstruction due to small bowel atresia in whom the bowel segment immediately distal to the obstruction opened directly into the peritoneal cavity. He advocates the use of water-soluble media delivered slowly.

Cecal perforation has been reported because of a slipping clamp on a barium enema tube in the presence of a competent ileocecal valve.[562]; if the valve is incompetent the same complication can result in filling of the small bowel, and stomach, with vomiting of barium and its aspiration into the lungs.[146, 660] Fatal perforation of the colon has also been reported following the use of a silicone foam diagnostic enema in a patient with an irradiation stricture.[17] These enemas were occasionally used in cases of sigmoid redundancy that did not allow visualization of that region, since they provided a three-dimensional montage of the area.

Ischemic Necrosis

This may occur by one of two mechanisms, the most common of which follows angiography (see p. 517), while the second may be a consequence of impacted contrast medium in the bowel, particularly in infants. Injury following angiography can be caused by a number of different mechanisms. Sometimes these result directly from attempts to achieve a therapeutic effect, such as embolization or from the infusion of pitressin.

Masses, Baroliths, and Acute Appendicitis

Gastrograffin is a widely used contrast medium consisting of 66 percent meglumine diatrizoate and 10 percent sodium diatrizoate in a lemon-flavored aqueous solution to which Tween 80, a detergent, is added. It is extremely hypertonic (about 1800 mOsm/l), and can therefore cause large fluid shifts into the intestine. In dilated loops of small intestine in infants, undiluted gastrograffin may cause necrosis of the bowel wall. It is uncertain whether this is the result of an irritative effect caused by the Tween 80, or a result of fluid shift in children with meconium ileus.[363] Cecal perforation, probably due to the same mechanism, has also been reported in adults.[553]

In acid solution, the water-soluble diatrizoate of gastrograffin may be precipitated out. Gastrograffin remaining in the stomach for more than about 24 hours can form a solid precipitate and even a cast of the stomach that can cause multiple gastric erosions. In one patient this appears to have caused massive hematemesis.[210]

It is noteworthy that masses of barium may form baroliths that adhere strongly to the gastrointestinal mucosa, and may resist purgation. However, such complications as obstruction, ulceration, and perforation are distinctly rare, and usually occur only when a partially obstructing mass such as a carcinoma is already present.[328, 559] In the appendix, baroliths may help precipitate an appendiceal obstruction, with subsequent acute appendicitis; however, examples of this are rare.[148, 429] The barium sulfate tablets formerly used may cause esophageal obstruction[541]; these tablets did not distintegrate for 3 hours in tap water at room temperature, whereas new tablets do so within 30 minutes.

Barium Granuloma

Barium granulomas are a consequence of the escape, through the mucosa into the submucosa, of contrast medium in an amount insufficient to cause full-thickness perforation. The resulting barium incites an inflammatory reaction that is polymorphic and includes histiocytes and sometimes foreign-body giant cells that contain the contrast medium. The granulomas are usually readily recognizable, in aggregates on H&E stained sections, as a whitish, crystalline material that is refractile but nonbirefringent. The granulomas tend to be found in the vicinity of the anal canal and rectum,[371] and much less frequently at other sites, such as the transverse colon[419]; they may vary from granulomas a few millimeters in size to large polypoid masses up to about 7 cm diameter. Some are ulcerated and may be mistaken clinically for a carcinoma.[488] They may also be associated with sinus or fistula tracts.[371]

A variety of other unusual effects have been noted following the escape of barium locally, including necrotizing proctitis[14] and ureteral occlusion by a barium granuloma.[174, 273] The entry of barium into the submucosal venous plexus may cause barium emboli; this has produced massive pulmonary emboli that were fatal[227, 523, 525] and a barium granulomatous hepatic abscess.[295]

OBSTRUCTION

Apart from the contrast material mentioned above, a variety of other agents can cause intestinal disease, and many of these may cause obstruction. At its simplest, this may involve the impaction of food—particularly meat—in the esophagus[345, 491] or, in the young, a lactobezoar in patients with cows' milk intolerance.[361] However, some drugs have been reported to form a physical mass that may ultimately give rise to obstructive symptoms; these include such substances as iron (see p. 565) and vitamin C,[642] the latter occurring in a patient who daily took 15 tablets of 300 mg each when getting a cold—a feat that was repeated 2 weeks later, when she developed abdominal pain. At laparotomy, numerous marble-like objects were removed, some of which appeared to be held up at, and obstructing, the ileocecal valve.

Ileocecal obstruction has also been reported from antacid tablets being inadequately chewed in a patient who already had partial obstruction at the valve secondary to Crohn's disease.[497] Obstruction in the transverse colon has been seen secondary to cholestyramine in a 10-month-old girl.[114] Rectal impaction and ensuing obstruction secondary to the ingestion of large quantities of bran, ultimately requiring manual evacuation under general anesthesia, has also been reported.[311]

SEQUELAE OF INSTRUMENTATION

A variety of complications of endoscopy adorn the medical literature. Some of these involve perforation,[344,675] hemorrhage (often as a result of biopsy or endoscopic polypectomy), and thermal injury to the bowel.[409,177] These are not within the scope of this chapter. However, one practice worthy of documention is that of preparing the bowel for colonoscopy by using mannitol solution. Bacterial degradation of mannitol results in the production of sufficient methane and hydrogen to produce a combustible mixture, and this has exploded in one patient, with lethal consequences, when colonoscopic polypectomy was being attempted.[61] The answer to the problem is to avoid this method of preparation and to use inert gases for insufflation. Injury caused by air pressure alone has also been reported.[344]

EXTRINSIC DAMAGE TO THE BOWEL

Intrauterine Devices

There are currently about 12 reports of intrauterine devices (IUDs) passing into the peritoneal cavity through the uterine wall and wreaking havoc with adjacent viscera, in this case the small or large intestine. Symptoms may vary from none to varying degrees of abdominal pain, depending on which part of the bowel is affected. At best, adhesions of the affected bowel with adjacent bowel may be found, but the device may also penetrate the bowel wall and either cause local perforation, actually pass into the lumen of the bowel,[324,652] or even cause gangrene.[34]

"Glove-powder" Peritonitis

Glove-powder may cause a granulomatous peritonitis, usually within 10 to 14 days postoperatively but, like any other form of peritonitis, the adhesions produced may later cause obstruction. Originally, when Halsted introduced rubber gloves, he found it necessary to use a lubricant in donning them. He used lycopodium-spore powder, and soon produced the first case of granulomatous peritonitis.[548] Talc (largely magnesium silicate) was then introduced, and produced similar complications, and even sinuses and fistula tracts.[171] This was followed by cornstarch, rice starch, and currently a cornstarch derivative treated with epichlorhydrin (a skin irritant) and 2 percent magnesium oxide,[593]—all of which can induce granulomatous peritonitis. However, with greater awareness of this complication, great care is now taken to ensure that excess starch is removed from the outside of surgical gloves, while low-starch gloves are made for the ultracautious. Sternlieb suggests that sodium bicarbonate might be a useful lubricant.[593] The morphologic appearance of "starch" granulomas is well known, comprising a classical foreign-body inflammatory reaction with giant cells that contain the starch, which birefringes, producing Maltese crosses when examined under polarized light. Clinically, affected patients have abdominal pain, ascites, and numerous granulomas that may be studded over the peritoneal surface or liver. These grossly resemble neoplastic or tuberculous disease, and their true cause is rarely suspected clinically at the time of their detection. They tend to respond well to either steroids or indomethacin. Interestingly, a similar pelvic disease has been described following the repeated use of condoms containing starch-powder.[540] There is also a report of hypersensitivity to cornstarch, with proctitis following a sigmoid resection for diverticulitis.[231]

Sclerosing Peritonitis

There have been several suggestions that beta-blocking agents may occasionally cause this condition. Practolol in particular has been invoked,[123] but single case reports suggest that other, related compounds may have a similar effect.[44, 161, 264] Nevertheless, the data in support of this causation are not strong,[24] and although it is reasonable to suggest that related compounds may have similar side effects, further evidence is required. Retroperitoneal fibrosis is discussed in Chapter 11. However, it should be remembered that methysergide-induced fibrosis can affect any part of the intestinal tract, including the esophagus and duodenum; ergot and its derivatives (including lysergic acid diethylamide) have all been implicated.[293]

Oleogranuloma and Sclerosants

Oleogranulomas in the intestinal tract are largely confined to the vicinity of the dentate line. However, sclerosants such as those used for esophageal varices may also cause a brisk acute and chronic inflammatory infiltrate (personal observation), although with relatively few foreign-body giant cells. In the rectum, oleogranulomas form as a result either of the local injection of hemorrhoids,[243, 602] or following repeated oil enemas for the treatment of constipation.[411, 460] Some rectal preparations now also contain hyaluronidase and heparinoid, as well as paraffin and wood alcohol; the former two substances may well enhance submucosal spread of the paraffin which, if it accidentally reaches the submucosa, may produce larger lesions.[245] Like barium granulomas, oleogranulomas may form large, tumorous masses that may even be annular and ulcerated, and may be clinically mistaken for carcinomas.[272, 607, 655] Histologically, mineral oils elicit the strongest reaction, followed by animal fats, while vegetable fats produce the least reaction.[447] Round droplets of oil that dissolve out during tissue processing are surrounded by a polymorphic inflammatory infiltrate that is predominantly of the chronic inflammatory type, but which also may include polymorphs and giant cells (Fig. 18-5).

SUBSTANCES ACTING PREFERENTIALLY ON PART OF THE TRACT

SALIVARY GLANDS

A variety of substances may produce painful enlargement of one or both parotid glands. These include iodide compounds, including contrast media; phenylbutazone and oxyphenbutazone; bretylium; guanethidine; and methyldopa; parotid enlargement may also follow endotracheal anesthesia and upper gastrointestinal endoscopy.[667] Isoprenaline may produce a painless enlargement of the glands. In all affected patients, sialography has been essentially normal, while tests for mumps and other infections have been negative. A few patients have had other associated immune phenomena. Withdrawal of the drug or steroid therapy provides effective treatment, although in some patients the lesion has recurred following challenge. Unfortunately, biopsy has been done in only one patient, with no inflammation being detected.[407] It appears likely that the swelling is the result either of spasm of the large ducts, causing the retention of secretions, or of edema within the gland, with a similar effect.

Radiation changes in the salivary glands are seen relatively frequently in patients with carcinomas of the head and neck region who have

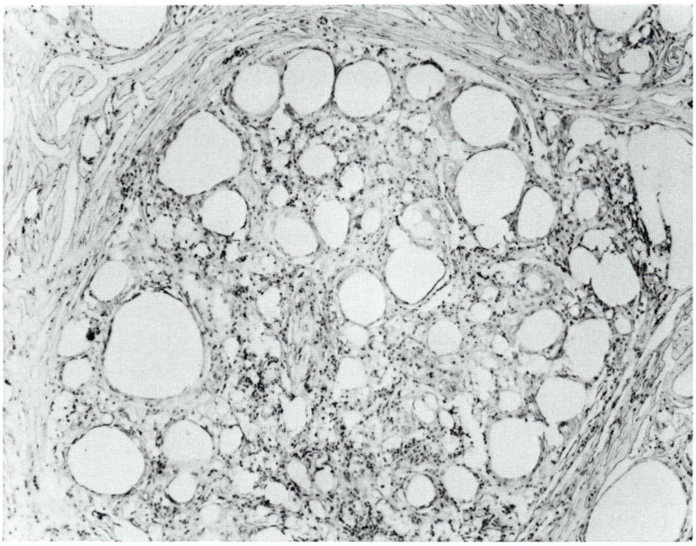

Fig. 18-5. Oleogranuloma following injection of sclerosant material. The empty spaces are surrounded by numerous foreign-body giant cells. (H&E, × 80).

radiotherapy followed by subsequent resection. The early glandular changes include a polymorph and eosinophil infiltrate, with desquamation of much of the large-duct epithelium and of serous glands; the mucous glands are relatively spared. Most of the glands encountered in pathology laboratories are examined at a later stage, when the ducts are distended with inspissated material. There is diffuse atrophy of the glands with intervening edema, fibrosis, and a predominantly plasmacytic infiltrate. Mucous glands and some of the smaller intercalated ducts remain relatively spared. Vascular changes and atypical fibroblasts are relatively uncommon. The entire subject has been reviewed by Fajardo and Berthrong.[180]

THE ESOPHAGUS

Although the statement that "Just about anything that can be put into the mouth will sooner or later be put into the mouth" is hardly original, it is certainly enough of a truism to pass unchallenged. Because of this, injury to the perioral region, oropharynx, and remainder of the intestinal tract will ultimately be seen to be the result of an incredible variety of solids, liquids, and even gases. Accidental pneumatic rupture of the esophagus has been reported due to anything from biting through the inner tubes of inflated tractor tires, to putting compressed air lines into various orifices, in this case the mouth.[218] However, most substances that injure the esophagus do so because of either a direct corrosive action, usually from chemicals that are accidentally or deliberately ingested, or from drugs that "stick" in the esophagus.

Some drugs, such as atropine and other cholinergics, nitrites, diazepam,[534] and oral contraceptive tablets[640] (as well as chocolate,[674] nicotine, coffee,[116,627] alcohol,[318] and peppermint[248]), reduce the lower esophageal sphincter pressure, thereby increasing gastric reflux and presumably the likelihood of the patient developing pathologic sequelae. Such sequelae in no way differ from reflux esophagitis in causing basal cell hyperplasia, elongation of the papillae, acute inflammation, ulceration, stricture, and possibly Barrett's esophagus; the effect is probably purely additive, and does not comprise any new or specific histopathologic features.

Some patients also have reflux of bile into the esophagus, and such cases show identical histologic features to those seen in peptic esophagitis (Fig. 18-6). It is perhaps relevant to point out that changes such as hyperplasia

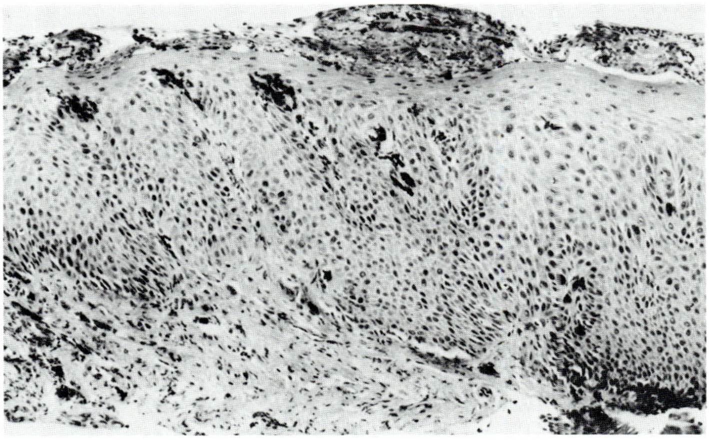

Fig. 18-6. Esophageal mucosa in a patient with bile reflux. There is mild hyperplasia of the basal layer, but the dermal papillae extend very close to the surface. (H&E, × 110).

of the basal layer, elongation of the papillae, polymorph infiltration, and so forth—while characteristic of reflux esophagitis—are not diagnostic; rather, these changes constitute a nonspecific reaction to any form of esophageal injury, and can be seen just as readily in patients with *Candida*-caused or other forms of esophagitis. The possibility that such changes are secondary to reflux should only be considered if they are found in abnormal mucosa that reaches down to the esophagogastric junction distally. It is positively misleading to report pathologic effects in a biopsy as being due to reflux if the clinical situation is unknown, or if the biopsy came from a localized abnormality in which the lower esophageal mucosa was normal. It should also be remembered that about 20 percent of patients show these changes in the 2 cm immediately proximal to the gastroesophageal junction,[296] and that biopsies from this region therefore should not be reported as showing "changes consistent with reflux." An abnormal gastroesophageal junction with histologic changes extending in continuity for more than 2 cm above the junction is required for changes to be considered secondary to reflux. Such thoughtless reporting does little to enhance relations with clinicians, and may lead to unnecessary surgery for the patient.

A variety of mechanisms may delay the passage of drugs from the oral cavity into the stomach. Among these may be simply the intake of insufficient fluid to ensure that a drug reaches the stomach. Many tablets contain a swelling agent that ensures their rapid disintegration upon contact with water. If this is insufficient, the hygroscopicity can cause the tablet to stick to the esophageal mucosa and damage it.[356] Mechanical effects may prevent tablets from passing easily into the stomach. These may take the form of a stricture of any cause, a motility disorder, a prominent aortic arch that may cause tablets to stick in the midesophagus, or an enlarged left atrium that causes hold-up in the lower esophagus just proximal to the esophagogastric junction.[664] Patients in the recumbent position are also prone to retain tablets in the esophagus, since they do not enjoy the additional aid of gravity in getting a tablet-plus-fluid into the stomach. Patients with acne are also predisposed to develop esophageal ulceration purely because the antibiotics most widely prescribed for acne (tetracyclines, clindamycin, and their derivatives) are those most likely to cause this condition. The final factor that plays a significant role is the nature of the tablet itself. Many tablets dissolve in water to form a relatively neutral solution, or they may be buffered. Others dissolve in small quantities of water to form a highly acidic solution that corrodes the esophageal mucosa. It is these that may produce ulceration which, if deep, may resolve with stricture formation or even be lethal.

An interesting study regarding the genesis

of esophageal ulceration from tablets was done by Evans and Roberts,[179] who at the time of routine radiologic studies of the upper intestinal tract gave patients two aspirin-sized barium sulfate tablets with about 15 ml of water (patients with symptoms suggesting organic esophageal obstruction were excluded). In 60 percent of the patients, the tablets remained within the esophagus for longer than 5 minutes, while in 5 of 57 patients they remained for longer than 20 minutes; in three-fourths the tablets held up in the lower esophagus, and this was particularly likely to happen if a hiatal hernia was present. In 10 of 57 patients the hold-up was at the level of the aortic arch, while in 4 of 57 it occurred at both this site and the lower esophagus.

There are three main categories of drugs that appear most likely to cause esophageal ulceration and its sequelae. These are emepronium bromide, potassium chloride (usually in the form of Slow K), and antibiotics, of which the most important are the tetracyclines and their derivatives.[129] However, other drugs have also been incriminated, and the list continues to grow. These include quinidine, ferrous salts, barbiturates, chloral hydrate, tolmetin, and phenylbutazone. Those drugs that produce highly acid solutions may also occasionally damage the gastric mucosa.

Emepronium Bromide

This quaternary ammonium anticholinergic agent increases bladder capacity, thereby delaying the desire to micturate; it is therefore particularly useful after prostatic or vesical surgery and urinary frequency of other causes. There have now been about 20 reports of esophageal ulceration related to emepronium bromide, most frequently in the midesophagus in middle-aged women.[117, 338, 560] Fortunately, most of these have healed either completely or with minimal scarring. It is uncertain whether this side-effect is the result of local irritation, lowering of the cardioesophageal sphincter pressure, allowing reflux, or perhaps both.

Potassium Chloride

Potassium chloride tablets were found to be a cause of "nonspecific" small-intestinal ulceration, particularly in the 1960s. For this reason, Slow K was introduced, in which the potassium chloride is released over approximately a 4-hour period. However, this preparation is usually given to patients with cardiovascular disease who are also on diuretics, and some of them, particularly those with mitral stenosis, will have marked enlargement of the left atrium, which compresses the esophageal lumen in its lower half and forms a potential site for these tablets to be retained.[382, 664] The potassium chloride may then be released over a period of time into the same small segment of the esophagus, causing ulceration and often stricture.[486] The local effects of potassium chloride appear far more damaging than those of emepronium bromide, and of the 12 patients summarized by Collins,[117] all developed either penetrating ulcers or strictures, and 5 died, 2 as a result of the stricture, 2 because of hemorrhage, and the other from mediastinitis. Similarly, 2 of Whitney's 6 patients died, the other 4 developing strictures.[664] However, such severe consequences do not always occur.[482] Teplick reports an esophageal stricture in a patient receiving 10 percent potassium chloride solution,[620] while Lambert's patient also developed a stricture.[350] Gastric ulceration as a result of potassium salts has also been reported.[299]

Antibiotics

Doxycycline. In 1975, Bokey and Hugh[70] described esophageal ulceration that seemed to be the result of a tablet of doxycycline that "did not go right down." Since then there have been several reports confirming this association.[133, 229, 338, 543] It was found that aqueous solutions of the drug have a very low pH, and that the direct effect of this causes injury to the esophageal mucosa. Large mucosal ulcers may result. Because doxycycline is green it may be more readily identified in the period immediately following injury, by the greenish-blue color of the exudate which may be seen during endoscopy.[472]

Tetracycline. Several tetracycline-treated patients have been described who developed symptoms very similar to those in patients taking doxycycline (pain on swallowing shortly after taking the tablet, together with the sensation that the tablet had lodged), with similar results.[133, 326, 595] The mechanisms of the tetracycline effect may also be similar to that with doxycycline, since tetracycline tablets, when dissolved in small quantities of water, produce a solution of pH 2.5 to 3.0.[595] Further reports of doxycycline and tetracycline-induced esophageal damage in the European literature may be found in the review by von Klingeren.[333]

Clindamycin. Discrete local ulcers in the midesophagus have been described, apparently as a result of ingestion of a capsule of clindamycin that stuck in the esophagus.[604] The injury healed completely in 2 weeks. Such injury may be more common than generally appreciated in view of the number of patients taking clindamycin on a long-term basis for acne.

Clinitest Tablets

Although the caustic effect of these tablets might better be included under the section on chemical corrosives (below), they are of sufficient importance to justify their inclusion here. The swallowing of these tablets is usually accidental, occurring in newly diagnosed diabetics in whom an oral hypoglycemic agent is also prescribed, although it is occasionally deliberate. As a result of some confusion, patients attempt to test their urine with the hypoglycemic tablet and ingest the Clinitest tablets, with disastrous results. The damaging ingredient is sodium hydroxide (NaOH) which, apart from being directly corrosive, particularly on squamous epithelium, also reacts with water exothermically, generating substantial heat. The injury sustained may therefore be the result of both mechanisms of action (Fig. 18-7). We have seen several patients with severe esophageal strictures as a result of Clinitest ingestion, and suspect that it is far more frequent than the literature suggests.[430, 625]

Antineoplastic Agents

The effects of antineoplastic agents, particularly Adriamycin or actinomycin when in combination with radiation therapy, have been discussed above. One paper reported lower esophageal necrosis in patients taking fluorouracil alone,[478] but this seems to have been an isolated report. However, 3 of 17 patients in the same study died as a result of the necrosis secondary to fluorouracil.

Barbiturates

Esophageal damage culminating in strictures has been seen at the University of Chicago as a result of phenobarbitone tablets sticking in the esophagus (C. Winans, personal communication), and another case has also been described.[648]

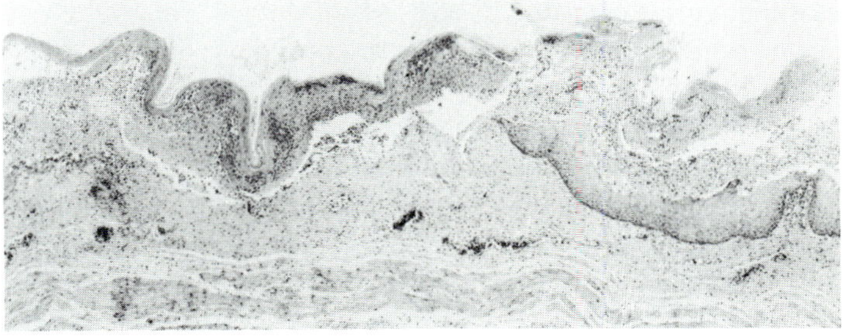

Fig. 18-7. Esophageal ulceration at the junction with normal mucosa (right) resulting from the ingestion of Clinitest tablets. Note the sloughing of the affected mucosa in the center and to the left (H&E, × 32).

Chloral Hydrate

This is an irritant in large quantities, affecting particularly the esophageal and gastric mucosa. In one patient, an esophageal stricture developed following the ingestion of a large amount of chloral hydrate. When she had been resuscitated from her comatose state, the patient complained of marked retrosternal burning.[233]

Compound Aspirin, Phenacetin, and Codeine Tablets

A single brief report describes a 5 cm-long, annular, midesophageal ulcer in a woman, posssibly as a result of these tablets. The ulcer appeared to have bled, but ultimately healed completely.[666]

Iron

Abbarah et al. report a woman who developed ulceration and marked swelling of the hypopharynx and cervical esophagus after a tablet of ferrous sulfate had become lodged in her hypopharynx.[1]

Nonsteroidal Anti-inflammatory Drugs

There are occasional reports of eosphageal ulceration caused by phenylbutazone in combination with prednisone,[308] although it is uncertain which agent was actually responsible. There are also reports in the European literature suggesting that indomethacin may cause both esophageal ulceration and hemorrhage.[9] Additionally, we have seen tolmetin-caused esophageal damage at this Institution (P. Frank, personal communication).

Quinidine

Teplick reported 2 patients who developed esophageal strictures as a result of ingesting quinidine tablets.[620] Both patients had cardiac disease. Although it is possible that esophageal compression by the enlarged heart may have played a part in the genesis of the stricture in one patient, the stricture in the other was in the cervical esophagus, and was probably unrelated to the enlarged heart.

Emetogenic Injury

It is difficult to know whether esophageal or gastric tears should be included in this chapter; nevertheless, the association between alcohol ingestion and the subsequent vomiting that actually produces the tear is worthy of mention as an indirect effect of alcohol. Some patients had also taken aspirin, although the exact role of this is uncertain; at worst, aspirin may cause some degree of gastritis that could make a tear more likely. Tears have also rarely been associated with vomiting induced by ipecacuana or methyl cellulose. If the tear is limited to the mucosa, the syndrome is named after Mallory and Weiss, while if it is of full thickness it is named after Boerhaave, who was the patient first described as having this condition. The Mallory-Weiss syndrome frequently presents as hematemesis, but the additional complications following perforation in Boerhaave's syndrome make the latter far more serious. The tears usually begin in the cardia and extend into the lower esophagus. There is an odd distribution to the tears, for which there is no satisfactory explanation. However, about half occur in the right quadrant, about a quarter in the left quadrant, and most of the remainder, posteriorly. Only about 7 percent occur anteriorly. Several good reviews on the subject are available.[91, 335, 654]

One report documents Mallory-Weiss syndrome following vomiting after an oral electrolyte solution was given as part of a bowel preparation for colonoscopy.[579]

Finally, it should be remembered that patients who vomit persistently, irrespective of the cause, may develop peptic esophagitis with all of its sequelae.

Injury Secondary to Ingestion of Chemical Corrosives

A variety of corrosive substances are ingested either deliberately, mistakenly by alcoholics, or accidentally by children—particularly those between 1 and 4 years of age. These substances are traditionally divided into four categories,[398] essentially comprising strong alkalis, strong acids, fixatives and weaker acids, and bases such as oxalic acid or weak ammoniacal solutions. The most commonly ingested of these are mainly alkalis containing sodium hydroxide, which is the basis of many household cleaners. In a series of 86 young patients who appear to be fairly representative,[625] virtually all cases of esophageal injury were related to alkali ingestion. The peak age in this group was between 1 and 4 years of age. Lye (NaOH or KOH, taken by 41 patients), and Drano (NaOH, taken by 30 patients) accounted for the vast majority of cases; perhaps the milky appearance of these substances accounted for the mistaken identity. Other ingested materials included Liquid Plumr (sodium hypochlorite and potassium hydroxide, taken by 3 patients), Clinitest (NaOH, taken by 2 patients; see above), Easy Off (NaOH, taken by 1 patient), and ammonia, taken by 3 patients. The remaining six ingested materials were unknown.

Conversely, in a series of adults from France,[155] over half of the patients (42 of 76) had ingested bleach (sodium hypochlorite), 12 had ingested acids, and 22 had ingested alkalis. Clearly there is a marked regional and age variation in the substances likely to be encountered. However, other seemingly innocuous products, most of which have been ingested at some time, also contain strong alkalis. Thus, dishwashing detergents used to contain alkaline phosphates, but the pollutant nature of the latter has prompted their replacement by highly alkaline agents, particularly sodium metasilicate.[347] Denture cleanser tablets and powders contain potassium monopersulfate and sodium perborate, and liberate vast quantities of hydrogen peroxide, which in itself may be corrosive. Some also contain pyrophosphate,[3] which is alkaline.

Relatively few acids are ingested, but most of the common acids have been ingested at some time. These include all of the common mineral acids (sulfuric, nitric, hydrochloric), phosphoric acid, glacial acetic acid and others.

Two other groups of compounds that are occasionally ingested are fixatives, such as formalin or Zenker's solution, and weak substances such as oxalic acid. While this broad classification covers the majority of corrosive esophageal injuries, other substances, such as boiling water and absolute ethanol, are also well recognized to be ingested, while a variety of unusual chemicals such as paraquat also frequently cause esophageal ulceration or perforation,[4] although the pulmonary effects of the latter drug are much better recognized.

The pathologic effects of the foregoing substances vary markedly, depending on the amount of the substance ingested, whether it was in solid or liquid form, and in the latter form, its concentration. Further, although occasional generalities can be made about the distribution of the lesions produced, it is imperative to realize that none of these are absolute, and that there is a very broad spectrum of injury that can exist for any substance or group of substances. Thus, one common generalization has been that injury due to alkalis affects the mouth and esophagus, while that resulting from acid ingestion affects the stomach. There are also logical reasons why this might be so, since strong alkalis can damage the oropharynx and esophagus, but on reaching the stomach may be neutralized by the hydrochloric acid in that organ, producing relatively less gastric damage. Nevertheless, 7 of 17 patients reported by Cello[104] demonstrated greater gastric than esophageal damage in a series that contained no patients with acid ingestion. The series was also of interest in confirming that some patients who had ingested alkali corrosives that caused severe esophageal or gastric damage failed to show oropharyngeal lesions. However, most of these patients did complain of glossopharyngeal pain and dysphagia. Conversely, the esophagus seems a little more resistant to the action of acid, while the stomach is surprisingly sensitive. Thus the generalization concerning the effects of acids and alkalis is reasonable, but there are so many exceptions that such generalizations are unreliable.

Alkalis. Because of their exothermic reaction with water, and their ability to combine with fats and proteins, alkali substances fix to the tissue and can therefore cause deep ulceration. They also tend to produce damage wherever they contact epithelium. Thus, burns may be found around the lips and on the hands, chest, face, and any other part of the anatomy on which a child will wipe its hands. Burns may also be present in the mouth, pharynx, and esophagus, and may damage the stomach, although rarely damaging the tract beyond this.[12] Although hydrochloric acid in the stomach may at least partially neutralize the alkali, thereby reducing any damage, severe gastric damage can still occur.

There is also variation depending on whether alkalis are ingested in solid or liquid form. Tablets tend to stick to the mucosa of the oropharynx and upper esophagus, and to produce severe local damage, sometimes with almost complete distal sparing.[3] Many of the affected patients vomit, which theoretically might be helpful in causing some neutralization by the vomited gastric acid as well as through eliminating residual, solid alkali. However, considerable local damage has invariably occurred. Conversely, if alkali is swallowed in liquid form, disease is induced over a much greater area and tends to involve much of the epithelium from the lips to the stomach, and occasionally the small intestine. Nevertheless, many children spit out the liquid as soon as it enters the mouth, so that the incidence of alkali-induced esophageal disease is perhaps lower than expected (35 of 86 cases in Tewfik's series[625]). Occasionally, tablets of an alkali-containing substance may be swallowed and enter the stomach directly, so that the brunt of the damage falls on the stomach. A Clinitest tablet in one patient had most of its effect in the gastric antrum[430] in the form of multiple ulcers. Another patient, ingesting potassium hydroxide and sodium hypochlorite, developed bullae in the gastric wall that were detected radiologically.[367]

Pathologically, the esophageal lesions induced by alkalis may be considered in three phases[136]: The acute necrotic phase involves coagulative necrosis of mucosa and underlying tissue to a variable depth, a heavy acute inflammatory infiltrate, thrombosis in the underlying blood vessels, often with local hemorrhage, and subsequent superficial infection, usually bacterial. This phase lasts for about the first 4 days, until the coagulum sloughs. Reparative efforts then become more apparent, granulation tissue filling in the slough and fibroblasts starting to proliferate. This reparative phase lasts from about the fifth to the seventh day, and is the phase at which the esophageal wall is weakest. After this there is progressive organization of granulation tissue, fibroblast proliferation with collagen deposition, further degeneration of the muscle layers and nerves, with extensive replacement by collagen, re-epithelialization of the surface, and further contraction of the collagen that has been layed down in the submucosa and muscle. This is therefore the time when strictures start to form. Once the surface has been re-epithelialized, the underlying inflammation rapidly resolves. The entire process may be completed between about 6 weeks and 3 months after the initial insult.

Ensuing fibrous strictures are most frequently seen in the retrocardiac portion of the esophagus, and have been divided into four grades[184]: Grade I includes strictures that are less than circumferential, and which occur only over a short segment, so that they produce "shelf" strictures. These never cause significant luminal narrowing. A grade II stricture is a localized annular stricture less than half an inch in length; since fibrosis rarely extends into the muscle, these strictures are relatively easy to manage. Grade III strictures are still less than half an inch in length, but are dense, presumably from muscle involvement. These may cause marked reduction in the lumen caliber, with a very narrow lumen. Grade IV strictures are tubular and dense, remain ulcerated within, and often have adhesions in the peri-esophageal tissue. These cause the most severe problems clinically. Patients with grade III or IV strictures usually require some form of operative intervention. However, it should be remembered that while surgical measures may be required for some esophageal lesions following alkali ingestion, antrectomy or even total gastrectomy has occasionally been required because of the severity of gastric damage.[143]

Acids. Although the ingestion of strong acids may also cause injury to any part of the upper gastrointestinal tract, squamous epithelium seems rather more impervious to its effects than glandular mucosa, possibly because of the slightly alkaline surface of the former. A relatively superficial coagulative necrosis is often seen in the esophagus, but large areas of ulceration, such as are seen with alkali ingestion, do not often occur. In the stomach, the brunt of the damage occurs in the antrum, with relative sparing of the acid-producing area. Antral damage is largely proportional to the quantity of acid ingested, its strength, the time it is in contact with the mucosa, and the gastric contents at the time of ingestion, the damage being less if the stomach is full.[6] Apart from the superficial coagulative necrosis and ulceration, submucosal vessels may also become thrombosed, thus potentiating the injury. If damage is severe there may be perforation and necrosis of large areas of the stomach, both of which may necessitate gastrectomy.[6,143] Late strictures may occur anywhere from the antrum to the small bowel, and may ultimately require resection. One patient developed severe stricturing of the jejunum as a result of nitric acid passing straight into the jejunum through a Billroth II anastomosis.[6]

Freezing

In the early 1960s, freezing the stomach was attempted in some centers for the treatment of duodenal ulcer.[417,485] This appeared to have little effect on the duodenal ulcer but did succeed in producing hemorrhagic necrosis of the gastric mucosa. However, this assault seems not to have had any long-term effects on the gastric mucosa.

Fixatives

Pathologic fixatives such as formalin are occasionally taken in suicide attempts. Their effectiveness depends very much on the amount and strength of the material ingested. Cello et al. describe a patient who ingested Zenker's fixative (which includes mercuric chloride and potassium dichromate), and who was found on endoscopy to have a mild diffuse esophagitis but severe distal gastritis.[104] Conversely, we have seen a patient who ingested 40 percent formalin solution that, apart from fixing the upper intestinal tract in situ, caused marked submucosal edema throughout. No inflammatory infiltrate was present.

Late Sequelae

Apart from strictures that may cause difficult problems in clinical management, any esophageal stricture if severe will cause marked hypertrophy of the muscularis propria immediately proximal to it, while the overlying epithelium becomes very acanthotic, often having a pearly white appearance. The most dangerous complication of any stricture is that of supervening squamous carcinoma. These neoplasms appear to be relatively uncommon, although the exact frequency with which lye ingestion is followed by esophageal carcinoma appears unknown. However, the converse data suggest that between 1 and 4 percent of all esophageal carcinomas occur as a result of corrosive ingestion (usually lye). All are squamous carcinomas, and there is a marked tendency for them to occur at the level of the tracheal bifurcation, about 80 percent of all lye-related carcinomas occurring in this region.[21] In Appelqvist's series, which virtually doubled the number of cases of lye-associated carcinoma in the literature, most patients ingested the lye at an average age of 6.2 years, while the average age of diagnosis of carcinoma was 38.7 years for men and 44.7 years for women—considerably below the national average for Finland. Despite the theoretical difficulties of diagnosing carcinoma in patients with permenant stricture symptoms, the prognosis was better in this group than for patients with esophageal carcinoma not associated with lye ingestion. Furthermore, although survival was still dismal overall (11 percent at 5 years), patients who had resectable disease had a 25 percent 5-year survival, while in those who were both resected and survived the operation, this increased to 33 percent. Occasionally, verrucose carcinoma—a tumor in which the long term prognosis is excellent if the patient survives esophagectomy—may complicate lye stricture.[479]

Other Causes of Chemically-induced Carcinoma

The relationship between alcohol and smoking, particularly if combined, is well documented in standard textbooks of pathology, and in the West these are the two most frequent, identifiable predisposing factors in esophageal carcinoma. In other areas of the world where the prevalence of esophageal carcinoma is high, tobacco and alcohol are relatively uncommon, and other substances may be responsible. Trace metals in the diet, or lack of them, may have some relationship to the disease. However, the possibility that residues of smoking may play a role has been suggested,[274] although it is controversial.[275] Hewar suggests that in Northeast Iran, the high incidence of esophageal carcinoma may be related to the chewing and swallowing of sukhteh, the crude residue from the opium pipe, while in the Transkei, injonga—the residue in the pipe-stem—and isixaxa, the residues in the pipe after smoking home-grown tobacco, are also sucked and chewed by pipe-smokers. Both substances are mutagenic by the Ames' assay, and both seem to bear some relationship to the frequency of esophageal carcinoma in the areas mentioned.

In other high-incidence areas, the possibility remains that esopheageal carcinoma may be related to the tannin content in tea (without milk, which binds the tannin).[448] Parenthetically, the theophylline content of tea may also cause constipation.[282] Clearly, nothing is "safe"!

THE STOMACH

Mechanisms of Damage

The effects of a variety of drugs on the stomach are both fascinating and frustrating. Being the main receptacle for all ingested compounds, the stomach, not surprisingly, is susceptible to mucosal injury; perhaps it is surprising that this does not happen with greater frequency. The subject is fascinating because of the light that is being thrown on the pathophysiology of gastric ulceration, but frustrating because some of the data inevitably conflict and each "answer" begs further questions. Much of the experimental data has been gathered from studies in animals, sometimes with doses that are closer to lethal than therapeutic, and also under a variety of artificial circumstances. Their extension to humans is therefore sometimes questionable. More recently, many drugs have been evaluated by giving them to volunteers and evaluating their effect endoscopically before and after therapy. Unfortunately, some of the descriptions are poor, and in many cases biopsies were not taken, so that the underlying pathology must be inferred. The terminology used is also a little unsatisfactory, since a variety of different terms are applied to endoscopic lesions on the basis of assumptions that may not be justified. Nevertheless, endoscopists are very prone to interpret endoscopic redness as "gastritis" when simple mucin depletion or hemorrhage into the lamina propria can cause a similar appearance. Similarly, "erosions" refer to mucosal breaks superficial to the muscularis mucosae, and "ulcers" to those breaks that extend through it. The observation of resected specimens for conditions such as acute hemorrhagic gastritis (a pathologic misnomer this time, since there is rarely much "itis" present) frequently show that the erosions are sometimes ulcers (as defined above).

There is relatively little that is specific about drug-induced pathology in the stomach. The lesions produced are basically gastric ulcers (and duodenal ulcers, which will be included here for convenience, as necessary), which may be single or multiple, and occur in any part of the stomach (or duodenum, although here they are usually proximal). Erosions or ulcers may occur against the background of a normal mucosa, a chronically inflamed mucosa, or hemorrhagic gastritis. These are essentially similar to the spontaneously occurring conditions, and it is unnecessary to repeat their pathology together with all of their possible sequelae in this chapter, since these are readily obtained in standard textbooks of pathology.

The single most characteristic histologic aspect of these lesions, from which a drug-induced etiology may often be suspected, is the lack of inflammation that may be present, particularly when anti-inflammatory drugs are being considered. The lesions themselves may occur rapidly after the administration of a drug. However, lack of time is not the reason for the lack of a surrounding chronic inflammatory infiltrate, since the latter is often absent months after a patient begins ingesting a drug. It is probably too simplistic to suggest that the absence of such an infiltrate is the result of the local anti-inflammatory properties of the drug, for if this were the case, one would expect chronic gastritis of any cause to become less severe in patients receiving anti-inflammatory drugs. This does not seem to be the case, although studies to determine this point have not been specifically done.

While the hallmark of drug-induced disease may well be its occurrence in the absence of any surrounding inflammation (allowing the correct diagnosis to be suspected pathologically), it is more correct to state that the pathology is that of any underlying gastric disease with the superimposed, drug-induced lesion. Thus, in a patient without gastric disease, aspirin may produce multiple antral erosions without inflammation in the surrounding mucosa. However, if the patient has chronic antral inflammation at the time the aspirin are taken, then the ulceration will clearly occur against the background of chronic inflammation. This does not mean that the erosions are not due to the aspirin, but that two diseases are present simultaneously. Questioning the patient or assaying for the presence of salicylates is required to suggest the true etiology of the disease. Other than indicating that two diseases may be present simultaneously every time one observes an ulcer or erosion against a background of chronic gastritis, there is currently no way to distinguish this from ulceration occurring in chronic gastritis, but which is unrelated to drug ingestion.

Similarity of Drug-induced Disease to "Stress" Ulcers

The similarity between "stress" lesions such as acute hemorrhagic gastritis and its drug-induced counterpart can hardly pass unnoticed—either clinically or histologically—raising the possibility that they may be very closely related. However, this must be treated with some caution, because it seems that the damage caused by most drugs is produced as a common final pathway yielding similar lesions for a variety of different reasons. Stress-induced disease, such as that occurring postoperatively or following accidental trauma or sepsis, may or may not be easily fitted into the pathway.[323] Sugawa showed that lesions induced by aspirin or alcohol appeared identical endoscopically, and that both are frequently observed in the antrum.[600] However, this was in contrast to the lesions in patients who developed acute hemorrhagic gastritis as a result of trauma or sepsis. In these patients the lesions always began in the body of the stomach, often close to the gastroesophageal junction, and swept down in a wavelike manner over the following 2 days to involve the remainder of the body of the stomach and sometimes the antrum, so that by the time the antrum was reached the first lesions in the upper body were already healing. In many patients these lesions never reached the antrum, and in no patient was disease found in the antrum in the absence of disease in the body of the stomach. This may prove a useful point, for it suggests that lesions confined to the antrum may be drug-related.

Pathophysiology

Experimental data on the genesis of stress ulcers in animals does provide a useful basis on which to consider the possible mechanisms of drug-induced disease, since it usually requires that a combination of factors be present for the disease to occur. These are (gastric) acid, bile (reflux), and hypoxia.[515] It is not unreasonable to suspect that a similar combination may be required in humans. There is strong evidence to suggest that the ultimate lesion is related to the back-diffusion of hydrogen ions into the gastric mucosa,[138] and that this is associated with a decrease in the potential difference across the mucosa and an outpouring of water, sodium, and protein into the gastric lumen. Bile can mediate these changes,[515] as can aspirin and alcohol, but not steroids or other nosteroidal anti-inflammatory drugs.[125] Large amounts of histamine are released, causing increased capillary permeability, so that plasma accumulates in the mucosa, while red cells may also be extruded into the lamina propria. Histamine also mediates gastric acid secretion. Thus the resulting pathology is indistinguishable from the early lesion of acute hemorrhagic gastritis (AHG). Furthermore, as in AHG, the experimental lesion may also be followed by superficial necrosis of the epithelium, usually occuring in numerous foci within a short period of time. Some of these remain as fairly superficial erosions that exude blood, but others may involve the entire epithelium and extend into the musclaris mucosae. However, the muscularis propria usually remains completely intact in both experimental and human AHG (Fig. 18-8).

The real question is exactly how human stress fits into this picture. A century ago, Beaumont[46] noticed that a patient of his with a gastrocutaneous fistula (one Alexis St. Martin) showed marked variation in both the appearances of the gastric mucosa and in its secretory pattern, and that these were related to the patient's emotional status as well as his alcohol intake. Emotional stress in humans studied in the laboratory has also been associated with increased acid secretion and motility[442]; the mechanism of these is uncertain, but is almost certainly multifactorial, with both a hormonal and neurogenic input. Experimentally, Brown et al.[89] found that gastric damage induced in rats either by aspirin or indomethacin was strongly related to the presence of stress (in this case, being kept at 5°C), and appeared to be of a synergistic nature. Interestingly, the ulceration induced by indomethacin was attenuated by both H_1 and H_2 receptor antagonists, while ulcers induced by aspirin were blocked only by H_2 receptor antagonists.

Steroids. Steroid therapy is interesting in that it also has effects on gastric acid secretion. These do not occur immediately, but take sev-

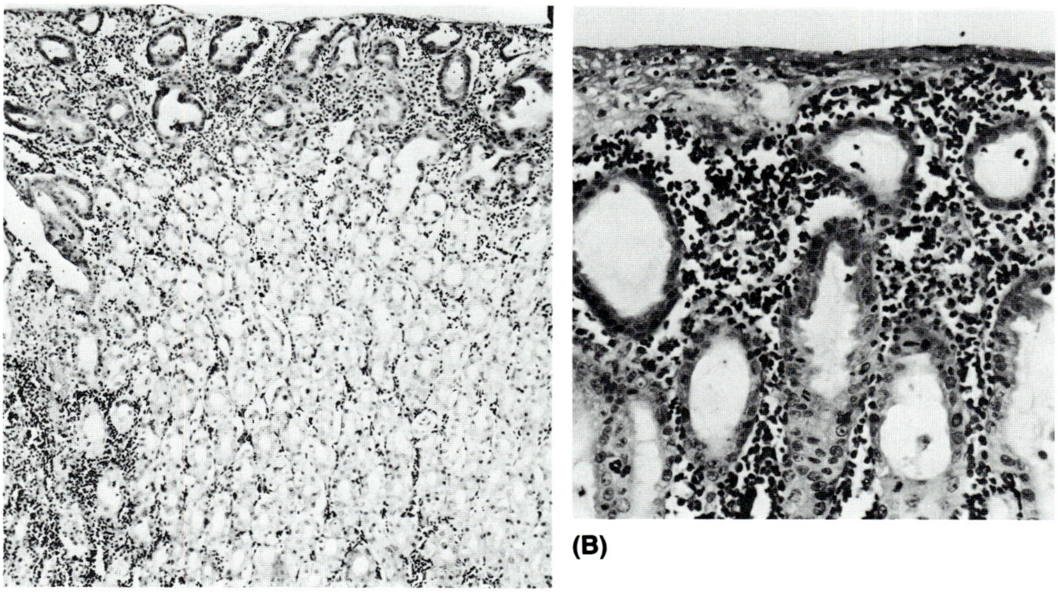

(B)

(A)

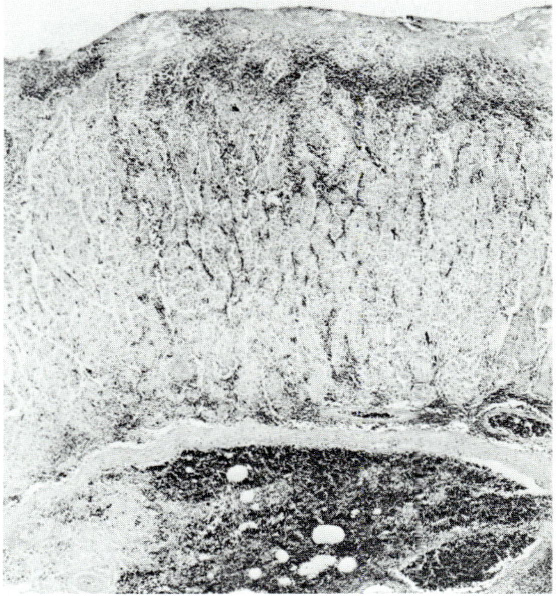

(C)

Fig. 18-8. Early acute hemorrhagic gastritis thought to be the result of aspirin ingestion. (A) There is extravasation of red blood cells into the superficial mucosa and also percolating down between the specialized glands of the corpus. (H&E, × 80). (B) Higher power view of (A), showing the marked mucin depletion in the gastric pits. The luminal epithelium has already been lost, but no polymorphs are visible. (H&E, × 200). (C) Same stomach from a more severely affected part of the mucosa. Note the hemorrhagic necrosis of the superficial mucosa. Red cells can be seen more diffusely between the columns of cells in the mucosa, while submucosal hemorrhage is also present. (H&E, × 40).

eral days to occur, and appear to be mediated by G-cell hyperplasia,[150] causing serum gastrin levels to rise a few days after steroids are administered. Steroids also potentiate the gastric response to feeding.[552] Patients with Cushing's syndrome show a similar phenomenon. The mechanism may result from the increased plasma amino acid level that results from steroid-induced protein catabolism. Some amino acids, such as arginine, are potent in promoting gastrin release.[309] These changes should be trophic for the parietal cell mass in the long-term, as well as causing increased acid secretion in the short-term. The latter may be sufficient to upset the delicate dynamic equilibrium in patients at risk of gastric ulceration, making them more susceptible to damage if other required factors are present. Experimentally, ulceration also correlates with decreased DNA and RNA synthesis, and is related to local gastrin concentration.[608] The latter, in turn, at least partially depends on the presence of solid food in the stomach, and depends strongly on somatomedin (gastric atrophy following hypophysectomy responds partially to somatomedin). Interestingly, lithium carbonate inhibits both basal and food-mediated gastrin secretion, probably through the adenylate cyclase system,[357] but the possible protective effect that this may have on psychiatric patients is unknown. Finally, cimetidine, an H_2-receptor antagonist, has also been found to reduce the incidence of aspirin-induced lesions in the stomach.[100] However, cimetidine probably also has a variety of other properties that are only gradually becoming recognized, so that pure reduction in acid output is unlikely to be the only mechanism involved.

Duodenogastric Reflux. The role of duodenogastric reflux in the genesis of gastric lesions is uncertain, but may well be crucial.[628] Bile probably has several different functions, one of which may be as a mucolytic agent or detergent, and the second a direct action on the mucosa. In isolated dog stomach, the transmucosal potential difference remains intact when both saline and hydrochloric acid are used as perfusates, but falls rapidly in the presence of bile, particularly when acid is also present; the latter immediately diffuses back into the mucosa. Bile therefore appears both to dissolve mucus and also to damage the epithelium when it is reached. Experimentally, the combination of bile and indomethacin produces extensive mucosal necrosis not seen with either agent individually.[665]

The sequelae of bile in the gastric antrum include hypergastrinemia and further acid production, and this may be mediated by somatomedin inhibition. Bile may also cause histologic mucin depletion and local chronic inflammation (Fig. 18-9). Indeed, one invariably sees superficial mucin depletion immediately proximal to any gastrointestinal anastomosis that allows the reflux of small-intestinal contents into the stomach. The refluxed activated pancreatic enzymes that are present may also have a role once they have access to the gastric mucosa. However, these seem to have received virtually no attention.

Hypoxia. The exact role of anoxia in damage to the gastric mucosa is also not fully documented, but there seems little doubt that its presence is required for stress ulceration to occur, while in many patients who develop "stress" lesions, an episode of shock, hypoxia, or circumstances readily predisposing to these can be identified. Erosive gastritis has been documented as a sequel to ischemia alone and in association with atheromatous emboli.[197] It is noteworthy that experimental attempts to increase the gastric blood flow have been accompanied by a reduction in the magnitude of the lesions produced by acid and aspirin.[415]

Prostaglandins and Nonsteroidal Anti-inflammatory Agents. Prostaglandins (PGs) are plentiful in normal gastric and duodenal mucosa, mainly in the form of prostaglandins E_2 (PGE_2) and I_2 (PGI_2), although they exist in reduced levels in patients with peptic ulcers. In the stomach, prostaglandin levels are highest in the fundus. Experimentally, PGE inhibits gastric secretion, increases mucus production and prevents peptic ulceration. The increased mucus production is marked.[163] Synthetic PG increases the healing of gastric[209] and duodenal ulceration,[225] and also prevents aspirin-induced fecal blood loss.[115] Aspirin itself causes a dose-dependent decrease in PG, but exogenous PG completely prevents the formation of aspirin ulcers.[341] Oral PGE_2 prevents the increased fecal blood loss associated with indomethacin therapy[306] as well as gastric damage produced by a variety of other substances—a phenomenon that is becoming known as cytoprotection.[254, 341, 436, 518]

Experimentally, the protective action of prostaglandins on the gastric mucosa is little

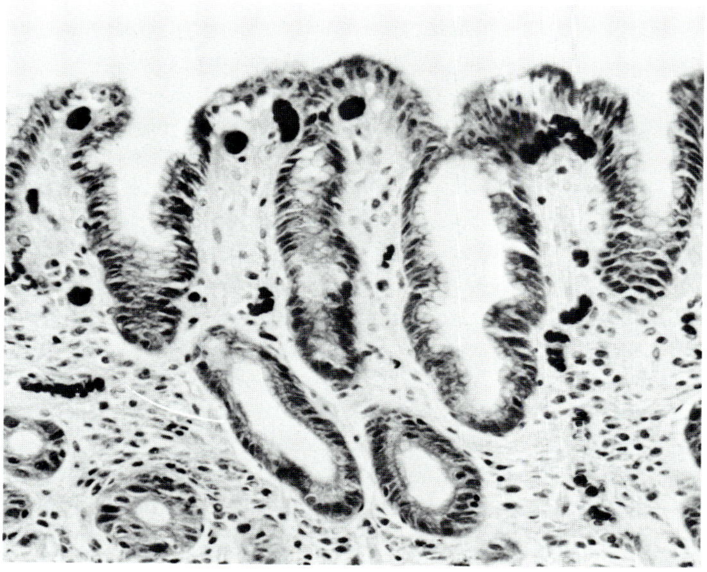

(A)

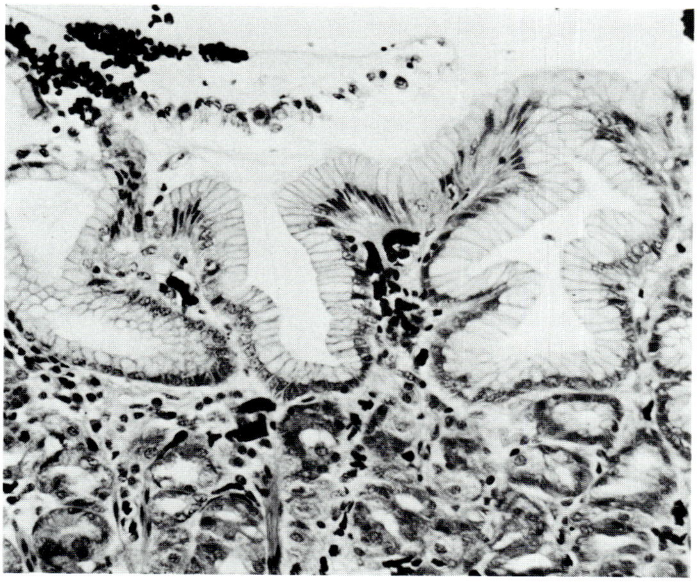

(B)

Fig. 18-9. Gastric mucosa in a patient with bile reflux into the stomach following a Billroth II anastomosis. (A) There is marked mucin depletion, but with no other significant changes. (B) Normal superficial gastric pits for comparison with (A). (Both, H&E, × 250).

short of phenomenal, shielding the latter against damage by boiling water, absolute ethanol, 0.6N hydrochloric acid (about four times the highest concentration of acid in gastric juice), 0.2M sodium hydroxide (also strong), and 25 percent sodium chloride.[517] Additionally, prostaglandins stabilize histamine in mast cells, inhibiting their inflammatory reaction, and have a variety of other actions associated with acute inflammation. Substances that block prostaglandin synthesis therefore upset the normal physiologic mechanisms that help maintain the stability of the normal gastric mucosa, rendering it susceptible to injury.

Aspirin, but probably not other nonsteroidal anti-inflammatory agents (NSAIAs), reduces the transmucosal potential difference that is necessary for the stability of the gastric mucosa, thus allowing the back-diffusion of hydrogen ions and the subsequent gastric damage that has been discussed above. It is possible that one of the modes of action of NSAIAs is to displace endogenous anti-inflammatory agents from their binding sites, with these agents then protecting tissues (such as those in the joints) from chronic inflammatory stimuli. A review of NSAIAs has been done by Simon and Mills.[568,569] A fascinating side effect of NSAIAs is that some tumors seem to produce more prostaglandins than their parent tissue, an effect that appears to be related to tumor spread and bone destruction; experimentally, especially when given with antineoplastic agents, NSAIAs seem to have a markedly beneficial action against tumors when compared to the effects seen with chemotherapy alone.[58]

SUBSTANCES IMPLICATED AS A MAJOR CAUSE OF GASTRIC INJURY

Alcohol

Acute Effects on the Stomach

Acute ingestion of alcohol has long been known to cause a variety of superficial gastric lesions, although minimal concentrations of alcohol, probably in the vicinity of 8 percent, are required before damage occurs. Apart from increasing the secretion of gastric juice,[457] alcohol also reduces the transmucosal potential difference, allowing back-diffusion of hydrogen ions.[103,216] This is of interest in that alcohol initially caused an increased mucosal blood flow in dogs, which was followed by a reduction in blood flow.[25] The morphologic counterpart of this may be the vasodilatation of capillaries, which reduces blood flow.[159] It is this relatively hypoxic period that is shared by other agents that cause the back-diffusion of hydrogen ions.[565] Additionally, alcohol has been shown to increase gastric mucosal permeability.[577]

Ultrastructurally, the initial changes in alcohol-induced lesions involve alterations in the cytoplasm and nucleus,[168] without disruption of the apical membrane or tight junctions. In dogs, it was shown that with increasing concentrations of alcohol there was a widening of the intercellular space, with focal separation of the tight junctions and disruption of the apical membrane.[159]

In humans, acute erosive gastritis has been repeatedly observed, and is important as a clinical cause of upper GI hemorrhage, in some studies being implicated in up to half the patients.[137,325] A major problem is that many patients have also taken aspirin; in practice, however, aspirin and alcohol may well be at least additive, since experimentally, damage may occur when both are given together in amounts that fail to produce damage independently.[519] Gottfried et al.[239] examined the effects of alcohol endoscopically in 7 alcoholic volunteers who had abstained from drinking for at least 2 weeks, were on a standard hospital diet, and had fasted for 12 hours before the experiment. They were endoscoped immediately before and 3 hours after ethanol ingestion. All were found to have moderate to severe antral erythema and friability, while 2 had patchy hemorrhage and erosions in the antrum and fundus. Five had duodenal erythema similar to that seen in the antrum. Microscopically, subepithelial hemorrhage was found in 4 of the volunteers, while another had frank mucosal hemorrhage—changes that were not present in prealcohol biopsies. Although it is easy to attribute these changes to trauma at the time of biopsy, we have seen them sufficiently frequently as the only explanation of an endoscopically red area with normal adjacent biopsies for them to be accepted as genuine. Further, Millan et al.[435] showed that alcohol increased the number of damaged villi, and also showed the villi to have subepithelial blebs that were probably the result of edema. Electron microscopy confirmed the surface abnormality.

Pathologically, alcohol-induced lesions tend to be localized to the antrum or body of the stomach, but may be diffuse in both.[137,565] However, there is no way histologically to distinguish these lesions from other drug-induced lesions. Nevertheless, patients with pure alcohol-induced lesions seem to fare less well clinically than those with their salicylate-induced counterparts.[137] The effects of alcohol are also far more severe in patients with either superficial or atrophic gastritis.[157] Experimentally, alcohol-induced gastric damage in the dog has been completely prevented by PGE_2 given intravenously, a response that was dose-related.[621]

Acute Effects on the Duodenum and Small Intestine

The effect of alcohol on the duodenum and small intestine has also been controversial. However, direct endoscopic examination in volunteers has shown marked erythema, and subepithelial bleeding.[239] Nevertheless, earlier studies by Pirola in patients that were active imbibers failed to reveal any abnormality.[493] The difference may lie in the time interval between alcohol intake and biopsy. In yet another study, Lev et al. compared duodenal biopsies from alcoholic and nonalcoholic patients. Although the number of mononuclear cells in the lamina propria was the same in both groups, goblet cell hyperplasia and gastric cell metaplasia were found almost exclusively in the alcoholics.[365]

Most studies of the small-intestinal mucosa show only minimal changes induced by alcohol.[346,399,432,435,493,531] Rubin's study involved electron microscopic observations on the small intestine in volunteers receiving isocaloric ethanol in place of carbohydrate. There was dilatation of the endoplasmic reticulum and cisternae of the Golgi apparatus, with irregular mitochondria.[531] Bode found a 20 percent decrease in the total mucosal surface in 9 chronic alcoholics, with twice as many intraepithelial lymphocytes as are usually seen.[68] The most striking small-bowel abnormalities have been seen in alcoholics with superimposed folate deficiency, who showed hypoplastic crypts with shortened villi, megaloblastic epithelial nuclei, and an increased inflammatory infiltrate in the lamina propria.[60,271] These changes responded to folate therapy. However, it should be pointed out that others have failed to find such changes,[200,669] so that there may be factors other than simple folate deficiency required to produce these changes.

Long-term Effects

The long-term effects of alcohol, and their relationship to chronic atrophic gastritis, are a little more clouded. Indeed, one study found that patients with normal gastric biopsies drank significantly more alcohol than controls with gastritis.[672] However, alcohol consumption was recorded only for the previous months, and some other unusual statistical data were present, including standard deviations of 2 to 3 times greater than the mean values. There is now growing evidence that alcohol does indeed cause superficial and chronic gastritis. Thus, Gobel found that 73 percent of 152 males and 21 percent of 96 females in his series of 248 patients with atrophic gastritis had a high alcohol intake.[235] Also, in a controlled, blinded, quantitated morphologic study, Parl et al. found a much higher incidence of chronic antritis, and a higher incidence of fundic inflammation in chronic alcoholics than in controls.[480] He also found that these conditions were present at a younger age in the alcoholic group; indeed, all of the gastritis patients under 45 years of age were alcoholics. However, it should be remembered that a low incidence of chronic gastritis can be found in young, apparently healthy volunteers.[348]

The studies by Debray, Dinoso, and Roberts[145,158,520] suggest that superficial gastritis is found in 25 to 43 percent of chronic alcoholics; atrophic gastritis was seen in 24 to 47 percent. In Dinoso's study, 10 percent of healthy controls had superficial gastritis and 3.6 percent had chronic gastritis.[158] Some alcoholics without gastritis seem to develop mucosal fibrosis in the absence of chronic inflammation, but the pathogenesis of this, although presumably the result of previous inflammation, is obscure. Conversely, Cheli concluded from his study comparing abstemious subjects, alcohol drinkers, drinkers with cirrhosis, and nondrinking cirrhotics that alcohol does not play an important part in the development of chronic gastritis.[107] However, his control group is questionable because 26 percent had superficial gastritis and 17 percent had chronic gastritis. Nevertheless, this appears to be a well-designed study that was controlled for age, so that the final answer remains open.

The relationship between chronic alcohol ingestion and peptic ulcer presents intrinsic difficulties because of the high incidence of ulcers in the cirrhotic population. In his excellent monograph on alcohol and the gastrointestinal tract, Bode[68] found that 8 percent of patients with alcoholic hepatitis, but 23 percent of those with hepatic fibrosis or cirrhosis of alcoholic etiology, had peptic ulcers. In his previous, unselected series consisting entirely of chronic alcoholics, the overall figure for peptic ulcers was 13.8 percent. The ulcers occurred both in the antrum and the duodenum. MacDonald illustrates diffuse loss of surface mucin without an increase in chronic inflammatory cells in a lesser-curve ulcer in a chronic alcoholic.[391]

Nonsteroidal Anti-Inflammatory Agents (NSAIAs)

Aspirin

Aspirin-induced damage to the gastrointestinal mucosa was first reported by Douthwaite in 1935, and involved hyperemia and submucosal hemorrhages in the stomachs of 13 of 16 patients who had taken aspirin.[165] This was 39 years after Bayer had introduced aspirin onto the market. However, the significance of Douthwaite's findings was not appreciated for some time.

Aspirin inhibits prostaglandin formation by the irreversible acetylation of cyclooxygenase, thus blocking the conversion of arachidonic acid to endoperoxides. Since the acetylated product is inactive, this prevents formation of the superoxides usually generated in this reaction, as well as the subsequent formation of prostaglandins, prostacyclin, and thromboxane A_2. The effect on platelet aggregation prevents normal coagulation, thus potentiating the actions of aspirin and resulting both in bleeding from a direct effect on the gastric mucosa and further blood loss as a result of the platelet abnormality. However, aspirin almost certainly also inhibits other enzyme systems, and this may contribute to its action.[182] Other salicylates, such as sodium salicylate, are much weaker inhibitors of cyclooxygenase than is aspirin.

In the stomach, NSAIAs reduce blood flow, causing a relative ischemia that may nevertheless be important in bringing about some of the side-effects of these agents. However, the effect of aspirin on the gastric mucosa is not a purely local phenomenon since gastric erosion have been stated to follow parenteral salicylate administration,[433] although other studies do not support this.[298] Experimentally, Kauffman[317] could produce lesions with intravenous aspirin only if there was acid in the stomach. Other nonacetylated salicylates, such as choline salicylate, choline magnesium salicylate, salsalate, and acetaminophen(paracetamol) cause less gastric irritation and have analgesic, and in some cases anti-inflammatory properties similar to those of aspirin.[568] They also have somewhat variable effects on the gastric mucosa experimentally.[208] Additionally, choline magnesium salicylate does not interfere with platelet cyclooxygenase.

Factors Influencing Aspirin Damage. The gastric side-effects of aspirin depend on high acid concentrations.[631] When the gastric pH is below 3.5 the drug exists in the lipid-soluble, undissociated from, and is readily absorbed, while if the pH is greater than 3.5 it is in the non-lipid-soluble dissociated form, and is less well absorbed. Bleeding as a side effect of aspirin is therefore largely acid dependent.[215] Neutralization of gastric acid may thus prevent acute damage, but also inhibits aspirin absorption. Paradoxically, it has been found that while gastric damage is occurring, the pH is high. This is because aspirin also reduces the transmucosal potential difference and allows the back-diffusion of acid.[39] But because this back-diffusion happens as fast as the acid is being formed, it does not reach the lumen. Particle size also affects the speed of absorption of aspirin,[215] smaller particles being absorbed more rapidly, causing a rapid rise in the serum salicylate level and therefore a rapid clinical action, but also at the price of greater gastric damage.

Bile reflux may also predispose to gastric damage by aspirin; aspirin damage is seen far more frequently in gastric operations in which gastroenterostomies allow the free reflux of intestinal contents into the gastric remnant.[53] Such damage is least in Billroth I gastrectomies, in which duodenogastric reflux is less common.[511] A correlation between bile reflux and bleeding in patients receiving aspirin has also been demonstrated.[98] Prostaglandins cause mucus production by the stomach, and this is markedly reduced by all cyclooxygenase inhibitors. Bile may further reduce the effectiveness of any mucus present, allowing a direct attack on the mucosa by aspirin, bile, and possibly by activated pancreatic enzymes in the duodenal juice that has been refluxed. Like aspirin, taurocholic acid has been shown to reduce the transmucosal potential difference[111]—a phenomenon associated with the back-diffusion of hydrogen ions.

Experimentally, alcohol potentiates the effects of aspirin in animals, the gastric mucosa being damaged by small-dose combinations of aspirin and alcohol which are inactive if given independently[520]; the combination is also dangerous in humans.[458] Apart from its own toxic effect, alcohol increases acid secretion (required for aspirin absorption) and enhances the solubility of aspirin. Experimentally, aspirin damage is also potentiated by shock[605] and hypoglycemia.[388] Conversely, aspirin damage may be reduced by glucagon,[611] bicarbonate,[78] and cimetidine.[394]

Clinical Effects. An indication of the amount of blood lost in patients taking aspirin may be gleaned from blood loss in the stool. Normally this is less than 1 ml. Two-thirds of aspirin users lose between 3 and 10 ml a day, while 11 percent lose more than 10 ml a day.[132] These losses are accentuated by ethanol and the use of unbuffered aspirin. The magnitude of this side effect of aspirin is hard to imagine. In one series it was noted that 54 of 166 patients admitted with hemorrhage had ingested aspirin within the previous 6 hours, and in 21 of these the aspirin appeared to be a major factor.[451] In a second study, 49 of 103 patients had ingested aspirin in the previous 24 hours, while only 7 of the matched controls had done so.[15] There also appears to be correlation between aspirin use and both newly diagnosed gastric ulcer and severe upper intestinal hemorrhage in the absence of duodenal ulcer[368]; however, Rees has suggested that aspirin ingestion rarely causes clinically significant gastric damage in normal subjects, and only then with large or frequent doses.[506]

Nevertheless, in endoscopic studies it has been found that buffered aspirin induces only slightly less gastric and duodenal mucosal damage than regular aspirin,[230] both causing multiple gastric erosions in 9 of 10 volunteers. Hemorrhages were observed in 9 volunteers with regular aspirin and in 7 with buffered aspirin, while duodenal erosions were present in 6 taking regular aspirin and 4 taking buffered aspirin. Acetaminophen (paracetamol), which was also studied, had effects essentially similar to those seen in the control group.[280,305,377] However, a real difference exists if enteric-coated tablets are used.[281] When compared with regular aspirin (which produced almost identical damage to that already described), the enteric-coated tablets caused a single antral erosion in 2 of 9 patients studied, while no duodenal lesions were observed. This difference was largely confirmed in long-term aspirin users; 25 percent of patients with rheumatoid arthritis taking regular aspirin had gastric ulcers, while less than 10 percent of enteric-coated users developed gastric ulcers over the same period.[566] Similar results were obtained by Lanza et al.[354]

Pathological Effects. As mentioned in the section on alcohol, it was impossible to distinguish endoscopically between the distribution of lesions in the stomach caused by different toxic substances; in Sugawa's series the effects produced by alcohol and aspirin were identical, but differed from those of acute hemorrhagic gastritis resulting from trauma or sepsis, in which the gastric body mucosa was always involved.[600]

The fact that damage produced by acute aspirin ingestion is not only superficial was shown by giving 5 patients, who were about to have a partial gastrectomy, soluble aspirin for several days immediately prior to the operation. In all of these patients, from 1 to 5 mucosal erosions were found, mainly on the lesser curve, and hemorrhage was also seen. Only one of the controls, a patient with carcinoma, exhibited similar changes. Microscopically the "erosions" were found to have penetrated the muscularis mucosae, and to therefore be "ulcers." Many were surrounded by a zone of hemorrhage.[132] Studies from Australia have strongly suggested a relationship between peptic ulcer and aspirin ingestion, particularly in young women.[106] Piper et al.[492] have reviewed the relationship between analgesics and chronic peptic ulcer.

Ulcer formation in long-term aspirin abusers has a characteristic appearance. In his classic paper, MacDonald examined 50 partial gastrectomy specimens with gastric ulcers. He found 44 ulcers occurring in the presence of pyloric gland inflammation that were on the lesser curve or posterior wall. Of these, 8 were in aspirin users. In the remaining 6 (plus 1 local excision of an ulcer), there was no pyloric gland inflammation. Five of these ulcers were on the greater-curve side of the antrum. All of these patients were chronic aspirin users.[391] These findings have been confirmed by Hamilton and Yardley, who examined biopsies of gastric ulcers in which there was no associated inflammation. All 6 of their patients so identified proved to be heavy aspirin users; 4 of the 6 ulcers they found were on the greater curve or posterior wall.[258] We have also seen biopsies of several patients with ulceration in the absence of chronic inflammation, and confirm the predictable association of these with the salicylates. Nevertheless, we have also seen what is clearly aspirin-induced disease clinically in patients with diffuse gastric inflammation. This is also in accordance with MacDonald's findings, but clearly the etiology cannot be inferred from the morphology in these cases.

Although the damage induced by aspirin is superficial in the acute phase, and the drug may cause ulceration after long-term abuse, there are virtually no reports of deep penetration or perforation. However, in two patients, a gastrocolic fistula was thought to be associated with long-term aspirin use.[127]

With light-microscopy, we have found that the most characteristic change in patients with endoscopic abnormality consists of areas of superficial mucin depletion that correspond to areas that are red endoscopically. In some patients this is virtually complete, and the foveolar cells are cuboidal or low-columnar rather than tall colomnar. Nuclear size is considerably enlarged, and there is mild nuclear pleomorphism and small nucleoli. In patients in whom the change is less severe, small apical mucin droplets are present in the foveolar cells. These changed appearances are in marked contrast to those of the usual surface cells, which have a large supranuclear mucin droplet in each cell, occupying up to about three-fourths of the cell (Fig. 18-10). There is also considerable variation in the inflammatory infiltrate, which may be virtually nil, be heavy and of a chronic inflammatory nature and part of a more diffuse gastritis, or sometimes be of an acute inflammatory nature and tend to affect the deeper portions of the mucosa, but only in the areas of damage.

Baskin studied the light- and electron microscopic appearances of acute gastric damage caused by aspirin. By light-microscopy, he

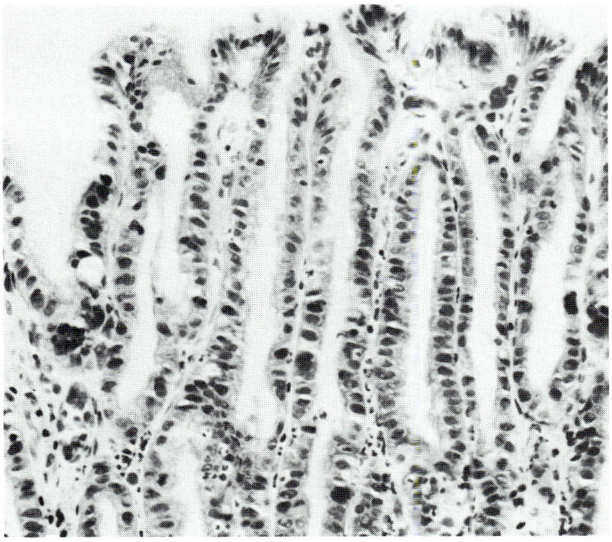

(A)

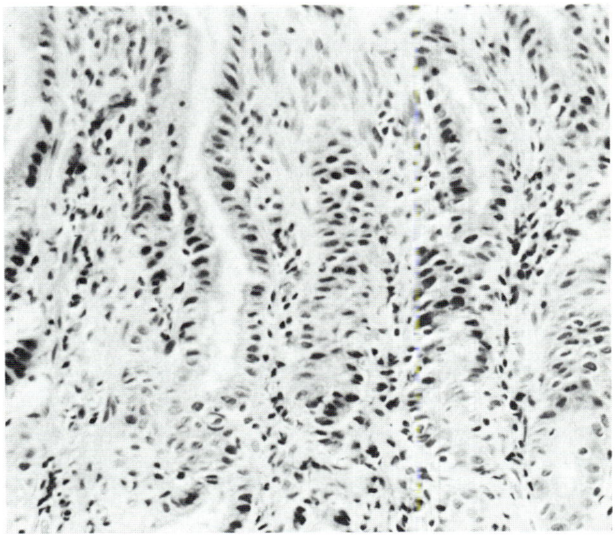

(B)

Fig. 18-10. Gastric damage from aspirin. (A) There is marked depletion of mucin with enlarged, hyperchromatic nuclei. The acute inflammation present is uncommon and may be unrelated to aspirin ingestion. (B) Aspirin damage similar to that seen in (A) in a patient who was also taking cimetidine. There is virtually no difference from (A). (Both, H&E, × 250).

noted focal disruption of cells, mucin depletion, and rupture of the apical membrane. Scanning electron microscopy showed damage to 25 percent of the cells within 10 minutes, although this had been reduced to 9 percent after an hour. Transmission electron microscopy confirmed the apical membrane rupture with cytoplasmic disruption, but the tight junctions remained intact.[39] Hahn saw similar changes, with the lysis of organelles,[257] while Rainsford also noted that in areas away from macroscopic disease, the parietal cells showed the greatest damage, which was seen in their mitochondra.[505]

Phenylbutazone and Its Derivatives

This group of drugs has now fallen into disrepute as an alternative to aspirin in patients with rheumatoid arthritis because of the high incidence of hematologic side effects (see

Chapter 5) and the availability of many good alternatives. Yet there remain some drugs, fortunately most of which have the suffix "zone" which are still used clinically. Carlson et al.[99] give an overview of drug-induced gastroduodenal disease in patients with rheumatoid arthritis.

The entire group of phenylbutazone-related drugs belong to the pyrazolones; amidopyrine was one of the first used, although it soon fell into disrespect because of the high incidence of side effects, particularly hematologic ones. Unfortunately, many amidopyrine derivates still present similar problems. Phenylbutazone and related compounds (such as oxyphenbutazone, ketophenylbutazone, feprazone, suxibuzone, trimethazone, clofezone, azapropazone, and pipebuzone) fall within this realm. Most give rise to constitutional gastrointestinal symptoms, but what they actually do to the human gastroduodenal mucosa is rather poorly documented, nor is it very certain whether the peptic ulcers that some of these drugs are alleged to have caused really occur in an incidence higher than that expected in a control population. Retrospective studies have suggested that peptic ulceration may occur in excess numbers of patients. Kern et al. found that 5 percent of males and 7.5 percent of females receiving phenylbutazone for rheumatoid arthritis developed peptic ulceration.[321] However, others reported either no ulcers[349] or very low levels that are probably no greater than those expected in the general population. Thus, Sperling[582] reported 562 patients treated for up to 10 years (mean 4.1 years), with either phenylbutazone or oxyphenbutazone, of whom only 3 developed peptic ulceration.

Azapropazone has been reported to cause a variety of gastrointestinal erosions with hemorrhage and perforations in many animal species.[8] Prescott[500] reports that one adverse reaction group considered a relationship between feprazone and bleeding duodenal ulcer causing melena, but another report suggested that this drug did not cause occult blood loss,[392] while yet another study suggested that it did, but much less than that associated with aspirin.[377]

Indomethacin

This was the prototype indole derivative that gradually replaced phenylbutazone and its derivatives, although it is chemically related to them. It inhibits both cyclooxygenase and phosphodiesterase activity, thus stabilizing lysozomal membranes and inhibiting leukocyte migration[191,198]; both of these actions inhibit superoxide formation.[568] However, indomethacin appears to have no effect on the transmucosal potential difference.[454] The first clinical trials of this drug produced some disasters in terms of gastric side effects. In one series, 5 of 14 patients developed gastric or duodenal ulcers, and 2 died, 1 following massive hemorrhage.[379] Three of these 5 patients had previously had peptic ulcer, suggesting that indomethacin might reactivate healed ulcers or be particularly troublesome in patients with an ulcer diathesis. However, reduction in the dose achieved more acceptable side effects, and in Rothernich's prospective study[528] the incidence of peptic ulcer was 2.8 percent, while a review of five series by Cooke[124] showed an overall peptic ulcer incidence of 5.5 percent. One patient reported by Taylor et al. was particularly interesting in that an ulcer healed following reduction in the dose of indomethacin.[614]

The acute effects of indomethacin on the gastric mucosa have been documented endoscopically. Although the damage produced was not as great as that occurring with aspirin, indomethacin given in doses of either 100 or 150 mg produced far more damage than a placebo, ibuprofen, or naproxen at 500 mg, but less damage than naproxen at 750 mg.[353] However, there was marked individual variation, some patients having no endoscopic abnormality while others had damage of a similar magnitude to that seen in the 3.6 g/day aspirin group, with numerous areas of hemorrhage and occasionally active bleeding.

Interestingly, as mentioned above, when 1 mg of oral PGE_2 was given three times daily, the fecal blood loss in patients with rheumatoid arthritis was reduced to normal levels. This was achieved without interfering with the beneficial effects of the drug clinically, and was also unrelated to gastric acid secretion.[306]

The question of whether indomethacin actually causes an excess of peptic ulcers remains virtually unanswered because of the paucity of well-controlled studies. Combining several studies produces an incidence of about 5½ percent but this is probably not greater than that expected in the general population.[124] In one study with dogs, it was noteworthy that while indomethacin produced erosions or ulcers, it failed to have any effect on, or to reactivate, partially healed artifically induced ulcers.[471] To further complicate our relative ignorance, the ulcerogenic effects of indomethacin can be inhibited experimentally by diflunisal,[122] while indomethacin may itself have a similar inhibitory effect on aspirin-induced damage.[524]

Other Nonsteroidal Anti-Inflammatory Agents

Because of the side effects of aspirin, phenylbutazone, and indomethacin, a myriad of other substances have been develoepd in attempts to keep the clinically useful properties of the first three substances while reducing toxic side-effects, especially those on the stomach. Perhaps the most important of these newer agents are the phenylpropionate or arylcarboxylic acid derivatives fenoprufen, ibuprofen, alclofenac, ketoprofen, fenoprofen, naproxen, and sulindac, and the anthranilic acid derivatives known as the fenamates, such as tolfenamic acid, niflumic acid, glafenine, diclofenac, floctafenine, and mefanamic acid. Tolmetin is a pyrrole-acetic acid derivative, although still chemically related to other compounds in the group.

Most studies continue to use patients with rheumatoid arthritis, and tend to test a variety of drugs. Invariably, aspirin, which is the local "gold standard," is included, and causes much damage, while indomethacin produces less, and some of the newer drugs such as sulindac seem to cause little more damage than a placebo when the latter is included.[102] However, the numbers of patients in studies such as these covering a variety of drugs, often in combination, are not very meaningful.

It is apparent that most nonsteroidal anti-inflammatory substances have some effect on the gastric mucosa that may well be the price that must be paid for inhibiting prostaglandin formation. However, there is clearly a gradient, and among these substances some appear to be less toxic overall to the gastric mucosa. Pemberton and Strand have reviewed the gastrointestinal side effects of many of these drugs, and include the blood loss per day in both their study and control groups. From their data it appears that ketoprofen and fenoprofen calcium cause the greatest blood loss, although even this is considerably less than that seen with aspirin, and much of it is no more than that seen in placebo control.[483]

From the clinical viewpoint it is largely unpredictable which of these drugs will work in a specific patient, and it seems to be in order to change the drugs almost on a weekly basis, until a drug is found that both produces the required clinical effect and is well tolerated by the patient. Even this may soon be unnecessary, for the gastric toxicity of many of these drugs appears preventable by the administration of oral synthetic prostaglandins without diminishing the clinical effect. It may be only a matter of time before this will become a widespread practice. Meanwhile, a brief summary of some of the effects of these drugs follows.

Alclofenac. This is a phenylacetic acid derivative that may cause gastrointestinal side-effects, but these are insufficient to require withdrawal of the drug; further information is required.[83]

Diclofenac. An endoscopic study of this drug in 20 volunteers revealed only minor changes in 4 patients, far fewer than the number found with naproxen, with which diclofenac was compared.[360, 474]

Diflunisal. This is a salicylate derivative that was initially thought not to lead to increased fecal blood loss. Some endoscopic studies reported low incidences of gastric disease following its ingestion.[487] However, there have been several individual case reports suggesting that diflunisal may occasionally cause significant hemorrhage from the upper gastrointestinal tract, and this will probably be a continuing problem,[7, 404, 547] while perforation possibly related to duflunisal has also been reported.[609] Experimentally, diflunisal protects against the ulcerogenic action of indomethacin.[122]

Fenoprofen. In a study that compared this propionic acid derivative to aspirin, and measured fecal blood loss, fenoprofen caused fewer lesions than aspirin but in a similar distribution, tending to affect the pyloric region, followed by the posterior antral wall, with the duodenum also occasionally being involved.[377,513] These changes were reflected in the fecal blood loss, which averaged 4.96 ml/day in the aspirin group, 2.46 ml/day in the fenoprofen group, and 0.79 ml/day in the placebo group.[108]

Naproxen. This drug appears to cause significant damage and also bleeding[262, 408] when compared with other available agents.[360, 474]

Piroxicam. This drug is unlikely to be popular unless the effective dose can be reduced, since one trial reported side effects severe enough to require stopping the drug in one-third of the patients. These effects included new peptic ulcers, which developed in 29 percent of the patients.[504]

Pirprofen. This drug is also associated with gastrointestinal side-effects, which have included gastric ulcer and gastrointestinal bleeding.[140, 530]

Sulindac. This is an indomethacin derivative that also suffers from many of the disadvantages of that drug. Nevertheless, it seems to have gained some degree of clinical acceptance, and in one study the fecal blood loss after 1 and 2 weeks of treatment with sulindac was the same as that with a placebo.[112] Reviews of this drug are available,[85] as are small endoscopic studies[495] suggesting relatively little immediate gastric damage.

Tolmetin. Although it is a pyrrole acetic acid derivative, the structure of tolmetin is similar to that of indomethacin. Occasional cases of both gastric and duodenal ulcer have been reported, usually in patients with an ulcer diathesis.[84, 170]

Steroids

There has been considerable simmering, and occasionally boiling controversy concerning the effects of steroids on the gastric mucosa since Bollet et al. noticed in 1955 that some patients taking glucocorticoids developed gastric ulcers. In 1958, Kammerer[310] reported that 31 percent of 117 patients with rheumatoid arthritis treated with steroids developed peptic ulcers, as compared with 9 percent in a control group of patients with rheumatoid arthritis not receiving steroids. Both groups had periodic barium meals over a 12 month period in order to assess the development of ulcers, but this was not done before the trial was started, in which case it could have been used to exclude the possibility that ulcers either were present or had been present at that time. The incidence of ulcers in the control group was high, raising the possibility that patients with rheumatoid arthritis were intrinsically at high risk for developing peptic ulceration.

The argument has raged since, and one notable paper summarizing the literature[120] argued that there may be very little or no association of steroids with ulceration, while this in turn was duly criticized as a misinterpretation of the original data.[247, 378] More recently, evidence has been forthcoming from neurologic sources that suggests a relationship between gastric bleeding and steroids. Thus, Cantu et al.[97] found the incidence of gastrointestinal bleeding to be four times as high following intracranial surgery in patients treated with steroids as compared with patients not receiving them. Teutsch[624] and Livathinopoulos[375] have suggested that the risk is raised even further in patients receiving either phenylbutazone and salicylates. Ottonella and Primavera[475] examined the intestinal tract at autopsy in patients dying of stroke, some of whom had been treated with steroids. In all of their subgroups there was a higher incidence of gastroduodenal disease in patients who had been receiving steroids (6 mg dexamethasone daily), although this did not reach statistical significance in all groups.

The problem with neurologic patients is that their tendency to develop gastric or duodenal ulcers is well documented, and it is likely that steroids in these patients have a potentiating effect in what is already a high risk group. Steroids also seem to potentiate the effects of other drugs associated with upper gastrointestinal hemorrhage, such as ethacrynic acid,[303] although in the same study the chances of patients bleeding while on steroids alone was low. Overall, the evidence suggests that steroids by themselves may have a relatively low risk of initiating gastric bleeding, but that they may potentiate the risk if other factors, known to predispose to bleeding, are also present. This conclusion also seems reasonable in view of the fact that steroids do not reduce the transmucosal potential difference (the so-called gastric mucosal barrier), nor are they inhibitors of prostaglandins synthesis. However, both ACTH and steroids reduce mucus secretion[278, 428] as do the nonsteroidal anti-inflammatory agents. This, plus their effect on gastrin secretion and those sequelae, offer at least a partial explanation for the action of steroids.

The pathology of steroid-associated ulcers is somewhat disappointing. Classically, these ulcers are shallow, multiple, and occur in the antrum.[584] However, one study of steroid ulcers in patients undergoing resection for benign gastric ulcer that was matched for age, sex, location and salicylate ingestion with controls revealed no differences in the ulcers, even multiple ulcers being similar in both groups.[213] The similarity also extended to histologic examination of the ulcers. Nevertheless, the clinical literature remains equivocal, mainly because so few well-controlled studies have been done, and because critical data such as the ingestion of other ulcerogenic drugs is not stated.

Other Substances that may Affect the Stomach

Bromocriptine

It has been suggested that patients receiving large doses of this drug, usually in the treatment of acromegaly, may be predisposed to gastrointestinal hemorrhage. Thus, among 96 patients treated with 10 to 60 mg of bromocriptine per day, 6 developed peptic ulcer while 3 had severe hemorrhage. Two of the patients, who were apparently in poor health, died as a result.[651] Similar results were not found in patients receiving much smaller doses of bromocriptine (7.5 mg/day) for hyperprolactinemia, nor in patients with Parkinson's disease also receiving large doses (60 to 100 mg/day). Further, it is likely that patients with acromegaly may be predisposed to peptic ulcer disease, as judged from 11 of 153 patients not treated with bromocryptine who developed ulcers.[152] It therefore requires much better documentation before bromocryptine can be incriminated causally in the genesis of peptic ulcers.

Ethacrynic Acid

There have been several suggestions that upper intestinal bleeding may follow treatment with ethacrynic acid.[303, 573] In Jick's study the figures are disconcerting, in that 5 of 111 patients (4.8 percent) receiving ethacrynic acid alone had major gastrointestinal bleeding (requiring transfusion), while the figure rose to 9.1 percent (2 of 22) in patients receiving steroids in addition. Although these numbers are small, the percentage figures involved are higher than any for the drugs usually associated with bleeding, including heparin, warfarin sodium, steroids, or aspirin, either alone or in any combination with each other. The three highest figures all involve ethacrynic acid (the third being with ethacrynic acid in combination with heparin). In Slone's paper, intravenous administration of the drug was required, to induce ulceration,[573] while Jick only mentions "exposure."[303] Neither the site of bleeding nor the mechanism are known. Fortunately, frusemide has largely replaced ethacrynic acid in most centers, so that bleeding associated with ethacrynic acid should be seen less frequently.

Erythromycin Estolate

One report suggests a temporal relationship between neonatal ingestion of erythromycin estolate and the subsequent development of pyloric stenosis.[537] Although fascinating, confirmation of this is clearly required.

H_2-Histamine Receptor Antagonists

This group of drugs blocks those effects of histamine that are not blocked by conventional antihistamines (H_1-receptor antagonists). The first H_2-histamine receptor antagonist was burimamide, which was succeeded by metiamide, while cimetidine is by far the most popular of these drugs currently in use. Others will undoubtedly follow. The major pharmacologic action of this group of drugs is to block gastric acid secretion, which it does effectively although not quite totally. It also reduces the output of pepsin. Reviews of both the effects[86] and side effects[416] of these drugs are available. It is becoming apparent that other groups of cells have H_2 receptors, one of which comprises T-cell suppressor cells. H_2 antagonists might therefore be expected to augment local immune responses, and some animal tumor models have benefited from treatment with cimetidine.

In contrast to bile, alcohol, and aspirin, cimetidine increases the gastric transmucosal potential difference, and prevents this from falling to the levels that permit injury by these substances. Cimetidine therefore effectively protects against all of these agents, and also reduces the incidence of bleeding from acute hemorrhagic gastritis resulting from stress, trauma, sepsis, or other causes. It is therefore widely used clinically in this capacity. We have had an opportunity to examine gastric biopsies from patients who have been on both aspirin and cimetidine. Interestingly, red lesions have been observed endoscopically which, when biopsied, appear indistinguishable from the typical mucin-depleted biopsies seen in patients taking aspirin but not cimetidine (Fig. 18-10B). It is easy to speculate that the cyclooxygenase blocking action of aspirin is still in effect in causing the changes shown, but that the cimetidine might be having a local physiologic effect that is not reflected in the morphology that is seen, or might simply have been locally overcome by the aspirin.

Nevertheless, the chief action of cimetidine is in the promotion of healing of gastric and duodenal peptic ulcers.[209,225,470] However, several side effects have been both reported or postulated,[416] and these are briefly discussed below.

Rebound Acid Hypersecretion. Soon after its introduction, there were several reports of patients treated for peptic ulcer disease with cimetidine, who returned with penetrating or perforating ulcers within days of being discharged from the hospital following healing of their original ulcers.[230,285,638,647] In one patient, perforation occurred while cimetidine was being taken.[175] A possibility in these cases was that the reduction in acid secretion caused an increased serum gastrin level, that in turn caused hypertrophy or hyperplasia of the parietal cell mass, so that when cimetidine was stopped, "rebound" hypersecretion occurred, causing an acute perforating ulcer. There is an animal precedent for this, since both parietal cell hyperplasia and serum gastrin elevation have been reported in rats fed antacids, as compared with a lack of these effects in a similar control group that did not receive antacids.[412] Some investigators were able to find increased gastrin levels in some patients receiving cimetidine[260, 343]; however, this may occur only in some patients, and the issue is far from settled. Nevertheless, many physicians now "tail off" the dose of cimetide rather than stopping it abruptly, in an effort to avoid this phenomenon. Whether such an action is justified is uncertain, but it is clear that the patients reported represented only a few cases among what is probably a rather more widespread complication of cimetidine. Since the nature of peptic ulcer disease is to recur whether treated with cimetidine or antacids,[134] there is always the question of whether these patients represented a true complication or simply the early-phase representatives of those in whom the ulcer will eventually recur.

Gastric Carcinoma. This problem arose following a report of 3 patients who developed gastric carcinoma within 10 weeks to 11 months of a course of cimetidine.[173] The underlying question was whether cimetidine was converted in the stomach to its *N*-nitroso derivative, which could then have been carcinogenic. Attention was drawn to the similarity of this derivative to *N*-methyl-*N'*-nitro-*N*-nitroso guanidine (MNNG), which is directly carcinogenic to the gastric mucosa in some animal species.[601] Nitrite-forming bacteria that may proliferate because of a cimetidine-induced increase in gastric pH may be involved. The criticism is fairly obvious, for many early gastric carcinomas may not be distinguishable from benign ulcers other than through biopsy, while it is well documented that early carcinomas may show evidence of healing on gastric ulcer regimens, including those that involve the use of cimetidine.[453, 613] Clearly, if these ulcers were assumed to be benign and showed evidence of healing, there may have been considerable delay until the symptoms reappeared and the correct diagnosis was reached. This complication must therefore be treated with some caution, at least in those patients in whom there is only a short interval between the diagnosis of the original ulcer and subsequent carcinoma. Long-term prospective studies will be required to determine the effect of cimetidine ingestion over extended periods of time.

Gastroduodenitis. There have been a few reports of gastric erosion or duodenitis occurring in patients taking cimetidine.[186, 373, 656] It is difficult to know how to interpret these cases, and more evidence is required.

Gastric Flora and *Candida* Peritonitis. It is perhaps not surprising that an increase in the gastric pH is followed by an increase in the number of organisms that can be grown from gastric juice[532] (including those that reduce nitrates to nitrites), and that this may in fact cause diarrhea as a result of bacterial overgrowth.[533] In one patient who perforated a peptic ulcer 3 days after starting cimetidine, the peritoneal fluid grew a pure culture of *Candida krusei.*[588] It is uncertain if this was an isolated event or, if genuine, whether the cimetidine allowed proliferation of the organism in the upper intestinal tract, or whether local immune responses had been modified by the cimetidine.

Iron

Ferrous salts appear capable of causing damage to most portions of the gastrointestinal tract, causing ulceration and sometimes hemorrhage. Ulcers appear to penetrate deeply into the wall of the bowel, and some are followed by stricture formation.[193, 644] One patient treated with iron in spansule form for dietary iron deficiency developed severe epigastric pain that was relieved when she vomited 70 plastic matrices. The possibility of pyloric obstruction was raised, but it is uncertain how much of this was already present and how much may have been induced or perpetuated by the iron.[101]

Potassium Supplements

Apart from their effect in the esophagus and small intestine, occasional cases of gastric ulcers following ingestion of potassium chloride have been reported, including enteric-coated tablets.[299, 421]

Reserpine

Reserpine and other rauwolfia alkaloids have been associated with peptic ulceration, particularly when given in large doses.[27, 283, 290, 671] In rats, reserpine produces gastric ulceration when given intraperitoneally, possibly by causing mast-cell degranulation, thereby releasing histamine and other substances that may be ulcerogenic. There is certainly a marked increase in the volume of gastric secretion when resperine is given.[329] Interestingly, this animal ulcer can be inhibited by the intraperitoneal injection of zinc sulfate.[469] In humans there is limited evidence that reserpine may either reactivate or cause new peptic ulcers, particularly in the duodenum.[396] In a further study, duodenal ulcers with a distinct tendency to bleed developed in 5 of 17 patients in coma who were given reserpine in the belief that it might promote a return to consciousness.[201] The evidence is therefore relatively strong that reserpine-induced ulcer is a genuine phenomenon.

Spironolactone

Possible cases of bleeding gastric ulcers in cirrhotic patients given spironolactone have been reported[237, 393]; as with many other drugs, mucus depletion may have been involved. However, confirmation of this is required before the association can be considered more than coincidental.

Zinc Sulfate

Moore[445] reported a 15-year-old girl who appeared to have lost a considerable amount of blood following a week of treatment with zinc sulfate tablets recommended for her acne. Endoscopy showed patchy areas of gastritis on the greater curve, and a healing erosion. This is almost predictable, in that zinc sulfate and hydrochloric acid can form zinc chloride, which has a powerful corrosive action.

Coffee

It has long been known that coffee stimulates the secretion of both acid and pepsin,[527] and that patients with duodenal ulcer have the greatest and longest response to coffee. In animals, coffee also delays the healing of stress ulcers. However, these effects of coffee do not seem to be due to caffeine. They may be mediated through gastrin, since both caffeinated and decaffeinated coffee cause gastrin release, while caffeine itself does not elicit this response.[77] Nevertheless, there are conflicting data concerning the ability of coffee to produce ulcer disease.[206, 476]

Tobacco

The role of smoking in the genesis of peptic ulcers[162] and in the delay of their healing[41, 162] is well documented in standard medical texts. The mechanism involved is not clearly understood, but may be through the enhanced histamine-mediated secretion of pepsinogen-1, which is increased in smokers.[646] Measurement of the duodenal bulb pH showed that it remained below 3.5 longer in smokers, and especially in gastric hypersecretors who smoked than in nonsmokers.[455] Persistent acidity may therefore be partly responsible for the deleterious effect of smoking on the gastroduodenal mucosa, although the precise relationship of smoking to duodenal ulcer remains questionable.[673] Experimentally, changes caused by nicotine have been described in the gastric mucosa.[302]

Cannabis

Unlike many of the other substances discussed in this section, the smoking of cannabis on more than a 2-days-per-week basis appears to cause a reduction in the amount of gastric acid secreted.[457] This may potentially increase the risk of developing bacterial diarrheas.

Red Pepper and Red Chili Powder

Many have wondered whether the indigestion suffered after a particularly "spicy" meal was anything more than a direct effect of the food on the gastroduodenal mucosa. Johnson et al.[307] found that in Ethiopia, where red peppers are a standard part of the diet, patients with duodenal ulcer, but not apparently normal controls, responded with maximal gastric acid secretion to meals containing these peppers, as compared to meals not containing this ingredient. The output of acid was actually significantly higher than the response obtained with pentagastrin! Red chili powder significantly increases gastric acid secretion in both control subjects and patients with duodenal ulcers.[153]

Pickled Gherkins and Fukujinzuke

The eating of 30 oz of vinegar-pickled midget gherkins or the Japanese salty pickle known as fukujinzuke over a 3-day period causes a typical drug-induced gastric injury, with depletion of superficial mucin and superficial injury in the absence of an inflammatory reaction; these changes were not seen in the controls who ate 30 oz of raw cucumber or carrots over the same period.[389] Interestingly, these changes could be prevented with carbenoxolone.[390] Judicious use of such pickles is therefore clearly desirable. It is not stated whether other undesirable side-effects were seen in either the pickle or control groups.

THE SMALL INTESTINE

Drugs Primarily Affecting the Stomach

Most of the drugs and other toxic substances that injure the stomach can cause similar although usually less marked disease in the small intestine. Thus aspirin, hydrochloric acid, and both combined can cause erosions of the tips of villi, with extravasation of red cells.[297] Indomethacin can cause inflammation and ulceration with subsequent stricture formation in humans[599] and ulceration in laboratory animals.[183] Alcohol is known to affect intestinal sodium transport in humans, offering at least a partial explanation for the diarrhea seen in chronic alcoholics (see also p. 581).[425] In animal studies, low concentrations of ethanol (2.1 to 4.8 percent) seemed to be accompanied by fluid blebs immediately beneath the enterocytes in the villi.[203] However, at least some of the illustrations of these look suspiciously like formalin-induced shrinkage of the villous core, and should perhaps be interpreted with caution. Phenylbutazone has been associated with small-bowel ulceration,[362] while some patients that developed small-intestinal ulceration probably due to potassium chloride were occasionally also taking either phenylbutazone or steroids.[139] However, the latter two drugs probably played little or no role in the genesis of these ulcers, which were otherwise typical. Some drugs which have been mentioned in the gastric section have more important effects in the small intestine. These are discussed below.

Hypersensitivity to Ingested Foods

Complete loss of villi may result from the ingestion of foods or substances that cannot be normally digested or absorbed. Some such losses, such as those occurring with lactose, are well documented as being the result of an enzyme defect, but are unaccompanied by injury to the underlying mucosa. Other substances, such as gluten, soy, eggs, or milk, in the appropriate individual, do cause severe mucosal damage, with partial or complete loss of villi and a marked increase in mitotic activity. Allergy to cow's milk protein is important as the major cause of chronic diarrhea of infancy and is seen in infants and children who tend to have other allergic disorders. Such enteropathies are dealt with in standard reference books of medicine, pediatrics, and gastroenterology, and will not be considered further here. A useful review on the adverse effects of milk is that by Eastham and Walker,[167] while the histologic appearances of milk enteropathy are described by Fontaine and Navarro.[196] Complete loss of villi secondary to soy protein hypersensitivity is described by Ament and Rubin.[19]

Drug-associated Malabsorption

Arsenic

An 8-year-old girl was reported to have developed a protein-losing enteropathy following the treatment of warts with arsenic trioxide. Rather dubious changes of lymphangiectasia were reported, which may have been artifactual, judging from the illustration provided.[337]

Biguanides

This group of drugs lowers the blood sugar not only by enhancing insulin action, but also by causing the malabsorption of glucose. Thus, phenformin decreases the hyperglycemic response to an oral but not to an intravenous glucose load,[135] and perfusion studies have shown that it may reduce glucose absorption by up to 50 percent.[23] Xylose absorption is impaired by phenformin[596] and metformin.[54] Examination by light-microscopy of jejunal biopsies from patients taking biguanides reveals no abnormality, although electron microscopically there is complete disappearance of the mitochondrial matrix.[23]

Methotrexate

The changes associated with methotrexate have been discussed in the section on antineoplastic drugs (see p. 530).

Methyldopa

A well-documented instance of loss of villi that was confirmed by challenge has been described in association with methyldopa.[563] In addition, a granuloma was said to be present, but the patient had no other evidence of Crohn's disease.

Neomycin

It is well known that neomycin can produce a malabsorption syndrome when administered in doses of 3 to 12 g/day. Small-intestinal biopsies in several studies have shown a partial loss of villi with increased mitoses and an excess inflammatory reaction in the lamina propria.[322] The light- and electron microscopic findings are described and reviewed by Dobbins et al.,[160] but essentially confirm those described by Jacobson et al. in 1960.[300] However, marked changes in the microvilli, which were ballooned and fragmented, were seen electron microscopically, while swelling of both the mitochondria and endoplasmic reticulum was observed. Apart from what appears to be direct damage to small-intestinal enterocytes, the cationic amino groups of neomycin bind the anionic groups of micelles in the intestinal lumen. The combined particles are precipitated, and are not available for absorption, with the result that there is loss of cholesterol, fatty acids, monoglycerides, and the fat-soluble vitamins.

ULCERATION

Neonatal Enterocolitis

This is considered only insofar as it is clear that feeding must occur for the disease to occur. Elemental formulas have been suspected of a relationship because of their hypertonicity, which causes an influx of fluid into the intestinal lumen.[76] This presumably causes both the distension of diseased bowel, increasing the likelihood of perforation, and reduces the blood volume, thereby decreasing blood flow to an already ischemic organ. However, the disease is related to feeding of any kind, including that with human milk.[332] The introduction of bacteria is also required for neonatal enterocolitis to occur; this presumably also occurs with feeding.[359] In one study, *Clostridium butyricum* was strongly implicated as the offending organism.[286] Exchange transfusion has long been recognized as a predisposing cause of this disease.[126, 473]

Digoxin-induced Ischemia

Although this could have been included in the general section on ischemia, it is included here because its effects appear to be almost entirely on the small bowel. It has been found that patients who are usually elderly and being treated with digoxin for cardiac failure develop abdominal pain, distension, vomiting, diarrhea, and melena. These features are usually associated with other, more typical clinical features of digoxin toxicity. Most of these patients succumb to their disease, and at autopsy have all been found to have hemorrhagic necrosis of the small intestine, although occasionally the stomach and even the esophagus have been involved.[95, 522] While digoxin may decrease splanchnic blood flow in patients with congestive failure,[190] stimulation of the renin-angiotensin system may cause further constriction and embarrassment of blood flow.

Potassium Salts

In the mid 1960s it was recognized that potassium salts, which were well known for causing severe gastrointestinal symptoms, were also causing small-bowel ulceration. Initially this was reported in patients taking KCl in combination with a diuretic, and it was uncertain which element was responsible, since the diuretic was in the outer core of the tablet and the KCl in the inner core. However, it was rapidly established experimentally that the potassium was the agent responsible, and it was thought that the delivery of high concentrations of potassium salts to a small area of intestine was the causative factor. The possible magnitude of this problem was suggested by Lawrason,[358] who did what was almost a worldwide search and received reports of 484 instances of small-intestinal ulceration, in 275 (57 percent) of which there was a history of taking potassium salts, a diuretic, or both. In attempts to solve this problem, "slow-release" or enteric-coated tablets were manufactured. Although this may have been helpful, it is apparent that ulceration as a result of potassium salts still occurs, as the 16 cases reported by Barbier[31] confirm. Further, ulceration can occur with relatively low doses.[659] Many more cases appeared to have occurred in the United States than in other parts of the world. However, to keep the problem in perspective, Davies found that 5 of 12 cases of small-intestinal ulceration at one British hospital over a 10-year period were associated with the use of potassium salts.[139] Some of these patients were also taking other medications, such as aspirin, steroids, or phenylbutazone, which could well have potentiated the effects of the injury. A similar study in the

United States showed similar cases occurring in patients who had taken potassium salts.[555] There is little characteristic about these ulcers, which present with symptoms either of obstruction or perforation. As mentioned in the esophageal section above, potassium salts are also known to damage the esophagus and stomach.

Iron

Ferrous ions appear capable of damaging most parts of the intestinal tract if they come in prolonged contact with it, and this has already been mentioned both with regard to the esophagus and the stomach. In the intestine, iron can cause ulceration and perforation, the latter occasionally occurring in diverticula, of both the jejunal[294] and Meckel's type.[11] The necrosis is sometimes more extensive, causing larger areas of gangrene.[336, 452] Iron encrustation has also been described in children (see Chapter 2).

Other Heavy Metals

Cadmium. Degenerative changes have been reported at both the light- and electron microscopic levels in the Japanese quail, but their applicability to humans is unknown.[512]

Mercury. Absorbable forms of this metal, such as methylmercury hydroxide, experimentally, cause inclusions and degeneration in Paneth cells, but quite how applicable this is to humans is uncertain.[449] Mercury within the lumen of the gut seems to be inert while in the metallic form. If a mercury balloon ruptures it may cause a foreign-body reaction in the peritoneal cavity, and this has led to enterocutaneous fistula formation.[169]

Zirconium. A cecal mass has been reported in a patient in whom radioactive zirconium phosphate was injected into the peritoneal cavity. The injection caused a dense fibroblastic mass, but it is uncertain whether this was the result of the relatively short-lived but intensive beta-irradiation or a reaction to the zirconium itself.[668]

Granulomatous Enteritis

Clofazimine, which is used in the treatment of leprosy, caused two cases of granulomatous enteritis involving both the ileum and the adjacent lymph nodes. There appears to be little doubt about the cause, since crystals of the drug were identified in the granulomas.[314]

Eosinophilic Enteritis

Clofazimine has also been reported to cause eosinophilic enteritis, which appeared as a nodular thickening, on this occasion in the upper ileum. Again, crystals of the drug, which are red, were identified in the wall of the bowel.[405]

THE APPENDIX

Apart from appendicitis that may have been related to contrast media, appendiceal agenesis has been reported as a result of maternal thalidomide ingestion.[81, 578]

THE LARGE BOWEL

Changes Secondary to Enemas

Some form of bowel preparation is usual before most endoscopies of the large bowel, and this may produce changes that may potentially be mistaken for mild inflammatory bowel disease.

Mannitol and Saline Enemas

These produce virtually no change in the bowel,[424] although the potential for mannitol to be converted into methane and hydrogen, and to be explosive, suggests that it should not be used for bowel preparation.[61]

Fleet's Enemas and Bisacodyl

Mucin depletion and sloughing of the surface epithelium may result, while bisacodyl may additionally produce a peculiar lack of staining by H & E in the upper part of the crypts. Also, occasional polymorphs may be present immediately beneath the luminal epithelium as well as passing through it, and this is often accompanied by mild edema in the same region. All of these changes resolve within a week after treatment.[424]

Hypertonic Saline Enemas

These tend to cause the epithelium to become separated, and also cause mucin depletion with extrusion of mucus into the lumen. An excess of erythrocytes may appear in the lamina propria.[364]

Soap and Other Enemas

Soap enemas are used with astonishing frequency both in and out of medical centers. In one study, 10 to 30 percent of hospitalized patients were given soapsuds enemas,[370] and patients have been known to feel "cleansed" after such enemas. Unfortunately, these enemas are far from harmless, and almost a third of patients experience irritative effects and may have abnormal bowel function for several months following their use.[277] Frank colitis has also been reported.[33, 490] The dangers can come at the time of insertion of the tube, which may lacerate the rectal mucosa and cause either hemorrhage or even perforation. Subsequent enema under pressure may further separate the mucosa from the submucosa, and either large sloughing ulcers or a peritonitis that is presumably both chemical and bacterial may result. On one occasion, a large rectal ulcer that sloughed and at the time was thought to be gangrenous was potentiated by the vigorous use of a Higginsons syringe.[50] Other injury may result directly from the pressure of the fluid injected. The old nursing dictum "high, hot, and a helluvalot" may not be without its risks. Pathologically, the most common effects of an enema are edema and chronic inflammation, but polymorphs and even occasional crypt abscesses may be present as an early development.

In one study among South African blacks, 8 percent admitted to the regular use of enemas over periods of years, while 2.7 percent used them daily. A variety of substances were used, including antiseptics, caustics, copper sulfate, potassium permanganate, potassium dichromate, and brown sugar. Perforations occasionally occurred following the use of the horn of a cow to administer the enema. The changes observed varied from mild acute and chronic inflammation to full-thickness necrosis of the bowel wall.[551]

We have seen one bizarre case in which a chemical necrosis of the mucosa was present, although the exact nature of the responsible chemical was unknown (Fig. 18-11).

Changes Due to Laxatives

Laxatives fall into several distinctive categories, including the anthracene derivatives such as cascara, senna, rhubarb, and aloes; a variety of salts—usually magnesium, or sodium sulfate, or sodium dihydrogen phosphate; the phenylmethanes such as phenolphthalein; substances that have a detergent action, such as dioctyl sodium sulfosuccinate; oily substances such as liquid paraffin or castor oil, and a variety of "bulk" laxatives including cellulose derivatives, bran, alginates, and mucilages. Although only pseudomelanosis is readily recognized histologically as a laxative effect, electron microscopic observations on specimens from patients chronically abusing laxatives have shown damage to the microvilli—both a reduction in numbers and abnormalities in cytoplasmic organelles, and an increase in the numbers of lysosomes and dense bodies.[514] Colonic perforation that ultimately proved fatal was reported in a man given a senna preparation before a barium enema. Although taking a regular dose of senna, he developed severe colic that finally perforated.[87]

Pseudomelanosis Coli (Melanosis Coli)

The deposition of this brown, or occasionally almost black pigment, is secondary to ingestion of the anthracene derivatives known as the anthraquinones.[670] The pigment produced is in fact lipofuscin-like, and has all of the staining reactions of that pigment (positive with PAS, acid-fast stains, Nile blue sulfate, and Schmorl's reaction, but negative with Perl's reaction). It is found primarily in the right colon and occasionally in the rectum. When more pronounced, the condition may extend to the left side of the colon or diffusely, throughout the entire large bowel. The appendix and occasionally the terminal ileum may be affected, but the same lesion occurring in the upper intestinal tract is probably unrelated to anthraquinone ingestion,[82, 130, 212] although one patient had an asociated gastric ulcer and folate deficiency, with the "melanosis" resolving with the ulcer and correction of the folate deficiency.[557]

The pigment in pseudomelanosis coli is found in macrophages in the lamina propria; however, unlike the macrophages normally found in the lamina propria of the colon, which occur in the superficial portion of the mucosa, those in pseudomelanosis coli tend to occur in the deeper part of the mucosa, and even in the submucosa if the condition is severe (Fig. 18-12A). Additionally an increased number of chronic inflammatory cells may be present in the lamina propria. Although thickening of the muscularis mucosae of the rectum has also been reported, this change is also seen in a variety of other inflammatory and noninflammatory conditions in the rectum. When pseudomelanosis is marked, macrophages may also be found in the sinuses of the mesenteric lymph nodes, usually in the subcapsular sinus (Fig. 18-12B).

The mechanism of formation of the pseudomelanotic pigment is poorly understood, but appears to require fecal stasis.[67, 580] Although many carcinomas are associated with the pigment (Fig. 18-12C) this is almost certainly

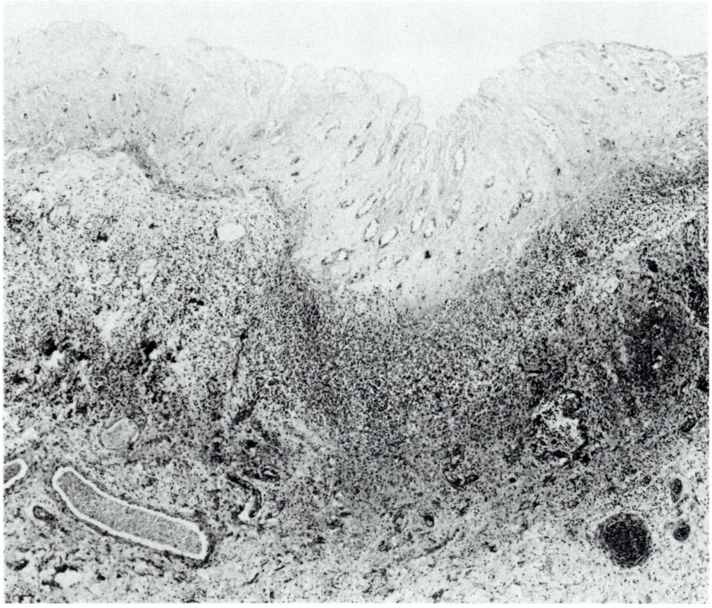

Fig. 18-11. Superficial coagulation necrosis of the colon, resembling an infarct with a peripheral zone of hemorrhage and acute inflammation. (H&E, × 35).

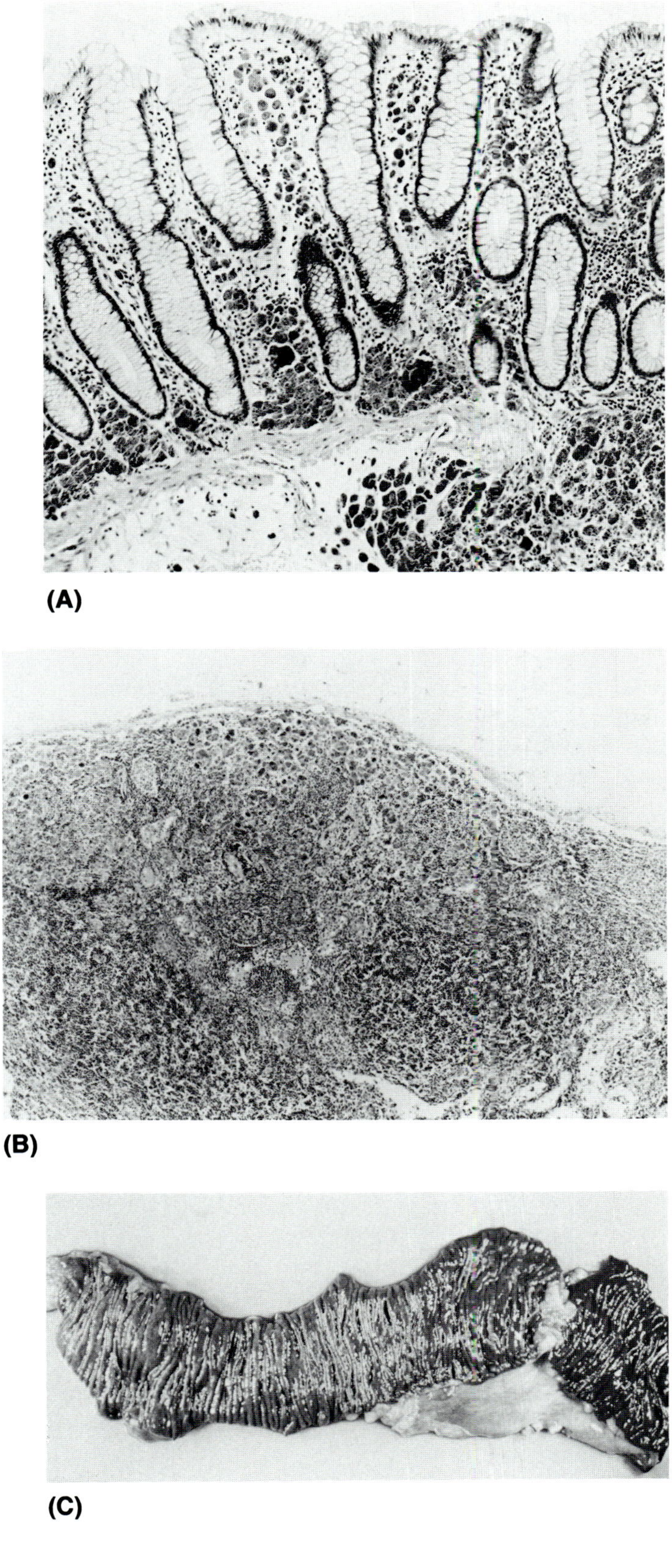

Fig. 18-12. Colon with pseudomelanosis. (A) Typical heavily pigmented macrophages are present, particularly in the vicinity of the muscularis mucosae, and even in the submucosa. (H&E, × 85). (B) Mesenteric lymph node from the same patient, showing pigmented macrophages in the sinuses (H&E, × 45). (C) Gross specimen from the same patient. The mucosa is a deep brown, while the carcinoma present may have caused the constipation, resulting in the patient taking large doses of laxatives.

the result of patients taking laxatives for their "constipation." Electron microscopic examination initially suggested that the pigment was formed from degenerating mitochondria or endoplasmic reticulum[222, 544] but more recent studies suggest a lysosomal origin.[589] Like many purgatives, the action of anthraquinones is not only exerted on the mucosa, but causes considerable damage to the myenteric plexus, with loss of neurons and Schwannosis.[576, 589] Ultimately, the large bowel may acquire the characteristics of a "cathartic colon."

Cathartic Colon

This is virtually an end-stage colon that cannot contract effectively, probably because of the extensive damage to the myenteric plexus. The mucosa may exhibit all of the changes of laxative abuse, including pseudomelanosis, while it also acquires a snake-skin like appearance and may have several small ulcers. The haustra are lost and the colon becomes converted into an irregular tube, although there may be areas of dilatation. The ileum and ileocecal valve are invariably affected; indeed, this is where the most marked radiologic changes tend to occur. The muscularis propria is invariably thinned and the submucosal fat is very prominent, seeming to bulge out from the cut edge of a resected specimen. In one patient, linear ulcers were present and a heavy infiltrate of eosinophils was also noted.[110]

Myenteric Plexus Damage, Pseudo-obstruction, Stercoral Ulceration

A variety of drugs are known to damage the myenteric plexus, causing loss of neurons and frequently Schwannosis.[577] These drugs may affect virtually any part of the intestinal tract, although the small and large bowel are the organs usually affected. The causative agents are especially likely to give rise to chronic constipation and pseudo-obstruction. Both of these, but especially the former, may be complicated by the formation of hard fecaliths which may cause local chronic inflammation, acute inflammation, ulceration, bleeding, and even perforation. These are commonly seen at autopsy, although many clinicians are surprised at the damage they can cause. In patients on antineoplastic or immunosuppressive drugs the ulceration constitutes a fine portal of entry for bacteria. A good review of pseudo-obstruction, including that caused by drugs, is given by Faulk et al.,[185] while stercoral perforation is reviewed by Gekas and Schuster.[217] Four major categories of drugs appear particularly likely to damage the myenteric plexus and cause pseudo-obstruction and its complications; these are anticholinergics, antidepressants, antineoplastic agents, and tranquilizers, particularly the phenothiazines.

Anticholinergic Drugs

While Parkinson's disease itself can cause pseudo-obstruction, drugs that are used to treat it, such as benztropine or trihexyphenidyl, can also cause a severe and exceedingly troublesome constipation.[585, 649]

Antidepressants

Following occasional suggestions that these compounds could affect the myenteric plexus,[92, 211] Milner[440] described 6 patients developing obstructive symptoms while taking amitriptyline, nortriptyline, or imipramine. This was rapidly confirmed. Some such patients concurrently take a variety of other psychotropic drugs, including the phenothiazines, that can also damage the myenteric plexus. The likelihood of pseudo-obstruction developing depends as much on the age of the patient as on the dose of drugs.

Antineoplastic Agents

Although it is relatively common to see some degree of ileus in patients dying following chemotherapy, most have been on combination chemotherapy regimens, making it difficult to know if a single specific agent is responsible or whether combinations are more potent in inducing this condition.[572] Of all antineoplastic drugs that might cause pseudo-obstruction, vincristine is the archetype. Since its first use it has been observed to cause colicky abdominal pain, constipation, and ileus as a result of direct damage to the myenteric plexus.[575] Almost half of all patients receiving this drug get colicky pain within 4 to 72 hours, and about 10 percent develop severe pain and radiologic evidence of ileus.[538]

Phenothiazines

This group of drugs is now well recognized as producing unwanted secondary effects because of its parasympatholytic action in patients who have been taking relatively high quantities of such drugs over long periods. It is therefore seen with greatest frequency in psychiatric patients, and has occurred with most members of the phenothiazine group including chlorpromazine,[142] trifluoperazine,[585] and thioridazine.[649] Clinically, this side-effect may be potentiated by alcohol.[440] In Warnes series,[649] 3 of 8 patients died as a result of adynamic ileus. ("Adynamic" ileus may be a misnomer in some instances of fecal impaction distally, when the ileus may be hyperdynamic.)

Ritama et al. did an autopsy study comparing the incidence of intestinal dilatation in a psychiatric unit with that in a local medical hospital. Both groups consisted largely of elderly patients. In the mental hospital group, intestinal dilatation was found at autopsy in 12 percent of the group compared with 2 percent for the control group. In the mental hospital group, all of the patients with ileus had been on phenothiazines for several years. The authors attributed the findings to the anticholinergic effects of the tranquilizers that had been used to treat all of the mental hospital patients with ileus. Unfortunately, no details are given as to the corresponding medication of patients in the psychiatric group who did not develop ileus.[516] The literature is reviewed in a further recent case report by Evans et al.[178]

Miscellaneous Substances

A variety of other substances have been associated with pseudo-obstruction, although whether or not they produce anything other than transient functional damage to the myenteric plexus is largely unknown. These will now be briefly mentioned.

Alcohol alone has been reported to cause intestinal obstruction, although the mechanism of this is unknown.[318] Both patients in the report were imbibing considerable quantities of alcohol at the time of their admission.

Amanita Poisoning. Four patients were reported to have developed an atonic, dilated small and large bowel following *Amanita* ingestion; in 3 the condition responded to conservative management.[259]

Clonidine. Pseudo-obstruction has now been reported in patients taking clonidine for hypertension; the condition seems to have a predeliction for the colon.[43, 45] However, simple discontinuation of the drug treatment produces relief.

Ganglion Blockers. These drugs are now rarely used in the treatment of hypertension; nevertheless, patients taking such agents as pentolinium or hexamethonium have frequently developed constipation requiring further laxative treatment.[205, 252] Occasionally, this has been complicated by pseudo-obstruction.[226, 228] Pseudo-obstruction has also affected the stomach.[49]

Narcotics. The potential for morphine and diamorphine to cause or potentiate ileus in the postoperative period is well documented, although the condition resolves spontaneously. There have been several reports of acute intestinal pseudo-obstruction occurring in heroin addicts,[94, 172, 192] and Spira et al. have described a similar phenomenon in patients treated with methadone for their heroin addiction.[583] The potential for narcotic drugs to destroy the myenteric plexus is well known.[575]

Others. Occasional instances of other drugs apparently producing paralytic ileus or pseudo-obstruction have been described. These have included duodenojejunal ileus following oxyprenolol[676] and colonic ileus following cimetidine.[653] Additionally, ileus has been described in young children given loperamide.[450]

Gaseous Distention and Pneumatosis Cystoides

We have observed two patients with both ulcerative colitis and severe liver disease (sclerosing cholangitis) who were treated with lactulose with good effect on their mental status but dangerous complications in the colon. In the face of active ulcerative colitis, the colon of one patient became very distended, mimicking toxic dilatation, and developed a small perforation; the second patient developed pneumatosis cystoides intestinalis, with marked dilatation of his colon that required colectomy (Fig. 18-13). The gas-filled cysts in this patient may well have been caused by the lactulose, and the relative lack of a giant-cell reaction around these cysts suggested that they were a very recent development. However, it should be remembered that pneumatosis develops very easily in children with any form of inflammatory bowel disease. Neither of the patients we treated was a child, but this association requires further confirmation.

A single case report also links high-dose practolol with pneumatosis cystoides intestinalis, but until further confirmation is received it is difficult to be certain that this was not coincidental, particularly since there is no obvious mechanism by which the drug and the condition could be linked.[626]

Pseudomembranous and Antibiotic-Associated Colitis

Pseudomembranous colitis (PMC) is a term that is today used almost synonymously with antibiotic-associated colitis (AAC). However PMC is almost certainly only the tip of the AAC iceberg; conversely, there are other causes of PMC, such as the early lesion of ischemia[413, 414] (including the changes seen in uremia) and mercuric compounds,[387,648a] while some forms of predominantly right-sided antibiotic-associated colitis may not be overtly pseudomembranous.

Antibiotics, irrespective of the route of their administration,[256, 489] are undoubtedly the most common factor implicated in PMC, although the disease may occur spontaneously. While occasional reports of an antibiotic-associated PMC can be found in the early 1950s literature, lincomycin was the first antibiotic to be incriminated and repeatedly confirmed as causing this condition,[51, 141, 494, 542, 546, 574, 633, 643] while its 7-chloro-7-deoxy derivative, clindamycin—developed largely because of this adverse side-effect—may also cause the same disease.[80, 113, 118, 141, 384, 438, 461, 494, 574, 597, 615, 633, 643] A variety of other antibiotics have now been incriminated, including penicillin derivatives such as amoxicillin,[567] ampicillin,[35, 40, 55, 80, 109, 253, 319, 384, 529, 542, 586, 633] and oxacillin,[207] as well as cephalosporins,[187, 292, 618, 637], chloramphenicol,[508] neomycin,[71] rifampicin,[5, 73, 202, 426] tetracycline,[334, 508, 542, 633] and metranidazole.[443, 629] Indeed, it is likely that most antibiotics, with the likely exception of vancomycin and any other antibiotic to which *Cl. difficile* is sensitive (see below), may cause AAC and PMC.

Many descriptions of PMC include antibiotics used in combination, such as co-trimoxi-

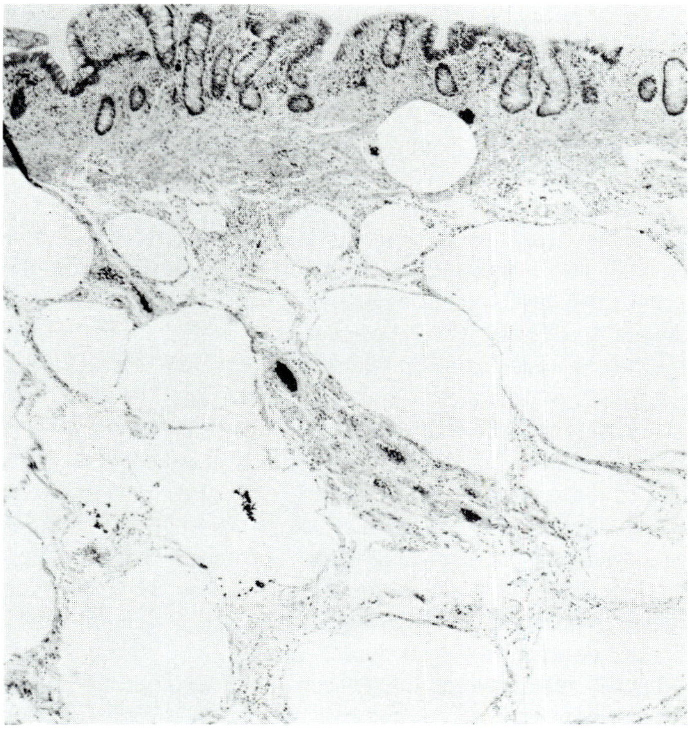

(A)

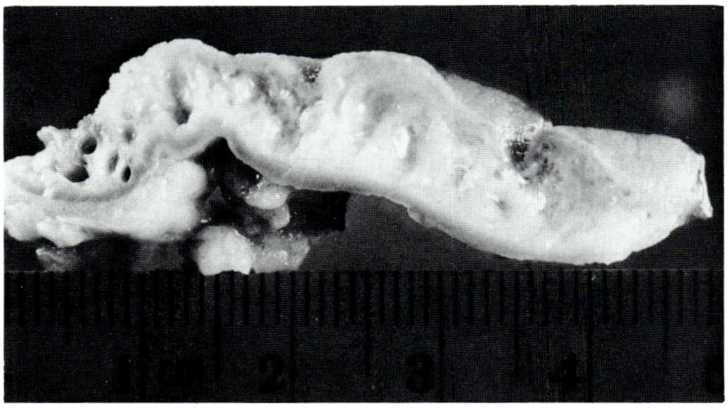

(B)

Fig. 18-13. Pneumatosis coli resulting from lactulose ingestion in the submucosa of the colon. (A) The mucosa shows typical regenerative features, as seen in ulcerative colitis, but the submucosa is distended by numerous gas-filled spaces. The lack of the giant cells usually seen around these cysts is due to inadequate time for their formation. (H&E, × 50). (B) Gross photograph of the specimen, showing marked thickening of the submucosa caused by the cysts present.

zole,[35, 96, 570] ampicillin with clindamycin,[80] tetracycline with streptomycin,[542] cephalothin with clindamycin,[633] clindamycin with erythromycin,[633] and clindamycin with gentamycin.[118] The fact that these combinations cause disease is hardly surprising, since most of the individual substances noted here are quite capable of inducing the disease by themselves. Nevertheless, it is of interest that in one series in which two such antibiotics, ampicillin and clindamycin, were given both separately and in combination, PMC was found in 3.8 percent of the patients given ampicillin alone, 4.2 percent of the patients given clindamycin aline, and 9 percent of the patients given both drugs simultaneously.[80]

An intriguing feature of both AAC and PMC is the tremendous variation in their incidence from one series to another, even when the same antibiotics are involved. Thus, when diarrhea alone is considered during clindamycin use, one study showed an incidence of 66 cases in 1,000 patients (6.6 percent),[606] while another study found 42 cases in only 200 patients (21 percent).[615] Both studies showed an increased incidence in women, and pointed out that oral administration is not a prerequisite for the development of disease. Similarly, the incidence of PMC has been variable, being 10 percent in one series in which clindamycin was used.[615] However, in a further series, investigating ampicillin, no PMC was found in 200 consecutive patients.[616] This variation is one of the unexplained features of AAC and PMC, even down to the point of some authors suggesting the occurrence of minor outbreaks of the disease[250, 439], implying either direct or indirect infection from patient to patient. Much more poorly documented is the incidence of inflammation alone, since biopsies are not done regularly in patients with antibiotic-associated diarrhea.

Etiology. The etiology of AAC and PMC has now been at least partly resolved, in what represents one of the great advances in medicine of the past few years. It is apparent that these conditions are caused by changes in the gut flora, and particularly the elimination of anaerobes[401] by antibiotics that preferentially allow the proliferation of at least one other organism that is unaffected by the antibiotic(s) used. Such proliferating organisms may include fungi—particularly *Candida*—and bacteria such as staphylococci (especially following the use of tetracycline)[13, 42, 144, 623] or pseudomonas.[189] However, in most patients with PMC, the offending organism is *Cl. difficile,* which produces the toxin causing the disease[36, 71, 219, 250, 320, 355, 374] and appears to be resistant to most antibiotics except vancomycin. For this reason it seems reasonable to suppose that antibiotics that are inactive against this organism and could therefore allow its proliferation are likely to be associated with PMC, while any other antibiotic to which *Cl. difficile* is sensitive is unlikely to be associated with the disease but should prove effective in its treatment. Nevertheless, rifampicin, which has only recently been added to the list of antibiotics apparently associated with PMC, is in fact quite active against *Cl. difficile,* while metronidazole, which has been implicated etiologically in PMC (see above), has also been used in its treatment.[71] Vancomycin and bacitracin appear to be the agents most useful in the treatment of PMC.[105, 221, 617, 619] Nevertheless, *Cl. difficile* may occasionally not be eradicated by apparently sufficient courses of appropriate antibiotics, and repeated courses may be required.[37, 220]

However, the advance made in treating PMC caused by *Cl. difficile* is not the end of the story. One report indicates that *Cl. perfringens* type C may occasionally be responsible,[545] although this can also be viewed in terms of being another organism that uncommonly causes the disease. Also, while *Cl. difficile* itself must be present in the intestinal flora to allow its proliferation under appropriate conditions, the frequency with which it is present in the general population is unknown. Indeed, like other toxin-producing clostridia, it may not be present in sufficient numbers to be cultured even while its toxin is causing the disease. Additionally, it is not known whether all strains of the organism are toxin-producing, or whether some strains are more capable than others of producing both the toxin and the disease.[320] In view of the marked variation in the incidence of clostridial PMC and in the apparent outbreaks of the disease,[250, 439] it seems likely that some strains not only are highly toxigenic, but that they may be readily transmissable from one patient to another. A further complicating factor is that while most patients developing PMC after antibiotics—and even those developing PMC spontaneously—exhibit the clostridial toxin in their stools,[287, 481] others have similar quantities of toxin but do not develop the disease.[36, 374] This may indicate individual sensitivity to the toxin. Conversely, not all patients with AAC have the toxin in their stools.[374] Since the acquisition or overgrowth of many organisms may be accompanied by temporary diarrhea (for example, travellers diarrhea), the lack of association between AAC and clostridial toxin is perhaps not surprising in view of the alteration in fecal flora that occurs during antibiotic administration.

Inflammatory Bowel Disease and *Cl. difficile*. An interesting interrelationship has become apparent between *Cl. difficile* toxin and exacerbations of inflammatory bowel disease, particularly ulcerative colitis, since a proportion of patients apparently suffering relapse of their disease are found to have the toxin in their stools.[38,72,351,431,636] Their symptoms respond to treatment with vancomycin, disappearing with disappearance of the toxin. In other respects the exacerbation resembles these patients' underlying disease, and true PMC seems not to develop in this group of patients despite the frequency with which they are treated with broad-spectrum antibiotics. The histology of toxin-induced relapses is virtually undocumented, and it is unknown whether this comprises the predominantly nonspecific increase in chronic inflammatory cells seen in some patients following antibiotics, or whether it resembles the underlying disease process. However, it should be emphasized that relapses of the disease attributable to *Cl. difficile* occur in only a minority of patients with inflammatory bowel disease and is not the cause of them.

Pathology

A variety of clinical and pathologic changes may be found in patients taking antibiotics. Symptomatically, these range from no change in bowel habit to varying degrees of diarrhea and ultimately to bloody diarrhea. Endoscopically there is a spectrum, from no abnormality at one extreme to erythema, friability, and PMC at the other. Histologically, these changes are almost undocumented other than in PMC. In a few examples seen personally, some patients on antibiotics clearly have no abnormality, while some with diarrhea show a fairly diffuse infiltrate consisting predominantly of lymphocytes and plasma cells in the lamina propria, with only occasional polymorphs seen superficially, and rare crypt abscesses. These changes resolve, with the mucosa returning to its former state. In contrast, the changes in PMC are well documented[240,422,501] and will therefore be only briefly described.

Macroscopically, and therefore endoscopically, PMC is a focal lesion, with plaques separated by apparently normal mucosa. Its appearance can be likened to a splashing of the mucosa with cream-colored paint. There is usually an abrupt transition to normal mucosa at the ileocecal valve, which is useful in distinguishing ischemic disease from PMC. Since the ileocolic artery serves the entire area, ischemic disease should therefore not stop completely at the ileocecal valve. Distally, PMC usually involves the rectum, so that sigmoidoscopy or proctoscopy are adequate for its diagnosis. However, some patients have a relatively normal rectal mucosa, with the characteristic lesions of PMC being found only more proximally with the colonoscope.[618]

Biopsy of the junction between plaque and normal colonic tissue is invariably diagnostic of PMC, and should be strongly encouraged to document that this was the original disease, lest the patient's disease subsequently recur and doubt be cast on the initial diagnosis. Microscopically, the lesion starts as a focal mushroom or volcano-like exudate from the luminal surface of the mucosa, with destruction of the most superficial part of the crypt, an occurrence that is consistent with damage caused by toxin to the luminal portion of the cells.[2] As the lesion develops, more of the mucosa is involved, leaving only the bases of the crypts intact (Fig. 18-14), and these may also be destroyed. The intervening mucosa shows at best a mild excess of chronic inflammatory cells, but mild submucosal edema is usually present.

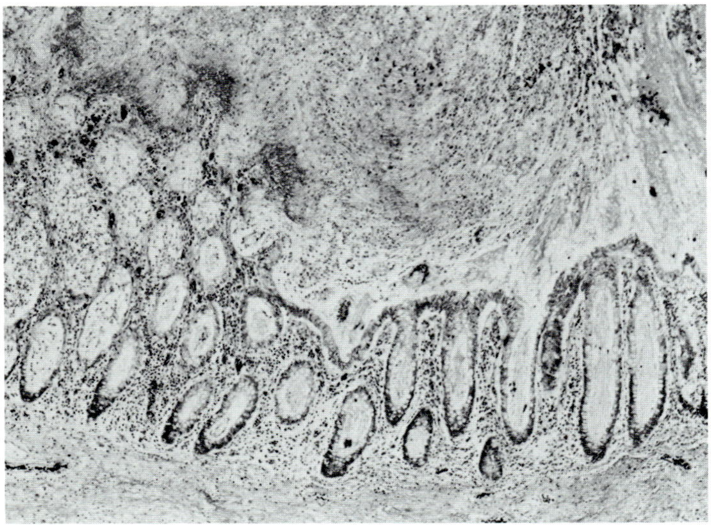

Fig. 18-14. Typical appearance of pseudomembranous colitis. The crypts on the right are relatively spared although containing inspissated mucus, while there is superficial destruction of the crypts on the left, only the crypt bases remaining intact. The characteristic volcano-like exudate is apparent in the lumen. (H&E, × 45).

A vasculitis is not found, but platelet thrombi may be found in capillaries, particularly just beneath the muscularis mucosae. However, this may well be a secondary rather than a primary phenomenon.

There is usually complete recovery, particularly when the condition is treated with vancomycin; however, it is apparent that in some patients, untreated PMC may progress to a stage that may be clinically difficult to distinguish from overtly active ulcerative colitis, and may occasionally progress to a stage of toxic dilatation[633] or even perforation.[574] The last two complications are indications for surgical intervention. In patients with severe, bloody diarrhea, a biopsy documenting the original disease proves invaluable, particularly if the patient is transferred to another hospital where the original proctoscopic diagnosis may be doubted.

The prognosis of PMC when recognized early and treated adequately is good, and recovery is the rule. However, in a small group of patients with neoplastic diseases,[164] particularly of a hematopoietic nature,[241, 438] and in those undergoing bowel resections, particularly for carcinoma,[320] this disease may be far more lethal as a result of its being unrecognized clinically. Under these circumstances, PMC produces a high mortality.

Right-sided Antibiotic-associated Colitis. Recently, it has become apparent that some patients developing an AAC have a predominantly right-sided disease that is not pseudomembranous and is not associated with *Cl. difficile* toxin.[420, 536, 632] The condition has been associated with ampicillin,[536] amoxicillin,[420] and erythromycin.[147] Its pathology and cause have yet to be described. The possibility that it may be a right-sided variant of PMC, caused by a different organism or toxin, cannot be excluded.

Granulomatous Colitis

There is a brief report of a patient developing a granulomatous colitis following the administration of naproxen, with the observation that this condition may be mistaken for Crohn's disease.[26] Further case reports would clearly be required to confirm any association.

Non-specific Colitis

A variety of drugs have occasionally been reported to be associated with either proctitis or colitis. Some of these associations might be expected, such as local proctitis in patients using suppositories containing indomethacin[369]; however, indomethacin has also been reported to be associated with perforation of a sigmoid diverticulum associated with inflammation and ulceration of the adjacent mucosa.[128]

Other drugs associated with a more diffuse colitis (other than those mentioned above, particularly in the section on antineoplastic drugs) are 5-flucytosine, gold, methyldopa, and penicillamine.

Alcohol

It is perhaps surprising that the effects of alcohol may occur in the distal intestinal tract, but one study utilizing rectal biopsies in patients who had recently imbibed heavily showed a surprising reduction in the number of goblet cells and an increased chronic inflammatory infiltrate in the lamina propria. Electron microscopically there were swollen and distorted mitochondria, with a dilated and vesicular endoplasmic reticulum. The changes persisted for up to 2 weeks. In view of the rapidity of absorption of alcohol from the upper intestinal tract, a direct effect seems unlikely unless large amounts of fluid are also ingested. These changes may help to explain the diarrhea seen in some alcoholics, irrespective of the mechanism.[90]

5-Flucytosine

This is an antifungal agent with a broad spectrum of activity. In several reports following its introduction in the early 1970s, there appeared to be a variety of side-effects, among which were diarrhea and colitis. The latter appears to have been severe, because in all papers there is mention not only of the colitis, but also of perforation, usually in the colon, but occasionally in the small intestine also.[52] Some of these complications proved fatal.[261, 521, 639]

Gold

Enterocolitis is one of the lesser-known complications of chrysotherapy, although it has been known for decades. Nevertheless, when it occurs it is severe, and bears considerable resemblance to ulcerative colitis[181, 224, 291, 591] (Fig. 18-15). Some of the reported episodes of gold-associated colitis have proven fatal.[564]

Methyldopa

Seven patients have been described in whom a relationship of colitis with methyldopa was postulated.[75, 242] The latter report included 4 additional patients in whom there was some question of the validity of the association because of other factors, although temporal eligibility was established. In all cases the disease remitted when the drug was stopped, while in 3 of the 6 cases in which the relationship seemed likely, it was confirmed by rechallenge. The authors draw an analogy with methyldopa-induced hemolytic anemia, and therefore suggest an autoimmune basis for the colitis.

Penicillamine

There has been a case report of colitis complicating penicillamine therapy,[276] but further cases are required to support the claim of an association.

Packing of the Rectum

A note should be added about the surgical practice of packing the rectum with gauze soaked in a substance such as Betadine to aid surgical dissection. This may produce superficial ischemic damage in the rectum. The association is unlikely to cause problems providing that it is recognized (Fig. 18-16).

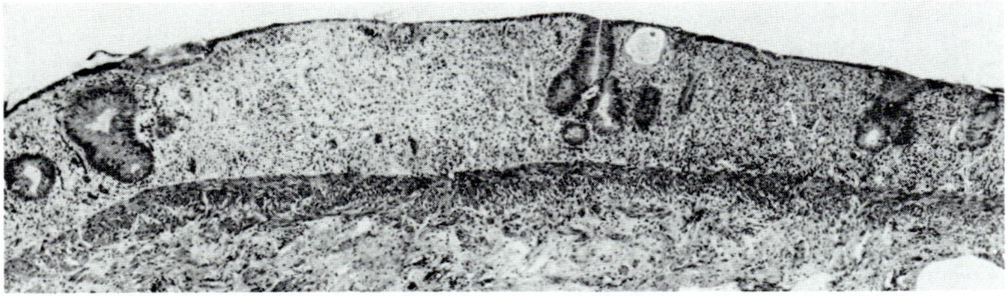

(A)

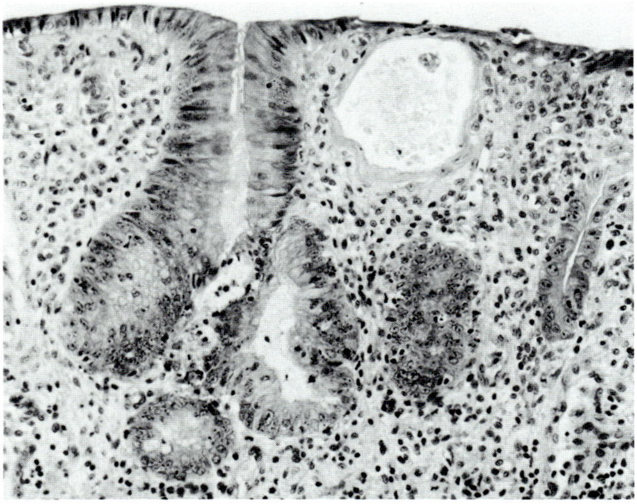

(B)

Fig. 18-15. Colitis following gold therapy in a 25-year-old woman with a long history of rheumatoid arthritis. (A) There is marked atrophy of the mucosa. (Saffronin, alcian blue, hematoxylin, × 30.) (B) Higher power view of crypts at center, showing active regeneration with a moderate acute and chronic inflammatory infiltrate. The disease at this stage could easily be mistaken for nonspecific ulcerative colitis. (Saffronin, alcian blue, hematoxylin, × 350.) (Courtesy of Dr. C. Rubin, Seattle, WA.)

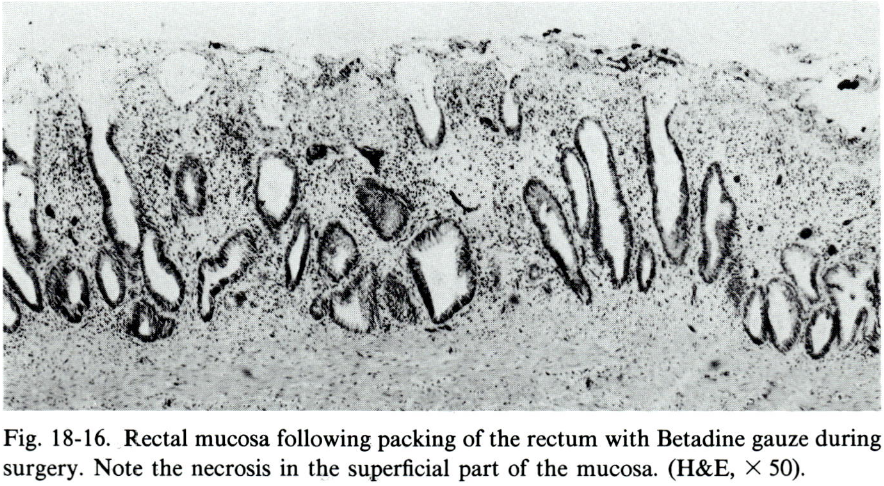

Fig. 18-16. Rectal mucosa following packing of the rectum with Betadine gauze during surgery. Note the necrosis in the superficial part of the mucosa. (H&E, × 50).

Ulcerative Colitis

While the cause of ulcerative colitis is unknown, it is worth mentioning that during active disease some drugs other than antibiotics (see above) may increase its clinical activity, leading to further complications. Thus anticoagulants may promote bleeding, although some, such as phenindione, can cause diarrhea or steatorrhea in their own right.[610] Toxic dilatation in ulcerative colitis can be precipitated by a variety of agents, including opiates, atropine and its derivatives, cathartics, barium enema, and colonoscopy—possibly as a result of preparation and also hypokalemia of any cause.[263, 331, 465] Loperamide has recently been reported to cause a similar complication.[88]

Elemental Diets

A variety of complications have arisen with elemental diets; in the GIT these include necrotizing enterocolitis[342] and bleeding, and in the pancreas of rats, acinar atrophy. Experimentally, such diets also cause atrophy of the colonic mucosa.[301] It is uncertain whether such disuse atrophy can be seen in humans, although it may be seen in defunctioned or bypassed loops of bowel. Although such analogies are always dangerous, it would seem more surprising if such an effect did not occur.

REFERENCES

1. Abbarah, T. R., Fredell, J. E., & Ellenz, G. B.: Ulceration by oral ferrous sulfate. J.A.M.A. 15:2320, 1976.
2. Abrams, G. D., Allo, M., Rifkin, G. D., et al.: Mucosal damage mediated by clostridial toxin in experimental clindamycin-associated colitis. Gut 21:493-499, 1980.
3. Abramson, A. L.: Corrosive injury to the esophagus: result of ingesting some denture cleanser tablets and powder. Arch. Otolaryngol. 104:514-516, 1978.
4. Ackrill, P., Hasleton, P. S., & Ralston, A. J.: Oesophageal perforation due to paraquat. Br. Med. J. 1:1252-1253, 1978.
5. Acocella, G., & Arioli, V.: Pseudomembranous colitis and rifampicin. Lancet 1:827, 1980.
6. Adams, J. T., & Skucas, J.: Corrosive jejunitis due to ingestion of nitric acid. Am. J. Surg. 139:282-285, 1980.
7. Admani, A. K., & Khaleque, D.M.N.F.: Gastrointestinal hemorrhage associated with diflunisal. Lancet 1:1247, 1979.
8. Adrian, R. W., Walker, F. S., & Noel, P. R. B.: Toxicological studies on azapropazone. Curr. Med. Res. Opin. 4:17, 1976.
9. Agdal, N.: Medicininducerede esophagusskader. Ugeskr. Laeger 141:3019-3021, 1979.
10. Aguilo, J. J., Zincke, H., Woods, J. E., & Buckingham, J. M.: Intestinal perforation due to fecal impaction and renal transplantation. J. Urol. 116:153-155, 1976.
11. Alaily, A. B.: Gangrene of Meckel's diverticulum in pregnancy due to iron tablet. Br. Med. J. 1:103, 1974.
12. Allen, R., Thoshinsky, M., Stallone, R., et al: Corrosive injuries of the stomach. Arch. Surg. 100:409, 1970.
13. Altemeier, W. A., Hummel, R. P., & Hill, E. O.: Staphylococcal enterocolitis following antibiotic therapy. Ann. Surg. 157:847-858, 1963.
14. Altobelli, A., Yamashita, T., & Kratzer, G. L.: Necrotizing proctitis caused by injection of barium into the wall of the rectum. Dis. Colon Rectum 13:333, 1970.
15. Alvarez, A. S., & Summerskill, W. H. J.: Gastrointestinal hemorrhage and salicylates. Lancet 2:920-925, 1958.
16. Alves, M., Patel, V., Douglas, E., & Deutsch, E.: Gastric infarction: a complication of selective vasopressin infusion. Am. J. Digest. Dis. 24:1252-1253, 1979.
17. Amberg, J. R.: A hazard of silicone foam diagnostic enema: report of a case of perforation of the colon. Am. J. Roentgenol. 99:96, 1967.
18. Amberg, J. R.: Complications of colonic radiography. Gastrointestinal Endoscopy 26:15S-17S, 1980.
19. Ament, M. E., & Rubin, C. E.: Soy protein—another cause of the flat intestinal lesion. Gastroenterology 62:227, 1972.
20. Amromin, G. D., & Solomen, R. D.: Necrotizing enteropathy. J.A.M.A. 182:23-29, 1962.

21. Appelqvist, P., & Salmo, M.: Lye corrosion carcinoma of the esophagus: a review of 63 cases. Cancer 45:2655-2658, 1980.
22. Aristizabal, S. A., Muller, R. C., Schlichtemeier, A. L., et al.: Adriamycin-irradiation cutaneous complications. Int. J. Radiat. Oncol. Biol. Phys. 2:325-331, 1977.
23. Arvanitakis, C., Lorenzsonn, V., & Olsen, W. A.: Phenformin-induced alterations of small-intestinal function and mitochondrial structure in man. J. Lab. Clin. Med. 82: 195-200, 1973.
24. Asbury, M. J.: Retroperitoneal fibrosis after treatment with atenolol (Letter). Br. Med. J. 1:492, 1979.
25. Augur, N. A.: Gastric mucosa blood flow following damage by ethanol, acetic acid, or aspirin. Gastroenterology 58:311, 1970.
26. Baas, E. U., Ewe, K., & Hohn, P.: Granulomatose kolitis nach naproxen. Dtsch. Med. Wochenschr. 101:1434, 1976.
27. Bachrach, W. H.: Reserpine, gastric secretion and peptic ulcer. Am. J. Digest Dis. 4:117-124, 1959.
28. Baird, G. M., & Dosseter, J. F. B.: Methotrexate enteropathy. Lancet 1:164, 1981.
29. Bank, S., Trey, C., Gans, I., et al.: Histoplasmosis of the small bowel with "giant" intestinal villi and secondary protein-losing enteropathy. Am. J. Med. 39:492-501, 1965.
30. Baratz, M., Werbin, N., Wiznitzer, T., et al.: Irradiation-induced colonic stricture and colitis cystica profunda. Dis. Colon Rectum 21:75-79, 1978.
31. Barbier, P., Pringot, I., Heimann, R., et al.: Ulcerations digestives induites par le chlorure de potassium. Acta Gastroenterol. Belg. 34:261, 1976.
32. Barcewicz, P. A., & Welch, J. P.: Ischemic colitis in young adult patients. Dis. Colon Rectum 23:109-114, 1980.
33. Barker, C. S.: Acute colitis resulting from soapsuds enema. Can. Med. Assoc. J. 52:285-286, 1945.
34. Barranco, C. J.: IUD gangrene of small intestine. Am. J. Surg. 135:717, 1978.
35. Bartle, W. R., & Saibil, F. G.: Antibiotic-associated pseudomembranous colitis. Can. Med. Assoc. J. 116:162, 1977.
36. Bartlett, J. G., Moon, N., Chang, T. W., et al.: Role of Clostridium difficile in antibiotic-associated pseudomembranous colitis. Gastroenterology 75:778-782, 1978.
37. Bartlett, J. G., Tedesco, F. J., Shull, S., et al.: Symptomatic relapse after oral vancomycin therapy of antibiotic-associated pseudomembranous colitis. Gastroenterology 78:431-434, 1980.
38. Bartlett, J. G.: Clostridium difficile and inflammatory bowel disease. Gastroenterology 80:863-865, 1981.
39. Baskin, W. N., Ivey, K. J., Krause, W. J., et al.: Aspirin-induced ultrastructural changes in human gastric mucosa. Correlation with potential difference. Ann. Intern. Med. 85:299-303, 1976.
40. Bass, J. W., Crowley, D. M., Steele, R. W., et al.: Adverse effects of orally administered ampicillin. J. Pediatr. 83:106-108, 1973.
41. Batterman, R. C., & Ehrenfeld, I.: The influence of smoking on the management of the peptic ulcer patient. Gastroenterol. 12:575-585, 1949.
42. Batts, D. H., Silva, J., Fekety, R.: Staphylococcal enterocolitis. Abstracts, 11th International Congress on Chemotherapy. Abstr. No. 181.
43. Bauer, G. E., & Hellestrand, K. J.: Pseudo-obstruction due to clonidine. Br. Med. J. 1:769, 1976.
44. Baxter-Smith, D. C., Monypenny, K. J., & Dorricott, N. J.: Sclerosing peritonitis in patient on timolol (Letter). Lancet 2:149, 1978.
45. Bear, R., & Steer, K.: Pseudo-obstruction due to clonidine. Br. Med. J. 1:197, 1976.
46. Beaumont, W.: Experiments and Observations on the Gastric Juice and the Physiology of Digestion. F. P. Allen, Plattsburgh, N.Y., 1833.
47. Beck, B., Brown, F., Fletcher, R., et al.: Indomethacin promotes healing of experimental esophagitis (Abstr.). Gastroenterology 74:1006, 1978.
48. Beck, J. C., Browne, J. S. L., Johnson, K. G., et al.: Occurrence of peritonitis during ACTH administration. Can. Med. Assoc. J. 62:423-426, 1950.
49. Becker, K. L., & Sutnick, A. I.: Paralytic ileus simulating acute intestinal obstruction due to pentolinium tartratre (Ansolysen). Ann. Intern. Med. 54:313-319, 1961.
50. Bendit, M.: Gangrene of the rectum as a complication of an enema. Br. Med. J. 1:664, 1945.
51. Benner, E. J., & Tellman, W. H.: Pseudomembranous colitis as a sequel to oral lincomycin. Am. J. Gastroenterol. 54:55-58, 1970.

52. Bennett, J. E.: Flucytosine. Ann. Intern. Med. 86:319-322, 1977.
53. Berardi, R. S., Siroospour, D., Ruiz, R., et al.: Alkaline Reflux Gastritis: a study in forty postoperative duodenal ulcer patients. Am. J. Surg. 132:552-557, 1976.
54. Berchtold, P., Bolli, P., Arbenz, V., & Keiser, G.: Disturbances in intestinal absorption following metformin treatment. Diabetologia 5:405-412, 1969.
55. Berkowitz, D., Bezahler, G., & Brandt, L. J.: Ampicillin-associated colitis. Am. J. Gastroenterol. 66:362-365, 1976.
56. Bernstein, W. C., Nivatvongs, S., & Tallent, M. B.: Colonic and rectal complications of kidney transplantation in man. Dis. Colon Rectum 16:255-263, 1973.
57. Bersack, S. R., How, J. S., & Rabson, A. S.: Inflammatory pseudopolyposis of the small and large intestines with the Peutz-Jeghers syndrome in a case of diffuse histoplasmosis. Am. J. Roentgenol. 80:73-78, 1958.
58. Berstock, D. A., Houghton, J., & Bennett, A.: Improved anticancer effect by combining cytotoxic drugs with an inhibitor of prostaglandin synthesis. Cancer Treat. Rev. 6:69-71, 1979.
59. Berthrong, M., & Fajardo, L. F.: Radiation injury in surgical pathology. Am. J. Surg. Pathol. 5:153-178, 1981.
60. Bianchi, A., Chipman, D. W., Dreskin, A., & Rosenweig, N. S.: Nutritional folic acid deficiency with megaloblastic changes in the small-bowel epithelium. N. Engl. J. Med. 282:859, 1970.
61. Bigard, M. A., Gaucher, P., & Lassalle, C.: Fatal colonscopic explosion during colonscopic polypectomy. Gastroenterology 77:1307-1310, 1979.
62. Billingham, M. E., Mason, J. W., Bristow, M. R., et al.: Anthracycline cardiomyopathy monitored by morphologic changes. Cancer Treat. Rep. 62:865-869, 1978.
63. Birns, M. T., Katon, R. M., & Keller, F.: Intramural hematoma of the small intestine presenting with major gastrointestinal hemorrhage. Gastroenterology 77:1094-1100, 1979.
64. Bischel, M. D., Reese, T., & Engel, J.: Spontaneous perforation of the colon in a hemodialysis patient. Am. J. Gastroenterol. 74:182-184, 1980.
65. Boal, D. K., Newburger, P. E., & Teele, R. L.: Esophagitis induced by combined radiation and adriamycin. Am. J. Roentgenol. 132:567-570, 1979.
66. Bock, Von J. U., & Schroeder, L.: Barium-pleuritis und mediastinitis nach iatrogener osophagus perforation. Zentralbl. Chirurg. 103:239-241, 1978.
67. Bockus, H. I., Willard, J. H., & Bank, J.: Melanosis coli: The etiologic significance of the anthracene laxatives: a report of 41 cases. J.A.M.A. 101:1, 1933.
68. Bode, J. CH.: Alcohol and the gastrointestinal tract. Adv Intern Med Pediatr 45:1-75, 1980.
69. Bogomoletz, W. V., Adnet, J. J., Pirembaut, P., et al.: Collagenous colitis: An unrecognized entity. Gut 21:164-168, 1980.
70. Bokey, L., & Hugh, T. B.: Oesophageal ulceration associated with doxycycline therapy. Med. J. Aust. 1:236, 1975.
71. Bolton, R. P.: Clostridium difficile-associated colitis after neomycin treated with metranidazole. Br. Med. J. 2:1479-1480, 1979.
72. Bolton, R. P., Sheriff, R. J., & Read, A. E.: Clostridium difficile associated colitis: a role in inflammatory bowel disease. Lancet 1:383-384, 1980.
73. Bommalaer, G., Larpent, J. L., Rumeau, J. L., & Ribet, A.: Pseudomembranous colitis and rifampicin. Lancet 2:1192, 1980.
74. Bonfils, S., Hervoir, P., Girodet, J., et al.: Acute spontaneously recovering ulcerating colitis (ARUC): report of 6 cases. Am. J. Digest. Dis. 22:429-436, 1977.
75. Bonkowsky, H. L., & Brisbane, J.: Colitis and hepatitis caused by methyldopa. J.A.M.A. 236:1602-1603, 1976.
76. Book, L. S., Herbst, J. J., Atherton, S. O., & Jung, A. L.: Necrotizing enterocolitis in low-birth-weight infants fed an elemental formula. J. Pediatr. 87:602-605, 1975.
77. Borger, H. W., Schafmeyer, A., Arnold, R., et al.: Der einfluss von kaffee und coffein auf den serumgastrinspiegel und die suresekretion beim menschen. Dtsch. Med. Wochenschr. 101:455-457, 1957.
78. Bowen, B. K., Krause, W. J., & Ivey, K. J.: Effect of sodium bicarbonate on aspirin-induced damage and potential difference changes in human gastric mucosa. Br. Med. J. 2:1052, 1977.
79. Bradley, E. L. III, & Goldman, M. L.: Gastric infarction after therapeutic embolization. Surgery 79:421-424, 1976.
80. Brause, B. D., Romankiewicz, J. A., Gotz,

V. et al.: Comparative study of diarrhea associated with clindamycin and ampicillin therapy. Am. J. Gastroenterol. 73:244-248, 1980.

81. Bremner, D. N., & Mooney, G.: Agenesis of appendix: a further thalidomide anomoly. Lancet 1:826, 1978.
82. Breslaw, L.: Melanosis of the duodenal mucosa. Gastrointest. Endoc. 26:45-46, 1980.
83. Brogden, R. N., Heel, R. C., Speight, T. M., et al.: Alclofenac: a review of its pharmacological properties and therapeutic efficacy in rheumatoid arthritis and allied rheumatic disorders. Drugs 14:241-259, 1977.
84. Brogden, R. N., Heel, R. C., Speight, T. M., & Avery, G. S.: Tolmetin: A review of its pharmacological properties and therapeutic efficacy in rheumatic diseases. Drugs 15:429-450, 1978.
85. Brogden, R. N., Heel, R. C., Speight, T. M., & Avery, G. S.: Sulindac: A review of its pharmacologic properties and therapeutic efficacy in rheumatic disease. Drugs 16:97-114, 1978.
86. Brogden, R. N., Heel, R. C., & Speight, T. M.: Cimetidine: a review of its pharmacological properties and therapeutic efficacy in peptic ulcer disease. Drugs 15:93-131, 1978.
87. Brouwers, J. R. B. J., & Schneider, H. S.: Bijwerkingen van eenmaal een hoge dosis laxeermiddel. Ned. Tijdschr. Geneeskd. 122:1098, 1978.
88. Brown, J. W.: Toxic megacolon associated with loperamide therapy. J.A.M.A. 241:501-502, 1979.
89. Brown, P. A., Sawrey, J. M., & Vernikos, J.: Aspirin- and indomethadin-induced ulcers and their antagonism by antihistamines. Eur. J. Pharmacol. 51:275-283, 1978.
90. Brozinsky, S., Fani, K., Grosberg, S. J., & Wapnick, S.: Alcohol ingestion-induced changes in the human rectal mucosa: Light and electron microscopic studies. Dis. Colon Rectum 21:329-335, 1978.
91. Bubrick, M. P., Lundeen, J. W., Onstad, G. R., et al.: Mallory-Weiss syndrome: Analysis of fifty-one cases. Surgery 88:400-405, 1980.
92. Burkitt, E. A., & Sutcliffe, C. K.: Paralytic ileus after amitriptyline ("Tryptizol") Br. Med. J. 2:1648-1649, 1961.
93. Buss, D. H., & Scharyj, M.: Herpesvirus infection of the esophagus and other visceral organs in adults. Am. J. Med. 66:457-462, 1979.
94. Butterfield, W. C.: Surgical complications of narcotic addiction. Surg. Gynecol. Obstet. 134:237, 1972.
95. Caldwell, J. L., & Thompson, C. T.: Intestinal hemorrhagic necrosis as a complication of digitalis intoxication. J. Okla. State Med. Assoc. 61:647, 1968.
96. Cameron, A., & Thomas, M.: Pseudomembranous colitis and co-trimoxazole. Br. Med. J. 1:1321, 1977.
97. Cantu, R. C., Prieto, A.: Evaluation of the increased risk of gastrointestinal bleeding following intracranial surgery in patients receiving high steroid dosages in the immediate postoperative period. Int. Surg. 49:325, 1968.
98. Capron, J-P., Dupas, J-P., & Lorriaux, A.: Duodenogastric reflux of bile and aspirin-induced damage in man. Lancet 1:601-602, 1977.
99. Carlson, D., Garber, E., Weinstein, W., et al.: Drug-associated gastroduodenal lesions in rheumatoid arthritis: An endoscopic and histologic study. Gastroenterology 78:1147, 1980.
100. Carmichael, H. A., Nelson, L. M., & Russell, R. I.: Cimetidine and prostaglandin: Evidence for different modes of action on the rat gastric mucosa. Gastroenterology 74:1229-1232, 1978.
101. Carne-Ross, I. P.: Pyloric stenosis and sustained-release iron tablets. Br. Med. J. 2:642-643, 1976.
102. Caruso, I., & Porro, G. B.: Gastroscopic evaluation of anti-inflammatory agents. Br. Med. J. 1:75-78, 1980.
103. Caspary, W. F.: Einfluf von aspirin, antacida, alkohol und gallensauren auf die transmurale elektrische potentialdifferenz des menschlichen magens. Dtsch. Med. Wochenschr. 100:1263, 1975.
104. Cello, J. P., Fogel, R. P., & Boland, C. R.: Liquid caustic ingestion: spectrum of injury. Arch. Intern. Med. 140:501-504, 1980.
105. Chang, T. W., Gorbach, S. L., Bartlett, J. G., & Saginur, R.: Bacitracin treatment of antibiotic-associated colitis and diarrhea caused by Clostridium difficile toxin. Gastroenterology 78:1584-1586, 1980.
106. Chapman, B. L., & Duggan, J. M.: Aspirin

and uncomplicated peptic ulcer. Gut 10:443-450, 1969.

107. Cheli, R., Giacosa, A., Marenco, G., et al.: Chronic gastritis frequency in alcohol drinkers. I.N.S.E.R.M. 95:373-376, 1980.
108. Chernish, S. M., Rosenak, B. D., Brunelle, R. L., & Crabtree, R.: Comparison of gastrointestinal effects of aspirin and fenoprofen. A double blind crossover study. Arthritis Rheum. 22:376-383, 1979.
109. Christie, D. L., & Ament, M. E.: Ampicillin-associated colitis. J. Pediatr. 87:657-658, 1975.
110. Clain, J., Novis, B. H., Bank, S., et al.: Cathartic colon with unusual histologic features. S. Afr. Med. J. 48:216-218, 1974.
111. Cochran, K. M., Mackenzie, J. F., & Russell, R. I.: Role of taurocholic acid in production of gastric mucosal damage after aspirin. Br. Med. J. 1:183-185, 1975.
112. Cohen, A.: Intestinal blood loss after a new anti-inflammatory drug, sulindac. Clin. Pharmacol. Ther. 20:238-240, 1976.
113. Cohen, I. E., McNeill, C. J., & Wells, R. F.: Clindamycin-associated colitis. J.A.M.A. 223:1379-1380, 1973.
114. Cohen, M. I., Winslow, P. R., & Boley, S. J.: Intestinal obstruction associated with cholestyramine therapy. N. Engl. J. Med. 280:1285-1286, 1969.
115. Cohen, M. M., Cheung, G., & Lyster, D. M.: Prevention of aspirin-induced faecal blood loss by prostaglandin E_2. Gut 21:602-606, 1980.
116. Cohen, S.: Pathogenesis of coffee-induced gastrointestinal symptoms. N. Engl. J. Med. 303:122-124, 1980.
117. Collins, F. J., Matthews, H. R., Baker, S. E., et al.: Drug-induced oesophageal injury. Br. Med. J. 1:1673-1676, 1979.
118. Condon, R. E., & Anderson, M. J.: Diarrhea and colitis in clindamycin-treated surgical patients. Arch. Surg. 113:794-797, 1978.
119. Conn, H. O., Ramsby, G. R., & Storer, E. H.: Selective intra-arterial vasopressin in the treatment of upper gastrointestinal hemorrhage. Gastroenterology 63:4, 1972.
120. Conn, H. O., & Blitzer, B. L.: Non-association of adrenocorticosteroid therapy and peptic ulcer. N. Engl. J. Med. 292:473, 1976.
121. Conrad, M. E., & Crosby, W. H.: Massive nitrogen mustard therapy in Hodgkin's disease with protection of the marrow by tourniquets. Blood 16:1089-1103, 1960.
122. Conti, P., & Continjenza, A.: Decreased ulcerogenic effect of indomethacin in the rat when given in association with diflunisal. J. Pathol. 131:357-361, 1980.
123. Cook, A. I. M., & Foy, P.: Sclerosing peritonitis and practolol therapy. Ann. R. Coll. Surg. Engl. 58:473-475, 1976.
124. Cooke, A. R.: Drug damage to the gastroduodenum. In: Sleisinger, M. H., & Fordtran, J. S., Eds. Gastrointestinal Disease 2nd ed., p. 813. W. B. Saunders, Philadelphia, 1978.
125. Cooke, A. R.: The role of the mucosal barrier in drug-induced gastric ulceration and erosions. Digest. Dis. 21:155-164, 1976.
126. Corkery, J. J., Dubowitz, V., Lister, J., & Moosa, A.: Colonic perforation after exchange transfusion. Br. Med. J. 2:345-349, 1968.
127. Coughlin, G. P., Willing, R. L., & Hamilton, D. W.: Gastro-colic fistula complicating benign gastric ulcer in analgesic abusers. Aust. N.Z.J. Med. 9:314-315, 1979.
128. Coutrot, S., Roland, D., Barbier, J., et al.: Acute perforation of colonic diverticula associated with short-term indomethacin. Lancet 2:1054-1055, 1978.
129. Cowan, R. E., Wright, J. T., & Marsh, F.: Drug-induced oesophageal injury. Br. Med. J. 2:132-133, 1979.
130. Cowen, M. L., & Humphries, T. J.: Pseudomelanosis of the duodenum. Gastrointest. Endosc. 26:107-108, 1980.
131. Craft, A. W., Kay, H. E. M., Lawson, D. M., et al.: Methotrexate-induced malabsorption in children with acute lymphoblastic leukemia. Br. Med. J. 4:1511-1512, 1977.
132. Croft, D. N., & Wood, P. H. N.: Gastric mucosa and susceptibility to occult gastrointestinal bleeding caused by aspirin. Br. Med. J. 1:137-141, 1967.
133. Crowson, T. D., Head, L. H., & Ferrante, W. A.: Esophageal ulcers associated with tetracycline therapy. J.A.M.A. 235:2747-2748, 1976.
134. Center for ulcer research and education (CURE): Is duodenal ulcer recurrence more common after cimetidine treatment? Gastroenterology 78:1152, 1980.
135. Czyzyk, A., Tawecki, J., Sadowski, J., et al.: Effect of biguanides on intestinal absorption of glucose. Diabetes 17:492-498, 1968.

136. Dafoe, C. S., & Ross, C. A.: Acute corrosive oesophagitis. Thorax 24:291-294, 1969.
137. Dagradi, A. E., Lee, E. R., Brosco, D. L., et al.: The clinical spectrum of hemorrhagic erosive gastritis. Am. J. Gastroenterol. 60:30, 1973.
138. Davenport, H. W.: Salicylate damage to the gastric mucosal barrier. N. Engl. J. Med. 276:1307-1312, 1967.
139. Davies, D. R., & Brightmore, T.: Idiopathic and drug-induced ulceration of the small intestine. Br. J. Surg. 57:134-139, 1970.
140. Davis, J. D., Struth, A. G., Turner, R. A., et al.: Pirprofen and aspirin in the treatment of rheumatoid arthritis. Clin. Pharmacol. Ther. 25:618, 1979.
141. Davis, J. S.: Severe colitis following lincomycin and clindamycin therapy. Am. J. Gastroenterol. 62:16-23, 1974.
142. Davis, J. T., & Nusbaum, M.: Chlorpromazine therapy and functional large bowel obstruction. Am. J. Gastroenterol. 60:635-639, 1973.
143. Davis, L. L., Raffensperger, J., & Novak, G. M.: Necrosis of the stomach secondary to ingestion of corrosive agents: Report of three cases requiring total gastrectomy. Chest 62:48-51, 1972.
144. Dearing, W. H., Bagenstoss, A. H., & Weed, L. A.: Studies on the relationship of *Staphylococcus aureus* to pseudomembraneous enteritis and post antibiotic enteritis. Gastroenterology 38:441-451, 1960.
145. Debray, C., Hardouin, J-P., Laumonier, R., et al.: La gastrite ethylique sous le controle de la gastrobiopsie. Arch. Mal. Appar. Dig. 55:925-935, 1957.
146. DeCarlo, J.: Complications associated with diagnostic barium enema. Surgery 47:965, 1960.
147. Decaux, G. M., & Devroede, C.: Acute colitis related to spiromycin. Lancet 2:993, 1978.
148. Dehart, O. W.: Barium appendicitis. Report of a case. J. Okla. State Med. Assoc. 63:570, 1970.
149. Deitel, M., & Vasic, V.: Major intestinal complications of radiotherapy. Am. J. Gastroenterol. 72:65-70, 1979.
150. Delaney, J. P., Michel, H. M., Bonsack, M. E., et al.: Adrenal corticosteroids cause gastrin cell hyperplasia. Gastroenterology 76:913-916, 1979.
151. Deller, D. J., Murrell, T. G. C., & Blowes, R.: Jejunal biopsy in malignant disease. Australas. Ann. Med. 16:236-241, 1967.
152. Del Pozo, E., & Maclay, W. P.: Gastrointestinal bleeding in patients on bromocriptine. Lancet 2:906, 1976.
153. Desai, H. G., Venugopalan, M., Philipose, M. P., et al.: Effect of red chili powder on gastric mucosal barrier and acid secretion. Indian J. Med. Res. 66:440-448, 1977.
154. Dewar, G. J., Lim, C. N. H., Michalyshyn, B., & Akabutu, J.: Gastrointestinal complications of acute and chronic leukemia. Can. J. Surg. 24:67-71, 1981.
155. DiCostanzo, J., Noirclerc, M., Jouglard, J., et al.: New therapeutic approach to corrosive burns of the upper gastrointestinal tract. Gut 21:370-375, 1980.
156. Dietz, M. W.: Ileocecal histoplasmosis. Radiology 91:285-289, 1968.
157. Dinoso, V. P., Meshkinpour, H., & Lorber, S. H.: Studies on the acute effects of ethanol on the gastric mucosa in man. Gastroenterology 62:843, 1972.
158. Dinoso, V. P., Chey, W. J., Braverman, S., et al.: Gastric secretion and gastric mucosal morphology in chronic alcoholics. Arch. Intern. Med. 130:715, 1972.
159. Dinoso, V. P., Chuang, J., & Murthy, S. N. S.: Changes in the mucosal and venous histamine concentrations during installation of ethanol in the canine stomach. Am. J. Digest. Dis. 21:93, 1976.
160. Dobbins, W. O., Herrero, B. A., & Mansbach, C. M.: Morphologic alterations associated with neomycin induced malabsorption. Am. J. Med. Sci. 255:63-77, 1968.
161. Doherty, C. C., McGeown, M. G., & Donaldson, R. A.: Retroperitoneal fibrosis after treatment with atenolol. Br. Med. J. 2:1786, 1978.
162. Doll, R., Jones, F. A., & Pygott, F.: Effect of smoking on the production and maintenance of gastric and duodenal ulcers. Lancet 1:657-662, 1958.
163. Domschke, W., Domschke, S., Hornig, D., & Demling, L.: Prostaglandin-stimulated gastric mucus secretion in man. Acta Hepatogastroenterol. (Stuttg.) 25:292-294, 1978.
164. Dosik, G. M., Luna, M., & Valdivieso, M., et al.: Necrotizing colitis in patients with cancer. Am. J. Med. 67:646-656, 1979.
165. Douthwaite, A. H., & Lintott, G. A. M.: Gas-

troscopic observation of the effect of aspirin and certain other substances on the stomach. Lancet 2:1222-1225, 1938.

166. Durward, Q. J., Cohen, M. M., & Naiman, S. C.: Intramural hematoma of the gastric cardia. Am. J. Gastroenterol. 71:301–305, 1979.
167. Eastham, E. J., & Walker, W. A.: Adverse effects of milk formula ingestion on the gastrointestinal tract. Gastroenterology 76:365-374, 1979.
168. Eastwood, G. L., & Erdmann, K. R.: Effects of ethanol on canine gastric epithelial ultrastructure and transmucosal potential difference. Am. J. Digest. Dis. 23:429, 1978.
169. Efrusy, M. E., & Dobbins, W. O.: Persistent enterocutaneous fistula associated with intraperitoneal metallic mercury. Am. J. Digest. Dis. 19:373-377, 1974.
170. Ehrlich, G. E., & Roth, S.: Rheumatoid arthritis: long-term therapy with tolmetin sodium. Orthop. Dis. 4:16-24, 1976.
171. Eiseman, B., Seelig, M. G., & Womack, N. A.: Talcum powder granuloma: a frequent and serious postoperative complication. Ann. Surg. 126:820-832, 1947.
172. Eiseman, B., Lam, R. C., & Rush, B.: Surgery on the narcotic addict. Ann. Surg. 159:748, 1964.
173. Elder, J. B., Ganguli, P. C., & Gillespie, I. E.: Cimetidine and gastric cancer. Lancet 1:1005-6, 1979.
174. Elliot, J. S., & Rosenberg, M. L.: Ureteral occlusion by barium granuloma. J. Urol. 71:692, 1954.
175. Ellis, D. J., Hamer, J. D., & Baker, S. E.: Perforation of chronic duodenal ulcer during treatment with cimetidine. Br. Med. J. 2:1538, 1977.
176. Eras, P., Goldstein, M. J., & Sherlock, P.: Candida infection of the gastrointestinal tract. Medicine 51:367-379, 1972.
177. Erdman, L. H., Boggs, H. W., Slagle, G. W.: Electrical ileal perforation: An unusual complication of colonoscopy. Dis. Colon Rectum 22:501-502, 1979.
178. Evans, D. L., Rogers, J. F., & Peiper, S. C.: Intestinal dilatation associated with phenothiazine therapy: a case report and literature review. Am. J. Psychiatry 136:970-972, 1979.
179. Evans, K. T., & Roberts, G. M.: Where do all the tablets go. Lancet 4:1237-1239, 1976.
180. Fajardo, L. F., & Berthrong, M.: Radiation injury in surgical pathology. Part III. Salivary glands, pancreas and skin. Am. J. Surg. Pathol. 5:279-296, 1980.
181. Fam, A. G., Paton, T. W., Shamess, C. J., & Lewis, A. J.: Fulminant colitis complicating gold therapy. J. Rheumatol. 7:479-485, 1980.
182. Famaey, J. P.: Recent developments about non-steroidal anti-inflammatory drugs and their mode of action. Gen. Pharmacol. 9:155-62, 1978.
183. Fang, W. F., Broughton, A., Jacobson, E. D.: Indomethacin-induced intestinal inflammation. Digest. Dis. 22:749-760, 1977.
184. Fatti, L., Marchand, P., & Crawshaw, G. R.: The treatment of caustic strictures of the esophagus. Surg. Gynecol. Obstet. 102:195, 1956.
185. Faulk, D. L., Anuras, S., & Christensen, J.: Chronic intestinal pseudoobstruction. Gastroenterology 74:922-931, 1978.
186. Fedeli, G., Anti, M., & Rapaccini, G. L.: Erosive duodenitis during cimetidine treatment. Br. Med. J. 1:853, 1978.
187. Fee, H. J., Ament, M. E., & Holmes, E. C.: Pseudomembranous colitis associated with Cephazolin therapy. Am. J. Surg. 133:247-248, 1977.
188. Fein, B. T.: Perforation and inflammation of diverticula of the colon secondary to long-term adrenocorticosteroid therapy for bronchial asthma and pulmonary emphysema. South. Med. J. 54:355-359, 1961.
189. Fekety, F. R.: Gastrointestinal complications of antibiotics. J.A.M.A. 202:144, 1968.
190. Ferrer, M. I., Bradley, S. E., Wheeler, H. O., et al.: The effect of digoxin in the splanchnic circulation in ventricular failure. Circulation 32:524, 1965.
191. Ferreira, S. H., & Vane, J. R.: New aspects of the mode of action of non-steroid anti-inflammatory drugs. Annu. Rev. Pharmacol. 14:57-73, 1974.
192. Fetterman, L. E.: Colonic fecal impaction in a young drug addict. J.A.M.A. 202:1056, 1967.
193. Filpi, R. G., Majd M., & LoPresto, J. M.: Reversible gastric stricture following iron ingestion. South. Med. J. 66 845-846, 1973.
194. Fishbein, P. G., Tuthill, R., Kressel, H., et al.: Herpes simplex esophagitis. A cause of upper-gastrointestinal bleeding. Am. J. Digest. Dis. 24:540-544, 1979.

195. Fisher, J. R., & Sanowski, R. A.: Disseminated histoplasmosis producing hypertrophic gastric folds. Digest. Dis. 23:282-285, 1978.
196. Fontaine, J. L., & Navarro, J.: Small intestine biopsy in cow's milk protein allergy in infancy. Arch. Dis. Child. 50: 357-362, 1975.
197. Force, T., MacDonald, D., Eade, O. E., et al.: Ischemic gastritis and duodenitis. Dig. Dis. Sci. 25:307-310, 1980.
198. Ford-Hutchinson, A. W., Walker, J. R., Connor, N. S., et al.: Separate anti-inflammatory effects of indomethacin, fluribiprofen and benoxaprofen. J. Pharm. Pharmacol. 29:372-373, 1977.
199. Foroozan, P., & Trier, J. S.: Mucosa of the small intestine in pernicious anemia. N. Engl. J. Med. 277:553-559, 1967.
200. Forshaw, J., Moorhouse, E. H., & Harwood, L.: Megaloblastic anemia due to dietary deficiency. Lancet 1:1004, 1964.
201. Fossatti, P., Caridroit, M., Pruvot, P., et al.: Action de la reserpine dans les comas post-traumatiques en neurologie. Presse Med. 73:2413, 1965.
202. Fournier, G., Orgiazzi, J., Lenoir, B., & Dechavenne, M.: Pseudomembranous colitis probably due to rifampicin. Lancet 1:101, 1980.
203. Fox, J. E., McElligott, T. F., & Beck, I. T.: Effect of ethanol on the morphology of hamster jejunum. Digest. Dis. 23:201-209, 1978.
204. Franzin, G., Novelli, P., & Fratton, A.: Histologic evidence of cytomegalovirus in the duodenal and gastric mucosa of patients with renal allograft. Endoscopy 12:117-120, 1980.
205. Freis, E. D., Partenope, E. A., Lilienfield, L. S., et al.: A clinical appraisal of pentapyrrolidinium (M&B 2050) in hypertensive patients. Circulation 9:540-546, 1954.
206. Friedman, G. D., Siegelaub, A. B., & Seltzer, C. C.: Cigarettes, alcohol, coffee and peptic ulcer. N. Engl. J. Med. 290:469-473, 1974.
207. Friedman, R. J., Mayer, I. E., Galambos, J. T., & Hersh, T.: Oxacillin-induced pseudomembranous colitis. Am J. Gastroenterol. 73:445-447, 1980.
208. Fuhro, R., & Fromm, D.: Effects of compounds chemically related to salicylate on isolated antral mucosa of rabbits. Gastroenterology 75:661-667, 1978.
209. Fung, W. P., & Karim, S. M. M.: Effect of 15 (R) methyl-prostaglandins E_2 on the healing of gastric ulcers. A double-blind endoscopic study. Med. J. Aust. 2:127-128, 1976.
210. Gallitano, A. L., Kondi, E. S., Phillips, E., et al.: Near-fatal hemorrhage following gastrograffin studies. Radiology 118:35-36, 1976.
211. Gander, D. R. & Devlin, H. B.: Ileus after amitriptyline. Br. Med. J. 1:1160, 1963.
212. Ganju, S., Adomavicius, J., Salgia, K., & Steigmann, F.: The endoscopic picture of melanosis in the duodenum. Gastrointest. Endosc. 26:44-45, 1980.
213. Garb, A. E., Soule, E. H., Bartholomew, L. G., & Cain, J. C.: Steroid-induced gastric ulcer. Arch. Intern. Med. 116:899, 1965.
214. Gardiner, G. A., & Bird, C. R.: Nonspecific ulcers of the colon resembling annular carcinoma. Radiology 137:331-334, 1980.
215. Gartner, A. H.: Aspirin-induced gastritis and gastrointestinal bleeding. J. Am. Dent. Assoc. 93:111-117, 1976.
216. Geall, M. G., Phillips, S. F., & Summerskill, W. H. J.: Profile of gastric potential difference in man. Effects of aspirin, alcohol, bile and endogenous acid. Gastroenterology 58:437, 1970.
217. Gekas, P., & Schuster, M. M.: Stercoral perforation of the colon: case report and review of the literature. Gastroenterology 80:1054-1058, 1981.
218. Gelfand, E. T., Fisk, R. L., & Callaghan, J. C.: Accidental pneumatic rupture of the esophagus. J. Thorac. Cardiovasc. Surg. 74:142-144, 1977.
219. George, R. H., Symonds, J. M., Dimock, F., et al.: Identification of *Cl. difficile* as a cause of pseudomembranous colitis. Br. Med. J. 1:695, 1978.
220. George, W. L., Volpicelli, N. A., & Stiner, D. B.: Relapse of pseudomembranous colitis after vancomycin therapy. N. Engl. J. Med. 301:414-415, 1979.
221. George, W. L., Rolfe, R. D., & Finegold, S. M.: Treatment and prevention of antimicrobial agent-induced colitis and diarrhea. Gastroenterology 79:366-372, 1980.
222. Ghadially, F. N., & Parry, E. W.: An electron-microscopic and histochemical study of melanosis coli. J. Pathol. Bacteriol. 92:213, 1966.
223. Ghidoni, J. J., & Campbell, M. M.: Karyolytic bodies: Giant lysozomes in the jejunum of proton-irradiated rhesus monkeys. Arch. Pathol. 88:480-488, 1969.

224. Gibbons, R. B.: Complications of chrysotherapy. A review of recent studies. Arch. Intern. Med. 139:343, 1979.
225. Gibinsky, K., Rybicka, J., Mikos, E., & Nowak, A.: Double-blind clinical trial on gastroduodenal ulcer healing with prostaglandin E_2 analogues. Gut 18:636-639, 1977.
226. Gibson, D. S.: A case of intestinal obstruction following the administration of pentapyrrolidinium bitartrate ("Ansolysen") Med. J. Aust. 2:860-861, 1957.
227. Giepel, A.: Todlicher zwischenfall nach kontrastmitteleinlauf des mastdarmes Dtsch. Z. Ges. gerichtl. Med. 59:225, 1967.
228. Gifford, R. W., Allen, E. V., & Birkhead, N. C.: Pentapyrrolidinium bitartrate (M&B2050A) in the treatment of hypertension: preliminary observations. Mayo Clin. Proc. 29:496-508, 1954.
229. Giger, M., Sonnenberg, A., Brandli, H., et al.: Das tetracyclin-ulkus der speiserohre. Dtsch. Med. Wochenschr. 103:1038-1040, 1978.
230. Gill, M. J., Saunders, J. B.: Perforation of chronic peptic ulcers after cimetidine. Br. Med. J. 2:1149, 1977.
231. Gill, P. G., & Piris, J.: Proctitis caused by cornstarch glove powder: Report of a case. Dis. Colon Rectum 21:207-208, 1971.
232. Gillespie, P., Riley, J., & Hunt, J.: Perforation of duodenal ulcer during barium meal. Australas. Radiol. 21:241, 1977.
233. Gleich, G. J., Mongan, E. S., & Vaules, D. W.: Esophageal stricture following chloral hydrate poisoning. J.A.M.A. 201:266-267, 1967.
234. Glenn, W., Wilson, S., & Long, W. B.: Surgical complications of adrenal steroid therapy. Ann. Surg. 165:1023-1032, 1967.
235. Gobel, D.: Die chronisch-atrophische gastritis aus klinischer sicht. Med. Klin. 72:1246, 1977.
236. Goldberg, H. I., & Moss, A. A.: Roentgenographic methods of colonic examination. p. 1574. In: Sleisinger, M. H., Fordtran, J. S., Eds. Gastrointestinal Disease. W. B. Saunders, Philadelphia, 1978.
237. Goodman, M. J.: Gastric ulceration induced by spironolactone. Lancet 1:752, 1977.
238. Goodman, Z. D., Boitnott, J. K., & Yardley, J. H.: Perforation of the colon associated with cytomegalovirus infection. Am. J. Digest. Dis. 24:376-380, 1979.
239. Gottfried, E. B., Korsten, M. A., & Leiber, C. S.: Alcohol-induced gastric and duodenal lesions in man. Am. J. Gastroenterol. 70:587–592, 1978.
240. Goulston, S. J. M., & McGovern, V. J.: Pseudomembranous colitis. Gut 6:207–212, 1965.
241. Goulston, S. J. M., & McGovern, V. J.: Clinical settings in pseudomembranous colitis. Aust. N.Z. J. Med. 10:139–145, 1980.
242. Graham, C. F., Gallagher, K., & Jones, J. K.: Acute colitis with methyldopa. N. Engl. J. Med. 304:1044–1046, 1981.
243. Graham-Stewart, C. W.: Injection treatment of haemorrhoids. Br. Med. J. 1:213, 1962.
244. Granger, D. N., Richardson P. D. I., Kvietys, P. R., & Mortillaro, N. A.: Intestinal blood flow. Gastroenterology 78:837–863, 1980.
245. Greaney, M. G., & Jackson, P. R.: Oleogranuloma of the rectum produced by Lasonil ointment. Lancet 2: 997, 1977.
246. Greco, F. A., Brereton, H. D., Kent, H., et al.: Adriamycin and enhanced radiation reaction in normal esophagus and skin. Ann. Intern. Med 85:294–298, 1976.
247. Green, S. B., Gail, M. H., & Byar, D. P.: Steroids and peptic ulcer. N. Engl. J. Med. 294:1291,1976.
248. Greenberger, N., Arvanitakas, A., & Hurwitz, A.: The esophagus. In: Drug Treatment of Gastrointestinal Disorders. p. 91. London, Churchill Livingstone, 1978.
249. Greene, F. L., Ariyan, S., & Stansel, H. C. Jr.: Mesenteric and peripheral vascular ischemia secondary to ergotism. Surgery 81:176-179, 1977.
250. Greenfield, C., Burroughs, A., Szawathowski, M., et al.: Is pseudomembranous colitis infectious? Lancet 1:371-372, 1981.
251. Greenwald, R. A., Rheingold, O. J., Chiprut, R. O., et al.: Local gangrene: A complication of peripheral pitressin therapy for bleeding esophageal varices. Gastroenterology 74:744-746, 1978.
252. Grimson, K. S.: Drugs recently introduced for hypertension. J.A.M.A. 158:359-367, 1955.
253. Groll, A., Vlassambrouk, M. J., Ramchand, S., et al.: Fulminating noninfective pseudomembranous colitis. Gastroenterology 58:88, 1970.
254. Grossman, M. I.: Protection of gastric mucosa

by prostaglandins. Gastroenterology 77:593-595, 1979.
255. Guice, K., Rattazzi, L. C., & Marchioro, T. L.: Colon perforation in renal transplant patients. Am. J. Surg. 138:43-48, 1979.
256. Gurwith, M. J., Rabin, H. R., Love, K., et al.: Diarrhea associated with clindamycin and ampicillin therapy: Preliminary results of a cooperative study. J. Infect. Dis. 135 (Suppl.): S104-S110, 1977.
257. Hahn, K.-J., Krischkofski, D., Weber, E., & Morgenstern, E.: Morphology of gastrointestinal effects of aspirin. Clin. Pharmacol. Ther. 17:330-338, 1975.
258. Hamilton, S. R., & Yardley, J. H.: Endoscopic biopsy diagnosis of aspirin-associated chronic gastric ulcers (Abstr.). Gastroenterology 78:1178, 1980.
259. Hanelin, L. G., & Moss, A. A.: Roentgenographic features of mushroom (Amanita) poisoning. Am. J. Roentgenol. 125:782-787, 1975.
260. Hansky, J., Stern, A. I., Korman, M. G., et al.: Effects of long-term cimetidine on serum gastrin in duodenal ulcer. Dig. Dis. Sci. 24:468-470, 1979.
261. Harder, E. J., & Hermans, P. E.: Treatment of fungal infections with flucytosine. Ann. Intern. Med. 135:231-237, 1975.
262. Hart, F. D.: Naproxen (Naprosyn) and gastrointestinal haemorrhage. Br. Med. J. 2:51-2, 1974.
263. Hartong, W. A., Arvanitakis, C., Skibba, R. M., et al.: Treatment of toxic megacolon. Am. J. Digest. Dis. 22:195-200, 1977.
264. Harty, R. F.: Sclerosing peritonitis and propranolol (Letter). Arch. Intern. Med. 138:1424, 1978.
265. Hawkins, C. F., Ellis, H. A., & Rawson, A.: Malignant gout with tophaceous small intestine and megaloblastic anemia. Ann. Rheum. Dis. 24:224-233, 1965.
266. Heckmann, G., Gura, C., & Voigt, G.: Fibrinolyse akuter und chronischer Verschlusse tiefer Venen. Intensivmed 13:56, 1976.
267. Heilman, K. L.: Reversible morphological changes of rectal mucosa in vitamin B_{12} deficiency. Pathol. Res. Pract. 163:261-266, 1978.
268. Hemstreet, M. P. B., Reynolds, D. W., & Meadows, J.: Oesophagitis—A complication of inhaled steroid therapy. Clin. Allergy 10:733-738, 1980.
269. Henson, D.: Cytomegalovirus inclusion bodies in the gastrointestinal tract. Arch. Pathol. 93:477-482, 1972.
270. Herbert, D. C.: Anticoagulant therapy and the acute abdomen. Br. J. Surg. 55:353-357, 1968.
271. Hermos, J. A., Adams, W. H., Liv, Y. K., et al.: Mucosa of the small intestine in folate-deficient alcoholics. Ann. Intern. Med. 76:957, 1972.
272. Hernandez, V., Hernandez, I. A., & Berthrong, M.: Oleogranuloma simulating carcinoma of the rectum. Dis. Colon Rectum 10:205, 1967.
273. Herrington, J. L.: Barium granuloma within the peritoneal cavity: ureteral obstruction 7 years after barium enema and colonic perforation. Ann. Surg. 164:162, 1966.
274. Hewer, T., Rose, E., & Ghadirian, P.: Ingested mutagens from opium and tobacco pyrolysis products and cancer of the oesophagus. Lancet 2:494-496, 1978.
275. Hewer, T. F.: Opium and oesophageal cancer in Iran. Lancet 1:45, 1979.
276. Hickling, P., & Fuller, J.: Penicillamine causing acute colitis. Br. Med. J. 2:307, 1979.
277. Hicks, E. S.: Observations regarding enemas. Can. Med. Assoc. J. 51:358, 1944.
278. Hirschowitz, B. I., Streeten, D. H. P., Pollard, H. M., & Boldt, H. A.: Role of gastric secretions in inactivation of peptic ulcer by corticotrophin (ACTH). J.A.M.A.: 158:27-32, 1955.
279. Hobson, R. W., Jervis, H. R., Kingry, R. L., et al.: Small bowel changes associated with vincristine sulfate treatment: an experimental study in the guinea pig. Cancer 34:1888-1896, 1974.
280. Hoftiezer, J. W., O'Laughlin, J. C., & Ivey, K. J.: Comparison of the acute effects of regular aspirin, bufferin, and acetaminophen on human gastroduodenal mucosa. Gastroenterology 78:1183, 1980.
281. Hoftiezer, J. W., Burks, M., Silvoso, G. R., & Ivey, K. J.: Comparison of the effects of regular and enteric-coated aspirin on gastroduodenal mucosa of man. Lancet 2:609-612, 1980.
282. Hojgaard, L., Arffmann, S., Jorgensen, M., & Krag, E.: Tea consumption: A cause of constipation? Br. Med. J. 282:864, 1981.
283. Hollister, L. E.: Hematemesis and malena

complicating treatment with raulwolfia alkaloids. Arch. Intern. Med. 99:218-221, 1957.

284. Hoover, R., & Fraumeni, J. F.: Drug-induced cancer. Cancer 47:1071-1080, 1981.
285. Hoste, P., Ingels, J., Elewaut, A., & Barbier, F.: Duodenal perforation after cimetidine. Lancet 1:666, 1978.
286. Howard, F. M., Flynn, D. M., Bradley, J. M., et al.: Outbreak of necrotising enterocolitis caused by Clostridium butyricum. Lancet 2:1099-1102, 1977.
287. Howard, J. M., Sullivan, S. N., & Troster, M.: Spontaneous pseudomembranous colitis. Br. Med. J. 2:356, 1980.
288. Hoyle, M., Kennedy, A., Prior, A. L., et al.: Small bowel ischaemia and infarction in young women taking oral contraceptives and progestational agents. Br. J. Surg. 64:533-537, 1977.
289. Hugon, J., & Borgers, M.: Ultrastructural and cytochemical studies on karyolytic bodies in the epithelium of the duodenal crypts of whole body X-irradiated mice. Lab. Invest. 15:1528-1543, 1966.
290. Hussar, A. E., & Bruno, E.: Acute duodenal ulcer associated with reserpine therapy. Gastroenterology 31:500-504, 1956.
291. Huston, G. J.: Gold colitis, therapy and confirmation of mucosal recovery by measurement of mucosal potential difference. Postgrad. Med. J. 56:875-876, 1980.
292. Hutcheon, D. F., Milligan, F. D., Yardley, J. H., & Hendrix, T. R.: Cephalosporin-associated pseudomembranous colitis. Digest. Dis. 23:321-326, 1978.
293. Hyson, E. A., Burrell, M., & Toffler, R.: Drug-induced gastrointestinal disease. Gastrointest. Radiology. 2:183-212, 1977.
294. Ingoldby, C. J. H.: Perforated jejunal diverticulum due to local iron toxicity. Br. Med. J. 1:949-950, 1977.
295. Isaacs, I., Nissen, R., & Epstein, B. S.: Liver abscess resulting from barium enema in a case of chronic ulcerative colitis. N.Y. State J. Med. 50:332, 1950.
296. Ismail-Beigi, F., Horton, P. F., & Pope, C. E.: Histological consequences of gastroesophageal reflux in man. Gastroenterology 58:163, 1970.
297. Ivey, K. J., Baskin, W. N., Krause, W. J., & Terry, B.: Effects of aspirin and acid on human jejunal mucosa. Gastroenterol. 76:50-56, 1979.
298. Ivey, K. J., Paone, D. B., & Krause, W. J.: Acute effect of systemic aspirin on gastric mucosa in man. Digest. Dis. Sci. 25:97-99, 1980.
299. Jacobs, E., & Pringot, J.: Gastric ulcers due to intake of potassium chloride. Am. J. Digest. Dis. 18:289-294, 1973.
300. Jacobson, E. D., Prior, J. T., & Faloon, W. W.: Malabsorption syndrome induced by neomycin: morphologic alterations in the jejunal mucosa. J. Lab. Clin. Med. 56:245-250, 1960.
301. Janne, P., Carpentier, Y., & Willems, G.: Colonic mucosal atrophy induced by a liquid elemental diet in rats. Digest. Dis. 22:808-812, 1977.
302. Jarvis, L. R., & Whitehead, R.: Effect of nicotine on the morphology of the rat gastric mucosa. Gastroenterology 78:1488-1494, 1980.
303. Jick, H., & Porter, J.: Drug-induced gastrointestinal bleeding. Lancet 2:87-89, 1978.
304. Jick, H., & Porter, J.: Thrombophlebitis of the lower extremities and ABO blood type. Arch. Intern. Med. 138:1566-1567, 1978.
305. Jick, H.: Effects of aspirin and acetaminophen in gastrointestinal hemorrhage. Arch. Intern. Med. 141:316-321, 1981.
306. Johansson, C., Kollberg, B., Nordemar, R., et al.: Protective effect of prostaglandin E_2 in the gastrointestinal tract during indomethacin treatment of rheumatic diseases. Gastroenterology 78:479-483, 1980.
307. Johnson, L. P., Girma, B., Zenabe, H. L., et al.: The effect of red pepper on gastric secretion in Ethiopia. Ethiop. Med. J. 16:111-113, 1978.
308. Juncosa, L.: Ulcus peptico yatrogeno del esofago. Rev. Esp. Enferm. Apar. Dig. 30:457-458, 1970.
309. Kalk, W. J., Vinik, A. I., Bank, S., et al.: Plasma gastrin responses to arginine in chronic pancreatitis. Diabetes 23:264-267, 1974.
310. Kammerer, W. H., Freiberger, R. H., Rivelis, A. L.: Peptic ulcer in rheumatoid patients on corticosteroid therapy: a clinical experimental and radiologic study. Arthritis Rheum. 1:122-141, 1958.
311. Kang, J. Y., & Foe, W. F.: Unprocessed bran causing intestinal obstruction. Br. Med. J. 1:1249-1250, 1979.

312. Kapadia, S. B.: Histiocytic lymphoma of the ileocecal region after chemotherapy for multiple myeloma. Cancer 43:435-439, 1979.
313. Karani, J., Veale, D., & Rake, M. O.: Intestinal pseudo-obstruction in alcohol abuse: report of two cases. Br. Med. J. 2:1400, 1979.
314. Karat, A. B. A.: Long-term follow-up of clofazimine (Lamprene) in the management of reactive phases of leprosy. Lepr. Rev. 46 (Suppl.):105-109, 1975.
315. Katz, J., & Vogel, R.: Abdominal angina as a complication of methysergide maleate therapy. J.A.M.A. 199:124-125, 1967.
316. Katzenstein, A. L. A., & Maksem, J.: Candidal infection of gastric ulcers. Histology, incidence, and clinical significance. Am. J. Clin. Pathol. 71:137-141, 1979.
317. Kauffman, G. L., & Grossman, M. I.: Prostaglandin and cimetidine inhibit the formation of ulcers produced by parenteral salicylates. Gastroenterology 75:1099-1102, 1978.
318. Kaufman, S. E., & Kaye, M. D.: Induction of gastro-oesophageal reflux by alcohol. Gut 19:336-338, 1979.
319. Keating, J. P., Frank, A. L., Barton, L. L., et al.: Pseudomembranous colitis associated with ampicillin therapy. Am. J. Dis. Child. 128:369, 1974.
320. Keighley, M. R. B., Burdon, D. W., Alexander-Williams, J., et al.: Diarrhoea and pseudomembranous colitis after gastrointestinal operations. Lancet 2:1165-1167, 1978.
321. Kern, F., Clark, G. M., & Lukens, G. J.: Peptic ulceration occurring during therapy for rheumatoid arthritis. Gastroenterology 33:25-33, 1957.
322. Keusch, G. T., Troncale, F. J., & Plaut, A. G.: Neomycin-induced malabsorption in a tropical population. Gastroenterology 58:197-202, 1970.
323. Kewalramani, L. S.: Neurogenic gastroduodenal ulceration and bleeding associated with spinal cord injuries. J. Trauma 19:259-265, 1979.
324. Key, T. C., & Kreutner, A. K.: Gastrointestinal complications of modern intrauterine devices. Obstet. Gynecol. 55:239-244, 1980.
325. Khadadoost, J., & Glass, G. B. J.: Erosive gastritis and acute gastroduodenal ulceration as source of upper gastrointestinal bleeding in liver cirrhosis. Digestion 7:129, 1972.
326. Khera, D. C., Herschman, B. R., & Sosa, F.: Tetracycline-induced esophageal ulcers. Postgrad. Med. 68:114-115, 1980.
327. Kies, M. S., Luedke, D. W., & Boyd, J. F., et al.: Neutropenic enterocolitis. Cancer 43:730-734, 1979.
328. Killingback, M.: Acute large bowel obstruction precipitated by barium X-ray examination. Med. J. Aust. 2:503, 1964.
329. Kim, K. S., & Shore, P. A.: Mechanism of action of reserpine and insulin on gastric amines and gastric acid secretion, and the effect of monoamine oxidase inhibition. J. Pharmacol. Exp. Ther. 141:321-325, 1963.
330. Kingry, R. L., Hobson, R. W., & Muir, R. W.: Cecal necrosis and perforation with systemic chemotherapy. Am. Surg. 39:129-133, 1973.
331. Kirsner, J. B.: Toxic megacolon complicating ulcerative colitis: current therapeutic perspectives. Gastroenterology 66:1088-1090, 1974.
332. Kliegman, R. M., Pittard, W. B., & Fanaroff, A. A.: Necrotizing enterocolitis in neonates fed human milk. J. Pediatr. 95:450-453, 1979.
333. von Klingeren, B.: Penicillins, cephalosporins and tetracyclines. In: Dukes, M. N. G., Ed. Side Effects of Drugs, Vol. 4. Exerpta Medica, Amsterdam 1980.
334. Klotey, A. P., Parker, W. L., & Kranes, J. B.: Aureomycin proctitis and colitis. A report of 5 cases. Gastroenterology 25:44-47, 1953.
335. Knauer, C. M.: Mallory-Weiss syndrome: Characterization of 75 mallory-weiss lacerations in 528 patients with upper gastrointestinal hemorrhage. Gastroenterology 71:5-8, 1976.
336. Knott, L. H., & Miller, R. C.: Acute iron intoxication with intestinal infarction. J. Pediatr. Surg. 13:720-721, 1978.
337. Kobayashi, A., & Ohbe, Y.: Protein-losing enteropathy associated with arsenic poisoning. Am. J. Dis. Child. 121:515-517, 1971.
338. Kobler, E., Buhler, H., Nuesch, H. J., et al.: Medikamentos induzierte osophagusulzera. Dtsch. Med. Wochenschr. 103:1035-1037, 1978.
339. Kodsi, B. E., Wickremesinge, P. C., Kozinn, P. J., et al.: Candida esophagitis. Gastroenterology 71:715, 1976.
340. Koep, L. J., Peters, T. G., & Starzl, T. E. Major colonic complications of hepatic trans-

plantation. Dis. Colon Rectum 22:218-220, 1979.

341. Konturek, S. J., Piastucki, I., Brzozowski, T., et al.: Role of prostaglandins in the formation of aspirin-induced gastric ulcers. Gastroenterology 80:4-9, 1981.
342. Koretz, R. L., & Meyer, J. H.: Elemental diets—Facts and fantasies. Gastroenterology 78:393-410, 1980.
343. Korman, M. G., Hansky, J., & Waugh, J.: The effect of cimetidine on gastrin release in ulcer disease. Aust. N.Z. J. Med. 9:367-369, 1979.
344. Kozarek, R. A., Earnest, D. L., Silverstein, M. E., & Smith, R. G.: Air-pressure-induced colon injury during diagnostic colonoscopy. Gastroenterology 78:7-14, 1980.
345. Kozarek, R. A., & Sanowski, R. A.: Esophageal food impaction: Description of a new method for bolus removal. Am. J. Digest. Dis. 25:100-103, 1980.
346. Krasner, N., Cochran, K. M., Russel, R. I., et al.: Alcohol and absorption from the small intestine. 1. Impairment of absorption from the small intestine in alcoholics. Gut 17:245, 1976.
347. Krenzelok, E. P., & Clinton, J. E.: Caustic eosphageal and gastric erosion without evidence of oral burns following detergent ingestion. J.A.C.E.P. 8:5-7, 1979.
348. Kreuning, J., Bosman, F. T., Kuiper, G., et al.: Gastric and duodenal mucosa in 'healthy' individuals. J. Clin. Pathol. 31:69-77, 1978.
349. Kuzell, W. C., Schaffarzick, R. W., Naugler, W., et al.: Phenylbutazone (Butazolidin) in gout. Am. J. Med. 16:212, 1954.
350. Lambert, J. R., & Newman, A.: Ulceration and stricture of the esophagus due to oral potassium chloride (slow release tablet) treatment. Am. J. Gastroenterol. 73:508-511, 1980.
351. LaMont, J. T., & Trnka, Y. M.: Therapeutic implications of clostridium difficile toxin during relapse of chronic inflammatory bowel disease. Lancet 1:381-383, 1980.
352. Lange, E. K.: A survey of complications of percutaneous retrograde arteriography. Radiology 81:257, 1963.
353. Lanza, F. L., Royer, G. L., Nelson, R. S., et al.: The effects of ibuprofen, indomethacin, aspirin, naproxen, and placebo on the gastric mucosa of normal volunteers. A gastroscopic and photographic study. Dig. Dis. Sci. 24:823-828, 1979.
354. Lanza, F. L., Royer, G. L., & Nelson, R. S.: Endoscopic evaluation of the effects of aspirin, buffered aspirin, and enteric-coated aspirin on gastric and duodenal mucosa. N. Engl. J. Med. 303:136-138, 1980.
355. Larson, H. E., Price, A. B., & Honour, P.: Clostridium difficile and the etiology of pseudomembranous colitis. Lancet 1:1063-1066, 1978.
356. Lauder, A. D.: Cetiprin and oesophageal ulceration. Br. Med. J. 2:211, 1979.
357. Lauritsen, K. B., Heltberg, J., Hornum, I., & Rehfeld, J. F.: Lithium inhibits basal and food-stimulated gastrin secretion. Gastroenterology 75:59-60, 1978.
358. Lawrason, F. D., Alpert, E., Mohr, F. L., & McMahon, F. G.: Ulcerative-obstructive lesions of the small intestine. J.A.M.A. 191:641-644, 1965.
359. Lahmiller, D. J., & Kanto, W. P.: Relationships of mesenteric thromboembolism, oral feeding, and necrotizing enterocolitis. J. Pediatr. 92:96-100, 1978.
360. Lehtola, J., & Sipponen, P.: A gastroscopic and histological double-blind study of the effects of diclofenac sodium and naproxen on the human gastric mucosa. Scand. J. Rheumatol. 6:97-102, 1977.
361. Lemoh, J. N., & Watt, J.: Lactobezoar and cows' milk protein intolerance. Arch. Dis. Child. 55:128-129, 1980.
362. Lennert, K. A., & Kootz, F.: Nil nocere. Arzneimittelbedingte dunndarmulzera. Munch. Med. Wochenschr. 109:2058-2062, 1967.
363. Leonidas, J. C., Burry, V. F., Fellows, R. A., et al.: Possible adverse effect of methylglucamine diatrizoate compounds on the bowel of newborn infants with meconium ileus. Radiology 121:693-696, 1976.
364. Leriche, M., Devroede, G., Sanchez, G., & Rossano, J.: Changes in the rectal mucosa induced by hypertonic enemas. Dis. Colon Rectum 21:227-236, 1978.
365. Lev, R., Thomas, E., Parl, F. F., et al.: Pathological and histomorphometric study of the effects of alcohol on the human duodenum. Digestion 20:207-213, 1980.
366. Levin, E., Clayman, C. B., Palmer, W. L., et al.: Observations on the value of gastric

irradiation in the treatment of duodenal ulcer. Gastroenterology 32:42, 1957.

367. Levitt, R., Stanley, R., & Wise, L.: Gastric bullae—An early roentgen finding in corrosive gastritis following alkali ingestion. Radiology 115:597, 1975.
368. Levy, M.: Aspirin use in patients with major upper gastrointestinal bleeding and peptic ulcer disease: a report from the Boston collaborative Drug Surveillance Program, Boston University Medical Center. N. Engl. J. Med. 290:1158-1162, 1974.
369. Levy, N., & Gaspar, E.: Rectal bleeding and indomethacin suppositories. Lancet 1:577, 1975.
370. Lewis, A. E.: Dangers inherent in soap enemas. Pacific Med. Surg. 73:131, 1965.
371. Lewis, J. W., Kerstein, M. D., & Koss, N.: Barium granuloma of the rectum: an uncommon complication of barium enema. Ann. Surg. 181:418-423, 1975.
372. Lightdale, C. J., Wolf, D. J., Marcucci, R. A., et al.: Herpetic esophagitis in patients with cancer: ante mortem diagnosis by brush cytology. Cancer 39:223-226, 1977.
373. Linaker, B. D., & Hughes, S.: Duodenal erosions on cimetidine therapy. Br. Med. J. 1:1278-1279, 1978.
374. Lishman, A. H., Al-Jumaili, I. J., and & Record, C. O.: Spectrum of antibiotic-associated diarrhoea. Gut 22:34-37, 1981.
375. Livathinopoulos, G.: L'effet de la cortisone sur le tractus gastrointestinal. Rev. Med. Moy. Or. 24:363, 1967.
376. Localio, S. A., Stone, A., & Friedman, M.: Surgical aspects of radiation enteritis. Surg. Gynecol. Obstet. 129:1163-1172, 1969.
377. Loebl, D. H., Craig, R. M., Culic, D. D. et al.: Gastrointestinal blood loss. Effect of aspirin, fenoprofen, and acetaminophen in rheumatoid arthritis as determined by sequential gastroscopy and radioactive fecal markers. J.A.M.A. 237:976-981, 1977.
378. Long, W. B., & Shiau, Y.: Steroids and peptic ulcer. N. Engl. J. Med. 294:, 1291, 1976.
379. Lovgren, O., & Alexander, E.: Side-effects of indomethacin. Br. Med. J. 1:118, 1964.
380. Lowe, P., Hoiseth, A., & Nordshus, T.: Spasm of the superior mesenteric artery complicating methysergide maleate therapy. Br. J. Radiol. 51:1014-1016, 1978.
381. Luban, N. L., Miller, D. R., & Mouradian, J.: Intestinal perforation during remission of acute lymphoblastic leukemia. J. Pediatr. 94:409-410, 1979.
382. Lubble, W. F., Cadogen, E. S., & Kannemeyer, A. H.: Oesophageal ulceration due to slow release potassium in the presence of left atrial enlargement. N. Z. Med. J. 14:377-379, 1979.
383. Lubitz, L., & Ekert, H.: Reversible changes in duodenal mucosa associated with intensive chemotherapy followed by autologous marrow rescue. Lancet 2:532-533, 1979.
384. Lusk, R. H., Fekety, F. R., Silva, J., et al: Gastrointestinal side effects of clindamycin and ampicillin therapy. J. Infect. Dis. 135 (Suppl.):S111-S119, 1977.
385. Lyon, D. C.: Intussusception complicating anticoagulant therapy. Br. Med. J. 2:345, 1968.
386. Lyon, D. T., Schubert, T. T., Mantia, A. G., & Kaplan, M. H.: Phycomycosis of the gastrointestinal tract. Am. J. Gastroenterol. 72:379-394, 1979.
387. MacCallum, W. G.: A Textbook of Pathology, 7th ed. p. 389. W. B. Saunders, Philadelphia, 1941.
388. MacDonald, A., DeKanski, J. B., Gottfried, S., et al.: Effects of blood glucose levels on aspirin-induced gastric mucosal damage. Digest. Dis. 22:909, 1977.
389. MacDonald, W. C., Anderson, F. H., & Hashimoto, S.: Histological effect of certain pickles on the human gastric mucosa. Can. Med. Assoc. J. 96:1521-1525, 1967.
390. MacDonald, W. C., & Stoller, L. J.: Protective action of carbenoxolone on pickle-induced gastric injury in man. Am. J. Digest. Dis. 18:941-945, 1973.
391. MacDonald, W. C.: Correlation of mucosal histology and aspirin intake in chronic gastric ulcer. Gastroenterology 65:381-389, 1973.
392. MacFarlane, J. D., Maisey, M. N., Grahame, R., Burry, H. C.: Gastrointestinal blood loss on phenylbutazone and feprazone. Rheumatol. Rehabil. 15:108-111, 1976.
393. Mackay, A., & Stevenson, R. D.: Gastric ulceration induced by spironolactone. Lancet 1:481, 1977.
394. MacKercher, P. A., Ivey, K. J., Baskin, W. N., et al.: Protective effect of cimetidine on aspirin-induced gastric mucosal damage. Ann. Intern. Med. 87:676, 1977.
395. Mahoney, T. J., Bubrick, M. P., & Hitchcock,

C. R.: Nonspecific ulcers of the colon. Dis. Colon Rectum, 21:623-626, 1978.

396. Mainguet, P., Bleiberg, H., & Tijs, O.: Les ulceres de la reserpine. Acta Gastroenterol. Belg. 29:503, 1966.
397. Makoui, C., Chakravorty, R. C., & Wilson, W. H.: Nonspecific ulcer of the ascending colon. Dis. Colon Rectum, 22:256-259, 1979.
398. del Marco, L. B.: Contribucion al estudio de la gastritis corrosiva: Estudio clinico y experimental. An Fac. Med. Montevideo 34:891, 1949.
399. Marin, G. A., Clark, M. L., & Senior, J. R.: Studies of malabsorption occurring in patients with Laennec's cirrhosis. Gastroenterology 56:727-736, 1969.
400. Markowitz, A. M.: The less common perforations of the small bowel. Ann. Surg. 152:240-257, 1960.
401. Marr, J. J., Sans, M. D., & Tedesco, F. J.: Bacterial studies of clindamycin-associated colitis. Gastroenterology 69:352, 1975.
402. Martins, A., Sternberg, S. S., & Attiyeh, F. F.: Radiation-induced carcinoma of the rectum. Dis. Colon Rectum 23:572-575, 1980.
403. Masel, H., Masel, J. P., and Casey, K. V.: A survey of colon examination techniques in Australia and New Zealand with a review of complications. Australas. Radiol. 15:140, 1971.
404. Mason, A. M., Bleeding massive gastric ulcer on diflunisal (Dolobid). Br. Med. J. 1:888, 1979.
405. Mason, G. H., Ellis-Pegler, R. B., & Arthur, J. F.: Clofazimine and eosinophilic enteritis. Lepr. Rev. 48:175–180, 1977.
406. Matek, W., Fruhmorgen, P., & Fuchs, H. F.: Barium enema with subsequent perforation of the rectum following rectoscopic biopsy. Endoscopy 10:132-136, 1978.
407. Matsuki, A., Wakayama, S., & Oyama, T.: Acute transient swelling of the salivary glands during and following endotracheal anaesthesia. Anaesthetist 24:25-28, 1975.
408. Matts, S. G. F.: Naproxen (Naprosyn) and gastrointestinal haemorrhage. Br. Med. J. 2:52, 1974.
409. Maudsley, R. F., & Qizilbash, A. H.: Thermal injury to the bowel as a complication of laparoscopic sterilization. Can. J. Surg. 22:232-234, 1979.
410. May, A. G., Betts, R. F., Freeman, R. B., and Andrus, C. H.: An analysis of Cytomegalovirus infection and HL-A antigen matching on the outcome of renal transplantation. Ann. Surg. 187:110-117, 1978.
411. Mazier, W. P., Sun, M. K., & Robertson, W. G.: Oil-induced granuloma (eleoma) of the rectum: report of four cases. Dis. Colon Rectum 21:292-294, 1978.
412. Mazzacca, G., Cascione, F., Budillon, G., et al.: Parietal cell hyperplasia induced by long-term administration of antacids to rats. Gut 19:798-801, 1978.
413. McDonald, G. S. A., & Hourihane, D. O'B.: Ischemic lesions of the alimentary tract. J. Clin. Pathol. 25:99-105, 1972.
414. McGovern, V. J., & Goulston, S. J. M. Ischaemic enterocolitis. Gut 6:213-220, 1965.
415. McGreevy, J. M., & Moody, F. G.: Protection of gastric mucosa against aspirin-induced erosions by enhanced blood flow. Surg. Forum 28:357-359, 1977.
416. McGuigan, J. E.: A consideration of the adverse effects of cimetidine. Gastroenterology 80:181-192, 1981.
417. McIlrath, D. C., & Hallenbeck, G. A.: Review of gastric freezing. J.A.M.A. 190:715, 1964.
418. McInerney, D. P., & Bullimore, J.: Reactivation of radiation pneumonitis by adriamycin. Br. J. Radiol. 50:224-227, 1977.
419. McKee, P. H., & Cameron, C. H. S.: Barium granuloma of the transverse colon. Postgrad. Med. J. 54:698-702, 1968.
420. McKinley, M., & Toffler, R. B.: Antibiotic-associated hemorrhagic colitis. Dig. Dis. Sci. 25:812-813, 1980.
421. McMahon, F. G., & Akdamar, K.: Gastric ulceration after "Slow K." N. Engl. J. Med. 295:733-734, 1076.
422. Medline, A., Shin, D. H., & Medline, N. M.: Pseudomembranous colitis associated with antibiotics. Hum. Pathol. 7 693-703, 1976.
423. Meisel, J. L., Perrera, D. R., Meligro, C., & Rubin, C. E.: Overwhelming watery diarrhea associated with Cryptosporidium in an immunosuppressed patient. Gastroenterology 70:1156-1170, 1976.
424. Meisel, J. L., Bergman, D., Graney, D., et al.: Human rectal mucosa: proctoscopic and morphological changes caused by laxatives. Gastroenterology 72:1274-1279, 1977.
425. Mekhjian, H. S., & May, E. S.: Acute and chronic effects of ethanol on fluid transport

in the human small intestine. Gastroenterology 72:1280-1286, 1977.
426. Melange, M., Vanheuverzwyn, R., & Fiasse, R.: Pseudomembranous colitis and rifampicin. Lancet 2:1192, 1980.
427. Menguy, R.: Surgical management of free perforation of the small intestine complicating regional enteritis. Ann. Surg. 175:178-189, 1972.
428. Menguy, R., & Masters, Y. F.: Effect of cortisone on mucoprotein secretion by the gastric antrum of dogs: pathogenesis of steroid ulcer. Surgery 54:19, 1963.
429. Merten, D. F., & Lebowitz, M. E.: Acute appendicitis in a child associated with prolonged appendiceal retention of barium (barium appendicitis). South. Med. J. 71:81-82, 1978.
430. Messersmith, J. K., Oglesby, J. E., Mahoney, W. D., & Baugh, J. H.: Gastric erosion from alkali ingestion. Am. J. Surg. 119:740-742, 1970.
431. Meyers, S., Mayer, L., Bottone, E., et al.: Occurrence of Cl.difficile toxin during the course of inflammatory bowel disease. Gastroenterology 80:697-700, 1981.
432. Mezey, E., Jow, E., Slavin, R. E., & Tobon, F.: Pancreatic function and intestinal absorption in alcoholism. Gastroenterology 59:657, 1970.
433. Mielants, H., Veys, E. M., Verbruggen, G., et al.: Salicylate-induced gastrointestinal bleeding: comparison between soluble buffered, enteric-coated, and intravenous administration. J. Rheumatol. 6:210-8, 1979.
434. Milgram, J. E.: Surgery of suppuration in the fascial spaces of the thigh. J.A.M.A. 98:117, 1932.
435. Millan, M. S., Morris, G. P., Beck, I. T., & Henson, J. T.: Villous damage induced by suction biopsy and by acute ethanol intake in normal human small intestine. Dig. Dis. Sci. 23:513-525, 1980.
436. Miller, T. A. & Jacobson, E. D.: Gastrointestinal cytoprotection by prostaglandins. Gut 20:75-87, 1979.
437. Milles, S. S., Muggia, A. L., & Spiro, H. M.: Colonic histologic changes induced by 5-fluorouracil. Gastroenterology 43:391-399, 1962.
438. Milligan, D. W., & Kelly, J. K.: Pseudomembranous colitis in a leukemia unit: a report of five fatal cases. J. Clin. Pathol. 32:1237-1243, 1979.
439. Mills, P. R., Main, A. N. H., Gemmell, C. G., et al.: Pseudomembranous colitis as infectious disease. Lancet 1:552, 1981.
440. Milner, G.: Gastro-intestinal side-effects of psychotropic drugs. Med. J. Aust. 2:153-155, 1969.
441. Misra, M. K., Pinkus, G. S., Birtch, A. G., et al.: Major colonic diseases complicating renal transplantation. Surgery 73:942-948, 1973.
442. Mittleman, B., & Wolff, H. G.: Emotions and gastroduodenal function: experimental studies on patients with gastritis, duodenitis, and peptic ulcer. Psychosom. Med. 4:5-61, 1942.
443. Mogg, G. A. G., Keighley, M. R. B., Burdon, D. W., et al.: Antibiotic-associated colitis—a review of 66 cases. Br. J. Surg. 66:738-742, 1979.
444. Moir, D. H., & Bale, P. M.: Necropsy findings in childhood leukemia, emphasising neutropenic enterocolitis and cerebral calcification. Pathology 8:247-258, 1976.
445. Moore, R.: Bleeding gastric erosion after oral zinc sulphate. Br. Med. J. 1:754, 1978.
446. Morrison, F. S., & Wurzel, H. A.: Retroperitoneal hemorrhage during heparin therapy. Am. J. Cardiol. 13:329-332, 1964.
447. Morson, B. C., & Dawson, I. M. P.: Gastrointestinal Pathology, 2nd Ed. p. 732. Blackwell, Oxford, 1979.
448. Morton, J. F.: Tea with milk. Science 204:909, 1979.
449. Mottet, N. K., & Body, R. L.: Primate Paneth cell degeneration following methylmercury hydroxide ingestion. Am. J. Pathol. 84:93-110, 1976.
450. von Muhlendahl, K. E., Bunjes, R., & Krienke, E. G.: Loperamide-induced ileus. Lancet 1:209, 1980.
451. Muir, A., & Cossar, I. A.: Aspirin and ulcer. Br. Med. J. 2:7-12, 1955.
452. Mullick, F. G., Drake, R. M., & Irey, N. S.: Morphologic changes in adverse drug reactions in infants and children. Human Pathol. 8:361-378, 1977.
453. Murray, C., Chapman, R., Isaacson, P., et al.: Cimetidine and malignant gastric ulcers (Letter). Lancet 1:1092, 1978.
454. Murray, H. S., Strottman, M. P., & Cooke, A. R.: Effect of several drugs on gastric potential difference in man. Br. Med. J. 1:19-21, 1974.
455. Murthy, S. N. S., Dinoso, V. P., Clearfield,

H. R., & Chey, W. Y.: Serial pH changes in the duodenal bulb during smoking. Gastroenterology 75:1-4, 1978.

456. Myren, J., Luketic, G. C., Ceballos, R., et al.: Effect of colchicine on intestinal mucosal dehydrogenases. I. Histochemical observations. Am. J. Digest Dis. 11:394, 1966.

457. Nalin, D. R., Levine, M. M., Rhead, J., et al.: Cannabis, hypochlorhydria, and cholera. Lancet 2:859-861, 1978.

458. Needham, C. D., Kyle, J., Jones, P. F., et al.: Aspirin and alcohol in gastrointestinal haemorrhage. Gut 12:19-21, 1971.

459. Nelson, N. A., Goodman, H. L., & Oster, H. L.: The association of histoplasma and lymphoma. Am. J. Med. Sci. 233:56-65, 1957.

460. Neshat, A. A., Stone, D. H., & Price, H. P.: Self-induced lipoid granuloma of the rectum: report of a case. Dis. Colon Rectum 17:696-699, 1974.

461. Neu, H. C., Prince, A., Neu, O. C., et al.: Incidence of diarrhea and colitis associated with clindamycin therapy. J. Infect. Dis. 135:S120-S125, 1977.

462. Newburger, P. E., Cassady, J. R., & Jaffe, N.: Esophagitis due to adriamycin and radiation therapy for childhood malignancy. Cancer 42:417-423, 1978.

463. Nielsen, V. T., Vetner, M., & Harslof, E.: Collagenous colitis. Histopathology 4:83-86, 1980.

464. Nime, F. A., Burek, J. D., Page, D. L., et al.: Acute enterocolitis in a human being infected with the protozoan *Cryptosporidium*. Gastroenterology 70:592-598, 1976.

465. Norland, C. C., & Kirsner, J. B.: Toxic dilatation of colon (toxic dilatation): etiology, treatment and prognosis in 42 patients. Medicine 48:229-250, 1969.

466. Northway, M. G., Libshitz, H. I., Osborne, B. M., et al.: Radiation in Esophagitis in the opossum: radioprotection with indomethacin. Gastroenterology 78:883-892, 1980.

467. Novak, J. M., Collins, J. T., Donowitz, M., et al.: Effects of radiation on the human gastrointestinal tract. J. Clin. Gastroenterol. 1:9-39, 1979.

468. O'Connor, T. W., Rombeau, J. L., Levine, H. S., & Turnbull, R. B.: Late development of colorectal cancer subsequent to pelvic irradiation. Dis. Colon Rectum 22:123-128, 1979.

469. Ogle, C. W., Cho, C. H.: Protection by zinc sulphate against reserpine-induced ulceration and other gastric effects in the rat. Pharmacology 17:254-261, 1978.

470. Okabe, S., Takeuchi, K., Urushidani, T., & Takagi, K.: Effects of cimetidine, a histamine H_2-receptor antagonist, on various experimental gastric and duodenal ulcers. Am. J. Digest. Dis. 22:677-684, 1977.

471. Okabe, S., & Tabata, K.: Does indomethacin activate healed gastric ulcers in the dog? Digestion 21:179-183, 1981.

472. O'Meara, T. F.: A new endoscopic finding of tetracycline-induced esophageal ulcers. Gastrointest. Endosc. 26:106-107, 1980.

473. Orme, R. L. E., Eades, S. M.: Perforation of the bowel in the newborn as a complication of exchange transfusion. Br. Med. J. 2:349-351, 1968.

474. Osnes, M., Larsen, S., Eidsaunet, W. & Thom E.: Effect of diclofenac and naproxen on gastroduodenal mucosa. Clin. Pharmacol. Ther. 26:399-405, 1979.

475. Ottonello, G. A., & Primavera, A.: Gastrointestinal complication of high-dose corticosteroid therapy in acute cerebrovascular patients. Stroke 10:208-210, 1979.

476. Paffenbarger, R. S., Wing, A. L., & Hyde, R. T.: Chronic disease in former college students. XIII. Early precursors of peptic ulcer. Am. J. Epidemiol. 100:307, 1974.

477. Palmer, T. H., Mason, P. J., & Adams, A. C.: Diverticulitis of the colon with perforation during cortisone and ACTH therapy. J. Maine Med. Assoc. 46:349-351, 1955.

478. Pannuti, F., Martoni, A., Pollutri, E., et al.: Studio dei principali parametri di biotollerabilita clinica ed ematochimica al 5-fluorouracil somministrato peros. G Med Ital. 132:303–315, 1973.

479. Parkinson, A. T., Haidak, G. L., & McInerney, R. P.: Verrucous squamous cell carcinoma of the esophagus following lye stricture. Chest 57:489-492, 1970.

480. Parl, F. F., Lev, R., Thomas E., & Pitchumoni, C. S.: Histologic and morphometric study of chronic gastritis in alcoholic patients. Hum. Pathol. 10:45-56, 1979.

481. Peikin, S. R., Galdibini, J., & Bartlett, J. G.: Role of Clostridium difficile in a case of nonantibiotic-associated pseudomembranous colitis. Gastroenterology 79:948-951, 1980.

482. Pemberton, J.: Oesophageal obstruction and

ulceration caused by oral potassium therapy. Br. Heart J. 32:267-268, 1970.

483. Pemberton, R. E., & Strand, L. J.: A review of upper-gastrointestinal effects of the newer nonsteroidal antiinflammatory agents. Digest. Dis. Sci. 24:53-64, 1979.
484. Perloff, L. J., Chon, H., Petrella, E. J., et al.: Acute colitis in the renal allograft recipient. Ann. Surg. 183:77-83, 1976.
485. Perry, G. T., Dunphy, J. V., Fruin, R. C., et al.: Gastric freezing for duodenal ulcer. a double blind study. Gastroenterology. 47:6, 1964.
486. Peters, J. L.: Benign oesophageal stricture following oral potassium chloride therapy. Br. J. Surg. 63:698-699, 1976.
487. Petrillo, M., Caruso, I., Fumagalli, M. et al.: Diflunisal, aspirin, and gastric mucosa. Lancet 2:638, 1979.
488. Phelps, J. E., Sanowski, R. A., & Kozarek, R. A.: Barium ulceration of the rectum resembling carcinoma. Gastrointest. Endosc. 26:74, 1980. (Abstr.)
489. Phillips, J. A., Lovejoy, F. H., & Matsumiya, Y.: Ampicillin-associated diarrhea: effects of dosage and route of administration. Pediatrics 58:869, 1976.
490. Pike, B. F., Phillipi, P. J., & Lawson, E. H.: Soap colitis. N. Engl. J. Med. 285:217-218, 1971.
491. Pillari, G., Bank, S., Katzka, I., & Fulco, J. D.: Meat bolus impaction of the lower esophagus associated with a paraesophageal hernia. Am. J. Gastroenterol. 71:287-289, 1979.
492. Piper, D. W., McIntosh, J. H., Ariotti, D. E. et al.: Analgesic ingestion and chronic peptic ulcer. Gastroenterology 80:427-432, 1981.
493. Pirola, R. C., Bolin, T. D., & Davis, A. E.: Does alcohol cause duodenitis? Am. J. Digest. Dis. 14:239, 1969.
494. Pittman, F. E.: Antibiotic-associated colitis: Lincomycin and clindamycin. Adv. Drug Reaction Bull. 63:220, 1977.
495. Porro, G. B., Petrillo, M., Fumagalli, M. & Carratelli, L.: Endoscopic evaluation of the effects of a new anti-inflammatory drug, Sulindac on the gastric mucosa. Eur. J. Rheumatol. Inflamm. 1:34-35, 1978.
496. Port, J., Levin, B., & Riddell, R. H.: Tegafor-induced colitis and neurotoxicity. (Submitted.)
497. Potyk, D.: Intestinal obstruction from impacted antacid tablets. N. Engl. J. Med. 283:134-136, 1970.
498. Powell, J. W., Moss, J. P., Nagar, D., et al.: Strongyloides in immunosuppressed hosts. Presentation as massive lower gastrointestinal bleeding. Arch. Intern. Med. 140:1061-1063, 1980.
499. Press, M. F., Riddell, R. H., & Ringus, J.: Cytomegalovirus inclusion disease. Its occurrence in the myenteric plexus of a renal transplant patient. Arch. Pathol. Lab. Med. 104:580-583, 1980.
500. Prescott, L. F.: Anti-inflammatory agents and drugs used in rheumatism and gout. In: Dukes M. N. G. Ed. Side Effects of Drugs Annual, 1. p. 86 Exerpta Medica. Amsterdam, 1977.
501. Price, A. B., & Davies, D. R.: Pseudomembranous colitis. J. Clin. Pathol. 30:1-12, 1977.
502. Prolla, J. C., & Kirsner, J. B.: The gastrointestinal lesions and complications of the leukemias. Ann. Intern. Med. 61:1084-1103, 1964.
503. Race, T. F., Paes, I. C., & Faloon, W. W.: Intestinal malabsorption induced by oral colchincine. Comparison with neomycin and cathartic agents. Am. J. Med. Sci. 259:32-41, 1970.
504. Rahman, M., Turner, R., Pisko, E., & Agudelo, C.: Long-term efficacy and safety of piroxicam in the treatment of rheumatoid arthritis. Clin. Pharmacol. Ther. 25:243, 1979.
505. Rainsford, K. D.: Electromicroscopic observations on the effect of orally administered aspirin and aspirin-bicarbonate mixtures on the development of gastric mucosal damage in the rat. Gut 16:514-527, 1975.
506. Rees, W. D., & Turnberg, L. A.: Reappraisal of the effects of aspirin on the stomach. Lancet 2:410-412, 1980.
507. Reimer, R. R., Hoover, R., Fraumeni, J. F., & Young, R. C.: Second primary neoplasms following ovarian cancer. J. Natl. Cancer. Inst. 61:1195-1197, 1978.
508. Reiner, L., Schlessinger, M. I., & Miler, G. M.: Pseudomembranous colitis following aureomycin and chloramphenicol. Arch. Pathol. 54:49-69, 1952.
509. ReMine, S. G., & McIlrath, D. C.: Bowel

perforation in steroid-treated patients. Ann. Surg. 192:581-586, 1980.

510. Renert, W. A., Button, K. F., Fuld, S. L., & Casarella, W. J.: Mesenteric venous thrombosis and small bowel infarction following infusion of vasopressin into the superior mesenteric artery. Radiology 102:299-302, 1972.

511. Reynolds, K. W.: Erosive gastritis with special reference to the role of aspirin and bile. Ann. R. Coll. Surg. Engl. 55:213-225, 1974.

512. Richardson, M. E., & Spivey, M. R.: Dietary cadmium and enteropathy in the japanese quail:histochemical and ultrastructural studies. Lab. Invest. 31:722, 1974.

513. Ridolfo, A. S., Rubin, A., Crabtree, R. E., et al.: Effects of fenoprofen calcium and aspirin on gastrointestinal microbleeding in man. Clin. Pharmacol. Ther. 14:226-230, 1973.

514. Riemann, J. F., Schenk, J., Ehler, R., et al.: Ultrastructural changes of colonic mucosa in patients with chronic laxative abuse. Acta Hepatogastroenterol. (Stuttg.) 25:213-218, 1978.

515. Ritchie, W. P., & Cherry, K. J.: Influence of hydrogen ion concentration on bile acid induced acute gastric mucosal ulcerogenesis. Ann. Surg. 189:637-642, 1979.

516. Ritama, V., Vapaatalo, H. I., Neuvonen, P. J., et al.: Phenothiazines and intestinal dilatation. Lancet 1:470, 1969.

517. Robert, A., Nezamis, J. E., Lancaster, C. & Hanchar, A. J.: Cytoprotection by prostaglandins in rats. Prevention of gastric necrosis produced by alcohol, HCl, NaOH, hypertonic NaCl, and thermal injury. Gastroenterology 77:433-443, 1979.

518. Robert, A.: Cytoprotection by prostaglandins. Gastroenterology 77:761-767, 1979.

519. Robert, A., Nezamis, J. E., Hanchar, A. J., & Lancaster, C.: Aspirin combined with alcohol is ulcerogenic. Gastroenterology 78:1245, 1980.

520. Roberts, D. M.: Chronic gastritis, alcohol and non-ulcer dyspepsia. Gut 13:768, 1972.

521. Robertson, D. M., Riley, F. C., & Hermans, P. E.: Endogenous Candida oculomycosis. Report of two patients treated with flucytosine. Arch. Ophthalmol. 91:33-38, 1974.

522. Robinson, B. F.: Drugs acting on the cardiovascular system. In: Dukes, M.N.G. Ed. Side Effects of Drugs Annual, 1. p. 152. Excerpta Medica, Amsterdam 1977.

523. Roman, P. W., Wagner, J. H., & Steinbach, S. H.: Massive fatal embolism during barium enema study. Radiology 59:190, 1952.

524. Rosenbaum, E. S., & Barbier, E. J.: Inhibition by aspirin of gastrointestinal toxicity induced by indomethacin in polyarthritic rats. Toxicol. Appl. Pharmacol. 49:535-541, 1979.

525. Rosenberg, L. S., & Fine, A.: Fatal venous intravasation of barium during barium enema. Radiology 73:771, 1959.

526. Rosenoer, V. M.: Radiologic contrast media. In: Meyler, L., & Herxheimer, A. Eds. Side Effects of Drugs, Vol. 7. p. 654. Excerpta Medica, Amsterdam, 1972.

527. Roth, J. A.: The effect of caffeine upon gastric secretion in the dog, cat and man. Am. J. Physiol. 126:814-819, 1944.

528. Rothernich, N.O.: An extended study of indomethacin. I. Clinical Pharmacology, J.A.M.A. 195:531, 1966.

529. Rothschild, B. M., Masai, A. T., & June, P. T.: Arthritis associated with ampicillin colitis. Ann. Intern. Med. 137:1605-1607, 1977.

530. Rowe, H. J.: Comparison of pirprofen with aspirin in rheumatoid arthritis: a multicenter study. Clin. Ther. 2:69, 1978.

531. Rubin, E., Rybak, B. J., Lindenbaum, J., et al.: Ultrastructural changes in the small intestine induced by ethanol. Gastroenterology 63:801-814, 1972.

532. Ruddell, W. S. J., Axon, A. T. R., Findlay, J. M., et al.: Effect of cimetidine on the gastric bacterial flora. Lancet 1:672-674, 1980.

533. Ruddell, W. S. J., & Losowskz, M. S.: Severe diarrhoea due to small intestinal colonisation during cimetidine treatment. Br. Med. J. 2:273, 1980.

534. Rushnak, M. J., & Leevy, C. M.: Effect of diazepam on the lower esophageal sphincter. Am. J. Gastroenterol. 73:127-130, 1980.

535. Rutter, K., & Riddell, R. H.: Solitary ulcer syndrome of the rectum. Clin. Gastroenterol. 4:505-530, 1975.

536. Sakurai, Y., Tsuchiya, H., Ikegami, F., et al.: Acute right-side hemorrhagic colitis associated with oral administration of ampicillin. Dig. Dis. Sci. 24:910-915, 1979.

537. SanFilippo, J. A.: Infantile hypertrophic pyloric stenosis related to ingestion of erythromycin estolate: a report of five cases. J. Ped. Surg. 11:177-180, 1976.

538. Sandler, S. G., Tobin, W., & Henderson,

E. S.: Vincristine-induced neuropathy. A clinical study of fifty leukemic patients. Neurology 19: 367-374, 1969.

539. Sawyerr, O. I., Garvin, P. J., Codd, J. E., et al.: Colorectal complications of renal allograft transplantation. Arch. Surg. 113:84-86, 1978.
540. Saxen, L., Kassinen, A., & Saxen, E.: Peritoneal foreign-body reaction caused by condom emulsion. Lancet 1:1295-1296, 1962.
541. Schabel, S, I., & Skucas, J.: Esophageal obstruction following administration of "aged" barium sulfate tablets—a warning. Radiology 122:835-836, 1977.
542. Schapiro, R. L., & Newman, A.: Acute enterocolitis. Radiology 108:263-268, 1973.
543. Schneider, R.: Doxycycline esophageal ulcers. Am. J. Digest. Dis. 22:805-807. 1977.
544. Schrodt, G. R.: Melanosis coli: a study with the electron microscope. Dis. Colon. Rectum 6:277-283, 1963.
545. Schwartz, J. N., Hamilton, J. P., Fekety, R., et al.: Ampicillin-induced enterocolitis: implication of toxigenic Clostridium perfringens type C. J. Pediatr. 97:661-663, 1980.
546. Scott, A. J., Nicholson, G. I., & Kerr, A. R.: Lincomycin as a cause of pseudomembranous colitis. Lancet 2:1232-1234, 1973.
547. Scott, B.: Bleeding massive gastric ulcer on diflunisal (Dolobid). Br. Med. J. 1:489, 1979.
548. Scully, R. E., Galdabini, J. J., & McNeely, B. U.: Case records of the Massachusetts General Hospital, Case 33-1975. N. Engl. J. Med. 923:296-399, 1975.
549. Seaman, W. B., & Wells, J.: Complications of the barium enema. Gastroenterology 48:728, 1965.
550. Searle, J., Lawson, T. A., Abbott, P. J., et al.: An electron-microscope study of the mode of death induced by cancer chemotherapeutic agents in populations of proliferating normal and neoplastic cells. J. Pathol. 116:129-138, 1975.
551. Segal, I., Tim, L. O., Hamilton, D. G., et al.: Ritual-enema-induced colitis. Dis. Colon Rectum. 22:195-199, 1979.
552. Seino, S., Seino, Y., Matsukura, S., et al.: Effect of glucocorticoids on gastrin secretion in man. Gut 19:10-13, 1978.
553. Seltzer, S. E., & Jones, B.: Cecal perforation associated with gastrograffin enema. Am. J. Roentgenol. 130:997-998, 1978.
554. Sewell, R. A., Killen, D. A., & Foster, J. F.: Small bowel injury by angiographic contrast medium. Surgery 64:459-465, 1968.
555. Shands, W. C., & Gatling, R. R.: Circumferential small bowel ulcers: a report of nine cases. Ann. Surg. 165:894-900, 1967.
556. Shapiro, N., Brandt, L., Sprayregan, S., et al.: Duodenal infarction after therapeutic gelfoam embolization of a bleeding duodenal ulcer. Gastroenterology 80:176-80, 1981.
557. Sharp, J. R., Insalaco, S. J., & Johnson, L. F.: "Melanosis" of the duodenum associated with gastric ulcer and folic acid deficiency. Gastroenterology 78:366-369, 1980.
558. Shaw, M. T., Spector, M. H., & Ladman, A. J.: Effects of cancer, radiotherapy and cytotoxic drugs on intestinal structure and function. Cancer Treat. Rev. 6:141-151, 1979.
559. Shehadi, W. H.: Orally administered water-soluble iodinated contrast media. Am. J. Roentgenol. 83:933, 1960.
560. Shepperd, H. W. H.: Iatrogenic reflux oesophagitis. J. Laryngol. Otol. 91:171-172, 1977.
561. Sherman, N. J., Williams, K., & Woolley, M. M.: Surgical complications in the patient with leukemia. J. Pediatr. Surg. 8:235-244, 1973.
562. Shlim, N.: Rupture of cecum during administration of an enema. Am. J. Surg. 87:798, 1954.
563. Shneerson, J. M., & Gazzard, B. G.: Reversible malabsorption caused by methyldopa. Br. Med. J. 2:1456-1457, 1977.
564. Siegman-Igra, Y., Yaron, M., Siletzki, M., et al.: Colitis and death following gold therapy. Rheumatol. Rehabil. 15:245, 1976.
565. Silen, W., & Skillman, J. J.: Stress ulcer, acute erosive gastritis and the gastric mucosal barrier. Adv. Intern. Med. 19:195, 1974.
566. Silvoso, G. R., Ivey, K. J., Butt, J. H. et al: Incidence of gastric lesions in patients with rheumatic disease on chronic aspirin therapy. Ann. Intern. Med. 91:517-520, 1979.
567. Simila, S., Kouvalainen, K., & Makaela, P.: Pseudomembranous colitis after amoxycillin. Lancet 2:317-318, 1976.
568. Simon, L. S., & Mills, J. A.: Drug Therapy: Nonsteroidal antiinflammatory drugs. N. Engl. J. Med. 302:1179-1185, 1980.
569. Simon, L. S., & Mills, J. A.: Drug Therapy:

Nonsteroidal antiinflammatory drugs. N. Engl. J. Med. 302:1237-1242, 1980.

570. Slagle, G. W., & Boggs, H. R.: Drug-induced pseudomembranous enterocolitis: a new etiologic agent. Dis. Colon Rectum 19:253, 1976.
571. Slavin, R. E., Millan, J. C., & Mullins, G. M.: Pathology of intermittent high dose cyclophosphamide therapy. Hum. Pathol. 6:693-709, 1975.
572. Slavin, R. E., Dias, M. A., & Sarai, R.: Cytosine arabinoside induced gastrointestinal toxic alterations in sequential chemotherapeutic protocols. A clinico-pathologic study of 33 patients. Cancer 42:1747-1759, 1978.
573. Slone, D., Jick, H., Lewis, G. P., et al.: Intravenously given ethacrynic acid and gastrointestinal bleeding. J.A.M.A. 209:1668-1671, 1969.
574. Smart, R. F., Ramsden, D. A., Gear, M. W. L., et al.: Severe pseudomembranous colitis after lincomycin and clindamycin. Br. J. Surg. 63:25-29, 1976.
575. Smith, B.: The Neuropathology of the Alimentary Tract. p. 80. Edward Arnold, London, 1972.
576. Smith, B.: Pathologic changes in the colon produced by anthraquinone purgatives. Dis. Colon Rectum 16:455-458, 1973.
577. Smith, B. M., Skillman, J. J., Edwards, B. G., Silen, W.: Permeability of the human gastric mucosa. Alteration by acetylsalicylic acid and ethanol. N. Engl. J. Med. 285:716-721, 1971.
578. Smithells, R. W.: Thalidomide, absent appendix, and sweating. Lancet 1:1042, 1978.
579. Sogge, M. R., & Butler, M. L.: Mallory-Weiss syndrome induced by the oral electrolyte overload technique for colonoscopy preparation. Gastrointest. Endosc. 26:51-52, 1980.
580. Speare, G. S.: Melanosis coli. Experimental observations on its production and elimination in 23 cases. Am. J. Surg. 82:631, 1951.
581. Sperling, H. V., & Reed, W. G.,: Herpetic gastritis. Digest. Dis. 22:1033-1034, 1977.
582. Sperling, I. L.: Adverse reactions with long-term use of phenylbutazone and oxyphenylbutazone. Lancet 2:906, 1976.
583. Spira, I. A., Rubenstein, R., Wolff, D., & Wolff, W. I.: Fecal impaction following methadone ingestion simulating acute intestinal obstruction. Ann. Surg. 181:15-19, 1975.
584. Spiro, H. M.: Stomach damage from aspirin, steroids and antimetabolites. Am. J. Digest Dis. 7:733, 1962.
585. Spiro, R. K., & Kysilewskyj, R. M.: Iatrogenic ileus secondary to medication. J. Med Soc. N.J. 70:565–567, 1973.
586. Stanley, R. J., Melson, G. L., & Tedesco, F. J.: The spectrum of radiographic findings in antibiotic-related pseudomembranous colitis. Radiology 111:519, 1974.
587. Stanton, P. E., Wilson, J. P., Lamis, P. A., & Letton, A. H.: Acute abdominal complications induced by anticoagulant therapy. Am. Surg. 40:1-14, 1974.
588. Stark, F. R., Ninos, N., Hutton, J., et al.: Candida peritonitis and cimetidine. Lancet 2:74, 1978.
589. Steer, H. W., & Colin-Jones, D. G.: Melanosis coli: studies on the toxic effects of irritant purgatives. J. Pathol. 115:199-205, 1975.
590. Steeves, R. A., & Bataini, J. P.: Neoplasms induced by megavoltage radiation in the head and neck region. Cancer 47:1770-1774, 1981.
591. Stein, H. B., & Urowitz, M. B.: Gold induced enterocolitis. Case report and literature review. J. Rheumatol. 3:21, 1976.
592. Sterioff, S., Orringer, M. B., & Cameron, J. L.: Colon perforation associated with steriod therapy. Surgery 75:56-58, 1974.
593. Sternlieb, J. J., McIlrath, D. C., van Heerden, J. A., & Harrison, E. G.: Starch peritonitis and its prevention. Arch. Surg. 112:458-461, 1977.
594. Stillman, A. E., Weinberg, M., Mast, W. C., & Palpant, S.: Ischemic bowel disease attibutable to ergot. Gastroenterology 72:1336-1337, 1977.
595. Stillman, A. E., & Martin, R. J.: Tetracycline-induced esophageal ulcerations. Arch. Dermatol. 115:1005, 1979.
596. Stowers, J. M., & Bewsher, P. D.: Studies on the mechanisms of weight reduction by phenformin Postgrad. Med. J. 45(Suppl.):13-16, 1969.
597. Stroehlein, J. R., Sedlack, R. E., Hofmann, H. N. II, et al.: Clindamycin associated colitis. Mayo Clin. Proc. 49:240-243, 1974.
598. Struiver, P. C., & Gould, T. J. L. M.: Corticosteroids and liver amoebiasis. Br. Med. J. 2:394-395, 1978.
599. Sturges, H. F., & Krone, C. L.: Ulceration and stricture of the jejunum in a patient on long-term indomethacin therapy: report of a

case. Am. J. Gastroenterol. 59:162-169, 1973.
600. Sugawa, C., Lucas, C. E., Rosenberg, B. F., Riddle, J. M., & Walt, A. J.: Differential topography of acute erosive gastritis due to trauma or sepsis, ethanl and aspirin. Gastrointest. Endosc. 19:127-130, 1973.
601. Sugimura, T., & Fujimura, S.: Tumour production in the glandular stomach of the rat by N-methyl-N′-nitro-N-nitro-soguanide. Nature 216:943-944, 1967.
602. Susnow, D. A.: Oleogranuloma of the rectum. Am. J. Surg. 83:496, 1952.
603. Sutherland, D. E., Chan, F. Y., Foucar, E., et al.: The bleeding cecal ulcer in the transplant patient. Surgery 86:386-397, 1979.
604. Sutton, D. R., & Gosnold, J. K.: Oesophageal ulceration due to clindamycin. Br. Med. J. 1:1598, 1978.
605. Svanes, K., Leiknes, K. A., Varhaug, J. E., & Soreide, O.: Aspirin damage to ischemic gastric mucosa in shocked cats. Scand. J. Gastroenterol. 14:633-639, 1979.
606. Swartzberg, J. E., Maresca, R. M., & Remington, J. S.: Clinical study of gastrointestinal complications associated with clindamycin therapy. J. Infect. Dis. 135(Suppl.):S99-S103, 1977.
607. Symmers, W. St. C.: Simulation of cancer by oil granulomas of therapeutic origin. Br. Med. J. 11:1536, 1955.
608. Takeuchi, T., Ensrud, E. R., & Steggerda, F. R.: The effects of large doses of aspirin and cortisone on the goblet cells and the mucosal membranes in the small and large intestine. Am. J. Digest. Dis. 17:49-53, 1972.
609. Talbot, R., & Rees, H.: Perforated duodenal ulcer on diflunisal (Dolobid). Br. Med. J. 2:1229, 1978.
610. Tanser, A. R., & Keat, E. C. B.: Phenindione-induced haemorrhagic ulcerative colitis. Br. Med. J. 1:388, 1966.
611. Tarnawski, A., Krause, W. J., & Ivey, K. J.: Effect of glucagon on aspirin-induced gastric mucosal damage in man. Gastroenterology 74:240, 1978.
612. Tarpila, S.: Morphological and functional response of human small intestine to ionizing radiation. Scand. J. Gastroenterol. 6(Suppl):9-48, 1971.
613. Taylor, R. H., Menzies-Gow, N., Lovell, D., et al.: Misleading response of malignant gastric ulcers to cimetidine. Lancet 1:686-688, 1978.
614. Taylor, R. T., Huskisson, E. C., Whitehouse, G. H., et al.: Gastric ulceration occurring during indomethacin therapy. Br. Med. J. 4:734-737, 1968.
615. Tedesco, F. J., Barton, R. W., & Alpers, D. H.: Clindamycin-associated colitis. A prospective study. Ann. Intern. Med. 81:429-433, 1974.
616. Tedesco, F. J.: Ampicillin-associated diarrhea—A prospective study. Am. J. Digest. Dis. 20:295-297, 1975.
617. Tedesco, F. J., Napier, J., Gamble, W., et al.: Therapy of antibiotic-associated pseudomembranous colitis. J. Clin. Gastroenterol. 1:51-54, 1979.
618. Tedesco, F. J.: Antibiotic associated pseudomembranous colitis with negative proctosigmoidoscopy examination. Gastroenterology 77:295-297, 1079.
619. Tedesco, F. J.: Bacitracin therapy in antibiotic-associated pseudomembranous colitis. Dig. Dis. Sci. 25:783-784, 1980.
620. Teplick, J. G., Teplick, S. K., Ominsky, S. H., & Haskin, M. E.: Esophagitis caused by oral medication. Radiology 134:23-25, 1980.
621. Tepperman, B. L., Miller, T. A., & Johnson, L. R.: Effect of 16, 16-dimethyl prostaglandin E_2 on ethanol-induced damage to canine oxyntic mucosa. Gastroenterology 75:1061-1065, 1978.
622. Teresa, E. de, Vera, A., Ortigosa, J., et al.: Interaction between anticoagulants and contraceptives: an unsuspected finding. Br. Med. J. 2:1260-1261, 1979.
623. Terplan, K., Paine, J. R., Sheffer, J., et al.: Fulminating gastroenterocolitis caused by staphylococci. Gastroenterology 24:476, 1953.
624. Teutsch, W., Gastroduodenale komplikationen der steriod- und phenylbutazon-behandlung aus chirurgischer sicht. Zentralbl. Chir. 93:926, 1968.
625. Tewfik, T. L., & Schloss, M. D.: Ingestion of lye and other corrosive agents—a study of 86 infants and child cases. J. Otolaryngol. 9:72-77, 1980.
626. Thein, S. L., & Asquith, P.: Pneumatosis coli: complication of practolol. Br. Med. J. 1:268, 1977.

627. Thomas, F. B., Steinbaugh, J. T., Fromkes, J. J., et al.: Inhibitory effect of coffee on lower esophageal sphincter pressure. Gastroenterology 79:1262-1266, 1980.
628. Thomas, W. E. G.: Duodeno-gastric reflux—A common factor in pathogenesis of gastric and duodenal ulcer. Lancet 2:1166-1168, 1980.
629. Thomson, G., Clark, A. H., Hare, K., & Spilg, W. G. S.: Pseudomembranous colitis after treatment with metronidazole. Br. Med. J. 282:864-865, 1981.
630. Thorpe, J. A. C., & Nysenbaum, A.: Co-trimoxazole fatality. Lancet 1:276-277, 1978.
631. Thorsen, W. B., Western, D. Tanaka, Y., et al.: Aspirin injury to the gastric mucosa. Gastrocamera observations of the effect of pH. Arch. Intern. Med. 111:499-505, 1968.
632. Toffler, R. B., Pingoud, E., & Burrell, M. I.: Acute colitis related to penicillin and penicillin derivatives. Lancet 2:707-709, 1978.
633. Totten, M. A., Gregg, J. A., Fremont-Smith, P., & Legg, M.: Clinical and pathological spectrum of antibiotic-associated colitis. Am. J. Gastroenterol. 69:311-319, 1978.
634. Trier, J. S.: Morphologic alterations induced by methotrexate in the mucosa of the human proximal intestine. I. Serial observations by light microscopy. Gastroenterology 42:295-305, 1962.
635. Trier, J. S.: Morphologic alterations induced by methotrexate in the mucosa of human proximal intestine. II. Electron microscopic observation. Gastroenterology 43:407-424, 1962.
636. Trynka, Y. M., & LaMont, J. T.: Association of Clostridium difficile toxin with symptomatic relapse of chronic inflammatory bowel disease. Gastroenterology 80:693-696, 1980.
637. Tures, J. F., Townsend, W. F., & Rose, H. D.: Cephalosporin-associated pseudomembranous colitis. J.A.M.A. 236:948-949, 1976.
638. Turkie, P. V.: Perforation of peptic ulcer after withdrawal of cimetidine. Br. Med. J. 2:1022-1023, 1977.
639. Utz, J. P.: Current and future chemotherapy of central nervous system fungal infections. Adv. Neurol. 6:127-132, 1974.
640. Van Thiel, D. H., Gavaler, J. S., & Stremple, J.: Lower esophageal sphincter pressure in women using sequential oral contraceptives. Gastroenterology 71:232-234, 1976.
641. Varki, A. P., Armitage, J. O., & Feagler, J. R.: Typhlitis in acute leukemia. Cancer 43:695-697, 1979.
642. Vickery, R. E.: Unusual complication of excessive ingestion of vitamin C tablets. Int. Surg. 58:422-423, 1973.
643. Viteri, A. L., Howard, P. H., & Dyck, W. P.: The spectrum of lincomycin-clindamycin colitis. Gastroenterology 66:1137-1144, 1974.
644. Vuthibhagdee, A., & Harris, N. F.: Antral stricture as a delayed complication of iron intoxication. Radiology 103:163-164, 1972.
645. Wagner, M. L., Rosenberg, H. S., Fernbach, D. J., & Singleton, E. B.: Typhlitis: A complication of leukemia in childhood. Am. J. Roentgenol. 109:341-350, 1970.
646. Walker, V., & Taylor, W. H.: Cigarette smoking, chronic peptic ulceration, and pepsin 1 secretion. Gut 20:971-976, 1979.
647. Wallace, W. A., Orr, C. M. E., & Bearn, A. R.: Perforation of chronic peptic ulcer after cimetidine. Br. Med. J. 2:865-866, 1977.
648. Walsh, J., & Kneafsey, D. V.: Phenobarbitone-induced oesophagitis: a case report. Ir. Med. J. 73:399, 1980.
648a. Wands, J. R., Weiss, S. W., Yardley, J. H., & Maddrey, W. C.: Chronic inorganic mercury poisoning due to laxative abuse. Am. J. Med. 57:92–101, 1974.
649. Warnes, H., Lehmann, H. E., & Ban T. A.: Adynamic ileus during psychiatric medication. Canad. Med. Assoc. J. 96:1112-1113, 1967.
650. Warshaw, A. L., Welch, J. P., & Ottinger, L. W.: Acute perforation of the colon associated with chronic corticosteroid therapy. Am. J. Surg. 131:442-446, 1976.
651. Wass, J. A. H., Thorner, M. O., Besser, G. M., et al.: Gastrointestinal bleeding in patients on bromocriptine. Lancet 2:851, 1976.
652. Watney, P. J. M.: Copper intrauterine devices and the small intestine. Brit. Med. J. 2:255-256, 1978.
653. Watson, W. C., Kutty, P. K., & Colcleugh, R. G.: Does cimetidine cause ileus in the burned patient? Lancet 2:720, 1977.
654. Watts, H. D., & Admirand, W. H.: Mallory-Weiss syndrome. A reappraisal. J.A.M.A. 230:1674, 1974.
655. Webb, A. J.: Oleocysts presenting as rectal tumours. Br. J. Surg. 53:410, 1966.

656. Webster, J., Petrie, J. C., & Mowat, N. A. G.: Erosive gastritis and duodenitis during continuous cimetidine treatment. Br. Med. J. 1:20-21, 1978.
657. Weisbrot, I. M., Liber, A. F., & Gordon, B. S.: The effects of therapeutic radiation on colonic mucosa. Cancer 36:931-940, 1975.
658. Weisburger, W. G., Hutcheon, D. F., Yardley, J. H., et al.: Cryptosporidiosis in an immunosuppressed renal transplant recipient with IgA deficiency. Am. J. Clin. Pathol. 72:474-478, 1979.
659. Weiss, S. M., Rutenberg, H. L., Paskin, D. L., & Zeren, H. A.: Gut lesions due to slow-release KCl tablets. N. Engl. J. Med. 262, 111, 1977.
660. Weissman, I.: Enterogastric regurgitation during barium enema examination. Am. J. Roentgenol. 88:637, 1962.
661. Weston, J. T., & Guin, G. H. Epithelial atypias with chemotherapy in 100 acute childhood leukemias. Cancer 8:179-186, 1955.
662. White, R. S., Fuqua, W. B., & Barrett, O.: The effect of 5-fluorouracil on small bowel mucosa. J. Surg. Oncol. 3:501-506, 1971.
663. Whitehead, R.: p. 98. Mucosal Biopsies of the Gastrointestinal Tract, 2nd ed. W. B. Saunders, Philadelphia, 1979.
664. Whitney, B., & Croxon, R.: Dysphagia caused by cardiac enlargement. Clin. Radiol. 23:147-152, 1972.
665. Whittle, B. J. R.: Mechanisms underlying gastric mucosal damage induced by indomethacin and bile-salts and the actions of prostaglandins. Br. J. Pharmacol. 60:455-460, 1977.
666. Williams, J. G.: Drug-induced oesophageal injury. Br. Med. J. 2:273, 1979.
667. Willoughby, J. M. T.: The alimentary system. In: D'Arcy, P. F., & Griffin, J. P., Eds. Iatrogenic Disease, 2nd ed. p. 141. Oxford University Press, Oxford, 1979.
668. Wilson, E.: A caecal mass due to the intraperitoneal injection of radioactive zirconium phosphate. Aust. N.Z. J. Surg. 35:237-238, 1966.
669. Winawer, S. J., Sullivan, L. W., Herbert, V., et al.: The jejunal mucosa in patients with nutritional folate deficiency and megaloblastic anemia. N. Engl. J. Med. 272:892, 1965.
670. Wittoesch, J. H., Jackman, R. J., & MacDonald, J. R.: Melanosis coli: general review and study of 887 cases. Dis. Colon Rectum 1:172-180, 1958.
671. Wofford, J. D., & Cummins, A. J.: Hemorrhage from duodenal ulcer during the administration of reserpine. N. Engl. J. Med. 255:1193-1194, 1956.
672. Wolff, G.: Does alcohol cause chronic gastritis? Scand. J. Gastroenterol. 5:289, 1970.
673. Wormsley, K. G.: Smoking and duodenal ulcer. Gastroenterology 75:139-142, 1978.
674. Wright, L. E., & Castell, D. O.: The adverse effect of chocolate on lower esophageal sphincter pressure. Am. J. Digest Dis. 20:703-707, 1975.
675. Wright, R. A.: Upper-esophageal perforation with a flexible endoscope secondary to cervical osteophytes. Dig. Dis. Sci. 25:66-68, 1980.
676. Young, D. W., Cottam, J., & Hoult, J. G.: Complications of oxyprenalol treatment. Lancet 2:1133, 1977.
677. Zheutlin, N., Lasser, E. C., & Rigler, L. G.: Clinical studies on the effect of barium in the peritoneal cavity following rupture of the colon. Surgery 32:967, 1952.

19

The Pancreas

Robert H. Riddell and Francis H. Straus II

ACUTE PANCREATITIS (AP)

The association between alcohol ingestion and acute pancreatitis has been recognized for decades. However, the possibility that acute pancreatitis could also be caused by drugs was first suggested by Zion et al.,[183] who in 1955 described acute hemorrhagic pancreatitis (AHP) associated with cortisone therapy. Since then a variety of other drugs have been implicated in the etiology of this disease, and the evidence is now sufficiently strong that some drugs can safely be included in the list of factors predisposing to the development of AP. However, the evidence for still others is less strong, while some substances have been implicated so infrequently or in so little detail that the association between them and AP may well be entirely coincidental.

Pathophysiology of Acute Pancreatitis

With the gradual increase in our knowledge of the pathophysiology of AP, at least a partial explanation exists as to why some drugs are associated with this disease. As a result it is possible to predict to some extent drugs that can occasionally be expected to be incriminated as a cause of this disease. Nevertheless, many cases inevitably remain idiopathic.

There is little doubt that the final common pathway is one that involves the release of enzymes from the exocrine pancreas, their activation, and the effects of activated enzymes both locally and systemically. The systemic manifestations of such enzyme activity may include hypovolemia, shock, myocardial and respiratory depression, and death. However, this is the most severe form of the disease, and very little is known of its less severe forms—especially from the pathologic viewpoint—and also of their sequelae. Thus it is generally thought that a relatively mild insult may cause only interstitial edema, or interstitial pancreatitis if the edema is accompanied by an inflammatory exudate. This may either resolve without trace or cause a degree of interstitial fibrosis. At this stage there may be evidence of enzyme release as indicated by local fat necrosis at autopsy or laparotomy, or by the presence of these enzymes in the blood or urine. Since the larger interlobular ducts run in the interstitial tissue between the pancreatic lobules, and in view of the apparent sparing of the pancreatic parenchyma, this stage of AP is likely to be the result of damage to these ducts, presumably something toxic within the large duct system. The disease may sometimes progress to more severe forms, with areas of hemorrhage that may eventually involve the whole pancreas.

Many of the difficulties in the clinicopathologic correlation of AP occur because of the relatively poor relationship between its symptoms, biochemistry, and pathology. Some patients may therefore exhibit hyperamylasemia and uria when challenged with a small quantity of a drug suspected of causing their disease, during which time no symptoms are present, but when damage to the pancreatic parenchyma is presumably occurring because of the release and detection of pancreatic enzymes in the urine or blood.

Factors known to predispose AP include alcohol, biliary-tract disease, hypercalcemia, local trauma, hyperlipemia, postoperative and ischemic states, viral diseases, hepatic disease, and drugs and other toxic substances; there are also hereditary forms of the disease. What then do these have in common that permits all of them to cause the end-stage picture of acute pancreatitis? It is relatively easy to speculate that when ampullary gallstones are present and there is a common opening of the pancreatic and common bile ducts that reflux of bile may occur into the pancreatic duct, but this would have to reach the parenchyma to cause damage. To do this the refluxing bile must either injure the epithelium in the pancreatic duct or reach the terminal ductules to exert an influence directly on the parenchymal cells, possibly by altering membrane permeability and thereby both injuring the parenchymal cells and allowing the release of enzymes.

It is not positively known whether bile or bile salts can activate pancreatic enzymes directly in humans. Under experimental conditions bile, bile salts, and duodenal contents may cause acute pancreatitis when injected directly into the pancreatic duct. However, such injection is frequently done under pressure, and it is uncertain whether these conditions are applicable to human disease. In one study in which sodium taurocholate injection was made directly into the pancreatic duct of Wistar rats,[1] it was apparent that the severity of the disease was proportional to the concentration of the salt, and that the first pathologic effect to occur appeared to be hemorrhage of the entire ductal tree, which occurred almost immediately following injection. Dissolution of the duct wall and adjacent parenchyma occurred within about 1 minute of the injection of 0.2 cc of a 5 percent solution of the salt. Intimal detachment also occurred in local vessels, with extravasation of red cells suggesting that the hemorrhage, at least in the initial phase of the model, was not elastase-induced, as had been previously supposed. Elastase released from the parenchymal cells had also been implicated in the blood-vessel damage in AHP. However, such release may clearly contribute in the later stages of the disease.

Physiologically, the pancreatic enzymes released in AP are secreted in an inactive form, and their conversion into active enzymes depends on the action of active trypsin and calcium. Nevertheless the problem remains that although it seems likely that bile salts can activate inactive enzymes released from the parenchyma, this has yet to be satisfactorily documented. The recognized association of AP with gallstones, including autopsy cases in which AHP was accompanied by a gallstone impacted in the ampulla of Vater,[53] adds strongly to the evidence suggesting that pancreatic enzymes may be activated directly by bile. However the means of enzyme activation in AP caused by other disease processes has still to be defined. It is likely that inappropriate enzyme activation may occur, since free trypsin has been recovered from the pancreatic juice of patients with acute pancreatitis.[58a] It is also possible that trypsin activation may be initiated by cathepsin B, a lysosomal enzyme.[60a]

In humans, the activation of pancreatic enzymes normally occurs in the gut lumen. The initial step is the activation of trypsinogen to trypsin, in the presence of calcium, by enterokinase, which is itself produced by the epithelium (absorptive cells only) of the duodenum and proximal 15 cm of jejunum.[72] Active trypsin then activates all other pancreatic enzymes. Clearly, duodenal contents refluxed into the pancreatic duct could include activated enzymes. Whether or not the cells of the sphincter of Oddi and the ampulla or Vater secrete enterokinase, and if they do whether it is present in sufficient quantities in the refluxed juice to initiate AHP, also remains unknown. Drugs causing either relaxation of the sphincter or causing an increase in intraluminal pressure, such as happens with vomiting or with the administration of morphine or bethanechol, might therefore be expected to predispose to the development of AP. Since this seems not to occur, it can only be supposed that enterokinase is either not present or is present in insufficient quantity to cause pancreatitis.

It is also known that calcium is required for trypsin activation. This is of interest in that hypercalcemia of any cause appears to predispose to the development of AP, and it is therefore likely that drugs causing hypercalcemia may similarly predispose patients to the development of the disease.

In patients with alcohol-induced AP there may be intraductal liberation of small amounts of activated trypsin, associated with disproportionately high concentrations of protein, a variety of zymogens, and trypsin inhibitor.[141] These abnormalities tend to remit when alcohol ingestion stops, raising the question of whether the trypsin activation is a result of the high levels of protein in the duct in this phase of the disease. Irrespective of the mechanism, these substances may be able to initiate the activation of other enzymes within the duct system. The secretion of trypsin inhibitors may also be reflected by an experimental decrease in serum antiprotease activity,[76] accompanied by a decrease in the levels of total hemolytic complement, C3, and C4 levels; also, serum from experimental animals was chemotactic for polymorphs. However, the AP induced by alcohol, and probably the familial form also, occur against a background of chronic pancreatitis, and are probably best not compared with other forms of AP unassociated with this lesion.

A further metabolic abnormality that appears to predispose to AP is hypertriglyceridemia. The mechanism involved in this is again unknown, but in many alcoholics it is well documented that episodes of AP occur when patients are hypertriglyceridemic, and this change appears to be a primary phenomenon. Some of these patients, when rendered hypertriglyceridemic artifically,[24] develop a clinical picture resembling AP; in many of them, hyperamylasemia is also present. It remains confusing that some patients with clinical AP have hyperamylasemia without hypertriglyceridemia, while the converse appears to be the case for other patients. Whether this is the result of mistiming in carrying out these estimations is not apparent. In the case of patients with an alcoholic background in whom chronic pancreatitis also probably exists, one can speculate that the finding of hypertriglyceridemia at the time of AP is incidental. However, many other diseases associated with hypertriglyceridemia are also associated with AP, so that the association is probably genuine. Such other diseases include familial hyperlipoproteinemias types I, II, and V and prostatic carcinoma treated by castration followed by estrogen therapy; the association is also seen in pregnancy and in women taking estrogens. The fact that several drugs that increase serum triglycerides may also be associated with AP is therefore less surprising.

In a review, Cameron[25] reported 19 patients with AP clinically, of whom only 5 exhibited hyperamylasemia, although all had hyperlipemia—which electrophoretically was usually of the types (I or V) associated with AP in patients with familial hypertriglyceridemia. He speculated that the mechanism of causation of the AP may have been the hydrolysis of triglycerides in the pancreatic capillaries, caused by lipase, and that this in turn released large amounts of free fatty acids which may have either damaged the acinar cells directly or produced microthrombi resulting in AP. However, it was found in a subsequent study that AP could exist with or without hyperlipemia, but that when the latter was present the triglyceride levels were over 400 mg/100 ml. Further investigation of 22 patients showed that 16 had fasting triglyceridemia. When given a 250 gm lipid load, 20 of the patients developed triglyceride levels greater than 500 mg/dl, while 2 whose levels rose over 3,000 mg/dl developed abdominal pain similar to, but less severe than, that experienced during their previous bouts of AP. Of even more interest was the fact that when 12 similar patients were given a diet to induce hypertriglyceridemia under carefully controlled circumstances in which alcohol could be excluded, 7 of 11 that became hypertriglyceridemic also developed abdominal pain within 36 hours, coinciding with their peak triglyceride level, while 4 simultaneously became hyperamylasemic. It is therefore apparent that alcohol can induce fasting hyperlipemia, and that within this group of patients either alcohol or dietary manipulation can further raise the triglyceride levels. Some of these patients will develop abdominal symptoms similar to those seen in AP, while a proportion of these will also show evidence of enzyme release into the blood. The mechanism involved in those patients who develop acute pancreatitis in the absence of hypertriglyceridemia remains to be determined. Similarly, the effects of these manipulations in a nonalcoholic population is also unclear.

Finally, the association between ischemia and AP is worthy of mention, despite being relatively poorly documented, since many of the agents associated with AP are potent diuretics. The fact that AP is sometimes associated with the postsurgical state raises the question of whether these cases are secondary to blood loss and ischemia, or whether hypovolemia itself might not somehow predispose to AP. Foulis[53] suggested that in AHP in which panlobular necrosis was not present, it might be possible to distinguish this group of patients morphologically. In a retrospective analysis of autopsy material he found that two distinct patterns of necrosis were present. One of these was primarily periductal and was associated with both alcohol abuse and cholelithiasis; this pattern was also associated with concretions within the duct together with polymorphs around the concretions (Fig. 19-1). A second pattern was one of perilobular necrosis in which the periphery of the lobules was involved rather than the periductal region (Fig. 19-2). The part of the lobule involved was the opposite to that in which the arterial supply was located. Since these arteries are probably endarteries, this is almost certainly the zone most prone to ischemic changes. In contrast to the case for the periductal necrosis group, the associated etiologies in the perilobular necrosis group were septic shock (5 of 9 patients), cardiogenic shock (2 of 9 patients), and "postoperative" pancreatitis in 1 patient. The ninth patient had no obvious association. This raises the inevitable question of whether patients given either antihypertensive drugs or vasodilators if bleeding from the gastrointestinal tract (as from esophageal varices) are

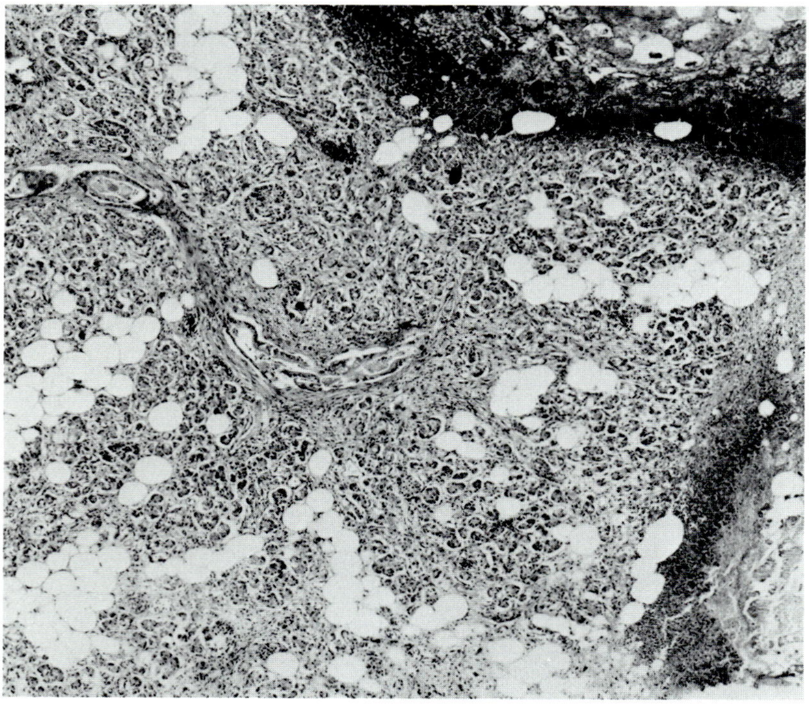

Fig. 19-1. Acute hemorrhagic pancreatitis involving primarily the periphery of a pancreatic lobule. H&E, × 40.

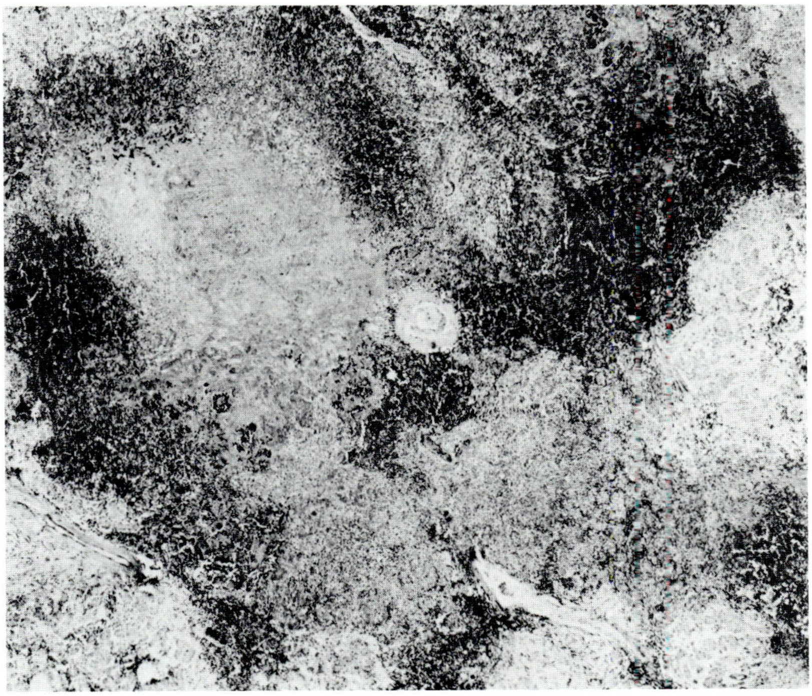

Fig. 19-2. Acute hemorrhagic pancreatitis involving primarily the periductal region of the pancreas. H&E, × 40.

predisposed to develop this pattern of AHP. It should certainly be expected.

There have been surprisingly few studies on the electron-microscopic appearances of AP in humans. In one good study, Helin et al.[71] examined areas of pancreas that were edematous by light-microscopy. Zymogen granules were increased in number, had lost the usual variability with osmium fixation, and showed peripheral dissolution. Increased autophagic activity was apparent. Acinar lumina were dilated and microvilli had been lost. The interstitium showed fibrillar material suggesting that it had been penetrated by secretory products.

SUBSTANCES CAUSING ACUTE PANCREATITIS

The substances causing AP will be considered under the major categories of hormones, diuretics, antibiotics, antimitotic agents, iatrogenic hypercalcemia, analgesics, and finally a miscellaneous group of substances including many for which the evidence of causation is rather limited. Alcohol is mentioned in the previous section and in the section dealing with chronic pancreatitis. Mechanisms will be considered where evidence is forthcoming.

Hormones

These are the estrogens (including contraceptives) and steroids.

Estrogens. Since the first suggestion in 1970 of this side-effect of estrogen therapy,[9] sufficient evidence has accumulated that the relationship between estrogens and AP can reasonably be accepted. Furthermore, estrogens are known to produce mild hypertriglyceridemia in many patients without lipid abnormalities,[70] and there also seems to be a degree of correlation between estrogen and triglyceride levels.[163] The latter effect may be marked in patients with lipid abnormalities,[58,184] when high triglyceride levels occur at the same time as the AP.[24,25] However, estrogen-induced pancreatitis is similar to alcoholic pancreatitis in that it has been reported in the absence of hypertriglyceridemia.[24,25] Nevertheless, the exact role of the latter remains uncertain. Further evidence of an association between estrogens and AP is a patient whose episodes of disease coincided with estrogen administration.[39]

Foster and Powell[52] reported a patient with multiple infarcts in a variety of organs due to thrombotic disease, suggesting an underlying ischemic basis, but while triglyceride levels were not reported for this case, there is a possibility that hypertriglyceridemic pancreatitis caused a defibrination syndrome resulting in systemic thrombosis.

Patients in whom estrogen-induced AP has been reported were taking estrogens either for contraception (usually with progestogens), menstrual disorders, menopausal symptoms, or for prostatic carcinoma. Most of the patients seem to have developed symptoms within the first 3 months of therapy, but the disease seems to be clinically mild, with only one reported fatality.[52]

Steroids. Despite the fact that steroids were the first drugs to be associated with AP, prompting numerous case reports, the evidence for steroid-induced pancreatitis[6,19,27,36,68,124,128,145,156] is more difficult to evaluate. In many of the cases reported the patients were receiving multiple drugs, some of which are now associated with AP, while others had debilitating diseases, being treated with steroids, that may also have predisposed to the development of AP. Nevertheless, there remain a sufficient number of patients in whom there is no good alternative explanation, including many cases affecting children,[6,128,145] to provide cause for justifying the association. The precise mechanism of causation is unknown, but in rabbits cortisol induces diffuse ductular hyperplasia similar to that seen following obstruction of the pancreatic duct,[14] while in humans ACTH reduces lipase and protein secretion without affecting volume or bicarbonate secretion.[63] It is unclear whether protein retention predisposes to AP under these circumstances.

Focal ectasia of pancreatic acini that is not dissimilar to that seen in uremia[8] and which may leave only a peripheral rim of cytoplasm, has been described[27] with inspissated secretions within the lumen. While this was seen in up to 60 percent of patients who had been treated with steroids, it was also seen in 24 percent of controls. However, within the same group of patients, 28 percent also had evidence of pancreatitis morphologically, compared with less than 4 percent of the control group.

Steroid-associated pancreatitis, unlike that associated with estrogens, appears to be a serious disease. Evaluable cases in the literature suggest that in over half of all fatal cases the disease was at least partly responsible for the patient's death. A variety of steroid preparations have been incriminated, including ACTH. However, both the dose and the time interval to the development of AP are extremely variable, the doses given varying between 8 and 200 mg of prednisone daily, and the latent interval average about 9 months, the shortest being 1 week and the longest appearing to be over 7 years. The credibility of such long intervals is questionable (see Chapter 1).

Diuretics

These include the thiazides, furosemide, chlorthalidone, ethacrynic acid, and diazoxide.

The association between diuretics and AP has been relatively tentative, however, two studies—one by Bourke,[18] the other by Moir[118]—have found that the frequency of diuretics ingested by the disease group was approximately two and one-half times that found in a control group.

Thiazides. This group of diuretics is derived from the sulfonamides (see below). Only a few reports have reached the literature, but the evidence that this group of drugs can cause pancreatitis is strong. Johnston et al.[82] reported both the first 4 patients, and subsequently found that 10 of 20 patients receiving chlorothiazide developed a 50 to 100 percent increase in serum amylase.[35] Several other papers suggest a relationship between thiazides and AP[2, 41, 115, 176] but the evidence is rather more flimsy. In two of the case reports[2, 115] the patients were also pregnant, and since pregnancy is associated with AP it is possible that the disease was caused by either pregnancy or thiazides, or that an additive or even potentiating mechanism was involved. However, work with mice given pharmacologic quantities of chlorothiazide also showed an increased incidence of AP. In an interesting study by Pickleman et al.,[136] 21 of 72 patients with AP were said to have idiopathic disease. However, on further evaluation, 6 of the 21 were found to have taken thiazides for between 3 weeks and 5 years. Although no patients in this subgroup were hypercalcemic, 3 were found to have parathyroid hyperplasia at autopsy. Hypercalcemia has been documented in patients taking thiazides, and the possibility that it may do so intermittently must be considered. This association is explored further in Chapter 20.

Thiazide-associated pancreatitis appears to be a severe disease, with a mortality of 75 to 80 percent. The mean latent interval varied from 2 weeks to 15 months with a mean of about 3 to 4 months. Some of these patients were found to have inspissated material within the pancreatic duct system at autopsy.

Furosemide (Frusemide). It is not surprising that this substance has also been reported to cause AP, since it is related both stucturally as well as functionally to the thiazides. Two patients have been independently described with this association,[23, 84] both of whom developed recurrent symptoms and hyperamylasemia upon challenge with furosemide. The patient reported by Call et al.[23] was also noted to be hyperlipidemic. Six further patients have been described,[21, 164, 181] substantiating this association, even though they were not challenged; several of these were also chronic alcoholics, raising the question of exactly which agent was responsible for the AP, whether potentiation is possible when more than one possible cause is present, and also whether a chronically diseased pancreas is more susceptible to the actions of substance that tend to cause AP.

Available data suggest the onset of furosemide-induced AP about a month after the drug was started. Although 2 of 4 patients died, the pancreatitis was not the major cause of death, but may have been contributory.

Chlorthalidone. This diuretic is related more closely to the sulfonamides than to the thiazides. While only a single case report of chlorthalidone-associated AP appears,[83] the fact that other sulfonamides are a well-documented cause of AP (see below) makes this association very likely. This patient recovered but was not challenged.

Ethacrynic acid. This association is based on a tenuous case report[155] of a patient developing severe upper abdominal pain within days of being given two separate courses of this drug. The serum amylase was normal after the first episode and was not recorded after the second. At autopsy, marked pancreatic edema was found, which may have represented the interstitial edema seen in early AP. However, no parenchymal damage was recorded, and it is unlikely to have contributed to the patient's demise. It is interesting that there is no structural relationship between ethacrynic acid and any of the other diuretics.

Diazoxide. This drug is included on the grounds of a single case report of a patient developing AP 4 months after being started on diazoxide for chronic renal failure and hypertension.[40] Since no further information was given, the relationship should be regarded as extremely tenuous.

Antibiotics

These include the sulfonamides, tetracycline, rifampicin, isoniazid (INH), and pentamidine.

Sulfonamides. Although only three case reports exist, in two of these the possible association was confirmed by challenge with the drug, which was sulfamethizole in one instance[10] and salicylazasulfidine in the other.[16] The third patient was receiving sulfisoxazole.[116] Symptoms began within 2 weeks of the initial therapy but recurred within hours of the challenge, together with a variety of other manifestations that raised the question of an allergic etiology. All patients recovered. While these three cases in themselves seem few to justify an association, it should be remembered that the sulfonamide-derived diuretics (chlorothiazide, furosemide, and chlorthalidone) have also been incriminated in the causation of AP (see preceding section).

Tetracycline. This is a difficult association to evaluate, since it occurs largely in that group of pregnant women who were given large doses of tetracycline, usually intravenously, and who also developed acute fatty degeneration of the liver (see Chapter 17). In one study of this disease all five patients were reported to have pancreatitis,[177] while in a second study[89] autopsy revealed AP in six of eight patients. In their excellent review of this entire subject, Mallory and Kern[109] note that not all have been pregnant women.[132, 158] Tetracycline-associated AP has also been described in nonpregnant women, men, and children. Mallory and Kern point out that the disease occurs predictably within 3 weeks of the onset of therapy, that either large doses are used or abnormally high serum tetracycline levels are obtained, and that all patients have had associated liver disease. The possibility therefore remains that, since pancreatitis is a complication of other forms of liver disease, tetracycline has a strong potentiating or initiating action in this situation.

Rifampicin. In a single study on the side effects of rifampicin therapy in a large group of patients with tuberculosis, it was reported that 2.7 percent developed abdominal pain accompanied by hyperamylasemia, while hyperamylasemia unaccompanied by pain was present in a further 3.7 percent.[111] While the study was uncontrolled and no patients were challenged, the results are nevertheless highly suggestive of an association, while the fact that rifampicin attains high concentrations in the bile adds weight to a possible association.

In their review of drug-induced AP until 1975, Nakashima and Howard showed that among 112 patients reported in the English literature until 1975, antibiotics were second only to steroids as a cause of AP, and that rifampicin headed the antibiotics, with 20 cases.[123] It has also been shown that rifampicin has potent microsomal enzyme-inducing properties. The authors suggest that concentration of the drug in lysosomes, or a deficiency of tissue inhibitors of these enzymes, may play a role in susceptible individuals.

Pentamidine. Two patients have been described who developed clinical evidence of AP soon after beginning treatment for *Pneumocystis* infection with pentamidine. In one patient the disease recurred following a second course.[121] However, further evidence is required for this possible association.

Isoniazid. An odd situation exists here, in that one source[62] quotes a second to the effect of there being an AP—isoniazid association,[93] but there is no such mention in the quoted source. It is therefore assumed that there is no association between isoniazid and AP.

Antimitotics

These include azathioprine, mercaptopurine, and L-asparaginase.

Azathioprine. There is no real doubt that azathioprine is associated with AP. Initially this was suggested in patients who were immunosuppressed following renal transplantation[49]; however, doubt persisted because a variety of other factors existed which might also have been responsible, such as steroids, possible viral infections, and even the transplantation surgery itself. But there are now several reports of patients developing AP while on azathioprine only,[78, 86, 125, 129] and in some of these patients the diagnosis was confirmed by challenge. Perhaps the strongest evidence of such an association comes from the National Cooperative Crohn's Disease Study, in which patients were randomized to either azathioprine, prednisone, sulfasalazine, or a placebo (no drugs were used in combination). Despite the fact that all active drugs used have been associated with AP, 7 of 116 patients (6.2 percent) on azathioprine developed clinical evidence of AP, a number that was statistically significant when compared to those for other groups. (None of the patients had duodenal Crohn's disease).[109,165] Additional cases of AP have been reported in patients with lupus and glomerulonephritis who were treated with azathioprine, although usually in combination with steroids.[68,73] It is not without interest that in one study in which a uniformly fatal AHP was produced in dogs, with a mixture of bile and trypsin injected directly into the major pancreatic duct, the only animals that survived were those receiving azathioprine![87]

Symptoms began within 13–21 days of a dose of 50 to 150 mg of azathioprine daily, but ceased when it was stopped. It appears to be a relatively mild form of the disease.

Mercaptopurine. Because mercaptopurine is the active metabolite of azathioprine, an increased incidence of AP might be expected with this drug. Nevertheless this seems not to be the case and only one possible instance of mercaptopurine-associated AP has yet appeared in the literature, in a child with steroid-resistant renal disease.[74]

L-Asparaginase. The evidence here is also highly suggestive of an association with AP, although less well documented than with azathioprine. The bulk of the evidence comes from a variety of studies of acute leukemia in which L-asparaginase has been used, frequently in combination.[12,69,80,90,101,127,137,138,175,179] (and sometimes including azathioprine). Virtually all of these report AP as a complication of therapy, although the actual incidence varies markedly from series to series, the highest being 7 percent. The inclusion of a variety of other medications in such a sick group of patients raises the inevitable speculation over the exact contribution of L-asparaginase to the disease. One study comparing the incidence of pancreatitis in acute leukemic patients receiving asparaginase with a group of similar patients not receiving asparaginase strongly supported the association of the drug with AP.[101] There seems to be adequate data implicating this drug, and pseudocyst formation complicating the drug-induced pancreatitis has also been described.[61]

A wide range of time intervals between receiving L-asparaginase and the onset of disease was reported, varying from about 2 days after the drug was begun to about 10 weeks after it had been discontinued. The severity of the disease and the role it played in the demise of the patients reported is difficult to assess; the AP was reported to have been a major cause of death in some patients, but in most instances it seemed relatively mild.

Iatrogenic Hypercalcemia

Iatrogenic hypercalcemia associated with AP has been reported with vitamin D, the calcium infusion test, hyperalimentation, and hemodialysis.

The association between hypercalcemia and AP was mentioned in the pathophysiology section of this chapter and also in the discussion of thiazide diuretics. Originally it was reported in patients with hyperparathyroidism,[54,88,107,117] but it has gradually been apparent that hypercalcemia from other causes may also be associated with AP.[112] However, documentation is rather patchy, with only rare or single papers implicating vitamin D,[97] the calcium infusion test,[75] hemodialysis,[45] hyperalimentation,[110,160] or total parental nutrition (TPN).[79] The last reference is of particular interest in that it documents hypercalemia and AP in six patients receiving TPN. In four of these the parathormone level was measured, and was found to be normal in 2 and not detectable in 2; calcium infusion was also not a cause of the disease. The authors speculate that vitamin D metabolites may interfere with bone calcification or mobilize calcium from bone, and have also observed that the withdrawal of vitamin D from the TPN solution sometimes corrects the hypercalcemia, hypercalciuria, and osteomalacia in some patients.[79] They also note that TPN may be used in the treatment of AP, and suggest that this may in fact cause further damage to the pancreas.

Analgesics and Anti-inflammatory Agents

The AP-associated drugs in this category are acetaminophen (paracetamol), indomethacin, opiates, propoxyphene, salicylates, and sulindac.

The evidence to incriminate any members of this group of substances is relatively sparse, frequently consisting only of a suggestive case report. It is most convincing in the cases of acetaminophen and the opiates. In the introductory section to this chapter, the possibility that opiates might cause AP because of reflux of bile into the pancreatic duct following spasm of sphincter of Oddi was considered. It is not known whether the pain occasionally evoked is in fact secondary to mild pancreatitis or increased pressure within the pancreaticobiliary tree. In some patients, the injection of opiates produce elevations of serum amylase and rarely abdominal pain mimicking AP.[109] Nevertheless, documented AP or AHP has yet to be reported with this group of substances. Yet morphine, as well as bethanocol, and cholecystokinin, cause an increase in the pressure in the pancreatic duct.[178]

Acetaminophen has been associated with AP on three occasions.[37,56,57] In all instances it occurred as a result of an overdose and in the face of severe liver disease that in two instances was also induced by acetaminophen. In the third case it was at least partly alcohol-associated. While AP related to acetaminophen may therefore be genuine, when it occurs it appears to be a secondary problem in the face of an overdose.

Indomethacin, propoxyphene and salicylates. Each have only single case reports of AP, without challenge to incriminate them.[50,62,166] The most interesting case was that associated with salicylates, which occurred in a 2-year-old boy admitted with salicylate poisoning but no other cause for the disease.[166] Mallory and Kern[109] point out that other diseases causing acidotic states, such as diabetes, lactic acidosis, and uremia, have also been reported in association with AP. It is apparent that experimentally, salicylates produce reproducible damage to the pancreatic duct that can be prevented by the administration of prostaglandin PGE_2[168] or cimetidine.[169] However, the clinical use of cimetidine in acute alcoholic pancreatitis proved unsuccessful.[113]

Sulindac. Five reports of AP associated with sulindac had been received by the U.S. FDA Division of Drug Experience by mid-1979[4]; the disease began from 3 to 90 days after starting the drug. Until further information becomes available this should be treated with caution.

Alcohol

The pathophysiology and pathology of AP following alcohol is discussed on page 609. The typical pathology in chronic alcohol abusers with underlying chronic pancreatitis is discussed on page 618.

Miscellaneous

Intravenous drug abuse (possibly amphetamine-associated), anticholinesterase intoxication, cholestyramine, cimetidine, clofibrate, contrast media, cyproheptidine, histamine, methyldopa, penicillamine, phenformin, procainamide, valproic acid, and warfarin have all been associated with AP.

Intravenous Drug Abuse. Some patients habitually abusing drugs intravenously have been described as developing AP in association with a necrotizing angiitis.[31] Since a variety of drugs are involved, frequently in combination, it is extremely difficult to incriminate any single drug.[7] Furthermore, in this population, hepatitis B is common, and it is possible that the polyarteritis-like lesions produced by deposition of hepatitis B surface antigen-antibody (HB_sAg-Ab) complexes might cause an ischemic pattern of AP (see above). Nevertheless, some have attempted to incriminate methamphetamines in this syndrome.[31, 66, 148] In one study there was a degree of success in reproducing the lesions in Rhesus monkeys.[148] However, further evidence is required before this association can be accepted.

Anticholinesterase Intoxication. A single case report exists[43] in which a patient accidentally ingested an anticholinesterase (O-ethyl-S-phenylethylphosphenodithioate). Following resuscitation and a stormy course, she developed an epigastric swelling on the ninth day that was drained 3 days later. The authors strengthened their case for the toxin being responsible for the pseudocyst by showing that experimentally in dogs, it caused a marked increase in intraductal pressure, an increased secretin-stimulated flow, and marked interstitial edema with hyperamylasemia and hyperlipemia. They postulated that the clinical syndrome was caused by hypersecretion and duct obstruction. Morphologically, only acinar cell vacuolization was demonstrated, with edema in the dogs, while the clinical diagnosis was presumptive. Nevertheless, it seems likely that this toxic anticholinesterase can cause pancreatitis of unknown morphology, with subsequent pseudocyst formation.

Cholestyramine. Four patients were described by Casdorph et al.[28] as developing AP as a side-effect of cholestyramine administration given to patients with type II or IV hyperlipidemia. Because details were not included, definitive conclusions cannot be drawn.

Cimetidine. Only one case report of cimetidine-associated AP has been identified,[5] in a patient that was also receiving furosemide; however, animal experiments also suggest a possible association.[81] Further evidence is clearly required.

Clofibrate. A single report documents two cases of AP developing 6 and 10 weeks after starting clofibrate.[161] The lack of confirmatory evidence since this report, which was published in 1968, suggests that the cases were most likely coincidental.

Contrast-media. AP may rarely follow a variety of techniques designed to display the pancreaticobiliary tree radiologically. Thus, it has been reported following operative, oral, and intravenous cholangiography; the latter two followed oral sodium ipodate and intravenous meglumine iodipamide.[119] AP has also been reported following transhepatic cholangiography,[140] but by far the greatest number of cases follows endoscopic retrograde cholangiopancreatography (ERCP). It has been estimated that about 1 percent of all such procedures are followed by clinical AP,[15] and that it has invariably followed the injection of contrast media into the pancreatic duct, usually with sufficient pressure to cause visible acinar filling. Interestingly, none of the reports were fatal, but two-thirds of the patients had had previous episodes of AP. While the mechanism of causation is not known, there is a suggestion that the contrast medium may prevent enzyme secretion. Experimentally, ERCP may be followed by a hypersecretory phase.[144]

Cyproheptidine. This has been reported to cause an increased serum amylase level,[42] but, as yet, not AP.

Histamine. Two patients have been reported with relapsing pancreatitis who developed either marked hyperamylasemia or frank AP within 2 hours of histamine injection for gastric analysis.[157] This association has not been reported in patients without pancreatic disease.

Methyldopa. One case report exists in which a methyldopa challenge reaction was extremely suggestive of AP, including marked elevations of both amylase and lipase in association with an appropriate clinical syndrome.[146]

Penicillamine. The evidence here is minimal, and only three possible cases have been described, with little detail.[114]

Phenformin. There are several case reports suggesting that either AP or hyperamylasemia may be associated with phenformin ingestion.[30, 33, 60, 99, 149, 180, 182.] Some of these reports are less than convincing, and none describe challenge tests. Nevertheless, the evidence seems to suggest an association that requires further proof.

Procainamide. A single case report documents a patient with clinical AP associated with procainaimide-induced lupus that recurred following challenge.[48]

Valproic Acid. Although few cases of valproic acid-associated AP have been reported,[11, 26, 130] these are relatively well documented, occurred in children, and were confirmed by rechallenge in two patients, suggesting a definite relationship that time will probably confirm.

Warfarin. Only a single report of warfarin-associated AP exists, written in 1962,[93] describing two patients who were also taking thiazide diuretics. In view of the lack of confirmation this association remains in serious doubt.

SUBSTANCES CAUSING CHRONIC PANCREATITIS (CP)

A real problem exists when considering drugs that may cause chronic pancreatitis (CP). It is apparent from the section on AP that much of the evidence is extremely flimsy, and this is compounded when CP is discussed. In fact, the practical problems are almost insurmountable, for if CP is found clinically or at autopsy, all of the usual common causes for it must be excluded. From among the residual "idiopathic" group, only a high degree of suspicion in patients of a relatively young age, could hope to be taken with any degree of seriousness as drug associated CP. Consequently, there is no good example of CP in the literature that can be attributed to the effects of drugs. Nevertheless, as physicians become increasingly aware of drug-induced AP, the opportunity to examine the pancreas of these patients will most surely arise. Such opportunities should be grasped, so that the long-term effects of these diseases are documented, with particular emphasis as to whether they heal without a trace or ultimately produce CP.

The single toxin known to cause CP is, of course, alcohol. So many good reviews are available regarding this subject[152] that only a short description will be given here, together with selected references. In the section on pathophysiology, mention has been made of alcohol in pancreatitis—as is appropriate. The numerous papers by Sarles and his co-workers in particular have emphasized that the initial effect of alcohol on the pancreatic parenchyma is a phase of stimulation, with the production of increased quantities of secretion.[151, 153] After a period of time usually measured in months, this gradually changes, and the secretions become thick, protein-rich, and inspissated in the acini and terminal ductules. This ultimately causes atrophy of those lobules of the pancreas affected, so that the end result of the process is a focal obliteration of small islands of pancreas, with subsequent fibrosis. The hallmark of the alcoholic pancreas is therefore the picture of patchy fibrosis that varies considerably from area to area within the gland, but contrasts markedly with the diffusely atrophic appearance found following ligation of the major duct. Sarles argues that all other sequelae, including AHP, are the result of the protein-rich deposits. This appears reasonable, in that in the section on AP (see above), it is apparent that protein plugs are frequently present. It also agrees with the dogma that in the alcoholic, AHP does not occur in a normal pancreas. The elegant three-dimensional work by Nakamura[122] confirms the part that these plugs play in the genesis of both the early disease, and also confirms their subsequent calcification, particularly within the duct system, to produce the calcified concretions that are the hallmark of the disease.

Perhaps the only feature not adequately explained morphologically is that in humans, although it is true that the early lesion tends to be associated with proteinaceous concretions, there is nevertheless at autopsy often a disproportionate amount of interlobular fibrosis in areas where there seems to be no evidence of intralobular disease. A variety of possibilities exist, but a plausable explanation for this is that the fibrosis is a sequel to the marked interstitial and interlobular edema that appears to present in the early phases of the disease. Particularly if recurrent, this could result in organization rather than just absorption of exudate.

MISCELLANEOUS PANCREATIC DISEASE

Atrophy

A single case report[159] exists of a child who, in addition to having AHP, also showed pancreatic atrophy, with an excess of interlobular adipose tissue, associated with thiazide use. In retrospect, the former claim has been confirmed but the latter has not. Until further evidence appears to confirm a possible association between thiazides and pancreatic atrophy, this claim must be treated with some degree of scepticism.

Nuclear Inclusions

Mullick[120] reports the death, following boric acid ingestion, of a child who had inclusions in the cells of the pancreas. However, no further details are given. Others have reported the presence of intracytoplasmic inclusions in the cells of patients dying of boric acid poisoning.[51a, 170] The intracytoplasmic inclusions may be either acidophilic or basophilic, or both in the same patient. In many infants dying of boron toxicity, absorption appears to have been from the skin following application for excoriation of the buttocks. Perrin (see Chapter 2) has seen one patient who did not have these inclusions.

Radiation Damage

When consideration is given to the frequency with which the pancreas is irradiated, it is surprising how little attention radiation-induced pancreatic disease has received. Only three reports appear to exist.[20, 29, 47] All report fibrosis, the second adds degeneration and necrosis of duct cells and atrophy of acini, while the third adds myointimal arterial proliferation, and stresses the patchiness of the atrophy and lack of parenchymal inflammation and necrosis.

ISLET TISSUE

The islets of Langerhans have been recognized as a separate entity in the pancreas since 1869.[92] Three functional cell types within the islets were described in the first three decades of this century.[17, 91] Elucidation of the function of these three cells has come more recently, and their function is still being characterized. Studies describing toxic effects on the islets of Langerhans are an even more recent scientific enterprise, beginning in 1943, when Dunn and co-workers first described the deleterious effects of a uric acid derivitive (alloxan) on rabbit islets.[44] Because the functional islet cell population is made up of three distinct cell types, the discussion of toxic effects on islet tissue must be subdivided in relation to each functional cell group.

The beta or insulin-secreting cells are the most numerous cells (60 to 90 percent of all cells) in the islets of Langerhans, and exert the most profound effect on the whole organism. "D" or somatostatin-secreting cells represent 2 to 8 percent of islet cells, and alpha or glucagon-secreting cells represent the difference.[59] The overproduction and release of insulin leads to life-threatening hypoglycemia; underproduction or diminished secretion of insulin causes life-threatening hyperglycemia, described in its more chronic state as diabetes mellitus. Most of the known toxic effects on the islets of Langerhans are effects on the beta cell population, but later in this section toxic effects on the alpha cells and D cells will be discussed.

Beta Cells

Alloxan, Streptozotocin, and Vacor. Alloxan toxicity to islet tissue was discovered in 1943, when renal toxicity studies were being done on several urea derivatives.[44] Besides its renal tubular effects and some milder Central Nervous System effects, it was found that alloxan had a profound and rapid effect on the pancreatic islet beta-cell cytoplasm within 5 minutes of its administration. At 15 minutes there is nuclear chromatin aggregation, followed by nuclear pyknosis and loss of nucleoli.[95] Later, there is vesiculation of the ergastoplasm, and karyolysis. If the dosage is sufficient, all beta cells are necrotic in sections taken 24 hours after the first exposure to alloxan. No leukocyte response to the necrotic cells is found, and the islets diminish in size, with the ensuing phagocytosis of necrotic beta-cellular debris. Recovery can only take place if initial toxic exposure is limited to the low-dosage range, and even then recovery is attributed to new formation of beta cells from acinar or ductal cells of the pancreas.[22,131] Sulfonylurea compounds may help induce the neoformation of beta cells.[104]

The toxic mechanism of alloxan action on islet tissue has been sought for three decades, without a clear explanation yet being accepted. Because of the rapid dissolution of secretory granules from the damaged beta cell, a cell-membrane effect leading to increased permeability was suspected. This indeed has proved to be the case. Alloxan-treated beta cells are very much more permeable to mannitol in tissue culture.[34] Also, insulin and protein levels increase in the supernatant fluid after alloxan treatment.

It is postulated that the glucose-like shape of the alloxan molecule allows it to be taken up by glucose receptors in the beta cell plasma membrane. Various sugars, nicotinic acid, nicotinamide, epinephrine, and ethanol are all protective against alloxan's toxic effect on beta cells.[51] The sugars may block the cell membrane receptor sites, and epinephrine and ethanol may raise blood glucose levels, accomplishing the same effect. Lazarow has proposed that once alloxan is in the glucose receptor site, it increases cell permeability by binding sulfhydryl groups.[94] Watkins suggests that binding to a single SH group is not enough, the binding agent (alloxan) must react and bind two adjacent sulfhydryl groups in order to change the cell membrane sufficiently to lead to the described increased permeability.[174] Alloxan has also been described as an inhibitor of adenyl cyclase, and can act as a block at some point in the Kreb's cycle.[64] Finally, alloxan has been shown to increase concentrations of hydrogen peroxide and superoxide anions, which might be damaging to the pancreatic beta cells.[32]

Streptozotocin exerts exactly the same effect upon the islet beta cells as does alloxan, but is not quite so rapid in its effect. Loss of secretory granules occurs only after several hours have elapsed, and chromatin aggregation can only be found 3 to 4 hours after exposure.[96] The methylnitrosoureido group in streptozotocin is thought to be the cytotoxic moiety, and may effect the beta cell by binding to the glucose receptor site, or may get into the beta cell and exert its toxic effect internally. Streptozotocin lowers cellular nicotinamide adenine dinucleotide (NAD) levels, and may adversely affect the beta cell by interrupting respiratory enzyme activity, leading to irreversable cellular necrosis.[154] Yet this is probably not the entire story, since streptozotocin also lowers hepatocyte NAD, but does not cause toxic necrosis of the liver. Nicotinamide 2-deoxy-glucose and pyrazinamide are protective against streptozotocin-induced islet cell toxicity, but the sugar molecules most effective against alloxan are not. This suggests that streptozotocin first acts deeper within the cell than the glucose receptor site. An interesting sidelight to this is that streptozotocin plus nicotinamide administration caused 64 percent of rats so treated to develop islet cell tumors in 18 months whereas, only a 4 percent incidence of islet cell tumors were found in the group fed streptozotocin alone.[139] There are no reports of human experimentation with alloxan or streptozotocin, although the latter has been utilized as an anti islet-cell-tumor chemotherapeutic agent.

A third compound vacor (*N*-3 pyridylmethyl—*N*^{1}-p-nitrophenylurea) or PNU for short, is a rodent poison that has been accidentally ingested by humans or used in suicide attempts.[100] Vacor antagonizes normal nicotinamide metabolism and causes diabetes mellitus along with some severe central nervous system affects. Of 12 individuals who swallowed varying amounts of vacor, 5 died, and full recovery was uncommon. Orthostatic hypotension and permanent, brittle diabetes mellitus were the main residual findings in patients who did not die of their vacor ingestion. This drug falls into the class of urea derivatives that damage or destroy pancreatic beta cells by biochemical toxicity.

Cyproheptadine, Cyclizine and Dihydromorphanthridine. These three drugs stimulate pancreatic islet beta cells to produce increased insulin secretion. After cyproheptadine administration to rats, light-microscopic analysis of beta cell cytoplasm shows a vesicular or vacuolar change of the rough endoplasmic reticulum (RER), and an increase in lysosome and myeloid bodies.[103, 143] Rabbits, hamsters, and mice are resistant to the effects of this drug, and humans are said to show an increase in appetite, but do not reveal any pathologic change in the appearance of their beta cells.[162] Beta cell necrosis is not seen, and complete, rapid reversal of the cytoplasmic vacuolization occurs after exposure to cyproheptadine is terminated. Oral drug administration is much more effective than parenteral administration.

Ultrastructural studies following cyproheptadine administration to rabbits reveal progressive secretory granule loss starting 15 hours after original exposure to the drug, and complete granule loss after 4 days. The rough endoplasmic reticulum becomes progressively dilated, with later vesiculation and finally vesicle fusion with vacuole formation.[103] Alpha cells and pancreatic acinar cells show no alteration from their normal morphology. Twenty-four hours after drug withdrawal, secretory granules reappear, and 2 weeks later, the vacuoles disappear.[103]

The effect of cyclizine on rat beta cells is very similar to that of cyproheptadine in rabbits, but is also reported to cause golgi hyperplasia.[77] Dihydromorphanthridine and 4-diphenylmethyl-piperidine cause a morphologic beta cell vacuolization in rats similar to that produced by cyclizine.[13]

The mechanism of action of these drugs on the beta cell population is not known, but may revolve around an unknown metabolite, possibly an epoxide, which stimulates and exhausts the islet cells involved. The beta cell cytoplasmic vacuolization and secretory granule loss are interpreted as the effects of hyperstimulation of the beta cells with concurrent damage to the natural formation and maturation of secretory granules.

Sulfonamides. Tolbutamide stimulates rapid insulin release in rabbits, dogs, and rats. Ultrastructural studies reveal strong stimulatory effects upon beta cell organelles, with cytoplasmic degranulation and vesiculation of the rough endoplasmic reticulum.[171] With the long-term administration of tolbutamine, light-microscopy shows islet hyperplasia and neoformation of islets.[3, 105]

Diazoxide, Tricholomethiazide, and Other Diuretics. These antihypertensive drugs are known to cause glucose intolerance through a strong action on the pancreatic beta cell, inhibiting the release of insulin.[46] The suggested mechanism is through beta cell calcium loss, leaving insufficient Ca^{++} ion for insulin release.[108] Ultrastructural studies show increased numbers of "multigranular sacs," which may represent fused secretory granules undergoing autophagocytosis. After longer (14-day) therapy with diazoxide, beta cells showed few secretory granules and small condensed nuclei suggestive of diminished activity.[38] The diabetogenic effect of these diuretics may be amplified by stimulation of epinephrine release simultaneous to the inhibition of insulin release.

Growth Hormone. Growth hormone excess antagonizes insulin action and may lead to beta cell exhaustion, as shown by progressive degranulation, hydropic degeneration, and later cell death.[173]

Glucagon. The long-term glucagon treatment of rabbits leads to degranulation, hypertrophy, and hyperplasia of beta cells, with glycogen infiltration.[102] This may lead to temporary diabetes mellitus. Alpha cell loss also occurs in glucagon toxicity.

Glucocorticoids. Large doses of glucocorticoids cause hyperglycemia, which stimulates insulin release with beta cell degranulation, later cytoplasmic vesiculation (smaller than cyproheptodine induced vacuoles), and developing prominence of the golgi apparatus.[172] Later changes may include a tendency to islet hyperplasia, but if stimulation is prolonged it will lead to beta cell exhaustion and death. Concurrent thiazide administration may potentiate the initial stimulation of islet hyperplasia, but also increases the likelihood of islet hemorrhage and beta cell cytolysis.[55]

Androgens. Androgen therapy for 40 to 60 months in human aplastic anemia has been reported to cause documented glucose intolerance, with secondary hypertrophy and hyperplasia of pancreatic islets[126] Pancreatic cell tumor formation, comprising both islet cell ductular elements, has also been described.[150] Beta cells remain the predominant cell type in the altered islets. Renal and hepatic tumors are described accompanying the islet changes.

Epinephrine. Epinephrine infused into dog pancreaticoduodenal arteries led to plasma membrane destruction, first at the vascular pole of beta cells and then among all beta cells adjacent to islet capillaries, and finally to widespread beta cell necrosis. All animals spontaneously recovered from their temporary diabetes.[106]

Zinc Chelators. Agents that bind zinc and reduce its availability for the crystallization of insulin in the beta cell secretory granule may cause beta cell necrosis and self-limited diabetes mellitus. Two such compounds are oxine (8-hydroxyquinoline)[147] and dithizone (diphenylthiocarbazone).[142] Oxine is diabetogenic only in rabbits, whereas dithizone adversely affects rats, mice, and cats. There is a triphasic blood glucose response, with initial hyperglycemia 2 to 4 hours after dithizone administration, followed by hypoglycemia after 5 to 20 hours, and remittent hyperglycemia after 24 hours in some of the treated animals. Morphologic changes include degranulation, vacuolization, nuclear pyknosis, and finally beta cell necrosis, occurring within 48 to 72 hours. The islets then showed a prominent alpha cell population.[85] Some other hydroxyquinoline compounds have a similar toxic effect on beta cells of the pancreatic islet.

Alpha Cells

Little is known about toxic compounds affecting the glucagon-secreting alpha cells of the pancreatic islet. Three agents—cobalt salts,[167] synthalin A (decamethylene diquaindine,[65] and phenylethyldiquanide—have a similar cellular exhaustive effect, leading to glucagonemia and cytoplasmic vacuolization of the alpha cells, which is reversible after withdrawal of the stimulating drug, and does not lead to alpha cell necrosis. On the other hand, excessive glucagon administration leads to alpha cell damage and loss.

D-Cells

The D-cell of the pancreatic islet is the least-well-understood functioning islet cell, and has only recently been recognized as the source of somatostatin secretion. Several diverse drugs—lithium chloride, pentagastrin, and streptozotocin—are all said to stimulate increased D-cell nuclear size,[133,134,135] which may be an indication of increased cellular activity, but this is as yet unproven. No known D-cell-destructive cytotoxic agent has been described.

There is a case report of a patient complaining of episodic watery diarrhea and weight loss at several periods in his life. Extensive work-up revealed little cause for these episodes, and finally a partial pancreatectomy was performed with the thought that the patient suffered from Verner-Morrison syndrome. The pancreas specimen revealed a remarkable islet hyperplasia (twice the amount of islet tissue found in two control pancreases), and most of the islet tissue was made up of D cells. Postoperatively the watery diarrhea and weight loss continued unabated until chemical metabolites of a phenolphthaline laxative were found in the patient's stool specimen. It was suggested to the patient that his problem centered around some toxic substance he was taking with his food. The symptoms then abruptly ceased, suggesting that laxative abuse was the main pathologic process.[98]

REFERENCES

1. Aho, H. J., Koskensalo, S. M. L., & Nevalainen, T. J.: Sodium taurocholate-induced acute hemorrhagic pancreatitis. Scand. J. Gastroenterol. 15:411-416, 1980.
2. Ances, I. G., & Mcclain, C. A.: Acute pancreatitis following the use of thiazide in pregnancy. South. Med. J. 64:267-269, 1971.
3. Anderson, A.: About islet cells from nonendocrine pancreatic cells with tolbutamide therapy. Endocrinology 96:1051, 1975.
4. Anonymous: Clinoril-Sulindac pancreatitis. ADR Highlights. August 17, 1979.
5. Arnold, F., Doyle, P. J., & Bell, G.: Acute pancreatitis in a patient treated with cimetidine. Lancet 1:382-383, 1978.
6. Baar, H. S., & Wolff, O. H.: Pancreatic necrosis in cortisone-treated children. Lancet 1:812-815, 1957.
7. Baden, M. M.: Angiitis in drug abusers. N. Engl. J. Med. 284:111-112, 1971.
8. Baggenstoss, A. H.: The pancreas in uremia: a histopathologic study. Am. J. Pathol. 24:1003-1011, 1948.
9. Bank, S. & Marks, I. N.: Hyperlipaemic pancreatitis and the pill. Postgrad. Med. J. 46:576-588, 1970.
10. Barrett, P. V. D., & Thier, S. O.: Meningitis and pancreatitis associated with sulfamethizole. N. Engl. J. Med. 268:36-37, 1963.
11. Batalden, P. B., Van Dyne, B. J., & Cloyd, J.: Pancreatitis associated with valproic acid. Pediatrics 64:520-522, 1979.
12. Beard, M. E. J., Crowther, D., & Galton, D. A. G., et al: L-Asparaginase in treatment of acute leukaemia and lymphosarcoma. Br. Med. J. 1:191-195, 1970.
13. Beliles, R. P.: The subchronic toxicity of 5-benzyl-11-,4-(N-methylpiperidylene)-5,6-dihydromorphanthridine hydrogen maleate. Toxicol. Appl. Pharmacol. 18:451, 1971.
14. Bencosme, S. A., & Lazarus, S. S.: The pancreas of cortisone-treated rabbits: a pathogenic study. Arch. Pathol. 62:285-295, 1956.
15. Bilbao, M. K., Dotter, C. T., Lee, T. G., & Katon, R. M.: Complications of endoscopic retrograde cholangiopancreatography. Gastroenterology 70:314-320, 1976.
16. Block, M. B., Genant, H. K., & Kirsner, J. B.: Pancreatitis as an adverse reaction to salicylazosulfapyridine. N. Engl. J. Med. 282:380-382, 1970.
17. Bloom, W.: A new type of granular cell in the islets of Langerhans in man. Anat. Rec. 49:363, 1931.
18. Bourke, J. B., Mead, G. M., McIllmurray, M. B., & Langman, M. J. S.: Drug-associated primary acute pancreatitis. Lancet 1:706, 1978.
19. Bourne, M. S., & Dawson, H.: Acute pancreatitis complicating prednisolone therapy. Lancet 2:1209-1210, 1958.
20. Brick, I. B.: Effects of million volt radiation on the gastrointestinal tract. Arch. Intern. Med. 96:26-31, 1955.
21. Buchanan, N., & Cane, R. D.: Frusemide-induced pancreatitis. Br. Med. J. 2:1417, 1977.
22. Bunnag, S. C., Warner, N. E., & Bunnag, S.: Microcirculation of islets of Langerhans in alloxan diabetes of mice. Bibl. Anat. 9:196, 1967.
23. Call, T., Malarkey, W. B., & Thomas, F. B.:

Acute pancreatitis secondary to furosemide with associated hyperlipidemia. Am. J. Digest. Dis. 22:835-838, 1977.
24. Cameron, J. L., Capuzzi, D. M., Zuidema, G. D., & Margolis, S.: Acute pancreatitis with hyperlipemia: evidence for a persistent defect in lipid metabolism. Am. J. Med. 56:482-487, 1974.
25. Cameron, J. L.: Lipid abnormalities in acute pancreatitis. Hosp. Prac.: 95-101, 1977.
26. Camfield, P. R., Bagnell P. Camfield, C. S., et al: Pancreatitis due to valproic acid. Lancet 1:1198-1199, 1979.
27. Carone, F. A., & Liebow, A. A.: Acute pancreatic lesions in patients with ACTH and adrenal corticoids. N. Engl. J. Med. 257:690-697, 1957.
28. Casdorph, H. R.: The efficacy and safety of cholestyramine therapy in hyperlipidemic patients (Abstr.). Ann. Intern. Med. 74:818, 1971.
29. Case, J. T., Warthin, A. S.: The occurrence of hepatic lesions in patients treated by intensive deep roentgen irradiation. Am. J. Roentgenol. 12:27, 1924.
30. Chase, H. S., Mogan, G. R.: Phenformin-associated pancreatitis. Ann. Intern. Med. 87:314-315, 1977.
31. Citron, B. P., Halpern, M., McCarron, M., et al: Necrotizing angiitis associated with drug abuse. N. Engl. J. Med. 283:1003-1011, 1970.
32. Cohen, G. & Heikklila, R. E.: The generation of hydrogen peroxide, superoxide radical and hydroxyl radical by 6 hydroxydopamine dialuric acid and related cytotoxic agents. J. Biol. Chem. 249:2447, 1974.
33. Coodley, E., Derasse, J., & Carver, J.: Phenformin and pancreatitis. Ann. Intern. Med. 78:307-308, 1973.
34. Cooperstein, S. J., Watkins, D., & Lazarow, A.: The effect of alloxan on islet tissue permeability. In: S. E. Brolin, B. Hellman and H. Knutson Eds. The Structure and Metabolism of the Pancreatic Islets p. 397. Pergamon Press Ltd., Oxford, England, 1964.
35. Cornish, A. L., McClellan, J. T., & Johnston, D. H.: Effects of chlorothiazide on the pancreas. N. Engl.J.Med.265:673-675,1961.
36. Cortese, A. F., & Glenn F.: Hypocalcemia and tetany with steroid-induced acute pancreatitis. Arch.Surg.96:119-122,1968.
37. Coward, R. A.: Paracetamol-induced acute pancreatitis.Br.Med.J.1:1086,1977.
38. Crentzfeldt, W., Crentzfeldt, C., Frerichs, H., et al: The morphological substrate of the inhibition of insulin secretion by diazoxide. Horm. Metab. Res.1:53,1969.
39. Davidoff, F., Tishler, S., Rosoff, C.: Marked hyperlipemia and pancreatitis associated with oral contraceptive therapy: N. Engl. J. Med. 289:552-555,1973.
40. DeBroe, M., Mussche, M., Ringoir S., et al: Oral diazoxide for malignant hypertension. Lancet 1:1397,1972.
41. Diamond, M. T.: Hyperglycemic hyperosmolar coma associated with hydrochlorothiazide and pancreatitis. N.Y. State J. Med. 72:1741-1742, 1972.
42. Drash, A., Elliott, J., Langs, H., et al: The effect of cyproheptadine on carbohydrate metabolism. Clin.Pharmacol.Ther.7:340-346,1966.
43. Dressel, T. D., Goodale, R. L., Arneson, M. A., et al: Pancreatitis as a complication of anticholinesterase insecticide intoxication. Ann. Surg. 189:199-204, 1979.
44. Dunn, J. S., Sheehan, H. L., & McLetchie, N. G.: Necrosis of islets of Langerhans produced experimentally. Lancet 1:484, 1943.
45. Evans, D. B., & Slapak, M.: Pancreatitis in the hard water syndrome. Br. Med. J. 3:748, 1975.
46. Fajans, S. S., Floyd, J. C., Knopf, R. F., et al: Benzothiadiazine suppression of insulin release from normal and abnormal islet tissue in man. J. Clin. Invest. 45:481, 1966.
47. Fajardo, L. F., & Berthrong, M.: Radiation injury in surgical pathology. III. Salivary glands, pancreas and skin. Am. J. Surg. Pathol. 5:279-296, 1981.
48. Falko, J. M., & Thomas, F. B.: Acute pancreatitis due to procainamide-induced lupus erythematosus. Ann. Intern. Med. 83:832-833, 1975.
49. Fernandez, J. A., Rosenberg, J. C.: Post-transplantation pancreatitis. Surg. Gynecol. Obstet. 143:795-798, 1976.
50. Fisch, H. P., Wands, J., Yeung, J. et al: Pulmonary edema and disseminated intravascular coagulation after intravenous abuse of d-propoxyphene (Darvon). South. Med. J. 65:493-495, 1972.
51. Fischer, L. J., & Rickert, D. E.: Pancreatic

islet-cell toxicity. C.R.C. Crit. Rev. Toxicol. 3:231-263, 1975.

51a. Fisher, R. S.: Intracytoplasmic inclusions in the pancreas due to boric acid poisoning. Am. J. Pathol. 27:745, 1951.

52. Foster, M. E., & Powell, D. E. B.: Pancreatitis, multiple infarcts and oral contraception. Postgrad. Med. J. 51:667-669, 1975.

53. Foulis, A. K.: Histological evidence of initiating factors in acute necrotising pancreatitis in man. J. Clin. Pathol. 33:1125-1131, 1980.

54. Fredell, C. H., McIver, M. A., & Fersebe, J. W.: Carcinoma of parathyroid gland and hyperparathyroidism: report of a case. Surgery 42:959-965, 1967.

55. Frenkel, J. K.: Dissecting aneurisms of the aorta and pancreatic islet cell hyperplasia with diabetes in corticosteroid and chlorothiazide-treated hamsters. Prog. Exp. Tumor Res. 16:300, 1972.

56. Gazzard, G. B., Portmann, B., Murry-Lyon, I. M., et al: Causes of death in fulminant hepatic failure and relationship to quantitative histological assessment of parenchymal damage. Q. J. Med. 176:615-626, 1975.

57. Gilmore, I. T., Tourvas, E.: Paracetamol-in duced acute pancreatitis. Br. Med. J. 1:753, 1977.

58. Glueck, C. J., Scheel, D., Fishback, J., et al: Estrogen-induced pancreatitis in patients with previously covert familial type V hyperlipoproteinemia. Metabolism 21:657-666, 1972.

58a. Goekas, M. C., & Rinderknecht, H.: Free proteolytic enzymes in pancreatic juice of patients with acute pancreatitis. Am. J. Dig. Dis. 19:591–598, 1974.

59. Gomori, G.: Pathology of the pancreatic islet. Arch. Pathol. 36:217-232, 1943.

60. Graeber, G. M., Marmor, B. M., Hendel, R. C., et al: Pancreatitis and severe metabolic abnormalities due to phenformin therapy. Arch. Surg. 111:1014-1016, 1976.

60a. Greenbaum, L. M., Hirshkowitz, A., & Schoichet, I.: The activation of trypsinogen by cathepsin B. J. Biol. Chem. 234:2885–2890, 1959.

61. Greenstein, R., Nogeire, C., Ohnuma, T., et al: Management of asparaginase induced hemorrhagic pancreatitis complicated by pseudocyst. Cancer 43:718-722, 1979.

62. Guerra, M.: Toxicity of indomethacin. Report of a case of acute pancreatitis. J.A.M.A. 200:222-223, 1967.

63. Gullo, L., Costa, P. L., Fontana, G., et al: Effect of adrenocorticotropic hormone on pure exocrine pancreatic secretion in man. Gastroenterology 73:762-764, 1977.

64. Gunnarsson, R., & Hellerstrom, C.: Acute effects of alloxan on the metabolism and insulin secretion of the pancreatic beta-cell. Horm. Metab. Res. 5:404, 1973.

65. Gunnarsson, R., Peterson, B., & Hellerstrom, C.: The two types of D-cells in the islets of langerhans of normal and synthalin treated guinea pigs. Acta Pathol. Scand. 76:184-192, 1969.

66. Halpern, M., Citron, B. P.: Necrotizing angiitis associated with drug abuse. Am. J. Roentgenol. 3: 663-671, 1971.

67. Ham, J. M., & Fitzpatrick, P.: Acute pancreatitis in patients with acute hepatic failure. Am. J. Digest. Dis. 18:1079-1083, 1973.

68. Hamad, I., Lindeman, R. D., & Czerwinski, A. W.: Acute pancreatitis following corticosteroid and azathioprine therapy. Am. J. Med. Sci. 276:211-219.

69. Haskell, C. M., Cannellos, G. P., Leventhal, B. G., et al: L-Asparaginase: therapeutic and toxic effects in patient's with neoplastic disease. N. Engl. J. Med. 281:1028-1034, 1969.

70. Hazzard, W. R., Spiger, M. J., Bagdade, J. D., et al: Studies on the mechanisms of increased plasma triglyceride levels induced by oral contraceptives. N. Engl. J. Med. 280:471-474, 1969.

71. Helin, H., Mero, M., Markkula, M., et al: Pancreatic acinar ultrastructure in human acute pancreatitis. Virchows Arch [Pathol Anat] 387:259-270, 1980.

72. Herman-Taylor, J., Perrin, J., Grant, D. A. W., et al. Immunofluorescent localisation of enterokinase in human small intestine. Gut 18:259-265, 1977.

73. Herskowitz, L. J., Olansky, S., & Lang, P. G.: Acute pancreatitis associated with long-term azathioprine therapy. Arch. Dermatol. 115:179, 1979.

74. Heuser, E., Lieberman, E., Donnell, G. N., et al: Subcutaneous fat necrosis with acute hemorrhagic pancreatitis: a case in a child with steroid-resistant nephrosis treated with 6-mercaptopurine. Calif. Med. 106:58-63, 1967.

75. Hochgelerent, E. L., David, D. S.: Acute pancreatitis secondary to calcium infusion in a dialysis patient. Arch. Surg. 108:218-219, 1974.
76. Horn, J. K., Ranson, J. H. C., Goldstein, I. M. et al: Evidence of complement catabolism in experimental acute pancreatitis. Am. J. Pathol. 101:205-216, 1980.
77. Hruban, Z., Rubenstein, A. H., & Slesers, A.: Alteration in pancreatic beta cells induced by cyclizine. Lab. Invest. 26(3):270-277, 1972.
78. Huizenga, K. A., Shorter, R. G., Phillips. S. F.: Pancreatitis: a specific complication of Azathioprine treatment of Crohn's disease (abstr). Gastroenterology 70:895, 1976.
79. Izsak, E. M., Shike, M., Roulet, M., et al: Pancreatitis in association with hypercalcemia in patients receiving total parental nutrition. Gastroenterology 79:555-558, 1980.
80. Jaffe, N., Traggis, D., Das, L., et al: Comparison of daily and twice-weekly schedule of L-asparaginase in childhood leukemia. Pediatrics 49:590-595, 1972.
81. Joffe, S. N., & Lee, F. K.: Acute pancreatitis after cimetidine administration in experimental duodenal ulcers. Lancet 1:383, 1978.
82. Johnston, D. H., & Cornish A. L.: Acute pancreatitis in patients receiving chlorothiazide. J.A.M.A. 170:2054-2056, 1959.
83. Jones, M. F., & Caldwell, J. R.: Acute hemorrhagic pancreatitis associated with administration of chlorthalidone: report of a case. N. Engl. J. Med. 267:1029-1031, 1962.
84. Jones, P. M., & Oelbaum, M. H.: Frusemide-induced pancreatitis. Br. Med. J. 1:133-134, 1975.
85. Kadota, I.: Studies on experimental diabetes mellitus, as produced by organic reagents; oxine diabetes and Dithizone diabetes. J. Lab. Clin. Med. 35:568-591, 1950.
86. Kawanishi, H., Rudolph, E., Bull, F. E.: Azathioprine-induced acute pancreatitis. N. Engl. J. Med. 289:357, 1973.
87. Kerstein, M. D., & Grabman, J.: Amelioration of pancreatitis with azathioprine. Am. J. Gastroenterol. 72:267-270, 1979.
88. Kleppel, N. H., Goldstein, M. H., & LeVeen, H. H.: Hypercalcemic crisis and pancreatitis primary hyperparathyroidism. J.A.M.A. 192:916-918, 1965.
89. Kunelis, C. T., Peters, J. L., & Edmondson, H. A.: Fatty liver of pregnancy and its relationship to tetracycline therapy. Am. J. Med. 38:359-377, 1965.
90. Land, V. J., Sutow, W. W., Fernbach, D. J., et al: Toxicity of L-asparaginase in children with advanced leukemia. Cancer 30:339-347, 1972.
91. Lane, M. A.: The cytological character of the islets of Langerhans. Am. J. Anat. 7:409, 1907.
92. Langerhans, P.: Beitrage zu-mikroskopischen anatomie der bauchspeicheldruse. Inaugural Dissertation G. Lange, Berlin, 1869.
93. Larsen, R. R., Sawyer, R. B., Sawyer, K. C., et al: Hemorrhagic pancreatitis complicating anticoagulant therapy. N.Y. State J. Med. 62:2397-2399, 1962.
94. Lazarow, A.: Alloxan diabetes and the mechanisms of beta cell damage by chemical agents. In: J. Hoet, F. Young, J. Delafresnage and G. Smith Eds. Experimental Diabetes: A Symposium. p. 49. Charles C Thomas, Springfield, Illinois.
95. Lazarus, S. S., & Shapiro, S. H.: Comparison of morphologic changes in nuclei of rabbit pancreatic islet beta-cell induced by streptozotocin alloxan and *in vitro* necrosis. Lab. Invest. 29:90, 1973.
96. Lazarus, S. S., & Shapiro, S. H.: Serial morphologic changes in rabbit pancreatic islet-cells after streptozotocin. Lab. Invest. 27:174-183, 1972.
97. Leeson, P. M., & Fourman, P.: Acute pancreatitis from Vitamin-D poisoning in a patient with parathyroid deficiency. Lancet 1:1185-1186, 1966.
98. Lesna, M., Hamlyn, A. N., Venables, C. W., et al: Chronic laxative abuse associated with pancreatic islet cell hyperplasia. Gut 18:1032-1035, 1977.
99. Levitan, A. A.: Phenformin and pancreatitis. Ann. Intern. Med. 78:306-307, 1973.
100. LeWitt, P.A.: The neurotoxicity of the rat poison vacor. N. Engl. J. Med. 302(2):73-77, 1980.
101. Loeb, E., Hill, J. M., Hill, N. O., et al: Treatment of acute leukemia with L-asparaginase. Rec. Res. Cancer Res. 33:204-218, 1970.
102. Logothetopoulos, J., Sharma, B. B., Salter, J. M. et al: Glucagon and metaglucagon diabetes in rabbits. Diabetes 9:278-285, 1980.
103. Longnecker, D. S., Wold, J. S., & Fischer, L. J.: Ultrastructural study of alterations in

beta cells of pancreatic islets from cyproheptadine-treated rats. Diabetes 21:71, 1972.

104. Loubetieres, A.: Therapeutic modification of islet function. In: Steiner, D., Freinkel, N., Eds. Handbook of Physiology. Sec. 7, Vol. 1. pp. 653. William and Wilkins, Baltimore, 1972.

105. Loubetieres, A.: Thesis doctorates Sciences Naturelles. Montsellier Sausse Graille et Castelnons, 1946.

106. Loubetieres, A., Mariani, M. M., Chapal, J., et al: Action Nocive de l'adrenaline pour la structure histologique des ilots de langerhans du pancreas. Action protectrice de la dihydroergotamine Diabetologia 1:13-20, 1965.

107. Ludwig, G. D., & Chaykin., L. B.: Pancreatitis associated with primary hyperparathyroidism. Med. Clin. North. Am. 50:1903-1918, 1966.

108. Malaisse, W. J., Pipeleers, D. G., & Mahy., M.: The stimulus-secretion coupling of glucose-induced insulin release XIII effects of diazoxide and gliclazide upon ^{45}Ca efflux from perfused islets. Diabetologia 9:1, 1973.

109. Mallory, A., & Kern., F., Jr.: Drug-induced pancreatitis: A critical review. Gastroenterology 78:813-820, 1980.

110. Manson, R. R.: Acute pancreatitis secondary to iatrogenic hypercalcemia: implications of hyperalimentation. Arch. Surg. 108:213-215, 1974.

111. Mattson, K.: Side effects of rifampicin: a clinical study. Scand. J. Resp. Dis. (Suppl) 82:8-52, 1973.

112. Meltzer, L. E., Florentino, P. P., Young, K. P., et al. Acute pancreatitis secondary to hypercalcemia of multiple myeloma. Ann. Intern. Med. 57:1008-1012, 1952.

113. Meshkinpour, H., Molinari, M. D., Gardner, L., et al: Cimetidine in the treatment of acute alcoholic pancreatitis. Gastroenterology 77:687-690, 1979.

114. Meyboom, R. H. B.: Heavy metal antagonists. In: Dukes, M. N. G., Ed. Side Effects of Drugs Annual. Vol. 2. pp. 215-221. Exerpta Medica, Amsterdam, 1978.

115. Minkowitz, S., Soloway, H. B., Hall, J. E., et al: Fatal hemorrhagic pancreatitis following chlorothiazide administration in pregnancy. Obstet. Gynecol. 24:337-342, 1964.

116. Minus, B. D., Field., M., & Rammelkamp, C. H.: Salivary gland enlargement caused by sulfisoxazole. Ann. Intern. Med. 63:663-665, 1965.

117. Mixter, C. G., Jr., Keynes, W. M., & Cope, O.: Further experience with pancreatitis as a diagnostic clue to hyperparathyroidism. N. Engl. J. Med. 266:265-272, 1962.

118. Moir, D. C.: Drug-associated acute pancreatitis. Lancet 2:369, 1978.

119. Muller, K., & Jorge, A.: Rezidive akuter pankreatitis nach cholezystographie. Med. Klin. 60:1693, 1965.

120. Mullick, F. G., Drake, R. M., & Irey, N. S.: Morphological changes in adverse drug reactions in infants and children. Hum. Pathol. 8:361-378, 1977.

121. Murphey, S. A., & Josephs, A. S.: Acute pancreatitis associated with pentamidine therapy. Arch. Intern. Med. 141:56-58, 1981.

122. Nakamura, K., Sarles, H., & Payan, H.: Three-dimensional reconstruction of the pancreatic ducts in chronic pancreatitis. Gastroenterology 62:942-949, 1972.

123. Nakashima, Y., & Howard, J. M.: Drug-induced acute pancreatitis. Surg. Gynecol. Obstet. 145:105-109, 1977.

124. Nelp, W. B.: Acute pancreatitis associated with steroid therapy. Arch. Intern. Med. 108:102-110, 1961.

125. Nogueira, J. R., & Freedman, M. A.: Acute pancreatitis as a complication of Imuran therapy in regional enteritis. Gastroenterology 62:1040-1041, 1972.

126. Novak, R., Wilimas, J., & Johnson, W.: Hypertrophy and hyperplasia of islets of Langerhans associated with androgen therapy. Arch. Pathol. Lab. Med. 103:483-485, 1979.

127. Oettgen, H. F., Stephenson, P. A., Schwartz, M. K., et al: Toxicity of *E. coli* L-asparaginase in man. Cancer 25:253-278, 1970.

128. Oppenheimer, E. H., & Boitnott, J. K.: Pancreatitis in children following adrenal corticosteroid therapy. Bull. Johns Hopkins Hosp. 107:297-306, 1960.

129. Paloyan, D., Levin, B., & Simonowitz, D.: Azathioprine-associated acute pancreatitis. Digest. Dis. 22:839-840, 1977.

130. Parker, P. H., Helinek, G. L., Ghishan, F. K., et al: Recurrent pancreatitis induced by valproic acid. Gastroenterology 80:826-828, 1981.

131. Patent, G. H., & Alfert, M.: Histologic changes in pancreatic islets of alloxan treated

mice, with comments on beta-cell regeneration. Acta. Anat. 66:504, 1967.
132. Peters, R. L., Edmondson, H. A., Mikkelson, W. P., et al: Tetracycline-induced fatty liver in nonpregnant patients: a report of six cases. Am. J. Surg. 113:622-632, 1967.
133. Petersson, B., Hellerstrom, C., & Gunnarsson, R.: Structure and metabolism of the pancreatic islets in streptozotocin treated guinea pigs. Horm. Metab. Res. 2:313, 1970.
134. Petersson, B.: The effect of pentagastrin on A_1 cells of the pancreatic islets in guinea pigs. Experientia 28:345, 1972.
135. Petersson, B., & Shopsin, B.: Effects of lithium chloride on the islets of Langerhans in guinea pigs. Acta Endocrinol. 70:731, 1972.
136. Pickleman, J., Straus, F. H., & Paloyan, E.: Pancreatitis associated with thiazide administration. Arch. Surg. 114:1013-1016, 1979.
137. Pratt, C. B., Choi, S., & Holton, C. P.: Low-dosage asparaginase treatment of childhood acute lymphocytic leukemia. Am. J. Dis. Child. 121:406-409, 1971.
138. Pratt, C. B., Simone, J. V., Zee, P., et al: Comparison of daily versus weekly L-asparaginase for the treatment of childhood acute leukemia. J. Pediatr. 77:474-483, 1970.
139. Rakieten, N., Gordon, B. S., Beaty, A., et al: Pancreatic islet cell tumors produced by the combined action of stretozotocin and nicotinamide. Proc. Soc. Exp. Biol. Med. 137:280, 1971.
140. Redman, H. C., & Joseph, R. R.: Hemobilia and pancreatitis as complications of a percutaneous transhepatic cholangiogram. Digest. Dis. 20:691-698, 1975.
141. Renner, I. G., Rinderknecht, H., & Douglas, A. P.: Profiles of pure pancreatic secretions in patients with acute pancreatitis: The possible role of proteolytic enzymes in pathogenesis. Gastroenterology 75:1090-1098, 1978.
142. Rerup, C. C.: Drugs producing diabetes through damage of the insulin-secreting cells. Pharmacol. Rev. 22:485, 1970.
143. Richardson, B. P., Turot-Lemay, L., McDaniel, M. L., et al: Pancreatic B cell changes induced by cyproheptadine in vitro. Lab. Invest. 33(5) 509-513, 1975.
144. Riemann, J. F., Stock, K. P., & Strunz, U. T.: Contrast-medium induced pancreatitis: in vivo experiments of the mechanisms involved. Gastroenterology 78:1244, 1980.
145. Riemenschneider, T. A., Wilson, J. F., & Vernier, R. L.: Glucorcorticoid-induced pancreatitis in children. Pediatrics 41:428-437, 1968.
146. Rominger, J. M., Gutierrez, J. G., Curtis, D., et al: Methyldopa-induced pancreatitis. Digest. Dis. 23:756-758, 1978.
147. Root, M. A., & Chen, K. K.: Experimental diabetes produced by 8-hydroxyguinoline. J. Pharmacol. Exp. Ther. 104:404, 1952.
148. Rumbaugh, C. L., Bergeron, R. T., Fang, H. C. H., et al: Cerebral angiographic changes in the drug abuse patient. Radiology 101:335-351, 1971.
149. Ryan, L. M., Hankwitz, P., & Banasiak, M.: Phenformin and pancreatitis. Ann. Intern. Med. 87:796, 1977.
150. Sale, G. E., & Lerner, K. G.: Multiple tumors after androgen therapy. Arch. Pathol. Lab. Med. 101:600-603, 1977.
151. Sarles, H.: Alcohol and the pancreas. Nutr. Metab. 21:175-181, 1977.
152. Sarles, H., & Sahel, J.: Pathology of chronic calcifying pancreatitis. Am. J. Gastroenterol. 66:117-139, 1976.
153. Sarles, H., & Tiscornia, O.: Ethanol and chronic calcifying pancreatitis. Med. Clin. North. Am. 58:1333-1347, 1974.
154. Schein, P. S., & Loftus, S.: Streptozotocin: Depression of mouse liver pyridine nucleotides. Cancer Res. 28:1501, 1968.
155. Schmidt, P., & Friedman, I. S.: Adverse effects of ethacrynic acid. N.Y. State J. Med. 67:1438-1442, 1967.
156. Schrier, R. W., & Bulger, R. J.: Steroid-induced pancreatitis. J.A.M.A. 194:564, 1965.
157. Schrogie, J. J., Holt, P., Hartley, R. C., et al: "Histamine-induced" pancreatitis. Gastroenterology 49:672-675, 1965.
158. Schultz, J. C., Adamson, J. S., Workman, W. W., et al: Fatal liver disease after intravenous administration of tetracycline in high dosage. N. Engl. J. Med. 269:999-1004, 1963.
159. Shanklin, D. R.: Pancreatic atrophy apparently secondary to hydrochlorothiazide. N. Engl. J. Med. 266:1097-1099, 1962.
160. Shike, M., Sturtridge, W. E., Harrison, J. E., et al: Metabolic bone disease in patients receiving long-term parental nutrition. Ann. Intern. Med. 92:343-350, 1980.
161. Smith, R. B. W., Prior, I. A. M., & Cooke,

N. J.: The effect of clofibrate on raised serum lipid levels. N.Z. Med. J. 68:231, 1968.
162. Stiel, J. N., Liddle, G. W., & Lacy, W. W.: Studies of mechanisms of cyproheptadine-induced weight gain in human subjects. Metabolism 19:192, 1970.
163. Stokes, T., & Wynn, V.: Serum-lipids in women on oral contraceptives. Lancet 2:667-680, 1971.
164. Strunge, P.: Frusemide-induced pancreatitis? Br. Med. J. 3:434, 1975.
165. Sturdevant, R. A. L., Singleton, J. W., Deren, J. J., et al: Azathioprine-related pancreatitis in patients with Crohn's disease. Gastroenterology 77:883-886, 1979.
166. Sussman, S.: Severe salicylism and acute pancreatitis. Calif. Med. 99:29-32, 1963.
167. Telib, M.: Effects of cobaltous chloride on laboratory animals I. The histological and electron/microscopical changes in the islets of rabbits. Endokrinologie 60:81, 1972.
168. Tweedie, J. H., Mosley, J. G., Austin, J. L., et al: Effect of 16,16 dimethyl prostaglandin E_2 on aspirin-induced permeability changes in the pancreatic duct. Am. J. Surg. 141:22-27, 1981.
169. Tweedie, J. H., Mosley, J. G., & Reber, H. A.: The cytoprotective effect of cimetidine on aspirin induced damage to the pancreas. Gastroenterology 78:1281, 1980.
170. Valdes-Dapena, M.A., Arey, J. B.: Boric acid poisoning. J. Peds. 61:531-546, 1962.
171. Volk, B. W., & Lazarus, S. S.: Beta-cell hyperfunction after long-term sulfonylurea treatment. Arch. Pathol. 78:114, 1964.
172. Volk, B. W., & Lazarus, S. S.: Ultramicroscopic studies of rabbit pancreas during cortisone treatment. Diabetes 12:162, 1963.
173. Volk, B. W., & Lazarus, S. S.: Ultramicroscopic evaluation of B-cell destruction in diabetic dogs. In: Brolin, S. E., Hellman, B., & Knutson, H. Eds. The Structure and Metabolism of the Pancreatic Islets. p. 144. Pergamon Press, Ltd., Oxford, England, 1964.
174. Watkins, D., Cooperstein, S. J., & Lazarow, A.: Effect of sulfhydryl reagents on permeability of toadfish islet tissue. Am. J. Physiol. 219:503, 1970.
175. Weetman, R. M., & Bachner, R. L.: Latent onset of clinical pancreatitis in children receiving L-asparaginase therapy. Cancer 34:780-785, 1974.
176. Wenger, J., Gross, P. R.: Acute pancreatitis related to hydrochlorothiazide therapy. Gastroenterology 46:768, 1964.
177. Whalley, P. J., Adams, R. H., & Combes, B.: Tetracycline toxicity in pregnancy: liver and pancreatic dysfunction. J.A.M.A. 189:357-362, 1964.
178. White, T. T., & Bourde, J.: A new observation on human intraductal pancreatic pressure. Surg. Gynecol. Obstet. 130:275-278, 1970.
179. Whitecar, J. P., Jr., Bodey, G. P., Harris, J. E., et al: L-Asparaginase. N. Engl. J. Med. 282:732-734, 1970.
180. Wilde, H.: Pancreatitis and phenformin. Ann. Intern. Med. 77:324, 1972.
181. Wilson, A. E., Mehra, S. K., Gomersall, C. R., et al: Acute pancreatitis associated with frusemide therapy. Lancet 1:105, 1967.
182. Wu, S., & Wolf, J. W.: Phenformin and pancreatitis. Ann. Intern. Med. 88:128, 1978.
183. Zion, M. M., Goldberg, B., & Suzman, M. M.: Corticotrophin and cortisone in the treatment of scleroderma: Q. J. Med. 24:215, 1955.
184. Zorrilla, E., Hulse, M., Hernandez, A., et al: Severe endogenous hypertriglyceridemia during treatment with estrogen and oral contraceptives. J. Clin. Endocrinol. Metab. 28:1793-1796, 1968.

20

The Endocrine System

Francis H. Straus II

Fortunately, the classic endocrine tissues of the body are quite resistant to toxic or tangential drug effects. On the other hand, endocrine tissues are exceedingly sensitive to stimulation by their physiologic trophic substances or analogs of these trophic substances. It is not the purpose of this chapter to relate the proliferative or atrophying effects on endocrine tissues of these trophic or inhibitory substances; in this discussion I will emphasize the effects, on endocrine tissue, of chemical substances which are not usually identified as direct trophic or antitrophic hormones or chemical imitators of these substances. Furthermore, I will not dwell upon the peripheral effects in the endocrine system of a drug under discussion that alters one aspect of hypothalamic or pituitary function which, in turn, has a predictable cascade effect down the endocrine system.

PITUITARY

Peptide Analogs of Hypothalamic Releasing and Inhibiting Hormones

Any peptide analogs of hypothalamic releasing or inhibiting hormones will produce a trophic or inhibitory effect on their target anterior pituitary cell population. If the stimulatory effect is long-term in nature, one could expect first an increased prominence of the responsive anterior pituitary cells, later an identifiable hyperplasia of that cell type, and finally, the possible formation of a pure cluster of these cells, leading to a pathologic diagnosis of pituitary adenoma (Fig. 20-1). Similarly, a steady exposure to inhibitory peptides would cause a decreased prominence of the affected anterior pituitary cell type, and often an apparent increase in the cell type that produces a balancing hormone. For example, a peptide mimicking the action of prolactin inhibitory substance would have an effect on the anterior pituitary like gonadotrophin releasing hormone (GNRH).

End-organ Feedback

Estrogen excess suppresses GNRH production, and directly suppresses follicle stimulating hormone (FSH) formation and release in the pituitary. This allows prolactin production to progress and increase in an unbalanced fashion. Prolactin-secreting acidophilic cells become more prominent.[28] The anterior pituitary slowly changes, and finally acidophile or chromophobe adenomas develop in rodents. Monkeys have only shown acidophile hyperplasia. Such changes in human pituitary morphology have not yet been described. Experimental animals and humans of both sexes with estrogen excess may develop the unwanted occurrence of galactorrhea due to the unbalanced excessive prolactin production.[13]

Testosterone generates a less powerful effect on the hypothalmus and pituitary, but will cause a similar depression of gonadatrophin secretion and an apparent stimulus to the prolactin system. Hyperplasia has been noted, but adenoma formation has not.[18]

Progesterone augments the effect of estrogen, amplifying the already described gonadatrophin inhibition and the prolactin stimulation. The higher-dosage oral contraceptives may have an effect on the anterior pituitary, leading to prolactin prominence.

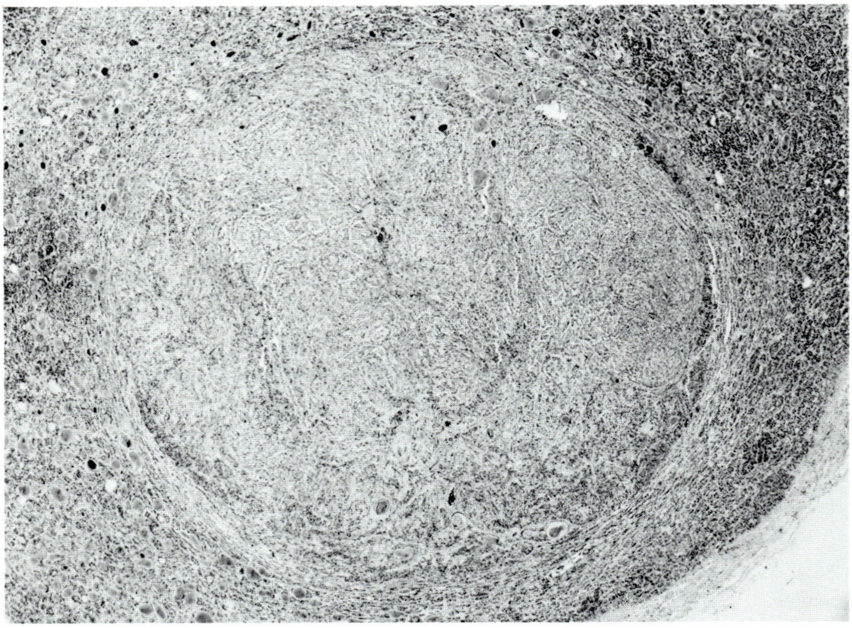

Fig. 20-1. Pituitary adenoma (chromophobe type). A spherical encapsulated group of morphologically similar cells. H&E, × 20.

Severe, long-standing thyroid deficiency working through the hypothalmus and causing excessive thyrotrophin releasing hormone (TRH)-stimulation of pituitary thyrotrophes, and the direct stimulation of these cells by diminished thyroid hormone, leads to their stimulation, hyperplasia, and in some cases basophile adenoma formation.[16] These basophiles stain positively with PAS, suggesting that they secrete a glucopeptide product similar to thyroid-stimulating hormone (TSH). The thyroid deficiency leading up to this may be due to several causes, such as iodine deficiency, ^{131}I, external radiation, surgical damage, or the administration of goitrogens. The aforementioned series of events has been well worked out in experimental animals, but only rarely documented in humans.

Similarly, interruption of the gonadal feedback loop by castration, or other diminution of androgen or estrogen feedback, can lead to excessive GNRH production and basophile hyperplasia or adenoma formation, or both, in the anterior lobe.

In Nelson's syndrome, after adrenalectomy and the absence of cortisol feedback, corticotrophin releasing factor (CRF) is produced excessively by the hypothalmus, leading to abnormal stimulation of corticotroph anterior pituitary basophiles, with consequent hyperplasia and sometimes adenoma formation in this cell population. Interestingly, excessive stimulation of these cells causes large amounts of melanin-stimulating hormone (MSH) to be generated, which leads to abnormal skin darkening in these individuals.

A rather special morphologic change occurs in anterior pituitary corticotrophs when there is excessive cortisol or other glucocorticoid feedback. This is the formation of pale, homogeneous cytoplasmic vacuoles in the cytoplasm of the corticotrophs, usually spoken of as Crooke's hyaline, after its original describer (Fig. 20-2).

Dopamine Receptor Agonists (Bromocriptine)

In clinical situations of proven prolactinemia, bromocriptine administration is very effective in reducing the high circulating levels

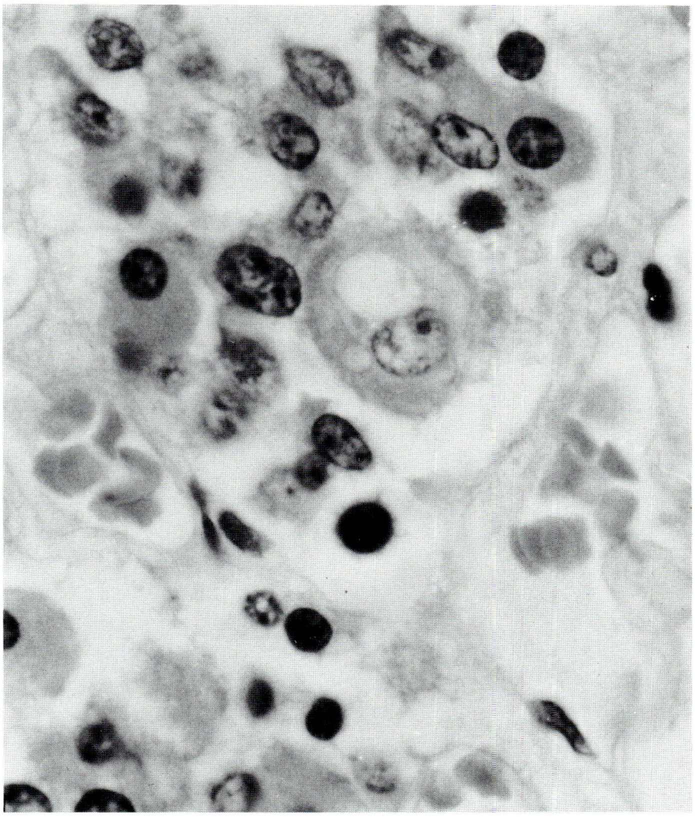

Fig. 20-2. An enlarged arterior pituitary showing basophilic cells with hyaline cytoplasm and vacuoles indicating Crooke's hyaline change. H&E, × 1250.

of prolactin down to normal levels. There has been little follow-up morphologic information about pituitary changes subsequent to such bromocriptine therapy. A diminished mitotic rate in anterior pituitary acidophiles has been reported, and there are several reports in the literature relating how bromocriptine has reduced the size or caused the complete regression of prolactin-secreting pituitary adenomas or recurrent malignant adenomas.[33,39] Dopamine, on the other hand, will increase the mitotic rate of anterior pituitary cells in organ culture.

Dopamine Receptor Blocker (Pimozide)

Here the primary effect on anterior pituitary cells is to enhance mitotic activity. This enhancement is lost when anterior pituitary cells are maximally stimulated toward mitotic activity by pretreatment with estrogens.

Carbon Tetrachloride

The toxic effect of CCl_4 on the mouse pituitary and pineal glands is total destruction and involution. No such destructive effect has been described in humans.

Lithium

Many people receiving lithium therapy experience polyuria and polydipsia compatible with a diagnosis of diabetes insipidus. Yet their polyuria is resistant to control by vasopressin administration. This clearly shows that the toxic effect of lithium is not at the level of the posterior pituitary, but is, in fact, a toxic blockade of renal tubular cyclic AMP, preventing its activation by vasopressin.

Lithium is said to sensitize the thyrotrophic cells of the anterior pituitary so that they respond in an exaggerated fashion to TRH stimulation, releasing excessive TSH. Return to a more normal response to TRH takes many months after discontinuing lithium exposure.[34]

Hexadimethrine

This organic bromide polymer causes anterior pituitary infarction. Heparin is protective by virtue of combining with hexadimethrine and rendering it ineffective. Histamine and serotonin may have roles in this drug's ischemic and toxic effects.[24]

THYROID

The follicular architecture of the thyroid gland, with cuboidal thyroid epithelial cells surrounding a medium-sized lake of colloid (thyroglobulin), is an excellent system in which to study various toxic effects, because flattened epithelial cells suggest inactivity and tall epithelial cells suggest increased activity. Unfortunately, most studies of thyroid toxicity do not histologically examine the tissue, but only relate patient symptoms or thyroid activity. Much more can be done in relating altered morphology to the chronic effects of therapeutically administered or inadvertently taken drugs.

Iodine

Excessive iodine intake has been recorded both from prescribed medication (KI for bronchial asthma) and in natural-food faddists (kelp ingestion), or from heavy commercial bread consumption (iodinated compounds used in the mixing process). Excessive iodine in biologic systems may have unpredictable effects, depending upon the balance present before the excessive influx. If the patient were severely hypothyroid and a heavy influx of inorganic iodine came into the system, it would immediately be trapped, organified, and put out as thyroid hormone. This would lead to transient hyperthyroidism. Because of the pre-existing strong TSH effect, the thyroid would show tall, active cells, watery colloid and, in short, the histology of a hyperactive gland. This would not change much with the addition of iodine, but eventually, as thyroid hormone is built up, it would feed back to the hypothalamus and anterior pituitary, turning off TSH, and the thyroid morphology would slowly revert to a "normal" pattern.

If, on the other hand, the thyroid function were normal at the outset of iodine excess, then the excess inorganic iodine circulating to the brain and anterior pituitary might be mistaken for thyroid hormone, and would thus help to turn down pituitary TSH secretion, so that under less pituitary drive the thyroid could shut down. In this "resting" state it might store iodine-poor colloid and form a symetric, nontoxic goiter. This proposed mechanism has been most sensitively shown in infants born of asthmatic mothers who used large amounts of potassium iodide during their pregnancy.[7]

The effect of inorganic iodine excess does not elicit the same response in everyone. The opposite reaction, of hyperthyroidism, may also occur in association with inorganic iodine excess. This was shown in the short report of an asthmatic who developed heat intolerance, an enlarged thyroid, and elevated circulating T_3 and T_4 levels. Taking her off inorganic iodine, plus the use of thyroid blocking agents, brought her thyroid function into the normal range within 2 months.[17]

Goitrogens (Cyanogenic Glucosides and Thioglucosides)

These naturally occurring chemicals are thought to block iodine trapping by the thyroid, and inhibit hormone synthesis in the thyroid. This in turn stimulates greater TSH formation, and the goitrogens seem themselves to increase the sensitivity of the thyroid to TSH. This lack of iodine and increased TSH stimulation causes diffuse enlargement of the thyroid, with the microscopic formation of many macrofollicles which store iodine-poor colloid (Fig. 20-3). Because of the epithelial cell hyperplasia (Fig. 20-4), such glands are thought to have an increased likelihood of developing thyroid carcinoma.[11]

Thyroid Blocking Agents (Propylthiouracil and Methimazole)

These agents prevent the organification of iodine—a necessary step in its storage as thyroglobulin or use in thyroid hormone. Animals treated with such blocking agents show little morphologic alteration in their thyroid histology, even though they are changed from a hyperthyroid to a euthyroid state, or from a euthyroid to a hypothyroid state (Fig. 20-5). Interestingly, if the conversion is from hyperthyroid to euthyroid and iodine is added to the treatment plan, the hyperplastic features of the thyroid are altered much more quickly from a microfollicular pattern with a tall follicular epithelium, engorged blood vessels, scanty watery colloid, and a crowded tufted follicular epithelium to normal-sized follicles lined by uncrowded cuboidal epithelium filled with even, protein-rich colloid, and with smaller interstitial blood vessels.

One report describes an increase in mitochondrial size, with elongation and the formation of dense, long cristae which are interpreted as intramitochondrial paracrystalloids in rat thyroid treated with propylthiouracil. These animals also showed depressed levels of T_3 in their circulation.[40]

A massive overdose of propylthiouracil occurred when a surgically treated hyperthyroid patient swallowed 5,000 to 13,000 mg of this drug. She showed no adverse effects. Her thyroid remained the same size, and although the circulating thyroxin levels dropped a little below normal and her TSH rose well above normal levels, no symptoms ensued.[21]

Irradiation

Low-dose (50 to 1,500 rads) irradiation in infancy and childhood causes diverse pathologic changes in the thyroid, although it may take a rather long latent period before these

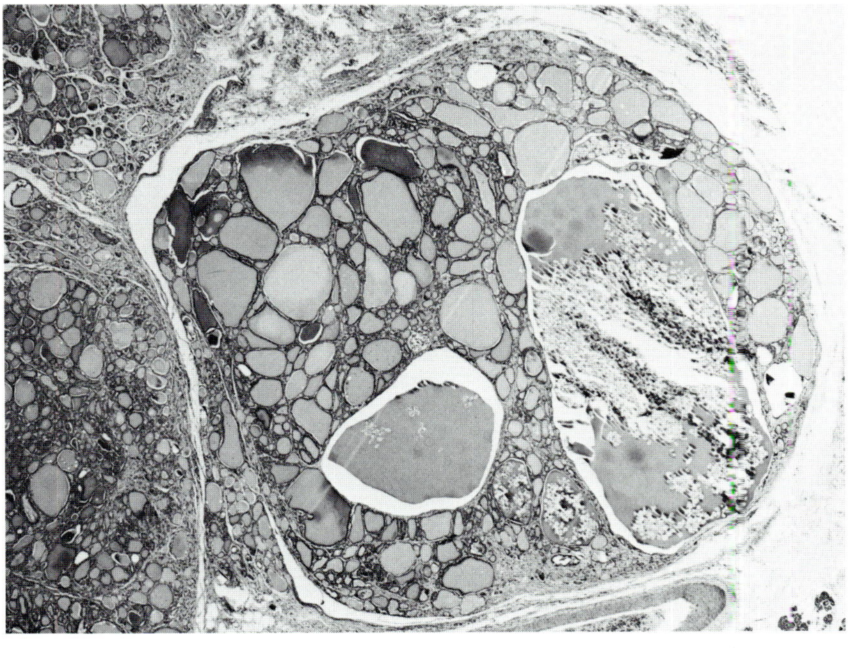

Fig. 20-3. Macrofollicular or colloid nodule showing some colloid phagocytoses (foamy cells in colloid) and focal hyperplasia elsewhere in nodule. H&E, × 23.

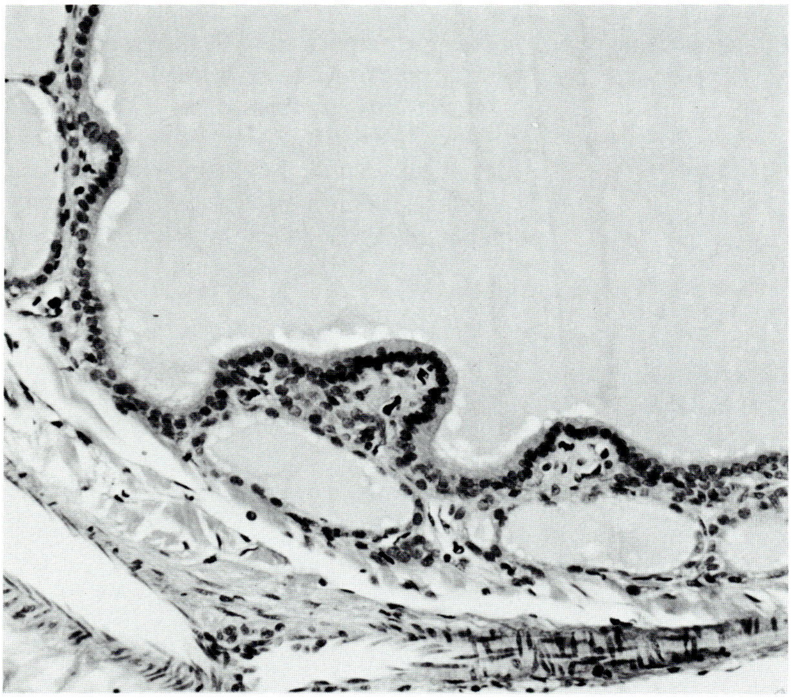

Fig. 20-4. Crowded tall thyroid epithelial cells push up into colloid forming "tuft" and representing focal hyperplasia. H&E, × 260.

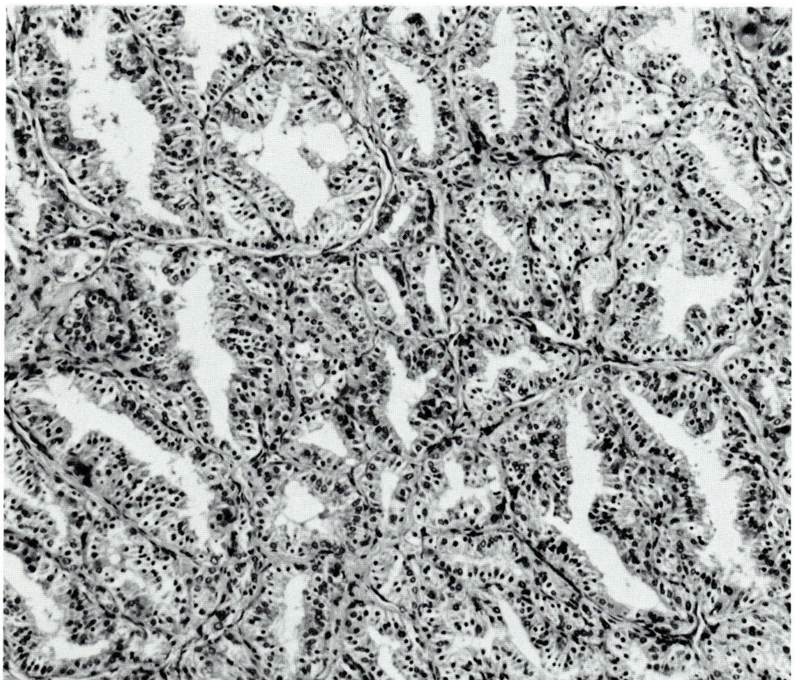

Fig. 20-5. Marked diffuse thyroid hyperplasia as seen in a patient with Grave's disease after use of thyroid blocking agent (propylthyrouracil) but without use of concurrent iodine. H&E, × 130.

changes become evident. The most consistent change is focal hyperplasia, identified by the focal proliferation of thyroid epithelial cells at one point in the circumference of a follicle. The crowded epithelium pushes up into the colloid, making a "tuft" and dropping new microfollicles into the immediately underlying interstitial space (see Fig. 20-4). Besides these foci, one might find increased colloid nodule formation, an increased likelihood of lymphocytic thyroiditis, increased occurrence of microfollicular adenomas, and increased occurrence of oxyphile nests.[49] One report states there is a 7 percent incidence of well-differentiated thyroid carcinoma 20 years after childhood head or neck low-dose irradiation for "thymic enlargement," tonsilar enlargement, or acne. This is far above the natural incidence of thyroid carcinoma, suggesting that childhood irradiation strongly predisposes to later carcinoma formation.[43]

The alarm generated by the concern over the relatively high incidence of malignant change occuring later in life after childhood irradiation was carried over to concern for what would happen to patients receiving thyroid irradiation from diagnostic or therapeutic ^{131}I exposure. It turns out that the risk for malignancy is much less, partly because such irradiation is seldom given in infancy, but also because the dosage to the effected cells is greater, with a greater likelihood for cell death instead of cell damage. Dobyns describes 19 thyroid malignancies in 19,186 patients treated with ^{131}I for hyperthyroidism as an incidence of 0.88 per 1,000 cases.[12]

The heavily irradiated thyroid will slowly undergo extensive fibrosis, with thyroid epithelial cell loss and atrophy of follicles, until it becomes an end-stage thyroid with a few scattered small epithelial cells in a dense collagenous stroma.

Thalidomide

This now seldom-used tranquilizing drug has an antithyroid action that can lead to lethargy, cold intolerance, rough dry skin, deepening of the voice, and myxedema. The mechanism of action is not known.[48]

Salicylates

These commonly used drugs do not directly alter the thyroid gland morphology, but occupy protein-binding sites in the blood stream, thereby effectively releasing T_4 and raising the free thyroxine index (FTI).[31] Hypothalamic and pituitary recognition of this greater free thyroxine causes diminished TSH production. In extreme cases this can lead to goiter with myxedema.[30]

Pyrazole

This drug is a known inhibitor of hepatic alcohol dehydrogenase, and was by chance found to damage the thyroid gland. When pyrazole is given to rats in a single dose of 140 mg/100 gm body weight by stomach tube, all of the animals show thyroid necrosis, and half of the animals will be dead after 5 days.[50] The thyroid changes start with focal necrosis and desquamation of thyroid epithelial cells into the follicular lumen. Cellular injury becomes more and more extensive until there is uniform necrosis throughout, and severe edema of the connective tissue. Almost no inflammatory infiltrate accompanies the epithelial cell necrosis. The thyroid hormone levels fall to unreadable levels and TSH increases in response to peripheral thyroxin depletion. The mechanism of this rather specific thyroid necrosis is not understood.

Sulfonylurea Compounds (Tolbutamide and Chlorpropamide)

Hypothyroidism was found in 30 of 220 patients being treated with sulfonylurea antidiabetic medication. Their basal metabolic rates were low, they had low protein-bound-iodine

(PBI) levels, and a diminished radioactive iodine uptake. It is suggested that sulfonylurea compounds somehow diminish TSH release from the pituitary thyrotrophs, causing hypothyroidism[20] but little morphologic change in the thyroid.[2]

Phenylbutazone

This antipyretic analgesic drug can cause thyroid gland enlargement without any derangement in thyroid control of metabolism. In this way phenylbutazone is sometimes responsible for the formation of nontoxic goiter.[42]

Lithium

Many manic-depressive patients put on lithium therapy develop diffuse thyroid enlargement. Some of these patients, when studied, are found to be hypothyroid, as indicated by low levels of circulating thyroid hormone. The thyroid gland returns to normal size and the FTI returns to normal levels a few months after discontinuing the lithium therapy.[5] One-third of patients receiving lithium show elevated plasma TSH levels, so it is not surprising to have a case report of thyroid cancer associated with lithium therapy.

This occurred in a 55-year-old manic-depressive woman who had had the psychosis for 7 years and was then started on 1,000 mg of lithium carbonate per day. After 1 year the patient had gained 28 lb and complained of tiredness. She was euthyroid upon testing, but showed right lobe enlargement. Three years later, a rapid increase in the size of the right thyroid lobe brought the patient to surgery. A 64 g multinodular right lobe was resected, including a 3-cm papillary follicular adenocarcinoma with associated calcospherites and one positive adjacent cervical lymph node.[3]

Resorcinol

This is another widely used skin medication that can lead to severe hypothyroidism with diffuse goiter, decreased PBI, decreased ^{131}I uptake and, in extreme cases, myxedema.[4]

Polychlorinated Biphenyls (Aroclor)

This toxic chemical all too frequently finds its way into human food for consumption. The Japanese call polychlorinated biphenyl (PCB) poisoning "Yusho," and have written about a series of cases caused by the ingestion of rice oil contaminated by a commercial brand of PCB. These patients have signs of hypothyroidism.[27]

When diets containing 500 PPM of aroclor were fed to rats for 42 days, their thyroids enlarged. There was a marked reduction in circulating thyroid hormone. Lowered thyroxin levels followed the activation of liver microsomal breakdown of thryoxin as well as the slowed thyroid production of thyroxin. Ultrastructural analyses of the thyroid epithelial cells showed inability of the colloid vacuoles to fuse with the intracellular lysosomes, which prevented acid hydrolysis of the thyroglobulin necessary to release the organified iodine for incorporation into thyroxin. Thyroid epithelial cell mitochondria were vacuolated and free surface microvilli were blunted and decreased in number. PCBs seem to have a direct toxic effect on thyroid epithelial cells.[23]

Anticancer Agents

Estradiol mustard, testosterone mustard, nitrogen mustard, and 5-fluorouracil all depress the thyroid gland weight when given to experimental animals. Nitrogen mustard depressed thyroid weights by one-third and 5-fluorouracil by two-thirds as compared to controls. Methotrexate increased the weight of the thyroid.[26] Ekholm suggests that these anticancer drugs somehow block the TSH stimulus of thyroid epithelial cells.[14]

Griseofulvin

This antifungal agent is known to induce mitotic arrests, and can potentiate the action of cholchicine. Rustia and Shubik describe griseofulvin as a goitrogenic substance because it leads to extensive colloid nodule formation in treated animals' thyroids.[45] As has been described, thyroids altered by goitrogens do not produce enough thyroxin, and pituitary TSH is thus remarkably increased. The net effect is overstimulation of thyroid epithelial cells, which cannot respond by generating thyroxin, and so multiply and eventually undergo neoplastic transformation, leading to the increased formation of adenomas and carcinomas. This occurred in these griseofulvin-treated rats, with approximately 37 percent of the animals having thyroid tumors in the highest-dose group. These were mainly follicular adenomas, with a few papillary and follicular carcinomas.[45]

Lead

Chronic plumbism is known to cause hypothyroidism. Sandstead describes 24 patients, 3 of whom developed lead poisoning from industrial exposure, and 21 of whom developed lead poisoning from drinking illicitly distilled moonshine whiskey. None of these patients exhibited thyroid enlargement, but most showed decreased ^{131}I uptake. It is proposed in this paper that lead interferes with the iodine trapping and concentrating mechanism at the level of the thyroid epithelial cell. TSH stimulus overcomes the trapping defect, allowing greater ^{131}I uptake to occur.[46] One case of a home painter describes such severe hypothyroidism that the painter had myxedema.[25]

PARATHYROIDS

The parathyroid glands are unusual in the classic endocrine system because they are not under direct pituitary gland influence. It seems that the trophic effect for parathyroid cell activity is the absence of calcium ion, which is recognized by cyclic AMP at the cell membrane, with the latter in turn stimulating the systhesis of parathyroid hormone (PTH), which in its way prompts renal tissue to conserve Ca^{2+} and bone to mobilize more Ca^{2+} from bone salt reservoirs. Any chemical that alters the serum calcium level will have a stimulating effect (if it lowers serum Ca^{2+}) or an inhibitory effect (if it raises serum Ca^{2+}) on the parathyroid parenchymal cell population.

Serum Calcium Lowering Agents (EDTA, EHDP, Cl_2MDP)

The calcium ion chelating agent edetate disodium binds calcium ions into a complex that is excreted by the kidney.[54] The lowered serum calcium ion levels that result stimulate the parathyroid parenchyma to increase PTH production. Ultrastructurally there is an increased prominence of rough endoplasmic reticulum (RER) and Golgi complexes. Secretory granules are dispersed into the blood, and glycogen storage becomes more prominent in the cell.[6] If the low serum calcium ion state is maintained for longer periods of time, parathyroid hyperplasia will ensue, with increased size of the parathyroids, less interspersed mature fat, and an increased mitotic rate of parenchymal cells.

Other agents, such as disodium etidronate (EHDP) and dichloromethane diphosphonate (Cl_2MDP)—which is ten times more potent than EHDP—inhibit bone reabsorption, thus effectively lowering serum calcium ion concentrations in animals, and necessitating more calcium than dietary sources can supply.[55] This is particularly true in the preparturent cow. Use of this drug under these special circumstances again causes stimulation of parathyroid parenchymal cells, with hyperplasia if the stimulus is prolonged.

Serum Calcium Elevating Agents (Vitamin D_3 and *Solanum malacoxylon*)

The use of 1,25-dihydroxycholecalciferol (in purified form or from the South American plant source *Solanum malacoxylon*) radically increases Ca^{2+} absorption from the intestinal tract, leading to hypercalcemia.[10] This increase in serum calcium levels turns off the parathyroid parenchymal cells, which ultrastructurally show increased secretory granule storage in their cytoplasm, a denser cytoplasm, straight plasma membranes, more lipid storage, and smaller Golgi complexes.[44] Continued hypercalcemia apparently does not hold all parenchymal cells in the resting state. Periodically and in rotation, some parenchymal cells will phase themselves into more active PTH synthesis, but will continue to store the hormonal product within the secretory granules still in their cytoplasm.

Hydrochlorothiazide

This substance has been used by large numbers (60 percent) of patients who were eventually recognized as hypercalcemic patients and given the diagnosis of hyperparathyroidism. At neck exploration many of these patients showed mixed parathyroid disease, with evidence of adenoma formation and hyperplasia in parathyroid tissue removed from the neck at the first operation. Attempts to cause parathyroid hyperplasia in dogs by giving hydrochlorothiazide were somewhat successful. No explanation of the mechanism by which this diuretic drug causes parathyroid hyperplasia has been put forward.[41]

L-Asparaginase

L-asparaginase has been reported to be toxic to the rabbit parathyroid. Administration of 1,000 IU/kg intravenously leads to profound weakness and seizures in half of the animals injected. Severe hypocalcemia was noted, along with hyperphosphotemia, uremia, and elevated creatinine levels. Histology of the rabbit parathyroid showed marked single cell oxyphilia and then necrosis. There were from 5 to 47 necrotic cells per high power field (HPF), with an average of 19. Of the most severely affected animals, most were dead within 48 hours.[8]

Ethyl Alcohol

There is one recent paper describing the effect on PTH and calcitonin secretion of the ingestion of 0.8 g/kg of ethanol within a 1-hour time span. Both circulating PTH levels and calcitonin levels were elevated. Serum calcium levels remained in the normal range. It is not clear whether the ethanol affects the parathyroid parenchymal cell directly or whether it lowers serum Ca^{2+} levels and the parathyroid hormone increase is a response to this. The fact that both the parathyroid parenchyma and the thyroid C cells responded positively suggests a direct cellular effect.[53] No morphologic changes of the parathyroid have been described.

Glucocorticoids (Triamcinolone Diacetate)

These steroid hormones are known to slowly cause osteoporosis if used over a long period of time, yet the mechanism of this action has not been well defined. Coleman and Silbermann have studied the mouse parathyroid after 21 days of triamcinolone diacetate therapy, and found that the chief cells show all the ultrastructural characteristics of turned on or active parathyroid parenchymal cells. They show complex interdigitated cell membranes with numerous microvilli, an increased, parallel RER, increased free ribosomes, large Golgi complexes, prominent mitochondria, and some vacuoles.[9] The authors did not report about changes in serum calcium or increased PTH levels, but it is expected that PTH would be increased.

ADRENAL CORTEX

The adrenal cortex has a limited number of morphologic responses to stimulation and injury. When stimulated by angiostensin II, the outer zona glomerulosa thickens and secretes the mineralocorticoid aldosterone. The cortex can form benign adrenal cortical adenomas or malignant cortical carcinoma, but these neoplastic proliferations are autonomously developed, and no drug action is known that initiates such neoplastic transformation.

The inner zones, the zona fasciculata and zona reticularis, are the source of cortisol, the glucocorticoid secretion. Adrenocorticotrophic hormone (ACTH), secreted by the corticotrophs in the anterior pituitary, is the trophic hormone for the inner zones of the adrenal cortex. Excessive prolonged stimulation of these zones leads to cell proliferation, with a remarkably uniform thickening of the zona fasciculata and reticularis, associated the with consumption of stored lipid and hyperplasia of the cytoplasmic smooth-walled endoplasmic reticulum (SER)—the steroid manufacturing organelle—which gives the cytoplasm an acidophilic appearance (Fig. 20-6). In contrast to the aforementioned diffuse hyperplasia is intermittent ACTH stimulation, which gives the picture of nodular hyperplasia. Nodules appear because at a given moment, some cortical cells are receptive to stimulation and consume their lipid and become acidophilic, while other groups remain refractory and maintain their lipid-laden appearance. Cell proliferation is similarly irregular, heaping up cells in one place but not in adjacent areas. (Fig. 20-7).

Glucocorticoids are the feedback hormones to the hypothalmus and anterior pituitary, turning off ACTH production and secretion. Use of large amounts of exogenous glucocorti-

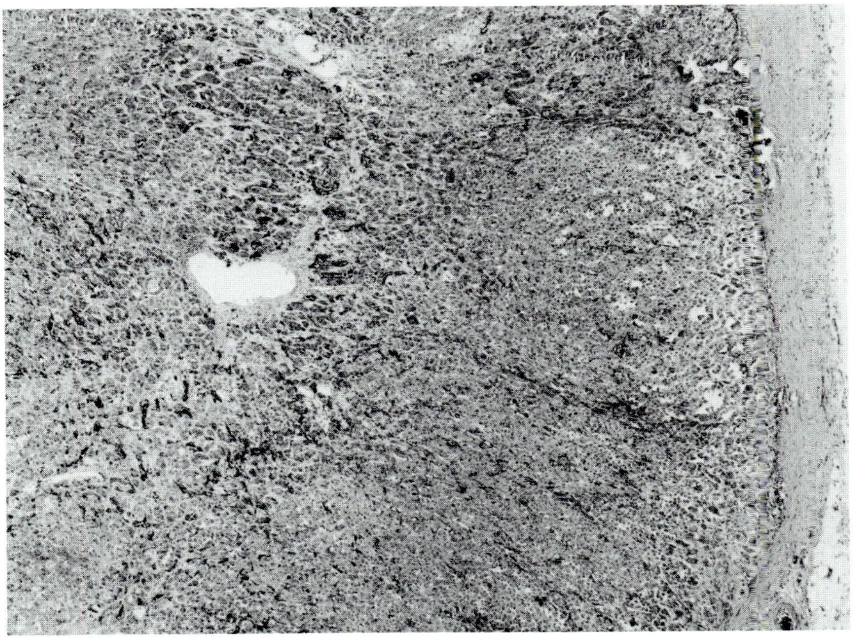

Fig. 20-6. Continuous strong ACTH stimulation of the adrenal cortex leads to diffuse cortical hyperplasia. This is a thickened cortex with conversion of lipid-rich cells to acidophilic compact cells. H&E, × 27.

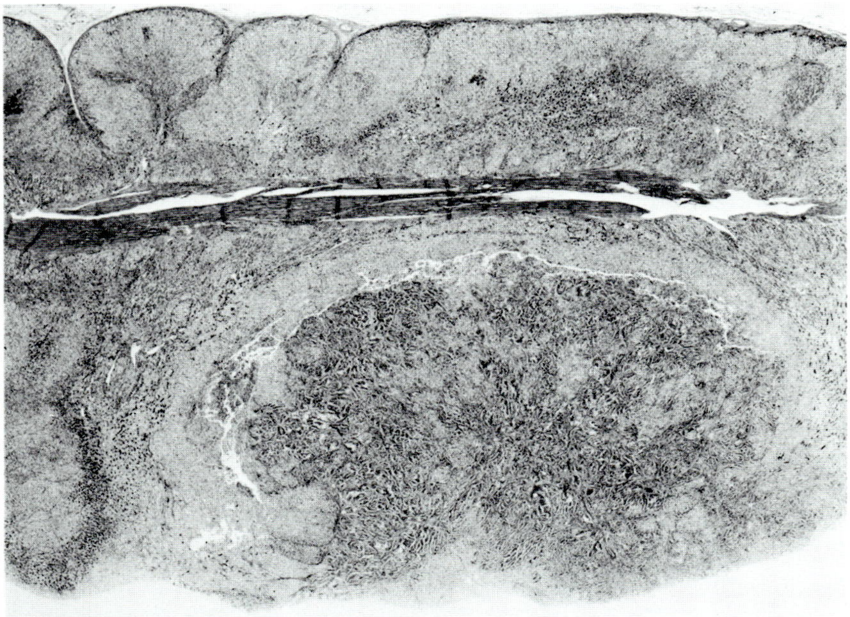

Fig. 20-7. Adrenal cortex exhibiting irregular thickening, which indicates nodular hyperplasia. Identification of cortical zones may be lost or maintained. H&E, × 10.

coids has the same effect on the adrenal cortex as does hypophosectomy, because it so thoroughly turns off ACTH production. The zona fasciculata and zona reticularis shrink down to much thinner layers, and the cells lose all of their SER and appear small, with stored lipid vacuoles. Such unstimulated adrenal cortex is resistant to rapid awakening, and needs time to be stimulated by ACTH back up to normal or stressful glucocorticoid production. During this recovery time the patient is very vulnerable to adrenal cortical insufficiency. Drugs such as cyproterone acetate mimic the steroid molecule enough to turn off pituitary ACTH, FSH, and LH, leading to hypocortisolism and hypogonadism.[37]

Spironolactone

This steroid molecule mimics the shape of aldosterone and lodges in the binding sites of the latter, but does not have a mineralocorticoid action, and thus, in effect, functions as an aldosterone blocking agent. Quite surprisingly it also leads to a morphologic change in aldosterone-secreting cells in the zona glomerulosa, or in tumor cells generating aldosterone. This change is the formation of spherical acidophilic lamellar bodies in the cytoplasm of these cells. These are called spironolactone bodies; their formation is not dose-dependent, and only about half of all patients receiving spironolactone show formation of the bodies. Ultrastructurally the spherical bodies appear to be densely rolled phospholipid membranes (Fig. 20-8), and are said to contain similar enzymes as those present in the SER.[1] Why they form has not yet been explained, but they might be interpreted as a special form of autophagosome.

Steroidogenic Blocking Agents

This is a group of complex organic molecules that block steroidogenesis at various points in the synthesis of adrenal steroid hor-

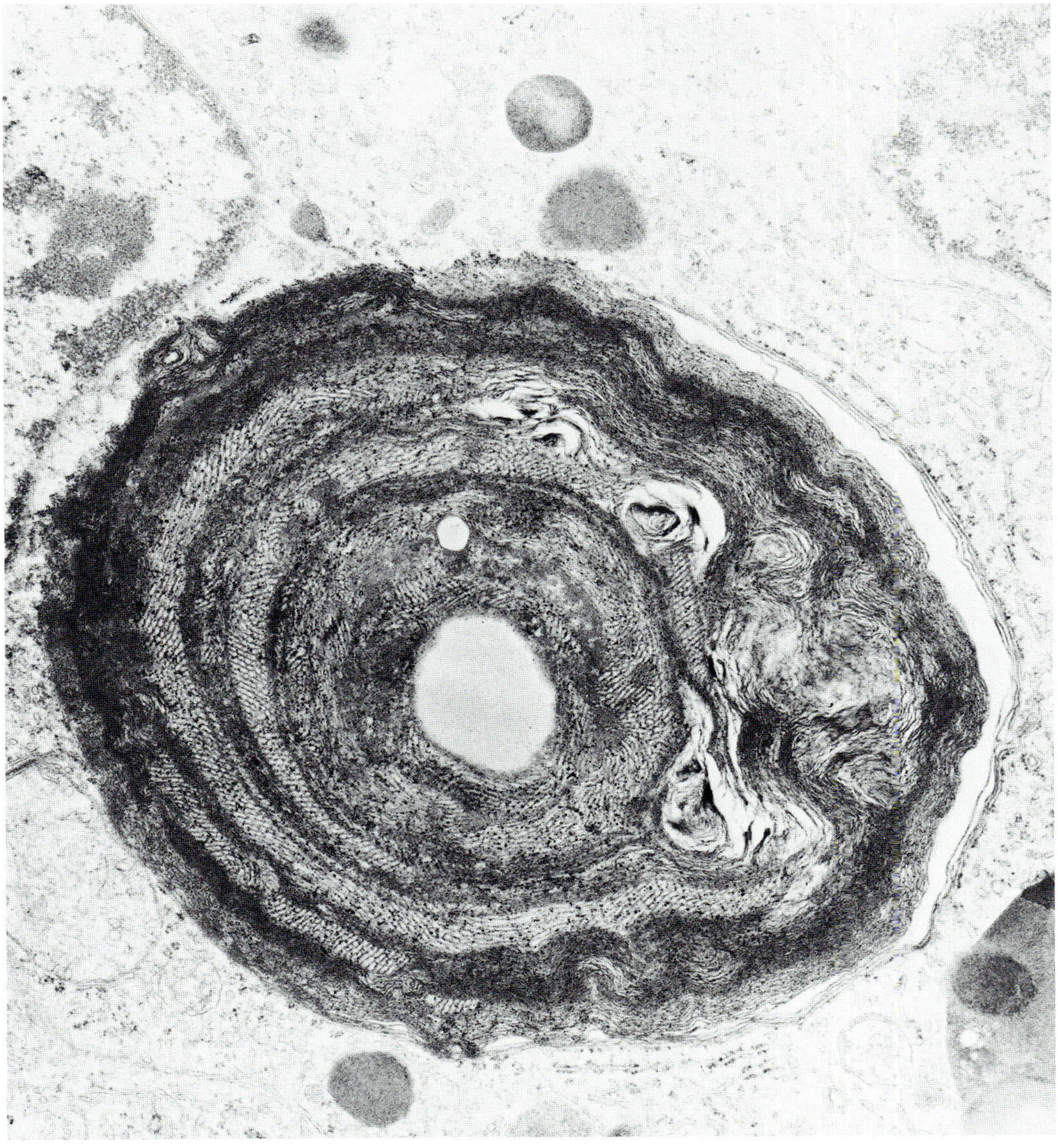

Fig. 20-8. Spironolactone body as visualized in human aldosterone-secreting adrenal cortical adenoma cell after treatment with 400 mg of aldactone per day for several months before adrenalectomy. ×21,000.

mones from their precursor, cholesterol. If blockade diminishes cortisol output, then ACTH levels rise and the histologic picture of hyperplasia develops, with thickened adrenal cortices.

Cyanoketone specifically inhibits 3-β hydroxysteroid dehydrogenase, leading to diminished cortisol production, increased ACTH stimulation of the adrenal inner cortex, and evidence of cortical hyperplasia. On ultrastructural examination, zona fasciculata cells reveal swollen mitochondria containing diminished cristae, large lipid droplets, and increased cytolysosomes. The drug effect is reversible, with normal steroidogenesis following the discontinuance of the cyanoketone.[15]

Amphenone is another glucocorticoid biosynthetic blocker that depresses adrenal cortical function. This drug causes an increase in mitochondrial size, the indentation of larger mitochondria by smaller adjacent ones, an increased density of mitochondrial matrix, vacuolization of mitochondria, prominent lipid vacuoles, fading and diminished prominence of lipid, and diminished SER.[29]

Su 4885 inhibits 11-β-hydroxylation, leading to diminished cortisol production, ACTH increase, and hyperplastic adrenal cortical changes. Lipid droplets become less dense and diminish in prominence. Mitochondria become more numerous, with some exhibiting a less dense matrix. Both of these ultrastructural changes are in keeping with an increased ACTH effect upon these organelles in the inner-cortex parenchymal cells.[29]

Triparinol blocks cholesterol and steroid synthesis, leading to decreased lipid storage in the zona fasciculata, with abnormal mitochondria and an increased SER.[29] These again are the changes of ACTH stimulation.

Aminoglutethimide is another steroidogenesis blocking agent. This drug was first developed as a anticonvulsant, but was found to cause adrenal insufficiency. It reversibly inhibits the conversion of cholesterol to pregnenolone. ACTH stimulation will override the blockade unless glucocorticoids are given concurrently.[47]

DDD (2:2-bis-p-chlorophenyl)-1:1 dichloroethane

This substance was first looked at as a possible substitute insecticide for DDT, and was first studied in the late 1940s for possible toxic effects; Nelson and Woodward described adrenal cortical atrophy in dogs in 1949.[38] The original technical grade DDD seemed specific for adrenal atrophy in the dog and rat, but with further purification and testing of isomers, more widespread species toxicity has been developed.

The atrophy is primarily limited to the zona fasciculata and zona reticularis, suggesting that DDD inhibits the ACTH effect on the adrenal cortex. But if this were the case, the atrophy would stabilize and the cortex could be restimulated at a later time. This atrophy is progressive, with eventual destruction of the inner cortex without any possibility of restimulation. Thus, DDD is toxic to the inner cortical cells, leading to their total destruction. Early in the toxic effect, mitochondrial changes are the most striking. Mitochondrial membrane outpouching filled with a pale matrix was noticed first, followed by the loss of all SER and by swollen mitochondria looking like empty sacs. Lipid droplets become crenated, cell membranes rupture, and fat droplets are found in intracellular spaces.[22,29] Even the zona glomerulosa can be affected if the dose level is raised high enough. Hypophysectomy is not protective from the toxic destruction caused by DDD.

The mechanism of action of DDD is not known on the cellular level. When destruction of cortical cells has progressed far enough, numerous lymphocytes accumulate at the site of the destroyed adrenal cortex. These eventually go away, and if the animal is supported on glucocorticoid replacement, fibrosis occupies the site of the old adrenal cortex.

Agents Causing Cortical Hemorrhagic Necrosis

Six agents are presented in this section, all of which cause hemorrhagic necrosis of the adrenal cortex. Most primarily affect the inner cortex, but if the reaction is severe the entire cortex becomes involved. It is also interesting that this pathologic process closely mimics the clinical and pathologic findings of the Waterhouse-Friederichsen syndrome first described in 1911.[52a]

Acrylonitrile (vinylcyanide) is one of the agents which cause rapidly progressive adrenal apoplexy. A 20 mg/100 g body weight dose delivered intravenously into the jugular vein of rats leads to hemorrhagic swelling of both adrenals within 2 hours. The first ultrastructural change is the loss of endothelial cell continuity in the adrenal cortical sinusoids within 30 minutes of drug injection. This is followed by extravasation of red blood corpuscles and plasma into the intercellular space. So much extravasation occurs that adrenal cortical cells are compressed and contorted out of their usual polyhedral shape. Clumped platelets are evident in the sinusoidal lumens, clustered around endothelial discontinuities. At this stage (3 to 4 hours) the animals die of acute adrenal insufficiency.[52]

Thioguanine is another of these agents causing hemorrhagic necrosis of the adrenal cortex. Here, five consecutive daily doses produce adrenal cortical changes that look very similar to what has been described with acrylonitrile. Endothelial blebbing was observed just before the loss of endothelial continuity and rupture of the capillary basement membrane. After cell extravasation, zona fasciculata cells are said to show the swelling of mitochondria and vesiculation of the SER. The parenchymal cells then rupture and necrose, and polymorphonuclear leukocytes migrate into the area. Hypophysectomy is totally protective, and it is impossible to develop hemorrhagic necrosis in treated animals after removal of the anterior pituitary.[51] **Thioacetamide** acts in a very similar manner to thioguanine, and **diphtheria toxin** also leads to sinusoidal rupture and hemorrhagic necrosis.

DMBA (7,12, dimethyl benz*(a)*anthacene) also causes adrenal cortical apoplexy. This was first described by Huggins in 1961.[19] This molecule mimics the shape of an adrenal steroid, and may gain entrance into the adrenal cortical endothelial cell by mascarading as a glucocorticoid; when there, however, it damages the endothelial cell beyond repair. Mazzocchi et. al. describe DMBA injury limited to the zona reticularis, and suggest that DMBA may bind to parenchymal cell nuclear and mitochondrial DNA and thus inhibit normal protein synthesis, eventuating in the cortical damage they describe.[32]

Hexadimethrine bromide has already been described as causing anterior pituitary infarction, and must now be relisted for its propensity to cause hemorrhagic infarction in the inner adrenal cortex, but also for its described toxic necrosis of the zona glomerulosa. Five milligrams given intravenously leads to toxic necrosis in the mineralocorticoid-secreting zone of the adrenal, and to toxic necrosis in the thick ascending limb of Henle's loop. About half of treated animals develop hemorrhagic infarction of the anterior pituitary and inner adrenal cortex.

Heparin is totally protective for all hexadimethrine lesions, and is said to bind directly with the drug molecule, rendering both substances inert. Hexadimethrine degranulates mast cells, and the release of serotonin is thought to initiate the hemorrhagic necrosis of the pituitary and adrenal glands. Pretreatment of target animals with Cpd 48/80 degranulates mast cells ahead of time, hexadimethrine then does not cause hemorrhagic infarction. Serotonin given with hexadimethrine potentiates pituitary and adrenal hemorrhagic lesions.[24]

Propylthiouracil

This thyroid blocking agent causes "brown degeneration" in the zona reticularis of mice treated for some weeks. These brown pigment granules are thought to be different from the commonly found lipochrome in the zona reticularis. Here, serial views at electron microscopic magnifications first show proliferation of the SER with a little RER; the mitochondria are larger and more variable in shape, and the cristae are short and tubular. Later, lysosomes become abundant, and appear to be closely associated with liposomes. Moore and Callas feel that these two organelles combine to form amorphous ceroid granules. The hypothyroid state is not thought to be important to the formation of the pigment granules unless abnormal cholesterol metabolism may be conducive to the ceroid granule formation. No abnormal function of the adrenal cortex is described.[35]

5-Fluorouracil

A number of antineoplastic medications have been studied for possible damaging effects on the adrenal cortex, but the only one that has showed such action is 5-fluorouracil, which caused an 80 percent reduction in cortisol production after 7 days of therapy.[12] Little morphologic change was noted on light-microscopy, but ultrastructural analysis showed some vesiculation of the SER, and abnormalities of mitochondrial cristae. No mechanism for this inhibitory effect on the adrenal cortex has been suggested.[36]

ACKNOWLEDGMENT

This chapter could not have been written without the generous aid of Jim Koch, a persistent, capable medical student.

REFERENCES

1. Aiba, M., Suzuki, H., Kageyama, K., et al. Spironolactone bodies in aldosteronomas and in the attached adrenals. Am. J. Pathol. 103(3):404–410, 1981.
2. Balodimos, M. C., Marble, A., & Rippey, J. Pathological findings after long term sulfonylurea therapy. Diabetes 17:503–508, 1968.
3. Brownlie, B. E., Turner, J. G., Millner, G. M. B., Perry, E. G., & Ding, L. Case report: Lithium associated thyroid cancer. Aust. N.Z. J. Med. 10:62–63, 1980.
4. Bull, G. M., & Russel-Fraser, T. Myxedema from resorcinol ointment applied to leg ulcers. Lancet 1:851–855, 1950.
5. Candy, J. Severe hypothryoidism in an early complication of lithium therapy. Br. Med. J. 3:277, 1972.
6. Capen, C. C. Fine structural alterations of parathyroid glands in response to experimental and spontaneous changes in calcium in extra cellular fluid. Am. J. Med 50:598–611, 1971.
7. Carswell, F., Kerr, M., & Hutchison, J. Congenital goiter and hypothyroidism produced by maternal ingestion of iodides. Lancet 1:1241–1243, 1970.
8. Chisari, F. V., Hochstein, H. P., Kirschstein, R. L., & Seligmann E. B. Parathyroid necrosis and hypocalcemia tetany induced rabbits by L. Asparaginase. Am. J. Pathol. 68(3):461–467, 1972.
9. Coleman, R., & Silbermann, M. Ultrastructure of the parathyroid glands in triamcinolone-treated mice. J. Anat. 126(1):181–192, 1978.
10. Collins, W. T., Capen, C. C., Dobereiner, J., & Tokarnia, C. H. Ultrastructural evaluation of parathyroid glands and thyroid C cells of cattle fed Solanum Malacoxylon. Am. J. Pathol. 87(3):603–614, 1977.
11. De Groot, L., & Stanbury, J. The thyroid and its external environment. In: The Thyroid and Its Diseases, 4th Ed. pp. 173. Wiley, New York, 1975.
12. Dobyns, B. M. Radiation hazard experience with therapeutic and diagnostic I^{131}. In: Radiation-Associated Thyroid Carcinoma. pp. 459. De Groot, L. J., Ed. Grune and Stratton, New York, 1977.
13. Draznin, B., & Maman, A. Estrogen-induced galactorrhea in man. Arch. Intern. Med. 139:1059–1060, 1979.
14. Ekholm, R., Erickson, L. E., Josefsson, J. D., & Melander, A. *In vivo* action of vinblastin on thyroid ultrastructure and hormone secretion. Endocrinology 94:641–649, 1974.
15. Finegold, M. J., & Basch, R. S. Inhibition of 3B-hydroxysteroid dehydrogenase in rat adrenal cortex: a metabolic and morphologic study. Lab. Invest. 26(6):767–777, 1972.
16. Griesbach, W. E., Chaikoff, I. C., Nichols, C. W., & Goldberg, R. C. Formation of adenomata in hypophyses of rats subjected to both subtotal thyroidectomy and administration of I^{131} and its prevention by feeding of dessicated thyroid. Cancer Res. 25:1804, 1965.
17. Gutknecht, D. R. Asthma complicated by iodine induced thyrotoxicosis. N. Engl. J. Med. 296(21):1236, 1977.
18. Hassani, M., Plas-Roser, S., Ros, J., & Aron, C. Action of testosterone proprionate on the gonadotrophic function of the pituitary gland in the cyclic female rat. Acta Endocrinol. 89(3):551–556, 1978.
19. Huggins, C., & Morii, S. Selective adrenal necrosis and apoplexy induced by 7-12 dimethylbenz (a) anthrocene. J. Exp. Med. 114:741–760, 1961.
20. Hunton, R. B., Wells, M. V., & Skipper,

E. W. Hypothyroidism in diabetes treated with sulfonylurea. Lancet 2:449–451, 1965.
21. Jackson, G. L., Flickinger, F. W., & Wells, L. W. Massive overdose of propyl thiouracil. Ann. Intern. Med. 91(3):418–419, 1979.
22. Kaminsky, N., Luse, S., & Hartroft, P. Ultrastructure of the adrenal cortex of the dog during treatment with DDD. J. Natl. Cancer Inst. 29:127,1962.
23. Kasza, L., Collins, W. T., Capen, C. C., Harthoff, L. H., & Friedman, L. Comparative toxicity of polychlorinated bipheryl and polybromated biphenyl in the rat thyroid gland. J. Environ. Pathol. Toxicol. 1:587, 1978.
24. Kovacs, K., Carroll, R., & Tapp, E. The pathogenesis of hexadimethrine necrosis of the pituitary and adrenal. Arzneim. Forsch. 16(4):516–519, 1966.
25. Kremer, H. U., & Frank, M. N. Coexisting myxedema and chronic plumbism. Ann. Intern. Med. 42:1130–1136, 1955.
26. Kuo, E., Esber, H., Taylor, J., & Bogen, A. Effects of cancer chemotherapeutic agents on endocrine organs and serum levels of estrogens, progesterone, prolactin and luteinizing hormone. Cancer Res. 35:1975–1980, 1975.
27. Kuratsune, M., Yosimura, T., Matsuzaka, J., & Yamaguchi, A. Epidemiologic study of Yusho, a poisoning caused by ingestion of rice oil contaminated with a commercial brand of PCB. Environ Health Perspect. 1:119, 1972.
28. Lacussagne, A., & Nyka, W. Difference de reaction de l'hypophyse a l'administration prolongee de substance oestrogenes dans diverses lignees selectionees de souris. C. R. Soc. Biol. (Paris) 126:1112, 1937.
29. Luse, S. Fine structure of adrenal cortex. In: The Adrenal Cortex. Eisenstein, A. B., Ed. pp. 40–42 & 47. Little Brown, Boston, 1967.
30. Marchese, M. J., Bartorello, M. C., & Cardozo, E. Mixedema en el curso de tratamiento antituberculoso. Rev. Asoc. Med. Argent. 77:542–544, 1963.
31. Marshal, J. S., Levy, R. P., & Lenardo, J. R. The acute effect of salicylate administration on human throxine transport. J. Lab. Clin. Med. 66:1001, 1965.
32. Mazzocchi, G., Belloni, A., Robba, C., & Nussdofer, G. High resolution autoradiographic investigation on the mechanisms of the adrenolytic effect of 7,12, dimethylbenzanthracene on the inner layers of the rat adrenal cortex. Virchows Arch [Cell Pathol.] 28:97–104, 1978.
33. McGregor, A., Scanlon, M., Hall, K., Cook, D., & Hall, R. Reduction in size of a pituitary tumor by bromocriptine therapy. N. Engl. J. Med. 300(6):291–293, 1978.
34. McLarty, D. C., O'Boyle, J H., Spencer, C. A., & Ratcliffe, J. C. Effect of lithium on hypothalamic-pituitary-thyroid functions in patients with affective disorders. Br. Med. J. 3:623–626, 1975.
35. Moore, N. A., & Callas, G. Observations on the fine structure of propylthiouracil-induced "brown degeneration" in the zona reticularis of mouse adrenal cortex. Anat. Rec. 183:293–302, 1976.
36. Morgan M., & O'Hare, M. Cytotoxic drugs and the human adrenal cortex: A cell culture study. Cancer 43(3):969–979, 1979.
37. von Muhlendahl, V., Kurth-Schutz, S., Miller-Hess, R., et al. Cyproterone acetate and adrenocortical function. Lancet 1:1160–1161, 28, 1977.
38. Nelson, A. A., & Landard, G. Severe adrenal cortical atrophy (cytotoxic) and hepatic damage produced in dogs by feeding 2,2-bix (parachloeophenyl) 1,1-dichloroethanine D.D.D. Arch. Pathol. 48:387–394, 1949.
39. Nillius, S. J., Bergh, T., Lundberg, P., Stahl, J., & Wide, L. Regression of a prolactin-secreting pituitary tumor during long term treatment with bromocryptine. Fertil. Steril. 30(6):710, 1978.
40. Nunez, E. A., Grief, R. L., & Gershon, M. D. Paracrystalloids from mitochrondria in thyroid follicular cells. Lab. Invest. 33(4):352, 1975.
41. Pickleman, J., Straus, F., & Paloyan, E. Pancreatitis associated with thiazide administration: A role for the parathyroid glands. Arch. Surg. 114:1013–1016, 1979.
42. Prescott, L. F. Antipyretic analgesic drugs. In: Side Effects of Drugs, Vol. VI. Meyler C., & Herxheimer, A. , Eds. Excerpta Medica, Amsterdam, 1968.
43. Refetoff, S., Harrison, J., Karanfilski, B., et al. Continuing occurrence of thyroid carcinoma after irradiation to the neck in infancy and childhood. N. Engl. J. Med. 292:171–175, 1975.
44. Roth, S. I., & Raisz, L. G. The course and reversability of the calcium effect on the ultrastructure of the rat parathyroid gland in organ culture. Lab. Invest. 15(7):1137–1211, 1966.

45. Rustia, M., & Shubik, P. Thyroid tumors in rats and hepatomas in mice after griseofulvin treatment. Br. J. Cancer 38:237–249, 1978.
46. Sandslead, H. H., Stant, E. G., Brill, A. B., Arias, L. I., & Terry, R. T. Lead intoxication and the thyroid. Arch. Intern. Med. 123:632–635, 1969.
47. Sanford, E., Drago, J., Rohner, T., et al. Aminoglutethimide medical adrenalectomy for advanced prostatic carcinoma. J. Urol. 115:170–174, 1976.
48. Simpson, J. A. Myxedema after thalidomide. Br. Med. J. 1:55, 1962.
49. Straus, F. H., & Spitalnik, P. F. Histologic parenchymal changes in the human thyroid after low dose childhood irradiation. In radiation associated thyroid carcinoma, De Groot, L. J., Ed. pp. 183. Grune and Stratton, New York, 1977
50. Szabo, S., Horvath, E., Kovacs, K., & Larsen, P. Pyrazole-induced thyroid necrosis: A distinct organ lesion. Science 199:1209–1210, 1978.
51. Szabo, S., Kovacs, K., Horvath, E., et al. Thioguanine induced adrenocortical necrosis and its prevention by hypophysectomy in the rat: Light and electron microscopic study. Exp. Mol. Pathol. 26:155–168, 1977.
52. Szabo, S., Reynolds, E., & Kovacs, K. Acrylonitrile-induced adrenal apoplexy. Am. J. Pathol., 82:653–656, 1976.
52a. Waterhouse, R. A case of suprarenal apoplexy. Lancet 1:577, 1911.
53. Williams, G. A., Bowser, E. W., Hargis, G. K., et al. Effect of ethanol on parathyroid hormone and calcitonin secretion in man. Proc. Soc. Exp. Biol. Med. 159:187–191, 1978.
54. Yarrington, J. T., Capen, C. C., Black, H. E., et al. Effect of Ethane-l-hydroxy-1,1-diphosphonate (EHDP) on the ulstrastructure of parathyroid glands and plasma immunoreactive parathyroid hormone in pregnant cows fed a low calcium diet. Lab. Invest. 36(4):402–412, 1977.
55. Yarrington, J. T., Capen, C. C., Black, H. E., et al. Effect of dichloromethane diphosphonate on calcium homeostatic mechanisms in pregnant cows. Am. J. Pathol. 87(3):615–632, 1977.

INDEX

Page numbers followed by t *indicate tables.*